MW01539092

The Art and Science of Diabetes Care and Education

Associate Editors
Susan Cornell, BS, PharmD, CDCES, FAPhA, FADCES
Cindy Halstenson, RDN, LD, CDCES
David K. Miller, RN, MSEd, BSN, CDCES, FADCES

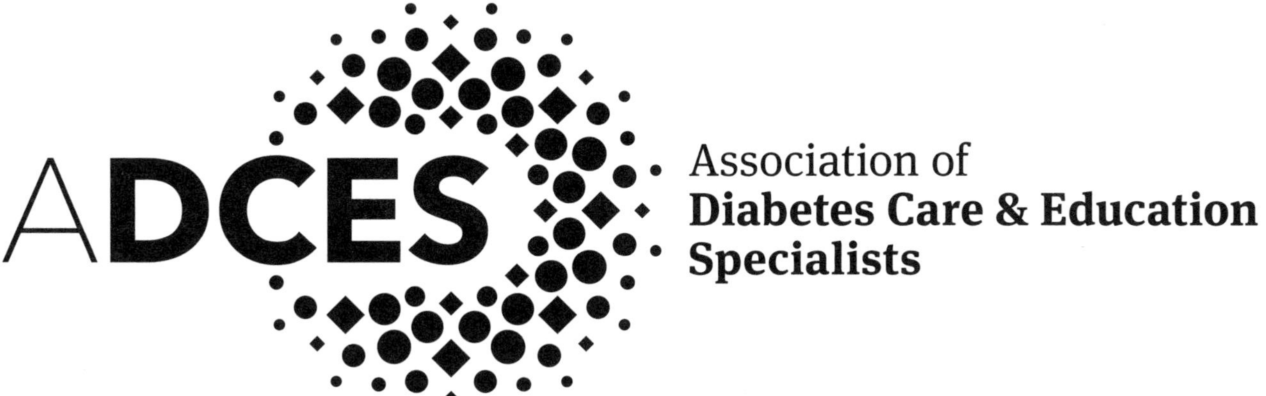

Previous Editions: 2017, 2014, 2011, 2006, American Association of Diabetes Educators, Chicago, Illinois.

10 9 8 7 6 5 4 3 2 1   20 21 22 23 24 25 26 27 28 29

TABLE OF CONTENTS

Acknowledgments . . . . *v*

Chapter 1 Diabetes Care and Education: Rich Past, Challenging Present, Promising Future 1
Sandra Drozdz Burke, PhD, RN, FADCES, FAAN, Janet Thorlton, PhD, RN, and Hiba Abbas, BSN, RN

Chapter 2 The Diabetes Self-Management Education Process 31
Barb Schreiner, PhD, RN, CDCES, BC-ADM

Chapter 3 Theoretical and Behavioral Approaches to the Self-Management of Health 97
Jan Kavookjian, MBA, PhD, FAPhA

Chapter 4 Healthy Coping 131
Janis Roszler, LMFT, RD, LD/N, CDCES, FAND, Melissa Brail, LMFT, and Eliot LeBow, LCSW, CDCES

Chapter 5 Healthy Eating 157
Cecilia Sauter, MS, RDN, CDCES, FADCES

Chapter 6 Being Active 183
Sheri R. Colberg, PhD, FACSM

Chapter 7 Taking Medication 241
Devra K. Dang, PharmD, BCPS, CDCES, FNAP

Chapter 8 Monitoring 263
Molly McElwee-Malloy, CDCES, RN

Chapter 9 Reducing Risks 285
Kimberly Coy DeCoste, RN, MSN, CDCES, MLDE, FADCES, and David K. Miller, RN, MSEd, BSN, CDCES, LDE, FADCES

Chapter 10 Problem Solving 307
Carolé Mensing, RN, MA, CDCES, FADCES

Chapter 11 Diabetes Education Program Management 327
Mary Jean Christian, MA, MBA, RD, CDCES

Chapter 12 Transitional Care. 351
Amy Hess Fischl, MS, RDN, LDN, BC-ADM, CDCES, and Christie A. Schumacher, PharmD, BCPS, BCACP, BC-ADM, CDCES

Chapter 13 Pathophysiology of the Metabolic Disorder. 379
Jane K. Dickinson, RN, PhD, CDCES

Chapter 14 Type 1 Diabetes Throughout the Life Span. 403
Carolyn Banion, RN, MN, CPNP, CDCES, and Virginia Valentine, APRN, BC-ADM, CDCES, FADCES

Chapter 15 Type 2 Diabetes Throughout the Life Span 431
Eva M. Vivian, PharmD, MS, CDCES, BC-ADM, FADCES

Chapter 16 Nutrition Therapy 451
Alison B. Evert, MS, RDN, CDCES

Chapter 17 Pharmacotherapy for Glucose Management 479
Lauren G. Pamulapati, PharmD, BCACP, and
Evan M. Sisson, PharmD, MSHA, BCACP, CDCES, FADCES

Chapter 18 Glucose Monitoring 533
Mary M. Austin, MA, RDN, CDCES, FADCES, and
Beth A. Olson, MHA, RN, CDCES

Chapter 19 Therapy Intensification: Technology and
Pattern Management 575
Debbie Hinnen, APN, BC-ADM, CDCES, FAAN, FADCES,
and Jennifer De Groot, MSN, APN, FNP-BC, CDCES

Chapter 20 Pharmacotherapy: Dyslipidemia and Hypertension
in Persons With Diabetes 613
John D. Bucheit, PharmD, BCACP, CDCES, and
Dave L. Dixon, PharmD, BCACP, BCPS, CDCES, CLS,
FACC, FCCP

Chapter 21 Dietary Supplements and Diabetes: A Focus on
Complementary Health Approaches 647
Skye McKennon, PharmD, BCPS, and
Jennifer Danielson, PharmD, MBA, CDCES

Chapter 22 Complementary Health Approaches and Diabetes Care 703
Diana W. Guthrie, PhD, APRN, BC-ADM, DCES,
FADCES, FAAN, AHN-BC (retired), and
Ethel Elkins, DHSc, MHA, MA (LCSW)

Chapter 23 Acute Hyperglycemia 721
Dace L. Trence, MD, MACE

Chapter 24 Pregnancy With Diabetes 747
Diane M. Reader, RD, CDCES, and Alyce Thomas, RD

Chapter 25 Cardiovascular Complications of Diabetes 783
JoAnn Sperl-Hillen, MD

Chapter 26 Eye Disease Related to Diabetes 817
Szilárd Kiss, MD

Chapter 27 Diabetic Kidney Disease 837
Elizabeth Van Dril, PharmD, BCPS, BCACP

Chapter 28 Diabetic Neuropathies 867
Eric L. Johnson, MD, Aaron I. Vinik, MD, PhD, FCP, MACP,
and Etta J. Vinik, MA (Ed)

Index *905*

ACKNOWLEDGMENTS

Associate Editors

Susan Cornell, BS, PharmD, CDCES, FAPhA, FADCES, is the associate director of experiential education and an associate professor in the department of pharmacy practice at Midwestern University Chicago College of Pharmacy in Downers Grove, Illinois. Dr. Cornell is also a certified diabetes care and education specialist, specializing in community and ambulatory care practice. She serves as the current Midwestern University American Pharmacists Association Academy of Student Pharmacists (APhA-ASP) faculty advisor. She also is faculty supervisor of the Collaborative Health Advocate Team (CHAT), an interprofessional team of students from the colleges of pharmacy, medicine, dental medicine, and health sciences that provides diabetes self-management education and training to people in underserved community clinics.

Dr. Cornell has served on the ADCES board of directors and is a past president and a past chair of the board of directors of the Illinois Pharmacists Association. She has received numerous awards and recognitions, including the 2019 Outstanding Faculty Advisor award, 2017 Outstanding Illinois Diabetes Educator of the Year, 2014 Bowl of Hygeia, 2010 Teacher of the Year Award, the 2010 American Association of Colleges of Pharmacy Student Engaged Community Service Award, the 2008 AADE Fellow Award, the 2008 American Pharmacists Association Fellow award, and the 2005 Midwestern University Golden Apple Teaching Award.

Dr. Cornell has given numerous presentations to various healthcare professionals and community groups and has published and contributed to many peer-reviewed, professionally written, and online publications.

Cindy Halstenson, RDN, LD, CDCES has specialized in diabetes care and education for more than 25 years, including clinical care, case and disease management, population health improvement, Medicare Stars Quality Improvement, and clinical program management.

She has served as Chair, as well as the Communications Coordinator, of the Diabetes Care and Education (DCE) dietetic practice group of the Academy of Nutrition and Dietetics; Chair and Director of the National Certification Board for Diabetes Educators; Chair of the MN American Diabetes Association Leadership Board; Chair, as well as Chair of the Professional Education Committee, of the AADE MN Network; and, President of the Board of the Minnesota Academy of Nutrition and Dietetics.

Ms. Halstenson served as the Food for Thought department lead for Association of Diabetes Care & Education Specialist (ADCES) *In Practice* magazine, and has been an editor for the 4 previous editions of *The Art and Science of Diabetes Care and Education.*

David K. Miller, RN, MSEd, BSN, CDCES, FADCES, is the CEO of Health Education and Life Promotion (HELP). He has worked with weight loss centers as well as pharmaceutical companies such as Eli Lilly, Roche, Johnson and Johnson, and Astra Zeneca Pharmaceuticals. He is currently the Diabetes Care Coordinator for Community Health Network.

Mr. Miller has developed and directed hospital-based diabetes self-management programs that have received American Diabetes Association (ADA) recognition and accreditation from the Association of Diabetes Care and Education Specialists. He is the past president for the Indiana Central Association of Diabetes Educators and a past Board of Director for the Association of Diabetes Care & Education Specialists (ADCES). He currently is a faculty member of the Core Concepts® Course, which prepares individuals to sit for the CDCES® exam. He is also an auditor for the Diabetes Education Accreditation Program (DEAP).

He has worked with numerous organizations including the National Council and Licensing Exam (NCLEX) for RN and LPN, Nursing 2000, Indiana University School of Nursing, J.B. Lippincott Publishing Company, Mosby Publishing Company, and the Nurse's Book Society, and PESI Continuing Education Company.

Mr. Miller has been published in national journals, authored chapters for textbooks, served as editor for several books, and presented at national conferences. He is also a Fellow of the Association of Diabetes Care & Education Specialists.

Reviewers

Jean Baumann, RN, BSN, CDCES
Diabetes Nurse Educator
Penrose Street Saint Francis Health Services
Colorado Springs, CO

Dana E. Brackney, PhD, MSN, RN, CNS, CDCES, BC-ADM
Associate Professor
Appalachian State University
Boone, NC

Johanna Cappelli, RN, RVS, CDCES
Director of Clinical Operations
Cardiovascular Medical Associates, a Winthrop University Hospital Affiliate
Mineola, NY

Mary Jean Christian, MA, MBA, RD, CDCES
Diabetes Program Coordinator
University of California, Irvine
Irvine, CA

Beth Ann Coonrod, PhD, MPH, RN, CDCES
The Center for Diabetes and Endocrine Health
Allegheny Health Network
Pittsburgh, PA

Lourdes Cross, PharmD, BCACP, CDCES
Assistant Professor
Sullivan University College of Pharmacy and Health Sciences
Louisville, KY

Kendra Durdock, BSN, RN, CDCES
Certified Diabetes Nurse Educator
Penn State Health/Penn State Hershey Medical Center
Hershey, PA

Cindi Goldman-Patin, RN, MSN, BA, CDCES
Integrative Diabetes Education Association
Pittsfield, MA

Carol Homko PhD, RN, CDCES
Seattle, WA

Tommy Johnson, PharmD, CDCES, BC-ADM, FADCES

Rosalyn Marcus, DPM, RN, CDCES
Inpatient Diabetes Educator
Stanford Healthcare
Indio, CA

Jennifer A. Markee, LMSW, CDCES
St. Louis, MO

AnnMarie McDade, MS, RD, CDCES
Hackensack Meridian Health Medical Group, Joslin Diabetes Center
Old Bridge, New Jersey

Molly McElwee-Malloy, RN, CDCES
Tandem Diabetes
Waynesboro, VA

Christine Memering, BSN, RN, CDCES, FADCES
Certified Diabetes Care and Education Specialist
CarolinaEast Medical Center
New Bern, NC

Britney Merchant, MA, RD, CDCES, LD, LDN
Certified Diabetes Educator and Diabetes Program Coordinator
Indiana University Health
Greenwood, IN

Diana G. Mercurio, BS Pharm, CDCES, CDOE, CVDOE
Ambulatory Care Clinical Pharmacist
Rhode Island Primary Care Physicians Corporation
Coventry, RI

Janet Meyer, DNP, RN, CDCES
Diabetes Educator/Memorial Hospital and Health Care Center
Memorial Hospital
Jasper, IN

Lois Moss-Barnwell, MS, RD, LDN, CDCES
Principal Diabetes, Nutrition & Regulatory Consultant
Diet Rx, Ltd.
Highwood, IL

Julie Pierantoni, MSN, RN, CDCES, BC-ADM
Diabetes Services Quality Coordinator
Sentara RMH Medical Center
Harrisonburg, VA

Michelle Phillips, MS, RCEP, CDCES
Exercise Physiologist
Oklahoma Heart Hospital
Oklahoma City, OK

Mary Powell, PhD, CRNP, CDCES
Associate Dean of Graduate Nursing and Associate Professor
Widener University
Chester, PA

Mara Schwartz, BSN, RN, CDCES, CPT
Self-Regional Healthcare
Greenwood, SC

Donna Stevens, APN, APRN, BC-ADM, CDCES
University of Alabama Medical Center
Birmingham, AL

Angela Thompson, DNP, FNP-C, BC-ADM, CDCES, FAANP
Endocrine Nurse Practitioner, Hendricks Regional Health
Hendricks Regional Health
Danville, IN

Bridget Turner Jennings, RN, BAS, CDCES
Orange Park, FL

Kirsten Ward, MS, RCEP, CDCES
Diabetes Consultant/Say Goodbye to Diabetes
Sudbury, MA

The editors of the fifth edition would like to acknowledge the contributions of the editors and the chapter authors of the four previous editions of *The Art and Science of Diabetes Self-Management Education Desk Reference*.

Anne J. Abbate, RN, CDCES
Samuel L. Abbate, MD, CDCES
Ann L. Albright, PhD, RD
Robert Anderson, EdD
Marilyn S. Arnold, MS, RD, LD, CDCES
Rodolfo M. Banda, MD
Joan K. Bardsley, RN, MBA, CDCES, FADCES
Jackie L. Boucher, MS, RD, BC-ADM, CDCES
Carol A. Brownson, MSPH
Dorothy Burns, PhD, RN
Laura D. Byham-Gray, PhD, RD, CNSD
Kiralee K. Camp, MS
Belinda P. Childs, MN, CNS, BC-ADM, CDCES
Ann Constance, MA, RD, CDCES, FADCES
Marjorie Cypress, MSN, C-CNP, CDCES
Mary de Groot, PhD
Linda Delahanty, MS, RD, LD
Michael M. Engelgau, MD, MS
Edwin B. Fisher, PhD
Marion J. Franz, MS, RDN, LD, CDCES
Janine Freeman, RDN, LD, CDCES, CDTP
Martha Funnell, MS, RN CDCES
Patti B. Geil, MS, RD/RDN, FAND, CDCES
Cindi Goldman-Patin, RN, MSN, CDCES, BA
Victor H. Gonzalez, MD
Connie Hanham-Cain, MSN, RN, CDCES
Felicia Hill-Briggs, PhD, ABPP
Tommy Johnson, PharmD, BC-ADM, CDCES, FADCES
Edna G. Johnson-Gutierrez, MSN, ANP-BC, RN, CDCES
Ginger Kanzer-Lewis, RN, BC, EdM, CDCES, FADCES
Kim L. Kelly, PharmD, BCPS, FCCP, CDTC, CPC, CEC
Amanda Kirpitch, MA, RD, LDN, CDCES, CSSD
Karmeen Kulkarni, MS, RD, BC-ADM, CDCES
Daniel Lorber, MD, FACP, CDCES
Gayle M. Lorenzi, RN, CDCES
Sarah L. Lovegreen, MPH
Michelle F. Magee, MD, MBBCh, BAO, LRCPSI
Susan D. Martin, RD, LD, CDCES
Melinda Maryniuk, MEd, RD, CDCES, FADA
Lois Maurer, MS, RD, LDN, CDCES
Susan McLaughlin, BS, RD, CDCES
Gail D'Eramo Melkus, EdD, C-ANP, FAAN
Carolé Mensing, RN, MA, CDCES, FADCES
Dara L. Murphy, MPH
K. M. Venkat Narayan, MD, MPH
Joseph B. Nelson, MA, LP, CST
Katherine I. Nelson Ward, MPH, CHES
Sherry Smith-Ossman, MS, ANP, RNCS, RN, CDCES
Gretchen A. Piatt, PhD, MPH
James W. Pichert, PhD

Margaret A. Powers, PhD, RD, CDCES
Robert E. Ratner, MD, FACP, FACE
Laurie Ruggiero, PhD
David G. Schlundt, PhD
Laura Shane-McWhorter, PharmD, BCPS, BC-ADM, CDCES, FASCP, FADCES
Linda Siminerio, PhD, RN, CDCES
Anne H. Skelly, PhD, ANP, RN, CS
Geralyn R. Spollet, MSN, ANP, CDCES
Condit F. Steil, PharmD, FAPhA, CDCES
Tricia S. Tang, PhD
Donna M. Tomky, MSN, C-ANP, RN, CDCES
Ann Vannice, MSN, APRN, CDCES
Jeffrey J. VanWormer, MS
Frank Vinicor, MD, MPH
Christopher J. Vito, PharmD
Julie Wagner, PhD
Elizabeth A. Walker, PhD, RN, CDCES, FADCES
Judith Wylie-Rosett, EdD, RD
Kristin M. Zimmerman, PharmD, CGP

CHAPTER 1

Diabetes Care and Education: Rich Past, Challenging Present, Promising Future

Sandra Drozdz Burke, PhD, RN, FADCES, FAAN
Janet Thorlton, PhD, RN
Hiba Abbas, BSN, RN

Key Concepts

- Diabetes is a relentless global public health emergency requiring a multilevel system response.
- The financial impact of diabetes management threatens the viability of healthcare systems across the globe.
- Continued rapid technological development is associated with improved diabetes-related outcomes.
- Recognizing expanded roles and responsibilities in pre-diabetes, diabetes, and cardiometabolic diseases, the diabetes educator changed to the diabetes care and education specialists.
- Diabetes care and education specialists possess unique skill sets essential to the interdisciplinary care team in diabetes and cardiometabolic disease states.
- Education is necessary to but not sufficient for behavior change. Diabetes care and education specialists possess the knowledge, skills, and abilities to facilitate effective self-management in persons with diabetes and cardiometabolic conditions.
- The diabetes care and education specialists should be encouraged to practice to the full extent of his or her education (training) and expertise.
- Updated competencies assist the diabetes care and education specialists to grow and advance.
- Barriers to equal access to diabetes care and education must be addressed.

Diabetes Care and Education: Challenges and Opportunities

"Change will not come if we wait for some other person, or if we wait for some other time. We are the ones we've been waiting for. We are the change that we seek."

Barack Obama

Definitions of Terms

- **Epidemic:** A disease that affects a defined group of people in a specific geographic location simultaneously
- **Pandemic:** An extremely widespread or globally occurring disease that affects many populations simultaneously
- **Syndemic:** A combination of health or social conditions that interact to increase the disease burden to a community, further developing a public health concern

Pandemic. Amid the fear and devastation associated with the outbreak of COVID–19, the word *pandemic* has become part of everyday language throughout the world. The rapid spread of this novel virus is impacting the daily lives of the nearly 8 billion people living in today's world.

As of January 2020, the American Association of Diabetes Educators (AADE) is known as the Association of Diabetes Care & Education Specialists (ADCES). Either the organization's full name or the acronym will be used in this chapter, regardless of whether the text is referencing activities prior to 2020.

Healthcare and financial resources are focused, rightly so, on mitigating the impact of the deadliest infectious diseases in living history. And, during the crisis, life goes on. Non-communicable diseases (NCD) that have the power to alter the lives of individuals are not taking a break. In the United States, more than 171 people are diagnosed with and 28 people die from diabetes every hour.[1] Diabetes, at pandemic levels for years, is now considered "one of the fastest growing global health emergencies of the 21st century."[2]

Certainly, there is a distinction, never more apparent than now, between communicable and non-communicable health emergencies. And, the importance of developing systems to rapidly respond to emerging health concerns cannot be minimized. At the same time, it is important not to lose sight of the needs of those with NCD. The negative impact exerted by diabetes mellitus on individuals and society is never-ending. The magnitude of impact will be most apparent in countries with fewest resources, but diabetes knows no boundaries. All segments of society in every corner of the world are affected by diabetes. Together, the quartet of diabetes, cardiovascular disease, cancer, and respiratory disease is responsible for 8 out of every 10 deaths attributable to NCD throughout the world.[3] Even within the wealthiest countries, including the United States, the effects of diabetes and prediabetes continue to exert significant effects on population health.[4] Without change, 15 million people are projected to die *prematurely* every year from NCD.[5] Fifteen million translates to more than 28 individuals every minute, of every day, 365 days of the year.

There are three primary forms of diabetes: type 1, type 2, and gestational diabetes. Each of these is addressed in detail in later chapters of this desk reference. Type 2 diabetes (T2DM) is the most common form, affecting up to 95% of all persons with the disease.[2,4] The development of type 2 diabetes is associated with genetics and epigenetics compounded by modifiable environmental risk factors including obesity, physical inactivity, and poor nutrition.[2,6] Although the onset of type 2 diabetes can be delayed or prevented by disrupting the association of 1 or more risk factors, continued worldwide growth makes it clear that type 2 diabetes has moved beyond pandemic levels into *syndemic* proportions.[3,7] Strong evidence shows the positive impact of healthy lifestyle behaviors on type 2 diabetes, and new data suggest that use of monoclonal antibodies may delay the onset of type 1 diabetes as well.[8,9] Once diagnosed, long-term complications of either type 1 or type 2 diabetes can be prevented or delayed with targeted diabetes management strategies.[4,7,10,11] These strategies include care, education, and ongoing support to facilitate healthy lifestyles aimed at achieving and maintaining target blood glucose levels.

Global Impact of Diabetes

In the *Atlas of Diabetes* published biennially, the International Diabetes Federation addresses the global impact of diabetes. According to 2019 data, the total estimated prevalence of diabetes in adults doubled during the past 20 years and currently affects 463 million worldwide.[2] Expected to rise another 25% over the next decade, the IDF is projecting a worldwide prevalence of diabetes over 700 million by 2045. This far surpasses previous projections. While growth is expected throughout the world, the largest increases are projected to occur in Africa (143%↑), the Middle East and North Africa (96%↑), South East Asia (74%↑), and South and Central America (55%↑). The largest increases are expected to occur as counties continue to develop and their economies improve.[2–4] Worldwide, type 2 diabetes continues to account for approximately 90% of all diabetes.[2] It is slightly more common in men than in women worldwide. In many countries, including the United States, T2D is far more common in nonwhite and older populations.[2,4,12] Type 2 diabetes is primarily a condition associated with aging. Whereas 9.3% of the overall adult population has diabetes, when the data are broken down according to age, nearly 20% of those over age 65 are shown to have diabetes.[2,4]

Across the United States, in addition to the estimated 34.2 million people with diabetes, another 88 million adults have prediabetes, bringing the total number of Americans with or at risk for diabetes to over 120 million.[4,13] In the United States, news is hopeful as examination of data collected between 2012 and 2017 reveals stability in prevalence rates as well as a reduction of incidence of diabetes in adults.[14] Even so, the impact of those who currently have or are at risk for diabetes combined with a continuing rise in worldwide prevalence rates are sobering and very serious. Assuming current projections are accurate, by 2050 as many as 1 in 3 adults throughout the world will have diabetes.[2,15,16] China, India, and the United States continue to lead the world in cases of diabetes, a situation that is not likely to change in the foreseeable future.[2]

Because diabetes affects all segments of society, the impact of this disease is far reaching. In 2010, an estimated 4 million deaths were attributed to diabetes worldwide, with the proportionate number of deaths from diabetes in middle-aged women sometimes reaching nearly 25%.[17] By 2017, the annual death rate attributable to diabetes had exceeded 4 million worldwide.[2] In the United States, diabetes is ranked as the seventh leading cause of death, and it is generally believed that estimates of mortality due to diabetes are greatly underestimated because the cause of death in persons with diabetes is often ascribed to other conditions.[3] Global targets to reduce premature death from non-communicable diseases 30% by 2030 have been established.[5] Despite unprecedented rapid advances in technology, healthcare systems in most countries are unprepared to deal with the consequences associated with a pandemic of this magnitude.[18] Public health initiatives promoting an understanding of the multifactorial nature of diabetes and its complications combined with targeted approaches to identify and treat diabetes and prediabetes appear to be helping to reduce the socioeconomic burden of this devastating disease. In the United States, for example, the National Diabetes Prevention Program (NDPP) is already demonstrating success.[13]

Incidence versus Prevalence

Health statistics often are expressed in terms of incidence and prevalence. The distinction between the two measurements is important when interpreting the data.

Incidence measures the risk of the target population developing the disease or condition being tracked over a specific time period. *Prevalence* measures the portion of the target population that has the disease or condition being tracked.

Incidence is calculated by taking the number of new cases of a disease or condition within a specific time frame—usually a year—and dividing by the size of the population.

Prevalence is calculated by dividing the number of individuals with the disease or condition at a particular point in time by the number of individuals examined.

There are differences in the incidence and prevalence of the primary types of diabetes. Many people are confused by the terms incidence and prevalence. The common definitions can be found in the sidebar, but there is an easy way to understand the difference. Think about prevalence as referring to those who are known to have the condition and incidence as those individuals who are newly diagnosed. Representing approximately 5% of all individuals with diabetes, the incidence of type 1 diabetes continues to rise. In other words, increasingly larger numbers of people are diagnosed with TID every year. The reasons for this persistent increase are unclear. While type 1 diabetes can be diagnosed at any point in the lifespan, it occurs most commonly in childhood and youth. Globally, 1,110,100 children and youth under age 20 years have type 1 diabetes, and more than 128,900 children develop type 1 diabetes annually.[2] In the United States, about 193,000 children and youth under age 20 years have type 1 diabetes with just over 18,000 new cases diagnosed each year.[4] Non-Hispanic whites in this age group have a relatively high incidence of type 1 diabetes compared with African-American, Hispanic, and Asian youth.[19,20] Data from the Search for Diabetes in Youth Study demonstrated an annual relative increase in incidence of 1.8% in the decade between 2002 and 20012.[21,22] Of note, these increases were seen in early school-age and mid- to late adolescent years, more often in boys, and in all racial/ethnic backgrounds except for Native Americans and Asian/Pacific Islanders.

Even though type 2 diabetes typically develops over many years and is more common in adults, type 2 is becoming much more common in children.[2,4] In the United States the incidence of type 2 diabetes in youth aged 10 to 19 years is increasing at an alarming 4.8% annually.[23] The increases are most pronounced in children of Native American and non-Hispanic Black ancestry, particularly among those who are overweight or obese. Ongoing reports from the SEARCH for Diabetes in Youth Study Group suggest that youth with type 2 diabetes have difficulty transitioning to adult care providers, experience higher levels of diabetes distress and depression, and demonstrate significant evidence of diabetes-related complications by the age of 21 years.[23]

Financial Impact of Diabetes

According to the most recent reports, the economic impact of diabetes continues to grow exponentially. In 2017, diabetes costs reached a level of $327 billion.[24] These costs rise to the level of $404 billion when prediabetes is added into the equation.[25] If analyzed on a state-by-state basis, the overall economic toll exerted by diabetes has been reported to be as high as $465 billion, with considerably higher indirect costs.[27] The cost of caring for diabetes far exceeds the cost of medical care in those without diabetes.[2,24] Several years ago, the cost of caring for diabetes in the United States was expected to be 20% of the gross domestic product (GDP) by 2016.[27] Currently, those with diabetes are responsible for 25% of the healthcare spending in the United States. Of that, 1 in every 7 healthcare dollars is used to pay for costs specifically linked to diabetes.[24] These costs include substantial direct medical expenses for inpatient care, outpatient care, emergency care, medications, and durable medical equipment, as well as indirect costs of absenteeism, reduced productivity at work, and lost productivity due to disability or premature death. Individuals with diabetes are more likely to be absent from work (absenteeism) and, while at work, suffer from fatigue or have reduced concentration; additionally, they may not be able to perform at a normal level (presenteeism). About 61% of all diabetes-related costs are attributed to the population over age 65 years.[24] Every day until 2030, 10,000 baby boomers will turn 65.[28] In 2009, Huang and colleagues estimated that 14.6 million people with diabetes would be Medicare eligible by 2034.[29] A more recent estimate of actual Medicare beneficiaries shows a diabetes prevalence rate of 31.6%, which translates to roughly 24.5 million people.[30] The price tag for medications to treat diabetes and diabetes-related complications accounts for about 30% of the direct costs of diabetes. Costs for antihyperglycemic medications have been steadily rising since 2001.[31] Taking inflation into account, the cost of all antihyperglycemic medications rose 45% between 2012 and 2017, but the cost of insulin during that time period rose 110%.[26] While the financial toll of diabetes will continue to adversely affect the ability of developed countries to finance their national healthcare systems, it will also have a considerable negative impact on the economic progress being made in developing countries.[2]

At the individual level, great disparities exist in the economic resources available to persons with diabetes in the United States. Prior to enactment of the Affordable Care Act (ACA), the number of uninsured in the United States was at 46.5 million. By 2016, that number dropped nearly 50% to 26.7 million. In 2017, the number of uninsured individuals in the United States began to rise. There are currently nearly 30 million uninsured in the country.[32] Medicare and Medicaid can be considered safety nets for older adults and those who meet or exceed the poverty threshold, but the working poor remain uninsured and continue to struggle. High deductibles that accompany insurance policies have an impact on a family's net income. When personal disposable income is limited, self-care practices can be significantly impacted

Diabetes Care and Education: A Brief History

Those familiar with Elliott P. Joslin's work will recall his passion for diabetes education and for involving individuals in their own care. As early as 1914, nurses were integral to Joslin's diabetes education model, serving as "diabetes wandering nurses," inpatient diabetes care specialists, and later as diabetes nurse educators.[33,34] In the 1950s and 1960s, diabetes teaching units were established at Deaconess Hospital in Boston and registered dietitians and "diabetes nurses" provided comprehensive diabetes education programs. The intended outcome of these programs was diabetes self-management for persons with diabetes and their families. Important and progressive, this level of diabetes care and education was uncommon. But around that same time in the mid-20th century, Donnell Etzwiler examined primary care practice patterns and the diabetes knowledge base of nurses and dietitians. In a 1967 paper, he concluded that diabetes teaching done in hospitals was provided by poorly prepared providers and that follow-up was rare.[35] Etzwiler, a prominent pediatric endocrinologist who was also passionate about the need for ongoing diabetes education and support, founded the International Diabetes Center (IDC) in Minneapolis in 1967.[37] Diabetes practices, clinics, and centers modeled after Joslin and the IDC soon appeared across the country, and diabetes education emerged as a specialty attracting primarily registered nurses and dietitians.[37,38] And, in 1974, a passionate multidisciplinary group of diabetes educators founded the Association of Diabetes Care and Education Specialists to serve the needs of this new and growing specialty.

Often occurring during hospitalization resulting from a diagnosis of diabetes, diabetes education in those early days might have been organized around the triad of diet, exercise, and medication management. In the 1980s home blood glucose monitoring became widely available and replaced urine glucose testing as the standard of care. "Control" of diabetes was the goal of care, and glycated hemoglobin testing became the gold standard for assessment. Debates about the use and frequency of self-monitoring of blood glucose (SMBG) were common. When federal regulations led to reduced hospital lengths of stay in the mid-1980s, out-patient diabetes education became more available. Insulin pump therapy (CSII) entered the field as a realistic alternative to multiple daily injections (MDI). Also in the 1980s, study sites for the proposed Diabetes Control and Complications Trial (DCCT) were selected and that (now epic) longitudinal study was initiated. In 1983, national standards and review criteria for diabetes education were developed and promulgated.[39] Using the new national standards, 39 diabetes education programs were awarded ADA recognition in 1986, and the first specialty certification exam for diabetes educators was offered that same year.[40–42]

Throughout the 1990s, diabetes care and education was marked by rapid scientific advancements. Human insulin was introduced to the market as the decade began, and insulin analogs entered the market shortly thereafter. Blood glucose monitoring and insulin pump technologies advanced rapidly. The Federal Drug Administration approved additional oral medications for the treatment of type 2 diabetes. Within the specialty, the term "diabetic diet" became obsolete as nutritional guidelines encompassed more successful strategies for healthy eating with diabetes. Results from the DCCT demonstrated the unequivocal value of targeting near-normal glucose levels in type 1 diabetes. The diagnostic cut-point for type 2 diabetes was lowered and the terminology characterizing diabetes changed to reflect pathophysiologic differences between the major variants of the disease. CSII or MDI combined with carbohydrate counting and frequent monitoring became the norm for management in T1D. The prevalence of overweight and obesity in children and adults was on the rise and type 2 diabetes began to appear in youth. As the evidence base grew and specialists were gaining more knowledge about diabetes management, the prevalence of diabetes was growing at an alarming rate of ~4.4% per year.[14] Greater numbers of diabetes educators were needed to serve a rapidly expanding population of people with diabetes. During this decade, the process and outcomes of diabetes education began to be increasingly person-centered.[43] And, in diabetes education, a paradigm shift was taking place.[44] Terminology began to reflect the change as educators moved from compliance to adherence to empowerment models. Reimbursement models were also shifting, and group sessions became increasingly more common in diabetes education.

It seemed that diabetes was on everyone's mind at the turn of the century. The first decade of the new millennium provided evidence supporting glycemic control for type 2 diabetes, and research linked healthy lifestyles with the delay or prevention of type 2 diabetes.[7–8,45,46] Incidence rates of diabetes, overweight, and obesity in the United States continued to surge. New classes of diabetes medications were added to the treatment arsenal. Incretin mimetics, DPP-4 inhibitors, long-acting insulin analogs, and an amylin analog were among the medications introduced to the market. Blood glucose monitoring, now ubiquitous to diabetes self-management, was faster and more reliable. Results were easy to download, analyze, and use during clinic appointments. Continuous glucose monitoring entered the market as a clinic-based option for complex care management. Terms like cultural competence, health literacy, diabetes distress, psychological insulin resistance, and empowerment became increasingly more common in the literature. The Chronic Care Model and the AADE7 Self-Care Behaviors® were adopted as organizing frameworks for diabetes education as the focus shifted toward active engagement and person-centeredness.[47,48] Evidence defining the value of diabetes education was published[27,49] but legislation requiring reimbursement for diabetes education services could not be realized. As the Association of Diabetes Care and Education Specialists (ADCES) identified the need for an advanced management credential, and the Board-Certified Advanced Diabetes Management® (BC-ADM®) was introduced to address the increasing complexities of diabetes education and management,[50–51] new provider categories such as community health workers emerged. Routinely reviewed and revised national standards for diabetes self-management education and support continued to reflect the evolving healthcare landscape. In 2009, the ADCES began offering program accreditation services. As of this writing, recognition through the American Diabetes Association or accreditation through the ADCES continue to serve as quality indicators for diabetes education programs.

If the first decade of the 21st century seemed like a whirlwind, the second decade has been nothing short of mind-boggling. At about the same time the world began to recover from a great recession, baby-boomers entered Medicare rosters at the rate of 10,000 new members per day. The twin epidemics of diabetes and obesity were still growing at an alarming pace. SGLT inhibitors, new combinations of diabetes medications, and new formations of insulins entered the market. New models of healthcare delivery systems such as Patient-Centered Medical Homes and Accountable Care Organizations were introduced. Reimbursement models focused on outcomes are the new norm. Duncan and colleagues published additional data about the value of diabetes education.[52] An ADCES-commissioned workforce analysis of diabetes educators appeared at about the same time as threats of an impending nursing shortage resurfaced. It became clear that the number of persons with and at risk for diabetes far exceeded the number and availability of existing diabetes educators. Programmatic costs and lack of reimbursement for services continued to plague diabetes education programs. And technology marched on. Real-time continuous glucose monitoring became an integral part of diabetes care for many persons with diabetes, especially those using insulin pump therapy. Telehealth, digital on-line communities, digital and mobile technologies, all grew and impacted diabetes education, care, and support in unprecedented ways. Research about locations of and providers for diabetes education is now common in the literature.[53–55] Individuals with diabetes can locate information about self-care and connect with like-minded others using any digital technology with access to the Internet. Community health workers, patient care navigators, health coaches, and care managers are now available and often used in, with, and by healthcare entities. And, along with sensitivity to the language used in health care, a focus on interprofessional care that includes the individual in shared decision-making models emerged. The "words matter" movement is gaining momentum as increasingly greater numbers of healthcare providers are learning how to use person-centered language in all encounters.

Diabetes Education: Profession or Specialty?

Diabetes education has been an important part of diabetes management since the early days of Elliott Joslin. Over the last half century, countless individuals devoted their professional careers to diabetes education. These early diabetes educators, mostly nurses and dietitians, are the recognized authorities in this field of expertise. They were trailblazers who understood that diabetes education involved more than distributing pamphlets. Many were involved in building the evidence base that supports current practice. Within today's diabetes community, clinicians know that structured diabetes self-management education and support (DSMES) results in better self-management knowledge and improvements in fasting blood glucose, A1C, lipid, and blood pressure levels in individuals across the lifespan, and that diabetes education with follow-up support delivered by diabetes educators also results in improved satisfaction and reductions in diabetes-related distress in persons with diabetes.[53,56,57] DSMES can lower A1C values by as much as 2.3%, and culturally appropriate diabetes education improves knowledge, healthy lifestyles, and A1C levels in ethnic minority groups.[58] There is no question that diabetes education is beneficial; arguably, it is critical to the success of the person with diabetes. Some leaders in the field have referred to diabetes education as a specialty, and others call it a profession. Which is it? Is diabetes education a profession or a specialty?

That very interesting question often causes considerable consternation and requires a little unpacking. What is a "profession"? Loosely defined, a profession can be any type of work, but many take a narrower approach and differentiate a "profession" from an occupation, trade, or industry. From an historical perspective, the first professions were law, medicine, and divinity (the Church.[59–61] Some say these three professions have been present from the start of time. Others identify periods in time that define social context and point to Ancient Greece, the Roman Empire, the time of Enlightenment, the Reformation, or even the Industrial Revolution. Most likely, the primary professions arose during the Middle Ages and were refined intermittently throughout more recent history.[60,62] A good understanding of the history of and criteria defining professions comes from the work of Abraham Flexner. Flexner was an academic in the early 20th century. Subsequent to his seminal report on the state of medical education in the United States and Canada, he presented a paper that detailed the characteristics of professions in 1917. Reprinted in 2001, his criteria of a profession have endured over time.[61] Flexner listed six essential characteristics of a profession. Consistent with more contemporary literature, these classic criteria can be distilled down to the following five characteristics.[60,62] First, professions must provide a service essential to human welfare. Next, each profession is responsible to develop, use, communicate, and grow a specialized, scientific body of knowledge. Third, admission to the profession requires formal education gained through institutions of higher learning at the conclusion of which members demonstrate competency through licensure and credentialing. Fourth, members practice autonomously. They develop and follow clear standards of practice for which they are legally and publicly accountable. Finally, members are bound to and guided by a strict code of ethics. This common set of values is typified by honesty, trustworthiness, and altruism. Over time, many more professions were added to list including, to name a few, accounting, architecture, journalism, nursing, nutrition and dietetics, social work, pharmacy, and the professorate. Experts continue to disagree about which disciplines have achieved professional status.

To answer the question of whether diabetes education is a profession, each criterion should be examined separately. The essential nature of diabetes education is debatable. Evidence clearly confirms the value of diabetes education and support when it is delivered by a qualified provider. Still, diabetes education is a recommended, not required strategy for those with newly diagnosed diabetes. And, many providers, both licensed and unlicensed, deliver what they believe to be diabetes education. Diabetes education is both an art and a science. The body of knowledge needed for diabetes education comes from related disciplines such as medicine, pharmacology, physiology, nutrition, exercise science, and more recently from health education, nursing, and other healthcare professions. Some diabetes educators conduct and disseminate research, particularly research specific to the process and outcomes of diabetes education. The body of knowledge specific to diabetes education is absolutely growing. Programs designed to prepare diabetes educators are uncommon. Rarer still are programs at the college or university level, but all programs of study in the primary clinical professions include course and clinical content specific to diabetes. In some disciplines, academic programs may offer diabetes as a specialty or provide fellowship opportunities. Licensure to practice as a diabetes educator is not required in most states, provinces, or countries, but certification does require licensure in a specified healthcare discipline.[63,64] Because certification is a voluntary activity, those who deliver diabetes education may or may not be certified. With respect to autonomy, there is considerable variability. Diabetes education practice is mostly collaborative, often directed, but seldom independent. Most importantly, diabetes educators are first educated in an established discipline, eg, medicine, nursing, nutritional science, pharmacy. Thus, each provider is responsible for knowing and following the state rules and regulations for their primary profession and is accountable to his or her state of residence for doing so. The standards of practice and codes of ethics to which most clinicians are accountable derive from their primary profession and state statutes. And, the Certification Board for Diabetes Care and Education requires that all who take the CDCES® exam agree to follow the cannon of ethics promulgated by the CBDCE Board.[65] See Table 1.1.

If diabetes education does not completely meet the Flexner benchmarks of a profession, it certainly qualifies as a clinical specialty. It is one that thousands of clinicians choose to practice and from which millions of individuals with diabetes benefit. Although 93% of today's diabetes educators have backgrounds in nursing, dietetics, or pharmacy, clinicians from a wide range of healthcare occupations, including social work, dentistry, podiatry, and exercise physiology choose to specialize in diabetes education.[66] Diabetes education has a long history punctuated by amazing successes. It is not only challenging and rewarding, it is genuinely interprofessional and characterized by a team approach that keeps the person with diabetes at the center of the care circle.

TABLE 1.1 Evaluating the Status of Diabetes Education as a Profession

	Yes	*No*	*Maybe*
Does diabetes education provide a service **essential** to human welfare?			X
Have diabetes education providers **independently** developed, used, communicated, and expanded a specialized, scientific body of knowledge?			X
Is an **academic degree** in the specialty required?		X	
Is licensure and/or **credentialing required** for practice?		X*	
Do diabetes educators have full control (**autonomy**) over their practice?		X	
Are members bound to and guided by a strict **code of ethics**?			X
Do members share a **common set of values** typified by honesty, trustworthiness, and altruism?	X		

*Licensure is required in Kentucky and Indiana.

From Diabetes Education to Diabetes Care and Education:

Many diabetes educators have been on the leading edge for decades, embracing new technologies and advocating for a clinical practice environment focused on person-centered care and support. In the 1980s and 1990s, educators had pivotal roles in the Diabetes Control and Complications Trials.[67–69] More than 20 years ago, Feste, Anderson, Funnell, and colleagues[44,70–72] first began publishing work about person-centered approaches using empowerment. And, in 2003, Mulcahy and colleagues identified behavior change as the unique outcome of diabetes education and introduced the world to AADE7®.[73] Now classic research demonstrated that while knowledge is an essential prerequisite for self-care, knowledge alone is not enough to promote behavior change.[44,74,75] In response to changes in diabetes management and a growing body of evidence, best practices for diabetes education evolved to focus on strategies that promote and support effective person-centered self-management.[72,76,77] From the beginning, person-centered empowerment approaches to DSMES have been successful because they are based on principles of self-determination and support for autonomy.[72,77]

In 2015, the Association of Diabetes Care and Education Specialists (ADCES), the Academy of Nutrition and Dietetics (AND), and the American Diabetes Association (ADA) published a joint position statement within which they collaboratively defined diabetes self-management education (DSME) as "the process of facilitating the knowledge, skill, and ability necessary for diabetes self-care" and diabetes self-management support as "the support required for implementing and sustaining the coping skills and behavior needed to self-manage on an ongoing basis.[75] The goal of diabetes self-management education and support (DSMES) encompasses improved quality of life, self-care behaviors leading to improvements in a wide variety of clinical attributes, and decreased healthcare costs.[46,76,78–80] To achieve this using a person-centered approach, diabetes educators need sophisticated skill sets built on a solid core of foundational knowledge. Self-management is continuous and often difficult, but effective diabetes education and support can lead to positive outcomes to satisfy all involved in the process.

The term "diabetes education," which served the specialty well for decades, no longer fully represents the educator's breadth of responsibilities. DSMES is not only effective for people with diabetes; it is instrumental in preventing type 2 diabetes in those with prediabetes.[49,52] In recent years, diabetes educators have been increasingly more knowledgeable about prediabetes, diabetes prevention programs, obesity management, and risk reduction for cardiometabolic disease. Whether through independent practice, collaborative direct care, or the referral process, a majority of diabetes educators are more involved in influencing practice.[66] So, in keeping with practice patterns, DSMES has most recently been defined as "the interactive, collaborative, ongoing process involving the person with diabetes or prediabetes and/or the caregivers and the specialist(s)."[81] This is an important change because despite an expanding evidence base that supports the legitimacy of its impact, diabetes education remains chronically underutilized.[56,66]

This begs the question: if it is so effective, why is diabetes education underutilized? A part of the answer can be linked with the Internet, where health information sources abound. People know that information is available at the touch of a button. A recent literature search revealed over 6,000 publications for the combined terms "health information" and "internet." The body of knowledge on this topic has been growing for years. The fifth iteration of the Health Information National Trends Survey (HINTS), supported by the National Cancer Institute, concluded in 2018. Data from HINTS can be generalized to identify all health information seeking trends on the Internet. Those who seek digital health information tend to engage with providers at a higher level, experience better quality of life, and be more satisfied with healthcare decision-making.[82] Information technology is so much a part of contemporary health care that use of the Internet to seek health information was identified as a goal for Healthy People 2020.* Not all, but increasingly more people are coming to healthcare appointments armed with information they downloaded from an Internet source. Still, digital disparities exist. The gaps in access to online technologies are consistent with actual (in-person) healthcare access issues. Individuals who are older, poorer, non-white, less well-educated, rural, and sicker are less likely to access on-line sources.[83,84] Other researchers suggest that the Internet is neither universally trusted nor used and conclude that healthcare professionals should not assume that everyone is comfortable with or ready for Internet use.[85]

Easy access to health information does not fully explain low attendance at diabetes education classes or appointments. In the UK, Canada, and the United States, low attendance rates have long been a concern.[86] In recent years, investigators have begun to seek explanations once again. Winkley and colleagues found that those at greatest risk for diabetes complications were not the ones attending classes.[87] Instead, attendees were more likely to be women, individuals who did not smoke, and those who had lower A1C levels at diagnosis. Horrigan and colleagues[88] conducted a systematic review of literature and concluded that there were two main categories of people who declined the opportunity to attend diabetes education classes: those who could not attend for medical, timing, or financial issues and those who, for many reasons, saw no personal benefit from attendance. Other researchers found similar themes. Length of course, competing health issues, individual experiences and opinions, and personal priorities topped the list of reasons for non-attendance. Similar findings for non-attendance were identified subsequent to the systematic review.[86,89–91] Various strategies to improve attendance are suggested, including individualized sessions and systems-based support of programs. All agree that further study is needed.

Giving consideration to the problems associated with this rapidly changing diabetes and healthcare landscape and armed with the results of a detailed environmental scan, the ADCES Board of Directors established Project Vision to address current and future needs of the diabetes educator. The definition of the specialty and the expanding role of the educator are of foremost concern.[92] The pillars associated with Project Vision are outlined in the blue sidebar.

ADCES Project Vision Pillars

Drive Integration: Understanding that our value is in offering care that is holistic and seamless, it's critical that we integrate the clinical and self-management aspects of care.

Include Related Conditions: Diabetes isn't isolated, and neither are diabetes care and education specialists. We will demonstrate our expertise in the full range of cardiometabolic conditions: diabetes, obesity, hypertension, and cardiac disorders.

Focus on Behavioral Health: Supporting the emotional well-being of the whole person with diabetes must be a foundational element of the care we provide.

Leverage Technology: Diabetes care and education specialists will be technology experts and data interpreters, trainers, and consultants driving care.

Promote Person-Centered Care: We will continue to advocate so that every individual with diabetes and cardiometabolic conditions has access to a diabetes care and education specialist.

Achieve Quadruple Aim: We strive to offer care that positively impacts quality and cost and enhances the experience for both the person with diabetes and the provider.

*As of this writing, Healthy People 2030 goals have not been finalized, but it is reasonable to expect to see goals for Health Information Technology.

From Diabetes Educator to Diabetes Care and Education Specialist

Diabetes educators have been defined as healthcare professionals who focus on helping people with and at risk for diabetes and related conditions achieve behavior-change goals which, in turn, lead to better clinical outcomes and improved health status. More than 20,000 healthcare providers from various professional disciplines, primarily nursing, dietetics, and pharmacy, were certified in the diabetes specialty in 2019.[93,94] Two mechanisms for certification in the specialty currently exist in the United States: the Certified Diabetes Care and Education Specialist® (CDCES®) credential awarded by the Certification Board for Diabetes Care and Education (CBDCE) and the Board Certified-Advanced Diabetes Management® (BC-ADM®) credential awarded by the ADCES. Criteria for certification, established by certifying bodies, typically include an educational background in health care, considerable experience in the specialty, and a comprehensive knowledge base. Other countries often have their own standards, processes, and names for the credentialed diabetes educator.

As noted previously, diabetes education involves more than information sharing. Diabetes educators use in-depth knowledge and skills in the biological and social sciences, communication, counseling, and education to provide self-management education and ongoing support to those affected by diabetes.[28,41] The title Diabetes Educator and its evolving definition served the specialty well for nearly 50 years. In 2019, the ADCES Board of Directors took a bold move and changed the title from Diabetes Educator to Diabetes Care and Education Specialist (DCES).[95] The name of the organization was changed to the Association of Diabetes Care and Education Specialists (ADCES) soon afterwards. As a result of these changes, the NCBDE changed its name to the Certification Board for Diabetes Care and Education (CBDCE) and the credential awarded to the Certified Diabetes Care and Education Specialist (CDCES).

Changing the title was neither taken lightly by the ADCES Board of Directors nor was it a quick process. It was a data-based, purposeful decision undertaken to reposition the educator as a critical resource within the healthcare team. Before taking this step, data from multiple sources were considered. For example, National Practice Surveys help to provide an understanding of the educator's role in the healthcare system. Eight biennial surveys have been undertaken by ADCES to date. Previous surveys demonstrated relatively stable demographics and practice changes consistent with the time frame.[94,96] While the most recent published data showed slight change in demographics, the results revealed shifting practice patterns, suggesting that the diabetes educator's role is expanding.[66] Depending on the setting and the educator's professional background and credentials, responsibilities might include DSMES, medical nutrition therapy, clinical management, disease management, counseling, and/or health professional education and research.[66,94] Diabetes care and education specialists practice in inpatient, outpatient, community, home care, academic, and other settings. They are involved in, among other things, direct care, program management, education of other healthcare professionals, research, social reform, and advocacy. And, as valued collaborators, they are becoming increasingly more involved with insulin initiation and titration, medication, device, and technology management.[66] Armed with this and other environmental scanning data, the ADCES Board outlined a vision that would allow for a diabetes educator to practice to the highest capacity of his or her license and to thrive in a dynamically changing environment. In December 2019, ADCES Board President Karen Kemmis stated that the role of the diabetes care and education specialist was envisioned as someone who could serve as an integrator for clinical management, education, prevention, and support. After formulating a comprehensive vision, the Board commissioned an external firm to gather additional data. At the conclusion of the process, the Board realized that the title "diabetes educator" adequately conveyed neither the educator's role within the integrated care team nor the breadth of the services they provided. An in-depth process to rename the specialty was undertaken, an outcome of which was the change in title. Various titles, including the current one, were tested among a broad base of stakeholders. The title Diabetes Care and Education Specialist was preferred by a majority. In December 2019, Kemmis noted that the title change moves the diabetes educator from a "knowledgeable and supportive advocate and coach who provides patient-centered education to people with diabetes" to "an expert who, as an integral member of the care team, provides collaborative, comprehensive and person-centered care and education to people with diabetes."

Diabetes Educator versus Diabetes Care and Education Specialist

Diabetes Educator

A knowledgeable and supportive advocate and coach who provides patient-centered education to people with diabetes

Diabetes Care and Education Specialist

An expert who, as an integral member of the care team, provides collaborative, comprehensive, and person-centered care and education to people with diabetes

Documents Supporting Practice

As the specialty evolved, so too did the documents supporting practice.[97–100] The earliest set of standards appeared in 1992. They were developed, in part, to accompany the National Standards for Diabetes Education and to assist educators to prepare for certification in the specialty. Definitions of diabetes education and the diabetes educator appeared in these initial guidelines. The role at that time was specifically limited to broad-based, comprehensive, and (ideally) interdisciplinary education. The 10 standards of practice (SOP) ranged from assessment through evaluation and included professional accountability and an ethical basis for practice.[97] Revised in 1999, the definitions of diabetes education and the diabetes educator broadened, and the six standards of educational practice were separated from the four standards of professional practice. The scope of practice continued to address the multidimensionality and multidisciplinary nature of the diabetes educator.[98] In the third version, the definition of DSME was broadened further.[99] The process now incorporated the AADE7 Self-Care Behaviors® and included group education and prevention. The six educational practice standards were rearranged, and the standards of professional practice, now called the standards of professional performance (SOPP), were expanded to include goals of care, professional performance appraisal, collaboration, and research. At about the same time, the ADCES began developing guidelines for the practice of diabetes self-management education (Guidelines) and competencies for diabetes care and education specialists (Competencies).[78,79] Initially intended to serve as companion documents to the Standards of Practice, the Guidelines incorporated much of the information from the SOP/SOPP and thus grew into the primary practice resource for people with diabetes, non–diabetes specialist providers, and other stakeholders.[78] In 2010, the SOP/SOPP were updated to reflect the new guidelines. Content of the SOP/SOPP were substantively unchanged, but the standards of professional performance were moved to an appendix.[100]

The Scope and Standards of Practice, Standards of Practice, and Standards of Professional Performance provided a framework for practice and guideline for excellence in diabetes education for more than 2 decades.[97–100] Importantly, scope of practice for diabetes education was always linked to state and/or national rules and regulations for the individual's primary profession. An intent of the original competencies and guidelines was to acknowledge the value of diabetes education providers across a broad continuum, from the community health worker to the advanced-level diabetes care and education provider. In the first version, the ADCES workgroup defined 5 levels of practice identifying a wide spectrum of practice ranging from the community health worker to the expert practitioner of diabetes education and/or management.[78] Revisions in 2013 and 2016 addressed the important contributions of all care providers, including the nontraditional and/or non-licensed healthcare worker and created a distinct category for the diabetes paraprofessional. Practice levels were condensed and competencies for each level of provider were developed and subsequently refined.[79,101]

Competencies for Practice

The first competencies for diabetes educators were published in 2009, and those for diabetes paraprofessionals were added several years later.[101,106] Competencies are intended to provide a road map for the development of the knowledge, skills, and abilities required for practice across the continuum of diabetes care.[79] The original competencies were organized according to provider level, using the Dreyfus Model and Bloom's revised taxonomy as organizing frameworks.[105,106] According to the Dreyfus model, experience is gained over time, and the individual moves from the level of advanced beginner to competent and then to proficient professional. With increasingly more time in the specialty, one moves through the levels of proficiency and gains an increasingly wider body of diabetes specialty knowledge and skills through achievement of competencies.[102,103] The knowledge base needed to provide quality diabetes education is multifaceted, so the competencies are structured into broad categories called domains. There were 292 original competencies, organized according to domain and level of practice, for the diabetes educator in the original document. In the most recent version, there were 126 competencies, sorted into two levels across five domains for the paraprofessional and 220 competencies for three levels of diabetes educator over the same five domains.[101]

Given the new vision and anticipated title change, in 2019 the ADCES Board of Directors recognized the need to revisit the Guidelines and Competencies. An inclusive, interprofessional, and geographically diverse workgroup was empaneled and charged with the task of reviewing and revising the existing practice documents. Work toward revision began in 2019 with a comprehensive review of the current practice documents followed by a review of literature specific to competencies in diabetes education as well as in related disciplines. Consistent with previous versions, the group decided to use the Dreyfus framework to organize competencies and Bloom's revised taxonomy to identify appropriate verbs for measuring the cognitive domain.[102,103] The group also decided to follow a Delphi technique to ensure rigor in the approach.[104] Using the Delphi technique provided a mechanism for the group to survey a larger group of experts in the field to ensure consensus with competency statements. A modified approach allowed for initial development of domains and competencies by the workgroup followed by input from selected experts. The draft document identifies six domains, crafted using this consensus methodology. The proposed domains compared with the existing domains can be found in Table 1.2. Updated competencies for the DCES and for others engaged in diabetes education and support will be published elsewhere when they become available.

Whether or not he or she is certified in the specialty, the diabetes care and education specialist will have achieved an advanced body of core knowledge and skills common to diabetes care and education above that which is required by their primary profession. The revised competency statements are intended to assist the DCES to build a foundation of knowledge and to grow as needed by his or her individual practice. Based on self-evaluation, each DCES will identify competencies appropriate for his or her practice, assess current knowledge in those areas, and seek educational opportunities where needed.

TABLE 1.2 Former and Proposed Domains for Diabetes Care and Education Specialists

	2016	*2020*	*Rationale for Change*
Domain 1:	Pathophysiology, Epidemiology, and Clinical Practice of Prediabetes and Diabetes	Clinical Management & Integration	Previously, this domain addressed the foundational knowledge of diabetes, including diabetes pathophysiology, epidemiology, and clinical guidelines. The updated Domain 1 focuses on clinical practice that integrates foundational knowledge.
Domain 2:	Culturally Competent, Supportive Care Across the Lifespan	Communication & Advocacy	Previously this domain encompassed competencies needed to provide culturally competent, supportive care across the lifespan. The updated Domain 2 focuses on communication competencies essential to optimize quality of care.
Domain 3:	Teaching and Learning Skills	Person-Centered Care & Education Across the Lifespan	Previously, this domain focused on aspects of teaching and learning and behavior change using aspects noted in the AADE7®. The updated Domain 3 identifies competencies necessary to partner with individuals to deliver care and education conducive to behavior change and improved quality of life for self-management of diabetes and cardiometabolic conditions across the lifespan.
Domain 4:	Self-Management Education	Research & Quality Improvement	Previously, this domain identified the competencies required to provide effective DSME while the updated version identifies research and QI competencies essential to guide research and quality improvement activities.
Domain 5:	Program and Business Management	Systems-Based Practice	Previously, the competencies in this domain enabled the educator to create a climate supporting successful self-management of diabetes. In the updated version of Domain 5, the focus is on application of business principles, population health management, and systems practice to positively impact outcomes of systems, providers, persons, and populations.
Domain 6:	N/A	Professional Practice	Domain 6 was added to address competencies related to lifelong learning and professionalism.

Source: Association of Diabetes Care & Education Specialists, *Competency Domains for Diabetes Care & Education Specialists* (Chicago: ADCES, 2020 (in review)).

Inclusivity: Others Engaged in Diabetes Care and Education

Recognizing that many individuals do not interface with a credentialed diabetes care and education specialist, ADCES has long held the position that all healthcare providers should have sufficient diabetes knowledge to provide safe clinical care for people with diabetes. Healthcare providers with a strong foundation in diabetes knowledge are more likely to choose to partner with diabetes care and education specialists and possibly even choose a diabetes specialty career path. With 122 million Americans already with or at risk for diabetes, clinicians, non-clinician providers, and peer supporters are all indispensable in the delivery of DSMES. Recognizing the importance of non-licensed and/or supportive personnel, several years ago ADCES created a separate category of provider called the diabetes paraprofessional. Competencies for the paraprofessional were developed and embedded into ADCES practice documents. The practice levels for the paraprofessional illustrated the important role of the wide variety of non-licensed health workers in the work associated with diabetes education and support. Moreover, physicians, nurses, dietitians, pharmacists, and other healthcare providers, such as a master certified health education specialist (MCHES), who may routinely connect with individuals who have diabetes, but who do not specialize in diabetes, previously were captured as Level I educators.[105,106] These point-of-care healthcare professionals have, at a minimum, completed the educational requirements for a specific health profession's degree. They are licensed and/or registered to practice in their primary professional discipline and/or are members of a professional registry. Many have the basic background knowledge of diabetes inherent to academic training in health professions but have yet to develop a deep, broad-based diabetes specialty practice knowledge base. People with diabetes commonly interface with these providers in hospitals, clinics, schools, home care, and pharmacy settings. It is essential for them to have sufficient knowledge to provide safe care and accurate information to the individual with diabetes. As such, a role exists for competencies specific to others engaged in diabetes care and education.

Barriers and Facilitators to Access

Indisputable evidence supports the need for and benefits of well-managed diabetes.[8,10–11,57,107] Ideally, all people with diabetes are referred to a qualified diabetes care and education specialist, but only an estimated 25% or fewer people receive formal diabetes education at diagnosis. Although this is a grim statistic, the parameters of education have changed. Individuals with diabetes no longer need to wait for clinic appointments to "receive" diabetes education. Many take a proactive role in seeking out diabetes self-management information. What was once accomplished only in face to face appointments can now be achieved using digital technologies, including distance learning, videoconferencing, mobile health applications, technology enhanced DSMES, and self-paced learning modules.[108–111] With over 120 million Americans with or at risk for diabetes, access to diabetes care and education is essential. Based on the amount of published literature, clinical interest in prediabetes, diabetes and its related conditions is at an all-time high. The relationship between diabetes and other cardiometabolic conditions is clear.[112–115] CDC-recognized diabetes prevention programs are widely available and there is continued national emphasis management of diabetes.[4,94,116] The time seems to be ideal for diabetes care and education specialists and programs to thrive. And yet, barriers to diabetes care and education nevertheless exist.

Well-known barriers to DSMES access align with healthcare inequities. Age, race/ethnicity, socioeconomic status, educational preparation, language, and geographic location are all connected with access … or lack thereof. Some of the more common access barriers to DSME were identified a decade ago in a national study of individuals with diabetes (who were primarily white, well educated, and insured), diabetes educators, and physicians.[117] The results of this still-relevant study showed that DSME is highly regarded among those who have participated in it, but less so among those who have not. Individuals with diabetes and physicians alike want easier access to quality diabetes education. Because most individuals value their doctor's opinions, it was not surprising that primary care physicians were found to be essential to the referral process. Some physicians reported struggles with the referral process, and others reported having limited access to local educators. Most participating physicians reported wanting their patients to have more self-management support, but some disagreed with the diabetes care recommendations provided by the educator.

Geographic barriers still exist. Practice settings for diabetes care and education specialists vary widely. The majority of diabetes educator practices are in urban/suburban areas and in the hospital outpatient/clinic settings.[66,96,118] In 2014, Zrebiec reported that just over 20% of CDCESs practice in the Great Lakes states.[116] The so-called diabetes belt that covers most of the southeast, now extends upward into the eastern Great Lakes area, but the states with the highest prevalence of diabetes are Mississippi, West Virginia, and Alabama, states that are mostly rural, suggesting continuing lack of access to the DCES.[4]

Demographic barriers continue to exist. Elders living in long-term care (LTC) settings represent a particularly vulnerable group. Neither the frail elder with diabetes in LTC nor his or her caregivers commonly use the services or expertise of diabetes educators.[119] On the other end of the age spectrum, type 1 and type 2 diabetes both occur in children. Because children spend most of their day in the school setting, they need access to appropriate resources in schools. Fewer than half of all schools currently meet national guidelines for having 1 nurse for every 750 students.[120] And, while some efforts are being made to improve diabetes competency of school nurses, school personnel in general are poorly prepared to support the needs of the child with diabetes.[71,120] Significant cultural barriers still exist. The largest-growing populations of individuals with diabetes are in non-white cultures, races, and ethnicities. Too few programs are tailored to meet the needs of these individuals.[109] There is room for improvement for diabetes educators to increase the diversity within their workforce to better reflect the populations that they serve.[66,96] And, clinical inertia continues to exist.[121]

An identified barrier in the public health space was inadequate reimbursement for DSMES.[122] While third-party payers may recognize the value of and be willing to underwrite or reimburse for quality DSMES, a challenge is to define quality measures associated with DSMES services. Willingness to support DSMES services will be a critical factor as healthcare delivery models continue to be redesigned. Programs demonstrating quality in delivery and outcomes are expected to be highly sought after. One way to ensure quality is by achieving and maintaining accreditation or recognition status. The ADCES and the ADA offer accreditation or recognition status to programs meeting established criteria. The Centers for Disease Control and Prevention (CDC) has established accreditation standards for diabetes prevention programs, and The Joint Commission (formerly JCAHO) provides accreditation for inpatient diabetes management. Morgan et al identified difficulty earning program recognition status in the public health arena. This latter point identifies an opportunity for the enterprising diabetes care and education specialist to partner with public health programs, articulating the depth and breadth of diabetes care and education specialist services available, assisting in the development of programs, and/or serving as an ongoing consultant.[122]

The diabetes care and education specialist can respond to these and other barriers by capitalizing on the rapidly expanding technology environment. For example, as work toward creating interoperable electronic health records (EHR) continues, the diabetes care and education specialist can develop community partnerships that link EHR systems to enable automated referrals. Because there are multiple modes of learning, there are individuals who may always prefer face-to-face programs, but even those who have reported valuing traditional DSMES sources and settings also like media-based education strategies. This finding is as true today as it was in 2009.[86,88,91] The DCES can also combine technology with more familiar strategies like promoting worksite and faith-based DSMES programs, developing statewide coalitions to address referrals, and identifying champion providers who understand the value of DSMES and are willing to refer.[122] The question is: to what will they refer? How will the evolving healthcare system and seemingly limitless advances in technology change DSMES? Diabetes information is everywhere. Perhaps nothing, as much as this, illustrates the need to move beyond diabetes education and toward diabetes care and education services. It will be up to the diabetes care and education specialist to find ways to add value and purpose to individual and shared visits, and to also find novel ways to incorporate person-centered technologies and resources into programs and services.

Evolving Healthcare Systems in the United States

Few observers would dispute the fact that the healthcare system in the United States remains fragmented and dysfunctional. Healthcare outcomes continue to be disappointing despite the allocation of nearly 18% of GDP to healthcare spending.[4,123] Although chronic diseases have supplanted acute illnesses as the primary reasons for seeking health care in the United States, the healthcare system continues to primarily use an acute care delivery model. Creative mechanisms are being explored in the hope of mitigating the impact of rising healthcare costs, and the fee-for-service model common to US health care is slowly being overtaken by alternative designs, including the patient-centered medical home (PCMH), integrated delivery networks (IDNs), and the accountable care organization (ACO).

mHealth and the 21st Century Cures Act

The *21st Century Cures Act* (*Cures Act*) was created to help streamline the process for drug and device approval and was signed into law in 2016 (Pub.L. 114 - 255, 2016), authorizing over $500 million in funding to be used by the FDA to carry out provisions in the *Act,* through the year 2025.[124,125] Title III of the *Cures Act* contains 10 subtitles; Subtitle F addresses Medical Device Innovations. Fast-tracking medical product development allows for faster, more efficient introduction of innovations and advances to those who need them. A certified full-text version of the *21st Century Cures Act* may be accessed through the Congress.gov Web site: https://www.congress.gov/bill/114th-congress/house-bill/34. The *Cures Act* discusses the use of various measures, user experience information, and observational data from standard clinical use (ie, "real-world evidence") to facilitate more rapid drug and device approval. However, "real-world evidence" is broadly defined and can be perceived as subjective.[126] Those opposed to the *Cures Act* have expressed concern that it would allow drugs and devices to be approved based on weak evidence, possibly bringing dangerous or ineffective devices to market.[126,127]

The US Food & Drug Administration (FDA) monitors reports of issues with medical devices, alerting the public and health professionals when indicated, to ensure proper use of devices and the health and safety of those using the devices.[124,125] The FDA asks device users and healthcare providers to report adverse events associated with the use of any diabetes management device to MedWatch, the FDA Safety Information and Adverse Event Reporting Program, by following the voluntary reporting guidelines described on their Web site (https://www.fda.gov/safety/medwatch-fda-safety-information-and-adverse-event-reporting-program/reporting-serious-problems-fda). Recently, the FDA warned persons with diabetes and healthcare providers against the use of devices for diabetes management not authorized for sale in the United States: FDA Safety Communication.[128]

The unprecedented spread of mobile technologies along with advancements in their innovative application to address health priorities has evolved into a field known as mHealth.[129] The World Health Organization defines mHealth as medical and public health practice supported by mobile devices (eg, mobile phones, monitoring devices, and other wireless devices). mHealth refers to the concept of mobile self-care such as smartphone and tablet apps that enable consumers to capture their own health data, with or without a clinician's assistance or interpretation. The most common application of mHealth is the use of mobile devices to educate consumers about preventive healthcare services. Consumers are increasingly using mHealth technology to meet their health information needs, for health self-management, and as a communication tool with their providers. It's important to evaluate the usability of mHealth technologies before they are made available to users.[129,130] Recent studies indicate a need for in-depth evaluation of user experiences with mHealth technologies.[129,131]

A variety of frameworks may be applied for evaluating mHealth technology, such as the *Health-IT Usability Evaluation Model (Health-ITUEM),* the *Think Aloud Usability Test,* the *Usability Problem Taxonomy (UPT),* the *Framework Analysis (FA) method,* and the *System Usability Scale (SUS)* described in several studies.[130–132] Furthermore, to help standardize the quality of mHealth evidence reporting, the mHealth evidence reporting and assessment checklist (mERA) has been developed.[129] The US FDA's Center for Devices and Radiological Health (CDRH) initiated the Fostering Medical Innovation: Software Precertification Pilot Program for the assessment of companies that perform software design and testing for digital health devices.[133] This program aims to balance the benefits and risks of digital health products and to speed the review process of marketing applications for software products. This voluntary pilot program is a transparent and open approach to provide continuous notice and solicitation of public input, by means of an open public docket, throughout the program development. Comments may be posted on the public docket available on the Regulations.gov Web site: https://www.regulations.gov/comment?D=FDA-2017-N-4301-0001.

Relevant to the Diabetes Care and Education Specialist

In this era of rapid technological growth and increasing an individual's interest in self-management of diabetes, the diabetes care and education specialist must be informed regarding usability ratings of new technologies and be apprised of any safety issues reported by the FDA. Meta-analyses and systematic reviews published in high-impact, peer-reviewed journals offer excellent recommendations. The *Journal of Medical Internet Research* is a peer-reviewed open-access source established in 1999 which covers eHealth and "healthcare in the Internet age," touting an impressive journal impact factor of 4.95 in 2018.

The diabetes care and education specialist must also consider real-time updates being shared on social media as a potential source of information. #OpenAPS is a worldwide movement with nearly 4000 followers who share an interest in making artificial pancreas (APS) technology available more quickly to persons with type 1 diabetes.[134] Using OpenAPS (open source) software and diabetes management devices (eg, continuous glucose monitors and insulin pumps), some followers of #OpenAPS have constructed their own artificial pancreas systems subsequently reporting lowered hemoglobin A1C levels and improved sleep quality.[134] This example illustrates valuable insight, data, and experiences that can help everyone (device manufacturers, healthcare providers, and individual users) to build better tools to better manage life with diabetes. Many persons with diabetes are interested in directly improving diabetes technology by donating their data and sharing their experiences of living with do-it-yourself closed-loop systems.[134] Since these hybrid systems are not sold as medical devices, they are not subject to FDA regulation, creating some ethical concerns as to their safety.[134] The diabetes care and education specialist must be aware that the FDA has not evaluated the safety and effectiveness of unauthorized diabetes management devices or systems that combine devices in unintended ways, and that these devices or systems may give incorrect results and introduce unknown risks. Diabetes care and education specialists may be interested in subscribing to FDA Medical Device Safety Communication email alerts, which include clinical recommendations for self-management, by visiting the FDA Web site at https://www.fda.gov/medical-devices/safety-communications/2019-safety-communications.

Diabetes care and education specialists are in an ideal position to engage individuals in research and product development opportunities. Furthermore, they are ideally suited to encourage medical device adverse event reporting to MedWatch and advise patients to use only diabetes management devices the FDA has authorized for sale in the United States and to use these devices according to manufacturer instructions. To inquire about the FDA regulatory status of any product, the manufacturer can be contacted directly, or the FDA Division of Consumer Education can be reached at DICE@FDA.HHS.GOV, or by calling 800-638-2041 or 301-796-7100.[133] In an era of rapidly emerging technologies, the DCES may witness in clinical practice that which has not yet been published or reported by the FDA. Social media, even with its challenges and limitations, can offer noteworthy, real-time information of interest to all stakeholders in diabetes care and education.[136]

Diabetes Care and Education Specialists and the Affordable Care Act*

Although individuals with diabetes benefit from DSMES, many persons with diabetes have not had the advantage of receiving diabetes management guidance from a DCES. As healthcare delivery and payment structures in the United States evolve, diabetes care and education specialists are wondering what patterns will change and how comprehensive changes to the healthcare system will affect persons with diabetes. Health insurance coverage constitutes an important first step in obtaining access to care, managing disease, preventing complications, and reducing the likelihood of developing related conditions.[138] Moreover, lack of health insurance coverage results in increased out of pocket costs and delays in treatment, thereby substantially impacting the US economy. The Patient Protection and Affordable Care Act[139] plays an important role in the evolving healthcare system.

The Patient Protection and Affordable Care Act, also known as the Affordable Care Act (ACA), is sometimes called "Obamacare" because is became public law during the Obama administration (Pub. L. No. 111-148, 2010). The law contains 2 parts: the Patient Protection and Affordable Care Act and the Health Care and Education Reconciliation Act. The official and consolidated (unofficial) versions of these Acts are available in PDF or HTML formats on the HealthCare.gov Web site. This ACA has 3 primary goals:[139]

- Make affordable health insurance available to more people.
- Expand Medicaid programs to cover adults with an income below 138% of the federal poverty level.
- Support innovative medical care delivery methods designed to lower the costs of health care.

When the ACA passed, it represented an opportunity to decrease the toll of diabetes in the United States.[140] Many of the ACA provisions did not go into effect until 2014. During the 116th Congress (2019-2020), over 1700 bills which directly pertain to the ACA have been introduced or resolved. Numerous bills have been introduced to repeal the ACA (eg, H.R. 2536). Additional bills have been introduced to protect Americans with preexisting conditions (eg, H.R. 986), for lowering prescription drug costs (eg, H.R. 987), restoring access to medication (S.1089), and for protecting individuals from higher insurance premiums (eg, H.R. 2447).

The ACA expanded insurance coverage, consumer protections, and access to primary care services. The law contains several provisions of specific interest to persons with diabetes, policymakers, and healthcare providers, including the DCES. These provisions directly address gaps in diabetes prevention, screening, and care, creating a comprehensive approach toward improved treatment.[139] The Catalyst to Better Diabetes Care Act of 2009, built

*The following information on the Affordable Care Act is current as of January 19, 2020. Ongoing healthcare reform news updates are summarized and may be viewed at Health Markets Web site at: (https://www.healthmarkets.com/resources/health-insurance/trumpcare-news-updates/).[137]

into the ACA, authorized the CDC to enhance surveillance of diabetes and to develop national quality standards for a national diabetes report card.[139] The *Diabetes Report Card* contains current information on the status of diabetes, gestational diabetes, prediabetes, preventive care practices, risk factors, quality of care, outcomes, and progress made toward meeting national goals.[4]

Diabetes-related provisions include wellness and prevention programs, Medicaid Health Homes for those with chronic conditions, the Medicaid Incentives to [illegible] Chronic Disease Program, and the Medic[illegible] dence at Home Demonstration Program [illegible] ACA contains 10 titles (or divisi[illegible] a particular aspect of reform. T[illegible] description of the 10 titles [illegible] mary of the contents [illegible] implications for th[illegible] The titles are su[illegible] mary is not intend[illegible]

Title I: Quality, A[illegible] for All Americans

Through shared responsibi[illegible] transform healthcare coverage, [illegible] Americans as it is introduced in[illegible] Persons with diabetes may particu[illegible] important federal legislation, given th[illegible] for preventive services included in the a[illegible]

the ACA is the National Diabetes Prevention Program, representing a partnership of public and private organizations working to reduce the growing problem of prediabetes and type 2 diabetes.[116,139]

This section discusses improvements in healthcare coverage for all Americans, including preventive health services. If the plan offers dependent coverage for an unmarried child, this coverage is available until the child turns 26. Wellness and prevention programs which include weight management, physical fitness, nutrition, [illegible]art disease, and diabetes prevention are specified. Sub[illegible] B of this section elaborates actions to preserve and [illegible]d insurance coverage for those with preexisting [illegible]ns. Subtitle C describes quality health insurance [illegible]or all Americans, prohibiting preexisting con[illegible]sions or other discrimination based on health [illegible]d essential health benefits include ambu[illegible] emergency services, hospitalization, pre[illegible]ab services, preventive/wellness services [illegible]se management, as well as oral and [illegible]ren. Levels of coverage for Bronze [illegible]ge), Silver, Gold, and Platinum [illegible]verage) are described. Flexibility [illegible]ment of exchanges is permit[illegible]tes may establish alternative [illegible]ction describes procedures [illegible] I addresses individual [illegible]dividual and employer [illegible]ellaneous provisions.

TABLE 1.3 The Affordable Care Act: Titles an[illegible]

Title	[illegible]	*[illegible]ctions of the ACA*
Title I	Quality, Affordable Health Care [illegible]	1001–2995
Title II	The Role of Public Programs	3001–3129
Title III	Improving the Quality and Efficiency [illegible]	3131–3602
Title IV	Prevention of Chronic Disease and Impr[illegible]n	4001–4402
Title V	Health Care Workforce	5001–5701
Title VI	Transparency and Program Integrity	6001–6801
Title VII	Improving Access to Innovative Medical Therapies	7001–7103
Title VIII	Community Living Assistance Services and Supports	8001–8002
Title IX	Revenue Provisions	9001–9023
Title X	Strengthening Quality, Affordable Health Care for All Americans	10101–10909

Source: Adapted from "An Act: The Patient Protection and Affordable Care Act." The Patient Protection and Affordable Care Act, Pub. L. No. 111-148, §2702, 124 Stat. 119, 318-319 (2010), US Government Printing Office. Because of myriad new bills and resolutions constantly occurring with the ACA, one may read the ACA by visiting this Web site: The Patient Protection and Affordable Care Act, 42 USC § 18001 (2010). US Government Printing Office. "HealthCare.gov" (cited 2020 March 12) on the Internet at: https://www.healthcare.gov/where-can-i-read-the-affordable-care-act/.

Health Insurance Exchanges

A health insurance exchange is an online store where consumers can compare and buy health insurance plans. Each US state had the option to run its own exchange, to work in partnership with the federal government to run an exchange, or to use a federal exchange. Since 2008, the Health Insurance Exchange has helped more than 16 million people find affordable health plans. Each exchange agrees to do the following:

- Present benefit options in a standard format so it's easy for consumers to compare plans
- Operate a toll-free hotline where consumers can ask questions and get help
- Set up a navigator program to help consumers understand and purchase health insurance
- Certify the health plans that sell policies through the exchange and make sure health plans comply with regulatory standards and requirements
- Provide an online calculator so consumers can determine their costs; the calculator will factor in tax credits or subsidies available to the consumer
- Interact with other computer systems and databases to determine whether consumers are eligible for tax credits or subsidies on the exchange or whether they qualify for Medicaid or the Children's Health Insurance Program (CHIP); this is called "no wrong door," and it will make it much easier for consumers to sign up for some kind of health coverage
- Certify which individuals are exempt from the individual mandate

Source: Healthinsurance.org, "What is a health insurance exchange?" (cited 2020, Jan 19), on the Internet at: https://www.healthinsurance.org/faqs/what-is-a-health-insurance-exchange/.[141]

The online marketplace for state insurance exchanges is also known as the Obamacare Health Insurance Exchange Marketplace. Consumers can locate their marketplace through the Obamacare Facts: State Health Insurance Exchange Web site available at: https://obamacarefacts.com/state-health-insurance-exchange/HealthCare.gov which was established to assist Americans in identifying coverage options, obtaining answers to questions, and enrolling in Platinum, Gold, Silver, or Bronze marketplace insurance programs. These plans offer different coverage levels, which differ by cost-sharing requirements.[139]

Relevant to the Diabetes Care and Education Specialist

This summary is intended to help the DCES obtain a general idea of what is contained in Title I. Being familiar with the contents of this section can facilitate communications with Case Managers and Social Workers who make up part of the interprofessional team charged with caring for persons with diabetes. A comprehensive summary of essential health benefits includes the following general categories that apply to diabetes coverage and treatment: ambulatory care, emergency services, hospitalization, maternity and newborn care, mental health and substance use disorders, behavioral health treatment, prescription drugs, rehabilitative and habilitative services and devices, laboratory services, preventive/wellness chronic disease management, and pediatric services, including oral and vision care.[142] The online National Diabetes Prevention Program Coverage Toolkit was developed to provide information about the mechanics of covering the year-long, evidence-based National Diabetes Prevention Program developed by the Centers for Disease Control.[143]

Title II: Role of Public Programs

Section 2703 outlines provisions for health homes for enrollees with chronic conditions. The term *health home* is defined as a designated individual provider or a health-care team selected by eligible individuals with chronic conditions. The term *chronic conditions* includes, but is not limited to, diabetes (Sec. 2703). Health home providers provide a cadre of services, including comprehensive care management, care coordination, and health promotion. Health services also encompass comprehensive transitional care (eg, follow-up from inpatient to other settings; patient and family support; referral to community and social support services, if relevant; and use of health information technology to link services, as feasible and appropriate). The ACA defines a "designated health provider" as a physician, clinical practice or clinical group practice, rural clinic, community health center, community mental health center, home health agency, or any other entity or provider (eg, pediatricians, gynecologists, obstetricians) that is determined by the state to be qualified to be a health home for eligible individuals with chronic conditions.

The ACA has improved access to Medicaid for the lowest-income populations, including coverage for children formerly place in foster care. Special adjustments are considered for certain states recovering from a major disaster. Enhanced support is available for the Children's Health Insurance Program (CHIP), and between fiscal years 2014 and 2019, states received a 23-percentage point increase in the CHIP federal match rate, subject to a 100% cap. Using authority described in the ACA, the Centers for Medicare & Medicaid Services (CMS) launched demonstration projects designed to better manage benefits and care for low-income and disabled Americans.[144] In an effort to improve the quality of Medicaid for both consumers and providers, various sections address fair health insurance premiums, adult health quality measures, payment adjustment for healthcare-acquired conditions, provision of health homes for enrollees with chronic conditions, and demonstration projects, such as the *Independence at Home Medical Practice Demonstration Program*. Under this demonstration, the CMS works with medical practices to test the effectiveness of comprehensive primary services delivery at home, and if doing so improves care for Medicare beneficiaries with multiple chronic conditions.[145] Of special note, the ACA has incorporated protections for American Indians and Alaska Natives containing special rules relating to Native Americans, including the elimination of sunset for reimbursement for all Medicare Part B services furnished by certain Indian hospitals and clinics.

Relevant to the Diabetes Care and Education Specialist

Subtitle F (Sec. 2501), Medicaid Prescription Drug Coverage, is of interest to the DCES as it addresses prescription drug rebates, the elimination of the exclusions of coverage for certain drugs, and provision of adequate pharmacy reimbursement. The DCES may wish to review the table of contents for the ACA, then query for specific items of interest by clicking ctrl + F and entering the topic of interest to quickly locate this information.

The DCES may also wish to monitor the timeline and updates for the *Independence at Home Medical Practice Demonstration Program*.[145] A model summary for this initiative is available on the Internet at https://innovation.cms.gov/initiatives/independence-at-home/. The demonstration rewards providers who deliver high-quality care while reducing costs.

Title III: Improving the Quality and Efficiency of Health Care

The ACA will make substantial investments to improve quality and delivery of care, supporting research to inform consumers about outcomes resulting from differing approaches to treatment and care delivery, via new care models. Payments will be linked to quality outcomes under the Medicare program, with a national strategy designed to improve healthcare quality through quality measure development, measurement, data collection, and reporting. Diabetes-specific information is available biennially through the Diabetes Report Card on the US Department of Health and Human Services, CDC Web site at: https://www.cdc.gov/diabetes/library/reports/reportcard.html.[4] Improvements in rural care and payment accuracy will occur, and the Medicare Part D prescription drug benefit will be expanded, with a reduction in the "donut hole" (a gap in prescription coverage that occurs once all deductibles and co-payments have been met).[146]

Relevant to the Diabetes Care and Education Specialist

Using cross-sectional data from the 2009 and 2016 National Health Interview Surveys (NHIS), Casagrande and colleagues (2018) examined national changes in costs and health insurance coverage before and after implementation of the ACA in a sample of US persons with diabetes, aged 18 to 64 (N=6,220).[138] They concluded that health insurance coverage increased significantly ($p<0.001$) after implementation of the ACA, and that medical costs decreased among lower-income families ($p=0.004$). DCESs are focused on improving outcomes. Current evidence already suggests that although Medicare recipients receiving diabetes care and education are more likely to receive preventive services, DSMES is an underutilized service.[142,147] Despite the discontinuation of many community-based public health programs, the Prevention and Public Health Fund continues to sustain the innovative National Diabetes Prevention Program.[148,149] Enterprising DCESs have an opportunity to partner with health home providers to address diabetes-specific quality measures (ie, DSMES, foot exams, eye exams, SMBG, A1C testing, and influenza vaccines).

Title IV: Prevention of Chronic Disease and Improving Public Health

Sections 4001 to 4402 of the ACA are designed to better position the nation's healthcare system toward disease prevention and health promotion. The ACA established the Prevention and Public Health Fund to provide expanded, sustained investments in prevention and public health, to improve health outcomes, and to enhance health quality. Since 2012, Congress passed several bills that cut these funds and redirect money to pay for non-public legislative proposals.[150] For fiscal year 2019, allocations for the Prevention and Public Health Fund have earmarked over 60 million dollars for chronic disease self-management and diabetes programs.[150] Additional planned activities include funding for a national resource center and awards for new competitive grants to help older adults and adults with disabilities from underserved areas and populations (including Tribal communities) better manage their chronic conditions by providing access to evidence-based chronic disease self-management programs, and to assist grantees with developing and implementing strategies for sustainable program funding beyond the scope of the grant period.[149] Nutrition labeling is required for standard menu items at chain restaurants, and funding will be available for the childhood obesity research.[151]

Section 4108 of the ACA, Incentives for prevention of chronic diseases, specifies that states shall be awarded grants to carry out initiatives to provide incentives to Medicaid beneficiaries who successfully participate in a program and, upon completion of such participation, demonstrate changes in health risks and outcomes, including the adoption and maintenance of health behaviors by meeting established measurable standards and health status targets. The purpose of these initiatives is to test approaches that may encourage behavior modification and determine scalable solutions. In general, a "program" is comprehensive, evidence based, widely available, easily accessible, and designed and uniquely suited to address the needs of Medicare beneficiaries; additionally, it has demonstrated success in helping individuals achieve one or more of the following from Section 4108:

- Cease use of tobacco products
- Control or reduce weight
- Lower cholesterol
- Lower blood pressure
- Avoid the onset of diabetes, or in the case of someone with diabetes, improve the management of the existing condition

In general, grants shall be awarded to state or local health departments and Indian tribes to carry out pilot programs to provide public health community interventions, screenings, and, where necessary, clinical referrals for individuals who are between 55 and 64 years of age (Sec. 4202). In addition to community-wide public health interventions, a state or local health department will be mandated to use funding received in conducting ongoing health screening to identify risk factors for cardiovascular disease, cancer, stroke, and diabetes among individuals in both urban and rural areas who are between 55 and 64 years of age (Sec. 4202). Individuals who are found to have chronic disease risk factors through these screening activities will receive clinical referral/treatment for follow-up services to reduce risk. With respect to individuals with risk factors for or having heart disease, stroke, diabetes, or any other condition for which they were screened, grantees shall determine whether these individuals are covered under a public or private health insurance program. Insured individuals will be referred to an in-network provider, with respect to the program involved. Uninsured individuals can be assisted in determining eligibility for available public coverage options and identifying other appropriate community healthcare resources and assistance programs (Sec. 4202).

Relevant to the Diabetes Care and Education Specialist

Diabetes care and education specialists have an opportunity to partner with state or local health departments as direct providers or as consultants. Community-based resources may need to be developed to serve the collective needs of individuals with or at risk for diabetes as they work to reduce risks and/or improve all aspects of control.

Title V: Health Care Workforce

The ACA originally promised to encourage innovation in healthcare workforce training, recruitment, and retention through the creation of the National Health Care Workforce Commission,[152] designed to support increasing the supply of healthcare workers. However, Congress has not allocated funding to the commission.[152]

Relevant to the Diabetes Care and Education Specialist

The CDC established the NDPP, targeted to adults at high risk for diabetes, to reduce or eliminate the consequences associated with type 2 diabetes. The NDPP includes a grant program for community-based diabetes prevention program model sites, a program which determines eligibility of entities to deliver community-based diabetes prevention services, a training/outreach program for lifestyle intervention instructions, evaluation, monitoring, technical assistance, and applied research carried out by the CDC. The CDC maintains a searchable national registry of recognized diabetes prevention programs that have agreed to follow standards and requirements for recognition as outlined in the CDC-approved curriculum.[116,153] Diabetes care and education specialists interested in offering a lifestyle change program to delay or prevent type 2 diabetes may be interested in learning more about the NDPP Diabetes Prevention Recognition Program (DPRP).[116,153] Training for lifestyle coaching is available through the Association for Diabetes Care and Education Specialists, https://www.diabeteseducator.org/prevention/lifestyle-coach-training).

The diabetes education specialty has long been populated primarily by nurses and dietitians. The former group is in a state of impending critical shortage. A workforce analysis commissioned by the ADCES projected a significant increase in the demand for diabetes care and education specialists through 2025.[147] The analysis identified all healthcare professions, including nursing, as continued sources of DCES. Therefore, having programs that support the education and training of nurses provides an ongoing source of trained professionals who can migrate into the field of diabetes care and education. To sustain and grow the specialty, current diabetes care and education specialists have an obligation to serve as models and mentors for new professionals entering the field. Preventive initiatives in the Affordable Care Act include increased loans and decreased fees associated with federal student loans for physicians, nurses, members of the National Health Service Corps, and the public health workforce.[154]

Title VI: Transparency and Program Integrity

Transparency implies open communication and accountability, thereby operating in a way that allows others to easily see actions being performed. Title VI addresses physician ownership, nursing home transparency of information, improving staff training, and patient-centered outcomes research and its coordinating council for comparative effectiveness research. Medicare, Medicaid, and CHIP program integrity provisions are described in Sections 6301 to 6607 of the ACA. The Elder Justice Act, enacted as part of the ACA, was the first piece of legislation passed to authorize funding to raise awareness for the prevention and elimination of elder abuse, neglect, and exploitation, particularly in long-term care facilities.

Relevant to the Diabetes Care and Education Specialist

According to the interpretation given by the Department of Health and Human Services, this section of the law is aimed, in part, at promoting more effective provider-patient relationships.[139] Improved transparency and improved communication can be linked to the engaged, activated patient. Diabetes care and education specialists, with their expertise in chronic care management, are well positioned to serve as resources and consultants for agencies working to bring more transparency into their processes.

Title VII: Improving Access to Innovative Medical Therapies

The ACA makes a provision for biologics price competition and innovation under Sections 7001 to 7003 and allows for more affordable medicines for children and underserved communities through the 340B program. Title VII of the ACA extends drug discounts to hospitals and communities serving low-income patients and makes a pathway for the creation of generic versions of biological drugs, improving access to effective, lower-cost alternatives.

Relevant to the Diabetes Care and Education Specialist

The intent of this section is to enhance access to medications by making them more affordable. Diabetes care and education specialists have long advocated, individually and in the aggregate, for underserved populations to have access to *all* diabetes medications and devices. Price competition brings with it a potential for compromised quality. Diabetes care and education specialists have an opportunity to serve as a watchdog group to ensure that as access to medications improves, quality does not deteriorate.

Title VIII: Community Living Assistance Services and Supports

The ACA established a national voluntary insurance program, the Community Living Assistance Services and Supports (CLASS) Independence Benefit Plan, for the purchase of community living assistance services and support. The intent was to provide a mechanism for beneficiaries to live as independently as possible in their own homes or a residential facility of choice. In 2011, the Obama administration elected to drop this long-term health program.[155]

Relevant to the Diabetes Care and Education Specialist

Title VIII is specific to development and enrollment issues rather than provider-linked services. However, diabetes care and education specialists who are actively engaged with the older adult population should be aware of Title VIII and its intent to ensure that beneficiaries have access to the equipment and services needed for independent living.

Title IX: Revenue Provisions

The ACA was designed to, when fully enacted, ultimately reduce the federal deficit. Title IX outlines tax cuts to citizens as well as the consequences for insurance companies and plan administrators, and it specifies the taxes and fees imposed on agencies and industry.

Relevant to the Diabetes Care and Education Specialist

Section 9003 is of specific interest to diabetes care and education specialists, in that it specifies distributions for medicine are qualified only if they are for prescribed drugs or insulin. An annual fee can be imposed on manufacturers and importers of branded pharmaceuticals and on medical devices. To remain informed about changes, the DCES may be interested in reviewing the complete law, latest statistics, and Republican counterproposals for additional updates.[156]

Title X: Strengthening Quality, Affordable Health Care for All Americans

Sections 10101 to 10909 address revisions, modifications, clarifications, expansions, and amendments made to the original ACA.

Relevant to the Diabetes Care and Education Specialist

Section 10407 may be cited as the Catalyst to Better Diabetes Care Act of 2009 and includes provisions for a national diabetes report card, prepared biennially in collaboration with the CDC. In general, each report card includes aggregate health outcomes related to individuals diagnosed with diabetes or prediabetes, including preventive care practices, quality of care, risk factors, and outcomes. Each report card includes trend analysis for the nation and, to the extent possible, for each state, for the purpose of tracking progress in meeting established national goals and objectives for improving diabetes care, costs, and prevalence and informing policy and program development. The report card is available to the public and is posted on the CDC's Web site (https://www.cdc.gov/diabetes/prevention/index.html).[4]

Also under this section is a mandate for improvement of vital statistics collection, which promotes the education and training of physicians on the importance of birth and death certificate data and how to properly complete these documents, including the collection of such data for diabetes and other chronic diseases. In carrying out this subsection, improvements may be promoted for the collection of diabetes mortality data, including the addition of a question for the individual certifying the cause of death regarding whether the deceased had diabetes. The National Academy of Medicine (formerly called the Institute of Medicine) and appropriate associations and councils will collaborate to conduct a study of the impact of diabetes on the practice of medicine in the United States, and the appropriate level of diabetes medical education that should be required prior to licensure, board certification, and recertification (Sec. 10407). Bright and Sakurada outline a population health approach, involving personal health care professionals and quality improvement interventions believed to be effective in improving diabetes care. These interventions include education and support and provider role changes such as expanding the role of pharmacists, nurses, multidisciplinary teams, and the use of telemedicine.[157]

Also under Title X, Section 10401: Centers of Excellence for Depression is a provision specifying that each national center shall collaborate with other centers to carry out general activities that foster communication with other providers attending to co-occurring physical health conditions such as cardiovascular disease, diabetes, cancer, and substance abuse disorders.

Summary

As a result of the ACA, persons with diabetes will not be penalized for having a preexisting condition and can expect reduced healthcare expenses due to annual caps for out-of-pocket spending. Individuals with diabetes are able to select a plan best suited to their needs, obtain coverage for preventive health screenings and, over time, experience fewer health disparities.

Relevant to the Diabetes Care and Education Specialist

These provisions include insurance components, diabetes prevention, chronic disease management, and improved standards and reporting mechanisms. Some of these provisions became effective in 2014 while others continue to be rolled out. The ACA is a comprehensive law that receives ongoing revision, modification, clarification, expansions, and amendments. To track the status of this law, readers are encouraged to query for updates on the Patient Protection and Affordable Care Act, Public Law 111-148 by visiting Congress.gov on the Internet at https://www.congress.gov. At the time of this writing, the Office of Disease Prevention and Health Promotion-National Clinical Care Commission is seeking comments about federal diabetes prevention and treatment programs. The Diabetes Care and Education Specialist may wish to monitor the activity of the Commission and review the final report—anticipated October 2021.The World Healthcare Organization defines health care policy as specific plans, actions, and decisions that are committed to attain health care goals within a society.[158]

Diabetes: Advocating for Policy Change

In the United States, the soaring costs linked to diabetes management make it imperative to adopt local and national policies addressing programs, plans, and services that can reduce the burden diabetes places on individuals and society at large.

Advocacy for diabetes can be broken down into four levels: (1) individual, (2) community, (3) national, and (4) international. The impact of policy work can be seen at each of these levels. In the community, a key goal is to improve situations for individuals locally who face barriers and challenges associated with diabetes management. Local challenges might be lack of access to food markets, school systems without nurses or other staff trained to assist children with diabetes, or lack of clean water. A current problem gaining considerable attention is the escalating cost of insulin.[159] Individuals can contact government officials at the state and federal levels about changes that need to be made in policies for people with diabetes.[160] While the battle surrounding the cost of insulin is far from over, an excellent example of local policy change can be found in the state of Colorado. Colorado was the first state in the nation to cap the cost of insulin in 2019 by passing House Bill 1216: Reduce Insulin Prices Bill.[161] This seemingly enormous task was accomplished through the efforts of community organizers and state legislators. At the federal level, advocacy is centered around influencing policies that impact individuals across the nation. As noted in the previous section, The Diabetes Prevention Act, launched in 2009, resulted in the establishment of the National Diabetes Prevention Program. This program aims to raise awareness of diabetes risk and assist people at high risk of developing diabetes to utilize evidence-based lifestyle change interventions.[162] Lifestyle change programs, now available in hundreds of locations throughout the nation, are frequently offered by DCES.[163]

An easy way to engage with federal representatives is to see whether they are members of the diabetes caucus, a large and influential body of legislators who are knowledgeable about diabetes.[164] An issue at the heart of diabetes care and education is the Expanding Access to DSMT Act, designed to reduce barriers and improve Medicare beneficiary access to DSMT services.[165–168] At the international level, advocacy has been seen to be focused on raising awareness on the impact that diabetes brings on a global scale. Financial efforts are made to bring resources to those who lack the resources to manage their diabetes. The International Diabetes Federation has been a global champion for advocacy. Some of their remarkable advocacy activities include the 2006 United Nations Resolution on Diabetes, and the 2011 IDF Road Map Programme. Both efforts challenged leaders to understand the devastation diabetes can cause by encouraging them to gain a more holistic understanding about the chronic disease as well as highlighting the urgency for funding proper resources.[160] It is easy to be overwhelmed by the enormity of what needs to be changed in diabetes. Former Speaker of the House, the late Tip O'Neill (1912–1994), coined the phrase "all politics is local," and while some may question the veracity of this statement in contemporary times, the impact of individual advocacy efforts cannot be minimized. At the individual level, advocacy can translate into improved care at the community, national, and international levels. One needn't look too far to find advocacy resources. Organizations such as the Academy for Nutrition and Dietetics, the American Diabetes Association, the Association for Diabetes Care and Education Specialists, and the JDRF (formerly the Juvenile Diabetes Research Foundation) all have advocacy arms, each with a focused agenda. There are also advocacy groups organized by and for persons with diabetes. One such group, the Diabetes Patient Advocacy Coalition (DPAC), is dedicated to the promotion and support of public policy initiatives that improve the health of people with diabetes (https://diabetespac.org/). The DCES is in a perfect position to keep informed about local, national, and international advocacy efforts and to use networking skills to engage with others.

Advocacy is crucial to promote change within a society, but it is imperative that the message being conveyed to legislatures, healthcare organizations, providers, professional groups, and other stakeholders is centered around strong evidence. To achieve and maintain a high level of evidence, continuous research is needed to evaluate how current policies and programs are impacting individuals with diabetes from a prevention, self-management, and healthcare utilization cost perspective.[169] Updated data highlighting best evidence is instrumental in supporting policies that are renewed on an annual basis, preferably through meta analyses and systematic reviews. While the highest level of evidence is essential for effective policy work, it is crucial for both professional and government organizations to align their evidence in order to fully translate research into practice.[162]

Focus on Education

Teaching Points

Diabetes can be viewed as a syndemic, a combination of health or social conditions that interact to increase the disease burden to a community, further developing a public health concern. A comprehensive approach to diabetes care is needed to minimize its negative social impact. Disease management strategies and the Chronic Care Model (CCM) might be used to improve access to diabetes care and education and provide systemic self-management support. Successful disease management includes diabetes care, education, and support to facilitate healthy lifestyle behaviors.

One in every 3 individuals born today will develop diabetes during his or her lifetime. Worldwide, the largest increases are expected in countries where resources are most limited. The incidence of type 2 diabetes is increasing in children of Native American, Hispanic, African American, or Pacific Islander ancestry, especially in those who are overweight or obese. Type 2 diabetes represents 90% to 95% of all cases of diabetes worldwide. Currently more than 1 in every 7 dollars from the US economy is used to pay for the costs linked to diabetes.

Diabetes self-management support refers to the activities that assist the person with prediabetes or diabetes in implementing and sustaining the behaviors needed to manage his or her condition on an ongoing basis beyond or outside of formal self-management training. The type of support provided can be behavioral, educational, psychosocial, or clinical.

Diabetes care and education specialists are the primary providers of DSMES. They are involved in direct care of those with diabetes, prediabetes, and related conditions; population health management, education of other healthcare professionals, research, social reform, and advocacy. Some educators obtain certification and are credentialed as a CDCES®, a BC-ADM®, or both. The work of the diabetes care and education specialist is supported by many others on the healthcare team. Competencies guide the development, practice, and career paths of healthcare professionals involved in diabetes care and education.

Healthy People 2020 targets related to diabetes remain essentially the same as the Healthy People 2010 targets because the percentage of individuals receiving formal diabetes education failed to reach the goal of 60%. Barriers to access continue to be a primary challenge in providing diabetes education.

Health Literacy

Health literacy is a multifactorial phenomenon that involves individuals, families, communities, and systems. When addressing health literacy, consider access to care and resources; the knowledge, skills, and abilities of everyone involved; the culture of healthcare providers and public health systems; and demographics.

The Patient Protection and Affordable Care Act of 2010 addresses health literacy both directly within 4 provisions and indirectly in the following broad themes:

- *Coverage expansion:* Enrolling, reaching out to, and delivering care to health insurance coverage expansion populations since 2014
- *Equity:* Ensuring equity in health and health care for all communities and populations
- *Workforce:* Training providers on cultural competency and diversifying the healthcare provider workforce
- *Patient information:* At appropriate reading levels in print and electronic media
- *Public health and wellness*
- *Quality improvement:* Innovation to create more effective and efficient models of care, particularly for individuals with chronic illnesses requiring extensive self-management

The Hospital Consumer Assessment of Healthcare Providers and Systems Survey—also known as Hospital CAHPS®, developed by the CMS, along with the Agency for Healthcare Research and Quality (AHRQ)—addresses health literacy and numeracy issues through survey questions on doctor and nurse communication, communication about medicines, and discharge information.

Focus on Practice

Improve care and enhance quality by facilitating and critically considering feedback from all individuals regarding coordination of their care. People with diabetes and related conditions choose where and how they want their DSMES and other services. Continuous quality assurance will allow program managers to evaluate the quality of systems and person-centered interventions.

Effectively communicate around all clinical care services. Use the title diabetes care and education specialist to communicate with stakeholders about DSMES and the breadth of services you can provide. Ensure follow-up with all persons involved in the process. Individually and collectively advocate for the services you provide.

References

1. National Institutes of Health. Current Burden of Diabetes in the U.S. (cited 2020, 9 Jan). On the Internet at: https://www.niddk.nih.gov/health-information/communication-programs/ndep/health-professionals/practice-transformation-physicians-health-care-teams/why-transform/current-burden-diabetes-us.
2. International Diabetes Federation. IDF Diabetes Atlas, 9th ed. 2019. Online version of IDF Diabetes Atlas (cited 2019 Dec 29). On the Internet at: www.diabetesatlas.org.
3. International Diabetes Federation. IDF Diabetes Atlas, 8th ed. 2017 (cited 2019 May 20). On the Internet at: http://www.diabetesatlas.org.
4. Centers for Disease Control and Prevention. National Diabetes Statistics Report, 2020. Atlanta, GA: Centers for Disease Control and Prevention, U.S. Dept of Health and Human Services; 2020. (cited 2020 Mar 20). On the Internet at: https://www.cdc.gov/diabetes/pdfs/data/statistics/national-diabetes-statistics-report.pdf.
5. World Health Organization. (2018). Noncommunicable diseases country profiles 2018. (License: CC BY-NC-SA 3.0 IGO). Geneva: World Health Organization.
6. Unnikrishnan R, Pradeepa R, Joshi SR, Mohan V. Type 2 diabetes: demystifying the global epidemic. Diabetes. 2017;66(6):1432.
7. Knowler WC, Barrett-Conner E, Fowler SE, et al. Reduction in the incidence of type 2 diabetes with lifestyle intervention or metformin. N Engl J Med. 2002;346:393-403.
8. UK Prospective Diabetes Study Group. Intensive blood glucose control with sulfonylureas or insulin compared with conventional treatment and risks of complications in patients with type 2 diabetes (UKPDS 33). Lancet. 1998;352:837-53.
9. Herold KC, Bundy BN, Long SA, et al. An anti-CD3 antibody, teplizumab, in relatives at risk for type diabetes. N Engl J Med. 2019;381(7):603-13.
10. The Diabetes Control and Complications Trial (DCCT)/Epidemiology of Diabetes Interventions and Complications Research Group (EDIC). Retinopathy and nephropathy in patients with type 1 diabetes four years after a trial of intensive therapy. N Engl J Med. 2000;342(6):381-9.
11. Diabetes Control and Complications Trial (DCCT)/Epidemiology of Diabetes Interventions and Complications (EDIC) Research Group. Beneficial effects of intensive therapy of diabetes during adolescence: outcomes after the Diabetes Control and Complications Trial (DCCT). J Pediatr. 2001; 6:804-12.
12. Geiss LS, Wang J, Cheng Y J, et al. Prevalence and incidence trends for diagnosed diabetes among adults aged 20 to 79 years, United States, 1980-2012. JAMA. 2014;312(12):1218-26. Doi:10.1001/jama.2014.11494.
13. Centers for Disease Control and Prevention. National diabetes prevention program (cited 2019 May 20). On the Internet at: http://www.cdc.gov/diabetes/prevention/index.htm.
14. Benoit SR, Hora I, Albright AL, Gregg EW. New directions in incidence and prevalence of diagnosed diabetes in the USA. BMJ Open Diabetes Research & Care. 2019;7((e000657)):1-6.
15. Boyle JP, Thompson TJ, Gregg EW, Barker LE, Williamson DF. Projection of the year 2050 burden of diabetes in the US adult population: dynamic modeling of incidence, mortality, and prediabetes prevalence. Population Health Metrics. 2010;8:29. doi: 10.1186/1478-7954-8-29.
16. Bullard KM, Cowie CC, Lessem SE, et al. Prevalence of diagnosed diabetes in adults by diabetes type—United States, 2016. MMWR Morb Mortal Wkly Rep. 2018;67:359–361. DOI: http://dx.doi.org/10.15585/mmwr.mm6712a2.
17. Roglic G, Unwin N. Mortality attributable to diabetes: estimates for the year 2010. Diabetes Res Clin Pract. 2009;87(1):15-9.
18. Dankwa-Mullan I, Rivo M, Sepulveda M, Park Y, Snowdon J, Rhee K. Transforming diabetes care through artificial intelligence: the future is here. Popul Health Man. 2019;22(3):229-42.
19. Hamman RF, Bell RA, Dabelea D, et al. The SEARCH for Diabetes in Youth Study: Rationale, Findings, and Future Directions. Diabetes Care. 2014;37(12):3336-44.
20. Pettitt DJ, Talton J, Dabelea D, et al. Prevalence of diabetes in U.S. youth in 2009: the SEARCH for Diabetes in Youth Study. Diabetes Care. 2014;37(2):402-8. Doi:10.2337/dc13-1838.
21. The Writing Group for the SEARCH for Diabetes in Youth Study Group. Incidence of diabetes in youth in the United States. JAMA. 2007;297(24):2716-24.
22. Imperatore G, Mayer Davis EJ, Orchard TJ, Zheng VW. Prevalence and incidence of type 1 diabetes among children and adults in the United States and comparisons with non-U.S. countries. In: Cowie CC, Casagrande SS, Menke A, et al, eds. Diabetes in America. Vol. NIH Pub No. 17-1468. 3rd ed. Bethesda, MD: National Institutes of Health; 2018.
23. Jensen ET, Dabelea D. Type 2 diabetes in youth: new lessons from the SEARCH study. Curr Diabetes Rep. 2018;18(6):36.
24. Mayer-Davis EJ, Lawrence JM, Dabelea D, et al. Incidence trends of type 1 and type 2 diabetes among youths, 2002–2012. N Engl J Med. 2017;376(15):1419-29.
25. American Diabetes Association. Economic costs of diabetes in the U.S. in 2017. Diabetes Care. 2018:dci180007.
26. Dall TM, Yang W, Gillespie K, et al. The economic burden of elevated blood glucose levels in 2017: diagnosed and undiagnosed diabetes, gestational diabetes mellitus and prediabetes. Diabetes Care. 2019;42(9):1661.
27. Shrestha SS, Honeycutt AA, Yang W, et al. Economic costs attributable to diabetes in each U.S. state. Diabetes Care. 2018;41(12):2526.
28. Boren SA, Fitzner KA, Panhalkar PS, Specker JE. Costs and benefits associated with diabetes education: a review of the literature. Diabetes Educ. 2009;35(1):72-96.
29. Pew Research Center. Baby Boomers Retire. (cited 2020 Jan 6). On the Internet at: https://www.pewresearch.org/fact-tank/2010/12/29/baby-boomers-retire/.

30. Huang ES, Basu A, O'Grady M, et al. Projecting the future diabetes population size and related costs for the US Diabetes Care. 2009;32(12):2225-29.

31. Andes LJ, Yanfeng L, Srinivasan M, et al. Diabetes prevalence and incidence among medicare beneficiaries - United States, 2001-2015. MMWR: Morbid Mortal Wkly Rep. 2019;68(43):961-6.

32. Hua X, Carvalho N, Tew M, Huang ES, Herman WH, Clarke P. Expenditures and prices of antihyperglycemic medications in the United States: 2002-2013. JAMA. 2016;315(13):1400-2.

33. Henry J. Kaiser Family Foundation. Key facts about the uninsured population. 2019 (cited 2019 May 26). On the Internet at: https://www.kff.org/uninsured/fact-sheet/key-facts-about-the-uninsured-population/.

34. Barnett DM. Elliott P. Joslin, M.D.: A Centennial Portrait. Boston, MA: Joslin Diabetes Center; 1998.

35. Allen NA. The history of diabetes nursing, 1914-1936. Diabetes Educ. 2003;29(6):976-989.

36. Etzwiler DD. Who's teaching the diabetic? Diabetes. 1967; 16(2):111-17.

37. Franz M. A tribute to Donnell D. Etzwiler, MD: Innovator, leader, educator. Diabetes Educ. 2003;29(6):969-75.

38. Ezzard NV, Deeb LC, Alogna M, Gettinger J. Profiles of diabetes education in 1979; results of three surveys. Diabetes Educ. 1980;6(2):11-15.

39. Siminerio LM. The diabetes education renaissance. Diabetes Spectr. 2006;19(2):76.

40. Fain JA. Developing the national standards. Diabetes Educ. 1995;21(3):175.

41. National Standards and Review Criteria for Diabetes Patient Education Programs: Quality Assurance for Diabetes Patient Education. Diabetes Educ. 1986;12(3):286-91.

42. Mensing C. Comparing the processes: accreditation and recognition. Diabetes Spectr. 2010;23(1):65.

43. National Certifying Board for Diabetes Educators. History (cited 2020 Jan 3). https://www.ncbde.org/about/history/.

44. American Association of Diabetes Educators. What is diabetes education. 2013.

45. Anderson RM, Funnell MM. Patient empowerment: reflections on the challenge of fostering the adoption of a new paradigm. Patient Educ and Couns. 2005;57(2):153-57.

46. Diabetes Control and Complications Trial (DCCT) Research Group. The effect of intensive control on the development and progression of complications in insulin dependent diabetes mellitus. N Engl J Med. 1993;329:977.

47. The DPP Research Group. The Diabetes Prevention Program (DPP). Diabetes Care. 2002;25(12):2165-71.

48. Siminerio LM, Piatt G, Zgibor JC. Implementing the chronic care model for improvements in diabetes care and education in a rural primary care practice. Diabetes Educator. 2005; 31(2):225-34.

49. Peeples M, Tomky D, Mulcahy K, et al. Evolution of the American Association of Diabetes Educators' Diabetes Education Outcomes Project. Diabetes Educ. 2007;33(5):794-817.

50. Duncan I, Birkmeyer, C., Coughlin, S., et al. Assessing the value of diabetes education. Diabetes Educ. 2009;35:752-60.

51. Tobin CT. A Rainbow of opportunities: advanced practices. Diabetes Educ. 2000;26(2):216-327.

52. Valentine V, Kulkarni K, Hinnen D. Evolving roles: from diabetes educators to advanced diabetes managers. Diabetes Spectr. 2003;16(1):27.

53. Duncan I, Ahmed T, Li QE, et al. Assessing the value of the diabetes educator. Diabetes Educ. 2011;37(5):638-57.

54. Norris SL, Chowdhury FM, Van Le K, et al. Effectiveness of community health workers in the care of persons with diabetes. Diabetic Med. 2006;23(5):544-56.

55. Siminerio L, Ruppert KM, Gabbay RA. Who can provide diabetes self-management support in primary care? Findings from a randomized controlled trial. Diabetes Educ. 2013;39(5):705-13. Doi:10.1177/0145721713492570.

56. Maryniuk MD, Mensing C, Imershein S, Gregory A, Jackson R. Enhancing the role of medical office staff in diabetes care and education. Clin Diabetes. 2013;31(3):116-22.

57. Chrvala CA, Sherr D, Lipman RD. Diabetes self-management education for adults with type 2 diabetes mellitus: a systematic review of the effect on glycemic control. Patient Educ Couns. 2015;99(6):926-43. Doi:10.1016/j.pec.2015.11.003.

58. Norris SL, Engelgau MM, Narayan KMV. Effectiveness of self-management training in type 2 diabetes: a systematic review of randomized controlled trials. Diabetes Care. 2001;24(3):561-87.

59. Creamer J, Attridge M, Ramsden M, Cannings-John R, Hawthorne K. Culturally appropriate health education for type 2 diabetes in ethnic minority groups: an updated systenatic review of randomized controlled trials. Diabet Med. 2016;33(2), 169-183. Doi:10.1111/dme.12865.

60. Larson MS. The Rise of Professionalism: a Sociological Analysis, Berkeley, California: University of California Press, 1978, p. 208.

61. Susskind RE, Susskind D. The Future of the Professions: How Technology Will Transform the Work of Human Experts. Oxford: Oxford University Press; 2017.

62. Flexner A. Is social work a profession? Res Soc Work Pract. 2001;11(2):152-65.

63. Joel LA, Kelly LY. Kelly's Dimensions of Professional Nursing. 10th ed. New York: McGraw-Hill Medical; 2011.

64. Association for Diabetes Care and Education Specialists (ADCES). Board Certified Advanced Diabetes Management (cited 2020 Jan 15). On the Internet at: https://www.diabeteseducator.org/practice/bc-adm-cdces-information.

65. National Certifying Board for Diabetes Educators. Eligibility Requirements. (cited 2020 Jan 10). On the Internet at: https://www.ncbde.org/certification_info/eligibility-requirements/.

66. National Certifying Board for Diabetes Educators. Canons of Ethics. (cited 2020 Jan 15). On the Internet at: https://www.ncbde.org/PosStatements/canons-of-ethics/.

67. Rinker J, Dickinson JK, Litchman ML, et al. The 2017 Diabetes Educator and the Diabetes Self-Management Education National Practice Survey. Diabetes Educ. 2018;44(3):260-68.

68. Ahern J, Grove N, Strand T, et al. The impact of the Trial Coordinator in the Diabetes Control and Complications Trial (DCCT). The DCCT Research Group. Diabetes Educ. 1993;19(6):509-12.

69. Ahern JA, Kruger DF, Gatcomb PM, Petit WA, Jr., Tamborlane WV. The diabetes control and complications trial (DCCT): the trial coordinator perspective. Report by the DCCT Research Group. Diabetes Educ. 1989;15(3):236-41.

70. Fain JA. DCCT: model of partnership. The Diabetes educator. 1994;20(1):9.

71. Feste C, Anderson RM. Empowerment: from philosophy to practice. Patient Educ Couns. 1995;26:139-44.

72. Anderson RM, Funnell MM, Fitzgerald JT, Marrero DG. The diabetes empowerment scale: a measure of psychosocial self-efficacy. Diabetes Care. 2000;23:739-43.

73. Funnell MM, Tang TS, Anderson RM. From DSME to DSMS: developing empowerment-based diabetes self-management support. Diabetes Spectr. 2007;20(4):221-6.

74. Mulcahy K, Maryniuk M, Peeples M, et al. Standards for outcomes measurement of diabetes self-management education. Diabetes Educ. 2003;29(5):804-16.

75. Coates VE, Boore JRP. Knowledge and diabetes self-management. Patient Educ Couns. 1996;29:99-108.

76. Glasgow RE, Eakin KG. Issues in diabetes self-management. In: Shumaker S, Schron E, Ockene J, McBee WL, eds. The Handbook of Health Behavior Change. New York: Springer; 1997.

77. Powers MA, Bardsley J, Cypress M, et al. Diabetes self-management education and support in type 2 diabetes: a joint position statement of the American Diabetes Association, the American Association of Diabetes Educators, and the Academy of Nutrition and Dietetics. Diabetes Educ. 2015;41(4):417-30. Doi:10.1177/0145721715588904.

78. Funnell MM, Brown TL, Childs BP, et al. National standards for diabetes self-management education. Diabetes Care. 2009;32 Suppl 1:S87-94.

79. American Association of Diabetes Educators. AADE guidelines for the practice of diabetes self-management education and training (DSME/T). Diabetes Educ. 2009;35 Suppl 3:S85-107.

80. American Association of Diabetes Educators. Competencies for diabetes educators and diabetes paraprofessionals. 2016 (cited 2020 Jan 15). On the Internet at: http://www.diabeteseducator.org/ProfessionalResources/position/competencies.html.

81. Neamah HH, Kuhlmann AKS, Tabak RG. Effectiveness of program modification strategies of the Diabetes Prevention Program: a systematic review. Diabetes Educ. 2016;42(2):153-65. Doi:10.1177/0145721716630386.

82. Association for Diabetes Care and Education Specialists (ADCES). Guidance for Becoming a Diabetes Care and Education Specialist (cited 2020 Jan 15). On the Internet at: https://www.diabeteseducator.org/practice/becoming-a-diabetes-care-and-education-specialist.

83. Finney Rutten LJ, Blake KD, Greenberg-Worisek AJ, Allen SV, Moser RP, Hesse BW. Online health information seeking among US adults: measuring progress toward a Healthy People 2020 Objective. Public Health Rep. 2019;134(6):617-25.

84. Estacio EV, Whittle R, Protheroe J. The digital divide: examining socio-demographic factors associated with health literacy, access and use of internet to seek health information. J Health Psych. 2019;24(12):1668-75.

85. Williams SL, Ames K, Lawson C. Preferences and trust in traditional and non-traditional sources of health information – a study of middle to older aged Australian adults. J Comm in Health. 2019;12(2):134-42.

86. Mc Sharry J, Dinneen SF, Humphreys M, et al. Barriers and facilitators to attendance at type 2 diabetes structured education programmes: a qualitative study of educators and attendees. Diabet Med. 2019;36(1):70-9.

87. Winkley K, Upsher R, Keij SM, Chamley M, Ismail K, Forbes A. Healthcare professionals' views of group structured education for people with newly diagnosed type 2 diabetes. Diabet Med. 2018;35(7):911-19.

88. Horigan G, Davies M, Findlay-White F, Chaney D, Coates V. Reasons why patients referred to diabetes education programmes choose not to attend: a systematic review. Diabet Med. 2017;34(1):14-26.

89. Bzowyckyj AS, Aquilante CL, Cheng A-L, Drees B. Leveraging the electronic medical record to identify predictors of attendance to a diabetes self-management education and support program. Diabetes Educ. 2019;45(5):544-52.

90. Coates V, Slevin M, Carey M, Slater P, Davies M. Declining structured diabetes education in those with type 2 diabetes: a plethora of individual and organisational reasons. Patient Educ Couns. 2018;101(4):696-702.

91. Lawal M, Woodman A, Fanghanel J. Barriers to structured diabetes education attendance: opinions of people with diabetes. J Diabetes Nurs. 2018;22(5):1-6.

92. American Association of Diabetes Educators. Project Vision: Shaping the future of our specialty (cited 2020 Jan 10). On the Internet at: https://www.diabeteseducator.org/about-adces/For-Diabetes-Care-and-Education-Specialists.

93. National Certifying Board for Diabetes Educators. Summary of the 2018 Certification Examinations and Renewal of Certification by Continuing Education (cited 2020 Jan 5). On the Internet at: https://www.ncbde.org/about/annual-reports/.

94. Sherr D, Lipman RD. The diabetes educator and the diabetes self-management education engagement: the 2015 national practice survey. Diabetes Educ. 2015;41(5):616-24.

95. Kemmis K. Repositioning the specialty. Elevating our role. Advancing care. AADE in Practice. 2019;7(5):10-11.

96. Martin AL, Warren JP, Lipman RD. The landscape for diabetes education: results of the 2012 AADE National Diabetes Education Practice Survey. Diabetes Educ. 2013;39(5):614-22.

97. American Association of Diabetes Educators. The scope of practice for diabetes educators and the standards of practice for diabetes educators: developed under the aegis of a multidisciplinary task force of the American Association of Diabetes Educators. Diabetes Educ. 1992;18(1):52-6. Doi:10.1177/014572179201800109.

98. American Association of Diabetes Educators. The 1999 scope of practice for diabetes educators and the standards of practice for diabetes educators. Diabetes Educ. 2000;26(3):519-25. Doi:10.1177/014572170002600316.

99. American Association of Diabetes Educators. The scope of practice, standards of practice, and standards of professional performance for diabetes educators. Diabetes Educ. 2005;31(4): 487-512. Doi:10.1177/0145721705279719.

100. American Association of Diabetes Educators. (2010). The Scope of Practice for Diabetes Educators, Standards of Practice and Standards of Professional Performance (cited 2020 Jan 15). On the Internet at: http://www.diabetesed.net/page/_files /Standards-of-Practice-ADA-2011.PDF.

101. American Association of Diabetes Educators. Competencies for diabetes educators and diabetes paraprofessionals. 2014 (cited 2020 Jan 20). On the Internet at: http://www.diabeteseducator .org/ProfessionalResources/position/competencies.html.

102. Benner P. From Novice to Expert: Excellence and Power in Clinical Nursing Practice. Upper Saddle River, NJ: Prentice-Hall; 2001.

103. Dreyfus HL. Mind Over Machine: The Power of Human Intuitive Expertise in the Era of the Computer. New York: Free Press; 1986.

104. Grove SK, Burns N, Gray Jr. The Practice of Nursing Research: Appraisal, Synthesis, and Generation of Evidence. 7th ed. St. Louis: Elsevier; 2013.

105. Burke SD, Thorlton J, Hall M. Diabetes self-management education: the art and science of disease management. In: Mensing C, ed. The Art and Science of Diabetes Education. 3rd ed. Chicago: American Association of Diabetes Educators; 2014:3-30.

106. Burke SD, Thorlton J. Diabetes self-management education: the art and science of disease management. In: Cornell S, Halstenson C, Miller D, eds. The Art and Science of Diabetes Self-Management Education Desk Reference. Chicago: American Association of Diabetes Educators; 2017:3-28.

107. Zhang Y, Dall TM, Mann SE, et al. The economic costs of undiagnosed diabetes. Popul Health Manag. 2009;12(2):95-101.

108. McLendon SF. Interactive video telehealth models to improve access to diabetes specialty care and education in the rural setting: a systemic review. Diabetes Spectr. 2017;30(2):124-36.

109. Clifton DC, Benjamin RW, Brown AR, Ostrovsky DA, Narayan AP. A tablet-based educational tool: toward more comprehensive pediatric patient education. Clin Ped. 2018;57(10):1176-82.

110. Yang S, Jiang Q, Li H. The role of telenursing in the management of diabetes: a systematic review and meta-analysis. Pub Health Nurs. 2019;36(4):575-86.

111. Smith KM, Baker KM, Bardsley JK, McCartney P, Magee M. Redesigning hospital diabetes education: a qualitative evaluation with nursing teams. J Nurs Care Qual. 2019;34(2):151-7.

112. Berkowitz SA, Hulberg AC, Standish S, Reznor G, Atlas SJ. Addressing unmet basic resource needs as part of chronic cardiometabolic disease management. JAMA In Med. 2017; 177(2):244-52.

113. Chang L-S, Vaduganathan M, Plutzky J, Aroda VR. Bridging the gap for patients with diabetes and cardiovascular disease through cardiometabolic collaboration. Cur Diabetes Rep. 2019;19(12):1-10.

114. Jardim TV, Mozaffarian D, Abrahams-Gessel S, et al. Cardiometabolic disease costs associated with suboptimal diet in the United States: a cost analysis based on a microsimulation model. PLoS Med. 2019;16(12):1-15.

115. Guo F, Garvey WT. Development of a weighted cardiometabolic disease staging (CMDS) system for the prediction of future diseasse. J Clin Endo Metab. 2015;100(10):3871-77.

116. Centers for Disease Control and Prevention. National Diabetes Prevention Program (cited 2020, Jan 19). On the Internet at: https://www.cdc.gov/diabetes/prevention/index.html.

117. Peyrot M, Rubin RR, Funnell MM, Siminerio LM. Access to diabetes self-management education: results of national surveys of patients, educators, and physicians. Diabetes Educ. 2009;35(2):246-63.

118. Zrebiec J. A national study of the certified diabetes educator: implications for future certification examinations. Diabetes Educ. 2014;40(4):470-5.

119. Burke S, Haas L, American Diabetes A. Diabetes Management in Long-term Settings: A Clinician's Guide to Optimal Elderly Care. Alexandria: American Diabetes Association; 2014.

120. Berget C, Nii P, Wyckoff L, Patrick K, Brooks-Russell A, Messer LH. Equipping school health personnel for diabetes care with a competency framework and pilot education program. J School Health. 2019;89(9):683-91.

121. Okemah J, Peng J, Quiñones M. Addressing clinical inertia in type 2 diabetes mellitus: a review. Advances in Therapy. 2018;35(11):1735-45.

122. Morgan JM, Mensa-Wilmot Y, Bowen S-A, et al. Implementing key drivers for diabetes self-management education and support programs: early outcomes, activities, facilitators, and barriers. Prev Chronic Dis. 2018;15:1-6.

123. Keehan SP, Poisal JA, Cuckler GA, et al. National health expenditure projections, 2015-25: economy, prices, and aging expected to shape spending and enrollment. Health Aff. 2016;35(8):1522-31. Doi:10.1377/hlthaff.2016.0459.

124. U.S. Food & Drug Administration. 21st Century Cures Act. (cited 2020, Jan 19). On the Internet at: https://www.fda.gov/regulatory-information/selected-amendments-fdc-act/21st-century-cures-act.

125. The 21st Century Cures Act, H.R. 34, 114th Cong. (2016). (cited 2020, Jan 19). On the Internet at: https://www.congress.gov/bill/114th-congress/house-bill/34.

126. Gabay M. 21st Century Cures Act. Hosp Pharm. 2017;52(4): 264–5. Doi:10.1310/hpj5204-264.

127. Lieberman, T. With media watchdogs on the sidelines, pharma-funded advocacy groups pushed Cures Act to the finish line. HealthNewsReview.org. 2016 (cited 2020, Jan 19). On the Internet at: http://www.healthnewsreview.org/2016/12/with-media-watchdogs-sidelined-pharma-funded-advocacy-groups-pushed-cures-act-to-the-finish-line/.

128. U.S. Food & Drug Administration. FDA warns people with diabetes and health care providers against the use of devices for diabetes management not authorized for sale in the United States: FDA Safety Communication (cited 2020, Jan 19). On the Internet at: https://www.fda.gov/medical-devices/safety-communications/fda-warns-people-diabetes-and-health-care-providers-against-use-devices-diabetes-management-not.

129. World Health Organization (2019). WHO Guideline: Recommendations on digital interventions for health system strengthening. Geneva, Switzerland: World Health Organization; 2019. License: CC-BY-NC-SA-3.0 IGO. (cited 2020, Jan 19). On the Internet at https://apps.who.int/iris/bitstream/handle/10665/311977/WHO-RHR-19.8-eng.pdf?ua=1.

130. Brown W, Yen P, Rojas M, Schnall R. Assessment of the Health IT Usability Evaluation Model (Health-ITUEM) for evaluating mobile health (mHealth) technology. J Biomed Inform. 2013;46:1080-7.

131. Georgsson M, Staggers N. An evaluation of patients' experienced usability of a diabetes mHealth system using a multi-method approach. J Biomed Inform. 2016. 59: 115-29.

132. Veazie S, Winchell K, Gilbert J, et al. Rapid evidence review of mobile applications for self-management of diabetes. J Gen Intern Med. 2018;33:1167. https://doi-org.proxy.cc.uic.edu/10.1007/s11606-018-4410-1.

133. U.S. Food & Drug Administration (2017, July 24). Fostering Medical Innovation: A Plan for Digital Health Devices; Software Precertification Pilot Program (cited 2020, Jan 19). On the Internet at https://www.regulations.gov/document?D=FDA-2017-N-4301-0001.

134. Lewis D, Leibrand S; #OpenAPS Community. Real-world use of open source artificial pancreas systems. J Diabetes Sci Technol. 2016;10(6):1411. Doi:10.1177/1932296816665635.

135. Farrington C. Hacking diabetes: DIY artificial pancreas systems. The Lancet. 2017; 5(5):332. Doi: https://doi.org/10.1016/S2213-8587(16)30397-7.

136. Thorlton J, Catlin AC. Data mining for adverse drug events: impact on six learning styles. CIN. 2019; 37(5), 250-9. Doi: 10.1097/CIN.0000000000000513.

137. Health Markets. Healthcare reform news updates (cited 2020 Jan 19). On the Internet at: https://www.healthmarkets.com/resources/health-insurance/trumpcare-news-updates/.

138. Casagrande SS, McEwen LN, Herman WH. Changes in health insurance coverage under the Affordable Care Act: a national sample of U.S. adults with diabetes, 2009 and 2016. Diabetes Care. 2018. 41(5), 956-62. Doi:10.2337/dc17-2524.

139. HealthCare.gov. Read the Affordable Care Act. (cited 2020 Jan 19). On the Internet at: https://www.healthcare.gov/where-can-i-read-the-affordable-care-act/.

140. Brown DS, Delavar A. The affordable care act and insurance coverage for persons with diabetes in the United States. J Hosp Manag Health Policy. 2018;2:17. 81? doi:10.21037/jhmhp.2018.04.07.

141. Healthinsurance.org, "What is a health insurance exchange?" (cited 2020, Jan 19). On the Internet at: https://www.healthinsurance.org/faqs/what-is-a-health-insurance-exchange/.

142. American Diabetes Association. 2019 state and federal legislative and regulatory priorities: Diabetes research and programs. 2019 Jan 11 (cited 2020, Jan 19). On the Internet at: http://www.diabetes.org/advocacy/advocacy-priorities/federal-state-priorities.html.

143. Centers for Disease Control and Prevention. National Diabetes Prevention Program Coverage Toolkit © 2020 (cited 2020, Jan 19).On the Internet at: https://coveragetoolkit.org/.

144. Centers for Medicare & Medicaid Services. Financial alignment initiative for Medicare-Medicaid enrollees. 2019 (cited 2020, Jan 19). On the Internet at: https://innovation.cms.gov/initiatives/Financial-Alignment/.

145. Centers for Medicare and Medicaid Services. Independence at home demonstration. 2019 May 23 (cited 2020, Jan 19). On the Internet at: https://innovation.cms.gov/initiatives/independence-at-home/.

146. Myerson R, Laiteerapong N. The Affordable Care Act and diabetes diagnosis and care: exploring the potential impacts. Curr Diab Rep. 2016;16(4):27. doi:10.1007/s11892-016-0712-z.

147. Burke SD, Sherr D, Lipman RD. Partnering with diabetes educators to improve patient outcomes. Diabetes Metab Syndr Obes. 2014;7(Feb 12):45-53.

148. Fraser, M.R. A brief history of the Prevention and Public Health Fund: implications for public health advocated. Am J Pub Health. 2019; 109, 572-77. https://doi.org/10.2105/AJPH.2018.304926.

149. US Dept. of Health and Human Services. Prevention and Public Health Fund. 2016 Dec 16 (cited 2020, Jan 19). On the Internet at: http://www.hhs.gov/open/prevention/.

150. American Public Health Association (APHA 2019). Prevention and Public Health Fund: Dedicated to improving our nation's public health. 2019 (cited 2020, Jan 19). On the Internet at: https://www.apha.org/-/media/files/pdf/factsheets/pphf_fact_sheet.ashx?la=en&hash=8AD9EFD10E474FC3DDFD5C750BBEDC85A424F35F.

151. Centers for Disease Control and Prevention. Childhood Obesity Research Demonstration (CORD) 1.0: Integrating Primary Care and Community Based Strategies to Prevent and Treat Childhood Obesity. (cited 2020, Jan 19). On the Internet at: https://www.cdc.gov/obesity/strategies/healthcare/cord1.html.

152. U.S. Government Accountability Office (GAO). Health care workforce: Comprehensive planning by HHS needed to meet national needs. 2015. GAO-16-17. (cited 2020, Jan 19). On the Internet at: https://www.gao.gov/assets/680/674137.pdf.

153. Centers for Disease Control and Prevention. Diabetes Prevention Recognition Program (DPRP) Standards and Operating Procedures. 2018. (Cited 2020, Jan 19). On the Internet at: https://www.cdc.gov/diabetes/prevention/pdf/dprp-standards.pdf.

154. Chait N, Glied S. Promoting prevention under the affordable care act. Annu Rev Public Health. 2018;39(1):507-24. https://doi.org/10.1146/annurev-publhealth-040617-013534. Doi:10.1146/annurev-publhealth-040617-013534.

155. CNN Politics. Obama drops long term health program 2011, Oct. 17. (Cited 2020, Jan 19) On the Internet at: https://www.cnn.com/2011/10/14/politics/health-care-program/.

156. White House, United States Congress. Obamacare: Complete law, latest statistics & Republican's counterproposal. 2017. Madison & Adams Press.

157. Bright R, Sakurada B. A population health strategy for diabetes: new partners, new opportunities. NAM Perspectives. Discussion Paper, National Academy of Medicine, Washington, DC. 2016. doi: 10.31478/201602d.

158. World Health Organization. (2020). Health Policy. (Cited 2020, Jan 15). On the Internet at: https://www.who.int/topics/health_policy/en/.

159. Diabetes Patient Advocacy Coalition. (cited 2020, Jan 18). On the Internet at: https://diabetespac.org/act-now/federal/).

160. Hilliard ME, Oser SM, Close KL, Liu NF, Hood KK, Anderson BJ. From individuals to international policy: achievements and ongoing needs in diabetes advocacy. Cur Diabetes Rep, 15(9). Doi: 10.1007/s11892-015-0636-z.

161. American Diabetes Association (2019, May 22). American Diabetes Association Applauds Colorado Governor and State Legislature for Passing HB 1216: Reduce Insulin Prices Bill. (cited 2020, Jan 19). On the Internet at https://www.diabetes.org/newsroom/press-releases/2019/colorado-reduce-insulin-prices-bill.

162. Golden SH, Maruthur N, Mathioudakis N, et al. The case for diabetes population health improvement: evidence-based programming for population outcomes in diabetes. Cur Diabetes Rep, 17(7). doi: 10.1007/s11892-017-0875-2.

163. Centers for Disease Control and Prevention. Recognized Lifestyle Change Program. (cited 2020, Jan 18). On the Internet at: https://nccd.cdc.gov/DDT_DPRP/Programs.aspx.

164. Congressional Caucus on Diabetes. (cited 2020, Jan 18). On the Internet at: https://diabetescaucus-degette.house.gov/.

165. Congress.gov. H.R.1840: Expanding Access to Diabetes Self-Management Training Act of 2019. 116th.

166. Congress (2019-2020). (cited 2020, Jan 18). On the Internet at: https://www.congress.gov/bill/116th-congress/house-bill/1840.

167. Congress.gov. S.814: Expanding Access to Diabetes Self-Management Training Act of 2019. 116th Congress (2019-2020). (cited 2020, Jan 18). On the Internet at: https://www.congress.gov/bill/116th-congress/senate-bill/814.

168. Association for Diabetes Care and Education Specialists. The Expanding Access to DSMT Act. (cited 2020, Jan 18). On the Internet at: https://www.diabeteseducator.org/advocacy/the-expanding-access-to-dsmt-act).

169. Konchak JN, Moran MF, O'Brien MJ, Kandula NR, Ackerman RT. The state of diabetes prevention policy in the USA following the Affordable Care Act. Cur Diabetes Rep, 16(6). doi: 10.1007/s11892-016-0742-6.

CHAPTER 2

The Diabetes Self-Management Education Process

Barb Schreiner, PhD, RN, CDCES, BC-ADM

Key Concepts

- Successful management of diabetes requires collaboration among the person with diabetes, the healthcare providers, and others in the support system.
- Components of diabetes self-management education (DSME) include assessment, goal setting, planning, implementation, and evaluation/monitoring, all of which focus on the individualized needs and goals of the person with diabetes.
- Review alternatives of what to ask and how to ask for information to individualize management and intervention plans.
- The plan for DSME must be individualized and sequenced to address objectives outlined in the medical plan, and include the personalized needs and capabilities of the person with diabetes.
- Effective plans differentiate between treatment, DSME learning objectives, and lifestyle behavioral goals. All are essential.
- Diabetes self-management education is a dynamic plan and a lifelong process.
- Diabetes care and education specialist competencies include refined assessment and clinical skills based in critical thinking; knowledge about diabetes, the chronic disease model, and the learning process; effective use of teaching tools and a variety of delivery methods; application of empowerment strategies and facilitation skills.
- Documentation provides data for collaboration, tracking person with diabetes outcomes, and overall program evaluation.

Introduction

Diabetes self-management education and support (DSMES), also known as diabetes self-management training (DSMT), is defined as a collaborative process through which people with or at risk for diabetes gain the knowledge and skills needed to modify behavior and successfully self-manage the disease and its related conditions.[1] Diabetes self-management education and support is an interactive, ongoing process involving the person with diabetes (PWD) (and support systems such as caregivers or family), a diabetes care and education specialist, and other members of the healthcare team.[1] The diabetes care and education specialist continues to be the recognized coordinator and is most often the provider of the diabetes knowledge, skills, and adjustment support for this chronic disease and its demands.

Diabetes self-management education is the cornerstone for the management of diabetes. In recent years, there has been a paradigm shift from the didactic (lecture) teaching style of self-management skills to a person-centered facilitation approach that encourages behavior change. It is critical that the person with diabetes have the knowledge, skills, and behaviors needed to successfully manage the disease. Measurable behavior change is the desired outcome of diabetes education.[2,3] Therefore, the intervention—the DSME process—aims to achieve optimal health status and better quality of life and reduce the need for costly healthcare.

The overall objectives of DSME are to support the following:[4]

- Informed decision making
- Self-care behaviors
- Problem solving
- Active collaboration with the healthcare team to identify individualized, targeted needs and to improve clinical outcomes, health status, and quality of life

Diabetes self-management education and support has drawn the attention of several groups in the past decade. Standards and algorithms have evolved not only for clinical care of diabetes but also for the education and support components. In 2007, the task force working on the National Standards for Diabetes Self-Management Education identified overriding principles based on existing evidence that were used to guide the review and revision of the standards. These principles were the following:[5]

1. Diabetes education is effective for improving clinical outcomes and quality of life, at least in the short term.
2. Diabetes self-management education has evolved from primarily didactic presentations to more theoretically based empowerment models.
3. There is no one "best" education program or approach; however, programs incorporating behavioral and psychosocial strategies demonstrate improved outcomes. Additional studies show that culturally and age-appropriate programs improve outcomes and that group education is effective.
4. Ongoing support is critical to sustain progress made by participants during the DSME program.
5. Behavioral goal setting is an effective strategy to support self-management behaviors.

These overriding principles support the efficacy of DSME and guide the development of sound DSME programs.

In 2012, the task force expanded the National Standards to include "support," underscoring the need for continued interaction with persons with diabetes after formal educational sessions have ended. The other addition to the National Standards was the inclusion of educating people with prediabetes, as this is an underserved population in need of content and support similar to that given to those with diabetes.[5]

In 2015 a joint position statement was published by the American Diabetes Association (ADA), the American Association of Diabetes Educators (AADE)–known as the Association of Diabetes Care and Education Specialists (ADCES) since January 24, 2020–and the Academy of Nutrition and Dietetics.[7] The writing group created an education algorithm to help providers, clinicians, and others identify critical times for self-management education and skill development for individuals with type 2 diabetes. There are 5 guiding principles at the foundation of the DSMES algorithm: engagement, information sharing, psychosocial and behavioral support, integration with other therapies, and coordination of care. Four critical times are delineated: at diagnosis, at annual assessment of needs, at time of complicating factors, and for transitions in care. Each of the critical times has a different focus for assessment and education. Clearly, at diagnosis, safety and survival information is most important. At times when complications develop, the focus turns to support and adapting current knowledge and skills to new physical or emotional demands. Finally, the authors recognized that as living conditions, resources, or provider changes occur, the person with type 2 diabetes will need yet another focus of DSMES. The DSMES algorithm of care and the 4 critical time points are found in Figures 2.1 and 2.2.

This chapter describes the 5-step process of DSME. The steps are as follows:

1. Assessment
2. Goal setting
3. Planning
4. Implementation
5. Evaluation/monitoring

Each step of this process is detailed in its own section. Skill builders, knowledge builders, and practice tips are included at each step. The educational process chart (Figure 2.3) graphically displays this process. It is important to note that the DSME process is presented in this chapter in a linear fashion for ease of comprehension. In practice, the 5 steps are not necessarily sequential, and often the diabetes care and education specialist finds it necessary to return to an earlier step in the process to address the individual needs of the person with diabetes.

Assessment

Assessment is the first, and arguably the most important, step in the process of DSME and includes collection and interpretation of relevant person with diabetes information. The diabetes care and education specialist and the person with diabetes use these data to mutually identify goals and then progress to implementation of an individualized education plan. Assessment is ongoing and involves reassessment throughout the process. Reassessment is ongoing as diabetes goals and care plans are updated to reflect changing priorities and progressive attainment of educational goals. Because of the chronic nature of diabetes, it is recognized that DSME is a lifelong process and that there may be life events that interrupt the learning process or cause the person's goals to be changed or put on hold.[8]

Assessment sets the foundation for helping people find their motivation to manage their diabetes and to adopt healthier lifestyle habits. The initial assessment is important for establishing rapport and developing trust between the diabetes care and education specialist and the PWD. The objective of the assessment is to gather

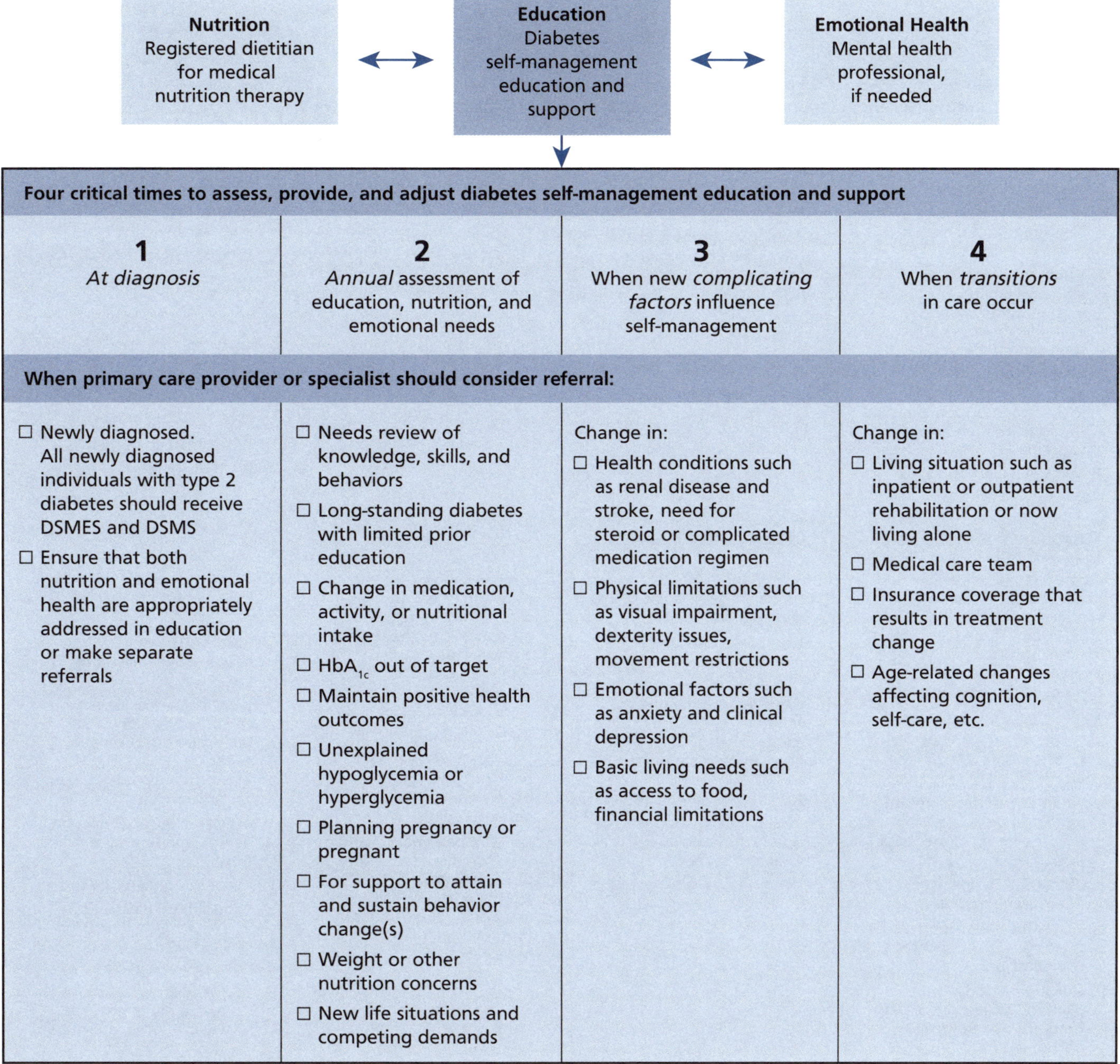

ADA *Standards of Medical Care in Diabetes* recommends all patients be assessed and referred for:
Nutrition
Registered dietitian for medical nutrition therapy
Education
Diabetes self-management education and support
Emotional Health
Mental health professional, if needed
Four critical times to assess, provide, and adjust diabetes self-management education and support
1
At diagnosis
2
Annual assessment of education, nutrition, and emotional needs
3
When new *complicating factors* influence self-management
4
When *transitions* in care occur
When primary care provider or specialist should consider referral:
☐ Newly diagnosed. All newly diagnosed individuals with type 2 diabetes should receive DSMES and DSMS
☐ Ensure that both nutrition and emotional health are appropriately addressed in education or make separate referrals
☐ Needs review of knowledge, skills, and behaviors
☐ Long-standing diabetes with limited prior education
☐ Change in medication, activity, or nutritional intake
☐ HbA_{1c} out of target
☐ Maintain positive health outcomes
☐ Unexplained hypoglycemia or hyperglycemia
☐ Planning pregnancy or pregnant
☐ For support to attain and sustain behavior change(s)
☐ Weight or other nutrition concerns
☐ New life situations and competing demands
Change in:
☐ Health conditions such as renal disease and stroke, need for steroid or complicated medication regimen
☐ Physical limitations such as visual impairment, dexterity issues, movement restrictions
☐ Emotional factors such as anxiety and clinical depression
☐ Basic living needs such as access to food, financial limitations
Change in:
☐ Living situation such as inpatient or outpatient rehabilitation or now living alone
☐ Medical care team
☐ Insurance coverage that results in treatment change
☐ Age-related changes affecting cognition, self-care, etc.

FIGURE 2.1 **DSME and DSMS Algorithm of Care**

Source: M Powers, J Bardsley, M Cypress, et al, "Diabetes self-management education and support in type 2 diabetes: a joint position statement of the American Diabetes Association, the American Association of Diabetes Educators, and the Academy of Nutrition and Dietetics," *Diabetes Educ* 41, no. 4 (2015): 421.

sufficient information, including the person's expectations, perceptions, and fears, so that the individual, along with his or her healthcare team, may identify goals and develop an individual education plan. The diabetes care and education specialist determines both the *scope* and the *content* of the assessments and manages the flow to allow for sufficient time to gather information needed to engage in goal setting and education planning.[9]

Four critical times to assess, provide, and adjust diabetes self-management education and support			
At diagnosis	*Annual* assessment of education, nutrition, and emotional needs	When new *complicating factors* influence self-management	When *transitions* in care occur
Primary care provider/endocrinologist/clinical care team: areas of focus and action steps			
☐ Answer questions and provide emotional support regarding diagnosis ☐ Provide overview of treatment and treatment goals ☐ Teach survival skills to address immediate requirements (safe use of medication, hypoglycemia treatment if needed, introduction of eating guidelines) ☐ Identify and discuss resources for education and ongoing support ☐ Make referral for DSMES, DSMS, and MNT	☐ Assess all areas of self-management ☐ Review problem-solving skills ☐ Identify strengths and challenges of living with diabetes	☐ Identify presence of factors that affect diabetes self-management and attain treatment and behavioral goals ☐ Discuss effect of complications and successes with treatment and self-management	☐ Develop diabetes transition plan ☐ Communicate transition plan to new healthcare team members ☐ Establish DSME and DSMS regular follow-up care
Diabetes education: areas of focus and action steps			
Assess cultural influences, health beliefs, current knowledge, physical limitations, family support, financial status, medical history, literacy, and numeracy to determine content to provide and how to provide it: ☐ Medications—choices, action, titration, side effects ☐ Monitoring blood glucose—when to test, interpreting and using glucose pattern management for feedback ☐ Physical activity—safety, short-term vs. long-term goals/recommendations ☐ Preventing, detecting, and treating acute and chronic complications ☐ Nutrition—food plan, planning meals, purchasing food, preparing meals, portioning food ☐ Risk reduction—smoking cessation, foot care ☐ Developing personal strategies to address psychosocial issues and concerns ☐ Developing personal strategies to promote health and behavior change	☐ Review and reinforce treatment goals and self-management needs ☐ Emphasize preventing complications and promoting quality of life ☐ Discuss how to adapt diabetes treatment and self-management to new life situations and competing demands ☐ Support efforts to sustain initial behavior changes and cope with the ongoing burden of diabetes	☐ Provide support for the provision of self-care skills in an effort to delay progression of the disease and prevent new complications ☐ Provide/refer for emotional support for diabetes-related distress and depression ☐ Develop and support personal strategies for behavior change and healthy coping ☐ Develop personal strategies to accommodate sensory or physical limitation(s), adapting to new self-management demands, and promote health and behavior change	☐ Identify needed adaptions in diabetes self-management ☐ Provide support for independent self-management skills and self-efficacy ☐ Identify level of significant other involvement and facilitate education and support ☐ Assist with facing challenges affecting usual level of activity, ability to function, health beliefs, and feelings of well-being ☐ Maximize quality of life and emotional support for the patient (and family members) ☐ Provide education for others now involved in care ☐ Establish communication and follow-up plans with the provider, family, and others

FIGURE 2.2 **Content for DSME and DSMS at 4 Critical Time Points**

Source: M Powers, J Bardsley, M Cypress, et al, "Diabetes self-management education and support in type 2 diabetes: a joint position statement of the American Diabetes Association, the American Association of Diabetes Educators, and the Academy of Nutrition and Dietetics," *Diabetes Educ* 41, no. 4 (2015): 422.

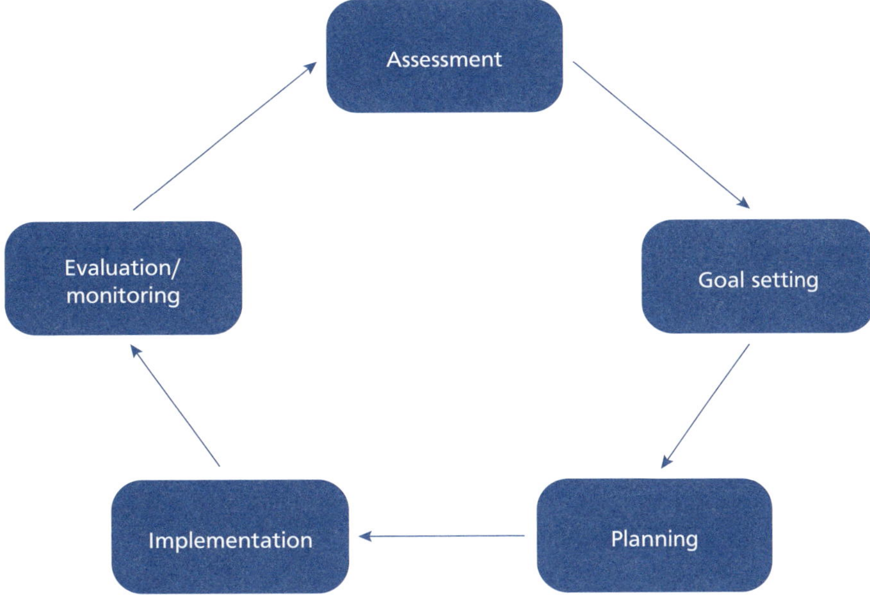

FIGURE 2.3 **The DSME Process**

Conducting an Effective Assessment

The diabetes care and education specialist conducts a thorough, individualized assessment of the person with or at risk for diabetes. The assessment process requires ongoing collection and interpretation of relevant data.[8] Assessment can be done by a variety of methods: face-to-face individual interview, group discussion, or a paper-based or electronic self-assessment tool. Detailed measurement criteria for assessment are included in *Competencies for Diabetes Care and Education Specialists*[8] and are summarized in Table 2.1.

Beginning an Assessment: Start With a Self-Assessment

When preparing to work with people with diabetes, the effective diabetes care and education specialist conducts a careful self-assessment. The self-assessment covers knowledge of population-based health, social determinants of health, and cultural competency. The diabetes care and education specialist should also have an appreciation of the impact of language when collaborating with people with diabetes.

Population-Based Health

How much do you know about the statistics about diabetes and its complications for your community? Knowing the greatest health risks in a community can help to set priorities for developing an education program and even an individualized education plan. For example, knowing that there is an increased incidence of type 2 diabetes among adolescents in your community might alert diabetes care and education specialists to add content to the program's curriculum about preventing type 2 diabetes in this population.

Social Determinants of Health

Social determinants of health (SDOH) are those "conditions in the places where people live, learn, work, and play [which] affect a wide range of health risks and outcomes."[10] Unstable housing, unsafe neighborhoods, food inequality and insecurity, poor access to health resources, and other social issues contribute to health disparities. Some SDOH may correlate with higher incidence of diabetes. For example, Dendup and colleagues[11] found an association between type 2 diabetes and environmental conditions such as air pollution, noise and lack of space for physical activity.

The Centers for Disease Control and Prevention (CDC) list 20 health conditions affected by SDOH, including obesity, type 2 diabetes, and cardiovascular disease. Diabetes care and education specialists, as members of local communities, have a role in supporting or participating in local initiatives to address SDOH in the community. For instance, diabetes care and education specialists might participate in health fairs to identify people at risk or advocate for improved lunches in schools. When developing education programs, diabetes care and education specialists could target "high-quality, evidence-based diabetes educational curricula across income levels, neighborhoods, or geographic regions."[12]

TABLE 2.1 Data Needed for Effective Assessment

Approach to Gathering Information
A systematic, organized, and holistic approach is called for, with data collected from the following sources: • Person with diabetes • Family members and members of the client's social support network, as appropriate • Existing medical records • Referring healthcare providers
Data to Be Collected
It is appropriate to gather information on the following topics: • Personal health history, family health history • Nutrition history and practices • Physical activity and exercise behaviors • Prescription and over-the-counter medications; use and practice of complementary and alternative therapies • Factors that influence learning, such as formal education and literacy levels, health beliefs, perceived learning needs, motivation to learn, preferred sources of information, and preferred learning source (eg, audio, visual, kinesthetic) • Diabetes self-management behaviors, including experience self-adjusting the treatment plan • Previous DSME, actual knowledge, and skills • Physical factors, including age, mobility, visual acuity, hearing, manual dexterity, alertness, attention span, and ability to concentrate; special needs or limitations requiring accommodations or adaptive support and use of alternative skills • Psychosocial concerns, factors, or issues, including family and social supports; experience with diabetes in friends or family; fears about diabetes or its complications • Current mental health status, including preferred stress management or coping strategies, history and treatment of eating disorders or depression • History of substance use, including alcohol, tobacco, and recreational drugs • Occupation; vocation; financial status; and social, cultural, and religious practices • Access to and use of healthcare resources
Data for Prediabetes Assessment
For an individual with prediabetes, gather the following information in addition to the above information: • Knowledge of prediabetes and risks: Evaluate person's understanding of prediabetes and the risks associated with it • Weight loss and weight management: Evaluate the person's understanding of the role of weight loss and weight management through nutrition modification and healthy eating in the management of prediabetes • Physical activity: Determine the individual's habits and behaviors associated with physical activity and the individual's understanding of the role of physical activity in management of prediabetes • Motivation: Assess the individual's motivation skills for maintaining positive behavioral change

Source: Adapted from JA Pichert, DG Schlundt, "Assessment: Gathering Information and Facilitating Engagement," in C Mensing, ed, *The Art and Science of Diabetes Self-Management Education: A Desk Reference for Healthcare Professionals* (Chicago: American Association of Diabetes Educators, 2006), 580.

Cultural Competency

The diabetes care and education specialist's self-assessment should also cover personal biases related to race, ethnicity, social status, education, body size, sexual orientation, and religion. By reflecting on personal biases and beliefs, the diabetes care and education specialist becomes more open to cultural sensitivity and more attuned to and accepting of individual differences. This self-awareness translates to a trusting environment.

Each adult learner comes for DSME with a unique set of experiences. These experiences affect the individual's ability to learn and the level of readiness to change behaviors. The individual's cultural, lifestyle, health beliefs, and even generation may be very different from those familiar to the health educator, and this needs to be acknowledged, honored, and respected. The impact of the steadily increasing diversity in the United States means that the diabetes care and education specialist must learn to manage differences in communication styles, attitudes, expectations, beliefs, and world views. The diabetes care and education specialist must use different approaches to remove barriers created by racial, ethnic, cultural, and linguistic differences. A large body of research underscores the existence of disparities in healthcare. The literature shows that in the United States, racial and ethnic minorities are less likely to receive routine medical procedures and more likely to experience a lower quality of health services compared with their counterparts in the white population.[13] In addition, the Office of Minority Health and Health Disparities has identified other vulnerable populations, including those defined by socioeconomic status, geography, gender, age, and disability.[14] The diabetes care and education specialist should expand his or her view of vulnerable populations as these also include people with physical and emotional disabilities as well as people from the lesbian, gay, bisexual, transgender, queer (LGBTQ) community.[15,16,17] Addressing health disparities is a core goal of the National Diabetes Education Program (NDEP).[18] In response to this need, the NDEP and its minority work groups have developed and adapted materials to reach audiences at highest risk for developing diabetes and with the highest prevalence of the disease. These materials address cultural issues like food choices and health literacy needs and can be accessed from the NDEP.[18] See Table 2.2 for more on the levels of cultural competence and how a diabetes care and education specialist can further develop those competencies.

Knowledge Builder: Health Disparities Linked to Ethnicity and Socioeconomic Factors

One example of health disparities tied to ethnicity is an analysis of a population in a large Federally Qualified Health Center in New York State.[19] In this population, a higher proportion of non-Hispanic blacks and Hispanic/Latinos had an A1C greater than 9% than non-Hispanic whites. Even engagement with DSME is associated with certain sociodemographic factors.[20] The authors analyzed data from the 2011–2013 Behavioral Risk Factor Surveillance System and discovered that non-Hispanic blacks were more likely than Hispanics to engage in DSME, females were more likely than males, older (greater than 66 years) more likely than younger (18–54 years), those with health insurance more likely than those without, and those with higher education and income. More recently, the goals for Healthy People 2020 address the known disparities across minority populations.[21]

TABLE 2.2 Cultural Competence in the Delivery of Healthcare Services: Foundation of the Practice Model

Competency	*Strategies to Promote the Competency*
Cultural awareness	Recognize personal prejudices and biases toward other cultures Understand personal cultural/ethnic background
Cultural humility	Commit to ongoing self-evaluation and self-critique Be willing to address power imbalances in person with diabetes-provider relationship Develop mutually beneficial partnerships with communities/organizations on behalf of defined populations
Cultural knowledge	Develop an education foundation that incorporates various world views of different cultures Identify and integrate knowledge regarding biological variations, disease and health conditions, and variations in drug metabolism
Cultural skill	Collect culturally relevant data regarding the individual's presenting problem and health history Conduct culturally based physical assessments in a culturally sensitive manner
Cultural desire	Commit to engage in the process of cultural competence Demonstrate compassion, authenticity, humility, openness, availability, and flexibility Provide care, regardless of conflict

Source: Adapted from L Pesta, CA Tucker, "The Teaching Learning Experience From a Generational Perspective," in MF Bradshaw, BL Hulquist, eds, *Innovative teaching strategies in nursing and related health professions* (7th ed) (Burlington, MA: Jones & Bartlett Learning) 39–58. http://samples.jbpub.com/9781284107074/9781284107074_CH03_039_058.pdf

A culturally sensitive and informed healthcare professional understands and addresses the cultural beliefs and myths that may influence the person with diabetes' ability and willingness to follow directions, ask questions, or seek additional information. When the diabetes care and education specialist understands the cultural factors and beliefs that can contribute to these differences, a tailored assessment is possible, a plan that reflects the needs of the individual can be developed, and effective interventions can be designed.

Language and Diabetes

Building trust also means appreciating the impact language can have on creating a collaborative relationship.

In completing a self assessment, consider the following questions: What words do I use to describe a person with diabetes? Do I find myself saying "diabetic," "compliant," "should," "must," "can't," or "don't"? Do I use such phrases as "I want you to" or "You need to"? Words are powerful and meaningful and very personal to the person with diabetes. Words can hurt and reinforce stigma. Dickinson and others [22,23] advocate for diabetes care and education specialists and all members of the diabetes team to use a "respectful, inclusive, and person-centered approach" to diabetes care and support. This is best accomplished when language is "person-first, strengths-based, [and] empowering."[22] For example, "compliance" and "adherence" should be replaced with "involvement" or "participation in medication taking." "Control" should be replaced with "manage." Finally, "diabetic" should never be used as a noun.

Setting the Tone for the Assessment

When starting an effective assessment, the diabetes care and education specialist examines the expectations of the person with diabetes for the visit. In the initial meeting, the diabetes care and education specialist builds trust and rapport with the person while creating an environment in which people feel comfortable talking about their needs, motivations, goals, problems, and feelings. One strategy for building rapport is to get to know the person by asking about his or her daily life and family, and what is most important in life. This builds a holistic assessment and demonstrates the diabetes care and education specialist's interest in both the person's diabetes and the nonmedical aspects of the person's life. Such an approach can also yield information about the person's affect and may uncover signs of emotional distress or depression. The diabetes care and education specialist uses a range of assessment strategies and interviewing skills to develop an understanding of clients and their specific problems.

The following list of steps provides an example of an effective opening:

1. Provide brief orientation. Introduce yourself and explain your role.
2. Share the objectives. Ask the person with diabetes what his or her goals are for the meeting. Share with the person with diabetes what you hope will happen in your time together.
3. Explain rationale. Help the person with diabetes understand why you are collecting this information and how his or her sharing will be of benefit.
4. Assess receptivity. Ask the person with diabetes for permission to move on with the assessment. Listen to the person with diabetes and observe the response. Does the person with diabetes find this acceptable, or does he or she express reluctance, dissatisfaction, or discomfort? Listen to what the person with diabetes says and observe nonverbal behaviors. Is the person with diabetes ready to engage in the assessment, or are more discussion and negotiation necessary?

Despite the fact that, ideally, an assessment is completed before an education plan is developed, the diabetes care and education specialist may encounter a person with diabetes for the first time in a group (class) environment with no prior information available from medical records or a referral form. A basic needs assessment of all persons with diabetes can be conducted efficiently by having each person with diabetes complete a short, written assessment tool and answer questions during group introductions. In addition to asking persons with diabetes to share some basic diabetes information, such as duration of diabetes, type of diabetes medication being taken, current A1C, target goal, and previous diabetes education, the diabetes care and education specialist might also ask, "What one question do you hope to have answered in this next hour?"

In a group setting it is important to respect each individual's privacy and invite people to participate at the level they feel most comfortable. It is also imperative to offer individual time if the person needs to share sensitive information.

When conducting a brief group assessment, the diabetes care and education specialist must also focus on anything that may be a risk for the class. Pay close attention to physical signs and symptoms that a person may be exhibiting. For instance, watch for signs of hypoglycemia.

In Practice: Tips for a Quick Assessment

Diabetes care and education specialists often are faced with groups of people, late arrivals, and tight time schedules. Assessing health literacy can easily fall away in the list of priorities. Following are a few key points on how to conduct a quick assessment of health literacy and safety:

1. Create an environment which recognizes health literacy challenges.[24] The following are key questions:
   - How often do you need to have someone help you when you read instructions, pamphlets, or other written material from your doctor or pharmacist?
   - What do you find most difficult in filling out medical forms by yourself?
   - Reading and understanding health information can be difficult. Has that been your experience?
2. Ask the person how he or she prefers to learn new information.
3. Ask about what he or she would like to learn: What part of living with diabetes is most difficult?

4. Ask about his or her feelings about having diabetes: How does (the situation described in the previous question) make you feel?
5. Ask about changes he or she has already tried and past experiences: How would this situation have to change for you to feel better about it?
6. Ask about support: Who in your family do you turn to for support with your diabetes? Which friend helps support you with your diabetes?

In summary, the diabetes care and education specialist is able to answer the following inquiries:

- Attitude: Do you understand enough about the person's needs and beliefs?
- Health: Do you have enough information about the person's physical and medical needs? What are the current medications and laboratory values?
- Psychosocial: Who supports the person with diabetes? What emotional needs does the person have? What cultural differences should be respected?
- Knowledge: Is the person ready to learn? What will support knowledge gain and behavioral change? What are the barriers to knowledge gain and behavioral change?

Due to time constraints related to group classes, have the person with diabetes complete a self-assessment prior to the initial face-to-face encounter. This may be done on paper or electronically. If there are literacy issues or if Internet access is not available, other arrangements can be made for completion. This self-assessment, combined with a short face-to-face assessment, assists the diabetes care and education specialist in understanding a person's individual needs.

Characteristics of Effective Assessments

Effective assessments give the diabetes care and education specialist the information needed to create an individualized approach to education and support. Effective assessments must be merged with critical thinking, clinical reasoning, and professional experience to best address the needs of a PWD. The following are characteristics of effective assessments:

- They reveal lifestyle issues and factors.
- They are person-centered, elicit sufficient participation, and promote honest self-disclosure.
- They involve family members and caregivers when appropriate.
- They identify the needs of those in special populations, searching for factors that interfere with an individual's activities of daily living.
- They respectfully honor cultural differences to garner cooperation, information, and trust.
- They identify pertinent social determinants of health.
- They uncover high-priority problems to be solved.

These characteristics are discussed more fully below.

Lifestyle Issues

Effective assessments address lifestyle as well as diabetes-specific content. Most diabetes care and education specialists are aware of and very knowledgeable about the diabetes-specific elements of an assessment. However, it is important that diabetes care and education specialists employ strategies to learn about both the diabetes- and the lifestyle-related components of assessments. The following is a quick summary of some lifestyle-related aspects to be addressed with sample questions:

- Current behaviors in terms of nutrition, exercise, medication, and monitoring. What is the most challenging aspect of diabetes self-care for you?
- Current desired health outcomes and goals. How do you envision your health in the next 5 years?
- Resources and barriers to achieving health outcomes. What seems to get in the way of your achieving your health goals?
- Psychosocial and cultural contexts. How does your culture view people with diabetes or chronic diseases? What is the most important thing you would like for me to know about your cultural, religious, or spiritual beliefs?
- Attitudes or health beliefs. What was it like to find out you have diabetes? How did you get diabetes? What are one or two things you want more of in your life?
- Knowledge, past experiences, stress, emotions, and values. How have you dealt with stress or emotional problems in the past?
- Psychomotor skills. What physical limitations do you have?

Skill Builder: Appreciative Coaching

Appreciative inquiry or appreciative coaching[25] approaches assessment with an attitude of curiosity. If you are truly curious, you behave less like an expert and more like a trusted facilitator or coach. Kimsey-House et al[26] said it well: "Asking questions for data will yield analysis, reasons, rationale, explanation. Asking questions out of curiosity will yield deeper—often more authentic—information about feelings and motivation."

Consider the different levels of responses from these questions:

- Why did you regain the weight? (asking for explanation)
- I am wondering what made it difficult to keep the weight off? (asking out of curiosity)

Family and Caregivers

Involving the family or caregiver of the person with diabetes can create both challenges and opportunities for self-management. In general, directing questions to the person with diabetes is best. Family members may agree or disagree with, elaborate on, or interrupt the responses of the person with diabetes or take over answering all the questions. Every one of these actions provides insight into family dynamics or cultural standards. It is important to understand the Individual's role in the family. This will often dictate who will participate with the PWD during an interview. One approach is for the diabetes care and education specialist to explain the purpose of the interview and the importance of hearing from each family member, including the PWD. What is important is reassuring each party that his or her input is valued.

Special Populations

Just as the education plan is individualized, the assessment takes into consideration unique or special needs. Assessment of a teenager, for instance, might include the HEEADSSS[27] list of questions, which focuses on the home environment, eating, education, activities, drugs, sexuality, suicide/depression, social media, and safety. For older adults and the elderly, the SPICES list of questions would be appropriate.[28] This tool focuses on sleep, problems with eating, incontinence, confusion, evidence of falls, and skin breakdown. Assessment should address the special challenges often faced by members of a particular population or cultural group. For example, assessing religious practices with a Muslim or Jewish individual will increase the diabetes care and education specialist's understanding of the impact of fasting or food preferences on diabetes management or blood glucose levels. When assessing a person from the LGBTQ community the diabetes care and education specialist should avoid assumptions and stereotyping.[29] Instead, listen carefully for the terms the person uses to describe himself or herself.[30] In addition, show respect for roles and how the individual defines family.

Practice Setting

Gear assessments to the demands of the practice setting and the individual's previous history in that setting:

- Initial inpatient: Assessments conducted on inpatient units for immediate "survival" skills training and/or discharge planning focus on those elements germane to the immediate safety needs for a successful transition to home.
- Repeat hospitalization: A person repeatedly hospitalized for diabetic ketoacidosis (DKA), on the other hand, will require a more specific, targeted assessment focused on the causes of DKA and barriers to care.
- Outpatient: Assessments conducted in outpatient clinics with a high probability of continuous follow-up visits may be more comprehensive and may be conducted in segments over time.
- Consultant: Assessments conducted by consultants who refer persons with diabetes back to other professionals in "shared care" arrangements may focus on previously negotiated goals and management approaches.

Structure the nature and depth of the assessment to both the person's needs and the boundaries and limitations imposed by the practice setting.

Activities of Daily Living

It is important to determine the individual's ability to safely and correctly perform self-care skills. Many persons with diabetes tell their diabetes care and education specialist that maintaining their independence is very important and is the reason that making behavior changes is something they want to do. On the other hand, the diabetes care and education specialist may need to ask about their ability to continue to live independently. Some questions to ask are:

- Do you require help in shopping or preparing your food, or with personal hygiene, medication, monitoring, or being active?
- Do you need assistance with transportation to medical appointments, social activities, or other important activities?
- Is assistance available from family, friends, colleagues, community, or social groups?
- Do you have daily living skills, such as cooking and doing laundry?

The diabetes care and education specialist should also make the following assessments:

- Is the person so anxious, disoriented, or depressed by the diagnosis of diabetes or the onset of a new complication that learning a new skill would be extremely difficult? If so, more time may be needed for learning or teaching diabetes skills.

- Does the person have adequate cognitive ability to learn new skills?
- Has the individual experienced short-term memory loss? If so, does he or she have adequate memory to learn new ways of performing reliable and safe diabetes self-care?

Cultural Considerations

Studies[31] confirm that culture influences the effectiveness of healthcare. Diabetes care and education specialists are encouraged to become familiar with the health-related cultural influences of the populations they serve. Culture is that constellation of values and beliefs, traditions and mores which define a group. Taking the broad view of culture, then, the diabetes care and education specialist may view even generations as having cultural differences. For instance, a baby boomer may have a very different learning style and preferences than a millennial.

For some ethnic cultures, the diabetes care and education specialist may want to consider incorporating community or lay health workers, also known as *promotoras*, as part of the assessment visit. Lay health workers are generally trusted and respected members of the community who act as a link between the healthcare system and the community.[32]

Effective diabetes care and education specialists also consider the culture of generations. The impact of diabetes spans generations, from the traditionalists to the baby boomers to generations X, Y, and Z. Just as in ethnic cultures, members of a generation share political and social influences, values, and characteristics. The impact of generation is addressed in detail later in this chapter.

Prioritizing Needs and Interventions

The assessment will likely reveal more than can possibly be covered in a single class or individual visit. The diabetes care and education specialist prioritizes the learning objectives into those that must be handled immediately for individual safety, such as hypoglycemia teaching or starting on insulin, and those that can wait. One technique to help engage a person during the assessment in setting priorities is to suggest a list of possible topic questions, recommend priorities, and negotiate on the teaching agenda.

Clinical judgment, knowledge of diabetes, and the experience of the person with diabetes will provide the framework for successfully identifying the most pressing needs. Several resources, including the following Skill Builder, can help the diabetes care and education specialist hone these clinical decision-making skills.[33,34]

Skill Builder: Applying Critical Thinking to Assessment of Person With Diabetes

Draw from your knowledge, experience, frame of reference, and intuition.

Listen to the person's story and consider a list of possible problems, making some reasoned assumptions to test out.

Gather data by asking powerful questions which promote insight.

Create an accurate representation of the problem.

Fill in information gaps by asking more questions and seeking more data.

Interpret the information and confirm with the individual what you believe or what you have heard.

Use evidence-based concepts, models, and theories to support or explain the data collected.

Develop conclusions and solutions.

Be open-minded and curious, applying a healthy skepticism as needed.

Later, learn from the experience through self-reflection.

Assessing Education Needs and Readiness to Change

While the education approach may be well matched to the person or population being served, if those on the receiving end are not ready to receive information or if the information is unimportant to them at the time, learning will likely be compromised.

Consider the following: An individual with type 2 diabetes has just been given a prescription for insulin. You are responsible for educating her. The information you have to share is important. Is the person agreeable, or is she angry and resistant to learning about insulin today? You are adamant that the information you have to share is important for the person to know and understand. However, the person you are trying to help may not agree with your assessment. You know that her history of glycemic stability has been suboptimal for years; however, she reports feeling "just fine." What are the chances that the information you have to offer her will be heard today? Will this onetime education session achieve your goals or meet the person's needs?

A key component of the assessment is determining not only the individual's education needs but also his or her willingness to learn and readiness to change. When the education method and message are not aligned with learner readiness, behavioral and educational goals will not be met.[35,36,37] Issues to consider when assessing educational needs and readiness to learn are summarized in Table 2.3.

TABLE 2.3 Assessing Education Needs and Readiness to Change

Assessment	*Issues to Consider*	*Probable Negative Impact if . . .*
Attitude, knowledge, psychomotor, and psychosocial background	• Attitude and health beliefs and feelings about diabetes: severity, susceptibility, costs, and benefits • Attitude toward participating in education program • Individual goals of treatment: A1C, blood pressure, weight, etc • Experience with diabetes to date • Presence of other confounding health conditions • Presence or absence of a support network	• Diabetes is viewed as unimportant, education is not desired, goals are different, diabetes is not a priority, prior negative experience with friend or family member, or support is lacking
Knowledge and practice of self-care or level of self-care	• Individual ability to perform complex tasks • Willingness to devote more time to management	• Individual not interested in being actively involved in self-management, attitude of "why bother"
Knowledge and preferred learning style	• Preferred method: read, listen, discuss • Usual method of acquiring new information: media, Internet, friends/family, etc • Preference for group vs. individual instruction	• Ability to learn depends on a method that is not available • Individual instruction is required but not available
Psychosocial status and level of stress	• Acute vs. chronic • Influence on ability to learn or make changes	• Stress is high enough to interfere with learning or prioritization of diabetes • Presence of depression may interfere with ability to learn
Psychosocial status and social, cultural, and religious preferences	• Influence on willingness to learn new behaviors • Potential conflict between treatment recommendations and cultural beliefs	• Education message or methods or treatment recommendations conflict with belief system
Health literacy	• Years of formal education • Learning style and ability to tolerate complexity • Directive teaching may be beneficial • Previous experience with diabetes education or diabetes care and educatio specialist	• Assumptions are made solely on years of education • Literacy level of education method and materials is not appropriate
Readiness for change	• Extent that need for change is recognized • Create conditions that stimulate desire to change or capitalize on readiness to change	• Expressed desire to change does not reflect willingness to change • Readiness for change is not aligned with education goals • Assumptions are made that the individual will never change

Source: Adapted from RM Anderson, "Applied Principles of Teaching and Learning," in MJ Franz, ed, *A Core Curriculum for Diabetes Education and Program Management,* 4th ed (Chicago: American Association of Diabetes Educators, 2001), 7-8.

Assessment Skills: Knowing What to Ask

A variety of strategies may be used to systematically gather information:[38–43]

- Direct questions
- Regimen or daily review
- Deviation review
- Specific examples
- Hypothetical situations
- Common obstacles

Direct Questions

Sometimes the best way to get information is to ask for it directly. Decide what information is needed and then formulate a question that will get at that information directly. Open-ended questions allow for general, descriptive answers, while closed-ended questions permit more focused, narrow answers.

Regimen or Daily Review

A regimen review asks individuals to summarize or describe what they typically do to take care of themselves. For example, "Please tell me what you do to care for your diabetes in the morning when you get up" or "Please walk me through a typical day, including what you do for your diabetes."

Deviation Review

When asking people to describe their typical routines, ask them also to describe times when they deviate from their routines. The diabetes care and education specialist benefits from knowing about both usual routines and exceptions to them. For example, "What happens on the weekend that is different from the weekday?"

Specific Examples

People often find it easier to provide details about a general problem or a behavior if asked to describe a specific example. Ask the person to recall a recent incident or day, and have them describe each episode in detail. For instance, "Please tell me about a time when you were able to follow your meal plan exactly" or "Tell me about a time when you successfully lost weight."

Hypothetical Situations

The diabetes care and education specialist can sometimes learn a great deal and have hypotheses confirmed or denied by posing a hypothetical situation. Hypothetical situations ask the person to consider what he or she would say, think, or do in a given situation. For example, the diabetes care and education specialist might ask the person to describe what he or she would do at a restaurant after suddenly realizing that insulin or blood glucose monitoring supplies were left at home. Hypothetical situations can provide a great deal of useful assessment information. The educator might pose what-if questions such as, "What if you accidentally left your meter in a hot car all day?"

Common Obstacles

Hypothesis testing offers diabetes care and education specialists opportunities to evaluate whether any common obstacles may be interfering with a person's self-care.[44–47] When the person's blood glucose level is not consistently in the target range, the diabetes care and education specialist might ask what could be contributing to this problem. Thoughtful diabetes care and education specialists will ask questions designed to reveal problems in areas such as these:

- Lack of knowledge or skill
- Competing priorities (lack of time)
- Treatment costs (money, social sacrifices)
- Habit patterns
- Family or social support
- Stress
- Unhelpful thoughts or beliefs
- Language-learning difficulties
- Other aspects

The obstacles to effective self care that are present or may arise often can be anticipated. When the diabetes care and education specialist sees potential trouble, assessing for its presence can minimize problems for the PWD. The assessment sets the stage for the diabetes care and education specialist and the PWD to develop both a plan for overcoming existing obstacles and plans for dealing with potential ones. The focus is on helping the person devise new and more effective ways of responding to situations that present self care obstacles. The person may be encouraged to practice or rehearse the plan to ensure success. For more on problem solving, see chapter 10.

Assessment Strategies

Give Time to Answer

Conducting an assessment can be difficult when the individuals is slow to respond or reticent. People have different response times, information processing rates, and social interaction styles. These factors vary widely from one culture to another. Trying to rush the discussion along may be perceived as disrespectful. Before moving on, be patient and provide enough time for the person to process and then answer the question.

Use Active Listening Skills

Most diabetes care and education specialists are aware of and employ one or more of 4 verbal and nonverbal behaviors generally referred to as active listening skills: clarifying, paraphrasing, reflecting feelings, and using minimal encouragers.

Clarifying Asking for clarification helps the diabetes care and education specialist ensure he or she understands what the PWD has said. The diabetes care and education specialist is checking the person's understanding of a particular word, phrase, or idea that has been used. For instance, "When you said you had 'high blood' did you mean blood sugar or blood pressure?"

Paraphrasing Paraphrasing tells the other person that he or she has been heard and understood. The diabetes care and education specialist restates what the person has said in slightly different words that have the same meaning. Paraphrasing responds to the factual or informational content of what the person is saying. Unlike clarification, paraphrasing does not involve asking a question. Instead, the diabetes care and education specialist confirms what was heard by restating it to the person. For example, "I think I heard you say that eating pizza really affects your blood glucose for hours after the meal."

Reflecting Feelings Reflecting feelings involves giving feedback to the PWD on the affective tone of what is being said. Thus, the emotion or feeling expressed in the person's verbal or nonverbal behavior is made explicit by reflecting feelings. Paraphrasing, in contrast, involves giving feedback on factual information. When a person is expressing an emotional reaction, reflecting this emotion back to the person is often helpful. Sometimes, people are not aware of their emotional reactions, so by reflecting feelings the diabetes care and education specialist is able to help them become more aware of how they appear to be reacting emotionally to a particular situation. Reflecting feelings can also be useful as a way for the diabetes care and education specialist to check whether he or she is accurately reading the person's feelings about a particular event or situation. Reflecting another's feelings might sound like, "You sound so sad when you describe what happened." Paraphrasing, on the other hand, sounds like, "What I hear you say is that checking your blood glucose is a hassle." Notice that both comments will encourage further dialogue, but reflecting feelings will foster further discussion at a deeper emotional level.

Using Minimal Encouragers Minimal encouragers are the verbal and nonverbal behaviors people use to signal to another person that they are listening and the person speaking should continue. The best way for educators to learn how well they use minimal encouragers is to watch one of their interviews on videotape. Examples of minimal encouragers include eye contact while listening, nodding the head, and saying short phrases like "yes," "continue," "uh-huh," and "ok."

One caveat: Avoid minimal encouragers if and when individuals engage in any kind of "jousting," such as blaming other healthcare professionals or family members for their poor management, for creating barriers to regimen participation, or for their complications. People may interpret minimal encouragers as agreement with their negative evaluations of others. In such cases, the diabetes care and education specialist must be especially attentive to listening carefully but studiously avoiding any appearance of agreeing. Otherwise, the educator may become an enabler or encourager of such behavior. The educator also may one day hear from colleagues or family members who were surprised to hear the diabetes care and education specialist had "accused" them of some wrongful behavior.

In conducting an individual or group assessment, a variety of practical strategies and skills can be used to gain a better understanding of a person with diabetes. A summary appears in Table 2.4.

Techniques for Closing the Assessment

Give Feedback At the end of an assessment, or when a portion of the assessment has been completed, the diabetes care and education specialist gives feedback to the PWD. Feedback involves not just a summary but an interpretation of what the diabetes care and education specialist learned in the assessment. Normalizing the person's problem and providing ideas that have been tried by others is a useful strategy. The person may find it reassuring to hear that he or she is not alone. As described in the Knowledge Builder, a careful assessment can help the diabetes care and education specialist understand how the individual is normalizing the experience of having diabetes.

TABLE 2.4 Effective Assessments at a Glance

Set the Tone • Decrease background sounds, especially for those who may have hearing or attention deficits • Avoid interruptions • Include family members and caregivers • When addressing an elderly adult, speak clearly and face-to-face • Avoid patronizing titles ("dear," "hon"); use formal salutations ("Ms. Jackson," "Dr. Jones") *Open and Close Effectively* Opening • Orientation • Objectives • Rationale • Receptivity Closing • Summary • Transitions *Build Trust and Encourage Honest Communication* Do: • Build trust • Encourage openness and honesty • Form a collaborative relationship, including caregivers as appropriate • Accept the person unconditionally • Express empathy • Be an active listener Don't: • Use fear or scare tactics • Be judgmental • Interrupt or hurry • Ignore feelings and emotion • Use jargon or unfamiliar terms • Underestimate people's desire and ability to learn • Appear distracted *Improve Skill in Information Gathering* • Use this checklist while reviewing videotaped assessments • Watch and emulate expert colleagues • Offer to teach these skills to others	*Ask Good Questions* • Pause and think • Be direct • Ask for specifics • Be persistent • Ask follow-up questions • Make mental notes • Ask for examples *Identify Sensory and Cognitive Deficits* Assess for: • Hearing deficits • Visual impairment • Literacy and language problems • Cognitive impairment *Know What Type of Questions to Ask* • Direct questioning: What do you want to know? • Regimen review: What do you usually do? • Deviation review: Tell me about exceptions or special circumstances. • Specific examples: Give me an example of when that happened. • Hypothetical situations: What would you do if . . . *Encourage Participation from the Individual* • Allow time to answer, recognizing individual and cultural differences • Use active listening skills • Summarize • Give feedback *Gather Information Using a Variety of Strategies* • Paper or online surveys • Physical and laboratory data • Self-monitoring (blood glucose, meal plan, activity) • Observe behavior (skills checks) • Solicit information from client, family, caregivers *Acknowledge Client's Feelings and Frustrations* • Listen to how it is said • Watch body language • Give feedback • Be sympathetic

Source: JA Pichert, DG Schlundt, "Assessment: Gathering Information and Facilitating Engagement," in C Mensing, ed, *The Art and Science of Diabetes Self-Management Education: A Desk Reference for Healthcare Professionals* (Chicago: American Association of Diabetes Educators, 2006), 592.

Knowledge Builder: Normalization and Chronic Disease

Due-Christensen and colleagues[48] discovered that as adults adapt to new onset type 1 diabetes, they progress through various stages. After the initial disruption in the physical and psychosocial elements of their lives, the adults began to construct their personal view of diabetes. Some recognized the seriousness of diabetes while others minimized it. Next, the adults set about restructuring their sense of self and how they now related to others. Finally, the adults were able to understand the boundaries imposed by the disease and to redirect needed resources. Planning and prioritizing the daily demands of diabetes led to a new normal for these individuals.

Diabetes care and education specialists can use the work of Due-Christensen et al to assess how their clients have normalized the experience of living with diabetes.

Summarize Summarizing is similar to paraphrasing in that the diabetes care and education specialist restates what the PWD has just said. A summary allows the diabetes care and education specialist to see whether he or she has accurately learned the gist of what the person has been talking about. A summary gives the person an opportunity to correct the diabetes care and education specialist's perception or to add information that has been omitted and also serves to create a smooth transition between topics. A large component of critical thinking involves interpreting the data and confirming with the PWD what was discussed. Using a summary can help the diabetes care and education specialist be ready for goal setting.

Summary for Assessment

To complete a comprehensive diabetes education assessment efficiently, the diabetes care and education specialist utilizes his or her well-developed interviewing skills and critical thinking skills. The diabetes care and education specialist also draws from a solid foundational knowledge of population health, social determinants of health, cultural competence, and appreciative questioning. Once the assessment is completed, the diabetes care and education specialist synthesizes the information and develops a sense of which topics and behavior targets need focus, while always remembering that DSME is person-driven and that the goals and plan are developed in cooperation with the individual with diabetes. The next step in the DSME process is goal setting.

Goal Setting

Goal setting is a critical component in successful DSME.[4] The process of developing goals is based on assessment and collaboration among the person with diabetes, the healthcare provider, other team members, and the person's support system. Goals can later serve as a method to evaluate progress.

Goals are defined in measurable terms stated in behavioral objectives.[3] These goals are monitored and measured throughout the DSME process. As defined by ADCES, the diabetes care and education specialist works with the person with or at risk for diabetes to identify person-centric DSME outcomes.[3] The goals reflect information obtained through the assessment process and also serve as a tool to evaluate progress toward individual, program, institutional, or community-level goals. The diabetes care and education specialist coordinates the delivery of the education with fellow healthcare team members to facilitate and support the person's goals.

Competencies for Diabetes Care and Education Specialists includes criteria to be considered in goal setting, and this step in the process includes the following:[8]

- Write desired goals in measurable terms.
- Define specific behavioral objectives and actions.
- Collaborate on goals that are consistent with diabetes practice guidelines and honor the role of the PWD.
- Incorporate consideration of risks and benefits of the proposed outcomes.
- Consider the resources available to increase the likelihood that the agreed upon behavior change will be adopted.
- Work together on goals that are tailored and appropriate to a person's state of health.
- Redefine goals as needed to meet the needs of the person.

In addition to the ADCES Scope of Practice (addressed later in this chapter), the National Standards for Diabetes Self-Management Education and Support include two directions for goal setting.[4] Standard 7 states that the assessment and education plan will be developed collaboratively by the participant and the instructor(s) to direct the selection of appropriate education interventions and self-management support strategies. This assessment and education plan and the intervention outcomes will be documented in the education record.[4] One of the indicators for meeting this standard is showing evidence of ongoing education planning and behavioral goal setting based on the assessed and/or reassessed needs of the person.

This standard reflects on the person's selected behavioral objective and measurable learning objectives. The objectives are mutually determined, but most important is that the person is involved in the process of the development and final selection of his or her goals.

Standard 9 states that the provider(s) of DSME and DSMS will assess each participant's personal self-management goals and progress toward those goals.[4]

This standard addresses the individual achievement of goals while Standard 10 addresses the program assessment of targeted goal achievement for the population served and actual goal achievement. This information can be used to reflect on the effectiveness of the program. For more on program management, see chapter 11.

Goal-Setting Theory

Goals have the power to both motivate and to discourage. It is the delicate balance of specificity and difficulty which sets successful goals apart.[49] For instance, a goal which is specific and moderately challenging is best for many people. Losing 10 pounds in a month may be too difficult and unrealistic. However, planning to walk 1 mile 4 days a week may be just the level of difficulty or challenge to motivate. In helping people set goals, diabetes care and education specialists should consider whether the goal is relevant to the needed behavior change, how much effort and persistence the goal will require, and specific strategies to achieve the desired outcome.

Goal-setting theory also reminds diabetes care and education specialists to consider ability, commitment, feedback, resources, and complexity.[49] To be successful, people with diabetes must have the requisite knowledge, skill, and resources to implement the behavioral actions. If the goal is to check blood glucose 2 times per day, the person must have access to the meter and strips, must know how to use the equipment, and must understand when to check. Commitment is important and can often be measured with questions such as "How important is it for you to do this?" Finally, successful goal achievement is often linked to feedback along the way. Diabetes care and education specialists have a key role as coach and cheerleader as individuals embark on goal setting for behavior change.

Goal-Setting Considerations

A person's goals are tailored to his or her attitude, knowledge, and behavioral skills. It is important to recognize where the person is in the learning process and the individualized needs for safety of persons with diabetes. For example, a person new to the disease may require basic information and "survival skills."

When working with the individual to develop goals, diabetes care and education specialists can do the following:

- Recognize that the goal belongs to the person, not to the diabetes care and education specialist.
- Identify options for achieving a goal, including the desired overall outcome(s).
- Choose the best agreed-upon option to start. Include a person's needs, skills, and learning preferences.
- Demonstrate respect for cultural, lifestyle, and health beliefs.
- Develop specific implementation of goals addressing strengths and barriers.
- Determine a person's commitment to his or her goals.
- Recognize goal setting as a lifelong process that evolves with changing needs, desires, and abilities of the person living with a chronic illness.
- Goal setting is iterative and dynamic. Expect goals to be refined, expanded, or even discarded as individuals form new behaviors, gain new knowledge, and set new priorities.

During the assessment process, it is common for a diabetes care and education specialist to discover that the person with diabetes has several needs. Where to begin in setting goals can be daunting. A simple approach is to ask the person, "Is there anything you would like to do this week to improve your health?" This encourages the individual to share a voice in the experience of goal setting and helps to boost interest and commitment.

Collaborating on Educational Goals

An important component in the process of program evaluation of outcomes is understanding the person's point of view, expectations, and desired outcomes as well as those of the referring provider. The educator may find that these don't always match. In addition, during the assessment a diabetes care and education specialist may discover additional behavioral and learning needs that should be included in the goals. A skilled diabetes care and education specialist will explore a variety of options for the person to select and to accomplish in a specific period of time.

Use the AADE7 Self-Care Behaviors® as a Guiding Tool to Goal Setting

The desired outcomes must be clearly defined and mutually agreed upon. Ideally, the diabetes care and education specialist has sufficient information from the person with diabetes, the family and others in the case of a child, and the referring provider. The AADE7 Self-Care Behaviors® provide a comprehensive framework for formulating goals. Because behavior change is a unique outcome measure for DSMES, the outcomes may focus on knowledge, behavior, or clinical results. Goals should be quantifiable so that behavior change can be measured and documented.

Obtain Buy-In

Goal setting is a collaborative activity which is built on rapport and trust. A large part of the initial visit and assessment is to establish a rapport with the person while setting up an agenda to include goals and follow-up plans. Essential to goal development is helping the person explore his or her commitment.[50,51] Asking a person to tell his or her story and share his or her perspective about diabetes helps the diabetes care and education specialist understand the individual's experience and get to the core of what that person with diabetes needs in terms of knowledge, skills, and a deeper understanding of his or her disease.

Understand and Respect Each Person With Diabetes as an Individual

Each person comes for DSMES with a unique set of experiences. The diabetes care and education specialist uses the person's initial information to further determine his or her level of conviction and confidence in goal setting. A person's conviction is his or her belief in how important it is to make a change. A conversation about the person's strengths and barriers can help the diabetes care and education specialist assess readiness to learn. A person's confidence is his or her belief in an ability to be successful and to overcome obstacles, and that sense of confidence is intimately linked to self-esteem, knowledge, and past experiences. For the diabetes care and education specialist, understanding a person's conviction and confidence offers a measure of the potential for successful behavior change and is a key factor in establishing appropriate, realistic behavior goals. A person's goals reflect his or her needs, skills, learning style, and preferences. The goals also respect a person's cultural, lifestyle, and health beliefs.

Keep the Client's Agenda in Mind

Diabetes care and education specialists often feel that they know what their clients need to do to improve their health, but working under this assumption is often counterproductive. It is not uncommon for diabetes care and education specialists to suggest that a person try something, only to receive a "Yes, but . . ." from the individual. This is what is called a "premature focus trap."[52] To be effective, goals need to be owned by the individual and supported by the diabetes care and education specialist.

Individualize the Goals

A key to successful goal setting is effective questioning. For example, if a person's goal is weight loss, some questions on past experiences with weight loss can be beneficial: What were the individual's most successful attempts and what were some barriers? What needs to be different this time to be successful? A simple tool used in motivational interviewing is the acronym DARN.[52]

> **D**esire: "What do you want, or like, or wish, hope, etc?"
> **A**bility: "What is possible?" or "What can or could you do?"
> **R**easons: "Why would you make this change?" or "What are the benefits and risks?"
> **N**eed: "How important is this change?" "How much do you need to do this?"

The more details generated by the person with diabetes, the more likely the chance for success. This helps not only the PWD but also the diabetes care and education specialist see difficulties or barriers with achieving the goal. For example, if a person's goal is meal planning, there may need to be a discussion around certain meals or snacks. It may turn out that the real issue is nighttime snacking, which narrows the goal and action plan.

Take a Step-by-Step Approach

The person should identify the first step in reaching his or her goal. The PWD may have a broad overall goal of reducing his or her A1C and a smaller goal to begin walking several times a week. The role of the diabetes care and education specialist is to help the person generate strategies for success. For example, in terms of the walking goal, there may need to be a discussion about when, where, and how long the person will walk. Sharing information such as "Studies show that people who exercise in the morning tend to stay with their program longer" can be very useful. Encouraging the person to keep a record of his or her walking to demonstrate success is another strategy to share for achievement of a goal.

Focus on the Behavior, Not on the Outcome

People are more likely to achieve improved outcomes such as lowering A1C or losing weight by focusing on incremental behavior changes. A behavior change is something a person can do that will influence the broader identified outcome.

Have a Written Agreement

Writing down a person's ideas for short-term goals and making an agreement to try new behaviors in the next week can prove effective. Both the diabetes care and education specialist and the PWD have a clear understanding of the plan. Publicly committing to a change plan is powerful and effective in initiating change.[1]

A well-written agreement is goal-specific, measurable, achievable, and timely. Between the diabetes care and education specialist and the PWD there may even be a discussion of a reward at the end of a specific time frame. Rewards don't have to involve money; a reward could be the person having time to pursue a hobby or a family member cooking dinner.

Involve Family Members and Friends

Diabetes may affect the lives of everyone who loves, lives with, or cares about the person with this disease. Family and friends can support the PWD in a number of ways. The diabetes care and education specialist may find it useful to learn more about the person's support system as goal setting is discussed. Perhaps a family member could volunteer to cook one meal a week and give the PWD the night off from that responsibility. Ideas for rewards and psychological support should be encouraged during the goal-setting process.

Keep Cultural Considerations in Mind

The diabetes care and education specialist must have a working understanding of the person's cultural preferences and practices. The diabetes care and education specialist should be open and curious to learn more. A community health worker may be a valuable resource in helping to understand cultural preferences when selecting attainable goals. Other diabetes care and education specialists who work with ethnically diverse people may also be a source of information and support. With social media outlets such as ADCES's membership network, access to diabetes care and education specialist colleagues is increasingly available.

A Word About Children

In the case of children, their readiness to learn can change considerably with age and maturation. Goals should be of short duration with frequent check points, rewards, and adjustments as needed. Included in the goal-setting process with children are other significant people in a child's life, such as parents, siblings, grandparents, extended family members, and teachers. A child's support system is usually much broader than that of an adult, and these other people must be included in the goal-setting process. The diabetes care and education specialist must also take into consideration age-specific behavioral and learning objectives.

Strategies for Developing Goals

Behavior-change counseling may be used to elicit participation in goal setting. By supporting the person's motivation, the diabetes care and education specialist is also helping the PWD make progress in identifying personal goals. During goal setting, the diabetes care and education specialist should continue to spend time building rapport.[53] Strategies include the following:

- Begin with open-ended questions: "So you would like to . . ."
- Reassure PWD of confidentiality: "This is just between us, talking out loud to try to come up with a plan."
- Show interest in what the person has to say: "I am happy to hear that you . . ."
- Be accepting and nonjudgmental: "You have really given this some thought."
- Be very slow to interrupt. Listen; try to allow time for a quiet pause for the person to think a little bit more and process information. Simply counting slowly (and silently) to 5 will show the diabetes care and education specialist's patience and encourage the PWD to be the one to break the awkward silence.
- Continue to explore what is most important for the person and what is most reasonable to work on.

Trust and Rapport

Ideally, an environment has been created during the assessment process that supports honest self-disclosure. Just as in the assessment process, honest self-disclosure of personal goals occurs only when people trust each other. The diabetes care and education specialist's task is to maintain an atmosphere of trust and nonjudgmental acceptance. This means listening, reflecting back what the person says, and asking for clarification, as described in the previous section.

Assess the Person's Skills at Planning Goals

The diabetes care and education specialist uses 4 critical skills to determine the abilities of the PWD for goal setting:[42]

1. **Interpret information gathering.** The diabetes care and education specialist uses data obtained from individuals during the assessment phase, including their attitude, knowledge, and skills related to their abilities, to assist with goal setting.
2. **Facilitating engagement.** These are skills the diabetes care and education specialist uses to create a

safe, trusting atmosphere in which the individual feels comfortable divulging details about personal health, self-management, and possible lifestyle changes. These skills include the following:

— Listening skills

— Empathy

— Making conversation easy and enjoyable

— Awareness of his or her own nonverbal behaviors that can discourage conversation and brainstorming (eg, crossing arms, pushing chair away from the person, and repeatedly checking the time)

3. **Hypothesis testing.** The process of identifying and understanding a person's ideas about problem solving is best accomplished via hypothesis testing. Effective and efficient interviewers develop hypotheses—educated guesses—about problems that are specific to a particular person. The diabetes care and education specialist asks questions designed to elicit information that will eliminate some hypotheses and confirm others. Using a hypothesis testing approach, the diabetes care and education specialist zeros in on a problem and develops an understanding of the issues in a relatively short period of time.
4. **Problem analysis.** Problem analysis refers to developing an understanding of the "whats and whys" of a person's medical and self-management problems. Understanding the kinds of problems typically faced and the most common obstacles to behavior change helps the diabetes care and education specialist develop reasonable hypotheses. These can then be tested by asking pertinent questions, analyzing the answers, and thereby increasing the understanding of the issues for subsequent problem solving. Each item addresses a specific event or behavior and employs multiple-choice responses, so the alternatives cover the range of possible responses.

Observe Behavior

Sometimes the diabetes care and education specialist has questions about a person's skills and abilities to do certain things. Observing the person performing the skill is often preferable to asking about self-perceived capabilities. For example, to assess someone's skill in using a particular blood glucose meter, give the person the meter and ask him or her to perform a blood glucose check. Use role-playing techniques, too. For example, give the person a restaurant menu and say, "Pretend I am a waiter at the restaurant and you are a customer. Order a meal that fits the meal plan you have chosen to follow."

In Practice Tip: Using Past Experiences With Self-Monitoring to Assist in Goal Setting

Self-monitoring involves asking people to keep a diary or record of a specific behavior. For example, the person can be asked to self-monitor (ie, count) the number of cigarettes smoked each day. A diary's purpose is threefold:

1. It provides the person with immediate feedback on his or her success at meeting the treatment goal.
2. It provides the healthcare professional with an ongoing record of behavior that can be used to identify specific problems.
3. It can promote self awareness, mindfulness, and behavior change.

Be sure to discuss the purpose of the self-monitoring activity with the person, as well as the specifics on how to report on the activity:

- Rationale: Give a clear rationale for keeping records. Explain how the data will be used and why a diary will be helpful. People who understand the importance of keeping good records are more likely to do so.
- Willingness: Make sure the person is willing to keep a diary.
- Report: The person and diabetes care and education specialist should be determining where to keep the record and when to complete it.
- Simplicity: Make the record-keeping task as simple as possible. For some people, using a smartphone app may be the best approach. Numerous apps are available that support diabetes behaviors.[54] For others, a handwritten log may be the best choice.
- Understanding: Ask the person to reiterate the plan. For example: "Tell me in your own words what you are going to record." Diabetes care and education specialists may assume the person understands; in fact, they are often surprised that how they interpreted the plan was viewed differently by the PWD.
- Receipt: Make a note in the medical record to ask for the diary at the next meeting. When the person shares a completed diary, recognize the effort and appreciate the collaboration. The data collected should inform next steps in the goal setting and action. Use the collected information in the teaching/counseling session. Help the person feel the effort was worthwhile.

Collaboratively Establishing Goals

In collaboration with each person with diabetes, the diabetes care and education specialist establishes and documents specific goals and objectives. The aim is to set goals and write specific behavioral objectives that are important to the individual and that the individual feels confident about achieving. It is important that the diabetes care and education specialist and the PWD are clear on what is meant by a goal, as well as the distinctions between a learning objective and a behavioral objective.

- Goal: This serves as a big-picture, directional guide; it is the focal point for the objectives and the end result of meeting the objectives.
- Learning objective: This is the knowledge or skills objective the individual with diabetes plans to meet at the end of the educational intervention. Examples of learning objectives are the following:
    - "Identify 3 foods with carbohydrate"
    - "Discuss sick-day treatment guidelines"
- Behavioral objective: Also referred to as "a behavioral goal," this is a planned, measurable change in behavior that is likely to achieve a positive health outcome over a period of time once the initial intervention is completed. Examples of behavioral objectives are the following:
    - "Eat 3 or 4 carbohydrate choices per meal"
    - "Monitor blood glucose 4 times per day before meals"

Both learning objectives and behavioral objectives are written as measurable, observable statements so the participant and the diabetes care and education specialist can clearly determine whether objectives have been met.[55] Table 2.5 gives examples of each type of objective. Table 2.6 is an aid, based on Bloom's Taxonomy, for writing both types of objectives.[55]

Since learning cannot be witnessed directly, objectives provide a basis for making the best possible inferences about whether learning has occurred. Objectives clarify the purposes and intent of instruction, and they enable the person with diabetes to know what the plan is, which helps improve communications.

Behavioral Objectives: Characteristics

A behavioral objective should have the characteristics described below.

A simple acronym to guide diabetes care and education specialists in assessing the completeness of their objectives is to determine whether they are SMART: specific, measurable, achievable, realistic, and time-bound (ie, stated in terms of a specific time when the behavior will happen).

TABLE 2.5 Differentiating Between Learning and Behavioral Objectives

Sample Learning Objectives
• Identify carbohydrate foods • List 4 treatments for hypoglycemia • Discuss differences between saturated and unsaturated fats
Sample Behavioral Objectives
• Record food intake and activity in a logbook 4 days per week for 1 month • Eat 4 carbohydrate servings at lunch and dinner and 1 carbohydrate snack for 2 weeks • Drink noncaloric beverages instead of sweetened ones until follow-up class

Source: JVC Hill, "Writing behavioral objectives: tips from an educator and auditor," *On the Cutting Edge* [DCE newsletter] 26, no. 2 (2005): 25-9.

SMART goal setting is defined as:

- Specific: What, why, and how? Encourage the person to be specific and identify details.
- Measurable: If the goal can't be measured, it can't be managed. Accurate tracking and the ability to identify progress are necessary components of goal achievement.
- Achievable: Help the individual identify what is important to him or her. The goal requires commitment and should stretch the person slightly, but it should not be too far out of reach. Success in goal achievement will help develop confidence and self-efficacy.
- Realistic: This doesn't mean easy, just doable. The diabetes care and education specialist can help the PWD evaluate how realistic the chosen goal is in the given situation. Work with the person to identify what he or she is or is not willing (or able) to do to meet the goal.
- Time-bound: Collaborate on a time frame for the goal. This gives a clear target to work toward. Setting very short-term goals such as "for the next week" allows for more immediate feedback.

Common Mistakes The following 3 examples represent behavioral objectives that are not SMART goals:

- "I will eat healthier foods."
    - *Explanation:* This is not a specific objective. What is a "healthier food"? Guide the person in making this more specific and measurable by asking, "What would this look

TABLE 2.6 Guide for Writing Learning and Behavioral Objectives

Sample Verbs	*Learning Objective*	*Behavioral Objective*
1. REMEMBERING Learner recalls or recognizes information, ideas, and principles in the approximate form in which they were learned.		
List Identify Record Recall	List 3 treatments of hypoglycemia.	Record how I treat hypoglycemia in my log for the next 2 weeks.
2. UNDERSTANDING Learner translates, comprehends, or interprets information based on prior learning.		
Describe Summarize Explain Compare	Describe steps in the 15–15 rule in hypoglycemia treatment.	Describe treatment of hypoglycemia to my husband and coworker within the next week.
3. APPLYING Learner selects, transfers, and uses data and principles to complete a problem or task with a minimum of direction.		
Demonstrate Choose Implement Complete	Choose food models of 15-g carbohydrate portion sizes.	Choose foods that match meal plan during the next month and discuss with registered dietitian at follow-up class.
4. ANALYZING Learner breaks material or ideas apart, determines how the parts relate to each other by organizing the material.		
Analyze Determine Summarize Organize	Determine carbohydrate foods that have a higher glycemic index based on case example information.	Analyze effect of different carbohydrate foods on blood glucose by keeping records for 1 month.
5. EVALUATING Learner originates, integrates, and combines ideas or parts into a whole idea, product, plan, or proposal that is new to him or her.		
Evaluate Order Prepare Critique	Evaluate a sample meal considering carbohydrate allowance and principles of healthy eating.	Prepare a set of sample menus for 1 week incorporating carbohydrate allowances and principles of healthy eating.
6. CREATING Learner puts elements together into a functional whole by reorganizing components in new ways.		
Generate Plan Produce	Create a meal from a list of preferred foods.	Create a week of breakfast meals, each containing 45 g of carbohydate, using a list of preferred foods.

Source: DR Krathwohl, "A revision of Bloom's Taxonomy: an overview," *Theory Pract* 41, no. 4 (2002): 212-8.

like to you?" A more specific goal in this case might be, "I will eat 5 servings of fruits and vegetables each day for the next month and reevaluate the goal at my next clinic visit."

- "I will lose 5 pounds."
  - *Explanation:* This is not an objective but an outcome of practicing healthy behaviors (such as eating less or exercising more). An objective is something the person can actually do that will result in weight loss. Help the individual create an objective by asking, "How will you lose 5 pounds?" The answer will often be phrased as an objective such as, "I will limit my meat servings at lunch and dinner to 4 oz at least 5 days per week."

- "I will join a gym and go for 1 hour every day."
  - o *Explanation:* Check with the person to see whether this is achievable. A daily, hour-long visit to the gym may be tough for even the most avid exercise enthusiast to meet. It is important to guide the person in setting small goals to ensure they can be met and to evaluate them after a short period to reward success.

Action Planning

Another form of goal setting is action planning. Action plans tend to use more informal goal setting. Behavioral goals are replaced with statements of intent, for example. Action planning has been found to be an effective component of health education programs.[54] Polonsky (written communication, January 2006) describes the critical elements of action planning to include the following:

- *Specificity:* The person with diabetes clearly understands exactly what he or she needs to do.
- *Reasonableness:* The person believes the plan for action is achievable.
- *Person-centered:* The person perceives some sense of personal ownership of the plan and its development; it is not merely a set of instructions delivered by the diabetes care and education specialist.
- *Meaningfulness:* The individual perceives that accomplishing the plan will be of personal value.

An excellent example of how action planning that meets these criteria can produce positive outcomes is illustrated in a study assessing implementation intentions in the following Knowledge Builder.

Knowledge Builder: Action Plans at Work

Sheeran and Orbell[56] asked a sample of 114 women to make appointments for cervical cancer screening. Half of the sample served as controls—that is, they were given no further instructions—while the remaining half were asked to specify in writing their intention to implement this recommendation. They were asked to write down when, where, and how they would make the appointment. Of this latter group, 92% attended screenings. In contrast, only 69% of the control group attended screenings. These data lend further support to the importance of personalized, specific behavioral objectives or action planning. When people have detailed their own "implementable" plan for action, they are equipped with a plan that is likely to be specific, reasonable, and, of course, person-centered. This enhances their intent to take action; therefore, behavior change is more likely to happen.

Preparing for Success The process of goal setting is fairly straightforward: Establish one or more SMART goals or an action plan and see what happens. Yet there are several considerations in predicting whether the goals are the most appropriate for the individual and the identified needs. Here are some questions to explore:[54]

- Does the person:
  - — Value the goal and perceive a need for it?
  - — Understand the steps needed to change the behavior?
  - — Have conviction (ie, believe) that changing the behavior is important and will improve his or her health or quality of life?
  - — Have confidence (ie, believe) that he or she has the necessary resources and is likely to be successful in both changing the behavior and overcoming the obstacles to behavior change?

Simple behavioral rulers can help answer these questions. Further described in chapter 6 rulers help gauge the person's conviction and confidence in launching new behavioral goals.

Tools for Goal Setting

Mobile applications are effective tools for people to gauge behavior change and to monitor outcomes.[59] The ADCES provides a comprehensive review of mobile apps to track diabetes goals. People with diabetes may track behaviors such as food and meals, blood pressure, blood glucose, medications, and activity.

Summary for Goal Setting

The person with diabetes owns his or her goals. A major role of the diabetes care and education specialist is to support people in their effort to establish goals that initiate and maintain healthy patterns of self-care. A diabetes care and education specialist is a facilitator in the change process, which also involves ongoing follow-up visits, communication, or support. The PWD's role is to implement the change and to share the results. The diabetes care and education specialist's skills are measured in the ability to ask the right questions and offer options rather than issue directives. The skilled diabetes care and education specialist has a firm understanding of the role the individual's view of diabetes, including health beliefs, locus of control, and self-efficacy, plays in motivating behavior change. Further, the effective diabetes care and education specialist understands how the person's support system of family, coworkers, and community enhances and sustains successful behavior change.

Self-care behaviors are assessed at baseline and at specific intervals during and after the education program.[3] Once the goals of the learning experience are established, the plan can be developed and implemented.

Planning

Planning is the third step in the DSME and training process. As described by ADCES in *Competencies for Diabetes Care and Education Speciaists*,[8] the diabetes care and education specialist develops the DSMES plan to help the person with his or her desired health outcomes. The plan integrates evidence-based diabetes care practices and established principles of teaching and learning. The plan is coordinated among the diabetes healthcare team members, the person with or at risk for diabetes, the person's family and other relevant support systems, and the referring provider. The plan for education must be individualized and appropriately paced and address not only the objectives outlined in the medical plan but also the needs and capabilities of the person with diabetes. Linked closely to the findings in the assessment, the most effective therapeutic plan is individualized and prioritizes the knowledge, skills, and behaviors required for desired behavior change and metabolic outcomes.

The planning process includes the following

- Development of a detailed intervention plan to address both clinical and behavioral goals established in the goal-setting process
- A learning plan to address gaps in knowledge and plan strategies for addressing identified barriers and referrals as needed

Planning is also described in Standard 7 of the National Standards for Diabetes Self-Management Education and Support[4] as well as in a standard in *Competencies for Diabetes Care and Education Specialists and Diabetes Paraprofessionals*.[8] Given the time limits of most education sessions, planning may be the one step which is abbreviated. However, planning serves as a road map or guide for the delivery of education. Planning is dynamic, changing as the needs of the person with diabetes change and as further assessment dictates.

According to the ADCES *Competencies* document,[8] the education plan includes the following:

- Specific outcomes
- Measurable, behaviorally focused terms
- Specific instructional strategies honoring the individual's cultural, lifestyle, and health beliefs
- Evaluation of the plan's effectiveness

In addition to guiding the service, an education plan is a required part of program accreditation/recognition. It must reflect collaboration and appropriate educational interventions and self-management support strategies.

The plan addresses issues identified in the multifaceted assessment, including gaps in knowledge and information and/or skills needed to address identified behavioral goals.[4] Barriers identified during the assessment, such as lack of transportation, difficulty in paying for medications or supplies, and psychosocial problems, must be considered when developing the plan.[4] The education plan, along with the outcomes, is documented in the record of the person with diabetes.[4]

In developing a successful education plan, the diabetes care and education specialist uses a number of important skills:

- Synthesizing information
- Using logical thinking
- Prioritizing interventions
- Developing objectives and targeting outcomes
- Maintaining engagement

It often can be challenging to analyze all the available assessment information and propose a realistic plan within the constraints of the individual or group visit. The diabetes care and education specialist prioritizes the learning objectives into those that must be handled immediately for the safety of the person with diabetes and those that can wait, while keeping in mind adult learning theory and the importance of responding to the priorities of the person with diabetes.

Program Curriculum Guides the Individual Education Plan

The curriculum for a DSMES program begins with a careful, thoughtful assessment of the target population, including demographic information and cultural factors. For instance, if a program aims to improve the health of women with gestational diabetes, then curriculum content and techniques must address this population. It is also important to understand the practice environment and local standards of care. For instance, a VA population will not have access to certain medications. Based on the population assessment, program designers then build program goals and objectives, mission, and vision. It is then time to create or purchase a curriculum. A well-constructed curriculum reflects current evidence and practice guidelines and is closely aligned with community and population needs. The structure of a curriculum includes content, teaching strategies and methods, appropriate learning resources, and outcome evaluation. The curriculum should also list current, credible references to confirm that the content is evidence-based.

At the program level, a curriculum provides a roadmap for content, teaching methods, approaches, and expected outcomes. The education program's curriculum guides the instructor through the implementation of DSME. A program curriculum may be a commercially prepared one which will need to be customized for the target population. A program curriculum may also be an original one, home-grown, so to speak. Either a purchased or home-grown curriculum will need to be evidence-based with attention to national standards of care. Mensing and Norris[60] suggest that new diabetes care and education specialists may find it useful to adapt an existing commercial curriculum to meet the standards, while more experienced diabetes care and education specialists may develop their own, focusing on unique delivery methods, creative alternatives, and a more interactive delivery style. Regardless of the source of the curriculum (commercially available or homegrown), the elements of the curriculum must link to the program's goals and to the population served. Even a commercially available curriculum will need to be adapted for the unique needs and goals of the diabetes education program.

An effective curriculum provides continuity of instruction for the education team. It also serves as a guidebook when diabetes care and education specialists must substitute for one another. Finally, the program curriculum is used by instructors to individualize a teaching plan. Figure 2.4 illustrates the intimate connection between a program's curriculum and the resulting teaching plan for an individual with diabetes, the learner.

Curriculum Content

Standard 6 of the National Standards for DSME and Support addresses the importance of having a written curriculum with measurable learning goals.[4] A curriculum meeting the needs of the person with diabetes must be maintained and updated to reflect current evidence and practice guidelines. Programs recognized by the Centers for Medicare and Medicaid Services (CMS), credentialed organizations (eg, the ADCES Diabetes Education Accreditation Program, and the ADA Education Recognition Program) should have a written set of lesson plans (curriculum) to guide instructors for information consistency.

Although the curriculum is comprehensive and extensive, the diabetes care and education specialist uses individual assessments to determine which content is appropriate for the particular learner. The content of the curriculum will include the principles and concepts of the AADE7 Self-Care Behavior® framework. In addition, content about the diabetes disease process will be included. More recently, the 2017 National Standards for Diabetes Self-Management Education and Support recommended including the following topics in the overall curriculum: immunizations, navigating the healthcare system, self-advocacy, patient-generated health data, and disaster planning and preparation.[4]

Finally, to increase the likelihood of success, the curriculum and educational materials used should take into account health literacy, cultural beliefs and attitudes, and practices of the target population. The effective curriculum also uses primarily interactive, collaborative, skill-based, person-centric teaching methods.

Initiating the Education Plan

Once the diabetes care and education specialist and person with diabetes have shared enough assessment information and collaborated on preliminary educational goals, planning can begin. To effectively develop an education plan, the diabetes care and education specialist must understand signals of readiness to learn, how to scaffold content, and how to engage learning preferences. Equally important is the diabetes care and education specialist's ability to prioritize content from the program's curriculum to avoid information overload for the person with diabetes.

Readiness to Learn

Learning is more likely to 'stick' when the adult learner is engaged and activated in the learning process. Powers and colleagues identified four critical times to provide DSME: at diagnosis, annual updates, at onset of complications, and when transitions in care occur.[7] See Figure 2.1. Beyond these critical times, adults will engage in learning when they have a problem to be solved, a skill to be learned (needed to solve a problem), or are simply inquisitive. The diabetes care and education specialist can easily assess readiness with a few questions: What are you interested in today about managing your diabetes? What is the most difficult or challenging thing about managing diabetes? What do you wish you could do better when thinking about your diabetes? What are you most curious about regarding your health or your diabetes? If you could change one thing about your diabetes, what would it be? Such questions provide insight into what is most salient or important for the person with diabetes.

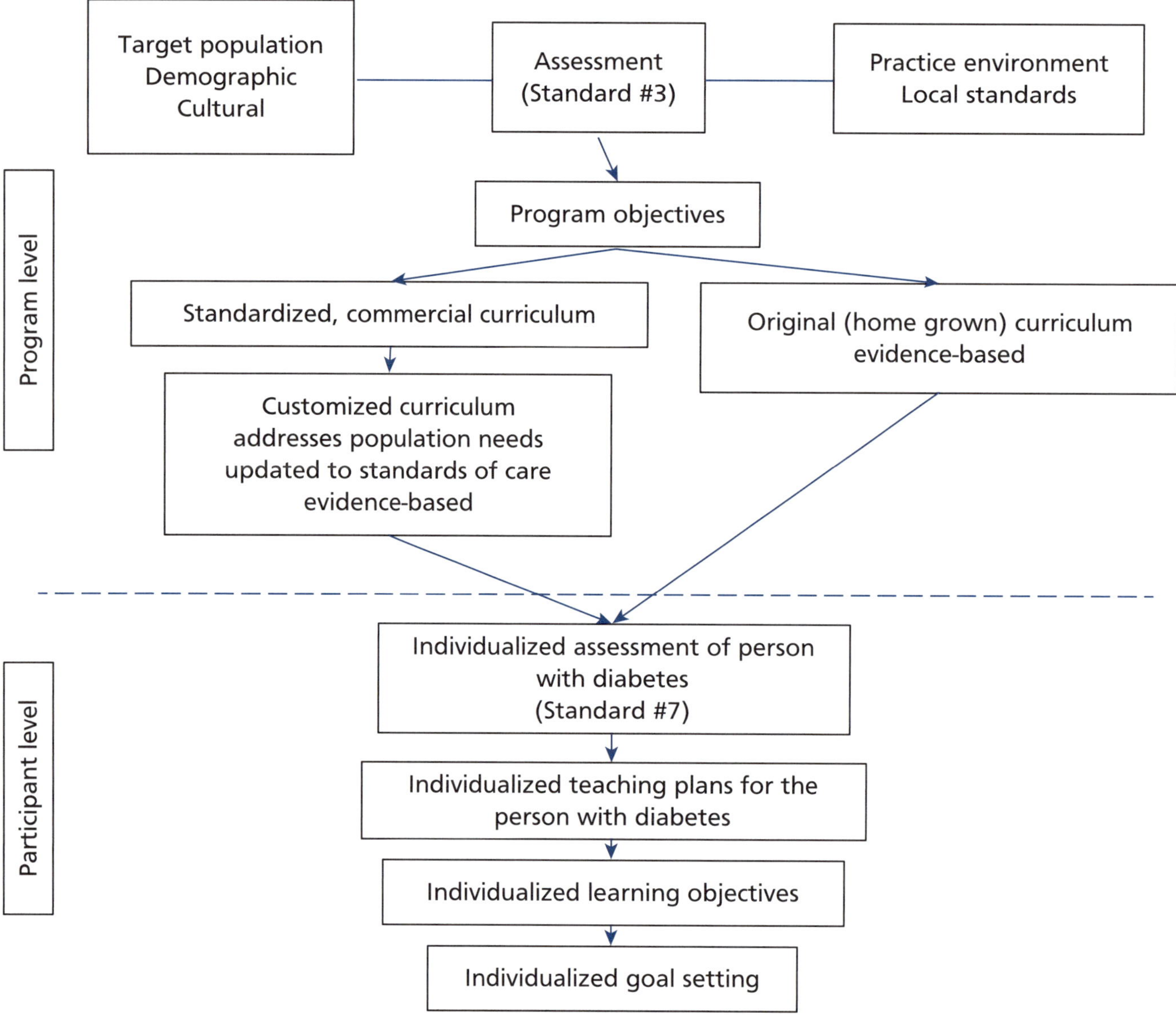

FIGURE 2.4 Model for Curriculum Design

Source: Barb Schreiner, PhD, RN, CDCES, BC-ADM

Prioritizing and Scaffolding Content Once the diabetes care and education specialist understands the person's interests and motivators, it is time to plan how and when the content will be provided. First, a little learning theory is in order. Each individual has a set of knowledge and skills which can be expanded with the help of others. In the early 1930s Lev Vygotsky, a Soviet psychologist, called this level of expertise the Zone of Proximal Development (ZPD).[61] Learning happens at the fringes of the ZPD. For the diabetes care and education specialist, ZPD helps define gaps in the learner's knowledge and skills. When the learner can build on existing knowledge, less cognitive energy is expended and deeper learning occurs. The diabetes care and education specialist uses "scaffolding" to gradually build from simple to more complex knowledge. Scaffolding means that the diabetes care and education specialist is supporting knowledge acquisition as it is occurring. For example, when teaching carbohydrate counting, begin with the number of carbs in a single food, then progress to analyzing carb content in a full meal. When teaching injections, begin with a simulated injection, and then move to how the pen is prepared and cared for.

Engaging Learner Preferences

Adults approach learning using several processing modes: verbal, visual, and doing. Some will like competition, games, and challenges. Others will want to observe before committing to action. Some will prefer to read pamphlets while others will want to see YouTube videos. Part of a thorough assessment is exploring how the person likes to learn new things. A simple question is: When you first buy a new phone (television, camera, etc), how do you go about learning how to use it? Some people will read the instruction book; others will use trial and error; still others will ask someone to show them how to use the new device. Once the diabetes care and education specialist has some idea of the person's preferred learning mode, the most effective teaching/learning strategies can be used.

Components of the Education Plan

Elements of the plan include specific desired outcomes, instructional approaches, and evaluation ideas. A template is provided in Table 2.7, and a sample completed plan is offered in Table 2.8.

Specific Outcomes

An important part of assessment is clarifying the individual's expectations and desired outcomes, as well as those of the referring provider. These may or may not be the same. In addition, during the assessment, the needs that should be addressed in the education plan are identified, including those of family members who are part of the visit. The skilled diabetes care and education specialist identifies all areas to be covered for comprehensive education and works with the individual and the education team to develop an education plan that includes learning objectives for the group or individual visit. Typically, behavioral objectives are determined at the end of the session. Learning and behavioral objectives are incorporated into the DSMES follow-up and reassessment.

Measurable, Behaviorally Focused Goals

Measurable, behaviorally focused goals are part of the plan. The mutually agreed-upon goals give direction to the DSMES plan. Utilizing the AADE7 Self-Care Behavior® framework for DSMES gives a behaviorally focused, action-oriented direction in the plan of care. See the section on goal setting for more information on creating measurable, behaviorally focused goals.

Content

Understanding what has gone awry in the body in the presence of diabetes is important. However, understanding how to manage the disease on a daily basis is critical to the individual's short- and long-term health and quality

TABLE 2.7 Template: Diabetes Education Plan

Person With Diabetes: Self-management goal(s): Behavioral objectives to achieve goal: Evaluation of goal achievement:			
Topic:			
Learning Objective	**Content**	**Teaching Strategies**	**Evaluation**
Topic:			
Learning Objective	**Content**	**Teaching Strategies**	**Evaluation**
Topic:			
Learning Objective	**Content**	**Teaching Strategies**	**Evaluation**

of life. Beyond the *what* and *why*, adequate attention must be paid to the *how*.

The challenge for healthcare diabetes care and education specialists is to effectively provide the individual with sufficient information to facilitate translation of new information into positive behavior change. An individual's management of diabetes requires integration of several skill sets: specific self-care skills, self-management skills, and coping skills. This content must be considered in the DSMES plan.

Current, evidence-based content should be readily available in the program's overall curriculum. The skillful diabetes care and education specialist will select the most appropriate content to include in the individual's education plan.

Self-Care Skills

Essential self-care skills include making food choices, monitoring blood glucose, taking medications (orally or by injection), adjusting for food or activity variations, and managing hyperglycemia and hypoglycemia. These are commonly referred to as "survival skills"; however, many people with diabetes have "survived" knowing less than this amount of information. Many self-care skills are psychomotor in nature. In this case, discussing the content will not be enough. Interactive strategies will be critical.

Self-Management Skills

Mastery of the essential self-management skills requires incremental learning that incorporates information and personal experience. Diabetes education is an ongoing process, not a once-in-a-lifetime experience. Development of self-management skills requires that learning be pushed to the next level. For this to happen, an individual must incorporate previously acquired information into situational decision-making. Utilization of anticipatory planning and problem solving promotes the development of self-management skills. For example, adjusting the insulin dose to compensate for pizza and beer involves

TABLE 2.8 Sample Diabetes Education Plan

Self-management goal(s): Decrease A1C 1%

Behavioral objectives to achieve goal:

Walk 15 minutes after breakfast and lunch for 2 weeks.

Decrease sugary drinks from 3 per day to 1 or less for 2 weeks.

Evaluation of goal achievement:

Short-term: Activity and diet logs and self-report

Long-term: A1C decreases 1% in 3 months

Topic: Exercise			
Learning Objective	**Content**	**Teaching Strategies**	**Evaluation of Learning**
Verbalize benefits of exercise	Benefits and risk of exercise	Handout Discussion	Actively involved in discussion
List preferred activities	Types of activities: aerobic, anaerobic, flexibility, strength	3-minute YouTube video	Lists and prioritizes preferred activities
Discuss safety and exercise	Blood glucose safety Foot safety Using a pedometer Clothing selection	Pedometer practice Options for blood glucose equipment Options for treating hypoglycemia	Practices with a pedometer Lists 1 or 2 safety issues and how to address
Topic: Nutrition			
Learning Objective	**Content**	**Teaching Strategies**	**Evaluation**
List favorite beverages and carbohydrate content	Hidden sources of sugar and carbohydrate	Handout Label reading examples	Reads label accurately
Select alternatives to sugary drinks	Fluid options Making non-sugary drinks flavorful	Web search for non-sugary drink alternatives	Describes a plan for locating other beverages

anticipatory planning. Evaluating the outcome of this adjustment using postmeal blood glucose data allows the individual to assess the effectiveness of the decision. In the DSMES plan, the content should include didactic information as well as practical application and problem solving. New knowledge sticks best when it is quickly applied in the real world. For example, when teaching a person how to count carbohydrates, the diabetes care and education specialist might use food models to make the experience closer to real life.

Coping Skills

Equally important to self-care is the identification and cultivation of appropriate coping skills. The presence of diabetes adds multiple stressors to the individual's life. The ability to manage the usual stressors (job, family, etc) will directly influence the individual's ability to manage the stressors associated with diabetes (inconvenience of daily care, potential for hypoglycemia, evolving complications, etc). Thus, helping the individual recognize and evaluate his or her usual coping strategies assists in the development of diabetes-specific coping behaviors. For example, if an individual typically responds to unplanned situations with frustration and agitation, helping him or her to anticipate and problem solve about delayed meals or unexpected schedule changes may decrease the frustration and agitation felt during these unplanned times. In this way, the event may be viewed as a learning opportunity rather than as a threat.

Finally, the person with diabetes needs to understand the goals and limitations of diabetes management. Maintenance of daily glycemic stability is a potential challenge. If the learner has access to self-management information and that information is presented in an effective manner, diabetes can be managed. In the DSMES plan, content related to coping and normalizing diabetes is important. This may be the perfect time to share stories of successfully living with diabetes.

Adding New Content to the Diabetes Education Curriculum

In 2017, Beck and colleagues recommended that several new topics be added to the diabetes education curriculum: immunizations, navigating the healthcare system, self-advocacy, patient-generated health data, and disaster planning and preparation.[4] These topics promote the holistic nature of diabetes education. Table 2.9 demonstrates the variety of topics and sample behavioral objectives.

Specific Instructional Strategies

Each individual has character traits, personality styles, and learning preferences that can affect the overall education intervention. Acknowledging that these differences exist is an important first step by the diabetes care and education specialist toward adapting and adjusting teaching styles.

TABLE 2.9 Adding New Content to the Curriculum

Categories	*Topics*	*Sample Objectives*
Immunizations	Recommendations Pros and cons	Participant will determine which immunizations are complete, needed Participant will determine when to schedule follow-up as needed.
Navigating the healthcare system/Self-advocacy	Health literacy Communicating with healthcare team Collaborating with healthcare team	Participant will suggest 2 ways to collaborate with the healthcare team. Participant will describe how best to share monitoring results with diabetes team.
Patient-generated health data	Managing personal health history Using health trackers Using patient portals	Participant will demonstrate accurate use of device.
Disaster planning and preparation	Local resources Weather alerts	Participant will describe details about planning for weather or other emergency. Participant will select location to post emergency checklist. Participant will add weather alert app to smartphone.

Instructional strategies used in a DSME encounter reflect the needs, skills, learning style, and preferences of the person with diabetes. Though a number of instructional methodologies are available to meet the needs of different learners, most individuals learn best when they are actively engaged (eg, through discussion groups, practice, and teaching others) rather than passively involved in learning (eg, listening to a lecture). Choosing the appropriate method of instruction is a critical determinant of effective education. While teaching and learning can occur informally, in person or remotely via phone or computer, more formal education requires planning to maximize success. Identification of content and skills to be learned, access to audiovisual materials, class size and composition, and time and available resources should all be considered when developing a teaching plan. Several teaching strategies can be considered, individually or collectively, to deliver information depending on the education needed for the expected outcome (see Table 2.10).

TABLE 2.10 Teaching Strategies and the Learning Experience

Teaching Format	*Goal*	*Learner's Experience*	*Attributes*	*Limitations*
Lecture	Present information	Passive—listens	Easy to implement and control content	Educator-centric; limited applicability of information to the individual
Discussion	Seek and acquire information	Active—asks questions, shares information and experiences	Person-centric; active participation and learning; ability to learn from others	Educator has less control over content and time; agenda may be influenced by outspoken few
Demonstration	Teach psychomotor or social skills	Active—if return demonstration included	Allows learner to observe, perform, and be evaluated	Takes more time; easier to do in small groups or one-to-one
Print materials	Provide and/or reinforce information	Passive—self-initiated	Augments in-person education and provides enduring resource	Does not replace in-person education; effectiveness influenced by congruence between materials and individual characteristics (literacy, language, readability, etc)
Audiovisual aids	Enhance presentation of information	Passive and active learning	Provides variety in presentation of information; assists those who are visual learners; adaptable to audience size and composition	Can decrease integration of information if used alone; complexity/simplicity needs to be balanced and targeted to audience
Computer-based or Web-based	Enhance self-directed education	Active learning—information resource with interactive potential	Provides opportunity for self-directed learning and problem-solving; 24-hour accessibility	Comfort with technology varies by age, socioeconomic status, and prior comfort and/or experience; questionable credibility and authority of some Web sites
Role-playing	Practice, express, explore, discuss, share	Active learning—facilitates sharing of information and exploration of what-if situations	Useful in individual or group setting	Requires cohesiveness of participants and instructor with good interpersonal skills; not palatable to some learners
Games	Enhance learning	Active learning—interactive	Can make learning more enjoyable or comfortable	Can detract from learning if not well planned or executed or if incongruent with content being taught

TABLE 2.10 Teaching Strategies and the Learning Experience (continued)

Teaching Format	*Goal*	*Learner's Experience*	*Attributes*	*Limitations*
Case study or stories	Explore, discuss, share	Active, applied learning and problem solving	Ability to learn from others and apply concepts to "real-life" experience; taps into the human preference for stories	Larger concepts may be lost in details of case studies; studies may have extraneous material
Conversation maps	Focus on health information most relevant to them	Active learning—interactive	Useful in individual or group settings; tool is colorful and engaging	Requires a skilled educator comfortable with content and with good interpersonal skills to keep the group engaged
Blended learning	Combination of a form of electronic learning and human interaction	Combination of the learning experiences listed above (computers, lecture, discussion)	Engages learners with a variety of learning styles; useful when resources or educators are limited	Requires a skilled educator comfortable with providing content in multiple technologies; lack of access to the technologies for both the person with diabetes and the educator

Source: Adapted from RM Anderson, "Applied Principles of Teaching and Learning," in MJ Franz, ed, *A Core Curriculum for Diabetes Education: Diabetes Education and Program Management*, 4th ed (Chicago: American Association of Diabetes Educators, 2001), 9-11.

No single format is conducive for teaching all components of diabetes self-management to all persons with diabetes. Using a combination of various media, tools, and materials can enhance integration of the information and skills needed to effectively self-manage diabetes. Creativity and ongoing assessment of the methods used to impart information to the learner will prevent monotonous delivery of outdated or irrelevant content—and make the education experience more rewarding for the teacher and the learner. In selecting effective teaching strategies, it is critical for the diabetes care and education specialist to consider health literacy and culture.

Health Literacy

Health information can be very confusing, and the amount of information needed to effectively self-manage diabetes can be overwhelming. Health literacy is defined as the ability to read, understand, and act on health information.[62] Because it includes the word *literacy*, people often assume it is concerned only with the inability to read. It includes the ability to not only read but also process numbers and navigate the healthcare system. The inability to understand and act on the health information can have a negative impact on health outcomes. Health information can be misunderstood for a number of reasons, including reading literacy, disability, age, language, culture, and emotion. Though everyone is at risk for low health literacy, limited literacy skills are the strongest predictor of health status—stronger than age, income, employment status, education level, and racial or ethnic group.[63] There are several screening tools available for assessing health literacy. The Newest Vital Sign, a new screening tool based on a nutrition label from an ice cream container, can be administered in as little as 3 minutes. The healthcare provider asks the person 6 questions about the nutrition label in order to assess the health literacy level.[64] The screening tool measures prose literacy, numeracy, and document literacy. Prose literacy allows the individual to follow medical instructions, while skills in numeracy mean the person can safely measure medication or evaluate a blood glucose value. Finally, document literacy means the person can determine a solution given a health problem. For instance, "What will you do with a BG value of 52 mg/dL?"

Understanding a person's health literacy is useful when developing the plan for DSME, and clearly communicating the health information is imperative to the success of the intervention. The words used to deliver the message, give directions, and present materials are all important. Identifying and incorporating health literacy into planning and implementation increases the possibility of influencing the person's actions and decisions. Osborne provides a working definition of health literacy as a shared responsibility in which people and providers must communicate in ways the other can understand.[63] Koh and colleagues have proposed a "Health Literate Care Model." In a health literate care system, individuals and their families have the knowledge and skills they need to make informed decisions to maximize their health and well-being and also to provide feedback that helps healthcare systems respond effectively to their evolving needs.[65]

In the Health Literate Care Model, prepared, the proactive, health literate healthcare team follows 'health literacy universal precautions. In essence, team members the assume that all clients are at risk of not fully understanding health conditions and interventions. Consequently, the professional must confirm and ensure understanding of health messages.

When planning DSME, it is important to consider the literacy level of the person with diabetes. In addition, the readability, appropriate adaptation, culture, personal relevance, and language should all be reviewed. A common misconception is that translation of educational materials from English to another language is sufficient for educating non-English-speaking individuals. Direct translation of words without an appreciation of the context or interpretation can create confusion. Practical guidelines to consider when choosing or creating educational materials include the following:[66]

- Use active voice; write the way you talk.
- Use short, simple sentences and common words.
- Give examples or tell a story to explain difficult words or concepts.
- Include the opportunity for interaction and informational review.

A checklist for evaluating handouts is found in Table 2.11.

Plan to use educational materials that have personal relevance. Does the material motivate readers and encourage them to take action? When creating materials, it is not adequate to rely strictly on the reading grade-level formulas included in word processing programs. These often look at the length of sentences and the number of syllables in words. Though they provide a start, other factors (such as those in Table 2.11) that are not assessed by these programs are important as well. Just because educational material is statistically readable doesn't mean it can be understood. Feedback from your clients may be the best judge of readability.

Most individuals are able to learn despite their literacy level, so long as the method of instruction is designed to recognize and compensate for the literacy deficits.[66] Within healthcare, there is a mismatch between the general literacy level and the literacy demands of healthcare instructions; this disparity impacts healthcare costs. Those with lower levels of literacy are more apt to put off preventive care measures or delay seeking medical assistance than those with high literacy levels, contributing to higher healthcare costs.[51] The diabetes care and education specialist incorporates aspects of assessing health literacy into individual and group plans. Communicate in whatever way works, applying the principles of "plain language" to all forms of communication. The University of Michigan provides the online "Plain Language Medical Dictionary," which helps diabetes care and education specialists select clear alternatives to medical jargon.[67] Remember, the diabetes care and education specialist's role as a health communicator is to translate difficult health information into words and concepts that individuals and their support team can understand and use in self-management.

TABLE 2.11 Checklist for Evaluating Handouts

	Yes	No
The purpose of the handout is clear		
Key messages are included		
Content is consistent with the lesson or curriculum		
Font is readable for the intended audience		
White space is used effectively so handout is uncluttered		
Design strategies make important text stand out		
Information is organized (tables labeled, pages numbered)		
Spelling and grammar are correct		
Pictures/graphics are relevant and realistic		
There is no commercial bias		
Content and graphics are culturally respectful		

In Practice Tip: Teaching Materials Address Literacy Needs

The education and clinical experts at Vanderbilt University have published a comprehensive series of 30 diabetes education modules to meet the needs of both English- and Spanish-speaking individuals.[69] Funded by a National Institutes of Health grant, the team created the PRIDE (*Partnership to Improve Diabetes Education*) toolkit. The tools address literacy and numeracy issues and include shared goal setting to support behavior change. The kit was designed to be used by the multidisciplinary members of the diabetes care team. Topics include general information, foot care, blood glucose monitoring, coping, oral health and men's and women's health. The modules may be accessed online at http://www.mc.vanderbilt.edu/root/vumc.php?site=CDTR&doc=37816.

In Practice Tip: Assess, Don't Assume

Consider the following example: You are covering the inpatient diabetes service and are scheduled to meet with a 45-year-old man to provide basic diabetes education before discharge. You go armed with all the pamphlets and handouts you can find, knowing that your time with him is limited to 45 minutes. Early in the conversation, he shares that he "doesn't read much." However, his medical record indicated he has a very successful business, and thus you expect he will be able to understand the new information in the written materials with minimal difficulty. He must be literate; after all, he runs a successful business. Is your assumption accurate? Could it be that he is successful in business because he has surrounded himself with individuals who provide oral reports? While literacy is one stepping stone to success, it is not the only one.

Teaching Across the Lifespan

When developing and implementing the diabetes education plan, it is important to consider how people learn at different stages of life. It is important that principles of learning be considered when identifying the individual's motivation to learn, in designing the curriculum to be taught, and in creating the learning environment.

Children and Adolescents

Readiness to learn in childhood changes considerably with age and maturation. A wide array of caregivers, including parents, siblings, grandparents, other family members, the primary care provider, school personnel, coaches, and babysitters, are included as part of the healthcare team, and considerable planning must occur for all to be included in the education process at relevant times. When educating the parents or caregivers of a child newly diagnosed with type 1 diabetes, it is important to remember that their ability to learn may be impacted by fear of the diagnosis. They must be reassessed regularly, along with the child, and the assessment information incorporated into the planning and implementation of DSME. In addition to imparting facts and teaching practical skills, diabetes education promotes desirable health beliefs and attitudes in the young person. This is often best accomplished in a setting where age-appropriate peer education can occur, such as at summer camps or on moderated Web site discussion boards. It is important that the child be included in education that is age appropriate. A recommended approach for a child with diabetes is for the child and the parent to attend several single-topic-focused sessions scheduled for no longer than 30 minutes. This will also offer the opportunity to reinforce learning, which is important in successfully achieving mutually defined self-management goals.[70]

Young children often learn best by example and simple explanation using words they are familiar with and incorporating play when possible. It is also important that at the appropriate stage in development, self-management responsibility begins to shift from the parent or caregiver to the individual with diabetes. This must be considered on an individual basis and will be guided by the child's developmental phase, intellect, ability, and willingness to assume responsibility. Understanding what the child is managing in his or her routine life can serve as a guide for encouraging increasing independence in diabetes management.[70]

Adolescents

Providing DSME to adolescents requires appreciating the developmental changes and challenges of that age group. While the adolescent still needs parental guidance, he or she is also evolving toward self-care and independence. Finding "teachable moments" can be quite effective. For instance, teens often exhibit an increased readiness to learn at key developmental times.[70] The adolescent will want answers for how to best live with diabetes in social situations, as hormones rage, and as developmental milestones are reached (eg, driving, employment). While safety topics are important, psychosocial and developmental concerns also need to be addressed. For the teen who was diagnosed as a young child, this may be the first time that education will be focused on his or her teen issues. Adolescents are avid learners—especially when the content directly meets their needs. They often prefer technology as the learning tool. Risky behaviors and risk taking is sometimes their method for learning. Therefore, problem solving becomes an important focus of DSME for teens. The curriculum for adolescents must include discussions about the impact of alcohol, smoking, drugs, and pregnancy on diabetes health. Finally, topics about transitioning to independence and adult care are warranted.[71–73]

Adults

In developing the plan for the adult learner, it is important to incorporate principles of learning.[67] These include the following:

- Adults are self-directed. They will decide for themselves what is important to be learned. The diabetes care and education specialist can only suggest and guide.

- Adults are task- or problem-oriented learners. The adult doesn't like to just sit back and listen. They prefer practical activities such as discussion, hands-on work, or a project related to a concept. Examples of this include interpreting a blood glucose log to identify patterns and using food models to build a plate with the appropriate amount of carbohydrates.
- Adults bring experience to the learning situation. This can be a rich resource for themselves and for others. Their experiences can be used effectively by connecting them to new learning.
- Adults are more likely to learn when learning has meaning for who they are and their social roles and responsibilities. This is sometimes described as WIIFM (what's in it for me). Adults' most teachable moments are "just in time learning" when they believe they need to learn something new or different.[74]
- Adult learners want to know why the content will be meaningful to them. New information must fit easily into an existing understanding of the world.

Quite simply, when working with adult learners, the diabetes care and education specialist should teach things worth learning.

Older Adults

There are special considerations when developing the individualized DSME plan for older adults. The plan incorporates assessment information related to the person's functional, cognitive, and psychosocial status, recognizing that these change over time.[74] It is important to consider comorbidities and the impact of coexisting conditions on the functional capacity of the individual. Quality of life and life expectancy must be considered when prioritizing the topics and content for the older adult. Older adults may require more time to assimilate the information and may benefit from a slower-paced education session. It may be necessary to involve a care partner in DSME if the older adult is unable to assume full responsibility for his or her self-care.[75–78]

Generational Differences in Learning

For the first time, adults in the United States come from 5 generations: veterans (born before 1946), baby boomers (born between 1946 and 1964), generation X (born between 1965 and 1980), generation Y or millennials (born between 1981 and 1995), and generation Z (born between 1996 and 2010). Imagine the world in which each generation was raised. The impact of the world and the early school experiences contribute to how each generation now approaches education and learning[79] (see Table 2.12).

TABLE 2.12 Generational Differences

	Veterans (born before 1946)	*Baby Boomers (born between 1946 and 1964)*	*Generation X (born between 1965 and 1980)*	*Generation Y or Millennials (born between 1981 and 1995)*	*Generation Z (born between 1996 and 2010)*
World events	WWII Great Depression	Vietnam Sexual revolution	Gulf War Fall of Berlin Wall *Challenger* disaster End of Cold War High divorce rates AIDS	Terrorism: local and global 9/11	Iraq/Afghanistan War Recession Hurricane Katrina
Technology	Radio Phones	Television Compact discs Handheld calculator Transistor radio Typewriter	Early computers	World Wide Web Cell phones Computers	Digital natives Gamification Globally connected

TABLE 2.12 Generational Differences (continued)

Education	Rote memorization Classroom Lectures	Classroom Participation in class	Games Role playing PowerPoint® presentations Educational videos and TV	Wikis Blogs Social media On demand	Crowd sourcing for solutions Mobile apps
Implications for diabetes education	Expect respect Formal relationship (Mr., Mrs.) Look to authority Prefer individual work, not groups	Want to be part of the solution Less impressed with authority figures	More informal Technologically able with devices Want relevant information delivered quickly	Sharing information is the norm Multitasking Social learning	Attention span is short Consume information in small packets
Teaching techniques	Traditional approaches (lecture, reading) Stories and sharing experiences Use large font size	Visual tools Interactive May not like role playing	Expect slides or video Group activities Use bullet points Provide ample feedback	Internet sources Smartphone apps Group work	Concise, readily usable information Social networking Distance or remote approaches

Source: Adapted from McCrindle Research, "Generations defined," 2012, on the Internet at: http://mccrindle.com.au.

Whether planning for group or individual education sessions, consider age as well as the individual's stage of life, as each presents unique issues and needs. Understanding generalizations about different groups broadens the diabetes care and education specialist's ability to explore differences with the individual with diabetes. Yet, broad generalizations do not replace a careful, comprehensive, individualized assessment. The individual is a uniquely blended person at the intersection of age, ethnicity, sexual preference, socioeconomic status, and social values. Regardless of age or stage of life, the education process must accomplish the following:

- Include information that is viewed as important to the individual
- Recognize the individual's experiences and integrate them into the learning process
- Foster the development of problem-solving skills
- Promote active participation in one's self-care
- Reinforce need for lifelong learning

The DSMES Plan Is Dynamic

In addition to recognizing that each plan must be individualized is that the plan is fluid and must be adjusted and updated to reflect the changing needs of the person with diabetes. This necessitates ongoing assessment and evaluation of the plan's effectiveness.

The DSMES Process Is Lifelong

Standard 8 of the National Standards for DSME and Support includes a collaboratively developed follow-up plan for ongoing DSMS.[4] It is recognized that to sustain behavior change at the level necessary to manage diabetes, most people need ongoing self-management support. Diabetes self-management support is a process of receiving education and motivation beyond the visits with the person's healthcare providers. The process of DSMS planning can begin during the assessment and may include discussion of complementary education opportunities while still in the DSME program or starting upon completion. Diabetes self-management support strategies may include support groups; disease management, case management, or care coordination programs; media or online support; medical nutrition therapy (MNT); and programs utilizing community health workers who work under the guidance of the diabetes care and education specialist.[7] Community initiatives can include health fairs, breakfast clubs, and social events for individuals and their families promoting self-management opportunities. Very important is that follow-up and support provide individuals with choices that meet their individual needs and are readily available and convenient. Personal connection or consistent contact with someone who knows them is also important.[7] In this era of mobile connectivity, social and treatment support can be as close as the nearest smartphone or tablet.[80]

DSME and Technology: The Diabetes Care and Education Specialist's Role

It is the 2020s. Your class roster for this week pops up on your smartphone. With a click on the button, you send a welcome message to your participants reminding them to bring their electronic log books to class. You include a link to the online courseroom and remind them to doublecheck the timezone for class to start. You answer several text messages and post a blog about analyzing CGM data.

The world of the diabetes care and education specialist is about to take an interesting turn. As technology becomes more pervasive in the daily lives of our clients, diabetes care and education specialists are finding new ways to use the power and benefits of a variety of engaging tools. Diabetes care, education, and support are being delivered remotely, virtually, and 24/7.

There are several ways in which the diabetes care and education specialist interfaces with the evolving, ever-connected digital world. People with diabetes are increasingly trying mobile apps to help with managing their diabetes. Greenwood and associates found that the most successful digital programs were those that provided interaction between the individual and the provider. When this 2-way communication was in place, A1C levels improved.[81]

Some educators are already providing DSME services remotely in a virtual environment. In such a world, diabetes care and education specialists serve as facilitators as learners engage in active learning such as gaming or chat rooms.[82] Such novel programs are emerging as a way to address access and scalability of education programs. What will this mean for the diabetes care and education specialist of the future. MacLeod and Peeples propose that the e-educator, because of expertise, must be at the table as technology is being created.[83]

Diabetes care and education specialists are indeed poised to enter the digital world of diabetes education and care. As lifelong learners themselves, educators will need to learn about the health technology tools and incorporate technology-based tools into their practice. Further, because these tools generate individual and population-based data, the educator will need to learn how to best interpret the information and take action to improve health outcomes.

In its current strategic plan, ADCES is exploring ways to leverage technology and prepare diabetes care and education specialists for future roles. Diabetes care and education specialists have a remarkable tool in the Diabetes Advanced Network Access (DANA), ADCES's one-stop healthcare resource that helps navigate the many new technologies people with diabetes and prediabetes can use to get and stay healthy. For the educator, DANA offers a product clearinghouse, professional courses, polls and focus groups, guidelines and resources, and ongoing reviews of mobile apps for diabetes care and education. DANA is available at https://www.danatech.org/.

Summary for Planning

Planning is the step in the DSMES process that involves the selection of specific content, teaching approaches, and goals that are based on a multifaceted assessment of the individual. Planning requires collaboration among the person with diabetes, their family members (as appropriate), the diabetes care and education specialist, the referring provider, and other members of the healthcare team to develop a mutually agreed-upon individualized, realistic, and effective plan for DSMES. The next step in the process is implementing the plan.

Implementation

The fourth step of the DSME process is implementation of the agreed-upon plan. Implementation involves interfacing with the person and various care providers and linking the individual to community and professional resources and services. Implementation involves recommendation and execution of the plan; ensuring that the person has the knowledge, skills, and resources necessary to follow through on the plan; and identification and assistance with removal of barriers identified throughout the process.

The DSME Team

One question that often arises is who should deliver DSME to the person with diabetes? Although reports on the effectiveness of different disciplines are mixed, registered nurses, registered dietitians, and registered pharmacists most commonly make up the DSME team. Standard 5 of the National Standards for DSME states that at least one of the instructors will be from one of these disciplines. Other health professionals (eg, behaviorist, exercise physiologist, nurse practitioners, and physicians) may be included as well.[4] The ADCES supports the role of the community or lay health worker serving as a bridge between the healthcare system and the people with diabetes.

Standards of Practice

Measurement criteria for implementation identified in *Competencies for Diabetes Care and Education Specialists* include the following:[8]

- Provides an accessible, safe, and appropriate environment for DSME

- Uses teaching materials and approaches appropriate to the learner's age, culture, learning style, and abilities
- Structures or scaffolds DSME to progress from basic safety and survival skills to advanced information for daily self-management and improved outcomes
- Addresses basic diabetes self-management skills, including safe medication use, meal planning, self-monitoring of blood glucose, and recognizing when and how to access professional services
- Provides increasingly advanced DSME, based on the client's needs and goals, on topics including preventing and managing chronic complications, psychosocial adjustment, developing problem-solving skills, managing physical activity, adjusting treatment regimens (including insulin and oral diabetes medications), stress management, travel situations, and pattern management
- Provides opportunities for peer support
- Integrates the DSME plan into the overall plan of care
- Shares the diabetes educational plan and progress with referring providers
- Establishes means for follow-up and continuity of DSMES, including referrals to other providers
- May provide a format of group education for DSME, if desired, to foster the support, encouragement, and empowerment of clients; group education can lead to behavior change as participants share ideas and experiences

Strategies for Implementing DSME

A frequently asked question when the Diabetes Control and Complications Trial (DCCT) ended was, "How was it done?" Specifically, healthcare professionals and people with diabetes were curious: What strategy was used to treat the intensive treatment group that resulted in achievement of the desired outcome? The DCCT illustrated the need for diabetes education, the importance of multidisciplinary team care, the value of incorporating regimens that were most consistent with the individual's lifestyle, and the importance of ongoing support. Various education strategies and tactics that recognized and capitalized on the individual's needs, attributes, and limitations were used. However, no universal strategy or education approach could be identified. So, what does this tell us about how to best educate people with diabetes? If there is no "right" way to do it, what factors should be considered to improve effectiveness?

Compliance and Empowerment Approaches to Education

While the compliance and empowerment approaches to education have specific attributes and limitations, they are not mutually exclusive, nor is one approach ideal for all individuals throughout the learning process. Consider the person recently diagnosed with diabetes. He will require basic information and instruction to prevent hospitalization and ensure safety. Adjusting insulin doses for eating out may not be relevant to him at this time. However, learning how and why he got diabetes, what has gone wrong in his body, how and when to take medication or give an injection, and why medication is needed every day are all vital pieces of information during these early weeks. Conversely, the individual who has had diabetes for several years may gain more from an interactive session about carbohydrate counting that allows opportunities to ask about adjustments that would be needed to cover her favorite foods or includes practice on making healthy choices at her favorite restaurant. Table 2.13 highlights distinct characteristics of the compliance and empowerment approaches to education of persons with diabetes.

The educator considers the order or sequence in which topics are to be presented. Are you planning to teach about diabetes the way you, as a healthcare professional, were taught, beginning with definitions, basics of diagnosis, pathophysiology, and treatment? Are psychosocial issues pushed to the very end? Consider switching the order around. In general, individuals are not interested in diabetes as an academic subject but in how it affects them in their day-to-day life. Funnell and Anderson have long described an empowerment model, making the experiences of the person with diabetes the basis for the curriculum.[84] Discussing the nature of a self-managed disease such as diabetes at the beginning of an education program helps participants understand why the interaction with the group and information presented are so important. Participants also then see that the role of the healthcare professional is to be a source of expertise, support, and inspiration rather than a teacher, caregiver, or sole decision-maker. This approach recognizes that the person living with diabetes has as important a contribution to make to the session as the diabetes care and education specialist. This view redefines the purpose of diabetes education, taking it from providing information so individuals will know why their behaviors need to change to providing information so individuals can make informed decisions about their behaviors. This empowerment-based approach for DSME has been effective in a variety of populations.[85,86]

TABLE 2.13 Approaches to Education of Persons With Diabetes

	Compliance Approach	*Empowerment Approach*
Assumptions	Healthcare professionals are the experts Person with diabetes comply with recommendations Person with diabetes must follow instructions for success	Persons with diabetes are capable of making complex decisions and joining in shared decision making Persons with diabetes have the right and responsibility to manage their diabetes Healthcare professionals provide guidance and support
Strategies	Healthcare professional identifies important aspects of care and provides education Instructions are directive and approach is often uniform over time	Basic understanding of disease and management tools needed Healthcare professional provides guidance regarding specific aspects of management, directed by the person with diabetes
Goal	Person with diabetes complies with treatment recommendations	Recommendations often replace standardized instructions Education focuses on self-care, self-management, and coping skills Person with diabetes assumes primary responsibility for daily decision-making
Usefulness of approach to person with diabetes	Early in disease process, beyond survival skills If unable to assume greater responsibility for personal healthcare decisions If unable to focus on specifics of self-care due to other life issues	After individual has a good understanding of diabetes survival skills If willing to actively participate in care decisions If able to make informed decisions and recognize when to seek assistance

Source: Adapted from RM Anderson, "Applied Principles of Teaching and Learning," in MJ Franz, ed, *A Core Curriculum for Diabetes Education: Diabetes Education and Program Management,* 4th ed (Chicago: American Association of Diabetes Educators, 2001), 9-11.

Fundamental to an empowerment approach is the concept of shared decision making. In shared decision making, the person tells his or her story, shares personal goals, and seeks clarification when needed.[87,88] The healthcare provider, in turn, offers expertise in managing the condition, listens to the individual's concerns, and explains the treatment options. Several tools are emerging to assist in this collaboration. For example, an interactive online decision aid for choosing medication is available through the Mayo Clinic at https://diabetesdecisionaid.mayoclinic.org. These tools are designed to be used during the encounter with the person with diabetes to guide both the person with diabetes and the provider in developing the person's medication plan. Wilkinson, Nathan, and Huang[46] reviewed similar tools to support personalized decision making.

Problem-Based Learning

One challenge to education or training is whether the learner ever transfers the knowledge or skill to practice. Another issue is how to teach a general concept yet keep it meaningful for each learner in the group. Problem-based or problem-focused learning is a strategy to address these concerns. In problem-based learning (PBL), the educator relies on case studies, stories, and what-if questions. Problem-based learning has been effective in diverse populations.[89,90] The Skill Builder provides tips for integrating PBL into diabetes education sessions.

Skill Builder: Using PBL

It is quite easy to incorporate PBL techniques into diabetes education sessions. Following these steps will integrate the problem-solving aspects of PBL:[90]

Invite a learner to share a problem or concern he or she is experiencing.

As a group, generate solutions to the problem.

Explore how easy or hard it would be to implement the possible solutions.

Discuss how relevant the problem is for each learner.

Create action plans based on the discussion.

Storytelling as a Teaching Strategy

One way to overcome some of the challenges of knowledge transfer to action is to use stories. Stories address a variety of learning styles and engage the individual at both cognitive and emotional levels. They create bonds, connections, and relationships between the educator and the learner.[91–93] Stories can help people make sense of their own journey with a chronic disease.[94] Stories bring meaning and help people uncover their own wisdom. Stories can help break down resistance and create trust. People with diabetes are already sharing stories informally through social media[95] and support groups. Storytelling can also be incorporated into the DSME plan. Most stories are a hero's quest: encountering an obstacle and overcoming the challenge. A simple outline for constructing an engaging story with a message includes the following:[91–93]

- Set the scene: Provide some background detail.
- Introduce the characters: Create a visual picture of the people involved in the story. What are their personalities, needs, and desires? Do you want the characters to share some of the characteristics of your learners?
- Begin the journey.
- Encounter the obstacle.
- Overcome the obstacle: Who helped in the journey?
- Resolve the story and reinforce the key message.
- Debrief the story and its meaning: Has this ever happened to you? What did you do?

In Practice Tip: Create a Story Catalog

Authentic stories are powerful teaching and communication tools. Diabetes care and education specialists hear the stories of people with diabetes every day, and over time, these stories could fill a book—or a catalog. Consider building a catalog of stories to share with people with diabetes. Of course, the stories should not divulge names or personal or identifying information. Tell stories about a person who:

- Was successful with weight loss
- Had a creative way to handle a challenge
- Changed behavior to achieve a goal
- Dealt with hypoglycemia safely
- Made a mistake with carb counting or with medication
- Taught you, the educator, something important
- Showed strength in dealing with adversity
- Used humor to deal with diabetes

Individual versus Group

Diabetes self-management education may be conducted in either group or individual counseling settings. Mensing and Norris describe how the process of group education has evolved over time.[60] Not long ago, diabetes group education might have been described as a set of didactic classes, presented lecture style, where the teacher would impart knowledge. Now, group education meetings are more interactive sessions or gatherings where the facilitator elicits discussion based on the participants' interests and needs. The shift to group education puts more responsibility on the individual to complete the assessment and the goal-setting activities with assistance and review by the educator.

Not only is group education the method required in most instances for Medicare reimbursement, the group setting has been found to be effective from both a clinical and cost perspective.[96] While many studies have demonstrated that group classes improve metabolic and behavioral measures,[97,98] other studies have found that individual classes are superior in achieving these goals.[99] Therefore, the educator must accurately determine which approach will best match the needs, preferences, and resources of the individual.

Knowledge Builder: DSME Outcomes Systematic Review

A systematic review of the literature is one of the most credible evidence-based tools. In 2015 the ADCES funded a review to better understand the impact of DSMES. Chrvala, Sherr, and Lipman conducted an extensive search of more than 3,700 scientific papers.[96] Sifting through these studies yielded 118 which met the criteria for sound scientific methodology. What is important for the diabetes care and education specialist to take away from the systematic review? First, DSMES has a favorable impact on A1C. Almost 62% of the studies reported significant changes in A1C with an average absolute reduction of 0.57. Second, when individual and group education approaches were combined, A1C reduction was even greater (0.88). Finally, when education time was 10 hours or more, 70.3% of programs reported a significant decrease in A1C.

In Practice Tip: Exceptions to the Medicare Requirement

Following are exceptions to the Medicare regulation requiring group instruction:

- No group session is available within 2 months of the date the education is ordered.

- The individual has severe vision, language, or hearing limitations.
- Other conditions are identified by the treating physician or nonphysician practitioner.
- If the education assessment indicates that individual instruction would better meet a person's needs, the diabetes care and education specialist should let the referring physician know this promptly so that the referring provider can document this request.
- Since rules and regulations change, check CMS for the most current information.

Managing Education Session Challenges

As important as it is to have a plan, having a backup plan is also important. Diabetes care and education specialists are flexible and spontaneous, and maintain a calm ride even through what may feel like stormy seas. Listed below are a couple of scenarios that diabetes care and education specialists may face from time to time, with suggestions for how to quickly make the best of the situation.

Inpatient Education: When Content Exceeds Time Available

The diabetes care and education specialist has unique challenges when providing DSME in an inpatient setting. Diabetes self-management education may be an afterthought to the attending physician and may not be ordered or considered until the day of discharge. Even if DSME is considered early in the admission, the individual may not be well enough to participate. Admittedly, hospitalization is not the ideal time to provide comprehensive DSME. The educator must carefully assess the person's needs to best plan the amount and depth of content to share. The most important content will be that which keeps the person safe. For example, the person going home using insulin will need instruction on use, dosing, timing, and precautions.

In some hospitals, the job of educating patients about diabetes is in the hands of the staff nurse. These nurses are faced with very limited time to provide focused, meaningful information. Several programs are being investigated to develop materials to help the inpatient nurse. For instance, Stotts Krall and colleagues developed the Nurse Education and Transition program, a series of short video vignettes for patients to view on an iPad.[100] The topics include nutrition, medication taking, activity, insulin administration, and hypoglycemia. The authors demonstrated that the merging of technology and DSME was effective in delivering survival content.

While the staff may be responsible for bedside education in some hospital settings, the diabetes care and education specialist may be coordinating and delivering education in other settings. One of the most important roles the inpatient diabetes care and education specialist has is participating in the transition to home care and outpatient education. To do this, the educator must further assess the barriers that may interfere with the individual obtaining more education or following through on appointments. One model which has been very effective in helping people make the transition from hospital to home is the Transition Care Model (TCM), developed and studied by the University of Pennsylvania.[101] The TCM is a nurse-led, multidisciplinary team which uses a case management approach. Hirschman and colleagues provide a full description of the model.

In Practice Tip: The Joint Commission's Certificate of Distinction for Inpatient Diabetes Care

The Joint Commission's Certificate of Distinction for Inpatient Diabetes Care recognizes those inpatient programs which have the critical components to affect long-term outcomes. The program is closely aligned with the ADA's Clinical Practice Recommendations. The following attributes are evaluated:

- Specific staff education requirements
- Written blood glucose monitoring protocols
- Plans for the treatment of hypoglycemia and hyperglycemia
- Data collection of incidences of hypoglycemia
- Patient education on self-management of diabetes
- An identified program champion or program champion team

For further information about the certification process and eligibility criteria, visit http://www.jointcommission.org.

Source: The Joint Commission, "Certification in inpatient diabetes" (cited 2019 Jun 1), on the Internet at: https://www.jointcommission.org/certification/inpatient_diabetes.aspx.

Outpatient Education

While the inpatient diabetes care and education specialist frequently experiences time pressures and challenges in transitioning the person's diabetes, the specialist in the outpatient setting must also plan for surprises. Small groups, large groups, and technical difficulties are some of the problems requiring flexibility and creativity.

A group will likely include different types of learners, eg, "the talker," the quiet one," "the distracted learner," and so on. specialist will need to guide all of them within the group setting.

A Group of One?

You have spent time preparing for class. You have content maps, slides, and handouts and are ready for a 1-hour session, but when you arrive at the classroom, 1 person is there. You are tempted to deliver the "class" you are accustomed to giving each week. Do not! Instead of delivering the class you had planned, treat the session as one-to-one counseling. Determine exactly what the person's needs are and individualize your messages to meet those needs directly. Although the person will not have the benefit of the group interaction, he or she will benefit from much more personal attention.

Attendance Exceeds Expectation

You enter the classroom expecting to encounter 8 individuals and instead you find 15. Acknowledging your surprise with the bigger group is fine, but avoid showing that you feel hassled or annoyed. Ask the group to assist you in making a few adjustments so that everyone with diabetes can be best accommodated. For example, guests who have accompanied class participants can be asked to sit in the outer circle behind their partners to give them priority at the table or inner circle. Ask participants to share materials and say that you will arrange to get everyone a set later. Use tools from effective group processes such as setting the ground rules for the session. Smile. Show a sense of humor, and all will be fine.

Technical Difficulties

Access to technology means an increased chance for equipment failure. Are you prepared if the projector does not work or your handouts do not get delivered from the copy center? Unless you have unlimited financial resources, you do not need two of everything "just in case." Instead, think about how you might get by on your own. If you are accustomed to using overheads or slides, have a handout set for yourself so you can at least use them as prompts to know what topic comes next. Use a flipchart or whiteboard to write down key points that may need emphasis. In fact, teach some classes without any audiovisual aids. Avoid overreliance on technology and ensure room for individualization and flexibility based on group needs.

Teaching Materials and Audiovisual Materials

Teaching materials must be available to support the curriculum. People with diabetes and their support system often find these materials very useful in their ongoing self-management and behavior-change efforts. The materials used should take into consideration previously discussed issues like health literacy and culture, attitudes, and health beliefs.

Audiovisuals such as PowerPoint® slides, electronic presentations, or videos are available alternatives. They may help support the educator in ensuring completeness of delivery of content. On the other hand, media can get in the way of learning. Software such as PowerPoint® packages an amazing array of graphical elements to enhance the visual appeal of slides. Dozens of fonts, animation options, and color palettes are available to the educator. It is easy to confuse attraction with education. Colorful slides with moving parts often overshadow the key message of the slide. This is one area where simpler truly is better (see Knowledge Builder for tips on cognitive overload).

Knowledge Builder: Cognitive Overload

Cognitive science reminds us that the human brain has 2 channels for taking information into working memory: an auditory channel and a visual channel.[102,103] Distractions from the visual channel (such as animated slides) can hinder the impact of information entering through the auditory channel. This is particularly true if the messages are incongruent. For instance, if the educator is discussing hypoglycemia and the slide has titles twirling and fireworks exploding, the learner's brain will expend unnecessary (and precious) cognitive energy trying to make sense of the messages. When an individual finds complex, animated, and overly designed presentations distracting, cognitive overload is at work.

What all this means for the educator is important:

- Keep your messages simple.
- Use media which best deliver the message in a clean and clear way.
- When tapping both cognitive channels, keep the message and media congruent.
- Avoid distractions when delivering a message.
- Just because a media tool *can* do something doesn't mean the educator *should* use it.
- Be prepared for technology failures (eg, power failures, device malfunctions) with a low-tech alternative (eg, handouts, whiteboards, flipcharts, drawings).

Educational materials from pharmaceutical companies and even government programs can be a huge boon to education programs with limited budgets. That is the good news—these materials are plentiful, very often Web based, and easily accessible. The challenge is when the materials are not consistent with the program's curriculum. Nuances in terms and procedures can be confusing to participants. Does the program use "blood glucose checks" where the materials use "blood sugar tests"? Other differences may be more philosophical. Does the program advocate the use of alcohol to clean the skin before injection, whereas the pamphlet eliminates this step? Materials used from sources outside the education program must be carefully scrutinized with these goals:

- Decrease as much inconsistency as possible.
- Ensure readability and language are appropriate for the program's target audience.
- Ensure ethnicity and culture portrayed in the materials are acceptable to the target audience.

Consider creating your own materials when feasible. Creating your own educational materials is much like cooking your own meal versus buying a frozen dinner: You will know what went into the final product.

Applying Learning Theory

Malcolm Knowles, often cited as the "father of adult learning theory," wrote, "The richest resources for learning reside in the adult learners themselves. Hence, the greater emphasis in adult education on experiential techniques—techniques that tap into the experience of the learners, such as group discussion, simulation exercises, problem-solving activities, case method, and laboratory methods—over transmittal techniques."[74] Adult learners come with a history, with experiences, with a need to know. These elements drive their readiness to learn.

Other learning theories such as Transformational Learning reinforce the importance of life experience as well as critical reflection on learning outcomes.[104] Effective educators tap into their participants' experiences and encourage self-reflection by keeping the learners involved in the learning. The following Skill Builder offers some examples of interactive learning strategies.

Skill Builder: Making Learning Active

Learning is most effective when the person is involved in making the content his or her own. The educator can use several strategies to make content informative and the learning interactive.

Topic menu: Create a list of topics (like a menu) for the class to choose from. Start with the first topic chosen and then move to another topic. You might keep all the topics within a certain category.

Interactive handouts: Create handouts that require filling in the blanks.

Each one teach one: Have partners teach each other the important concepts or a specific subject they have just learned.

Matching activities: Using flashcards, have participants match a concept to a definition, or a symptom to a condition, or a treatment to a condition.

Skill sequence: Take photos of the key steps in a particular skill and print them. Mix up the photos and ask learners to put the photos in the correct order of the steps in the skill.

Create a meal: Using photos, food models, or information from nutrition Web sites, ask learners to create a meal of 30 g (or any number) of carbohydrate.

Applying Cognitive Science

Learning theory can support the curriculum and the type of teaching tools used. So can cognitive science. Part of the role of the diabetes care and education specialist is to build expertise in persons with diabetes. While experts have developed extensive knowledge, they are also able to organize information, remember details, and solve problems.[105] This means that diabetes education should incorporate plenty of opportunities to learn new information, remember and retrieve that information, and apply that knowledge in practical ways to solve problems.

Memory becomes an important cognitive concept for educators to understand. The human brain takes in information through sensory pathways. While all experiences are registered in the brain, many are not remembered. Memory depends on the meaning the experience has for the individual. If a person is taking oral medications, for instance, will a class on insulin therapy be remembered? Memories become linked to emotions as well. What do you remember of your first kiss, for example? Because of the emotional impact, persons with diabetes will often remember what their healthcare team said on the day of diagnosis.

Helping learning to stick is all about creating enduring memory. Here are some practical ways to help persons with diabetes remember content:[106]

- Use a variety of approaches that engage the senses. Cooking classes are a great way to teach nutrition concepts.

- Encourage discussion about the emotional impact of the new information being presented.
- Repeat important concepts in varied ways. Repetition is a key way that the brain settles new information into long-term memory.
- Use a teach-back approach. Ask the participant to teach another learner to content or skill just covered.
- Recognize that memory is enhanced when blood glucose levels are normal. Hypoglycemia and hyperglycemia can both interfere with learning and attention.
- Because content at the beginning and the end of a session is remembered best, keep sessions of content short, with adequate breaks, so there are many beginnings and endings.
- Ask participants to summarize what they have learned. For example, "What are the 3 things you will probably remember about today's session?" "What are 2 things that you still wonder about?"
- Allow learners to make mistakes and problem solve when they are learning a new skill. Balance self-discovery with careful coaching to avoid too much frustration (a memory killer).

Thoughtful Use of Technology

Technology-based instruction can be appealing and enticing to an education team. Who doesn't want to use the best videos, the most colorful slides, and the best teaching software? These all have a place in teaching individuals but they must be thoughtfully selected and judiciously used. Some learners will crave the technology aspect of a tool; others will find it distracting or confusing. Assess the learner and that learner's preferred mode of learning. Teaching can be just as effective when done with a flipchart as with a set of slides or videos. Technology is a tool, and the instructor's role is to carefully integrate technology into the curriculum. Remember, the message should not be lost in the medium.

Teaching Environment

Controlling and modifying the learning environment is another way to promote memory. Careful consideration of the teaching environment is a component of a diabetes care and education specialist's ability to effectively lead a group or individual education session. In a group, when possible, create a room arrangement that encourages interaction and discussion. Alternatives to traditional classroom style should be considered. Will the educator be sitting in a circle with the class, standing in the front, or moving around, or will it be a blend of all three? Generally, a combination works best for most kinds of groups. In individual education sessions, people often discuss very personal healthcare matters that can become emotional. The interaction can be more difficult in a setting that feels cold and impersonal or lacks adequate privacy. Whether providing a group or individual intervention, consider the lighting, color, sound, movement, artwork, and clutter; also make sure that the facilities are accessible for people with physical disabilities.[91] The environment should be inviting and elicit curiosity while minimizing distractions.

Create an inviting space by posting a welcome message on the door or as the first slide. Elicit curiosity by posting your key message with some of the words missing. For example, the message might state: "The best way to lose weight is . . ." People will naturally wonder what is missing and will stay engaged as they listen for the message to be completed. When teaching a class on foot care, place paper cutouts of footprints around the room, perhaps ending at a key message posted. Enlist the whole environment as a teaching tool.

The environment should support your teaching. Plan ahead so that handouts and materials to be distributed are well organized for easy referencing and accessibility. Be prepared. Before leading a group, you might consider practicing delivering a mini-presentation to colleagues to confirm that the use of audiovisual aids, lighting, sound, your voice projection, and other elements all work well in a particular room. Safety is a priority. Have supplies available to treat emergencies such as a hypoglycemic reaction.

Disabilities

People with disabilities may actually be another population experiencing health disparities.[107] The Standards of Care[4] suggest that it is incumbent on the provider to ensure that DSME is available for all people with diabetes. Diabetes care and education specialists can play a key role in the care of individuals with disabilities and diabetes by providing DSME in a way that enables them to achieve behavioral change goals similar to those of persons with no current disability.[91] Disabilities do not necessarily preclude effective diabetes self-management.

People who have disabilities and diabetes are usually capable of caring for themselves when they are provided with appropriate adaptive DSME tools and techniques. Physical factors identified in the assessment—mobility, visual acuity, hearing, manual dexterity, alertness, attention span, ability to concentrate, mental health status (including depression), and other special needs or limitations, either physical or psychological—must be considered when implementing DSME. The process and the content must be both accessible and meaningful for the person with diabetes with disabilities. The ADCES supports application of universal design to DSME programs in general and to consumer medical products.[108]

In Practice Tip: Definition of Universal Design

The design of products, environments, and services to be effectively and efficiently used by persons with a wide range of abilities to the greatest extent possible, without adaptation or specialized design.[108]

In 1990, the Americans with Disabilities Act was enacted to offer protection to those with disabilities in the workplace, healthcare setting, and general community.[109] Specifically, the act prohibits discrimination against those with disabilities and ensures they are afforded the same opportunities related to employment, services, commercial and public facilities, and transportation as those without disabilities. This act further defines the rights of those with disabilities:

- A right to reasonable accommodations to make goods, services, and facilities available
- Access to the goods, services, facilities, accommodations, privileges, and advantages available to those without disabilities, provided this is appropriate for the individual

The presence of a disability must be incorporated into the entire education process. Assessment of individual capability, planning that incorporates accommodations specific to the person, implementation of the plan that includes ongoing evaluation, and subsequent modification as needed are key components of an education intervention designed for success. Additionally, including others who assist in the care of the person with a disability can provide helpful insight about the person's capabilities and challenges, while also educating the person about appropriate diabetes management. Community and professional organizations that support the needs of those with disabilities can be excellent resources for materials, adaptive devices, and general information about the issues to be considered in dealing with a particular disability. In addition, several of these organizations offer support resources for both the person with diabetes and his or her support network.

Working With a Special Population: Hearing Impaired

- Arrange the room in a way that does not block the view of the ASL (American Sign Language) interpreter. All participants must be able to view the interpreter whenever you and the interpreter are speaking.
- Write out medication names and other medical terms and keep them posted during the class so the interpreter can simply point to them rather than having to spell out each name and term letter by letter.
- Be sure to address questions and answers to the participant and not to the interpreter.
- Visual tools are extremely important for this population. These include props, handouts, slides, freehand drawings, and well-written instructions for completing paperwork.

Identifying and Addressing Barriers

Barriers are factors that interfere with disease self-management, for example, stress, lack of social support, and environmental factors such as unavailability of grocery stores or parks in the neighborhood.

In Practice Tip: Addressing Barriers

A simple question, "What's standing in the way of your taking care of your diabetes?" is a great lead-in to help the person with diabetes identify barriers to achieving his or her goals.

Barriers to successful implementation of the DSME plan and achievement of identified goals may appear at each step of the process. For instance, a person's lack of follow-through with a plan may be misinterpreted by a provider as a lack of engagement when it is actually related to a barrier to achieving DSME goals.[110] Ngo-Metzger and colleagues studied the relationship of financial burden, medication costs, and glucose management in more than 1,000 low-income white, Latino, and Asian individuals with type 2 diabetes.[111] Thirty percent to 50% of the study participants "reported taking less medication than prescribed because of cost." In this study, poor medication participation seemed to be the mediating factor between the person's perceived financial burden and poor glucose management.

Barriers related to access to care, finances, limitations on number and frequency of visits, functional health literacy, comorbid conditions (ie, depression or chronic pain), acute illness or hospitalization, and disability have been identified, along with social or cultural barriers. Issues related to access may be more prevalent in rural areas versus urban settings. When implementing DSME it is important to work with the individual, the individual's support system, and outside resources and providers for assistance in removing the barriers. Common barriers and tips for addressing them are listed in Table 2.14.

Being an Agile Educator

Imagine the following scenario: Four people sit around the table listening to the diabetes care and education specialist discuss the possible complications from diabetes. Suddenly one person begins to cry. The educator hands the person a tissue and continues to flip through the slides, recognizing that the session must cover this content to be able to move to the next lesson. There is also a curriculum checklist that must be completed.

Whose agenda was addressed? What would you have done? Is this an opportunity for additional education and support, or is it a distraction that is interfering with the planned lesson?

Educators frequently must find a balance between the volume of information and skills to be addressed and the constraints of time and participant needs. Being an agile educator means using highly refined assessment skills, even after the assessment stage. It also means reacting to situations and shifting priorities as needs change.

In this scenario, how different it would have been if the educator had stopped to explore the impact of the lesson on the individual. How powerful it would have been to take the chance to debrief what diabetes means, how to achieve a new normal, how fears might become barriers to care, and how to overcome those barriers. How much richer the learning experience might have been for all the participants.

Being an agile educator means putting the learner's needs ahead of the planned lesson or curriculum. It means assessment skills continue throughout the education process.

Being an agile educator also means being a lifelong learner about education tips and techniques. It means cross-pollinating with other teaching disciplines to adapt approaches to the education of adults, adolescents, and children. So where might a diabetes care and education specialist go for inspiration? Look beyond the diabetes literature to adult learning, professional training, or continuing education. Even resources from higher education can provide ideas that the educator can adjust and modify for a diabetes education class. Table 2.15 provides some possible resources to get you started.

TABLE 2.14 Addressing Barriers to DSME

Barrier	*Tips for Addressing the Barrier*
Access to care: may include a lack of referral or availability of DSME, lack of transportation, financial issues	Outreach to providers about importance of DSME; link patient to community resources; support availability of diabetes education in provider's office. Include key messages in community campaigns (eg, NDEP's ABC message).
Finances	Link patient to community resources; several pharmaceutical companies and diabetes education supply companies have uninsured and underinsured patient assistance programs. Develop a plan with the patient that works within his or her means.
Comorbid conditions (depression, chronic pain)	Work collaboratively with primary care provider and other care providers related to the comorbidity. Individualize strategies related to the comorbidity.
Acute illness or hospitalization	Sessions should be short. Give small segments over several days. Prioritize content to what is necessary for the patient to learn to be safely discharged.
Health literacy	Assume low level of health literacy when choosing materials for DSME; simplify information; use additional strategies other than print; use clear and plain language.
Cultural beliefs and attitudes	Individualized approach. Recognize and respect social and cultural barriers. Help patient develop an action plan for working within these cultural boundaries. For example, in some cultures not being willing to eat traditional foods may be a sign of disrespect. Help the patient develop and implement an action plan with this in mind.
Disabilities	Make programs accessible without needing special adaptations if possible; communicate among all healthcare team members, sharing the effects of the disability on DSME; help patient acquire assistive devices and/or appropriate self-management supplies if necessary.
Time constraints and competing priorities	Make sessions short and accessible. Consider technology as a tool, using webcasts or conference calls. Make timing of sessions flexible by working around the schedules of patients.

TABLE 2.15 Education Resources to Inspire the Diabetes Care and Education Specialist

Teaching resource	*Web site*
Creative training techniques	https://www.bobpikegroup.com/
Brain-based teaching strategies	https://bowperson.com/
"How to captivate an motivate adult learners"	https://www.cdc.gov/trainingdevelopment/pdf/AdultLearningGuide_508.pdf
Teaching strategies from higher education	https://www.facultyfocus.com/
Technology tools for teaching adults and children	https://www.freetech4teachers.com/
Adding games to teaching	http://www.thiagi.com/
Training magazine	https://trainingmag.com/

Source: On the Internet. Last accessed 14 Jan 2020.

Providing Support Following DSME

As part of DSME a personalized follow-up plan is developed by the person with diabetes and the diabetes care and education specialist[4] (Standard 8). In practice, in addition to educating persons with diabetes on and promoting the importance of the Standards of Care and Clinical Practice Recommendations, the diabetes care and education specialist may be the one who helps facilitate access to important aspects of care like a dilated eye exam or flu shot or important risk reduction resources like smoking cessation or weight loss classes. As previously discussed, ongoing self-management support is necessary to sustain behavior change and is now an emphasis of the National Standards for Diabetes Self-Management Education and Support.[4] The type of support provided can include behavioral, psychosocial, or clinical. The diabetes care and education specialist should advocate for access to diabetes support groups, camps, and other community resources. Communication back to the referring provider includes the person's goals and the plan for ongoing self-management support. While the primary responsibility for DSME rests with the diabetes education team, it is very helpful to the individual to receive ongoing reinforcement and support for his or her evolving self-management plan from the entire healthcare team.[4]

One example of DSMS is the use of "Graduate School," a support group of people who have completed DSME classes. They choose topics based on their interests and needs. The group is interactive and offers opportunities for discussion and sharing. Celebrations are shared each month and are primarily tied to success in behavior change. This support group could take place face-to-face or through social media interest groups.[112–114]

Community approaches to diabetes awareness, prevention, and advocacy can be a successful approach to DSMS. Health fairs are excellent for reaching out into the community and providing basic diabetes information and awareness. Additionally, they serve as a link to diabetes education services. Information about DSME programs and the importance of DSME for successful diabetes management is shared. School-based interventions are an opportunity to make an impact at an early age. Age-specific programs related to diabetes prevention and awareness can be presented to most any school-aged child.

Examples of Community Approaches

- School Walk for Diabetes, ADA: In addition to the fund-raising efforts for diabetes research, the children participate in interactive classes and a walk or physical activity highlighting the importance of physical activity in diabetes prevention. The ADA provides lesson plans and teaching materials in its School Walk campaign.[115]
- Workplace or faith-based community diabetes programs are offered as an employee benefit or as part of faith community health initiatives.

Diabetes care and education specialists are often called on to participate in advocacy related to diabetes prevention and awareness, and barriers to care or systems changes. Examples include the following:

- Advocate for the removal of barriers that stand in the way of children self-administering insulin or checking blood glucose during the school day.
- Speak to the mayor of the person with diabetes' community about building sidewalks in neighborhoods so that persons with diabetes (and all community members) can successfully meet their behavior goal related to being active.
- Meet with legislators and ask them to include reimbursement for certified diabetes care and education specialists to improve access to care for the many Medicare recipients.

Such examples demonstrate how diabetes care and education specialists provide DSMS at an organizational level. These examples are also concrete ways that educators meet the competencies identified in the ADCES *Competencies for Diabetes* and Education Specialists[8]

Summary for Implementation

A key to effective implementation of DSME and DSMS is building relationships with the person with diabetes and his or her support persons, identifying and individualizing appropriate goals and a realistic time frame, and implementing the plan. This sets the stage for supporting the individual's quest to achieve goals established in the collaboratively developed plan, leading to improved care and evaluation of both individual and program outcomes.

Evaluation/Monitoring

Evaluation/monitoring is the fifth step in the DSME process. The diabetes care and education specialist documents each step in the DSME process, from assessment to goal setting, planning, and implementation. Recording of this ongoing education process supports each step of the DSME process and provides data for individual and program evaluation. Standard 9 of the National Standards for Diabetes Self-Management Education and Support states that "the provider(s) of DSMES services will monitor and communicate whether participants are achieving their personal diabetes self-management goals and other outcome(s) to evaluate the effectiveness of the educational intervention(s), using appropriate measurement techniques."[4] To facilitate evaluation, educators must document the individual's assessment, education plan, intervention, and follow-up status in his or her permanent confidential education record.[4,7,116] The more complete the documentation, the more accurate and actionable the individual or program evaluation will be.

Evaluation should be considered throughout the education process. Whether the educator is evaluating an individual's outcomes or the success of a program, the approaches and processes are similar.

Understanding What to Document

Clear documentation provides the necessary data to make decisions about individual and program outcomes. Quality documentation is relevant, accurate, and timely. Table 2.16 describes the information to be included at each step to ensure accurate, quality documentation throughout the DSME process.

Documentation might be organized around the AADE7 Self-Care Behaviors®.[3] These standards complement the National Standards for Diabetes Self-Management Education and Support by recognizing that behavior change is the unique outcome measurement for DSME. These measures can be used to determine the effectiveness of DSME at the individual, group, and population levels:

- Healthy coping
- Healthy eating
- Being active
- Taking medication
- Monitoring
- Reducing risks
- Problem solving

Diabetes self-care behaviors should be evaluated at baseline and then at regular intervals following the initial education program. The continuum of outcomes, including learning, behavioral, clinical, satisfaction, and health status, should be assessed to demonstrate the inter-relationship between DSMES and behavior change in the care of individuals with diabetes (see Figure 2.5). Individual outcomes are used to guide the intervention and improve care for that individual. The aggregate population outcomes are used to guide programmatic services and continuous quality improvement (CQI) activities for the DSME program and the population it serves.

Evaluation

Diabetes care and education specialists are in a position to promote healthy lifestyles. Educators participate in health behavior change by integrating disease-state knowledge, educational theories, and health behavioral models. The educator role includes behavior-change facilitator, goal-setting coach, organizer of the learning environment (space, sequence, and materials), and evaluator. As an evaluator, the educator ensures educational programs are accountable to the learner and his or her family and to consumers in the health service community. This accountability is ensured by evaluation in the form of individual objectives and health outcomes for DSME as step 5 of the educational process. Evaluation is a process that provides evidence that what is done makes a value-added difference in the service/care provided. Evaluation is defined as a systematic process by which the worth or value of something—in this case, teaching, learning, and support—is judged. The outcome of education for the learner must be measurably effective.

It is the diabetes care and education specialist's responsibility to ensure that the evaluation is based on

DSMES Core Outcome Measures (Diabetes Self-Care Behaviors)	*Outcomes Measurement Process*			
	Measurement/ Assessment		*Monitoring*	*Management*
	Immediate Outcome Learning and Barrier Resolution	*Intermediate Outcome/Behavior Change*	*Recommended Interval Between Measurement*	*Outcomes Information Used to Drive Decision Making and the Delivery of Care*
	• Knowledge • Skills • Barriers	• Measures • Methods of Measurement	• Learning Outcomes • Behavioral Outcomes	• Behavior • Barrier Identification • Barrier Resolution • Behavior Change

Source: Adapted from Association of Diabetes Care and Education Specialists (ADCES). An effective model of diabetes care and education: revising the AADE7 self-care behaviors®. Published online ahead of print, Feb 2020. Diabetes Educ. doi: https://doi.org/10.1177/0145721719894903.

FIGURE 2.5 DSMES Outcome Measures (Diabetes Self-Care Behaviors)

TABLE 2.16 Documentation of the DSME Process

DSME Process	*What to Document*
Step 1: Assessment	• Date and time of assessment • Pertinent medical history from referring providers, person with diabetes, and family members/ support persons • Comparison of data collected with standards • Person's attitude, health beliefs, values, perceptions, and readiness to change • Knowledge or level of understanding, expectation of learning self-care behaviors, and pertinent clinical or functional outcomes • Psychosocial status • Psychomotor skills
Step 2: Goal setting	• Date and time • Specific treatment and behavioral goals and expected outcomes as identified as part of the assessment process
Step 3: Planning	• Date and time • Recommended interventions and instructional strategies to be used, and who on the care team will provide those interventions
Step 4: Implementation	• Date and time interventions provided • Description of interventions provided, including educational materials used, and receptivity/ understanding of the person with diabetes • Referrals made, resources used, and communication with referring provider (if appropriate) • Rationale for discharge/discontinuation of care, if appropriate
Step 5: Evaluation/ monitoring	• Date and time • Specific outcomes measured (ie, learning, behavioral, clinical, and health status) and results • Progress toward goals and/or barriers to achieving goals

Source: Adapted from Association of Diabetes Care and Education Specialists, *Competencies for Diabetes Care and Education Specialists* (Chicago: Association of Diabetes Care and Education Specialists, Forthcoming).

objective assessment of collecting quantitative and qualitative data. The more the process is rooted in evaluation principles, the greater the confidence in the objectivity, meaningfulness, and usefulness of the evaluation. The timing of the evaluation determines the type of evaluation used. The 2 types are formative (or process) and summative (or outcomes) evaluation.

Formative Evaluation

The purpose of formative or process evaluation is to make adjustments in the educational process as they are needed. Process evaluation is integral to the education process and is an ongoing component of assessment, planning, and implementation. The scope is limited to a learning experience such as a class or workshop. Formative evaluation is used for the person's experience as well as the program's outcomes. Sample questions for each are included in Table 2.17.

Summative Evaluation

The purpose of summative or outcomes evaluation is to determine the effects or outcomes of teaching or program efforts. Its intent is to sum what happened as a result of education or support. Some guiding questions in outcomes evaluation are listed in Table 2.17.

Both process (formative) and outcomes (summative) evaluation should be used for diabetes self-management education.

It is worthwhile to note that while assessment and evaluation are interrelated and often used interchangeably, they are not synonymous. The process of assessment is to gather, summarize, interpret, and use data to determine a direction for action. The process of evaluation is to gather, summarize, and interpret data to determine the extent to which an action was successful. Evaluation is a value judgment that attaches meaning to the data obtained by measurement and gathered through assessment. It is guided by professional judgment and involves interpreting the accumulated information and how it can be used.

Formative and summative evaluations provide the educator with data to make decisions and to make needed changes in the curriculum. With systematic collection of information about the activities, characteristics, and outcomes of programs, judgments can be made about the program to improve its effectiveness and/or enable informed decision making for future program development.[4] While program evaluation is discussed in detail in chapter 11, this chapter will address evaluation as applied to the individual person with diabetes.

Individual Evaluation

Evaluation is the final step in the DSME process, before the process cycles again into reassessment, goal setting, planning, and implementation. At the individual level, assessment and evaluation examine processes and outcomes to determine whether an individual has achieved his or her behavior-change goals and health outcomes.[7,96] Together at each encounter the educator and the person with diabetes review the progress toward the individual's established goals. Individuals receive feedback and support. The purpose of individual evaluation is not to find weakness or fault in the plan or the execution. Rather, individual evaluation is a time for feedback, reflection and further planning. It holds an element of lifelong learning and goal adjustment.

TABLE 2.17 Distinguishing Between Forms of Evaluation

Type of Evaluation	*Participant Experience*	*Program Results*
Formative (or Process)	• Is there enough time for participants to ask questions? • Is the information in class consistent with information included in handouts? • Should additional opportunities be given for return demonstration? • Is the session honoring multiple learning preferences?	• How many people were scheduled for the session and how many attended the session? • Are participants satisfied with the sessions?
Summative (or Outcomes)	• Did the individual(s) learn? • Were behavioral goals achieved? • Did the learner learn the skill taught and use it correctly?	• Was teaching appropriate? • What was the aggregate decrease in weight or A1C? • How many people completed the program? • What was the cost to run the program?

Based on data from groups of individuals, programs can then aggregate the outcome data to make decisions about program changes and upgrades. Aggregate data also contribute to requirements for maintaining program recognition or accreditation.

What Should Be Evaluated?

Guidelines for documentation and evaluation are outlined in Outcome Standards 9 and 10 of the National Standards.[4] These include a structured educational process based on the critical elements of diabetes care that address the critical self-care activities. Elements include educational, behavioral, and psychological elements which target lifestyle change and factors of self-efficacy and empowerment. Behavioral goal setting is an effective strategy to support diabetes self-care.

Of course, goal setting is preliminary to behavior change and outcome evaluation. Goal setting helps the person with diabetes to define what a current behavior is and what a desired behavior would be. People and educators can use individual outcome data to make comparisons against expected or desired results. They can then decide which interventions are most effective and which will need to be adjusted.

Setting goals and monitoring/evaluating progress provide both the educator and the person with diabetes with information on what is working and what is not. Evaluation is based on individual variables but allows others (such as accrediting bodies or program administrators) to see the bigger picture.

Evaluating learner or individual outcomes should consider 3 components: knowledge, skills, and satisfaction. Knowledge involves remembering and applying critical self-care information. Skills include mastering the necessary psychomotor tasks for diabetes self-care. Satisfaction involves the sense of fulfillment with attending the education session or program. Satisfaction can be a powerful motivator in self-care behavior.[117,118]

Use of forms or checklists can help the educator and the PWD track different behaviors, assess progress toward goals, and see how achievement or lack of achievement of those goals impacts treatment outcomes. Forms can be used for both individual-level interventions and group classes. Lorig[119] cautions that in any evaluation it is important to ask yourself 2 questions: "What do you want to know?" and "What difference does it make?" Ask thoughtful evaluation questions that make sense with the goals. In essence, has the intervention changed knowledge, behaviors, attitudes, health status, or healthcare utilization?

Individual outcomes within the AADE7 Self-Care Behaviors® may also be considered in terms of immediate or intermediate outcomes. Documentation should ultimately capture immediate, intermediate and post-intermediate, and long-term outcomes.[3]

- *Immediate outcomes* are those that can be measured at the time the intervention is delivered. Teaching and learning, for example, are immediate outcomes.
- *Intermediate and post-intermediate outcomes* result over time. Behavior change and clinical improvements are examples of intermediate outcomes.
- *Long-term outcomes* result from multiple variables over an extended period of time. Reduction in healthcare costs or complications, and improvements in quality of life are examples of possible long-term outcomes.

Approaches to measuring immediate and intermediate outcomes are listed in Table 2.18.

In addition to measuring knowledge and skills, educators should ascertain whether people are satisfied with their education. One method of determining satisfaction is to provide the person with a brief satisfaction survey. Content includes items related to education and may use a Likert scale (in which information is ranked from 1 to 10). In setting up a satisfaction survey, consider what elements of the education session or program are important in pleasing a person. Do you believe that the environment should be pleasant and conducive to learning? Do you want to learn whether the diabetes care and education specialist's style is facilitating learning? Some typical satisfaction questions are listed in Table 2.19.

The satisfaction survey may be in a paper-and-pencil format that is given at the end of the session or it may be an online survey. Online surveys are inexpensive (even free) and are easy to set up. SurveyMonkey and Zoomerang are 2 examples.

TABLE 2.18 Outcomes for the AADE7 Self-Care Behaviors®

	*Immediate Outcome**			*Intermediate Outcome†*	
	Knowledge	*Skill*	*Barriers*	*Measures*	*Methods of Measurement*
Healthy Coping living with diabetes (psychosocial adaptation)	• Internal and external motivators • Benefits of solution focused problem solving • Active self-management • Value of nurturing support system (peers, online, family, friends) • Individual empowerment • Role as partner with other members of healthcare team	• Goal setting • Problem solving • Coping strategies • Self-efficacy	• Physical • Financial • Emotional • Competing priorities • Lack of support network • Psychosocial distress including diabetes distress • Cognitive including mental health disorders	• Depression score • Stress level • Quality of life (perceived self-efficacy, perceived disease severity, perceived interference of chronic disease) • Functional measurement • Treatment self-efficacy • Level of empowerment • Absenteeism • Presence of support	• Self-report • Skills, Confidence, and Preparedness Index (SCPI)[188–189] Problem Areas in Diabetes (P.A.I.D) • Quality of Life (QOL) tools, such as SF-36 or SF-12 with Appraisal of Diabetes Scale (ADS)[191] • Depression/diabetes distress tools, such as Diabetes Distress Scales (DDS), Parents-DDS, Partners-DDS, T1-DDS or DDS[192]; Beck-Depression-Inventory (BDI); PHQ-9 Cognitive Impairment tools, such as Saint Louis University Mental Status (SLUMS)[193]; Mini-Mental Status Exam (MMSE)
Healthy Eating	• Effect of foods/beverages on metabolic parameters (including blood glucose, lipids, blood pressure, weight, etc) • Sources and distribution of nutrients (nutrient-dense carbohydrates, lean proteins, healthy fats) • Eating Patterns (frequency of meals, timing, portions, etc) • Resources to assist in food choices • Macronutrient composition (quality, quantity, combination, substitutions)	• Meal planning • Portion awareness and management • Planning Strategies (Carb counting, Exchanges, Plate Method, Mindful Eating) • Nutrition Facts Label comprehension • Special situations and problem solving (planning, shopping, meal delivery/kits, eating away from home at work/school/restaurants)	• Environmental factors • Cultural and family Influences • Food and health beliefs • Financial (food security) • Cognitive • Health literacy and numeracy • Emotional • Meal pattern sustainability	• Types of food choices • Amounts consumed • Timing of meals and snacks • Alcohol (with or without food, amount, frequency) • Fluids (adequate hydration) • Effect of food/beverages on metabolic parameters • Progress toward goal achievement	• Observation • Self-report (24-hour recall, typical day, food frequency, food diaries) • Monitoring tools with associated records • Goal setting

(continued)

TABLE 2.18 Outcomes for the AADE7 Self-Care Behaviors® (continued)

	*Immediate Outcome**			*Intermediate Outcome†*	
	Knowledge	*Skill*	*Barriers*	*Measures*	*Methods of Measurement*
Being Active	• Planned exercise (type, duration, intensity, frequency, progression) • Daily movement • Breaking up sedentary time • Safety precautions, such as obtaining pre-participation medical clearance and/or exercise stress testing prior to unaccustomed vigorous activity • Special considerations, such as appropriate footwear	• Appropriate daily movement and physical activity plan • Adjustment of activity with food and medication to maintain glycemic balance • Monitoring of cardiometabolic parameters, data stream, and feedback	• Physical (health conditions, injuries) • Perceived lack of time • Environment, facilities • Fear (hypoglycemia) • Self-efficacy • Lack of enjoyment • Lack of social support	• Type, frequency, duration, and intensity of planned activities • Daily movement • Progress toward goal achievement • Quality of life, health improvement	• Self-report • Goal setting • Monitoring tools and their associated records including digital health tracking and wearable technologies • Quality of life and health assessments • Exercise vital sign (EVS) to evaluate whether weekly goals for physical activity have been met:[194] o On average, how many days per week do you engage in moderate to strenuous exercise (like a brisk walk)?' o On average, how many minutes do you engage in exercise at this level? • Physical activity vital sign (PAVS)[194] when individual is physically active for at least 30 minutes per day: o How many days during the past week have you performed physical activity where your heart beats faster and your breathing is harder than normal for 30 minutes or more? o How many days in a typical week do you perform activity such as this?

Taking Medication	• Name, dose, frequency, and optimal timing of medications • Medication mechanism of action • Common side effects, toxicity • Action for adverse effects • Action for missed dose • Storage, travel, safety, and disposal • Recognition of efficacy, optimal outcomes, and therapeutic goals	• Maintenance of a medication list • Preparation, technique, administration • Safe handling, disposal of equipment • Dose adjustment • Recognition, treatment, prevention of common adverse effects	• Plan complexity (greater than 1 medication or dose daily) • Physical (vision or dexterity) • Financial (medication cost, copay) • Health beliefs (skeptical of benefit, worried about side effects) • Health literacy and numeracy • Cognitive (dose recall, refill initiation) • Psychological (depression, fear, or embarrassment) Change in schedule or work status	• Medication-taking • Prescription filling • Dose accuracy • Glycemic trends • Metabolic trends • Emergency department and hospital utilization • Weight change	• Self-report and medication records • Review of pharmacy refill history • Pill count • Return demonstration (observation, role playing) • Labs (A1C, Total cholesterol, LDL cholesterol, etc) Monitoring tools with associated records (such as records for blood glucose, blood pressure, weight, medication use, etc)

(continued)

TABLE 2.18 Outcomes for the AADE7 Self-Care Behaviors® (continued)

		*Immediate Outcome**		*Intermediate Outcome†*	
	Knowledge	*Skill*	*Barriers*	*Measures*	*Methods of Measurement*
Monitoring	• Monitoring plan/schedule (structured, episodic, continuous, etc) • Appropriate lifestyle data to track • Target values • Safety issues including disposal of lancets • Use of data for decision making • Awareness of body's symptoms (eg, blurred vision, shortness of breath) and/or physical changes (eg, teeth, skin, gums)	• Equipment use and technical care (blood glucose meter, continuous glucose monitor, blood pressure cuff, wearable, mobile app, etc) • Record keeping with note taking • Tracking and reporting body symptoms and physical changes • Interpretation of patient-generated health data	• Physical • Financial • Cognitive • Emotional • Time • Inconvenience • Treatment burden • Health literacy and numeracy • Limited understanding of value of data and how to use it • Lack of interest/ability to use equipment and other tools for self-monitoring	• Frequency of self-monitoring • Schedule of monitoring • "Unscheduled" monitoring (triggered by symptoms, etc) • Number of devices/apps used to support monitoring • Blood glucose values • Time in range (TIR) • Glucose management indicator (GMI) • Blood pressure values • Hours of sleep • Mood status • Amount of time performing physical activity, number of steps • Medication use/insulin doses • Amount of carbohydrate consumed, meal size • Presence of notes that add context to tracked data • Presence of organized data that allows for decision making	• Monitoring tools and their associated records (log book, device memory review, printouts) • Self-report responses to questions/surveys

Reducing Risks	• Safety (sick day plan, driving/machine operation precautions, emergency preparedness) • Standards of care • Therapeutic goals • Symptoms that require attention or follow-up (hypoglycemia, hyperglycemia, rapid weight fluctuation, stroke, heart attack, bleeding gums, vision changes, skin changes) • How to decrease risks/prevent harm (pre-pregnancy counseling, smoking cessation, etc)	• Planning • Monitoring of blood glucose (self, continuous) • Maintaining personal care record • Performing self-foot exam • Performing self-skin exam • Self-monitoring of blood pressure • Use of health apps and web portals • Ability to adjust food, medication, and activity (to increase the amount of time glucose is in range) • Recognition of concerning symptoms or changes in health • Ability to determine when health requires care from healthcare team (emergency vs. non-emergency)	• Financial (lack of personal resources; insurance barriers such as high deductible, underinsured, step therapy requirements; insufficient monitoring supplies; food insecurity) • Unawareness of disease process and its seriousness • Lack of access to DSMES services or healthcare providers • Therapeutic inertia • Physical (hypoglycemia unawareness) • Cognitive • Emotional • Lack of self-efficacy and coping strategies • Poor support network including lack of rapport with provider • Perceived lack of time	• Glycemic trends • Frequency of low or high blood glucose • Frequency of contact with healthcare provider for problem resolution • Missed days from work, school, or related activities • Number of visits to the emergency department or hospitalizations • A1C • Lipids • Blood pressure • Kidney tests (urine albumin excretion and serum creatinine for eGFR, urine albumin creatinine ratio) • Weight and Body Mass Index (BMI) • Scheduled vs. attended visits with healthcare team • Dilated eye exam • Immunization status (flu vaccine, pneumonia vaccine, hepatitis B) • Screening for hearing loss • Dental exam • Sleep study • Smoking status • Frequency of foot self-exam • Comprehensive foot exam • Screening for sexual dysfunction • Neuropathy • Aspirin therapy • Frequency of medication adjustment • Sick day plan	• Self-report • Chart or exam code audit • Review of monitoring records • Demonstration of self-care activities

(continued)

TABLE 2.18 Outcomes for the AADE7 Self-Care Behaviors® (continued)

		*Immediate Outcome**		*Intermediate Outcome†*	
	Knowledge	*Skill*	*Barriers*	*Measures*	*Methods of Measurement*
Problem Solving	• Complexity and challenges of diabetes • Changes in diabetes throughout the lifecycle • Changes in diabetes as it progresses • Relevant diabetes self-management education and support knowledge items (see other behaviors)	• Relevant diabetes self-management education and support skill items • Ability to recognize/identify problem • Ability to generate potential solution • Ability to transfer past experience(s) • Ability to finalize solution • Ability to measure/monitor results	• Cognitive • Health literacy and numeracy • Lack of self-efficacy and coping strategies • Financial • Time • Emotional • Lack of/limited support network • Physical	• Glycemic trends including TIR and GMI • A1C • Other health indicators (weight, blood pressure, etc) • Frequency of phone calls/visits to provider • Quality of life indicators (Missed days of work/school, frequency of hypoglycemia, etc) • Confidence level (in situational problem solving) • Progress towards goal achievement • Level of diabetes distress • Frequency of acute complications • PAID score • Frequency of medication • adjustment • Self-report • Return demonstration/Teach-back • Goal setting	• Self-report • Return demonstration/Teach-back • Goal setting • Monitoring tools and associated records (data from meter, continuous glucose monitor, device, app, lab) • Health Problem Solving Scale (HPSS) • Summary of Diabetes Self-Care Activities scale (SDSCA)

*Immediate outcomes are those that can be measured at the time of the intervention (eg, learning).

†Intermediate outcomes result over time (eg, behavior change) and require more than a single measurement.

Source: Adapted from Association of Diabetes Care and Education Specialists (ADCES). An effective model of diabetes care and education: revising the AADE7 self-care behaviors®. Published online ahead of print, Feb 2020. Diabetes Educ. doi: https://doi.org/10.1177/0145721719894903.

TABLE 2.19 Sample Statements in a Satisfaction Survey

Environment	The classroom was comfortable. The registration process was easy. There was adequate parking.
Educators	The educator was effective in teaching me to use my pump. The educator provided enough time to practice the skill.
Education	As a result of the education, I am better able to take care of my diabetes. The handouts were easy to follow.
Value	I received good value for my money. I would recommend this program to other people with diabetes.

Case: The DSME Process

LC, a 60-year-old man, was diagnosed with type 2 diabetes less than a year ago. Upon referral from his primary care provider (PCP), he was scheduled to meet with the diabetes care and education specialist. Information provided includes the following:

- A1C: 7.8%
- Metformin 500 mg twice a day

Assessment

At the initial DSME visit, the educator began with an assessment of LC's learning needs, self-management behaviors (including current nutrition, physical activity, and medication-taking practices), and current treatment plan. The educator also assessed health literacy and physical and psychosocial factors impacting learning. LC indicated he was motivated to learn what he needed to know to prevent complications, because his mother had "bad diabetes." LC has not received previous diabetes education. He looked for information on a few Internet sites but found it overwhelming. He has not had a dilated eye exam in over 4 years. He is willing to monitor but is a little unsure of how to use the equipment and when he should perform the blood glucose checks.

Goal Setting and Plan

At LC's initial DSME visit, the diabetes care and education specialist used the information provided by LC's PCP and gathered in his assessment to develop an education plan to meet his needs. The diabetes care and education specialist engaged LC in shared decision making, and it was mutually decided to begin with some basic diabetes information and a review of self-monitoring of blood glucose. They also agreed on the importance of scheduling an eye exam.

His overall stated goal was to "decrease risk of complications."

Learning Goal

Review blood glucose monitoring including correct use of meter, frequency, and timing of testing.

Goals

AADE7 Self-Care Behavior®: Monitoring

- Monitor once a day at alternating times (fasting, before meals, 2 hours after meals, and before bed) for 2 weeks and write down results in a glucose logbook.
- Call diabetes care and education specialist to report blood glucose results in 2 weeks.

AADE7 Self-Care Behavior®: Reducing risks

- Within the next week, call to schedule an appointment for an eye exam.

Implementation

The educator shared basic information about diabetes, promoting a healthy lifestyle, and reducing risks of complications, including healthy checkups and recommended tests and exams. LC also was educated on the importance and significance of monitoring, including guidelines for frequency, keeping records, meaning of results, and reporting results to his healthcare team. He demonstrated appropriate monitoring technique. Below is a sample of a piece of documentation from the education record.

For his DSMS plan, LC chose to subscribe to a popular diabetes magazine. To extend his learning, he was given a

(continued)

Case: The DSME Process (continued)

diabetes self-care workbook, which had additional references. LC agreed to the plan that he would call the educator with his blood glucose results in 2 weeks, and a return visit was scheduled in 1 month.

Communication Back to the Referring PCP

The communication back to the referring PCP included a summary of the visit, goals of the person with diabetes, and the plan for ongoing self-management support. The communication was sent through the electronic medical record with an alert to notify the PCP that the visit had been completed.

Follow-Up Phone Call

LC phoned the diabetes care and education specialist 2 weeks after the initial visit with monitoring results as planned. During the phone call he reported his blood glucose records, and he also mentioned that he noticed some high numbers after a meal of spaghetti and meatballs. He learned that exercising on his treadmill lowered his blood glucose levels. He was pleased to report that his weight had dropped 2 lb over the last 2 weeks. His educator agreed that he was doing well. LC said that at the next visit, he would like to learn more tips that will help him avoid complications like his mother had. He would especially like more help with choosing what to eat and learning how his food affects his blood glucose. He also reported that he has not had a chance to schedule his eye exam.

Evaluation of the Goals of the Person With Diabetes

AADE7 Self-Care Behavior®: Monitoring

- Monitor once a day at alternating times (fasting, before meals, 2 hours after meals, and before bed) for 2 weeks and write down results in a glucose logbook.
- Call diabetes care and education specialist to report blood glucose results in 2 weeks.

AADE7 Self-Care Behavior®: Reducing risks

- Within the next week, call to schedule an appointment for an eye exam.

Monitoring Behavior Evaluated

Blood glucose records shared with the educator showed that LC had checked his blood glucose at least once a day at different times of the day. He called to report the results as planned. His goal of monitoring once a day will continue, and he will bring his blood glucose log to the follow-up visit.

Reducing Risks Behavior Evaluated

LC did not schedule his eye exam within the week, so he and the educator adjusted his goals to state the following: Prior to next appointment with the diabetes care and education specialist, schedule an appointment for an eye exam.

Follow-Up Visit

LC brought his blood glucose logbook to his follow-up visit. He and the educator reviewed the logbook together, and LC again mentioned that he noticed that certain foods affect his blood glucose more than others. He is interested in learning more about carbohydrate counting and getting help with his personal meal plan. The educator updated LC's assessment and provided him with some basic carbohydrate information. He was able to identify a list of foods containing carbohydrate. A referral to a registered dietitian (RD) for medical nutrition therapy (MNT) was arranged with his PCP's office. He would like to get additional

Assessment Summary Date: 5/19/20	*Behavioral Objectives*	*Instruction Given*					*Goal Reached*
		Insert total time spent with person with diabetes					
		90 min					
		Date: 5/19/20	*Date:*	*Date:*	*Date:*	*Date:*	*Date/Initial*
	Monitoring						
1 2 3 0	Demonstrates monitoring skills						5/19/20 LM
1 2 3 0	Monitors BG according to plan						
1 2 3 0	Uses results of monitoring						

1 = completed, 2 = review needed, 3 = full education needed, 0 = not applicable

Case: The DSME Process (continued)

DSME from a diabetes class since he enjoys participating in groups. A referral to a group class was made as well. LC wondered whether there were other things he should be tracking to decrease his risk of complications. The educator reviewed the impact of blood pressure and weight on long-term health and suggested that LC monitor these things routinely. The educator showed LC how to accurately check his blood pressure. LC decided to weigh himself every week and check his blood pressure each evening. In addition to communicating a summary of the visit to LC's PCP, information was shared with the RD and the diabetes education team leading the classes.

Learning Goal

LC's learning goal is to use carbohydrate counting in his meal planning.

AADE7 Self-Care Behavior®: Healthy eating

- Practice carbohydrate counting for at least 1 meal a day by identifying and writing down foods that contain carbohydrate.

AADE7 Self-Care Behavior®: Reducing risks

- Check weight weekly on Friday and record.
- Check blood pressure each evening and record.

TABLE 2.20 Data Collection Tools

Method	*Examples of Outcomes Collected*	*Easy to Use?*	*Yields Reliable Data?*	*High Response Rate?*
Survey Method used to question individuals in writing, face-to-face, by phone, by mail, or online	Learning; behavior change; quality of life; satisfaction	Yes; can be designed to be simple and easy to use	Yes; although respondents' interpretation of survey questions can vary; surveys more reliable if surveyor is not the diabetes care and education specialist	Depends; telephone and face-to-face surveys can have a high response rate while mail and online surveys tend to have low response rates
Chart/File Audit Review of closed, open, or computerized medical records to retrieve information	Lab data (A1C, lipids); process data (eye or foot exam)	Depends; paper chart review can be labor intensive and time intensive	Depends on skill of individuals doing the review	Yes
Checklist Data collection sheet for gathering concurrent information during a study	Behavior change; process and implementation tasks	Yes; can be designed to be simple and easy to use	Depends; all people who will be completing the checklist during the data collection must be trained on how to use the data collection instrument	Depends on the cooperation and availability of the personnel completing the forms
Time Study Concurrent information about time to complete a process such as turnaround time	Cycle time to schedule a person with diabetes for a visit	Usually very time intensive and labor intensive	Depends; all people who will be completing the time study during the data collection must be trained on how to use the instrument	Depends on the cooperation and availability of the personnel completing the study

Source: Adapted from K Mulcahy, "Management of Diabetes Education Programs," in MJ Franz, ed, *A Core Curriculum for Diabetes Educators*, 5th ed (Chicago: American Association of Diabetes Educators, 2003), 203.

Tools to Track Progress

In addition to tools for tracking satisfaction, there are a variety of means for collecting information about knowledge and skills outcomes. These are listed in Table 2.20

Making Use Evaluation Data of Person With Diabetes

Once evaluation information is collected, it is time to sift through the data and make follow-up decisions. The educator first revisits the person's goals and then asks a series of questions.[73]

What is the individual's assessment of the goal?

- Did the person feel he or she achieved the goal?
- How would the person rate his or her progress?

What is your collaborative assessment of the goal?

- Was the goal appropriate for the person?
- Did the person have adequate time to achieve the goal?
- Did the goal achieve the expected outcome?
- Did that outcome impact the diabetes treatment plan?
- If so, does therapy need to change?

What should the next steps be?

- Should the goal be changed or continued?
- Should additional goals be added or other goals changed?
- When will new goals be evaluated?
- What other changes in the diabetes treatment plan need to occur to support the goal(s)?

Answers to open-ended questions provide detail and depth. For some of the questions, the educator might also use a rating scale. For example, the person can be asked to rate his or her progress on a Likert scale from 1 to 10 (1 = did not meet goal; 10 = achieved goal) or given word choices (eg, met goal most of the time, met goal some of the time, did not meet goal, or changed goal).

Once the analysis is complete, the educator and the person with diabetes establish the next goal and implement the next set of tactics to reach the goal. In doing this, the educator models for the person one form of problem solving and how future decisions can be based on past experience.

Finally, the educator sends a summary of the individual's outcomes and recommendations for future DSME and medical follow-up to the referring provider. The information can also be reviewed by the educational team and summarized (without identifying details) and presented to the advising group, directors, or administrators for use in program reviews and program outcome studies.

Evaluation/Monitoring Summary

Documentation and evaluation are critical components of the DSME process. Both are considered standards of diabetes care.[4] The information is needed to evaluate both outcomes related to the individual and a DSME program's progress toward achieving its goals. Without such documentation, providing ongoing education that evolves to match the changing needs of the person with diabetes is difficult.

For individuals and programs to be successful, the following elements are required:[3]

- Outcomes measurement: consistent measurement of specific indicators
- Outcomes monitoring: measurement of those indicators at specified intervals
- Outcomes management: use of those outcomes to drive educational and clinical decision making

Standardized tools and methods to track and report outcomes can help the educational process and improve the health of individuals and the quality of programs when the documentation is reviewed regularly.

Conclusion

Diabetes self-management education is a critical component of care for people with diabetes. There is building evidence that DSME is effective in reducing A1C.[96] It is not a singular event but an ongoing process of facilitating knowledge, skill, and ability necessary for self-care leading to improved health outcomes and quality of life. The process outlined in this chapter includes assessment, goal setting, planning, implementation, and evaluation/monitoring that is based on the DSME process outlined in the National Standards for Diabetes Self-Management Education and Support.

The DSME process described in this chapter begins with assessing an individual with diabetes or prediabetes to determine understanding, knowledge, and experiences of the person. Assessment is the cornerstone of diabetes education and management and relies on critical thinking and clinical judgment. Next, empowerment models are employed to explore the needs and goals of the individual. An empowerment approach also engages the person's family or caregivers in support of the individual's self-management efforts. The process is dynamic and ongoing. A variety of healthcare professionals are responsible for assessing, planning, and implementing appropriate healthcare education that promotes longevity and productivity for the people served. Appropriate education incorporates information from a comprehensive curriculum of content areas that is tailored to the individual and delivered in a manner that both facilitates learning and honors cultural and learning preferences. Those implementing the plan to provide diabetes education must then adapt teaching tactics, methods, and materials to be sensitive to the learning capability, readiness, needs, and cultural influences of the learner.

Diabetes self-management education incorporates educational, behavioral, and psychosocial strategies to implement the plan. For this reason, DSME is ideally delivered collaboratively by a multidisciplinary team with a comprehensive plan of care. Team members work toward collaborative objectives using expertise in clinical care of diabetes, MNT, learning and teaching strategies, and psychosocial and behavioral aspects of diabetes self-management.

Competencies for Diabetes Care and Educations Specialists address the process of assessment, goal setting, planning, implementation, and evaluation of DSME.[8] The components and issues to consider when implementing an education plan were addressed throughout this chapter. In summary, to implement diabetes education successfully, confirm the individual's readiness to learn, identify teaching methods appropriate for the person's literacy level, recognize the importance of cultural influences, and integrate these factors into the education process. Additionally, strive to motivate the people with diabetes you serve by understanding what is important to them and why, helping them identify barriers they may encounter, and working with them to address those barriers. Keep in mind that you cannot "make" someone learn, but inability or unwillingness to learn is not a permanent state.

Documentation and evaluation are critical components of the DSME process. Both are considered to be standards of diabetes care. To maintain continuity of care, it is important to document the person with diabetes' progress in attaining the mutually determined goals. Progress in achieving goals leads to effective reassessment or evaluation. Individual outcomes are the most important elements of DSME.

This chapter considered self-management behaviors as the key outcomes for DSME and thus ideal for evaluation. These self-care behaviors include physical activity, healthy eating, medication taking, monitoring blood glucose, diabetes self-care-related problem solving, reducing risks of acute and chronic complications, and psychosocial aspects of living with diabetes. Standardized tools such as the AADE7 Self-Care Behaviors® Goal Sheet are useful for tracking and reporting outcomes.

Finally, this chapter emphasized the crucial role of the diabetes care and education specialist in applying a systematic process to providing diabetes education and support. Effective care of people with diabetes is dependent on a clinician or educator who continually assesses changes in the individual, the family, and the environment to make the best collaborative decisions about care and support.

Focus on Education

Teaching Strategies

Foster an atmosphere of trust. Maintaining a nonjudgmental attitude improves identification of other teaching opportunities.

Prioritize. A person's goals, interests, and needs guide what to cover and when. There are always more topics and more information to discuss than there is time. Focus on the person's ability to make safe and informed decisions.

Be flexible. Plan to deliver information in several ways, adjusting the teaching plan to accommodate the learner's needs at that time. Avoid information and cognitive overload. Be practical in collaborating on actionable behaviors. It will increase the likelihood of improved outcomes.

Keep the pace. Allow time to discuss goals, application, and next steps. Covering fewer topics and having a behavioral action plan is preferable to covering many topics with no discussion or implementation intentions.

Use novel, engaging approaches to educate. Use effective strategies, not just the latest technology. Low-tech options (drawings, handouts, etc) can be as effective as high-tech options and are an important tool in the diabetes care and education specialist's toolkit. Use technology judiciously and effectively.

Messages for People With Diabetes

Permission to ask as well as answer. No question or answer is silly or dumb. Clarify what each person on the care team needs and ask for help so you have a clear path to progress.

Education is ongoing and lifelong. Diabetes education is not just a onetime event. Take as much time as you need to understand the information and make choices.

Rights and responsibilities. You have the right and responsibility to ask questions, seek clarification, and make decisions and changes in managing your diabetes and overall health. You have the right to know all the choices, alternatives, and potential outcomes of your choices. You have the right to a second opinion, to ask your family or others for advice, and to take as much time as needed.

Health Literacy

Learning principles. Consider learning preferences, learner readiness, and special needs of the learner (vision, concentration, physical health, etc) when determining educational content and delivery. Health literacy is different from reading literacy or mental capacity.

Educational content. Ensure that materials and methods are at the appropriate literacy level. Build on existing knowledge. Move in sequence from simple to more complex information. Materials should reflect sensitivity and awareness of cultural differences. Adjust teaching options to fit the person's style.

Tune in to culture. Be sensitive to differences in cultural, generational, and ethnic backgrounds during assessment. Appropriate tone of voice, rate of questioning, and nonverbal cues are critical in establishing rapport and the success of future educational encounters.

Focus on Practice

Documentation is critical and an ongoing process. Documentation chronicles past care and outcomes and serves as a road map for future encounters and expected outcomes. Create documentation that allows multiple team members to accumulate information and data to foster reinforcement of the self-management plan and to evaluate the program.

Evaluation. Data can be captured, reviewed, and evaluated more easily when tools are consistent. Behavioral outcomes, along with program data, are used to update curriculum, educational materials, delivery methods, and instructors to enhance effectiveness of care in meeting program goals.

References

1. Burke SD, Sherr D, Lipman RD. Partnering with diabetes educators to improve patient outcomes. Diabetes Metab Syndr Obes. 2014;7:45-53. doi:10.2147/DMSO.S40036.
2. Association of Diabetes Care and Education Specialists (ADCES). An effective model of diabetes care and education: revising the AADE7 self-care behaviors®. Published online ahead of print, Feb 2020. Diabetes Educ. doi: https://doi.org/10.1177/0145721719894903.
3. American Association of Diabetes Educators. Standards for outcomes measurement of diabetes self-management education. Diabetes Educ. 2003;29:804-16.
4. Beck J, Greenwood DA, Blanton L, et al. 2017 National standards for diabetes self-management education and support. Diabetes Educ. 2017; 43(5):449-64. DOI: 10.1177/0145721717722968.
5. Haas L, Maryniuk M, Beck J, et al. National standards for diabetes self-management education and support. Diabetes Care. 2014;37(1):S144-53.
6. Funnell MM, Brown TL, Childs BP. National standards for diabetes self-management education and support. Diabetes Educ. 2007;33(4):599-614.
7. Powers M, Bardsley J, Cypress M, et al. Diabetes self-management education and support in type 2 diabetes: a joint position statement of the American Diabetes Association, the American Association of Diabetes Educators, and the Academy of Nutrition and Dietetics. Diabetes Educ. 2015;41(4):417-30.
8. Association of Diabetes Care and Education Specialists. Competencies for Diabetes Care and Education Specialists. Chicago: American Association of Diabetes Educators; Forthcoming.
9. Pichert JA, Schlundt DG. Assessment: gathering information and facilitating engagement. In: Mensing C, ed. The Art and Science of Diabetes Self-Management Education: A Desk Reference for Healthcare Professionals. Chicago: American Association of Diabetes Educators; 2006:578-9.
10. Centers for Disease Control and Prevention. Social determinants of health: Know what affects health. 2018 (cited 2019 Jun 2). On the Internet at: https://www.cdc.gov/socialdeterminants/index.htm.
11. Dendup T, Feng X, Clingan S, Astell-Burt T. Environmental risk factors for developing type 2 diabetes mellitus: A systematic review. Int. J. Environ. Res. Public Health. 2018; 15(1):78. doi: 10.3390/ijerph15010078.
12. Haire-Joshu D, Hill-Briggs F. The next generation of diabetes translation: a path to health equity. Annu Rev Public Health. 2019 Apr 1;40:391-410. doi: 10.1146/annurev-publhealth-040218-044158.

13. Centers for Disease Control and Prevention. Strategies for reducing health disparities. 2016 (cited 2019 Jun 2). On the Internet at: https://www.cdc.gov/minorityhealth/strategies2016/index.html.

14. Agency for Healthcare Research and Quality. 2017 national healthcare quality and disparities report. Rockville, MD: Agency for Healthcare Research and Quality; 2018 September. AHRQ Pub. No. 18-0033-EF. (cited 2019 Jun 2). On the Internet at: https://www.ahrq.gov/sites/default/files/wysiwyg/research/findings/nhqrdr/2017nhqdr.pdf.

15. Lim FA, Brown VR Jr, Justin Kim SM. Addressing health care disparities in the lesbian, gay, bisexual, and transgender population: a review of best practices. Am J Nurs. 2014; 114(6), 24–34. quiz 35, 45. doi:10.1097/01.NAJ.0000450423.89759.36.

16. National LGBT Health Education Center. (n.d.). *Providing quality care to lesbian, gay, bisexual, and transgender patients: An introduction for staff training*. (Cited 2019 Jun 1). On the Internet at: https://www.lgbthealtheducation.org/lgbt-education/learning-modules/.

17. Margolies L, Brown CG. Increasing cultural competence with LGBTQ patients. Nursing. 2019;49(6):34-40. doi: 10.1097/01.NURSE.0000558088.77604.24.

18. National Institute of Diabetes and Digestive and Kidney Diseases. National Diabetes Education Program. (cited 2019 Jun 2). On the Internet at: https://www.niddk.nih.gov/health-information/communication-programs/ndep/health-professionals.

19. Calman N, Hauser D, Schussler L, Crump C. A risk-based intervention approach to eliminate diabetes health disparities. Primary Health Care Research & Development. 2018; 19(5): 518-22. doi:10.1017/S1463423618000075.

20. Adjei Boakye E, Varble A, Rojek R, Peavler O, Trainer A K, Osazuwa-Peters N, Hinyard L. Sociodemographic factors associated with engagement in diabetes self-management education among people with diabetes in the United States. Public Health Reports. 2018;133(6):685–91. https://doi.org/10.1177/0033354918794935.

21. Healthy People 2020. Diabetes (cited 2019 Jun 2). On the Internet at: https://www.healthypeople.gov/2020/topics-objectives/topic/diabetes.

22. Dickinson JK, Guzman SJ, Maryniuk MD, O'Brian CA, Kadohiro JK, Jackson RA, D'Hondt N, Montgomery B, Close KL, Funnell MM. The use of language in diabetes care and education. Diabetes Care. 2017; 40:1790–9 https://doi.org/10.2337/dci17-0041.

23. Aldred C, Scibilia R. Changing the way we talk about diabetes complications. The Plaid Journal. 2018;4(1):26-9. DOI: http://dx.doi.org/10.17125/plaid.2018.111.

24. Cornett S. Assessing and addressing health literacy. Online J Issues Nurs. 2009;14(3, Manuscript 2). DOI: 10.3912/OJIN.Vol14No03Man02.

25. Orem SL, Binkert J, Clancy AL. Appreciative Coaching: A Positive Process for Change. San Francisco: Jossey-Bass; 2007.

26. Kimsey-House H, Kimsey-House K, Sandahl P. Co-Active Coaching. 3rd ed. Boston: Nicholas Brealey Publishing; 2011.

27. Klein DA, Goldenring JM, Adelman WP. HEEADSSS 3.0: The psychosocial interview for adolescents updated for a new century fueled by media. 2014 (cited 2019 Jun 2). On the Internet at: http://contemporarypediatrics.modernmedicine.com/contemporary-pediatrics/content/tags/adolescent-medicine/heeadsss-30-psychosocial-interview-adolesce?page=full.

28. Fulmer T. How to try this: Fulmer SPICES. Am J Nurs. 2007;107(10):40-8.

29. Garnero TL. Providing culturally sensitive diabetes care and education for the lesbian, gay, bisexual, and transgender (LGBT) community. Diabetes Spectrum. 2010;23(3):178-82. https://doi.org/10.2337/diaspect.23.3.178.

30. Landry J. Delivering culturally sensitive care to LGBTQI patients. J Nurs Prac. 2017;13(5): 342-7. DOI: https://doi.org/10.1016/j.nurpra.2016.12.015.

31. Zeh P, Sandhu HK, Cannaby AM, Sturt JA. The impact of culturally competent diabetes care interventions for improving diabetes-related outcomes in ethnic minority groups: a systematic review. Diabet Med. 2012;29(10):1237-52. doi:10.1111/j.1464-5491.2012.03701.x.

32. Palmas W, March D, Darakjy S, Findley SE, Teresi J, Carrasquillo O, Luchsinger JA. Community health worker interventions to improve glycemic control in people with diabetes: a systematic review and meta-analysis. J Gen Intern Med. 2015; 30:1004. https://doi.org/10.1007/s11606-015-3247-0.

33. Benner P, Hughes RG, Sutphen M. Clinical reasoning, decision-making, and action: thinking critically and clinically. In: Hughes RG, ed. Patient safety and quality: An evidence based handbook for nurses. Rockville, Md: Agency for Healthcare Research and Quality; 2008 (cited 2019 Jun 5):1:87-109. On the Internet at: http://archive.ahrq.gov/professionals/clinicians-providers/resources/nursing/resources/nurseshdbk/nurseshdbk.pdf.

34. Koharchik L, Caputi, L, Robb, M, Culleiton, A. Fostering clinical reasoning in nursing students. Am J Nurs. 2015;115(1): 58-61. DOI: 10.1097/01.NAJ.0000459638.68657.9b.

35. Anderson RM. Applied principles of teaching and learning. In: Franz MJ, ed. A Core Curriculum for Diabetes Education: Diabetes Education and Program Management. 4th ed. Chicago: American Association of Diabetes Educators; 2001:3-18.

36. Rubin RR, Napora JP. Behavior change. In: Franz MJ, ed. A Core Curriculum for Diabetes Education: Diabetes Education and Program Management. 4th ed. Chicago: American Association of Diabetes Educators; 2001:72-92.

37. Weinger K, McNeil T, Greenlaw SJ. Behavioral strategies for improving self-management. In: Childs B, Cypress M, Spollet G, eds. Complete Nurse's Guide to Diabetes Care. 3rd ed. Alexandria, Va: American Diabetes Association; 2017: 317-29.

38. Bosworth HB, Fortmann SP, Kuntz J, et al. Recommendations for providers on person-centered approaches to assess and improve medication adherence. J Gen Intern Med. 2017;32(1):93-100. DOI:10.1007/s11606-016-3851-7.

39. Abu Sabha R. Interviewing clients and patients: improving the skill of asking open-ended questions. J Acad Nutr Diet. 2013;113(5):626-33. doi:http://dx.doi.org/10.1016/j.jand.2013.01.002.

40. Søndergaard Jakobsen N, Kaufmann, L, Hennesser, Y, Kristensen, ST. Narrative Dietary Counseling: a new approach for the dietitian that strengthens the relationship and collaboration with clients. Topics in Clinical Nutrition. 2017;32(3): 229-42. doi: 10.1097/TIN.0000000000000111.

41. Barnes RD, Ivezaj V. A systematic review of motivational interviewing for weight loss among adults in primary care. Obes Rev. 2015;16(4):304–18. doi:10.1111/obr.12264.

42. Bos-Touwen I, Dijkkamp E, Kars M, Trappenburg J, De Wit N, Schuurmans M. Potential for self-management in chronic care: nurses' assessments of patients. Nurs Res. 2015;64(4):282-90. doi:10.1097/NNR.0000000000000103.

43. Doas M. Are we losing the art of actively listening to our patients? Connecting the art of active listening with emotionally competent behaviors. Open J Nurs. 2015;5:566-70. doi: 10.4236/ojn.2015.56060.

44. Mansyur CL, Rustveld LO, Nash SG, Jibaja-Weiss ML. Social factors and barriers to self-care adherence in Hispanic men and women with diabetes. Patient Educ Couns. 2015;98(6):805-10. doi:10.1016/j.pec.2015.03.001.

45. Saunders T. Type 2 diabetes self-management barriers in older adults: an integrative review of the qualitative literature. J Gerontol Nurs. 2019;45(3):43-54. DOI:10.3928/00989134-20190211-05.

46. Wilkinson A, Whitehead L, Ritchie L. Factors influencing the ability to self-manage diabetes for adults living with type 1 or 2 diabetes. Int J Nurs Stud. 2014;51(1):111-22. doi:10.1016/j.ijnurstu.2013.01.006.

47. Anderson BJ, Rubin RR, eds. Practical Psychology for Diabetes Clinicians: Effective Techniques for Key Behavioral Issues. 2nd ed. Alexandria, Va: American Diabetes Association; 2003.

48. Due-Christensen, M, Zoffmann, V, Willaing, I, Hopkins, D, Forbes, A. The process of adaptation following a new diagnosis of type 1 diabetes in adulthood: a meta-synthesis. Qualitative Health Research. 2018;28(2):245–58. https://doi.org/10.1177/1049732317745100.

49. Miller CK, Bauman J. Goal setting: an integral component of effective diabetes care. Curr Diab Rep. 2014;14:509-16. doi:10.1007/s11892-014-0509-x.

50. Rollnick S, Miller WR, Butler CC. Motivational Interviewing in Health Care: Helping Patients Change Behavior. New York: Guilford Press; 2008.

51. Steinberg MP, Miller WR. Motivational Interviewing in Diabetes Care. New York: Guilford Press; 2015.

52. Miller WR, Rollnick S. Motivational Interviewing: Helping People Change. 3rd ed. New York: Guilford Press; 2013.

53. Stoeckel M, Duke D. Diabetes and behavioral learning principles: often neglected yet well-known and empirically validated means of optimizing diabetes care behavior. Curr Diab Rep. 2015;15(7):1-8. https://doi.org/10.1007/s11892-015-0615-4.

54. Gutnick D, Reims K, Davis C, et al. Brief action planning to facilitate behavior change and support patient self-management. J Clin Outcomes Manag. 2014;21(1):17-29.

55. Krathwohl DR. A revision of Bloom's Taxonomy: an overview. Theory Pract. 2002;41(4):212-8. doi:10.1207/s15430421tip4104_2.

56. Sheeran P, Orbell S. Using implementation intentions to increase attendance for cervical cancer screening. Health Psychol. 2000;19(3):283-9.

57. Park L, Howie-Esquivel J, Dracup K. A quantitative systematic review of the efficacy of mobile phone interventions to improve medication adherence. J Adv Nurs. 2014;70(9):1932-53. https://doi.org/10.1111/jan.12400.

58. El-Gayar O, Timsina P, Nawar N, Eid W. Mobile applications for diabetes self-management: status and potential. J Diabetes Sci Technol. 2013;7(1):247-62. doi:10.1177/193229681300700130.

59. Kebede MM, Pishke CR. Popular diabetes apps and the impact of diabetes app use on self-care behaviour: a survey among the digital community of persons with diabetes on social media. Front. Endocrinol. 2019, March 1. https://doi.org/10.3389/fendo.2019.00135. (Cited 2019 Jun 2). On the Internet at: https://www.frontiersin.org/articles/10.3389/fendo.2019.00135/full.

60. Mensing CR, Norris SL. Group education in diabetes: effectiveness and implementation. Diabetes Spectr. 2003;16:96-103. https://doi.org/10.2337/diaspect.16.2.96.

61. Clapper TC. Cooperative-based learning and the Zone of Proximal Development. Simulation & Gaming. 2015;46(2): 148–58. DOI: 10.1177/1046878115569044.

62. U.S. Department of Health and Human Services. Quick guide to health literacy. (n.d.) (cited 2019 Jun 2). On the Internet at: https://health.gov/communication/literacy/quickguide/quickguide.pdf.

63. Osborne H. Health Literacy From A to Z: Practical Ways to Communicate Your Health Message. 2nd ed. Lake Placid, NY: Aviva Publishing; 2018.

64. Pfizer. The Newest Vital Sign: a health literacy assessment tool for patient care and research. 2011 (cited 2019 Jun 5). On the Internet at: https://www.pfizer.com/files/health/nvs_flipbook_english_final.pdf.

65. Koh HK, Brach C, Harris LM, Parchman ML. A proposed "Health Literate Care Model" would constitute a systems approach to improving patients' engagement in care. Health Affairs. 2013;32(2): 357-67. DOI:10.1377/hlthaff.2012.1205.

66. Doak CC, Doak LG, Root JH. Teaching Patients With Low Literacy Skills. Philadelphia, Pa: JB Lippincott Co; 1996 (cited 2019 Jun 2). On the Internet at: http://www.hsph.harvard.edu/healthliteracy/resources/teaching-patients-with-low-literacy-skills/.

67. Levy H, Janke A. Health literacy and access to care. J Health Commun. 2016;21Suppl1:43-50. doi:10.1080/10810730.2015.1131776.

68. University of Michigan. Plain Language Medical Dictionary. 2015 (cited 2019 Jun 2). On the Internet at: http://www.lib.umich.edu/taubman-health-sciences-library/plain-language-medical-dictionary.

69. Wolff K, Chambers L, Bumol S, White RO, Gregory BP, Davis D, Rothman RL. The PRIDE (Partnership to Improve Diabetes Education) Toolkit: development and evaluation of novel literacy and culturally sensitive diabetes education materials. Diabetes Educ. 2015;42(1):23-33. DOI: 10.1177/0145721715620019.

70. Schreiner B, Ponder S. Self-management education for the child with diabetes mellitus. UpToDate. 2019 Apr 4. (cited 2019 Jun 3). On the Internet at: www.uptodate.com.

71. Phelan H, Lange K, Cengiz E, et al. ISPAD Clinical Practice Consensus Guidelines 2018: Diabetes education in children and adolescents. Pediatric Diabetes. 2018;19(Suppl. 27):75–83. https://doi.org/10.1111/pedi.12762.

72. Juvenile Diabetes Research Foundation. Teen Toolkit. 2013. (cited 2019 Jun3). On the Internet at: http://www.jdrf.org/wp-content/uploads/2013/10/JDRFTEENTOOLKIT.pdf.

73. Grey M. Coping skills training for youths with diabetes. Diabetes Spectr. 2011;24(2):70-5. http://dx.doi.org/10.2337/diaspect.24.2.70.

74. Knowles M. Adult Learner: A Neglected Species. Houston, Tex: Gulf Publishing Co; 1990.

75. Young-Hyman D, de Groot M, Hill-Briggs F, Gonzalez JS, Hood K, Peyrot M. Psychosocial care for people with diabetes: a position statement of the American Diabetes Association. Diabetes Care. 2016;39(12):2126-40. DOI: 10.2337/dc16-2053.

76. American Association of Diabetes Educators. Special considerations in the management and education of older persons with diabetes. 2016 June (cited 2019 June 5). On the Internet at: https://www.diabeteseducator.org/docs/default-source/default-document-library/special-considerations-in-the-management-of-older-persons-with-diabetes.pdf?sfvrsn=0.

77. Shatto B, Erwin K. Moving on From Millennials: Preparing for Generation Z. The Journal of Continuing Education in Nursing. 2016;47(6):253-254. On the Internet at: https://doi.org/10.3928/00220124-20160518-05.

78. McCulloch DK, Munshi M. Treatment of type 2 diabetes mellitus in the older patient. UpToDate. 2016 May 9 (cited 2019 Jun 5). On the Internet at: http://www.uptodate.com/contents/treatment-of-type-2-diabetes-mellitus-in-the-older-patient.

79. Pesta, L., & Tucker, C. A. (2017). The teaching-learning experience from a generational perspective. In M. J. Bradshaw & B. L. Hultquist (Eds.), Innovative teaching strategies in nursing and related health professions (7th ed., pp. 39-58). Burlington, MA: Jones & Bartlett Learning. (cited 2019 Jun3). On the Internet at: http://samples.jbpub.com/9781284107074/9781284107074_CH03_039_058.pdf.

80. Capozza K, Woolsey S, Georgsson M, et al. Going mobile with diabetes support: a randomized study of a text message–based personalized behavioral intervention for type 2 diabetes self-care. Diabetes Spectr. 2015;28(2):83-91. http://dx.doi.org/10.2337/diaspect.28.2.83.

81. Greenwood DA, Gee PM, Fatkin KJ, Peeples M. A systematic review of reviews evaluating technology-enabled diabetes self-management education and support. J Diabetes Sci Technol. 2017;11(5):1015-27. doi: 10.1177/1932296817713506.

82. Reagan L, Pereira K, Jefferson V, Evans Kreider K, Totten S, D'Eramo Melkus G, Johnson C, Vorderstrasse A. Diabetes self-management training in a virtual environment. Diabetes Educ. 2017;43(4):413-21. doi: 10.1177/0145721717715632.

83. MacLeod J, Peeples M. Are you ready to be an eEducator? AADE in Practice. 2017;5(5):30–35. doi: https://doi.org/10.1177/2325160317722163.

84. Funnell MM, Anderson RM. Empowerment and self-management of diabetes. Clin Diabetes. 2004;22(3):123-7. https://doi.org/10.2337/diaclin.22.3.123.

85. Ricci-Cabello I, Ruiz-Perez I, Nevot-Cordero A, et al. Health care interventions to improve the quality of diabetes care in African Americans. Diabetes Care. 2013;36(3):760-8. http://dx.doi.org/10.2337/dc12-1057.

86. Marrero DG, Ard J, Delamater AM, et al. Twenty-first century behavioral medicine: a context for empowering clinicians and patients with diabetes. Diabetes Care. 2013;36(2):463-70. On the Internet at: http://dx.doi.org/10.2337/dc12-2305.

87. Rodriguez-Gutierrez R, Gionfriddo MR, Ospina NS, et al. Shared decision making in endocrinology: present and future directions. Lancet Diabetes Endocrinol. 2016;4(8):706-16. doi:http://dx.doi.org/10.1016/S2213-8587(15)00468-4.

88. Tamhane S, Rodriguez-Gutierrez R, Hargraves I, Montori VM. Shared decision-making in diabetes care. Curr Diab Rep. 2015;15(12):112. doi:10.1007/s11892-015-0688-0.

89. Hill-Briggs F, Lazo M, Peyrot M, et al. Effect of problem-solving-based diabetes self-management training on diabetes control in a low income patient sample. J Gen Intern Med. 2011;26(9):972-8. doi:10.1007/s11606-011-1689-6.

90. Mamykina L, Heitkemper EM, Smaldone AM, Kukafka R, Cole-Lewis H, Davidson PG, et al. Structured scaffolding for reflection and problem solving in diabetes self-management: Qualitative study of mobile diabetes detective. J Am Med Inform Assoc. 2016;23(1):129–36. https://doi.org/10.1093/jamia/ocv169.

91. Stevenson D. Story Theatre Method. Colorado Springs, Colo: Cornelia Press; 2008.

92. Baldwin C. Storycatcher: Making Sense of Our Lives Through the Power and Practice of Story. Novato, Calif: New World Library; 2005.

93. Caminotti E, Gray J. The effectiveness of storytelling on adult learning. J Workplace Learn. 2012;24(6):430-8. https://doi.org/10.1108/13665621211250333.

94. Haigh C, Hardy P. Tell me a story—a conceptual exploration of storytelling in healthcare education. Nurse Educ Today. 2011;31(4):408-11. https://doi.org/10.1016/j.nedt.2010.08.001.

95. Partridge SR, Gallagher P, Freeman B, Gallagher R. Facebook groups for the management of chronic diseases. J Med Internet Res. 2018;20(1):e21. DOI: 10.2196/jmir.7558.

96. Chrvala CA, Sherr D, Lipman RD. Diabetes self-management education for adults with type 2 diabetes mellitus: a systematic review of the effect on glycemic control. Patient Educ Couns. 2015 (Epub ahead of print). doi:http://dx.doi.org/10.1016/j.pec.2015.11.003.

97. Steinsbekk A, Rygg L, Lisulo M, et al. Group based diabetes self-management education compared to routine treatment for people with type 2 diabetes mellitus. A systematic review with meta-analysis. BMC Health Serv Res. 2012;12:213. doi:10.1186/1472-6963-12-213.

98. Odgers-Jewell K, Ball LE, Kelly JT, Isenring EA, Reidlinger DP, Thomas R. Effectiveness of group-based self-management education for individuals with Type 2 diabetes: A systematic review with meta-analyses and meta-regression. Diabet. Med. 2017;34, 1027–1039. https://doi.org/10.1111/dme.13340.

99. Sperl-Hillen J, Beaton S, Fernandes O, et al. Comparative effectiveness of patient education methods for type 2 diabetes: a randomized controlled trial. Arch Intern Med. 2011;171(22):2001-10. doi:10.1001/archinternmed.2011.507.

100. Stotts Krall J, Calabrese Donihi A, Hatam M, Koshinsky J, Siminerio L. The Nurse Education and Transition (NEAT) model: educating the hospitalized patient with diabetes. Clin Diabetes Endocrinol. 2016;2:1. doi:10.1186/s40842-016-0020-1.

101. Hirschman KB, Bixby MB. Transitions in care from the hospital to home for patients with diabetes. Diabetes Spectr. 2014;27(3):192-5. doi: 10.2337/diaspect.27.3.192.

102. Gooding HC, Mann K, Armstrong E. Twelve tips for applying the science of learning to health professions education. Med Teach. 2017;39(1):26-31, DOI: 10.1080/0142159X.2016.1231913.

103. Medina J. Brain Rules. 2nd ed. Seattle, Wash: Pearl Press; 2014.

104. Merriam SG, Caffarella RS, Baumgartner LM. Learning in Adulthood: A Comprehensive Guide. 3rd ed. San Francisco: Jossey-Bass; 2007.

105. Bransford JD, Brown AL, Cocking RR, eds. How People Learn: Brain, Mind, Experience, and School. Washington, D.C.: National Academy Press; 2000 (cited 2019 Jun 3). On the Internet at: http://www.nap.edu/catalog/9853/how-people-learn-brain-mind-experience-and-school-expanded-edition.

106. Jensen E. Brain-Based Learning: The New Paradigm of Teaching. 2nd ed. Thousand Oaks, Calif: Corwin Press; 2008.

107. American Association of Diabetes Educators. Diabetes and disabilities (practice paper). 2017. (cited 2019 Jun 3). On the Internet: https://www.diabeteseducator.org/docs/default-source/practice/practice-documents/practice-papers/diabetes-and-disabilities.pdf?sfvrsn=4.

108. Krahn GL, Walker DK, Correa-De-Araujo R. Persons with disabilities as an unrecognized health disparity population. American Journal of Public Health. 2015;105(S2):S198-206. doi:10.2105/AJPH.2014.302182.

109. Americans with Disabilities Act of 1990: Public Law 101-336, 101st Congress. Washington, D.C.: US Government Printing Office; 1990.

110. Rendle SGM, Uy V, Tietbohl CK, et al. Persistent barriers and strategic practices: why (asking about) the everyday matters in diabetes care. Diabetes Educ. 2013;39(4):560-7. doi:10.1177/0145721713492218.

111. Ngo-Metzger Q, Sorkin DH, Billimek J, et al. The effects of financial pressures on adherence and glucose control among racial/ethnically diverse patients with diabetes. J Gen Intern Med. 2012;27(4):432-7. doi:10.1007/s11606-011-1910-7.

112. Toma T, Athansiou T, Harling L, et al. Online social networking services in the management of patients with diabetes mellitus: systematic review and meta-analysis of randomised controlled trials. Diabetes Res Clin Pract. 2014;106(2):200-11.

113. Zhang Y, He D, Sang Y. Facebook as a platform for health information and communication: a case study of a diabetes group. J Med Syst. 2013;37:9942. doi:10.1007/s10916-013-9942-7.

114. Merkel RM, Wright T. Parental self-efficacy and online support among parents of children diagnosed with type 1 diabetes mellitus. Pediatr Nurs. 2012;38(6):303-8.

115. American Diabetes Association. School walk for diabetes. 2018. (cited 2019 Jun 3). On the Internet at: http://schoolwalk.diabetes.org/site/PageServer?pagename=SW_teach.

116. Wang J, Siminerio LM. Educators' insights in using Chronicle Diabetes: a data management system for diabetes education. Diabetes Educ. 2013;39(2):248-54. doi:10.1177/0145721713475844.

117. Al Shahrani A, Baraja M. Patient satisfaction and its relation to diabetic control in a primary care setting. J Family Med Prim Care. 2014;3(1):5-11. doi:10.4103/2249-4863.130254.

118. Doyle C, Lennox L, Bell D. A systematic review of evidence on the links between patient experience and clinical safety and effectiveness. BMJ Open. 2013;3:1e001570. doi:10.1136/bmjopen-2012-001570.

119. Lorig K. Patient Education: A Practical Approach. 3rd ed. Thousand Oaks, Calif: Sage Publications, 2001.

CHAPTER 3

Theoretical and Behavioral Approaches to the Self-Management of Health

Jan Kavookjian, MBA, PhD, FAPhA

Key Concepts

- Be familiar with prevailing behavioral theories, models, and approaches that support self-management of health in current and emerging contexts. These individual and social theories/models include the Health Belief Model, Social Cognitive Theory, the Theory of Reasoned Action and Theory of Planned Behavior, the Transtheoretical Model (sometimes referred to as the stages of change model), and Self-Determination Theory.
- Be aware that some models and approaches go beyond explaining or predicting psychosocial factors and health behavior of persons with or at risk for diabetes to also inform actions practitioners can take in addressing resistance or ambivalence to health behavior change. Person empowerment and motivational interviewing include the values, skills, and proficiency practitioners need to effectively engage in person-centered, collaborative diabetes care, education, and support.
- Learn the importance of assessing whether a theory/model will assist in understanding the intended goals and purpose in a specific situation, for example, applications in program design or for individual person encounters.
- Think critically about depending entirely on models that focus only on behavior of persons with or at risk for diabetes, or their caregivers, versus including one of the models or approaches that also addresses the skills, expertise, and values necessary to actively engage in person-centered, collaborative diabetes care and education.
- Be able to choose an approach that also incorporates the emotional, psychosocial, cultural, and health literacy factors that can significantly influence self-management behaviors and quality of life for an individual person.
- Be aware of the emerging vision and contexts in the self-management behavior support realm of diabetes care and education, including a significant focus on prevention of diabetes among persons with prediabetes, the use of technology to augment in-person encounters and provide efficient means of support, care for the related conditions person with diabetes are likely to experience (eg, cardiometabolic conditions), the use of person-first language to help reduce stigma, and the rapidly growing role of online peer support communities, among others.

The purpose of this chapter is to provide an overview of prevailing behavior theories/models that can help practitioners within the specialty of diabetes care and education understand the impact of thoughts, feelings, motivations, barriers, and behaviors of persons with or at risk for diabetes. Taking into account a person's unique psychosocial motivators and barriers for health behavior change is a first step towards providing person-centered care for management and/or prevention of diabetes and its complications.

Introduction

The mission of diabetes self-management education and support (DSMES) is to help individuals with diabetes acquire the knowledge, skills, attitudes, and behaviors needed to optimize both self-management of their diabetes and their quality of life. The specialty of diabetes care and education has advanced substantially over the past 30 years. Originally, diabetes education focused on helping a person with diabetes acquire knowledge and skills. More recently, diabetes education focused on behavior change as both a strategy and an outcome. Knowledge and behavior change strategies are necessary components of DSMES, but they are not enough to ensure that persons with diabetes and their families are fully prepared to live well with a lifelong chronic illness. Because diabetes-related distress and other psychosocial challenges profoundly affect self-management behaviors, these issues also must be addressed as part of the process for those practicing within the specialty of diabetes care and education.[1,2] In addition, a 2017 joint position statement by the American Diabetes Association, the American Association of Diabetes Educators–known as the Association of Diabetes Care and Education Specialists since January, 2020–and the Academy of Nutrition and Dietetics describes the importance of providing DSMES on an ongoing basis across the lifespan of a person with diabetes, and specifically recommends referral to DSMES at four critical times including at new diagnosis, at annual health maintenance appointments, when new complications arise, and at transitions in care.[3] Theories and approaches to support self-management behaviors should adapt or evolve across these four critical times to address an individual's changing needs, emotions, psychosocial factors and challenges.

Ideally, modern diabetes education programs focus on helping people with diabetes or at risk for diabetes identify and adopt the behaviors and coping strategies that will optimize their diabetes self-management or prevention and overall well-being. These education programs address knowledge and skill acquisition, and they often include much more. For example, they facilitate persons with diabetes learning for how to solve problems and set goals; they address the psychosocial and the clinical aspects of having diabetes, prediabetes, and/or additional cardiometabolic conditions; they help the person with diabetes define and acquire social support; and they provide the knowledge and skills necessary for effective coping and managing or preventing diabetes in challenging social situations and personal relationships.

The role of those practicing within the specialty of diabetes care and education has evolved as well. To be effective, the modern practitioner within this specialty needs to have the interpersonal skills, expertise, and values necessary to effectively engage in person-centered, collaborative diabetes care and education. Because of the need for ongoing support throughout a lifetime of diabetes, providing ongoing diabetes self-management support (DSMS) programs as follow-up to initial DSME is now a prominent component of the National Standards for DSMES, as is a focus on prevention in persons with prediabetes.[4] Practitioners within the specialty of diabetes care and education also need the skills required to provide DSMS, which can include psychosocial, behavioral, educational, and clinical support.[2–5] Additionally, practitioners are being increasingly called upon to train others (peer leaders, community health workers, *promotoras de salud*, National Diabetes Prevention Program [DPP] Lifestyle Coaches, etc) in these skills in order to deliver effective DSMS.[6] The purpose of this introduction is not to list all the attributes of modern DSMES or DPP, or to address all of the variables that influence behavior, but to illustrate how complex and sophisticated this specialty has become.

Before presenting several major theoretical approaches related to self-management behavior of those with or at risk for diabetes, this chapter outlines considerations pertinent to choosing theories for application in diabetes care, education, and support at the program- or individual-level. The chapter next gives a brief overview of each theory that has demonstrated value in understanding an individual's health behavior and will then describe 2 theory-based approaches shown to be effective in facilitating self-directed behavior change to illustrate how to put theories into practice. It should be noted that many theories, models, and approaches from across health professions, as well as from the fields of education and psychology, are relevant for specific or general contexts for those practicing within the specialty of diabetes care and education. The theoretical approaches chosen for this chapter were selected because of their sustained and/or growing evidence base and frequent use by diabetes care and education specialists. In addition, most other context-specific theories have a basis in the included theories or their components. This chapter is meant to be illustrative rather than definitive and will overview the following:

- Health Belief Model
- Social Cognitive Theory
- Theory of Reasoned Action and Theory of Planned Behavior
- Transtheoretical Model, specifically the construct of stages of change
- Self-Determination Theory
- Patient empowerment
- Motivational interviewing

The chapter will conclude with a brief summary of implications for the future vision for DSMES via emerging contexts and tools currently being developed and studied for their role in augmenting those practicing within the specialty of diabetes care and education.

Selecting and Applying Theory in Diabetes Care and Education

The words *theory*, *model*, and *approach* are often used interchangeably, and yet, they are somewhat different. A *theory* is a set of assumptions or facts that attempt to provide an explanation or link for an observed phenomenon. A *model* is a representation of a phenomenon and is sometimes used to explain or apply the components of a theory. This chapter includes 2 *theory-based approaches* to behavior change a diabetes care and education specialist or might using in practice (ie, the empowerment approach and motivational interviewing).

To be effective, practitioners within the specialty of diabetes care and education need to carefully choose the theories and approaches to behavior and education they will apply—both for individual practice and in the design, conduct, and evaluation of care, education and support programs.[7] With a clear conception of what theories and approaches to behavior change are and how they can be used in program design and individual practice, diabetes care and education specialists are then prepared to compare the relative merits of each and choose those most suitable to their situation. Behavioral and educational theories are usually selected for use in educational program design and individual practice based on how well they meet 1 or more of the following 4 purposes: describing, explaining, predicting, and influencing health behavior.[9–11]

Describing

The first purpose of a theory is describing the phenomena of interest. The theory tells us the way things are, but not why they are the way they are or how they are likely to change. The value of descriptive theory is largely dependent on how coherent and thorough it is. For example, suppose you noticed that persons with diabetes graduating from the diabetes education program on the east side of town got consistently higher scores on the same knowledge test than persons with diabetes graduating from another program on the west side of town. You could begin theory building by developing a thorough description about what you observed. How many observations were involved? Were the differences in test scores always in the same direction and similar in magnitude? Were the participants in both programs demographically similar (eg, age, gender, socioeconomic status)? Were the diabetes care and education specialists in both programs certified diabetes care and education specialists? Do both educational programs meet the National Standards for DSMES? Do both programs provide DSMS? Are families included in the education program? Who delivers DSMS? The answers to these and similar questions would constitute your descriptive theory.

Explaining

The second purpose of a theory is explanation. Your descriptive theory has answered the question "What is happening?" Now attention turns to the question "Why is it happening?" You want to know what is causing the differences in the knowledge test scores. You could carefully examine the descriptions of the 2 programs you observed to determine whether you could enhance your theory by incorporating an explanation of what you observed. If the only significant difference you found between the 2 programs was that the east-side program provided 60% more instructional time than the other, you might theorize that increasing the amount of time spent on instruction accounted for the better test results.

Predicting

The third purpose of a theory is prediction. Building on the same example, your new educational theory would be considered robust if it proved to be true in other settings (ie, other diabetes programs). Consistent correlations, in the expected direction between instructional time and educational achievement, derived from data found in other studies would support a prediction of similar results based on these factors.

Influencing

Your new educational theory would be viewed as even more robust and useful if you conducted experiments that demonstrated that you could increase instructional time to produce better educational outcomes. The ability of your theory to influence educational achievement in this example could be contrasted with a theory that is less useful (eg, a theory about IQ and learning) because it cannot be manipulated to produce better outcomes.

Choosing a Theory That Fits

When choosing a theory and/or approach to apply to a program design or for working with individual persons, 3 areas of inquiry are important to consider: how well the theory resonates with you, how the theory extends your thinking, and how useful the theory has been shown to be, particularly in the context of education or support for persons with or at risk for diabetes.

The first area of inquiry addresses the compatibility between the theory and your sense of how people learn and behave. Questions to ask are, "Does this theory fit with my experiences of how I learn and change?" "Does this theory resonate with what my participants will accept and respond to?" "Does it fit with how I define success when I provide diabetes education?" Those working in diabetes education and support are unlikely to make effective use of a theory unless they feel an affinity for values and vision embedded in it.

The second area of inquiry considers whether the theory helps organize and/or coherently expand your ideas and observations. Questions to ask are, "Does this theory provide a thorough description of the phenomena of interest?" "Does this theory offer a plausible explanation for why things happen the way they do?" "Does this theory help me to better understand and relate to my particpants?" In other words, is the theory consistent with your perspective on learning and health behavior change, and does it help enhance your perspective and practice?

The third area of inquiry should address the utility of the theory. Questions to ask are, "Can this theory be translated into specific practice behaviors or strategies (approach) that will help me become a more effective diabetes care and education specialist?" "Does this theory help me design and evaluate my education program?" "Will my participants benefit from this approach?"

Choosing a Theory or Approach That Can Be Measured

A theory's usefulness is very much related to the user's ability to measure its main attributes.[9] The user will need to answer the following questions: "What measures/instruments exist to evaluate this theory?" "Have these measures/instruments been shown to be valid and reliable in similar populations?" "Are they sensitive to change?" "Have applications of the measures been reported as successful in the evidence base for diabetes education?"

Questions to Answer to Ensure the Theory Is Appropriate to the Specific Practice or Program:

- Is there a convincing evidence base indicating that this theory can be used to facilitate learning and behavior change, and to positively impact quality of life?
- Is it a good fit with the kind of diabetes care, education, and support provided by our team?
- Can this theory help guide our interactions with persons with or at risk for diabetes and program design in one or more of these ways: Can I visualize how I would apply this theory in one-to-one interactions with persons? Can I visualize how I would apply this theory when group teaching? Can I incorporate this theory into the design of my program?
- After conducting some sessions or programs, will it be apparent whether this theory has improved my practice or programs?
- After conducting some sessions or programs, will it be apparent whether this theory is viewed positively by my participants?
- Does this theory fit the cultural, demographic, and medical history characteristics of the persons seen in our program?
- Do I possess the knowledge, skills, and experience to use this theoretical approach to practice person-centered, collaborative DSME and/or DSMS?

At both the individual practitioner and program levels, theories and approaches to behavior change can be important tools for the design, understanding, and conduct of DSME, DSMS, and DPP. Theory-based practice and evaluation add to professionals' understanding of how to be effective and enhance the credibility of the diabetes care and education specialty.

Theoretical Approaches to Behavior Change

Health behavior theories/models that have explored self-management behaviors of persons with or at risk for diabetes are described in this section. Tables are included to summarize theory/model components and include case examples for illustrating applications of the components, elucidating pertinent issues, and comparing and contrasting theory/model components. A fictitious person, "MG," is included in the case examples across theories and their tables. The theories/models and their primary components include:

- Health Belief Model
- Social Cognitive Theory
- Theory of Reasoned Action and Theory of Planned Behavior
- Transtheoretical Model, specifically the construct of stages of change
- Self-Determination Theory

Health Belief Model

The Health Belief Model (HBM) has been widely used as a theoretical framework to understand health behavior change initiation and maintenance.[8,10,12] The model was first introduced in the 1950s when behavioral scientists at the US Public Health Service sought to understand the low participation rates in government-sponsored, cost-free, and easily accessible screening, detection, and immunization programs.[13] As the model matured, the nature of events underlying beliefs about health problems was extended to include diagnosed conditions, such as diabetes.[14] The HBM underscores the importance of an individual's perceived risk and perceived seriousness as part of his/her health beliefs and determines the likelihood of adopting preventive health behaviors.[8,10,15] The more an individual perceives himself or herself to be at a particular health risk and considers this risk to be serious and important, the more likely it is that he or she will make the necessary changes to prevent health problems from occurring.

Under this model, a person with diabetes's decision to perform a "target" health behavior is influenced by the following factors:[8,10]

- Level of personal vulnerability the person feels about developing the illness
- How serious the person believes the illness is or has the potential to be
- Efficacy of the behavior, in the person's view, in preventing the development, or minimizing the consequences, of the illness (eg, diabetes)
- The person's perceptions of the costs or barriers associated with performing the behavior compared to the benefits that can be achieved as a result

When it was determined that self-efficacy fit conceptually within the HBM framework and was a strong predictor of health behaviors, an expanded HBM that incorporates readiness and self-efficacy was developed to provide a more powerful approach to understanding health-related behavior.[10,16] The Expanded Health Belief Model (EHBM) has become the most frequently used theoretical model to predict health behaviors.[8,17] The 2 additional constructs are the following:[8,10]

- Cues to action
- Self-efficacy

Table 3.1 provides definitions of the expanded model's constructs and examples of these constructs in relation to diabetes self-management and support. Of these, beliefs about treatment effectiveness and seriousness of the disease and consequences are most important in diabetes self-management, although the emotional response to diabetes may influence the relationship between beliefs and behaviors.[12]

TABLE 3.1 Health Belief Model: Constructs and Application to Diabetes Self-Management

Construct	*Definition*	*Case Example*
Perceived susceptibility	Estimate of personal vulnerability of developing an illness	MG's A1C levels have been high for 5 years, and her father had gone blind as a result of diabetes. Therefore, she believes her risk level for developing diabetes-related complications is high.
Perceived severity	Perception of how serious an illness and its complications are and can be if diagnosed	MG thinks that if she does not keep her blood glucose closer to normal she will experience severe complications like going blind or losing a leg because of her diabetes.
Perceived benefits	Perception of how a specific action will lead to a positive outcome	MG believes that checking her blood glucose frequently and taking her diabetes medication as prescribed will result in the benefit of substantially minimizing the long-term chances of her going blind or having her leg amputated.
Perceived barriers	Perception of the deterrents to engaging in a behavior or the costs associated with a behavior	MG feels that checking her blood glucose several times a day is a burden. She also does not want her coworkers to find out she has diabetes because she is worried they will start monitoring what she eats throughout the day.
Self-efficacy	Level of confidence one has for engaging in the identified health behavior	MG is fairly confident that she can find a private place to check her blood glucose during the workday.
Cues to action	External stimulus that activates engaging in the health behavior	MG sees her blood glucose monitor and remembers to check her own blood glucose.

Evidence Base

A substantial body of US research has utilized the HBM components for explaining diabetes self-care behaviors.[15–41] A brief summary of select studies using the HBM as a theoretical basis for health behavior change intervention in persons with or at risk for diabetes includes:

- impactful applications in physical activity among African American women with type 2 diabetes,[1]
- insulin taking according to guidelines among persons with type 1 diabetes,[24]
- a text message application for self-management behaviors for African Americans with type 2 diabetes,[25]
- a framework for developing educational materials for weight management for African-American women,[26]
- the Diabetes and Healthy Eyes Toolkit,[27]
- addressing reproductive behaviors and metabolic stability in teens with type 1 diabetes,[16]
- college students with type 1 diabetes living away from home for the first time,[28]
- foot care behavioral intervention for amputation prevention in African Americans with diabetes,[29]
- promoting physical activity in primary care settings in persons with prediabetes and type 2 diabetes,[33]
- exploring medication taking motivations and confidence in persons with diabetes who also had comorbid conditions,[34] and
- understanding young children's health beliefs and diabetes regimen participation.[16]

These US contributions to the evidence base have spanned the traditional contexts for self-management behavior support like applications across the lifespan and diabetes types, and also modern realms like culturally tailoring interventions in diverse segments of the population, applications in prevention of diabetes in persons with preiabetes, and use of technology to support the intervention, among others.

The HBM has also been the theory-basis of diabetes self-management research conducted outside the United States.[34–41] Studies have been reported that used aspects of the HBM to explain, predict, and/or impact outcomes that included medication taking in persons with type 2 diabetes in Saudi Arabia,[34] healthy eating behaviors in persons with type 2 diabetes in Iran,[35] complication prevention behaviors in persons with type 2 diabetes in China,[36] predictors of self-care impact on glycemic stability in aboriginals with type 2 diabetes in British Columbia,[37] appointment keeping with their dietitian in persons with type 1 and type 2 diabetes in the Netherlands,[38] impact of a culturally tailored HBM-based DSME program on persons with diabetes in Malaysia,[39] impact on general self-care in persons with diabetes in Iran,[40] and effect on health beliefs of genetic counseling on adult children of persons with type 2 diabetes in Japan,[41] among others. As in the select US studies briefly highlighted above, this sample of recent international studies that applied the HBM also addressed diverse groups, target behaviors, diabetes types, and other impactful factors or predictors of outcomes from self-management of diabetes.

Social Cognitive Theory

Social Cognitive Theory (SCT) evolved from Bandura's Social Learning Theory, which states that individuals learn not only from their own personal experiences but also from observing and interacting with the behaviors and behavioral consequences of others.[8,10,42–48] Social Cognitive Theory is built upon an array of multiple constructs that contribute individually to understanding health behavior change and have formed stand-alone intervention strategies in themselves. For example, the concept of Social Support, which is an active ingredient in diabetes support groups, online peer support communities, and often in group DSME or diabetes prevention program (DPP) classes, derives from the SCT. This section describes the major SCT constructs and applies them to diabetes self-management. Social Cognitive Theory addresses 2 primary areas:[8,10]

- Psychosocial factors that influence health behavior
- Methods of stimulating behavior change

Table 3.2 presents and defines the concepts of SCT and applies them to case examples in diabetes self-management.

Evidence Base

Social Cognitive Theory has been widely used to study diabetes care and education practices and to design intervention programs. The theory has been applied to people with type 1 diabetes or type 2 diabetes and across different target behaviors, settings, and age groups, including adolescents and adults.[36,44–68] Self-management interventions based on SCT have focused on a variety of target health behaviors, but have demonstrated a predominance in increasing physical activity, improving healthy eating choices and patterns, promoting frequent blood glucose testing, or a combination of self-management behaviors or preventive behaviors.

A few recent literature reviews have been conducted with a basis specific to SCT as a whole or in components as an intervention focus or as a predictor of outcome.

TABLE 3.2 Social Cognitive Theory: Concepts, Definitions, and Application to Diabetes Self-Management

Concept	*Definition*	*Case Example*
Reciprocal determinism	Behavior influences and is influenced by both personal factors and social environment	MG wants to take better care of her diabetes, so she cooks lower fat, low carbohydrate dinners. Her family complains that the meals do not taste good. Additionally, fresh produce is very costly at the local grocery. Given these environmental challenges, after 2 weeks MG returns to her previous style of cooking.
Environment	The external factors of and interactions with an individual	MG's home/family, work, community, neighborhood, social circle, etc.
Behavioral capability	The knowledge and skills required to perform a specific behavior	MG recently attended a DSMES program in which she learned a method for checking her blood glucose in a way that does not invite attention or disrupt her workday. As a result, she increases her capability to perform this behavior.
Expectations	The outcome that an individual anticipates as a result of performing a specific behavior	MG believes that if she starts being active by playing tennis regularly, her A1C will probably be lower at the next physician visit.
Modeling	Utilizing the experiences of others' performance of a behavior as a way to acquire that specific behavior	During MG's DSMES class, another person with diabetes demonstrated how to check her blood glucose, and MG sees and is now able to test her own blood glucose.
Reinforcements	The responses an individual receives that facilitate or deter the future performance of a specific behavior	Three weeks after starting tennis, MG noticed her clothes were fitting better. This tangible evidence of increased fitness and potential weight loss served as a positive reinforcement for her to continue playing tennis 3 times per week.
Self-efficacy	The level of confidence an individual has with regard to performing a behavior successfully	Given that MG enjoys playing tennis and sees her skill level and stamina improving has progressively increased her confidence that this will remain a permanent part of her lifestyle.

An integrative literature review conducted by Allen examined research that studied the role of SCT, specifically the construct of self-efficacy, in explaining and predicting physical activity and the long-term maintenance of activity among people with diabetes.[43] Of the 13 retained studies that met pre-established inclusion criteria, all studies with a correlational design found a significant positive association between self-efficacy and physical activity, and all studies with a predictive design found self-efficacy to be a significant predictor for physical activity. The studies that specifically examined physical activity maintenance found that self-efficacy predicted a person's ability to sustain physical activity over the study follow-up period. Other recent systematic reviews that either focused directly on SCT in diabetes self-management or focused on theory-based interventions that included impact of SCT have included Lepard and colleagues (2015) examining diabetes self-management interventions in rural adults with type 2 diabetes,[44] Theng and colleagues (2015) examining use of videogames and other technology-based diabetes self-management interventions,[45] an integrative review by Hilliard and colleagues (2016) that reported an array of diabetes management strategies that included SCT in populations from across the age spectrum and diabetes types,[46] and Zhao and colleagues' (2017) systematic review and meta-analysis of theory-based self-management interventions, including SCT, in persons with type 2 diabetes.[47]

Some individual studies have specifically used SCT as a framework to predict or directly impact healthy eating choices and patterns. Some of the seminal works include Miller and colleagues (2002), who applied the SCT principles of expectations and self-efficacy in developing a 10-week intervention aimed at increasing food label knowledge and skills among 93 older individuals recently diagnosed with type 2 diabetes,[48,49] Glasgow and colleagues (2006), who created an SCT-based, brief computer-assisted intervention focused on healthy eating and weight loss for persons with type 2 diabetes,[50] and Toobert and colleagues (2002), who used an SCT-guided intervention aimed at prevention of heart disease in women with type 2 diabetes.[51] More recently, Hansen and colleagues (2015) reported a cross-sectional study of children's self-report of fruit and vegetable knowledge and consumption.[52]

Most published studies with a focus on SCT as a predictor of or impact on outcomes have focused on varied behavior targets within diabetes self-management and/or prevention. Recent SCT-based studies approaching general self-management include Lorig and colleagues' (2010) online diabetes self-management program,[53] a culturally adapted, brief overall DSME program for Native Hawaiians and Pacific People—Partners in Care,[54] and Steed's (2014) exploration of general self-management intervention in adults with type 2 diabetes.[54] Utilization of SCT-based interventions have also used the theory to promote physical activity[36,56,57] in persons with type 2 diabetes and also had a focus on prevention of type 2 diabetes in teens or young adults using online and mobile interventions.[58,59] All of the aforementioned studies demonstrate the effectiveness of utilizing SCT as a theoretical framework for predicting or impacting behavioral and self-management outcomes for people with or at risk for diabetes.

Among the SCT components that have been studied as stand-alone intervention strategies, self-efficacy and social support have demonstrated that they are key mechanisms for improving and maintaining self-care behaviors in diabetes self-management or prevention. Several self-management behaviors are required for glycemic stability and complications prevention in diabetes; self-efficacy has a long history as a predictor of an individual person engaging in and sustaining a target self-management behavior.[60] Self-efficacy and social support, both components/derivatives of SCT, were both primary components for the development and implementation of a standardized peer-based program in diabetes: the Stanford Diabetes Self-Management Program, offered in-person[61] or online.[53] Another recent study conducted in China by Shao and colleagues (2017) examined the significant mediating roles among social support, self-efficacy, taking medication according to the prescription, and glycemic stability in 532 adults with type 2 diabetes. Structural equation modeling analysis revealed that greater reported social support was significantly associated with higher self-efficacy, which then associated with medication taking according to prescription, which was next associated with improved glycemic levels.[62] In addition, Jiang and colleagues (2019) conducted a systematic review and meta-analysis of self-efficacy-focused education in persons with diabetes and reported that even though the retained studies were heterogeneous in study designs, populations, and measures, outcomes for persons with diabetes may benefit from a self-efficacy focus within a DSME program.[63]

While the impact of social support is also sometimes named as a derivative of other behavior theories/models like the one discussed next, the social influence on health that can be learned through observation and positive interactions with familiar or unfamiliar others has been studied extensively and recently in applications in diabetes[64–66] including via the use of peer coaches in rural communities in a section of the US with high prevalence of type 2 diabetes[67] and in applications described in an integrative review of social support from eHealth interventions.[68] This has important implications for the current state of DSMES where diabetes education is frequently delivered via group classes and for the current state of the traditional support group impact being increasingly experienced through online peer support communities.

Theory of Reasoned Action and Theory of Planned Behavior

The Theory of Reasoned Action (TRA), developed by Fishbein, was extended by Azjen in the Theory of Planned Behavior (TPB).[69,70] This combined model (TRA/TPB) of behavior change operates through 3 primary contributing constructs:

- Attitude and beliefs the individual has toward the target health behavior
- How the individual thinks important or public others view the health behavior (subjective norm)
- Extent to which the individual believes he/she is equipped with the knowledge, skills, and accessibility needed to perform the behavior (perceived behavioral control)

These 3 constructs work together to formulate how strong an individual's intention is related to performing the health behavior, which, consequently, leads to the likelihood that the individual will demonstrate the health behavior.[8,10] The individual's intention to engage in the target behavior has been a strong predictor of persons actually initiating the behavior and has been studied extensively in health behaviors and other behaviors outside the realm of self-management and prevention.[71] Table 3.3 defines the elements of the TRA/TPB model and applies them to a diabetes-specific case example.

Evidence Base

The TRA/TPB is another major theory that has included the framework of social support for understanding how people decide to make behavior changes. This derives

TABLE 3.3 Theory of Reasoned Action/Theory of Planned Behavior: Concepts and Application to Diabetes Self-Management

Concept	*Case Example*
Attitude	MG believes that physical activity is an effective method of managing blood glucose levels.
Subjective norm	MG values the opinion of her healthcare team (physician, nurse educator, and dietitian) and peers, who have all recommended that engaging in some type of physical activity will help manage her diabetes.
Perceived behavioral control	MG would like to play tennis as her physical activity. She took tennis lessons in the past so she knows the rules and how to play; she also knows there are tennis courts near her house, and has 2 friends who have offered to play with her.
Behavioral intention	Each of the factors above contribute to MG's strong intention to start playing tennis as 1 way of managing her diabetes.
Behavior	MG regularly incorporates tennis playing into her schedule 3 times a week for at least 60 minutes.

from the subjective norm component of the TRA/TPB and how others can have a positive influence on an individual's engagement in self-management behaviors.[72] In general applications for the TRA and/or TPB in diabetes self-management behavior interventions, Syrjala and colleagues[73] utilized the TRA/TPB to examine the relationship between dental care practices and diabetes self-management among people diagnosed with type 1 diabetes and found a significant positive relationship between attitudes toward and normative beliefs related to tooth brushing and tooth brushing intentions and behavior. Additionally, individuals with better attitudes and greater intentions to brush demonstrated better diabetes self-management and had lower A1C levels, respectively.

Components of the TRA/TPB have been integrated into a proposed prevention program targeting minority children at risk for developing type 2 diabetes. Specifically, Burnet and colleagues (2002) outlined the TRA/TPB–related constructs, including beliefs and knowledge, attitudes, normative beliefs, and behavioral intention, as critical aspects of prevention behavior.[74] The researchers theorized that a child's beliefs and knowledge about an illness or associated health behaviors influence the child's attitudes about the health behavior. In turn, attitudes in combination with a child's belief about the public perception of the health behavior (normative beliefs) factor into the child's intention to perform the behavior. Finally, a child's level of intention to take action will ultimately determine the actual occurrence of the health behavior. In addition, Akbar and colleagues (2015) conducted a systematic review of the intentions construct of the TPB for general self-management in persons with or at-risk of diabetes and even though retained studies were heterogeneous in study designs, populations, and target self-management behaviors, outcomes mostly supported use of the intention construct for predicting those likely to engage in the target self-management behavior.[75]

In recent years, the TPB has in general been more widely used in the diabetes literature[76–79] than the TRA; however, in 2014, Didarloo and colleagues[80] evaluated the efficacy of the TRA, along with self-efficacy to predict dietary behavior in Iranian women with type 2 diabetes. The authors demonstrated that self-efficacy was the strongest predictor of intentions and dietary practice and the relative importance of the TRA constructs on behavioral intentions. The researchers emphasized the need to utilize the TRA when designing educational interventions to increase dietary self-care behaviors in people with diabetes.[80] Most recently, Burch and colleagues (2019) published a research protocol for an ongoing TPB-based study examining how a diagnosis of type 2 diabetes impacts dietary habits among persons newly diagnosed.[81]

Transtheoretical Model

The Transtheoretical Model (TTM) was first introduced by Prochaska and DiClemente as a framework for understanding general behavior change in smoking cessation[82] and evolved to studies of multiple behavior targets[83] with an eventual strong focus in diabetes self-management behaviors.[84] Although the model includes decisional balance (ie, weighing the individual's salient pros and cons), self-efficacy, and 10 identified processes of change that naturally occur at specific stages and facilitate movement from one stage to the next, the major construct used in diabetes education research and practice is the stages of change. Within the stages of change construct, the behavior-change continuum has traditionally included

5 distinct stages of motivational and behavioral readiness for change, with the sixth "termination" stage added in recent years.[85] The 6 stages include:

- Precontemplation
- Contemplation
- Preparation
- Action
- Maintenance
- Termination

Behavior change, viewed in the TTM with a temporal perspective, is seen as an ongoing process rather than as a specific outcome. During the process, an individual has different levels of motivation to change a behavior. Relapsing or "recycling" is considered a natural part of the change process and not a failure, as movement through the stages is not necessarily a linear process. The final, ongoing stage—termination—occurs when the change is a permanent part of the person with diabetes's lifestyle. It is important to recognize that individuals will exhibit different levels of readiness for different behaviors—some may report maintenance for medication taking and precontemplation for being active, for example. The TTM stages of change have been used in behavior change interventions to not only measure the outcome of change in behavioral readiness but to also inform the tailoring of intervention strategies to the readiness level of an individual. For example, a person with diabetes in the precontemplation stage who is not ready to start blood glucose monitoring due to lack of knowledge about the need to monitor is more likely to consider starting monitoring if receiving an intervention aimed at informing or raising awareness about monitoring, rather than an intervention strategy that goes directly to giving advice about how to start doing it. Awareness-raising is one of the 10 TTM processes of change that have been shown to naturally occur at particular stages of change and facilitate movement to the next stage—awareness-raising is a process that has been shown to help transition a person from precontemplation to contemplation.[86]

Table 3.4 lists and defines the stages of change in the TTM and applies them to a diabetes-specific case example.

TABLE 3.4 Transtheoretical Model: Stages of Change Definitions and Application to Diabetes Self-Management

Stage	*Definition*	*Case Example*
Precontemplation	Individual may not be aware of the problem, or is intentionally resistant to change; has no intentions of changing his or her health behavior	MG was diagnosed with type 2 diabetes 5 years ago. At that time, she was not aware of the long-term risks for complications and didn't think it would be important to change health behaviors to lower her blood glucose.
Contemplation	Individual is aware of the problem and intends to change the behavior in the long run; knows the benefits associated with the health behavior change but also is acutely aware of the drawbacks; often exhibits a state of ambivalence	Last year, MG started to understand that if she did not take care of her diabetes, she could eventually develop kidney or vision problems. She also knew that self-management involved a set of responsibilities including regularly checking her blood glucose, and she was unsure that she wanted to take on these responsibilities.
Preparation	Individual is motivationally ready and makes plans to engage in the health behavior change in the short-run	This month, MG is starting to look for diabetes education and support groups. She also joined a tennis club and has contacted friends who play tennis so that she can actively start playing tennis.
Action	Individual consistently engages in the behavior change and has been doing so for less than 6 months	MG has been consistently checking her blood glucose before and 2 hours after every meal for several months (but less than 6 months).
Maintenance	Individual consistently engages in the behavior change and has been doing so for more than 6 months	MG continues to check her blood glucose prior to and 2 hours following every meal and has been doing so for more than 6 months so that the blood glucose monitoring behavior has become a sustained habit.
Termination	Individual has been consistently engaging the target behavior for a year or more and is no longer at risk for relapse.	MG continues to check her blood glucose in the same time and pattern; the habit is ingrained and she is not tempted to skip.

Evidence Base

In diabetes management, the TTM has been studied:

- To understand motivations and readiness for diabetes self-management behaviors[87,88]
- To customize self-care interventions aimed at promoting physical activity,[89–92] healthy dietary habits,[93–96] and blood glucose testing,[93] among others

Researchers have examined the stages of change in relation to metabolic stability after a DSME intervention was delivered.[97,98] Kavookjian[87] found that although a person with diabetes may become ready for action toward self-care, a decrease in A1C levels might happen more slowly. Peterson and Hughes[97] found that persons with diabetes in the preparation and action stages achieved a significantly larger reduction in A1C levels in a shorter time than persons with diabetes in the precontemplation and contemplation stages. The authors concluded that stages of change were significantly associated with clinical improvement in A1C levels at 3 months after an educational intervention, and these significant differences in clinical improvement between groups were sustained for at least 12 months. However, it should be noted that although study persons with diabetes had significant reductions in A1C levels, none achieved an A1C level of ≤8%.[97]

Kirk and colleagues conducted a series of studies using stages of change for physical activity where a TTM-based exercise consultation was tailored to the stage of physical activity readiness in which subjects were classified. Intervention groups significantly increased the number of minutes of moderate activity per week and the number of times per week they engaged in physical activity compared to the control group. A greater number of participants from the intervention group advanced across a stage of change. Similarly, a 12-week stage-matched intervention to promote physical activity among Korean individuals with type 2 diabetes was developed by Kim and colleagues[90] and resulted in intervention group participants progressing to more advanced stages of change, increasing physical activity levels, and decreasing fasting blood glucose levels and A1C. Other studies addressing physical activity in persons with diabetes have used impactful staged-matched interventions that were delivered via print materials[91] and, more recently, via a mobile health intervention.[92]

Studies evaluating the usefulness of the TTM for understanding readiness to change dietary behaviors have been mixed, although reviews have been hampered by significant heterogeneity in study designs, interventions, populations and measures, as well as a limited number of methodologically rigorous studies.[88,95] In a sample of 768 overweight participants enrolled in a diabetes self-management trial, Vallis and colleagues (2003) identified participant-specific factors associated with different stages of changing dietary behavior.[93] Among those subjects diagnosed with type 2 diabetes, the subjects classified in the action stage were significantly more likely to be female, report a higher quality of life, and engage in healthy dietary habits than those in other stages. It is also important to note that stage of change for healthy eating has been linked to literacy and glycemic stability in persons with type 2 diabetes in 1 recent study.[96]

Studies using the TTM in diabetes self-management have often examined combinations of focus on physical activing and healthy eating[92] and on an array of self-management behaviors, including the study conducted by Jones and colleagues[98] comparing a TTM-based intervention (Pathways to Change) with usual care in improving 3 self-care behaviors: blood glucose testing, dietary habits, and smoking cessation[98]; Kavookjian's study that included medication taking/insulin use, healthy eating, being active, and blood glucose monitoring[87]; and the TTM interventions used by 14 sites in the Robert Wood Johnson Foundation Diabetes Initiative,[99] among others. Other target behaviors important to outcomes in diabetes include smoking cessation; Perez-Tortosa and colleagues (2015) demonstrated that an intensive intervention adapted to the individual's stage of change was feasible and effective at improving smoking cessation rates in people with diabetes at 1-year follow-up.[100] In addition, in a diabetes prevention initiative, Benitez and colleagues (2015) demonstrated that an intervention based on the TTM and the SCT was effective at producing increases in self-efficacy and cognitive and behavioral processes of change in 24 Latina adults at risk for developing diabetes.[57] As with the other theories, TTM applications in the literature are being increasingly conducted within the rapidly emerging and growing contexts (eg, technology, prevention, and others) relevant to the specialty of diabetes care and education.

Self-Determination Theory

Self-Determination Theory (SDT) is a macro theory of human motivation concerned with the development and functioning of personality within social contexts. The theory focuses on the degree to which human behaviors are self-determined—that is, the degree to which people endorse their actions at the highest level of reflection and engage in the actions with a full sense of choice.[101–103]

Within SDT, the components for healthy development and functioning are specified using the concept of basic psychological needs, which are innate, universal, and essential for health and well-being. Basic psychological needs are a natural aspect of human beings that apply to all people, regardless of gender, group, or culture. To the extent that the needs are continually satisfied, people will function effectively and develop in a healthy way, but to the extent that they are dissatisfied, people will show evidence of ill-being or non-optimal functioning.[102,104–107] Ryan and Deci[101] identified these psychological needs as the need for competence, relatedness, and autonomy. These needs are essential for facilitating optimal functioning, growth, and integration.[101]

Self-Determination Theory provides an example of how a theoretical analysis of motivation improves upon the TTM and other theories, as well as both approaches addressed in this chapter (ie, empowerment and motivational interviewing). For example with the TTM and HBM, lack of motivation to make a behavior change (precontemplation stage of change) can be due to a number of reasons, such as the person not valuing the activity, low self-efficacy, or the belief that change will not yield a desirable outcome (perceived benefits of consequences of action from the HBM). Different underlying reasons for lack of motivation at any point in the process of changing a behavior may require different interventions. Self-Determination Theory also considers not only the level of motivation but also the degree to which the motivation is extrinsic or intrinsic.[101] The theory proposes a continuum of motivation ranging from external regulation to intrinsic motivation, reflecting different degrees of autonomy or self-determination. The greater the person's autonomy or intrinsic motivation, the greater his or her likelihood of learning and sustaining a behavioral change.[101] Self-Determination Theory also considers the extent to which significant others in a person's social context are autonomy supportive, which means that they understand the person's choices, and provide relevant information. According to the theory, a person will develop and maintain an increased level of autonomous motivation to the extent that significant others are autonomy supportive.[102] Table 3.5 lists and defines the concepts of SDT and applies them to a diabetes-specific case example.

Evidence Base

Over the past 15 years, SDT, an alternative way of being for a practitioner than a compliance and adherence approach, emerged in the diabetes literature. The application of SDT to diabetes is somewhat different than the application of the HBM or the TTM.[103] Self-Determination Theory views motivation as psychological energy that is directed toward particular goals.[108] Studies using SDT hypothesize that people with diabetes have greater motivation if their healthcare provider supports their psychological needs, autonomy, competence, and relatedness. Studies also test the hypothesis that if a person with diabetes feels more autonomous and competent, he or she will have better glycemic stability and better quality of life.[108] Williams and colleagues[108–110] and Senecal and colleagues (2000)[111] pioneered the study of SDT concepts in relation to diabetes self-care behavior and to DSMES. They use the term *autonomy motivation* to refer to the psychological process that drives behavior change of a person with diabetes, and the term *autonomy support* to refer to actions by healthcare professionals that enhance a person with diabetes autonomy motivation.

In Williams's first study,[110] the objective was to explore factors related to persons with diabetes becoming more motivated for long-term glucose stability, building on the results of the Diabetes Control and Complications Trial (DCCT). Persons with diabetes in the DCCT who perceived their healthcare providers to be more autonomy supportive (provides choices, listens to and acknowledges perspective of the person with diabetes, and provides clear rationale for behavior change) improved their glycemic

TABLE 3.5 Self-Determination Theory: Definitions and Application to Diabetes Self-Management

Concept	*Definition*	*Case Example*
Autonomy support	Actions by those in the patients' social network that enhance patient autonomy motivation	MG attends a diabetes support group led by a peer leader. The peer leader actively listens to MG's barriers to getting more exercise and reflects back, paying special attention to what is important to MG at this time. The peer leader facilitates MG setting her own short-term goal and MG decides to walk 3 days per week for 15 minutes.
Autonomy motivation	Psychological process that drives patient behavior change	Following MG's autonomy supporting time with her peer leader, she feels more confident in her ability to walk for just 15 minutes 3 days per week and achieves her goal during the next week. MG feels autonomous in her achievement and is very proud to share her accomplishment with her peer leader the following week.

stability over 12 months and reported greater autonomous regulation of their treatment regimen in comparison with those who did not perceive their provider as supportive.[110] The authors concluded that when a person with diabetes is provided choices and information about the problem, and experiences a healthcare practitioner who acknowledges the person's emotions with minimal pressure to behave in a particular way, persons may achieve improved metabolic outcomes.

Similar to Williams, Senecal and colleagues[111] examined constructs drawn from SDT in relation to dietary self-care and life satisfaction among people with diabetes. The results demonstrated that self-efficacy was significantly more associated with improvements in dietary habits, whereas autonomous self-regulation was significantly more associated with life satisfaction. Based on the model, the authors concluded that interventions for dietary self-care and life satisfaction in people with diabetes should focus on increasing self-efficacy and autonomous self-regulation.[111]

Over the years, a growing body of literature[111–123] developed based on the seminal studies described above. Williams and colleagues (2007)[112] continued their work in SDT by determining whether a person-centered, computer-assisted diabetes care intervention increased perceived autonomy support and perceived competence and whether these constructs mediated the effect of the intervention on recommended diabetes outcomes based on the American Diabetes Association Standards of Medical Care. Williams and colleagues (2009)[113] also studied the application of SDT to predict medication adherence, quality of life, and other diabetes-related outcomes. Patrick and Williams (2012) also published an important integrative review of the association between SDT and motivational interviewing, an approach included in this chapter.[114]

Similar to the work of Williams,[112,113] many additional researchers set out to examine the relationship between autonomous motivation and diabetes self-care behaviors. Following a series of analyses, autonomous motivation was the only variable that was significantly associated with maintaining diet and self-monitoring of blood glucose, or an array of self-management behaviors. As changes in self-care behaviors are traditionally difficult to maintain, these studies demonstrated the positive potential for tailoring interventions from a basis of autonomous motivation in order to sustain improvements in diabetes outcomes.

The person empowerment approach to diabetes education, developed by Anderson, is rooted in SDT and has been prevalent in the diabetes literature since the early 1990s. Multiple studies using the empowerment approach have been conducted and published over the past 20 years, demonstrating the efficacy and effectiveness of the empowerment approach for DSMES.[124] In addition, there is also recognition that the SDT-based autonomy support, which is a foundational strategy within the motivational interviewing approach, contributes significantly to the effectiveness of motivational interviewing.[114]

Combining Theories and Approaches to Behavior Change

Even as the chapter presented individual theories, models, and approaches, there is often overlap in components of these as noted above; while a practitioner in the specialty of diabetes care and education may have selected a particular theory, model, or approach to intentionally employ and measure, it is frequently seen that in whole or part, more than one theory or approach to behavior change is often engaged in encounters with individuals as well as in developing DSMES and DPP programs. It is also true that the evidence-based approaches described next are applications that were developed from one or more theories or their components. When using a combination of theories/approaches, compatibility is important; the theories must embody the same values and world view. For example:

- *The empowerment approach posits:* Individuals will carry out self-management tasks more consistently and over a longer period of time if those tasks were freely chosen by the individual to help reach his/her own goals.[9,10]
- *The Health Belief Model posits:* The health-related choices people make are a function of their beliefs about their susceptibility to the disease (diabetes, in this instance) and its complications, the severity of diabetes and its complications, the efficacy of available treatments, and the ability to carry out those treatment options.[8,10]
- *In combination, these 2 frameworks could accomplish this:* Empowerment of participants could be used as the program's overall approach to facilitating self-directed behavior change and healthy coping, and the Health Belief Model could be used to order and sequence the educational content of the program.

Systematic Approaches to Facilitating Self-Directed Behavior Change

Person Empowerment and Behavior-Change Theories

The differences between person empowerment and the theories discussed above (with the exception of SDT) are crucial and have the potential to have a significant impact on practice within the specialty of diabetes care and education. These differences and their significance are discussed next.

Effective diabetes education involves a combination of art and science. The design of DSME and DSMS programs should be based on scientifically derived evidence and standards of education and care. However, communicating effectively with persons with diabetes in the context of a positive human relationship is an art. Central to empowerment is the development of a less hierarchical relationship and a collaborative approach to DSMES and behavior change.[4] Practitioners in the specialty of diabetes care and education have their own interpersonal skills, personal values, and character traits that play an important role in their practices. They can feel and express compassion, empathy, and warmth. They can establish relationships with persons with diabetes that are characterized by trust, respect, and acceptance. Such relationships create an environment of psychological safety and caring that nurtures persons with diabetes. Furthermore, such relationships facilitate high levels of candor and self-disclosure by persons with diabetes, laying the groundwork for growth and behavior change.[11]

Counseling psychology defines this relationship as a therapeutic alliance. Establishing a therapeutic alliance is an art. It's an art because it is dynamic and fluid and cannot be reduced to a set of algorithms, particularly within the objective of being patient- or person-centered. It involves the creativity, values, and personalities of practitioners within the specialty of diabetes care and education as well as their ability and willingness to respond to the unique needs and personality of each person with diabetes or caregiver.[70] Although published research has demonstrated the science of empowerment approach effectiveness, the art of diabetes care and education has been established for over two decades as a fundamental component of the empowerment approach and is based on fundamental elements from several behavior change theories.[11,125–130]

Patient Empowerment and Diabetes Education and Support

Patient empowerment has been incorporated into a variety of DSME and DSMS programs for over 20 years.[131–144] Empowerment grew out of the traditions of community psychology, adult education, and counseling psychology. Empowerment is defined "as helping patients discover and develop their inherent capacity to be responsible for their own lives and gain mastery over their diabetes."[126] The empowerment approach is based on 3 characteristics of diabetes that differentiate this disease from an acute illness.[4,11]

1. The choices that have the greatest effect on metabolic and other outcomes are made by persons with diabetes, not health professionals.
2. Individual persons with diabetes are in charge of their self-management.
3. The consequences of self-management decisions accrue first and foremost to persons with diabetes; thus, it is both their right and their responsibility to be the primary decision-makers.

Strategies implemented in a repeatedly impactful empowerment-based diabetes self-management education program included the following:[135,137]

- Affirming that the person with diabetes is responsible for daily self-management of diabetes
- Educating persons with diabetes to promote informed decision making rather than adherence/compliance
- Teaching how to set goals and providing weekly experience in setting, implementing, and evaluating action plans
- Integrating clinical, psychosocial, and behavioral aspects of diabetes into education
- Affirming participants in a DSMES or DPP program as experts in their own learning needs
- Affirming the ability of participants to determine an approach to diabetes self-management that will work for them
- Affirming the innate capacity of individuals to identify and learn to solve their own problems
- Creating opportunities for social support
- Providing ongoing self-management support following diabetes self-management education

Empowerment-Based Behavior-Change Protocol Example

To illustrate what an empowerment-based behavior change protocol might look like, the case for MG in the box below is provided as an example of what an empowerment-based protocol might look like. The protocol includes a logically sequenced set of questions to identify problems/challenges, address emotions influencing the problems/challenges, facilitate the person's movement toward his/her own solution, and evaluate the outcome. The protocol questions elicit an empowering process but should not be used as a rigid sequence or script for interacting with persons with or at risk for diabetes since a natural flow in an interaction could bring a different order and/or the addition or deletion of some questions.[125,135]

This protocol is meant to guide or facilitate a person in considering how he/she can make self-management changes in the contexts of his/her own routine. There may be instances when the health professional needs to provide information about diabetes care, may be helping facilitate the person to focus on short-term goals, or may be guiding the persons with diabetes to information or resources that will help in developing necessary skills and/or make informed choices. The protocol may also focus on addressing the emotions or barriers hindering the person's ability to reach his/her goal. These questions are meant to help support a process of person-centered decision making.

The empowerment protocol is equally effective in an individual or group situation. In a group situation, the diabetes care and education specialist can ask participants to think about or write down a response as each question is read to the group. In addition, participants can be asked to volunteer their perspectives on a common problem (eg, handling an upcoming holiday, stress) or can be asked to volunteer to share their experience with a real problem in a group discussion. The participant then works through the process with the practitioner and the other participants to create an action plan as part of the group session.[135,137]

In traditional care, health professionals often evaluate a person's health behaviors and offer positive or negative feedback based on their judgment of the person's success or failure. When using the empowerment approach, it is essential that the person with or at risk for diabetes, rather than the professional, be encouraged to evaluate and reflect on the outcome. This reinforces the concepts that persons with or at risk for diabetes are responsible for their own efforts and decisions and that the health professional is not the judge of their efforts or behaviors.

Evidence Base

Empowerment has been used as the theoretical basis for DSME and DSMS provided to both individuals[132,133,140,142] and groups.[132,133,136–138,141,143] Studies have reported impact on an array of outcomes from empowerment-based DSMES programs in varied populations, settings, and

Case: Applying Empowering Behavioral Approaches in Diabetes Care and Education

MG is a 48-year-old woman who was diagnosed with type 2 diabetes 5 years ago. She is a mother of 2 children, ages 13 and 16. For the past 12 months, MG has been working as a receptionist at the internal medicine outpatient clinic affiliated with a hospital. Prior to this position, she worked as an office assistant at a small advertising agency. Her current job provides healthcare benefits, whereas her previous position did not.

- MG does not check her blood glucose regularly during her workday because she feels self-conscious about coworkers discovering she has diabetes.
- She encounters difficulty when making food choices because her husband and children prefer high-fat and high-sugar foods.
- Until several months ago, she had not been exercising regularly.

Within the empowerment approach, the purpose of education is to enable participants to gain more power over their lives, increase the number of choices available in their decision-making, and enhance their ability to influence the individuals and organizations around them.[11] A 5-step behavior-change model was developed as a fundamental component of this approach and a systematic method to use when working with people who have diabetes, both one-to-one and in groups.[11,108] Each step is important; however, defining the problem and identifying emotions are the most critical to the process. Once the problem is fully explored, it will be easier for the participant to identify a solution and establish meaningful and relevant goals. The 5 steps are as follows:

1. Define the problem
2. Identify feelings
3. Identify long-term goals
4. Identify a short-term behavior-change experiment (I-SMART)
5. Experiment with and evaluate the short-term behavior-change plan

The purpose of the 5-step model is to assist participants in identifying behaviors they wish to address, and then create a self-directed behavior-change plan. The role of the diabetes care and education specialist is to ask questions and actively listen to MG's responses so that she learns and gains commitment through hearing herself and through reflection prompted by the diabetes care and education specialist's questions. The participant uses this information to create both a long-term goal and a short-term behavioral experiment as a first step toward achieving this goal. Table 3.6 elucidates the steps in the protocol, and Table 3.7 illustrates the use of this protocol with a participant.

(continued)

Case: Applying Empowering Behavioral Approaches in Diabetes Care and Education (continued)

TABLE 3.6 Example of an Empowerment-Focused Behavior-Change Protocol
What part of living with diabetes is the most difficult or unsatisfying for you?
(Would you tell me more about that? Would you give me some specific examples? Would you paint a picture of the situation for me?) The purpose of this question is to focus the discussion on the person with diabetes' concerns about living with and caring for diabetes. Diabetes care and education specialists and persons with diabetes often have different priorities about the most important issues related to diabetes care. Persons with diabetes are most likely to make changes that will solve problems that are personally meaningful and relevant to them.
How does that (the situation described above) make you feel?
(What are your thoughts about this issue? Are you feeling [insert the feeling, eg, angry, sad, confused]? Are you feeling [insert the feeling] because [insert the reason]?) As mentioned earlier, patients seldom make and sustain changes in situations unless they care deeply about solving the problem or improving the situation. It is very common for people to repress uncomfortable emotions, and repressed emotions reduce the energy and clarity necessary for effective problem solving. Discussing the feelings associated with a particular diabetes care situation can energize patients. When patients experience the depth of their anger, sadness, or dissatisfaction by talking about their feelings, they are much more likely to take action.
How would this situation have to change for you to feel better about it? What do you think will happen if you don't make any changes?
(Where would you like to be regarding this situation in [insert specific time, eg, a month, 3 months]?) The purpose of this question is to help patients concretely identify how the situation would appear if it were improved. This means imagining the particulars of the situation if it were to be changed and imagining how patients would feel if the situation improved. It is also useful to help patients imagine how they would feel if things did not improve. This question helps patients focus on tangible elements in the situation that must change for them to feel better.
What are some steps that you could take to bring you closer to where you want to be?
(What could you do to help solve this problem? Are there any barriers you would have to overcome? Are there other people who could help you?) This question helps patients develop a specific plan that will operationalize their commitment to change. It is useful to consider the various actions that could be taken, barriers to those actions, and potential resources, personal and otherwise, that patients could employ to help themselves.
Is there one thing that you will do when you leave here to improve things for yourself?
This question helps patients focus on the first thing they will do to begin to improve the situation. It is useful to end the session by having identified at least 1 immediate step the patient will take to begin the behavior-change process. Creating an I-SMART plan—1 that is important and inspiring, specific, measurable, achievable, relevant to their long-term goals, and time-specific—is 1 approach that can help patients learn the behavior-change process. Writing down the action serves as a reminder for subsequent visits to begin with a discussion of how the problem-solving process proceeded. Patients may wish to take a written copy of their commitment home with them. Participants in a group class can tell others in the group what they will do. Commitments tend to be more binding when they are expressed publicly and/or documented.
How did the plan we discussed at your last visit work out?
(What happened when you tried the behavior? Why do you think that it worked (or didn't work)? What did you learn? Would you do anything differently next time? Based on this experience, what action would you like to take or what goal would you like to set for next time?) The purpose of this question is to help patients view the behavior and the behavior-change efforts as experiments. The purpose of experiments is to try something new and to learn from the experience. Whether the effort is successful or not, learning can still occur. In fact, some of our best lessons come from experiments that did not accomplish what we had planned.

Case: Applying Empowering Behavioral Approaches in Diabetes Care and Education (continued)

TABLE 3.7 Empowerment-Based, Self-Directed Behavior-Change Model: Steps and Example Questions

Step	*Questions*	*Case Example*
Define problem	What part of diabetes is the most difficult or unsatisfying? What is hardest for you? What is causing you the most distress?	MG has struggled with losing weight and making changes in her eating habits since her diabetes was diagnosed. She identifies the "real" issue as her family and their limited support for her efforts.
Identify feelings	How do you feel about this situation?	MG is very afraid that if she does not lower her blood glucose levels she will go blind or lose a leg. She also feels angry at her family that they do not seem concerned about her future health. She does not feel she can be open about her diabetes at work because she has heard other staff members make negative comments about "noncompliant" persons with diabetes seen in the practice. She is worried the other staff members will judge her eating and other choices just as harshly. During the discussion, she comes to realize that feeling alone in managing diabetes is the hardest thing for her.
Identify a personal short-term behavior-change experiment	What are some steps that you could take to bring you closer to where you want to be? Is there one thing that you will do when you leave here to improve things for yourself?	MG feels that the first step is to write down exactly how she feels and what she wants so that she can do a better job of asking her family for their help. She decides for herself that she will complete this during the next week.
Implement and evaluate plan	How did the plan we discussed at your last visit work out? What did you learn? What would you do differently next time? What will you do when you leave here today?	Upon reviewing what she had written, MG recognizes that while she cannot force her family to change, she also has not asked for their support or told them what she needs. She decides to speak with her husband next Wednesday when their schedule will allow for a private conversation. In addition, she will attend a weight-loss support group with her friend on Monday evening and see whether it is helpful.

communities, including success in diabetes education programs in urban setting,[136,140] for a culturally tailored community-based program for African Americans,[128] in a community-based program for homeless persons,[144] in a telephone-based intervention,[145] and in studies that have implemented the Chronic Care Model for improvements in diabetes care and outcomes in primary care settings.[138,139,142,148] The empowerment approach has been used as the basis for studies in Europe as well. X-PERT was a person-centered, group-based diabetes self-management program in the UK.[141] In addition, improved A1C and psychosocial variables were reported from an empowerment-based education program for individuals with type 2 diabetes that was tested in a randomized trial in Germany.[149]

Many intervention studies demonstrate short-term impact on target outcomes from any type of psychosocial/behavioral intervention for diabetes self-management behaviors. In thinking about sustaining self-management behavior changes, the empowerment approach has also been designed into provision of DSMS to sustain changes resulting from DSME through ongoing support.[145] A study providing weekly DSMS groups for African Americans demonstrated significant improvements in diabetes-specific quality of life, healthy eating that included spacing carbohydrates throughout the day, and using insulin as recommended.[146] One year after the conclusion of the program, participants not only had sustained the behavioral improvements but demonstrated significant improvements in glycemic stability, serum cholesterol, and LDL levels.[147] Although the sessions were guided by participants' self-management questions and emphasized experiential learning, coping, goal setting, and problem solving, the process for each session consisted of 5 key interactive activities:

1. Reflecting on diabetes self-management experiments: Sessions began with a discussion of participants' experiences over the past week.
2. Discussing the emotional impact of living with diabetes: Discussion of psychosocial aspects of diabetes was integrated with clinical content and behavior-change discussions.
3. Solving problems systematically in the group: Primary focus of program was participant-driven, based on their problems and concerns.
4. Responding to diabetes self-management questions: Clinical content typically provided by lecture was instead given in response to questions raised by participants.
5. Choosing a personal diabetes self-management experiment: Participants were encouraged to create a specific action plan working toward one of their own long-term goals as a behavioral experiment for the next week.

Diverse recent research efforts in empowerment are continuing a focus on peer-based DSMS in community settings as well as other areas of focus. A curriculum[150] was recently developed and tested in a pilot study to determine whether an empowerment approach was effective for training African-American adults to provide group-based peer support. The training program was found to be effective for providing potential peer leaders with the necessary communication, group facilitation, and behavior-change skills needed to provide effective DSMS.[151] In addition, a recent study by Shin and Lee (2018) was reported in the Journal of Advanced Nursing that implemented a mediation analysis of psychosocial and self-management behavior variables among a population of older adults with type 2 diabetes; results suggest that the link between health literacy and diabetes self-management behaviors is significantly mediated by empowerment, particularly for healthy eating and being active.[152] These results contribute to the consistently growing evidence base supporting the importance of including an empowerment-basis in the structure of modern DSMES programs.

Motivational Interviewing

Motivational interviewing (MI) is characterized as a person-centered communication skills set and way of being[153–156] that has a rapidly expanding presence in the literature across a variety of target conditions, behaviors, populations, settings, study designs, and interventionists[157–162] and has demonstrated significant impact on outcomes when practitioners or interventionists have been appropriately trained in MI.[163–165] Motivational interviewing originated in the alcohol and substance abuse fields and has evolved to chronic disease management, particularly in diabetes.[166,167]

The underlying assumption of the MI way of being, known as the "Spirit of MI," includes the primary objective of building a positive, empowering relationship with the person, a therapeutic alliance as described in a previous section of this chapter. In the interest of this premise, assumptions for MI include that the practitioner, while directing, guiding, and following the person in the conversation, will also be making a mindful decision to be caring, non-judgmental, collaborative, and eliciting of the person's knowledge, ideas, and goals first, before giving information or advice. Important MI assumptions also include the need for the practitioner to use active listening and empathic responding in helping a person feel understood and supported in an alliance toward change. The autonomy-supporting aspects of MI are particularly important in not only empowering a person in change ideas, goal setting, and efforts, but also to reinforce movement toward change by giving the person the opportunity to learn by hearing him/herself make the arguments for the change.[153–156] The Spirit of MI is characterized as the relational component of MI.

A major focus and distinguishing feature of MI is interviewing the person in a way that elicits change talk[153,155,168–170] to assist individuals in working through their ambivalence about behavior change and resolving discrepancies between actual behaviors and stated goals.[4] Practitioners using an MI approach intentionally decide to be person-centered and to establish a supportive, guiding rapport in which persons feel comfortable expressing both positive and negative aspects of their current behavior. Motivational interviewing also employs other more common communication techniques and strategies, such as reflective listening, use of open-ended questions to explore and support autonomy, and others.[153–156,168]

Traditional communication strategies in health care have tended to involve an advising, autonomy-violating approach, known as the Righting Reflex[153–156] that can do more harm than good in behavior change outcomes. When persons are told what to do, or that what they are currently doing is wrong, they are likely to feel autonomy-violated and tend to become defensive. **The very act of hearing oneself defend the reasons why they have not or will not change only brings *reinforcement for the reasons not to change* and brings about the**

opposite of what is hoped for in change for the target behavior.[154,155] The Righting Reflex is a human instinct that is a natural part of all people and is engaged by many clinically trained practitioners who value their role as a problem-solver; becoming aware of one's Righting Reflex is an important first step for a practitioners in the specialty of diabetes care and education who aim to learn the MI skills, strategies, and way of being in order to conduct constructive and autonomy-motivating problem-solving.

The MI approach encourages individuals to make fully informed and deeply contemplated life choices, even if the decision is not to change.[170–173] Any appropriately trained health professional can successfully use MI, even in brief encounters[132] and with group classes.[174] However, learning about MI through self-study or in short 1- or 2-hour workshops is generally not adequate to master the necessary skills.[155,163–165,167,170,172,175] Although the concepts in the MI approach make intuitive sense, particularly in light of the theoretical foundations of MI which were developed from several strengths of the behavior theories presented earlier, most health professionals have not had extensive background and training in psychology and counseling, particularly with a multidimensional, person-centered skills set like MI. Most practitioners will need repeated practice with feedback and encouragement from MI-knowledgeable guides to adopt the practice behavior changes that MI requires for person-centered encounters.[155,163–165,170]

Motivational Interviewing Skills and Micro Skills

The MI approach to behavior change rests on active ingredients that are characterized as relational (Spirit of MI) and technical (MI skills, micro skills, and strategies). These are based on primary communication principles, overarching skills, and micro skills described next; an example dialog tying these together is provided in Table 3.8. Because the person-centered nature of MI is at the heart of its effectiveness, it is important to focus on following the person's desired direction in a guided conversation and not rely on a practitioner-centered script or protocol for how to engage the self-management behavior change conversation. While most of the examples and applications given within this chapter refer to interactions with individual persons with or at risk for diabetes, the reader is encouraged to reflect on how each of these strategies and skills can be also be engaged with groups in DSMES or DPP classes, and even via online peer support communities. It is also important to reflect on how each of these strategies and skills are relevant for application with caregivers of persons with or at risk for diabetes. This includes use with children/adolescents as well as their parents; the practitioner may also find him/herself interacting with child and both parents and will need to engage MI and group management strategies to be sure each participant's views and feelings are respected.

The Primary Communication Principles of MI

The foundational communication principles of MI include expressing empathy, rolling with resistance/avoiding arguments, developing discrepancy, and supporting self-efficacy.

Expressing Empathy is: deciding to put oneself in the shoes or perspective of another by carefully listening for what the individual is feeling and then reflecting that feeling back to him or her. Sometimes the underlying feeling will be obvious by what the person said (eg, "I'm so discouraged"). Other times, the underlying feeling is implied by what they say ("I am so tired of all this self-management work and seeing that nothing I do seems to be helping my numbers"). An ideal empathic response would demonstrate a simple attempt at expressing understanding of the feeling a person is expressing (eg, "You sound discouraged, Mrs. Smith"). Expressing empathy is a foundational, person-centered communication skill that is a key in making a connection and building a therapeutic alliance with a person with or at risk for diabetes. There are several types of empathic responding beyond the scope of this narrative, so the reader desiring further study in various and more complex empathic responding is referred to additional sources.[153,154]

Rolling with Resistance/Avoiding Arguments is: mindfully deciding not to get drawn into an argument, not creating defensiveness, not arguing a person's point of view. It is about recognizing that resistance is information to be explored for problem-solving. Resistance may come in the form of logical resistance regarding facts or issues (eg, "I don't have transportation to get to my diabetes class so I'm not coming") or in the form of psychological resistance regarding something that is happening in the relationship or the current exchange (eg, "You people need to quit bugging me about not getting any exercise."). An optimal first response to either type of resistance is to first express empathy (early empathy), and next explore with an open-ended question. Examples might include, "You're clear that you won't be able to get there unless transportation is available" for the person with diabetes's first statement, and "It sounds like you're frustrated with the way people are talking with you about getting physical activity" for the second example. Each of these early empathic statements should be followed by an

TABLE 3.8 A Motivational Interviewing Dialog Example With a Person With Type 2 Diabetes

Mary Gibson, T2D

Mary Gibson is a 48-year-old female who is overweight. Her A1C is 9.0%. She doesn't like taking medicine. She works, has two teenaged children, and has a very busy and stressful life. She often eats food "on the run."

MG: I just can't keep up with all of this…taking medicine, exercising, changing my diet….I know my blood sugar is up, but I feel okay most of the time.

Practitioner: It really does take a lot of effort to control your diabetes. You really do need to do a better job though. Your blood glucose is too high. **[absolute "control" is impossible to achieve; "though" negates early empathy, is judgmental, and stigmatizing]**

Rewrite of the Practitioner's Statement

Mrs. Gibson, you sound discouraged by all that you're being asked to keep up with. **[early empathy]** I am concerned that your A1C has been on the rise. What do you know about the things that can happen from having high blood sugar? **[open-ended lead into information giving]**

What would MG say next?

I guess I don't know the specifics, but I really do feel okay most of the time.

What would the Practitioner say next?

It's the times that you don't feel okay that I'm worried about. May I share with you some of my concerns about the complications you may be at risk for if your blood sugar remains high? **[asking permission to give information empowers MG and shows respect]**

[MG agrees to hear the concerns]

What would the Practitioner say next?

For every A1C percentage point above 7.0%, the risk rises significantly for developing complications like losing your eyesight, having serious kidney problems requiring dialysis, or losing circulation and feeling in your feet and hands. In addition, your risk for a heart attack or stroke rises also. What are your thoughts about fitting just a few small steps into your busy schedule that might help lower your blood sugar? **[open ended question, encouraging by using a focus on small steps]**

What would MG say next?

I really should; if it was just a few small steps, I think I could manage something.

What would the Practitioner say next?

That's great that you're thinking about taking some steps. **[supporting the self-efficacy of change talk]** You mentioned taking medication, getting activity, and changes in some of the foods you eat. Which of these would you like to talk about first today **[agenda setting]**? [MG chooses medication taking since she has been forgetting lately]

Great, tell me any things you can think of that you could do to remember to take your medication at the prescribed times? **[this engages the eliciting component in MI – eliciting MG's ideas first before asking permission to give information or advice]** [MG expresses that she can't think of anything]

Do you mind if I share with you some ideas that other people with type 2 diabetes have said worked for them? **[asking permission to give ideas empowers MG, and she is interested in hearing what relatable others – other persons with type 2 diabetes – have found useful]**

open-ended question to explore (eg, "Tell me more about that" or "What could be done differently?").

Developing Discrepancy is: an advanced MI skill that is intended to gently and caringly confront an individual to ask questions that help bring to light differences between what the person is doing or not doing and the goals he or she set previously. This might be done by contrasting the pros and cons the person stated for the change, or by illustrating the difference between goals and behaviors. Examples might include the following statements: "So on the one hand you want to prevent the diabetes complications you mentioned and on the other hand you don't like to take medication. What are your thoughts about that?" or "What are your thoughts about how not taking your medication will affect the goal you made last time for keeping your blood sugar levels at target levelsl?" This strategy can feel confrontational, so a key to using this strategy while maintaining the therapeutic alliance is to mindfully use engaged nonverbal strategies like maintaining caring eye contact and a conversational, non-judgmental voice tone. An additional conversational strategy to consider for developing discrepancy is to ask a thought-provoking question. (eg, "What will your life be like if your blood sugar remains high and complications begin?" "What would have to happen for you to think about checking your blood sugar?").

Supporting Self-efficacy is: focusing on encouragement by noticing and praising the person for things they are doing or saying toward change, even if they are just thinking about considering a change (eg, "That's great that you know that smoking is not good for your diabetes and other conditions," or, "That's great that you're willing to hear options for healthy choices you can make at a lunch buffet."). It is important to look for progress that can be noticed; it is also important not to over-praise as this can sound insincere and can dilute the effects. Encouragement and self-efficacy support also come from the language we use. Words that imply incremental change are encouraging and are especially important for those who are ambivalent toward change and repeatedly struggle to make a change and make it stick even though they have expressed that they want to. The AADE7 self-care behaviors® are phrased in a self-efficacy supporting way—"healthy eating" instead of "changing your diet," "being active" instead of "get exercise" both imply change that is more feasible than their big-change alternatives. It can be seen that the former in these two example contrasts implies incremental, doable change that can encourage and build confidence through small successes that can build upon themselves and support confidence for progressive goals and actions.

Additional Motivational Interviewing Principles, Skills, and Strategies

The MI originators and ongoing scholars in MI have used acronyms to organize expression of the MI guiding principles and micro-skills. The RULE and OARS acronyms are often seen to characterize these, with RULE standing for Resist the Righting Reflex, Understanding the Person's Perspective, Listen, and Empower[154] and OARS standing for Open-Ended Questions, Affirm, Reflect, and Summarize.[153] Motivational interviewing emphasizes active listening as well as creating a safe and accepting environment in which the person can express personal thoughts, feelings, and experiences, and the skills represented by these acronyms are intended to support these psychological needs. Giving facts or advice or direct teaching without first asking permission are in contrast to the Spirit of MI. These approaches can be autonomy-violating, not autonomy-motivating, and can result in defensiveness. As noted earlier, when a person hears him/herself defend why not to change, this reinforces the reasons why not to change and makes it much less likely that the person will be making a change for the target behavior.

There are a few specific MI communication or conversation skills that are intended to support autonomy, and these include using open-ended questions, using permission-asking before giving information or advice, using agenda-setting to support the person's autonomy to decide which topics to discuss in an encounter, and also, to a degree, eliciting change talk.

Open-Ended Questions: are important ways to explore and gather information. Because of the open-ended nature of the question, the individual is less likely to feel interrogated or judged, and less likely to get defensive. Many practitioners have been trained and rewarded to gather information through closed-ended yes/no questions that start with "Would you…" or "Have you…" or "Is there…." or "Do you…," among others (eg, "Do you know how eating that affects your blood sugar?"). Closed-ended questions like this impose an authoritative position for the practitioner and may undermine the therapeutic alliance when the person then feels violated for competency or autonomy by the authority in the encounter. An open-ended alternative, "Tell me what you've been told about how eating pasta can affect blood sugar," removes violations of competence and autonomy because it assumes that someone should have told them and it makes the assumption that they do know something (rather than the yes/no scenario where there is a right or wrong, all or none answer). In addition, while "why" questions aren't technically closed-ended, people often get immediately defensive when they hear the practitioner ask "why." The practitioner may have simply been attempting to explore or find out more, but the person hears him or her ask "why" and perceives this is a set-up for arguing the person with diabtes's point of view. Consider this contrast: "Why aren't you taking your medication as prescribed?" versus "Tell me more about what challenges you are facing in taking the medication as prescribed." Examples of other open-ended questions are included here:

- What did your doctor tell you about what the lab values mean?
- Tell me what you know about how food choices at a lunch buffet can affect your blood sugar.
- Many of my particpants have said they have challenges taking this many medications according to the directions. Tell me about any challenges you've been having with it?

- What types of physical activity do you get during a typical week?
- What concerns you most about [any topic]?
- What have you tried already for getting more activity into your routine?
- About how many snacks do you eat during a typical day?
- What are some things you can think of to do to bring the numbers down?
- Which of these strategies sounds like something you could try?
- What are your thoughts about trying one of the changes we've discussed today?
- What questions do you have for me? (Instead of, Do you have any questions?)

Asking Permission to Give Information or Advice: is a hallmark of MI. The strategy is autonomy-supporting and puts the person with diabetes at an equal position of power and autonomy in the behavior change alliance. When a practitioner realizes there is a knowledge deficit or intentional detrimental behavior the person is exhibiting, the mindful decision to first ask permission before giving the needed information or advice is somewhat of a "treatment" for the practitioner's own Righting Reflex. Practitioners who realize that the instinct to give information or advice is rising within themselves can decide to give the needed information or advice, but to first ask permission to do so in order to preserve the individual's autonomy. It is highly unlikely that a person will respond with a "no" to a respectful, autonomy-supporting permission-asking. Examples of ways to ask permission are included here:

- May I give you some additional information about that?
- I'd like to share some information with you about how eating late night ice cream can affect your blood sugar, if that's okay with you.
- Do you mind if I make a suggestion?
- Can I tell you what concerns me/what I'm worried about?
- If it's okay with you, I'd like to share with you some things that other persons with diabetes have told me worked for them for how to fit blood glucose monitoring into their schedule at work.

Using Agenda-Setting: gives a person with or at risk for diabetes choices about which topics to discuss first in an encounter. The strategy is actually a form of permission asking but presents to the person up front the topics that can be discussed and then asks him or her to choose which one first (and then next, and next, and so on). A traditional agenda-setting might look like this example with a person newly diagnosed with type 1 diabetes: "Today we can talk about changes you can make in the foods you eat, what to do about getting physical activity, using insulin, or monitoring blood sugar. Which of these would you like to talk about first?" The practitioner returns to the agenda after completing the first topic, using it to continue supporting autonomy by offering a choice of topics but also to organize the conversation and transition between topics while also being person-centered (eg, "Now that we've talked about monitoring, which of the other topics would you like to talk about next?"). One important advantage to using agenda setting is that the practitioner can put into the list of topics some difficult topics that need to be discussed, or that he/she knows the person is resistant to, and are hard to introduce into a conversation. The person first selects the topics he or she is most interested in or most concerned about/comfortable with, and these are usually the least difficult to discuss. This gives the practitioner an opportunity to build rapport and trust in the encounter with the easier topics so that eventually when the difficult topics on the list are reached, a trusting rapport has been built, making it much smoother to navigate through difficult topics while trying to maintain the therapeutic alliance. It's also important to note that if the individual is most concerned or anxious to talk about a particular topic and the practitioner decides something different will be discussed first, it is likely that the person will not be fully listening but rather, will be waiting for the practitioner to finish so they can get to the topic he/she is most interested in.

There are other ways of using agenda-setting to set expectations in a conversation while being person-centered and maintaining support for the person's autonomy to choose. If there is a specific objective, this can be stated first as an option. For example, "I have been asked by your doctor to talk with you today about your medication taking, but I want to be sure to address your concerns first. So, which topic would you like to talk about first?" Or, if there is a time limitation, the practitioner can state it up front: "Since we only have about 5 minutes left to talk today, we can probably cover 1 or 2 more topics; which would you like to talk about first?" It is much easier to smoothly end a conversation if needed when the expectation for a time limit has been expressed up front. Agenda setting also represents acknowledgment that individuals will exhibit different levels of readiness for different behaviors as noted in the section for the TTM.

Eliciting Change Talk: is not specifically an autonomy-supporting strategy in MI, but it is a powerful, evidence-based conversation strategy that accomplishes several key objectives in an MI encounter, including autonomy support. This strategy asks open-ended questions to first elicit the person's ideas, inputs, values, vision, and goal setting for change on the target behavior. It holds a premise that the individual person is the expert for how behavior change will fit into his/her life, and therefore the practitioner should embrace this assumption and explore from this expert source what might work for making change on a target behavior. The primary objective for change talk is that "we tend to believe what we hear ourselves say."[154] As noted in the SDT section of this chapter and in the MI section, among other things, people learn about change, about what will work, and even what won't work, through the things they hear themselves say. A person with or at risk for diabetes who hears him- or herself talk about his or her desire, abilities, reasons or needs for change is more likely to actually make those changes.[153,168–170] It is very important when a practitioner hears a person express change talk to praise the change talk to reinforce the self-efficacy for the movement on the change continuum that it represents.

Eliciting change talk may include a focus on benefits of change, future vision of what life would be like with the change, things that the person can do to make the change, or may use the readiness ruler to guide a change talk conversation. Examples of change talk eliciting questions and tools are included here:

- What do you see as the benefits (pros) of changing?
- What would you like about your life if this changed?
- What would you like to change in order to reach your long-term vision for managing your diabetes?
- How ready/important/confident are you for this change?
- The readiness ruler: On a scale from 1 to 10, with 10 being most, how ready are you to take your medication according to the prescription? [person says 7]
    - 1) A 7, that's great! Why a 7 and not a 1?
    - 2) What would have to happen for that 7 to become an 8 or 9?

The ruler can ask how ready, how important, how confident, how willing the person is. It is important to anchor the scale and also to support the self-efficacy for any change talk that is expressed to reinforce that for the person. It is also important to note that the first follow-up question elicits change talk (comparing where they are to a 1) and also supports self-efficacy (by comparing to a 1, the practitioner recognizes that the person is higher than a 1).

There are other MI skills and micro-skills that could be explored beyond the scope of this narrative.[153–156] While most of the principles, skills, and micro-skills that have been presented here in examples represent conversations with individual persons, MI has been increasingly used in groups[174] that could include diabetes education classes and support groups, and within DPP classes for persons with prediabetes. In fact, MI is a premise within the DPP PreventT2 curriculum the Centers for Disease Control and Prevention (CDC) has developed and disseminated for the National DPP Lifestyle Coach training program.[176] The CDC's National Diabetes Education Program also hosted a national webinar for Motivational Interviewing in diabetes care in varied settings and programs.[177]

Evidence Base

Motivational interviewing has gained increasing attention as an evidence-based set of skills and strategies, as well as a way of being, as noted in several recent systematic reviews for applications in self-management behaviors across populations, target behaviors, settings, and diseases, including diabetes.[157–163,165–167] Each of these reviews retained studies that demonstrated impact of MI-based intervention when interventionists were appropriately trained and intervention fidelity was evaluated. Early published literature examining MI as an intervention in diabetes was reported by Stott, Rollnick, and colleagues (1995 and 1996) just a little over a decade after MI first emerged in the alcohol and substance use literature.[178,179]

Smith and colleagues (1997) soon followed with a diabetes-focused investigation of the unique benefit that MI might add to standard behavioral intervention aimed at improving self-care practices and promoting weight loss.[180] Twenty-two women over the age of 50 with type 2 diabetes were randomly assigned to either a standard 16-week group weight-control program (instruction in healthy eating and being active behavior modification) or the standard program plus 3 personal MI sessions. Compared with the control group, the MI group performed significantly better with regard to maintaining food diaries and documenting blood glucose. While there were no differences in the amount of weight lost between the 2 groups, the mean A1C for the MI group was significantly lower than for their counterparts.

There have also been studies involving MI provided by specific groups of trained health professionals working with persons with type 2 diabetes.[181–185] Welch and colleagues (2011) found that MI delivered by diabetes care and education specialists was less effective than DSME alone for reducing A1C among adults with poorly controlled type 2 diabetes.[181] In a study of MI provided by nurse case managers working with high-risk type 2 diabetes, Gabbay and colleagues (2013) found improvements in systolic blood pressure and complications screening for the case manager group compared with the usual care control group. Both the case management and the usual care participants demonstrated reduced A1C levels (1.0% vs 1.1%), which were therefore not statistically different.[182] In addition, pharmacists have expanded practice services to include diabetes management/prevention and are an increasing practitioner segment achieving the Certified Diabetes Care and Education Specialists (CDCES) credential. A few key studies positively impacting medication taking were conducted by MI-trained pharmacists; these included the DOTx.Med pilot project funded by the American Pharmacists Association Foundation (2011)[183] which was a national randomized controlled trial of pharmacist/pharmacy resident pairs talking with persons with diabetes at refill pickup in varied types of practice settings, the Pennsylvania Project (2014)[184] conducted in community pharmacy settings, and the study by Ekong and Kavookjian (2017)[185] that included MI-trained pharmacists talking with persons with diabetes about medication taking/insulin use in a hospital-based worksite wellness program.

The MI approach has been evolving for use in varied population segments, interventionists, and settings as described above. Practitioners within the specialty of diabetes care and education are increasingly working with prevention as a priority, and this also includes working with pediatric/adolescent persons with or at risk for diabetes; this is a segment of the population receiving increased focus for self-management behavior interventions during an important developmental life stage when forming positive self-management habits can impact future outcomes.[46,186]

In closing out this brief survey of the vast evidence base for Motivational Interviewing, it is relevant to point out that scholars are studying the active ingredients in MI, or the components demonstrating most significant contribution to the changes and sustained changes persons exhibit after encounters with well-trained MI interventionists. While many aspects of MI derive from pieces of the theories and models discussed earlier in the chapter that already have a history of evidence base contributions, one MI skill or strategy that has received significant attention, with endorsement from MI originator William Miller,[170] is the process of eliciting change talk. A few studies have examined the role of change talk in these objectives and found that the more change talk a person expresses, the more likely they are to make movement on the change continuum, compared with persons expressing sustain talk (ie, the reasons why not to change).[169,170] Studies by Apodaca and colleagues (2016)[187] and Villarosa-Hurlocker and colleagues (2019)[188] suggest that both the technical and relational components of MI are important contributors to outcomes in MI interventions, but Villarosa-Hurlocker reported that while the technical component of MI was a stronger contributor than the relational in eliciting more change talk over sustain talk, the relational and technical components of MI have a synergistic effect on facilitating more change talk, and that the self-efficacy support, open-ended questions, and reflections were significant contributors to presence of change talk in MI-based encounters.

Motivational Interviewing and Person Empowerment

Motivational interviewing and person empowerment share the same vision and values and have many similarities, and yet a few differences as well. Similarities include that both approaches are person-centered, embrace a priority for autonomy support, and are built from Self-Determination Theory as well as components from Social Cognitive Theory and the Health Belief Model. In addition, both approaches strongly avoid persuasive tactics and instead engage active listening and empathy with priorities in recognizing these are critical to building a therapeutic alliance. Both approaches also interview the person using some of the same or similar general communication skills, and also require training and practice in specific communication skills and strategies. There are also some minor differences between the empowerment and MI approaches. The empowerment approach considers goals and changes as steps on the way to achieving an overall purpose; for MI goals are focused on building a therapeutic alliance to support specific behavior changes that are often viewed as ends in themselves. In addition, the general approach for person empowerment starts with problem-solving and challenges by asking questions to elicit goal setting by the participant. Motivational Interviewing starts with a focus on rapport-building and eliciting change talk so that the participant hears him/herself make the argument for change and then moves to problem-solving and goal setting after rapport and positive impact from hearing his/her own change talk have resulted. Motivational Interviewing and empowerment both have their own language and terms and yet also have similar language and terms.

Motivational Interviewing and person empowerment are both person-centered communication strategies that have some structure and even suggested protocols in person empowerment, but are intended to carefully discern the needs of the individual and respond accordingly. This requires flexibility and adaptation, particularly when providing care and education for persons from other cultures or who may have literacy limitations. Motivational interviewing, in particular, has extensive international implementation with presence in many countries and languages. A key conclusion for either approach is the notion that no two conversations will be alike if the practitioner is truly being person-centered in each encounter. And, while the MI approach includes a significant focus in autonomy support and asking permission to give information or advice, it should be remembered that some persons may be of culture or established mindset that they want the practitioner to tell them what to do. Being truly person-centered means the practitioner will adapt the approach to the preferences of the individual.

In addition, both approaches have long held high the importance of person-centered communication that should also include person-first language that supports awareness, respect, and positive attitudes toward a person with diabetes (eg, "She has diabetes" instead of "She is a diabetic") and strengths-based language that focuses in a positive direction and strengths or what a person can do or does know, rather than focusing on what they don't know or have not done (eg. "She takes her medication 50% of the time because she has limited income" instead of "She misses her medication doses 50% of the time."). A task force representing the American Association of Diabetes Educators (since January 2020, known as the Association of Diabetes Care and Education Specialists) and the American Diabetes Association published a consensus statement in 2017 with the overarching premise that the language we use in talking with and about persons with diabetes matters in encouraging or discouraging self-management and in preventing or propagating stigma.[189] Stigma is problematic in that those perceiving stigma from others or in a setting are less likely to seek care or treatment and less likely to stick with it if they do. This is an important common commitment across psychosocial and theoretical bases for talking with persons with or at risk for diabetes about self-management behaviors; the details of the recommendations are beyond the scope of this chapter and readers are encouraged to explore this important topic further through the consensus statement.[189]

Implications for Education

Teaching Strategies

Select and employ theories that will effectively guide practice. Establish a framework, define an approach and purpose, and provide a common language for the healthcare team and persons with diabetes. This philosophy is then reflected in the program design and implementation.

Base outcomes on evidence. Use valid and reliable measures of self-management behavior, metabolic status, and diabetes-related distress and quality of life, and then compare and contrast the results with expectations.

Match the content and educational materials to the particular characteristics of your audience. Of particular importance in person-centered approaches are different cultures, ethnicities, ages, and levels of health literacy.

Know yourself and play to your strengths. Some diabetes care and education specialists are comfortable with participant-driven discussions that move from topic to topic. Others need a more structured approach to education of persons with diabetes. Take the time to reflect on your educational efforts and interactions with individual persons. Do they reflect your values and your philosophy of diabetes care and education?

It is easy to underestimate the power of listening. There are many situations where it would be more effective for the diabetes care and education specialist to listen than to talk. Experiment with reducing the time you spend talking and increasing the time you spend listening.

Recognize that changing how you communicate with and relate to persons with diabetes can be challenging and represents behavior change in itself in the practice behaviors that require adjusting. It is hard to change old habits and the influence of the Righting Reflex. It takes training, practice, and reflection. Think about your own health behavior change challenges as you think about trying to understand the perspective of your participant.

Messages for Persons With or at Risk for Diabetes

Make decisions. Gather as much information as is available. Learn the skills necessary to make decisions and create and implement behavior-change goals and plans. Identify options and discuss them with the healthcare team, family, and diabetes care and education specialists to create a plan that will be most effective in helping you reach your goals. Be kind to yourself in this; it is often optimal to start with small goals with a plan for progression toward achieving the overall vision you have for your future.

Learn about yourself. Recognize that your emotional responses to diabetes, your culture, your family, your sources of support, your other priorities, and your values all influence your self-management and behavior-change efforts. While knowing about diabetes in general is helpful, it is more important to understand your own diabetes within the context of your life.

Be involved in planning your care. Be clear on what you plan to do and the criteria upon which you will judge your own success. Know that the plan can be altered and that every step forward is a step in the right direction. It's okay to ask questions when your healthcare team makes recommendations or plans for your care and treatment. You are the expert for how these recommendations or changes will fit into your life, so your input in these is very important to the likelihood for success. Most practitioners welcome questions and inputs from persons with diabetes when a plan or change to a plan needs to be made.

Involve family members, as they have a very specific and important role to play. They share the burden of diabetes and provide the support needed to manage this complex disease that greatly impacts your day-to-day life as well as theirs. Invite them to attend diabetes education and support sessions with you. If they are struggling with how to be supportive, tell them specifically how they can help you. In return, ask what you can do to ease their burden.

Realize how much impact your self-management has on your current and future health and well-being. It is true that you are responsible for your own self-management. But remember that the other side of the responsibility coin is freedom. You have the freedom to adapt your self-management to the unique characteristics and needs of your life. Yes, you are responsible, but you can also take charge and take control over your own decisions.

Implications for Practice

Be part of an organization's stewardship and acculturation for person-centered communication. The culture in which diabetes care and education specialists practice is reflective of the professional credibility and theoretical and behavioral approaches that are used. Realize that you set an important example; diabetes care and education specialists model the interpersonal skills, expertise, and confidence that are needed by persons with diabetes in directing their own learning.

Create a person-focused services mission statement, with clear communication of that mission in interactions from the reception desk to discharge planning. Provide in-service education to colleagues on health literacy, prevalent cultural differences in your community, and what it takes to help persons with diabetes change behaviors. Modify behavioral and psychosocial strategies to accommodate persons with special literacy and learning needs.

Reflect on growth and development in delivering person-centered education. No matter which theoretical and behavioral approaches you learn, in order to facilitate change among persons, practitioners within the specialty of diabetes care and education need to put theory into practice. Teaching skills are as important as clinical skills. Partner with other practitioners within the specialty of diabetes care and education to regularly discuss best practices, successes, and challenging encounters, and practice these approaches in all of your professional encounters with persons with diabetes and colleagues.

References

1. Skovlund SE, Peyrot M; for the DAWN International Advisory Panel. The Diabetes Attitudes, Wishes, and Needs (DAWN) program: a new approach to improving outcomes of diabetes care. Diabetes Spectr. 2005;18:136-42.
2. Young-Hyman D, deGroot M, Hill-Briggs F, Gonzalez JS, Hood K, Peyrot M. Psychosocial care for people with diabetes: a position statement of the American Diabetes Association. Diabetes Care. 2016;39:2126-40.
3. Powers MA, Bardsley J, Cypress M, et al. Diabetes Self-management education and support in type 2 diabetes: a joint position statement of the American Diabetes Association, the American Association of Diabetes Educators, and the Academy of Nutrition and Dietetics. Diabetes Educator. 2017;43(1):40-53.
4. Beck J, Greenwood DA, Blanton L, et al. 2017 Standards Revision Task Force. 2017 National standards for diabetes self-management education and support. Diabetes Care. 2017;40:1409-19.

5. Marrero DG, Ard J, Delamater AL, et al. Twenty-first century behavioral medicine: a context for empowering clinicians and patients with diabetes: a consensus report. Diabetes Care. 2013;36:463-70.

6. Tang TS, Nwankwo R, Whiten Y, Oney C. Training peers to deliver a church-based diabetes prevention program. Diabetes Educ. 2012;38(4):519-25.

7. Fain J, Nettles A, Funnell MM, Charron-Prochownik D. Diabetes patient education research: an integrative literature review. Diabetes Educ. 1999;25Suppl 6:7-15.

8. U.S. Department of Health and Human Services, National Institutes of Health, National Cancer Institute. Theory at a Glance: A Guide for Health Promotion Practice, 2nd ed. NIH publication no. 05-3896;2005.

9. Fawcett J. Criteria for evaluation of a theory. Nurs Sci Q. 2005;18:131-5.

10. Glanz K, Rimer BK, Marcus-Lewis F, eds. Theory, Research, and Practice. 4th ed. San Francisco: Jossey-Bass; 2008.

11. Anderson RM, Funnell MM. The art and science of diabetes education: a culture out of balance. Diabetes Educ. 2008;34(1):109-17. doi:10.1177/0145721707312398. PubMed PMID:18267997.

12. Harvey JN, Lawson VL. The importance of health belief models in determining self-care behaviour in diabetes. Diabet Med. 2009;26(1):5-13. doi:10.1111/j.1464-5491.2008.02628.x.

13. Rosenstock IM. Historical origins of the Health Belief Model. Health Educ Behav. 1974;2(4):328-35. doi:10.1177/109019817400200403.

14. Kirscht J. The Health Belief Model and prediction of health actions. In: Gochman D, ed. Health Behavior: Emerging Research and Perspectives. New York: Plenum Press; 1988:27-41.

15. Bond GG, Aiken LS, Somerville SC. The health belief model and adolescents with insulin-dependent diabetes mellitus. Health Psychol. 1992;11:90-8.

16. Charron-Prochownik D, Becker MH, Brown MB, Liang WM, Bennett S. Understanding young children's health beliefs and diabetes regimen adherence. Diabetes Educ. 1993;19:409-18.

17. Charron-Prochownik D, Sereika SM, Becker D, et al. Reproductive health beliefs and behaviors in teens with diabetes: application of the Expanded Health Belief Model. Pediatr Diabetes. 2001;2:30-9.

18. Koch J. The role of exercise in the African-American woman with type 2 diabetes mellitus: application of the health belief model. J Am Acad Nurse Pract. 2002;14(3):126-30. doi:10.1111/j.1745-7599.2002.tb00103.x.

19. Aljasem LI, Peyrot M, Wissow L, Rubin RR. The impact of barriers and self-efficacy on self-care behaviors in type 2 diabetes. Diabetes Educ. 2001;27(3):393-404.

20. Pham DT, Fortin F, Thibaudeau M. The role of the Health Belief Model in amputees' self-evaluation of adherence to diabetes self-care behaviors. Diabetes Educ. 1996;22(2):126-32.

21. Swift CS, Armstrong JE, Beerrman KA, Dorothy RK, Pond-Smith D. Attitudes and beliefs about exercise among persons with insulin-dependent diabetes. Diabetes Educ. 1995;21(6):533-40.

22. Polly RK. Diabetes health beliefs, self-care behaviors, and glycemic control among older adults with non-insulin-dependent diabetes mellitus. Diabetes Educ. 1992;18(4):321-7.

23. Kurtz SM. Adherence to diabetes regimens: empirical status and clinical applications. Diabetes Educ. 1990;16(1):50-6.

24. Cerkoney KAB, Hart LK. The relationship between the health belief model and compliance of persons with diabetes mellitus. Diabetes Care. 1980;3(5):594-8.

25. Nundy S, Dick JJ, Solomon MC, Peek ME. Developing a behavioral model for mobile phone-based diabetes interventions. Patient Educ Couns. 2013;90(1):125-32. doi:10.1016/j.pec.2012.09.008. PubMed PMID:23063349; PubMed Central PMCID:PMC3785373.

26. James DC, Pobee JW, Brown L, Joshi G. Using the health belief model to develop culturally appropriate weight-management materials for African-American women. J Acad Nutr Diet. 2012;112(5):664-70.

27. Ammary-Risch NJ, Aguilar M, Goodman LS, Quiroz L. Diabetes and Healthy Eyes Toolkit: a community health worker program to prevent vision loss and blindness among people with diabetes. Fam Community Health. 2012;35(2):103-10. doi:10.1097/FCH.0b013e3182464fc0. PubMed PMID:22367257.

28. Wdowik MJ, Kendall PA, Harris MA, Keim KS. Development and evaluation of an intervention program: "Control on Campus." Diabetes Educ 2000; 26(1):95-104. doi:10.1177/014572170002600110.

29. Scollan-Koliopoulos M. Theory-guided intervention for preventing diabetes-related amputations in African Americans. J Vasc Nurs. 2004; 22(4):126-33. doi:10.1016/j.jvn.2004.09.003. PubMed PMID:15592343.

30. Ferranti EP, Narayan KM, Reilly CM, et al. Dietary self-efficacy predicts AHEI diet quality in women with previous gestational diabetes. Diabetes Educ. 2014; 40(5):688-99. doi:10.1177/0145721714539735. PubMed PMID:24942530; PubMed Central PMCID:PMC4260266.

31. Tang JW, Foster KE, Pumarino J, Ackermann RT, Peaceman AM, Cameron KA. Perspectives on prevention of type 2 diabetes after gestational diabetes: a qualitative study of Hispanic, African-American and White women. Matern Child Health J 2015;19(7):1526-34. doi:10.1007/s10995-014-1657-y. PubMed PMID:25421329.

32. Fischetti N. Correlates among perceived risk for type 2 diabetes mellitus, physical activity, and dietary intake in adolescents. Pediatr Nurs. 2015;41(3):126-31. PubMed PMID:26201170.

33. Rossen J, Yngve A, Hagstromer M, et al. Physical activity promotion in the primary care setting in pre- and type 2 diabetes—the Sophia step study, an RCT. BMC Public Health. 2015;15:647. doi:10.1186/s12889-015-1941-9. PubMed PMID:26164092; PubMed Central PMCID:PMC4499440.

34. Williams A, Manias E. Exploring motivation and confidence in taking prescribed medicines in coexisting diseases: a qualitative study. J Clin Nurs. 2014. 23(3-4):471-81. doi:10.1111/jocn.12171. PubMed PMID:24028554.

35. Alatawi Y, Kavookjian J, Ekong G. A pilot study of medication adherence beliefs in patients with type 2 diabetes. Res Soc Amin Pharm. 2016.12(6):914-25.

36. Mohammadi S, Karim NA, Talib RA, Amani R. The impact of self-efficacy education based on the health belief model in Iranian patients with type 2 diabetes: a randomised controlled intervention study. Asia Pac J Clin Nutr. 2018;27(3):546-55.

37. Tan MY. The relationship of health beliefs and complication prevention behaviors of Chinese individuals with type 2 diabetes mellitus. Diabetes Res Clin Pract. 2004;66(1):71-7.

38. Daniel M, Messer LC. Perceptions of disease severity and barriers to self care predict glycemic control in aboriginal persons with type 2 diabetes mellitus. Chronic Dis Can. 2002;23:130-8.

39. Spikmans FJM, Brug J, Doven MMB, Kruizenga HM, Hofsteenge GH, Van Bokhorst-van der Schueren MAE. Why do diabetic patients not attend appointments with their dietitian? J Hum Nutr Diet. 2003;16(3):151-8. doi:10.1046/j.1365-277X.2003.00435.x.

40. Ahmad B, Ramadas A, Kia Fatt Q, Md Zain AZ. A pilot study: the development of a culturally tailored Malaysian Diabetes Education Module (MY-DEMO) based on the Health Belief Model. BMC Endocr Disord. 2014;14:31. doi:10.1186/1472-6823-14-31. PubMed PMID:24708715; PubMed Central PMCID:PMC4005520.

41. Dehghani-Tafti A, Mazloomy Mahmoodabad SS, Morowatisharifabad MA, Afkhami Ardakani M, Rezaeipandari H, Lotfi MH. Determinants of self-care in diabetic patients based on Health Belief Model. Glob J Health Sci. 2015;7(5):33-42. doi:10.5539/gjhs.v7n5p33. PubMed PMID:26156902; PubMed Central PMCID:PMC4803867.

42. Nishigaki M, Tokunaga-Nakawatase Y, Nishida J, Kazuma K. The effect of genetic counseling for adult offspring of patients with type 2 diabetes on attitudes toward diabetes and its heredity: a randomized controlled trial. J Genet Couns. 2014;23(5):762-9. doi:10.1007/s10897-013-9680-5. PubMed PMID:24399094.

43. Allen NA. Social cognitive theory in diabetes exercise research: an integrative literature review. Diabetes Educ. 2004;30(5): 805-19. PubMed PMID:15510532.

44. Lepard MG, Joseph AL, Agne AA, Cherrington AL. Diabetes self-management interventions for adults with type 2 diabetes living in rural areas: a systematic review. Current Diabetes Reports. 2015;15:37. https://doi.org/10.1007/s11892-015-0608-3.

45. Theng Y-L, Lee JWY, Patinadan PV, Schubert SBF. The use of videogames, gamification, and virtual environments in the self-management of diabetes: a systematic review of evidence. Games for Health Journal. 2015; 4:5. https://doi.org/10.1089/g4h.2014.0114.

46. Hilliard ME, Powell PW, Anderson BJ. Evidence-based behavioral interventions to promote diabetes management in children, adolescents, and families. American Psychologist 2016;71(7): 590-601.

47. Zhao FF, Suhonen R, Koskinen S, Leino-Kilpi H. Theory-bsed self-management educational interventions on patients with type 2 diabetes: a systematic review and meta-analysis of randomized controlled trials. J Advanced Nursing. 2016; 73(4). https://doi.org/10.1111/jan.13163.

48. Miller CK, Edwards L, Kissling G, Sanville L. Evaluation of a theory-based nutrition intervention for older adults with diabetes mellitus. J Am Diet Assoc. 2002;102(8):1069-81. PubMed PMID:12171451.

49. Miller CK, Edwards L, Kissling G, Sanville L. Nutrition education improves metabolic outcomes among older adults with diabetes mellitus: results from a randomized controlled trial. Prev Med. 2002;34(2):252-9.

50. Glasgow RE, Nutting PA, Toobert DJ, et al. Effects of a brief computer-assisted diabetes self-management intervention on dietary, biological and quality-of-life outcomes. Chronic Illn. 2006;2(1):27-38. PubMed PMID:17175680.

51. Toobert DJ, Strycker LA, Glasgow RE, Barrera M, Bagdade JD. Enhancing support for health behavior change among women at risk for heart disease: the Mediterranean Lifestyle Trial. Health Educ Res. 2002;17(5):574-85.

52. Hansen AR, Alfonso ML, Hackney AA, Luque JS. Preschool children's self-reports of fruit and vegetable knowledge, preference, and messages encouraging consumption. J Sch Health. 2015;85(6):355-64. doi:10.1111/josh.12260. PubMed PMID:25877432.

53. Lorig K, Ritter PL, Laurent DD, et al. Online diabetes self-management program: a randomized study. Diabetes Care. 2010;33(6):1275-81. doi:10.2337/dc09-2153. PubMed PMID:20299481; PubMed Central PMCID:PMC2875437.

54. Sinclair KA, Makahi EK, Shea-Solatorio C, Yoshimura SR, Townsend CK, Kaholokula JK. Outcomes from a diabetes self-management intervention for Native Hawaiians and Pacific People: Partners in Care. Ann Behav Med. 2013;45(1):24-32.

55. Steed L, Barnard M, Hurel S, Jenkins C, Newman S. How does change occur following a theoretically based self-management intervention for type 2 diabetes. Psychol Health Med. 2014;19(5):536-46. doi:10.1080/13548506.2013.845301. PubMed PMID:24111492.

56. Plotnikoff RC, Lubans DR, Penfold CM, Courneya KS. Testing the utility of three social-cognitive models for predicting objective and self-report physical activity in adults with type 2 diabetes. Br J Health Psychol. 2014;19(2):329-46. doi:10.1111/bjhp.12085. PubMed PMID:24308845.

57. Benitez TJ, Cherrington AL, Joseph RP, et al. Using Web-based technology to promote physical activity in Latinas: results of the Muevete Alabama Pilot Study. Comput Inform Nurs. 2015;33(7):315-24. doi:10.1097/CIN.0000000000000162. PubMed PMID:26049367; PubMed Central PMCID:PMC4506230.

58. Muzaffar H, Castelli DM, Scherer J, Chapman-Novakofski K. The impact of web-based HOT (Healthy Outcomes for Teens) Project on risk for type 2 diabetes: a randomized controlled trial. Diabetes Technol Ther. 2014;16(12):846-52. doi:10.1089/dia.2014.0073. PubMed PMID:25127372.

59. Cha E, Kim KH, Umpierrez G, et al. A feasibility study to develop a diabetes prevention program for young adults with prediabetes by using digital platforms and a handheld device. Diabetes Educ. 2014;40(5):626-37. doi:10.1177/0145721714539736. PubMed PMID:24950683; PubMed Central PMCID:PMC4169327.

60. Beckerle CM, Lavin MA. Association of self-efficacy and self-care with glycemic control in diabetes. Diabetes Spectrum. 2013; 26(3):172-78.

61. Lorig K, Ritter PL, Villa FJ, Armas J. Community-based peer-led diabetes self-management: a randomized trial. Diabetes Educ. 2009;35(4):641-51. doi:10.1177/0145721709335006. PubMed PMID:19407333.

62. Shao Y, Liang L, Shi L, et al. The effect of social support on glycemic control in patients with type 2 diabetes mellitus: the mediating roles of self-efficacy and adherence. J Diabetes Research. 2017; article 2804178. https://doi.org/10.1144/2017/2804178.

63. Jiang X, Wang J, Lu Y, et al. Self-efficacy-focused education in persons with diabetes: a systematic review and meta-analysis. Psychology Research and Behavior Management. 2019;12:67-79. https://doi.org/10.2147/PRBM.S192571

64. Shaya FT, Chirikov VV, Howard D, et al. Effect of social networks intervention in type 2 diabetes: a partial randomised study. J Epidemiology and Community Health. 2014;6894: 326-32.

65. Rankin D, Barnard K, Elliott J, et al. Type 1 diabetes patients' experiences of, and need for, social support after attending a structured education programme: a qualitative longitudinal investigation. J Clinical Nursing. 2014;23(19-20): 2919-27.

66. Bowen PG, Clay OJ, Lee Lt, et al. Associations of social support and self-efficacy with quality of life in older adults with diabetes. J Gerontol Nurs. 2015;41(12): 21-29.

67. Safford MM, Andrae S, Cherrington AL, et al. Peer coaches to improve diabetes outcomes in rural Alabama: a cluster randomized trial. Annals of Family Medicine. 2015;13(S1):18-26.

68. Vorderstrasse A, Lewinski A, Melkus GD, et al. Social support for diabetes self-management via eHealth interventions. Curr Diab Rep. 2016;16:56. https://doi.org/10.1007/s11892-016-0756-0.

69. Azjen I, Fishbein M. Understanding Attitudes and Predicting Social Behavior. Englewood Cliffs, NJ: Prentice Hall; 1980.

70. Madden TJ, Ellen PS, Ajzen I. A comparison of the theory of planned behavior and the theory of reasoned action. Pers Soc Psychol Bull. 1992;18(1):3-9.

71. Predicting Intentions and behaviors in populations with or at-risk of diabetes: A systematic review. Preventive Medicine Reports. 2015;2:270-82. https://doi.org/10.1016/j.pmedr.2015.04.006.

72. Lee LT, Bowen PG, Mosley MK, Turner CC. Theory of planned behavior: social support and diabetes self-management. J for Nurse Practitioners. 2016;13(4):265-70.

73. Syrjala AM, Niskanen MC, Knuuttila ML. The theory of reasoned action in describing tooth brushing, dental caries and diabetes adherence among diabetic patients. J Clin Periodontol. 2002;29(5):427-32. PubMed PMID:12060425.

74. Burnet D, Plaut A, Courtney R, Chin MH. A practical model for preventing type 2 diabetes in minority youth. Diabetes Educ. 2002;28(5):779-95.

75. Akbar H, Anderson D, Gallegos D. Predicting intentions and behavours in populations with or at-risk of diabetes: a systematic review. Prev Med Rep. 2015;2:270-92. https://doi.org/10.1016/j.pmedr.2015.04.006.

76. Watanabe T, Berry TR, Willows ND, Bell RC. Assessing intentions to eat low-glycemic index foods by adults with diabetes using a new questionnaire based on the theory of planned behaviour. Can J Diabetes. 2015;39(2):94-100. doi:10.1016/j.jcjd.2014.09.001. PubMed PMID:25439502.

77. Boudreau F, Godin G. Participation in regular leisure-time physical activity among individuals with type 2 diabetes not meeting Canadian guidelines: the influence of intention, perceived behavioral control, and moral norm. Int J Behav Med. 2014;21(6):918-26. doi:10.1007/s12529-013-9380-4. PubMed PMID:24442932.

78. Jennings CA, Vandelanotte C, Caperchione CM, Mummery WK. Effectiveness of a web-based physical activity intervention for adults with type 2 diabetes—a randomised controlled trial. Prev Med. 2014;60:33-40. doi:10.1016/j.ypmed.2013.12.011. PubMed PMID:24345601.

79. Muzaffar H, Chapman-Novakofski K, Castelli DM, Scherer JA. The HOT (Healthy Outcome for Teens) project. Using a web-based medium to influence attitude, subjective norm, perceived behavioral control and intention for obesity and type 2 diabetes prevention. Appetite. 2014;72:82-9. doi:10.1016/j.appet.2013.09.024. PubMed PMID:24099704.

80. Didarloo A, Shojaeizadeh D, Gharaaghaji Asl R, Niknami S, Khorami A. Psychosocial correlates of dietary behaviour in type 2 diabetic women, using a behaviour change theory. J Health Popul Nutr. 2014;32(2):335-41. PubMed PMID:25076670; PubMed Central PMCID:PMC4216969.

81. Burch E, Williams LT, Makepeace H, et al. How does diet change with a diagnosis of diabetes? Protocol of the 3D longitudinal study. Nutrients. 2019;11:158. https://doi.org:10.3390/nu11010158.

82. Prochaska J, DiClemente C. Transtheoretical therapy: Toward a more integrative model of change. Psychotherapy: Theory, Research & Practice. 1982;19(3):276-88.

83. Prochaska JO, Velicer WF, Rossi JS, et al. Stages of change and decisional balance for 12 problem behaviors. Health Psychology. 1994;13(1):39-46.

84. Ruggiero L, Prochaska JO. Readiness for change: application of the transtheoretical model to diabetes. Diabetes Spectrum. 1993; 6(1):21-60.

85. Cardinal BJ. Extended stage model of physical activity behavior. J Hum Movement Stud. 1999;37:37-54.

86. Marcus BH, Rossi JS, Selby VC, et al. The stages and processes of exercise adoption and maintenance in a worksite sample. Health Psychology. 1992;11(6): 386-95.

87. Kavookjian J, ed. Does readiness for self-care behaviors predict glycemic control? Diabetes. 2002;51Suppl3:A437.

88. Riemsma RP, Pattenden J, Bridle C, et al. A systematic review of the effectiveness of interventions based on a stages-of-change approach to promote individual behaviour change. Health Technol Assess. 2002;6(24):1-231. PubMed PMID:12433313.

89. Kirk AF, Mutrie N, Macintyre PD, Fisher MB. Promoting and maintaining physical activity in people with type 2 diabetes. Am J Prev Med. 2004;27(4):289-96. doi:10.1016/j.amepre.2004.07.009. PubMed PMID:15488358.

90. Kim CJ, Hwang AR, Yoo JS. The impact of a stage-matched intervention to promote exercise behavior in participants with type 2 diabetes. Int J Nurs Stud. 2004;41(8):833-41. doi:10.1016/j.ijnurstu.2004.03.009. PubMed PMID:15476756.

91. Dutton GR, Provost BC, Tan F, Smith D. A tailored print-based physical activity intervention for patients with type 2 diabetes. Prev Med. 2008;47(4):409-11. doi:10.1016/j.ypmed.2008.06.016. PubMed PMID:18652840.

92. Holmen H, Wahl A, Torbjornsen A, et al. Stages of change for physical activity and dietary habits in persons with type 2 diabetes included in a mobile health intervention: the Norwegian study in RENEWING HEALTH. BMJ Open Diabetes Research & Care. 2016; 4:1. https://doi.org:10.1136/bmjdrc-2016-000193.

93. Vallis M, Ruggiero L, Greene G, et al. Stages of change for healthy eating in diabetes: relation to demographic, eating-related, health care utilization, and psychosocial factors. Diabetes Care. 2003;26(5):1468-74. PubMed PMID:12716806.

94. Kavookjian J, Berger B, Grimsley D, et al. Patient self-efficacy and decision-making: strategies for diet intervention. Research In Social and Administrative Pharmacy 2005;1(3):389-407.

95. Salmela S, Poskiparta M, Kasila K, Vahasarja K, Vanhala M. Transtheoretical model-based dietary interventions in primary care: a review of the evidence in diabetes. Health Educ Res. 2009;24(2):237-52. doi:10.1093/her/cyn015. PubMed PMID:18408218; PubMed Central PMCID:PMC2654060.

96. Tseng HM, Liao SF, Wen YP, et al. Stages of change of the transtheoretical model for healthy eating links health literacy and diabetes knowledge to glycemic control in people with type 2 diabetes. Primary Care Diabetes 2017;11(1):29-36.

97. Peterson KA, Hughes M. Readiness to change and clinical success in a diabetes educational program. J Am Board Fam Pract. 2002;15(4):266-71. PubMed PMID:12150458.

98. Jones H, Edwards L, Vallis TM, et al. Changes in diabetes self-care behaviors make a difference in glycemic control: the Diabetes Stages of Change (DiSC) study. Diabetes Care. 2003;26(3):732-7.

99. Highstein GR, O'Toole ML, Shetty G, Brownson CA, Fisher EB. Use of the transtheoretical model to enhance resources and supports for diabetes self management: lessons from the Robert Wood Johnson Foundation Diabetes Initiative. Diabetes Educ. 2007;33Suppl 6:193S-200S.

100. Perez-Tortosa S, Roig L, Manresa JM, et al. Continued smoking abstinence in diabetic patients in primary care: a cluster randomized controlled multicenter study. Diabetes Res Clin Pract. 2015;107(1):94-103. doi:10.1016/j.diabres.2014.09.009. PubMed PMID:25444354.

101. Ryan RM, Deci EL. Self-determination theory and the facilitation of intrinsic motivation, social development, and well-being. Am Psychol. 2000;55(1):68-78.

102. Deci EL, Ryan RM. The "what" and "why" of goal pursuits: human needs and the self-determination of behavior. Psychol Inq. 2000;11(4):227-68.

103. Velicer WF, Prochaska JO, Fava JL, Norman GJ, Redding CA. Smoking cessation and stress management: applications of the Transtheoretical Model of Behavior Change. Homeostasis. 1998;38:216-33.

104. Ryan RM, Deci EL. The darker and brighter sides of human existence: basic psychological needs as a unifying concept. Psychol Inq. 2000;11(4):319-38.

105. Vinicor F, Jack LJ. 25 years and counting: Centers for Disease Control and Prevention identifies opportunities and challenges for diabetes prevention and control. Ann Intern Med. 2004;140(11):943-4.

106. Wagner EG. Meeting the needs of chronically ill people. BMJ. 2001;323:945-6.

107. Bodenheimer T, Wagner EH, Grumbach K. Improving primary care for patients with chronic illness: the Chronic Care Model, part 2. JAMA. 2003;288(15):1909-14.

108. Williams GC, Zeldman A. Patient-centered diabetes self-management education. Curr Diab Rep. 2002;2(2):145-52.

109. Williams GC, McGregor HA, Zeldman A, Freedman ZR, Deci EL. Testing a self-determination theory process model for promoting glycemic control through diabetes self-management. Health Psychol. 2004;23(1):58-66.

110. Williams GC, Freedman ZR, Deci EL. Supporting autonomy to motivate patients with diabetes for glucose control. Diabetes Care. 1998;21(10):1644-51.

111. Senecal C, Nouwen A, White D. Motivation and dietary self-care in adults with diabetes: are self-efficacy and autonomous self-regulation complementary or competing constructs? Health Psychol. 2000;19(5):452-7.

112. Williams GC, Lynch M, Glasgow RE. Computer-assisted intervention improves patient-centered diabetes care by increasing autonomy support. Health Psychol. 2007;26(6):728-34. doi:10.1037/0278-6133.26.6.728. PubMed PMID:18020845.

113. Williams GC, Patrick H, Niemiec CP, et al. Reducing the health risks of diabetes: how self-determination theory may help improve medication adherence and quality of life. Diabetes Educ. 2009;35(3):484-92. doi:10.1177/0145721709333856. PubMed PMID:19325022; PubMed Central PMCID:PMC2831466.

114. Patrick H, Williams GC. Self-determination theory: its application to health behavior and complementarity with motivational interviewing. Int J Behavioral Nutrition and Physical Activity. 2012;9:18.

115. Juul L, Maindal HT, Zoffmann V, Frydenberg M, Sandbaek A. Effectiveness of a training course for general practice nurses in motivation support in type 2 diabetes care: a cluster-randomised trial. PLoS One. 2014;9(5):e96683. doi:10.1371/journal.pone.0096683. PubMed PMID:24798419; PubMed Central PMCID:PMC4010512.

116. Fleming SE, Boyd A, Ballejos M, et al. Goal setting with type 2 diabetes: a hermeneutic analysis of the experiences of diabetes educators. Diabetes Educ. 2013;39(6):811-9. doi:10.1177/0145721713504471. PubMed PMID:24081301.

117. Gillison F, Standage M, Verplanken B. A cluster randomised controlled trial of an intervention to promote healthy lifestyle habits to school leavers: study rationale, design, and methods. BMC Public Health. 2014;14:221. doi:10.1186/1471-2458-14-221. PubMed PMID:24592967; PubMed Central PMCID:PMC3944885.

118. Gatwood J, Bailey JE. Improving medication adherence in hypercholesterolemia: challenges and solutions. Vasc Health Risk Manag. 2014;10:615-25. doi:10.2147/VHRM.S56056. PubMed PMID:25395859; PubMed Central PMCID:PMC4226449.

119. Nouwen A, Ford T, Balan AT, Twisk J, Ruggiero L, White D. Longitudinal motivational predictors of dietary self-care and diabetes control in adults with newly diagnosed type 2 diabetes mellitus. Health Psychol. 2011;30(6):771-9. doi:10.1037/a0024500. PubMed PMID:21707174.

120. Murphy K, Chuma T, Mathews C, Steyn K, Levitt N. A qualitative study of the experiences of care and motivation for effective self-management among diabetic and hypertensive patients attending public sector primary health care services in South Africa. BMC Health Serv Res. 2015;15:303. doi:10.1186/s12913-015-0969-y. PubMed PMID:26231178; PubMed Central PMCID:PMC4522057.

121. Blackford K, Jancey J, Lee AH, et al. A randomised controlled trial of a physical activity and nutrition program targeting middle-aged adults at risk of metabolic syndrome in a disadvantaged rural community. BMC Public Health. 2015;15:284. doi:10.1186/s12889-015-1613-9. PubMed PMID:25885657; PubMed Central PMCID:PMC4419409.

122. Seo YM, Choi WH. A predictive model on self care behavior for patients with type 2 diabetes: based on self-determination theory. J Korean Acad Nurs. 2011;41(4):491-9. doi:10.4040/jkan.2011.41.4.491. PubMed PMID:21964224.

123. Karlsen B, Bruun BR, Oftedal B. New possibilities in life with type 2 diabetes: experiences from participating in a guided self-determination programme in general practice. Nurs Res Pract. 2018; 2018:6137628. doi: 10/1155/2018/6137628.

124. Funnell MM, Anderson RM. Patient empowerment: a look back, a look ahead. Diabetes Educ. 2003;29(3):454-60.

125. Anderson RM, Funnell MM. The Art of Empowerment: Stories and Strategies for Diabetes Educators. 2nd ed. Alexandria, Va: American Diabetes Association; 2005.

126. Funnell MM, Anderson RM, Arnold MS, et al. Empowerment: an idea whose time has come in diabetes education. Diabetes Educ. 1991;17:37-41.

127. Anderson RM, Funnell MM. Patient empowerment: myths and misconceptions. Patient Educ Couns. 2010;79(3):277-82.

128. Anderson RM, Funnell MM. Ten things patient empowerment is not. Treat Strategies Diabetes. 2010;2(1):185-92.

129. Funnell MM, Anderson RM. Patient empowerment: from revolution to evolution. Treat Strategies Diabetes. 2011;3:98-105.

130. Funnell MM, Anderson RM. Empowerment and diabetes: why bother? J Diabetes Nurs. 2012;16Suppl 1:2.

131. Arnold MS, Butler PM, Anderson RM, Funnell MM, Feste C. Guidelines for facilitating a patient empowerment program. Diabetes Educ. 1995;21(4):308-12. PubMed PMID:7621733.

132. Davis ED, Vander Moor JM, Yarborough PC, Roth SB. Using solution-focused therapy strategies in empowerment-based education. Diabetes Educ. 1999;25(2):249-57.

133. Dijkstra R, Braspenning J, Grol R. Empowering patients: how to implement a diabetes passport in hospital care. Patient Educ Couns. 2002;47(2):173-7.

134. Pibernik-Okanovic M, Prasek M, Poljicanin-Filipovic T, Pavlic-Renar I, Metelko Z. Effects of an empowerment-based psychosocial intervention on quality of life and metabolic control in type 2 diabetic patients. Patient Educ Couns. 2004;52(2):193-9. PubMed PMID:15132525.

135. Funnell MM, Anderson RM. Empowerment and self-management of diabetes. Clin Diabetes. 2004;22(3):123-7.

136. Anderson RM, Funnell MM, Nwankwo R, Gillard ML, Oh M, Fitzgerald JT. Evaluation of a problem based empowerment program for African Americans with diabetes: results of a randomized controlled trial. Ethn Dis. 2005;15:671-8.

137. Funnell MM, Nwankwo R, Gillard ML, Anderson RM, Tang TS. Implementing an empowerment-based diabetes self-management education program. Diabetes Educ. 2005;31(1):53,55-6,61. PubMed PMID:15779247.

138. Siminerio LM, Piatt GA, Emerson S, et al. Deploying the Chronic Care Model to implement and sustain diabetes self-management training programs. Diabetes Educ. 2006;32(2):253-60.

139. Siminerio LM, Ruppert K, Emerson S, Solano F, Piatt G. Delivering diabetes self-management education (DSME) in primary care. Dis Manage Health Outcomes. 2008;16(4):267-72.

140. Anderson RM, Funnell MM, Aikens JE, et al. Evaluating the efficacy of an empowerment-based self-management consultant intervention: results of a two-year randomized controlled trial. Ther Patient Educ. 2009;1(1):3-11.

141. Deakin T, Whitham C. Structured patient education: the X-PERT Programme. Br J Community Nurs. 2009;14(9): 398-404. doi:10.12968/bjcn.2009.14.9.43916. PubMed PMID:19749659.

142. Piatt G, Anderson RM, Brooks MM, et al. Three-year follow-up of clinical and behavioral improvements following a multifaceted diabetes care intervention. Diabetes Educ. 2010;36(2):301-9.

143. Tol A, Alhani F, Shojaeazadeh, et al. An empowering approach to promote the quality of life and self-management among type 2 diabetic patients. J Educ Health Promot. 2015:4:13. doi: 10.4103/2277-9531.154022.

144. Davis S, Keep S, Edie A, et al. A peer-led diabetes education program in a homeless community to improve diabetes knowledge and empowerment. J Community Health Nursing. 2016; 33(2):71-80.

145. Funnell MM, Tang TS, Anderson RM. From DSME to DSMS: developing empowerment based self management support. Diabetes Spectr. 2007;20:221-6.

146. Tang TS, Funnell MM, Noorulla S, Oh M, Brown MB. Sustaining short-term improvement over the long term: results from a 2-year diabetes self management (DSMS) intervention. Diabetes Res Clin Pract. 2011. [Epub ahead of print.]

147. Tang TS, Funnell MM, Oh M. Lasting effects of a 2-year diabetes self-management support intervention: outcomes at 1-year follow-up. Prev Chron Dis. 2012;9:e109. doi:10.5888/pcd9.110313.

148. Siminerio L, Piatt G, Zgibor J. Implementing the chronic care model for improvements in diabetes care and education in a rural primary care practice. Diabetes Educ. 2005;31(2):225-34.

149. Kulzer B, Hermanns N, Reinecker H, Haak T. Effects of self-management training in type 2 diabetes: a randomized, prospective trial. Diabet Med. 2007;24(4):415-23. doi:10.1111/j.1464-5491.2007.02089.x. PubMed PMID:17298590.

150. Tang TS, Funnel MM, Gillard ML, Nwanko R, Heisler M. The development of a pilot training program for peer leaders in diabetes. Diabetes Educ. 2011;37(1):67-77.

151. Tang TS, Funnell MM. Peer Leader Training Manual. Brussels, Belgium: International Diabetes Federation; 2011.

152. Shin KS, Lee EH. Relationships of health literacy to self-care behaviors in people with diabetes aged 60 and above: empowerment as a mediator. J Advanced Nursing. 2018;74(10): 2363-72.

153. Miller WR, Rollnick S. Motivational Interviewing, 3rd Edition: Helping People Change. New York: Guilford Press; 2013.

154. Rollnick S, Miller WR, Butler CC. Motivational Interviewing in Health Care. New York: Guilford Press; 2008.

155. Kavookjian J. Motivational Interviewing. In Richardson M, Chant C, Chessman KH, et al, eds., Pharmacotherapy Self-Assessment Program, 7th ed. Book 8: Science and Practice of Pharmacotherapy. Lenexa, KS: American College of Clinical Pharmacy; 2011;1-18.

156. Steinberg MP, Miller WR. Motivational Interviewing in Diabetes Care. New York: Guilford Press; 2015.

157. Rubak S, Sandbæk A, Lauritzen T, Christensen B. Motivational interviewing: a systematic review and meta-analysis. Br J Gen Pract. 2005;55(513):305-12.

158. VanWormer JJ, Boucher JL. Motivational Interviewing and diet modification: a review of the evidence. Diabetes Educator. 2004;30(3):404-419.

159. Martins RK, McNeil DW. Review of motivational interviewing in promoting health behaviors. Clin Psychol Rev. 2009;29(4):283-93. doi:10.1016/j.cpr.2009.02.001. PubMed PMID:19328605.

160. Hill S, Kavookjian J. Motivational Interviewing as a behavioral intervention to increase HAART adherence in patients who are HIV+: a systematic review. AIDS Care. 2012; 24(5):583-92.

161. Teeter B. Kavookjian J. Telephone-based motivational interviewing for medication adherence: a systematic review. Translational Behavioral Medicine. 2014; 4(4):372-81.

162. Schaefer MR, Kavookjian J. The impact of motivational interviewing on adherence and symptom severity in adolescents and young adults with chronic illness: a systematic review. Patient Education and Counseling. 2017; 100(12):2190-9.

163. Madson MB, Loignon AC, Lane C. Training in motivational interviewing: a systematic review. J Substance Abuse Treatment. 2009;36:101-9.

164. Madson MB, Landry AS, Molaison EF, et al. Training MI interventionists across disciplines. Motivational Interviewing Training Research Implementation Practice. 2014;1(3) 20-24.

165. Schwalbe CS, Oh HY, Zweben A. Sustaining motivational interviewing: a meta-analysis of training studies. Addiction. 2014;109:1287-94.

166. Christie D, Channon S. The potential for motivational interviewing to improve outcomes in the management of diabetes and obesity in paediatric and adult populations: a clinical review. Diabetes, Obesity and Metabolism. 2014;16:381-7.

167. Ekong G, Kavookjian J. Motivational interviewing and outcomes in adults with type 2 diabetes: a systematic review of the literature. Patient Education and Counseling. 2016;99(6): 944-52.

168. Glynn LH, Moyers TB. Chasing change talk: the clinician's role in evoking client language about change. J Subst Abuse Treat. 2010;39(1):65-70.

169. DiLillo V, West DS. Incorporating motivational interviewing into counseling for lifestyle change among overweight individuals with type 2 diabetes. Diabetes Spectrum. 2011; 24(2):80-4.

170. Miller WR. From the desert: confessions of a recovering trainer/ what about decisional balance? Motivational Interviewing Training Research Implementation Practice. 2013;1(2):2-5.

171. Miller WR, Rose GS. Toward a theory of motivational interviewing. American Psychol. 2009;64(6):527.

172. Miller WR, Rollnick S. Ten things that motivational interviewing is not. Behav Cogn Psychother. 2009;37(2):129-40.

173. Carino JL, Coke L, Gulanick M. Using motivational interviewing to reduce diabetes risk. Prog Cardiovasc Nurs. 2004;19(4):149-54.

174. Wagner CC, Ingersoll KS. Motivational Interviewing in Groups. New York: Guilford Press; 2013.

175. Spears J, Erkins J, Misquitta C, Cutler T, Stebbins M. A pharmacist-led, patient-centered program incorporating motivational interviewing for behavior change to improve adherence rates and star ratings in a Medicare Plan. J Manag Care Spec Pharm. 2020;26(1):35-41.

176. US Department of Health and Human Services/ Centers for Disease Control and Prevention. Prevent T2: A Proven Program to Prevent or Delay Type 2 Diabetes.

177. National Institutes of Health and the Centers for Disease Control and Prevention. Motivational Interviewing: how and Why It Works for People With Diabetes. National Diabetes Education Program Webinar Series. 2015. https://www.cdc.gov/diabetes/ndep/pdfs/ndep_motivational_interviewing_webinar_slides.pdf.

178. Stott NC, Rollnick S, Rees MR, Pill RM. Innovation in clinical method: diabetes care and negotiating skills. Fam Pract. 1995;12(4):413-8. PubMed PMID:8826057.

179. Stott NC, Rees M, Rollnick S, Pill RM, Hackett P. Professional responses to innovation in clinical method: diabetes care and negotiating skills. Patient Educ Couns. 1996;29(1):67-73. PubMed PMID:9006223.

180. Smith DE, Heckemeyer CM, Kratt PP, Mason DA. Motivational interviewing to improve adherence to a behavioral weight-control program for older obese women with NIDDM. A pilot study. Diabetes Care. 1997;20(1):52-4. PubMed PMID:9028693.

181. Welch G, Zagarins SE, Feinberg RG, Garb JL. Motivational interviewing delivered by diabetes educators: does it improve blood glucose control among poorly controlled type 2 diabetes patients? Diabetes Res Clin Pract. 2011;91(1):54-60. doi:10.1016/j.diabres.2010.09.036. PubMed PMID:21074887; PubMed Central PMCID:PMC3011053.

182. Gabbay RA, Anel-Tiangco RM, Dellasega C, Mauger DT, Adelman A, Van Horn DH. Diabetes nurse case management and motivational interviewing for change (DYNAMIC): results of a 2-year randomized controlled pragmatic trial. J Diabetes. 2013;5(3):349-57. doi:10.1111/1753-0407.12030. PubMed PMID:23368423; PubMed Central PMCID:PMC3679203.

183. American Pharmacists Association. DOTx.MED: Pharmacist-delivered interventions to improve care for patients with diabetes. J Am Pharm Assoc. 2012;52:25-33.

184. Pringle JL, Boyer A, Conklin MH, et al. The Pennsylvania Project: pharmacist intervention improved medication adherence and reduced health care costs. Health Affiars. 2014;33(8):1444-52.

185. Ekong G, Kavookjian J. Pharmacist-delivered motivational interviewing for diabetes medication adherence in a hospital-based worksite wellness program. J Am Pharm Assoc. 2017: 57(3):e477.

186. Naar-King S, Suarez M. Motivational Interviewing With Adolescents and Young Adults. New York: The Guilford Press; 2011.

187. Apodaca TR, Jackson KM, Borsari B, et al. Which individual therapist behaviors elicit client change talk and sustain talk in motivational interviewing? J Substance Abuse Treatment. 2016; 61:60-5.

188. Villarosa-Hurlocker MC, O'Sickey AJ, Houck JM, Moyers TB. Examining the influence of active ingredients of motivational interviewing on client change talk. J Substance Abuse Treatment. 2019;96:39-45.

189. Dickinson JK, Guzman SJ, Maryniuk MD, et al. The use of language in diabetes care and education. Diabetes Care. 2017; 40:1790-9.

CHAPTER 4

Healthy Coping

Janis Roszler, LMFT, RD, LD/N, CDCES, FAND
Melissa Brail, LMFT
Eliot LeBow, LCSW, CDCES

Key Concepts

- Understanding healthy coping within the context of diabetes helps healthcare professionals work collaboratively while utilizing a person-centered approach when helping individuals living with diabetes, their families, and caregivers toward successful diabetes self-management.
- Mental health, stress, illness adjustment, and coping, as well as related concepts of self-efficacy, perceived control, and coping styles, are important for diabetes care and education specialists to understand.
- Successful self-management of diabetes depends on mastery of the medical regimen as well as coping with the emotional and social demands of living with diabetes.
- A person-centered educational approach contributes to positive medical outcomes and psychological well-being.

Introduction

The AADE7® model defines healthy coping as "A positive attitude toward diabetes and self-management, positive relationships with others, and quality of life." which is critical to master the other 6 behaviors.[1]

The diagnosis of a chronic disease, such as diabetes mellitus, is often an unanticipated life event for an individual and their family. Even when known risk factors exist, such as a family history of type 2 diabetes or gestational diabetes, most individuals are caught off guard when they are diagnosed with diabetes. The initial response is often one of disbelief or doubt regarding the accuracy of the diagnosis.

Individual responses to chronic disease are varied and depend on multiple personal, interpersonal, cultural, and environmental factors. According to the biopsychosocial model of adaptation to illness, individuals with a chronic disease experience change in 3 areas of their lives—biological, psychological, and social. The biological area refers to physical changes that occur, the psychological area is how persons with diabetes perceive these changes, and the social area focuses on the impact the disease has on their ability to relate to loved ones, the community, and the spiritual or "life-meaning" part of their world.[2] Persons with diabetes who struggle with any or all of these areas will require additional support so these issues don't distract or discourage them from participating in diabetes self-management.

Because diabetes requires daily self-management behaviors and decision making, individuals and families may require help coping in order to make necessary lifestyle adjustments. The Association of Diabetes Care and Education Specialists (ADCES) lists healthy coping as one of its AADE7 Self-Care Behaviors® for successful diabetes self-management.[3] Learning and implementing healthy coping skills helps individuals with diabetes overcome barriers and successfully engage in self-management behaviors.[3] The goal of developing coping and problem-solving skills involves regularly assessing these skills in the person with diabetes and determining whether there is a need for intervention.

Mental Health Concerns

Clinical care and research have helped us understand that all individuals with diabetes regardless of type are at greater risk for mental health issues such as depression, diabetes distress, anxiety, and eating disorders.[3–5] While children diagnosed with type 1 diabetes during their developmental years are also at risk for developing attention-deficit/hyperactive disorder (ADHD).[7] These issues are often mistaken for behavioral problems in diabetes; consequently, if these issues are not identified and treated, they may affect one's coping, diabetes management, behavior change, and diabetes outcomes. It is important that people with diabetes be screened regularly to identify whether these concerns need to be addressed.

Cognitive Impairment

Any impairment to a person's ability to focus, process, retain, and recall information can impact their ability to perform self-care behaviors, causing poor diabetes self-management and related glycemic outcomes.[8–12] Mental health issues, such as diabetes distress, ADHD, depression, diabulimia, and addiction, also cause cognitive impairment.[13]

Hyperglycemia and hypoglycemia also cause cognitive impairment impacting a person's ability to manage diabetes effectively. Hypoglycemia is very easy to recognize and resolved quickly. Diabetes care and education specialists must pay attention to hyperglycemia, as it is challenging to identify and plays a significant role in hindering effective diabetes management. "Hyperglycemia causes many physical issues, particularly if blood glucose is high for extended periods, but both short and long periods of elevated blood glucose levels can cause drastic cognitive issues that often go unattended too."[14] Cognitive impairment also affects knowledge and skill transfer, and the ability to learn and apply new information, impacting self-care management, especially problem solving.[15]

According to several studies, individuals with type 1 diabetes diagnosed before 17 years old, have cognitive impairment as a result of severe hypoglycemia, chronic hyperglycemia, and diabetic ketoacidosis during early brain development. This causes brain damage to the frontal lobe along with reduced gray and white matter, negatively impacting mental efficiency, psychomotor speed, executive functioning, and intelligence.[8–10] Studies on type 2 diabetes show that cognitive impairment stems from obesity, insulin resistance, hypertension, dyslipidemia, poor diabetes self-management, and associated glycemic outcomes.[11–12]

Cognitive impairment is one of the factors diabetes care and education specialists need to assess for when they start working with an individual living with diabetes regardless of the person's age or diabetes type. When assessing for cognitive impairment, the Mini-Mental Status Exam (MMSE) provides a foundation for developing effective and individualized, person-centered treatment plans. Recently a more sensitive instrument than the MMSE has been developed called the Saint Louis University Mental Status (SLUMS).[16] The advantage of utilizing the SLUMS evaluation is its ability to detect mild cognitive impairment and dementia. Once assessed, person-centered treatment plans providing individualized support along with a referral to a mental health specialist help reduce the impact of cognitive impairment, improving DSM.

One important note for diabetes care and education specialists to pay attention to is the co-morbid relationship between type 1 diabetes and Attention Deficit Hyperactivity Disorder (ADHD). A referral to a mental health provider that specializes in ADHD is recommended when both are present.[7]

Diabetes Distress

Diabetes distress is the emotional burden of diabetes, the constant demands from diabetes self-management, the possibility of developing complications, and the lack of support and access to care.[17–20] The present research has shown that diabetes distress negatively impacts the physical and emotional well-being of the person living with diabetes.[21]

In 2013, the findings of the second Diabetes Attitudes, Wishes, and Needs study (DAWN2) confirmed and deepened the understanding of how often people with diabetes experience distress linked to having and managing diabetes. The study was conducted in 17 countries and included 8,596 adults with diabetes. The results of DAWN2 showed that diabetes distress was reported by 44.6% of the participants, but only 23.7% reported that their healthcare team asked them how diabetes affected their life.[20]

The DAWN2 study also surveyed and reported on how much diabetes affects family members. Supporting a family member was perceived as a significant burden by 35.3%, and 61% reported high levels of distress.[20] DAWN2 confirmed that psychosocial problems of family members are barriers to their effective involvement in self-management. In addition, it showed how person-centered care and support is not being adequately delivered in clinics and through health systems.[20]

Despite not being in the Diagnostic and Statistical Manual of Mental health, diabetes distress is a mental health issue that impacts all areas of a person's psychosocial picture. So much so that diabetes distress has been shown to appear in the person with diabetes support network: Parents,[22] and Partner.[23] Several studies have shown a direct correlation between elevated diabetes distress and poor glycemic management.[18,23–26] Assessment of diabetes-related distress can be clarified by using one of the following Diabetes Distress Scales: Parents-DDS, Partners-DDS, T1-DDS or DDS (T2).[27,28] SMES has been shown to reduce diabetes distress for mild to moderate symptoms; however, according to Fisher, diabetes distress–specific interventions could be needed for persons with high levels of diabetes distress. Referring persons with diabetes to appropriate and qualified mental health professionals is necessary if they present with high levels of diabetes distress[13,18,29] and would be beneficial for individuals who have moderate symptoms.

Depression

Depression is characterized by depressed mood, loss of interest in activities usually found pleasurable, poor energy, difficulty concentrating and sleeping, appetite problems, catastrophic thinking, and, often with diabetes, difficulty in following through with self-management behaviors. The assessment of depression is complicated by the fact that the neurovegetative signs of depression are very similar to symptoms of poorly managed diabetes, and, thus, depression is often confused with diabetes distress. For example, an individual with diabetes who is depressed will probably not be able to engage in healthy diabetes behaviors. But the term *diabetes distress* actually covers an even greater experience that includes the worries, fears, and concerns people with diabetes may develop as they struggle with the demands of this chronic and progressive disease.[26]

Due to recent research that indicates a bidirectional relationship between diabetes and depression, the need to assess and offer treatment for depression is essential.[30, 31–32] Different types of depression include persistent depressive disorder, which affects care but is usually not disabling, and major depressive disorder (MDD), which is often disabling and highly likely to make life with diabetes very difficult. Some individuals may also be more depressed during certain times of the year, which can affect diabetes care during those times.

Often in conversation, the diabetes care and education specialist may sense that the person with diabetes is experiencing "the blues" or that the person is not feeling well. At times "the blues" can be normal, but unless the diabetes care and education specialist asks, it can be difficult to discern whether the person with diabetes is experiencing a temporary down period or if it is a more serious, longer-term problem. If it appears more complicated and possibly related to depression, the Patient Health Questionnaire-9 (PHQ9) could be used to conduct a preliminary screening for depression. Table 4.1 is the PHQ9 Screen tool used to help diabetes care and education specialists assess for depression.

Each question is scored on a 0 to 3 scale: 0 for not at all, 1 for several days, 2 for more than half the days, and 3 for nearly every day. If the total is greater than 9 with at least one of the first 2 questions answered "more than half the days" or "nearly every day" in the past 2 weeks and the tenth question is answered "somewhat difficult" or more than further assessment should take place with referral to a qualified mental health professional.

Helping the person with diabetes with the referral process is critical. This might include contacting a professional or assisting in making the appointment. Keep in mind that someone who is depressed may lack the energy or focus to follow up on seeking this help, even if they want to get better. For this reason, one should refer individuals to a mental health professional as soon as possible after diagnosis, before crises arise. If and when one develops, individuals are often more willing to open up to someone they already know and trust. That established relationship can help them enjoy better results.[33] Additional reasons to refer early are listed in Table 4.2.

Mental health professionals may suggest different approaches, such as counseling, medication, exercise, or meditation. By helping those who suffer from depression to access this treatment, the diabetes care and education specialist is helping them move closer to better diabetes management. It is essential to consult with person with diabetes' mental health professional to explain diabetes-specific issues the person may face and inform them if diabetes distress is present along with providing assessment tools for diabetes distress.[28]

Self-Efficacy

Self-efficacy is an individual's confidence in their ability to exert control over their behavior and social environment as well as their ability to execute actions necessary to accomplish self-beneficial tasks, including diabetes self-management tasks. Psychological issues like depression, attention-deficit/hyperactivity disorder, diabetes distress, and other psychiatric conditions can negatively influence self-efficacy. Research states that high levels of self-efficacy, along with increased social support and positive attitudes toward self-care behaviors, are associated with good diabetes self-management.[13,34]

When properly incorporated into treatment, goal setting can increase self-efficacy while improving the person's ability to cope with diabetes.[35] Goal setting has a positive effect on healthy living, helping individuals living with diabetes create a sense of purpose while increasing positive solution-based thinking. SMART, an acronym which stands for Specific, Measurable, Achievable, Reasonable, and Timely, is used to help persons with diabetes set obtainable goals with reasonable objectives. The findings from research show improvement in disease management,

TABLE 4.1 Patient Health Questionnaire (PHQ9)

PHQ9				
Over the last 2 weeks, how often have you been bothered by any of the following problems?	*Not at All*	*Several Days*	*More Than Half the Days*	*Nearly Every Day*
1. Little interest or pleasure in doing things	0	1	2	3
2. Feeling down, depressed, or hopeless	0	1	2	3
3. Trouble falling or staying asleep, or sleeping too much	0	1	2	3
4. Feeling tired or having little energy	0	1	2	3
5. Poor appetite or overeating	0	1	2	3
6. Feeling bad about yourself or that you are a failure or have let yourself or your family down	0	1	2	3
7. Trouble concentrating on things, such as reading the newspaper or watching television	0	1	2	3
8. Moving or speaking so slowly that other people could have noticed or the opposite—being so fidgety or restless that you have been moving around a lot more than usual	0	1	2	3
9. Thoughts that you would be better off dead or of hurting yourself in some way	0	1	2	3

(For office coding: Total Score ________ = ________ + ________ + ________)

If you checked off any problems, how difficult have these problems made it for you to do your work, take care of things at home, or get along with other people?

Not difficult at all	Somewhat difficult	Very difficult	Extremely difficult
☐	☐	☐	☐

From the Primary Care Evaluation of Mental Disorders Patient Health Questionnaire (PRIME-MD PHQ). The PHQ was developed by Drs. Robert L. Spitzer, Janet BW Williams, Kurt Kroenke, and colleagues. For research information, contact Dr. Spitzer at rls8 @columbia.edu. PRIME-MD is a trademark of Pfizer Inc. Copyright 1999 Pfizer Inc. All rights reserved. Reproduced with permission.

TABLE 4.2 Rationale for Therapist Referral

Diabetes care and education specialists can share the following messages with persons with diabetes when discussing the need for therapy referral:

—**I refer all person with diabetes to a therapist.** A therapist is a vital part of every diabetes team. If you have no emotional, social, family, or behavioral concerns right now, this referral can help you develop a relationship with someone who can assist you in the future.

—**How you think about your health can make a difference.** Your blood glucose can affect your mood and vice versa. A therapist can help you learn how to think about your health in a more positive way.

—**Living with diabetes can be stressful.** Your therapist can help you learn skills that enable you to interact with others better and handle stress, worries, and fears more effectively.

—**A therapist can help you embrace yourself as a complete person,** not just as a person with diabetes.

Source: J Roszler, WS Rapaport, *Approaches to Behavior* (Alexandria, Va: American Diabetes Association, 2015).

lifestyle change,[36] and emotional well-being when utilized across multiple areas of health.

Problem Solving

Studies have linked deficits in problem solving to various psychological problems, including anxiety and depression. Impairments in problem solving are also linked to difficulties coping with chronic illnesses. Problem solving is a core skill for diabetes self-management education and contributes to healthy living for people living with diabetes.[37] Problem solving is a process where a person finds adaptive solutions for everyday problems. Consult chapter 10 for more on problem solving.

Anxiety

Anxiety is healthy in moderation and a normal part of life. It is normal to feel anxious before taking a test, facing a problem at work, or when facing an important decision. Anxiety helps us study for our test and problem-solve solutions to issues we face. It is normal to have some amount of anxiety due to diabetes-specific issues, such as low glucose, high glucose, or long-term complications. These types of issues help motivate people living with diabetes to perform self-care behaviors needed for diabetes management, like how they eat, exercise, and monitor their glucose. With anxiety disorders the anxiety doesn't go away and causes symptoms that can interfere with daily activities like work or school or cause problems in their relationships,[38] and for people living with diabetes this includes diabetes management. Individuals with heightened levels of anxiety are more likely to have greater fear of these issues and exhibit more extreme behavior. Examples include people who intentionally allow their blood glucose level to run high to prevent lows, or those who ignore their diabetes completely so they don't feel the anxiety related to developing long-term complications. On the other end of the anxiety continuum are those who check their glucose excessively out of fear of having hypoglycemia. Those with anxiety might also intentionally maintain a very low blood glucose level, to try to avoid the development of long-term complications. This often prompts them to experience frequent episodes of severe hypoglycemia. Brief anxiety measures can be used to detect generalized anxiety, but for diabetes-specific distress, the Diabetes Distress Scale[39] or the Problem Areas in Diabetes (PAID)[40] can be used to measure these concerns and to stimulate discussion about how one is dealing with diabetes overall. If you believe an anxiety disorder is present, a referral to a qualified mental health professional for further assessment is necessary.

Stress

Stress is the body's response to any demand made on it. Stress can be perceived as positive or negative. Stressors are expected and unexpected events that upset our balance. The crises of the diagnosis of diabetes and the resulting demands of disease self-management place numerous stressors on the individual and his or her family.

Stress not only affects individuals psychosocially but also includes a biochemical response in the body. The biochemical (hormonal) stress response can significantly impact metabolic stability in persons with diabetes, which is why learning to manage and cope with stress is so important.

Common diabetes-related stressors occur on 3 levels:

1. Personal
2. Interpersonal
3. Environmental

Stress, whether temporary or chronic, results in physiological and behavioral reactions that can affect diabetes self-management. Behavioral responses can have a positive or negative influence on eating, testing, exercise, and self-care activities. The consequences will have an impact on physiological measures like glucose stability as well as psychosocial well-being.

Table 4.3 offers helpful questions in screening for depression and diabetes distress. Referring persons with diabetes to appropriate and qualified mental health

TABLE 4.3 Diabetes-Related Stress, Depression, and Anxiety Disorders: Informal Screening Questions
Depression In the past 2 weeks, did you consistently feel depressed or down? Have you had difficulty with feeling sad or blue? Has your mood interfered with taking care of your diabetes?
Anxiety Disorders *Anxiety* What concerns do you have about your diabetes? Tell me about the aspects of diabetes you worry about. *Avoidance* What parts of your diabetes self-care are the hardest for you to do? Are there situations or activities you avoid because of your diabetes? *Fear* What is scary about diabetes for you? Are there things about diabetes that frighten you? *Worry* What do you worry about regarding your diabetes? Tell me some of the thoughts that run through your head about diabetes.
Diabetes-Related Stress *Identification of Specific Stressors* What drives you crazy about your diabetes? Describe your typical day for me, starting when you wake up and ending when you go to sleep. What stressors do you face on a typical day? *Assessment of Stress Levels* How high has your stress level been since our last appointment? On a scale from 0 to 10, with 0 being no stress and 10 being the worst stress imaginable, what number would you give your stress level today? *Assessment of Diabetes Distress* Do you ever feel frustrated, fed up, overwhelmed, or burned out by diabetes? I've noticed that lately you've had a hard time managing your diabetes. Do you think stress may play a role?

professionals may be necessary after you have covered these questions.

Diabetes, Drugs, and Alcohol

It would seem obvious that a metabolic disease like diabetes mixed with mind- and body-altering substances would be counteractive to self-care. The temptation for people who have diabetes is no less than it is for anyone else who desires an altered state of consciousness. In fact, some who have not adjusted well to having diabetes may be more likely to have a desire for something different. The consequences for such behavior, however, are likely to be more dangerous. Alcohol abuse can cause difficulties with tracking blood glucose, unpredictable fluctuation in glucose, and potentially serious lows that could be mistaken for alcohol intoxication. These side effects could result in hospitalization or potential death if the individual does not receive proper care. Regular and chronic abuse of alcohol can lead to overall poor self-care, lack of follow-up to diabetes treatment, and a self-destructive attitude. Significant others and families can also be dramatically affected. Alcoholism has a serious effect that is much broader than just the individual and needs to be addressed with proper treatment and follow-up.

Drug use can be harmful as well. Recreational drugs such as methamphetamine, cocaine, and heroin take a toll on the individual's way of thinking, significantly impacting self-care. They also have no known medicinal or therapeutic use and have a high potential for abuse, addiction, and dependence. Marijuana can also have a negative effect with unpredictable eating binges as well as forgetful behavior, leading to poor self-care.

Moderate alcohol use in adults with no history of alcohol abuse is considered to be reasonable. However, it needs to be accompanied by planful behavior that includes eating, testing, and self-monitoring of amounts. The legalization of marijuana use in some states is likely to introduce a similar recommendation for its use as well. A mindful approach to moderating alcohol and marijuana use may in fact be appropriate to avoid creating an "all or nothing" type of thinking.

For people with diabetes it's appropriate to discuss the use of these substances, particularly if their diabetes management seems questionable. Additionally, it's important to simply check in as part of the education process.

Eating Disorders

The diabetes care and education specialist needs to be aware of symptoms of eating disorders and the potential need for assessment and referral for treatment. What are the major eating disorders?

The American Psychiatric Association has 3 diagnostic categories for eating disorders:[41]

- Anorexia nervosa
- Bulimia nervosa
- Binge eating disorder

Anorexia Nervosa

The primary clinical features of anorexia nervosa are the following:[41]

- Restriction of energy intake relative to requirements
- Intense fear of becoming fat even though underweight
- Body image issues

In addition, people with anorexia may display unusual eating habits, such as cutting their food into very small pieces or not eating in front of others, and they often obsess about food.[41]

Bulimia Nervosa

The primary clinical signs of bulimia nervosa include the following:[41]

- Repeated episodes of binge eating involving a sense of loss of control and an amount of food consumed in a 2-hour period that is larger than what would be typical for most people in a similar amount of time
- Compensatory behaviors to prevent weight gain, such as self-induced vomiting, fasting, excessive exercise, and/or misuse of diuretics, laxatives, enemas, or other medications for weight-loss purposes
- The binge eating and compensatory behaviors occur on average once a week for 3 months
- Body image issues
- The behavior does not occur during episodes of anorexia nervosa

Binge Eating Disorder

While purging is not associated with binge eating disorder (BED), many of the challenges that someone with BED faces are similar to those of bulimia nervosa. Unwanted weight gain is often a symptom of the disorder. Many people live in a combination cycle of bingeing and starving, so they do not quite meet the criteria for anorexia nervosa but are still doing serious damage to their physical and mental health.

Table 4.4 lists diagnostic criteria for anorexia nervosa, bulimia nervosa, and BED.

TABLE 4.4 Anorexia Nervosa, Bulimia Nervosa, and Binge Eating Disorder: Diagnostic Criteria

Anorexia Nervosa	*Bulimia Nervosa*	*Binge Eating Disorder*
A Restriction of energy intake relative to requirements leading to a significant low body weight in the context of age, sex, developmental trajectory, and physical health. Significantly low weight is defined as a weight that is less than minimally normal, or, for children and adolescents, less than that minimally expected. B Intense fear of gaining weight or becoming fat, or persistent behavior that interferes with weight gain even though at a significantly low weight. C Disturbance in the way in which one's body weight or shape is experienced, undue influence of body weight or shape on self-evaluation, or denial of the seriousness of the current low body weight. D *Specify Type:* *Restricting Type:* During the last 3 months, the person has not regularly engaged in recurrent episodes of binge-eating or purging behavior (ie, self-induced vomiting or misuse of laxatives, diuretics, or enemas). *Binge-Eating/Purging Type:* During the last 3 months, the person has regularly engaged in recurrent episodes of binge-eating or purging behavior (ie, self-induced vomiting or misuse of laxatives, diuretics, or enemas).	A Recurrent episodes of binge eating. An episode of binge eating is characterized by both of the following: 1. Eating, in a discrete period of time (eg, within any 2-hour period), an amount of food that is definitely larger than most people would eat during a similar period of time and under similar circumstances. 2. A sense of lack of control over eating during the episode (eg, a feeling that one cannot stop eating or control what or how much one is eating). B Recurrent inappropriate compensatory behavior in order to prevent weight gain, such as self-induced vomiting; misuse of laxatives, diuretics, enemas, or other medications; fasting; or excessive exercise. C The binge eating and inappropriate compensatory behaviors both occur, on average, at least once a week for 3 months. D Self-evaluation is unduly influenced by body shape and weight. E The disturbance does not occur exclusively during episodes of anorexia nervosa.	A Recurrent episodes of binge eating. An episode of binge eating is characterized by both of the following: 1. Eating, in a discrete period of time (eg, within any 2-hour period), an amount of food that is definitely larger than most people would eat during a similar period of time and under similar circumstances. 2. A sense of lack of control over eating during the episode (eg, a feeling that one cannot stop eating or control what or how much one is eating). B The binge-eating episodes are associated with at least 3 of the following: 1. Eating much more rapidly than normal 2. Eating until feeling uncomfortably full 3. Eating large amounts of food when not feeling physically hungry 4. Eating alone because of being embarrassed by how much one is eating 5. Feeling disgusted with oneself, depressed, or very guilty after overeating C Marked distress regarding binge eating. D The binge eating occurs, on average, at least once a week for 3 months. E The binge eating is not associated with the recurrent use of inappropriate compensatory behaviors and does not occur exclusively during the course of bulimia nervosa or anorexia nervosa.

Source: Reprinted with permission from the American Psychiatric Association, *Diagnostic and Statistical Manual of Mental Disorders,* 5th ed., text revision (Washington, D.C.: American Psychiatric Association, 2013). Copyright 2013. American Psychiatric Association.

Eating Disorders and Diabetes

Several aspects of diabetes and its treatment may make people with diabetes more vulnerable to eating disorders.[32] For example, the initial weight loss associated with the onset of type 1 diabetes followed by weight gain with the initiation of insulin may increase the risk of an eating disorder. This is especially true in those who have body image issues or weight concerns. In addition, routine dietary recommendations may challenge the vulnerabilities of those prone to eating disorders. Such individuals may interpret recommendations in an extreme manner. For example, a recommendation to monitor intake of simple carbohydrates may be interpreted as "never eat sweets," and a recommendation to get regular physical activity may be interpreted as "exercise every day for 2 hours."

Diabulimia

Over time some individuals with type 1 diabetes learn they can alter their weight through omitting insulin injections or reducing the amount they take, and thereby discover a unique way to purge. This is often referred to as "diabulimia." While not accepted in the fifth edition of the *Diagnostic and Statistical Manual of Mental Disorders* as a specific eating disorder, it clearly meets the criteria. This is especially true when used in combination with bingeing behavior. The consequences can be quite dramatic, with an increased risk of hospitalization from diabetic ketoacidosis (DKA) and the risk of chronic complications. The elevated glucose levels also contribute to difficulty in performing daily tasks and an increased risk of depression. Diabulimia is also more difficult to treat because persons with this disorder experience the sensations of hypoglycemia when they begin taking the required insulin, in spite of having a more normalized glucose level. They are then tempted to reduce insulin again to rid themselves of the physical discomfort of hypoglycemia and bloating from water weight gain.

Table 4.5 provides questions that can be used to screen for eating disorders in people with diabetes. Diabetes care and education specialists can facilitate referrals to qualified mental health professionals if an eating disorder is suspected.

Table 4.6 is the Screen for Early Eating Disorder Signs (SEEDS) tool. Scoring guidelines are provided in the full paper,[42] along with broad suggestions for intervention based on the level of eating disorder risk.

TABLE 4.5 Eating Disorders: Informal Screening Questions
Weight Concerns How do you feel about your weight? Do you think you are overweight or worry about becoming overweight? Do you avoid getting on the scale? Would you weigh yourself in front of others? What is your ideal body weight?
Body Image Issues How do you feel about your appearance? Shape? Body size?
Binge Eating Are there certain foods you try to totally avoid eating? (Ask for details.) How often do you binge eat? (May need to define.) Describe your last binge episode. Do you ever feel as though you cannot control your eating?
Compensatory Behaviors Have you ever induced vomiting or taken laxatives, diuretics, or enemas to lose weight? Have you ever reduced or skipped an insulin dose for weight purposes? Do you exercise regularly? (Ask for details.)
Weight History What was your lowest and highest adult weight? (Ask about weight during adolescence when appropriate.) At what weight are you happiest? Have you experienced any rapid weight changes? (Ask for details.)
Unusual Eating Behaviors Are you uncomfortable eating in front of others? Do you have any eating habits your friends or family have told you were unusual?

Coping

Successful self-management of diabetes depends on mastery of the medical regimen as well as coping with the emotional demands of living with a chronic disease.

Illness Adjustment

The process of healthy coping involves actions that are needed to restore order and a sense of well-being. For self-management to occur, integration of the chronic illness has to be incorporated into the individual's self-awareness. For the person with diabetes, the question is, "How do I take this new information and apply it to what I know about my life in order to live the way I want?"

Frequently, however, such adjustment is difficult due to societal or self-imposed stigmas that are often associated with having a chronic condition. This gets at the core of an individual's personal identity.

TABLE 4.6 Screen for Early Eating Disorder Signs (SEEDS)

SEEDS

These questions ask about you, your life, and your health. Please read each question carefully and answer honestly. Mark your answer by filling in one circle.

1. How do you usually feel?	Very sad							Very happy
	O_7	O_6	O_5	O_4	O_3	O_2	O_1	
2. How would *your friends* describe you?	Grumpy							Cheerful
	O_7	O_6	O_5	O_4	O_3	O_2	O_1	
3. How often do you compare how you look to those around you?	All the time							Not at all
	O_7	O_6	O_5	O_4	O_3	O_2	O_1	
4. How well do you fit in with your friends?	Not very well							Very well
	O_7	O_6	O_5	O_4	O_3	O_2	O_1	
5. How often do you feel in control of your life?	Never							Always
	O_7	O_6	O_5	O_4	O_3	O_2	O_1	
6. How satisfied are you with how you look?	Very dissatisfied							Very satisfied
	O_7	O_6	O_5	O_4	O_3	O_2	O_1	
7. How satisfying is your life?	Very unsatisfying							Very satisfying
	O_7	O_6	O_5	O_4	O_3	O_2	O_1	
8. How well do *you* handle your feelings?	Poorly							Very well
	O_7	O_6	O_5	O_4	O_3	O_2	O_1	
9. How would *your family members* describe your mood most of the time?	Grumpy							Cheerful
	O_7	O_6	O_5	O_4	O_3	O_2	O_1	
10. How often do you feel your life is valuable?	Never							Always
	O_7	O_6	O_5	O_4	O_3	O_2	O_1	
11. How well do *you* manage your stress?	Poorly							Very well
	O_7	O_6	O_5	O_4	O_3	O_2	O_1	
12. How often do you think about your body shape and size?	All the time							Not at all
	O_7	O_6	O_5	O_4	O_3	O_2	O_1	
13. How do *you* describe your mood?	Grumpy							Cheerful
	O_7	O_6	O_5	O_4	O_3	O_2	O_1	
14. How satisfied are you with your body *shape*?	Very dissatisfied							Very satisfied
	O_7	O_6	O_5	O_4	O_3	O_2	O_1	
15. How satisfied are you with your body *size*?	Very dissatisfied							Very satisfied
	O_7	O_6	O_5	O_4	O_3	O_2	O_1	
16. How do you describe your moods?	Up and down							Steady
	O_7	O_6	O_5	O_4	O_3	O_2	O_1	
17. How much do you think you matter to your family?	Not at all							Very much
	O_7	O_6	O_5	O_4	O_3	O_2	O_1	

(continued)

TABLE 4.6 Screen for Early Eating Disorder Signs (SEEDS) (continued)

18. How do you feel when others around you talk about body shape and size?	Uncomfortable						Comfortable
	O_7	O_6	O_5	O_4	O_3	O_2	O_1
19. How much do you think you matter to your friends?	Not at all						Very much
	O_7	O_6	O_5	O_4	O_3	O_2	O_1
20. How often do you think you meet the expectations your family has for you?	Never						Always
	O_7	O_6	O_5	O_4	O_3	O_2	O_1

Sources: MA Powers, SA Richter, DM Ackard, C Craft, "Development and validation of the Screen for Early Eating Disorder Signs (SEEDS) in persons with type 1 diabetes," *Eating Disord: J Treatment Prev,* 2015 Oct 14; MA Powers, SA Richter, DM Ackard, C Cronemeyer, "Eating disorders in persons with type 1 diabetes: a focus group investigation of early eating disorder risk," *J Health Psychol,* published online ahead of print 2015 Jun; MA Powers, S Richter, D Ackard, S Critchley, M Meier, A Criego, "Determining the influence of type 1 diabetes on two common eating disorder questionnaires," *Diabetes Educ* 39, no. 3(2013):387-96.

Personal Identity

Personal identity comprises the following: the material self, the psychological self, the cognitive-affective self, the social self, and the ideal self.[43] Each of these components focuses on specific aspects of the self and is affected by coping with a chronic illness and is potentially redefined by the individual's responses. The components of personal identity are defined as follows:

- *Material self:* The physical body
- *Psychological self:* Attitudes, beliefs, judgments
- *Cognitive-affective self:* Thinking, imagining, experiencing
- *Social self:* Roles and labels
- *Ideal self:* Aspirations

Table 4.7 shows the types of questions and concerns a person with diabetes might have and to which component of personal identity these questions and concerns are related.

Further, one's cultural identity, affiliation, and spiritual values often provide the foundation for personal identity and subsequent behaviors. Cultural identity is composed of the learned and shared beliefs, values, and lifestyle norms of a given group that have been passed down from one generation to another, which influences the thinking and behaviors of its members.[44] For instance, spiritual and/or religious traditions often foster distinct healthcare practices and beliefs across and within ethnic groups affected by diabetes. Such beliefs may cause individuals to ask why they have been burdened with the diagnosis of diabetes or diabetes-related complications despite their adherence to spiritual and religious beliefs and practices.[45] Many religions are based on a belief in a higher power, and some members believe and accept that this higher power has ultimate control over their lives.[45] Such beliefs can sometimes result in a less proactive coping style, so perceived control over diabetes self-management outcomes can be low. Diabetes care and education specialists can acknowledge the beliefs and devise strategies to facilitate a higher level of self-management.

When working with individuals from diverse cultural backgrounds, obtain some or all of the following information to help determine their specific needs: where they were born, their family structure, the language they speak at home, their ability to understand English, their financial situation, social status and education level, how well they have adapted to this country's culture, their traditions, religious affiliation, and social patterns.[46] The diabetes healthcare professional should acknowledge different views and beliefs and incorporate them into motivational strategies for diabetes self-management education (DSME) that will assist with restoring balance between the individual and the environment.

The Diabetes Care and Education Specialist's Role in Coping

The diabetes care an education specialist can play a major role in guiding a person with diabetes through coping and stress management. This role begins with assessing and identifying mental health issues early in the treatment process. Once these issues are managed, the diabetes care and education specialist can begin working with a person with diabetes to generate a diabetes self-management plan that includes various coping strategies.

Assessment

Perceptions of how to fit daily diabetes self-management into an already busy or demanding life may cause emotional distress, anxiety, or depressive symptoms. Perceptions of "fit" affect all aspects of personal identity and in particular the *social self.* Because stress responses and

TABLE 4.7 Personal Identity and Concerns About Diabetes

Component of Personal Identity	*Aspects of Component*	*Questions/Concerns*
Material self	Physical body	Individuals may have concerns or questions about their body. For those diagnosed with type 1 diabetes, the question may be: Why is my body not functioning as it should? For children and adolescents with type 1 diabetes, the question may be: How can I be "normal" with my insulin pump? For individuals diagnosed with type 2 diabetes, the question may be: Why is my body not working as it used to?
Psychological self	Attitudes	Individuals may have concerns, and questions can range from the healthcare system to the reactions of their family and friends to the diagnosis. Kids and adolescents may have attitudes about receiving help from parents, teachers, and friends. Adults may have attitudes toward accessing medical care. Ask: What do they feel toward doctors? People who have diabetes? Has anyone in their family had diabetes and what are their attitudes toward this person?
	Beliefs	Individuals may question their beliefs. Are they going to suffer the same fate as the person in their family who had diabetes? Do they believe they are different and will have a different fate? What are their beliefs about the need for them to control their food?
	Judgments	Individuals may blame themselves for having the disease. "I deserve this because I'm fat." "I can't tell anyone about this because they will treat me differently." "I can't be honest with the diabetes care and education specialist or she will know how bad I've been."
Cognitive-affective self	Thinking	Individuals may have concerns about how their diabetes will affect their plans for the future. "I have to be perfect or diabetes will kill me." "I can't be perfect so why even try?"
	Imagining	Individuals may have concerns about how their diabetes will affect their plans for the future. "I planned on serving in the military, and I guess I can't now. I might go blind." "What does this mean if I want to have children? Can I have children? Will my children have diabetes?"
	Experiencing	Individuals may have concerns about how their diabetes will affect their current activities and interests. "I have to be more responsible than everyone else." "Why can't I go to the sleepover?" "Do I have to quit scuba diving because I use insulin?"
Social self	Roles and labels	Individuals may have concerns about how their diabetes will affect their relationships with their family, friends, colleagues, or classmates. "My family is always watching what I eat." "I feel so out of control when I have a low reading." "I don't want the people at work to know that I have diabetes because they'll treat me differently." "I hate it when my children have to help me out of a low."
Ideal self	Aspirations	Individuals may have concerns about how their diabetes will affect their view of themselves. "This really changes how I see myself as a healthy person." "I hate having to depend on anything, even insulin." "This really changes how we see our son. We know he's not different, but somehow how we see him has changed."

coping strategies are based on a complex set of personal health beliefs, perceptions, motivations,[46,47] and support relationships, it is important to assess these issues to determine how they impact the individual.

Developmental Age and Stage

It is critical to understand and appreciate how developmental stages play a role in the way an individual adapts to the demands of diabetes. For example, a school-aged child may take pride in being able to do their own injections even though the child's healthcare team is encouraging the parents to give the injections. Teenagers may seem willing to do all of their own injections, but not do so when peers are present. All are normal behaviors, but without understanding this, parents can become quite distressed.

The most obvious aspect of life stage interacting with diabetes care occurs in the ages between infancy and early adulthood. This is a time of growth and change that is most dramatic for human growth physically, mentally, socially, and emotionally.

When considering the developmental challenges of the infant and toddler—trust and mistrust coupled with autonomy and dependence—having parents be the source of physical pain can challenge a positive resolution. The need exists to not only understand how the stage of development might interact with the necessary aspects of diabetes care, but also give careful thought to how the diabetes care an education specialist or parent might approach the child with awareness of these issues. This can be complicated by the fact that parents have their own feelings about their child having diabetes, which also need to be in balance so they can communicate this acceptance to the child. While some of these developmental stages can be challenges, some can be used as resources. The opportunity for a family to join together in support of the infant or toddler by changing familial behaviors can provide support for the child and the parents, ultimately strengthening the family bonds.

School-aged children's developmental focus is to be industrious, and they are interested in performing to please parents and teachers. This energy might be guided toward focusing on their diabetes and their own courage to deal with it as something positive and potentially teach others.

The teen years can be a bit more complicated, as the development task has to do with identity and intimacy. Given the very nature of diabetes, which requires a focus on the body and how it doesn't work quite perfectly, this is not exactly something of which the teen wants to be more aware. Teenagers prefer to go through life automatically, and diabetes requires far more thought than they want to give. While negotiation is not an automatic strength for the teen, it can be an opportunity for both parent and teen to get their needs met. This stage can be difficult given the risky behavior common to teens. However, it is critical to keep the developmental stage in mind as a normal aspect of growing up.

Often young adulthood is an opportunity for the person with diabetes to accept responsibility for the disease and sort out how to live with it. This is also an opportunity for the diabetes care an education specialist to open a dialogue that is appropriate for someone who can take full responsibility and may be willing to look honestly at how diabetes can fit into their life.

Adults between the ages of 25 and 55 will be different depending on the type of diabetes as well as where they are with their overall developmental process. Each individual will be influenced somewhat differently by their developmental stage, and also by the physical, emotional, and social impact of diabetes.

The personal and developmental aspects of older individuals will be moderated by who they are and how they have lived their lives; overall health, complications from the disease, and degree of needed support will all have an effect. Ultimately, questions for this group include how they feel about their level of involvement in their world, and if diabetes negatively impacts their ability to have an active social life. Their responses can influence their diabetes self-care if it is viewed as interfering or as not affecting them at all. In either case, it is important to address how they perceive diabetes and whether this perception needs to be altered.

The bottom line is that the developmental life stage will interact with diabetes. It might be negative or positive, and diabetes care and education specialists can influence this by being aware of it and encouraging those involved to use this awareness to facilitate a positive approach.

Psychosocial Factors of Social Support

Social support may be one of the most influential aspects of dealing with diabetes. Support systems may include friends, classmates, family members, significant others, and support group members. The AADE7® highlights peer support as having the benefits of including social, emotional, and cultural support.[1] There are various models of peer support that can improve self-efficacy, mood, self-care behaviors, and health-related outcomes.[49] A support system that addresses the demands of diabetes and provides the support that the person with diabetes requests serves a helpful purpose. People who take on a social support role should ask themselves the key question, "What does the person with diabetes want in the way of support?" If the person with diabetes verbalizes their needs clearly, does the support system provide the requested support? This type of honest communication is necessary for both the person with diabetes and the people who support them. Diabetes care and educations specialists can facilitate this discussion.

The Family System and Related Roles and Responsibilities

Family systems vary dramatically. The system can range from being too close (enmeshed) to being too distant (disengaged). Family systems also involve levels of structure that are provided by the parents, which can range from rigid (inflexible) to overly flexible. The points of balance here have to do with levels of structure that use rules and guidelines in a clear fashion that the family understands. With diabetes it is important to have family systems that have useful structure and caring that is clear and present. Without the proper structure for a child or adult, diabetes can be lonely and very confusing.

Financial Resources and Insurance Coverage

Diabetes can be a costly disease, so it is important for diabetes care and education specialists to ask about and understand each person's or family's financial situation. Families that struggle financially may need help accessing resources.

Process of Coping With a Chronic Disorder

Some describe the stages of denial, anger, bargaining, depression, and acceptance that Kübler-Ross[50] described for the process of grief in dying as being similar to what an individual facing a new diagnosis of diabetes may feel. Table 4.8 describes how these stages, which are synonymous with the stages of loss, may appear in some individuals with a chronic disease. Basic to both of these demanding life situations—living with a chronic illness or living with dying—is the process of coping. It is important to keep in mind that the process of coping has no set order as to when and how each task of coping is

TABLE 4.8 Adaptation to the Emotional Stages of a Chronic Disease: Therapeutic Approaches

Stage	*Presentation*	*Approach*
Denial	May question diagnosis and treatment, especially if asymptomatic. Attempts to seek alternative diagnosis or may "doctor shop."	Work with person to help him or her see the connection between the medical data and his or her beliefs. If possible, let the person come to his or her own conclusion. Limit teaching to survival skills and reinforcement of basic principles. Denial is a coping defense, usually needed until the person is emotionally ready to deal with the crisis.
Anger	Anger, blame, and guilt are common. Cognitive confusion results in the need for repeated instructions. Family conflict may arise. "Why me?" "I don't want to change my routine." Anger is often suppressed, and it may be important to give the person opportunities to identify it.	Indicates that awareness is taking place. Learning begins at this stage. Provide clear, concise instructions. Persons with diabetes may need to talk about the existential question of "Why" and have opportunities to talk about feelings about this new issue. Reading children stories about other children with diabetes may be helpful.
Bargaining	May involve magical attempts to cure diabetes. Compulsive behavior to "make up" for prior behavior is common. "If I lose 20 pounds, can I go off insulin?"	Identifies with others; group classes and support groups may be helpful. Education needs to focus on what the person wants to know. Person with diabetes may need to have small, safe experiments to test the reality of diabetes mellitus (eg, have a treat and then test 1 and 2 hours afterward).
Depression and frustration	Can occur at any time. Difficulty establishing or maintaining self-management. Feelings of anxiety, hopelessness, and loss of control. "I can't handle this. No matter how hard I try, my blood sugar stays high." If this becomes protracted a referral to therapy may be required.	Person reaches a point of resignation to diabetes diagnosis and treatment; there are no vacations or breaks. Make mental health referrals as needed. Emphasize positive changes and accomplishments but appreciate the sadness that comes with this resignation.
Acceptance and adaptation	Becomes actively involved in management plan. asks questions and seeks more information. "I never realized this." "What do you mean by that?" "What should I do?"	Indicates acknowledgment of condition and a sense of responsibility for care/self-management. This is not a permanent state, as new challenges always come along. Grief is a cycle; expect its return.

accomplished. It is also important to note that not everyone goes through these stages. They may, in fact, react with other emotions that may include feelings of "disbelief, hope, terror, bewilderment, rage, apathy, calm, anxiety, and others." However they respond, their feelings should be respected.[50]

Methods of Measurement

Measuring a person with diabetes' level of healthy coping is a difficult task and has relied heavily on self-report in the past. This leave the diabetes care and education specialist at a disadvantage when documentation is needed to guide treatment and determine how effective the treatment has been. There are several tools that can be implemented at the beginning and during treatment to obtain a baseline and improvement of patient functioning. The Skills, Confidence and Preparedness Index is a brief and easy to administer scale used to assess self-management, optimize, and individualize resources as well as determine educational and clinical management needs.[51,52] There is strong evidence the Short Form-36 provides accurate information on patients quality of life (QoL), but in a recent review of QoL tools, the Short Form-12 (SF-12)[53] has shown a good correlation with its more extended version Short Form-36.[54] The shorter length of SF-12 makes it more practical in the busy clinical setting. There are some concerns about its reliability in smaller sample sizes. It's recommended that the Appraisal of Diabetes Scale is used in conjunction with the SF-12.[55]

The Beck-Depression-Inventory is a clinically relevant tool for assessing depression in patients, but the PHQ-9 also has good clinical validity for detecting depression and has the advantage of being easy to use and can be completed by the patient in minutes as well as administered repeatedly, reflecting improvement or worsening of depression in response to treatment.[56] Depression and diabetes distress are very similar, and that is why it is critical to administer one of the following Diabetes Distress Scales: Parents-DDS, Partners-DDS, T1-DDS, or DDS.[28] Cognitive impairment requires a mental status exam and requires experienced mental health providers to administer, but recently an instrument more sensitive than the MMSE[57] was created for the Department of Veterans Affairs, the SLUMS Examination for Detecting Mild Cognitive Impairment and Dementia.[16]

Coping Styles

Newly diagnosed persons with diabetes and those who have lived with diabetes for years face numerous challenges. According to the Diabetes Attitudes, Wishes, and Needs study, 85.2% of newly diagnosed persons with diabetes felt shock, anger, guilt, depression, anxiety, and helplessness. Those who had diabetes for up to 15 years continued to struggle with these same feelings as well as those related to worries about developing complications and the emotional burden of taking care of their diabetes.[58] Individuals who adapt well despite serious stress or stressors usually possess a "growth mind-set" that enables them to embrace challenges as they arise. Those who lack this mind-set tend to view challenges as obstacles rather than opportunities.[59]

Of numerous coping styles, optimism has been studied most extensively and has been shown to affect behavior-change outcomes.[60] In addition to optimism, information-seeking and avoidance coping styles have also determined coping outcomes. Depending on their coping style, some individuals will need to avoid or minimize the extent of information seeking in order to cope with the stress confronting them. Initially, this can be a healthy coping response that eases an individual forward in the process. This type of coping also happens to fit with what was identified earlier as denial, a defense that helps prevent one from becoming overwhelmed emotionally. However, if continued for an extended period, such avoidance or minimizing can be maladaptive and affect diabetes self-management and related outcomes.

Problem-Focused Coping

Problem-focused coping can be characterized as a style that involves identifying various problem areas that need solutions. This often involves what has been identified as a problem-solving approach. This is a useful approach when there are specific issues that need to be addressed and a resolution that will solve the concern. This style tends to be consistent with the acute care medicine view that diagnoses the problem, identifies the best solution, applies the solution, and resolves the problem.

How to Work With This Style

The problem-focused coping style is conducive to working with a problem-solving approach. This style is particularly useful when there is a "best response" to a problem area, and it is easily taught since diabetes care and education specialists can usually help the person with diabetes identify life experiences in which they successfully resolved a problem. With this style, the diabetes care and education specialist may be able to do more guiding and coaching rather than directing, and this often feels very collaborative and cooperative to both the diabetes care and education specialist and the person with diabetes. Consult chapter 10 for more on the problem-solving approach.

Emotion-Focused Coping

The emotion-focused coping style can be characterized as using emotion-based decision making (ie, choosing what feels right). The person with diabetes may be doing what feels best rather than using a more thought-out, logical process. This can be frustrating for diabetes care and education specialists, who are trained to think through the problem and come to a rational decision that can be planned and measured. Emotion-focused copers may not be able to provide a clear explanation as to why they act the way they do. They will need to process their feelings about diabetes and the issues associated with it.

How to Work With This Style

Emotion-focused copers will likely need to process their feelings about diabetes before they can conduct the problem solving needed to achieve better self-management. This style requires that the diabetes care and education specialist be willing to listen to the person with diabetes and validate their emotions. By doing so, the diabetes care and education specialist is not confirming that this is how to make decisions regarding treatment. Rather, the diabetes care and education specialist is simply confirming that these emotional experiences are normal and that it is acceptable to have these emotions. This may open the door to a collaborative approach and invite a discussion of how the person can use their emotions to work with the problem to be addressed. For example, the diabetes care and education specialist might say, "That anger is very strong. I wonder how you might use that energy to work with diabetes struggles?" The main challenge for the diabetes care and education specialist is to acknowledge the person's emotions but not acquiesce to this style as the only way to cope with the challenges of self-management.

Information-Seeking Coping

Some diabetes care and education specialists and persons with diabetes prefer the information-seeking style of coping since it is primarily a question-and-answer process, which supports the traditional roles of the diabetes care and education specialists as the expert and the person with diabetes as the student. Persons with this style may look at diabetes as primarily a disease for which there are always right answers. They often seek information online, so this may challenge the diabetes care and education specialists, particularly when the person gets poor or contradictory information from the Internet that can confuse and overwhelm them. While persons with diabetes with this coping style often treat the diabetes care and education specialist as the expert, this can be a setup for the diabetes care and education specialist to simply give information and the person with diabetes to passively receive it.

How to Work With This Style

The information-seeking style is likely to be the most used coping style early in the diagnosis since most of the information will be new and the person with diabetes is more likely to be passive. As time passes, this style can become difficult if the person does not assume responsibility and do some of their own thinking and problem solving. It becomes important for the diabetes care and education specialist to be prepared to not only give information but also elicit interaction and responses from the person's perspective. By using the approaches described in motivational interviewing, the person's involvement becomes part of the educational goal, and this coping style can be used appropriately. (See chapter 3 for more on motivational interviewing.)

Avoidance Coping

The avoidance coping style is characterized as doing only the bare minimum and ignoring or blocking additional information that is beyond the scope of survival skills alone. Avoidance is often attached to the emotion-focused coping style. The avoidance of diabetes tasks and information is primarily associated with the emotional discomfort that comes with fear, anxiety, the inability to be perfect, anger, shame, or any number of uncomfortable feelings the person with diabetes may have. If the person learns to manage the discomfort associated with these feelings, they will be more likely to be open to expanding the scope of their information base. Some persons with diabetes may develop an avoidance strategy commonly known as "psychological insulin resistance." This is the emotional barrier many persons with diabetes put up when faced with the need to take insulin. These individuals avoid this option because they fear needles, see insulin as a punishment, feel like failures, worry about gaining weight, worry that their diabetes has gotten worse, or don't want to deal with their fear of hypoglycemia.[61]

How to Work With This Style

Avoidance coping can be a difficult style with which to work because the mere fact that the diabetes care and education specialist may broach the topic of diabetes creates discomfort in the person with diabetes. The approach here is one of combining honesty about the issue with some work on self-soothing skills needed to help calm the person's anxiety or fears. An open discussion of what the person is feeling is a first step in working with an avoidance coping style. It is important to keep in mind that the strong feelings the person with diabetes has are not the diabetes care and education specialist's problems to solve. These feelings are information that is acting as a barrier to the person getting the care required. It is ultimately the person with diabetes' responsibility to deal with these emotions. The diabetes care and education specialist can listen, validate, and help show the person how to manage the anxiety associated with these feelings. Part of anxiety management can be helpful for diabetes care (eg, using breathing techniques to relax). Diabetes care and education specialists also may make a referral to a mental health professional. It is important to remember that the person with diabetes will act only when they are ready. If diabetes care and education specialists push too hard too soon, they may lose any follow-up with that person with diabetes.

Summary: Coping Styles

The coping style a person uses is likely due to what has worked in the past. If being optimistic and using a problem-focused style of coping worked before, the person will likely move in that direction first. If it was helpful to use denial and avoidance to get past the early stage of fear at another time in life, the person may do this again until emotionally ready to address the issues related to their self-management. Whatever style of coping people use initially is not necessarily what they will continue to use as they learn to manage their diabetes. Diabetes care and education specialists need to be careful not to judge any particular style as bad or inappropriate. It is likely that most persons with diabetes do not use just one style of coping. The style may change given different situations. People likely have patterns in their life of when and how they have used these different coping processes. Uncovering these patterns will be useful for the diabetes care and education specialist in planning how to work with the person with diabetes.

Stress Management

The association between stress and diabetes self-management is multilayered. The first layer has to do with the direct impact of stress on the person's glucose. It is typical for one's glucose level to rise during or after a stressful event. Long-term stress may also have a longer-term effect of causing problems with glycemic management. The second layer is that stress can act as a distraction, which may take away from the focus or energy necessary to deal with diabetes management tasks. The third layer is that the behaviors used to manage stress may work against optimal glycemic levels. Overeating, drinking alcohol, watching too much TV, or playing video games may be used to combat the effects of stress but will not help with diabetes management. It is clear that stress has a negative impact on diabetes self-care. It will be helpful early in the relationship for the diabetes care and education specialist to discuss what stress is, how the person with diabetes usually experiences stress (symptoms the indvidual has), the impact of stress on diabetes, and whether the person with diabetes knows how stress affects their own diabetes and self-care. It is helpful to ask about the usual stressors in an individual's life and to revisit this question at least once every 6 months. It is important that the diabetes care and education specialist be able to assess for stress, help the person with diabetes identify the impact that stress has on them, and identify helpful methods to manage stress that lower the impact on diabetes management.

Assessing for Stress

Stress shows up in most people as the following symptoms:

1. Physical symptoms, such as headaches, gastrointestinal concerns, muscle tension, teeth grinding, fatigue, elevated glucose, lower glucose, and loss of appetite or increased appetite
2. Emotional symptoms, such as increased anger or hostility, sadness, increase in fears or anxiety, frustration with diabetes, and a feeling of just being burned out with managing the disease
3. Interpersonal symptoms, such as lack of patience, more arguments, distancing from usual contacts, lack of interest in sex, avoidance of follow-up with healthcare providers, and missing meetings

In assessing for diabetes distress, the Diabetes Distress Scale[9] and PAID[40] are useful in identifying specific areas where the person with diabetes is having difficulty. Use of these questionnaires can also help initiate a conversation with the person with diabetes about the nature of stress and how it impacts diabetes care. These questionnaires can be given annually to keep this type of communication open and to note any changes.

Diabetes care and education specialists who don't want to use these questionnaires may assess diabetes distress by asking simple, open-ended questions such as the following:

- "What emotions have you been experiencing lately?"
- "How would you describe your energy level over the past week/month?"

- "What noticeable physical problems have you experienced lately that might be connected to stress (eg, stomachaches, headaches, or pain in the neck or lower back)?"
- "What changes in your glucose have you noted when you are under stress?"
- "Describe recent feelings of tenseness or irritability—what was the trigger for these feelings?"

All of these questions are specific to symptoms, but if the person is attuned to their own stress-related symptoms, a simple question like "How has your stress been?" might suffice as an assessment. If a diabetes care and education specialist sees that stress is having an impact and the person with diabetes agrees and would like some help dealing with it, the next question is "What are your stress triggers?" This may seem like an easy question, but as with problem solving, diabetes care and education specialists need to continue to drill down to find the origin of the stress. Since the stress associated with diabetes cannot be eliminated, it needs to be balanced. Once the diabetes care and education specialist knows what the stressor is and the current impact of the stress on the person with diabetes, the diabetes care and education specialist will have a better idea of what type of intervention will be most useful.

Physiologic Reaction to Stress

Often the physiology of stress can prevent people from dealing with the circumstance rationally. If a person is angry, heart rate and blood pressure rise and brain chemistry hormones are elevated in a way that inhibits clear thinking. The rule of thumb is if your heart rate is above 80 (or above your natural resting heart rate), step away from the battle and settle down first, get your heart rate back to normal, consider the circumstance and methods to manage it, and then go back to the discussion. Because stress affects the mind/body process, learning to first lower the physical reactivity and then identify what to do about the stressor is a helpful skill for persons with diabetes.

Methods to deal with physical reactivity include deep breathing, mindfulness, self-hypnosis, meditation, deep muscle relaxation, rational self-talk, acupressure points, yoga postures, and biofeedback. Many of these techniques use the breath to establish calmness.[62–64] These techniques have the ability to calm the brain and the body's reactivity when a person becomes stressed. They are generally simple to do, but do require practice in order to be useful.

Another method of dealing with physiological reactivity is to do something physical, such as the following:

- Walking or running
- Swimming, riding a bike, lifting weights
- Yoga, Tai Chi, Qigong, Pilates
- House cleaning, gardening

These stress management activities can have the added benefit of helping the person with diabetes manage their weight and the prolonged impact of diabetes on the body. Persons with diabetes should, of course, get clearance from their healthcare team prior to starting any physical activity.

Identifying and Managing Stress

The next series of questions is designed to get at the nature of the stressor and identify methods to deal with it and what the diabetes care and education specialist can do to help.

Can something be done to deal with or eliminate the stressor? This question has implications with problem solving, and a problem-solving approach might be used here. (See chapter 10 for more on problem solving.)

It also may be as simple as identifying how to make a stressor go away by changing the situation. For example, "I'm worried about what my blood glucose is. I'm feeling a little funny." Stress solution: check blood glucose. In essence, if something can be done to change the situation that is causing stress and the person can take charge of it, then direct action is fitting here.

If something cannot be done to directly affect the stressor, can the person with diabetes change their judgment, opinion, or feelings about the stressful situation? If so, this would be a good place for cognitive restructuring (CR), an approach that helps individuals identify negative thoughts and adopt a more positive thought process that helps reduce stress and anxiety.[65] For example, "John" thinks the following: "My friends will think I'm weird and won't hang out with me if I tell them I have diabetes." He experiences anxiety because he believes this is what his friends think, regardless of whether there is any evidence to support the belief. The diabetes care and education specialist may take this opportunity to help John explore alternative possible thoughts he could have in response to his fear to help reduce his stress and anxiety. The diabetes care and education specialist may ask, "How can you confirm or deny what your friends actually think? How could you educate them about diabetes, so they might become more supportive? What would you do if they did think you were weird? What would they do if they supported you? A referral to a mental health professional trained in cognitive behavioral therapy (CBT) could be very helpful for persons with diabetes suffering with catastrophic thinking, cognitive distortions, and irrational beliefs.

Stress management process:

- Assess for diabetes-specific distress every 6 months
- Assess for general stress issues every 6 months
- Increase person with diabetes' awareness of stress symptoms
- Educate as to stress awareness
- Identify stressors

If a stressor cannot be changed or if a person cannot change their view of the stressor, the next option is to explore "letting it go." This requires the ability to accept that the stressor cannot be altered or is something that is simply out of one's control. The diabetes care and education specialist can help the person with diabetes focus on what they *can* do instead of what they can't do or change.

This is an appropriate time to seek support from a group of peers. Those who live with diabetes will from time to time feel exhausted by the effort it takes to keep doing what needs to be done. To sit in a group with others who are experiencing the same issues can be reassuring. It also may be a place to share ideas for coping with the challenges of managing diabetes. People can benefit from being in a support group where they can express themselves and not feel judged when they are struggling with self-care issues.

Relapse Prevention Strategies

Persons with diabetes who have successfully changed their behavior can benefit from learning relapse prevention strategies. One component of prevention is self-awareness. For behavior change to occur, one must be aware of and acknowledge their risky behavior, such as knowing they tend to overeat or smoke when stressed. Next, the person with diabetes should have a plan to deal with stressful situations—for example, combating negative thinking with positive thoughts, or calling a friend or family member when they feel tempted to engage in risky behavior. Substituting positive thoughts or behaviors can be a useful prevention strategy.

Using these strategies, individuals who are stressed or anxious can find new ways of responding to stressors. It is important to keep in mind that these new responses may require extraordinary commitment and planning for persons with diabetes to change their behavior, because they may be used to automatically respond in another way.

The stress management techniques described earlier are particularly helpful because the physiological arousal when stressed leads to a desire for immediate relief. Negative behaviors such as overeating, drinking alcohol, and smoking may have given the person with diabetes immediate relief from stressors in the past. Practicing and using the stress management strategies can help in reducing the physiological reaction and may also allow the person to make better choices.

The following are ways to deal with risky behavior:

- Acknowledge the risky behavior and when it is most likely to happen
- Identify what is likely to happen (ie, what is the person with diabetes' scenario)
- Identify factors that contribute to this risky behavior (eg, stress, conflict, fatigue, hunger, being alone)
- Find ways to combat these behaviors at higher risk times (eg, alternative solutions like finding support)
- Develop a plan to follow
- Refer to a mental health professional, self-help groups such as Overeaters Anonymous or Alcoholics Anonymous, addiction clinics, etc.

Considerations for Special Populations

Age: Children and Adolescents

Anxiety is the most common mental health disorder among children and adolescents in the general US population.[66] It is unclear whether youth with diabetes are at greater risk for anxiety disorders, but it is known that anxiety is associated with poor metabolic stability. In addition, youth with type 1 diabetes have significantly higher rates of depression compared with the general US population.[67] Both anxiety and depression play a significant role in the ability of children and adolescents to cope with diabetes stressors. Eating disorders, such as anorexia nervosa, bulimia nervosa, binge eating disorder, and diabulimia, often co-occur with anxiety and/or depression. Diabetes care and education specialists should be able to recognize the signs and symptoms of eating disorders and make appropriate referrals, as eating disorders can negatively impact one's ability to manage diabetes. (See assessment of eating disorders earlier in this chapter.) Anxiety, depression, and eating disorders are serious mental health conditions that require help from a qualified mental health professional.

Children and adolescents are exposed daily to stressors in school and at home, and youth with diabetes have the added stress of managing their disease. For the diabetes care and education specialist, helping youth cope with these stressors may begin with understanding the importance of peer relationships. Peer conflict has been shown to increase the likelihood of poor metabolic management among girls with type 1 diabetes, whereas positive peer interactions are associated with fewer depressive symptoms and better self-care behaviors.[66]

There are 2 mental health conditions that may affect a person's lifelong ability to effectively cope with the daily stressors associated with diabetes: attention-deficit hyperactivity disorder (ADHD) and autism. These conditions are among the most common mental disorders in children and adolescents in the general population,[68] and there is evidence showing a link between ADHD and diabetes.[69] It should be noted, however, that certain ADHD medications can cause a lack of appetite, which can have significant implications for blood glucose levels in youth with diabetes. Attention-deficit hyperactivity disorder primarily affects an individual's ability to focus, which can be quite challenging for a diabetes care and education specialist. For this reason, one should address ADHD-related issues first, so the individual can focus more easily on diabetes management concerns. Autism is a spectrum disorder, meaning it is a group of disorders with common features (ADHD is on this spectrum), and no 2 people have the same symptoms.[67] Autism typically affects an individual's ability to communicate and connect emotionally with others. With all of the conditions listed above, youth with diabetes and their families face several challenges of coping with both diabetes and another serious, lifelong condition.

Age: Adults

About 7% of all adults in the United States have been diagnosed with major depressive disorder (MDD).[67] Depression, which often co-occurs with anxiety disorders, affects adults with diabetes significantly more often than the general population.

Age: Elderly Adults

In working with elderly persons with diabetes, diabetes care and education specialists should be cognizant of the impact of dementia and Alzheimer's disease. Both dementia and Alzheimer's disease affect an individual's memory, problem-solving ability, and management of their moods. Therefore, individuals with dementia or Alzheimer's disease may struggle significantly with self-care behaviors. Diabetes care and education specialists may need to work with these individuals in coping with their frustrations and their emotional distress. Recent research has shown that cognitive training may improve self-management behaviors in older adults with diabetes.[70]

Increasing age is the greatest risk factor of both dementia and Alzheimer's disease, with onset most commonly occurring after the age of 65. People with type 2 diabetes are at an elevated risk for developing Alzheimer's disease,[71] so it is important for diabetes care and education specialists to be able to identify early signs and symptoms of the disease among the aging persons with diabetes with whom they work.

Veterans

A mental disorder commonly occurring in adulthood, although it can manifest earlier, is posttraumatic stress disorder (PTSD). Posttraumatic stress disorder is more common among combat veterans than among the general population[72] and affects veterans of all ages and sexes. Studies have found a link between PTSD and diabetes, but it is unclear which one precedes the other. The comorbidity of diabetes and PTSD is especially prevalent among veterans.[73] Posttraumatic stress disorder in veterans is commonly accompanied by depression, substance abuse, or other anxiety disorders, all of which can contribute to poor glycemic stability.[73]

Gender

Gender identity should be considered when working with persons with diabetes. Diabetes care and education specialists can demonstrate greater respect for those who don't identify as male or female by bringing a nonjudgmental attitude to the counseling session. Ask people for their preferred pronouns and use them. Some may want to be addressed as him, her, they, or something else. Offer a "____" or "other" along with "Male" and "Female" categories on data collection forms. Note that gender identity—how people perceive themselves—is separate from sexual identity, which refers to the type of people they find sexually attractive.

Both anxiety disorders and MDD affect women twice as much as men, in addition to PTSD and eating disorders affecting women disproportionately.[67]

Eating disorders commonly co-occur with anxiety or depression. About half of those with BED are depressed. Women with diabetes are 2.4 times more likely than women without diabetes to develop an eating disorder.[4]

Diabetes during pregnancy puts both the mother and the baby at risk of negative health outcomes. In addition, self-management is complex and behaviorally demanding. For those with preexisting diabetes, the management of diabetes may be intensified with additional glucose self-tests and insulin shots.[74] For those who are newly diagnosed, there is the need to learn all about diabetes and its management as well as engage with the complex daily self-care regimen. The regimen, either intensified or new, may be accompanied by emotional and behavioral challenges. To date, however, few controlled studies have focused on psychosocial aspects of diabetes during pregnancy.

Pregnant women with diabetes, especially those newly diagnosed with gestational diabetes, may experience an initial increase in certain emotions, such as sadness, anger, and frustration.[75] In one study, mothers with gestational diabetes had nearly double the odds of experiencing depression during pregnancy compared with those without diabetes and with women with preexisting diabetes.[76]

More information on pregnancy complicated by diabetes can be found in chapter 24.

Ethnicity

Ethnic minorities commonly experience economic inequality, racism, and discrimination, all of which increase the risk for anxiety and depression. People in the lowest strata of income, education, and occupation are 2 to 3 times more likely to have a mental disorder compared with those in the highest strata.[77] Many ethnic minority groups in the United States are less likely than Caucasian Americans to seek care for mental health disorders due to financial and/or cultural and linguistic barriers, causing mental health disorders to be underreported in many minority communities. In many cultures, mental health problems are seen as shameful, have different symptom manifestations, and are attributed to the spiritual world.

African Americans

There is no significant difference between African Americans and Caucasians regarding rates of depression and anxiety.[67,77]

Native Americans and Alaska Natives

Native Americans and Alaska Natives have the highest prevalence of diabetes of any minority group. While currently there is little evidence linking diabetes and mental health disorders in this particular minority group, it should be noted that Native Americans and Alaska Natives have a suicide rate that is 50% higher than the national rate.[67,77] Diabetes care and education specialists working with this population should become familiar with the warning signs of suicide.

Asian Americans and Pacific Islanders

Asian Americans and Pacific Islanders have a relatively low incidence of mental health disorders. However, elderly Asian-American women have the highest suicide rate among all women over the age of 65. Diabetes care and education specialists working with refugees from Southeast Asian countries such as Cambodia, Vietnam, or Laos should be mindful that PTSD is very common among immigrants from these war-torn countries.[67,77]

Hispanic Americans

Hispanic Americans are the fastest-growing minority group in the United States. On average, Hispanic-American adults are known to have fewer reported mental health disorders due to a cultural stigma against mental illness.[78] Hispanic-American youth, however, experience higher rates of depressive and anxiety disorders, suicide ideation, and suicide attempts compared with White youth.[67,77]

Case: A Maladaptive Coping Strategy

LP is a 56-year-old woman who has had diabetes for 10 years. She came into the diabetes center because her blood glucose management had worsened over the past 6 months. Her daughter, a nurse, accompanied her. LP lives alone, but her daughter lives nearby in the same city. LP admitted to poor dietary intake, skipping meals, and eating whatever was available when she did eat. While LP was reporting her dietary intake, her daughter encouraged her to give more details about what she was eating and drinking. With some hesitation, LP reported that she drinks alcohol and asked if that was a problem.

Assessment

The diabetes care and education specialist could have responded to the question by providing knowledge about how alcohol can increase blood glucose and predispose one to hypoglycemia. However, an approach that will help the diabetes care and education specialist know best what knowledge to impart and to facilitate coping will be the most helpful in understanding the drinking behavior.

- Is this something new, or did LP drink in the past?
- How much and what is LP drinking?

Case: A Maladaptive Coping Strategy (continued)

- When does the drinking occur, daily or episodically?
- Does LP drink with others or alone?
- Can LP recall a time when the drinking began to increase? If so, was there any reason that triggered the increased drinking?

Understanding the Behavior

One or more of these assessment questions might lead to an understanding of the issues LP was attempting to address.

LP responded to the questions, saying that in the past she only drank socially, but now drinks when she is alone. She stated that she begins drinking in the afternoon and continues into the night, usually skipping lunch but having some supper. She stated that her drinking increased in the past year, since her husband, sister, and mother had died.

LP is clearly trying to cope, but using a maladaptive strategy of alcohol abuse. It will be important to either discuss whether LP thinks she is depressed or ask the 2-question assessment. The drinking has resulted in increased isolation and disengagement from others as well as lack of motivation for diabetes self-management. Before LP can achieve better diabetes stability, she needs to deal with her grief. The diabetes care and education specialist needs to ascertain whether LP is depressed and whether she wants to change her drinking behavior. If so, LP can be referred for further assessment of her depression or alcohol consumption to identify whether she needs treatment. Discussion of her grief process may help determine whether a support group or therapy might be helpful in getting through her losses. LP should meet with the diabetes care and education specialist more frequently until optimal glucose levels can be achieved and LP demonstrates she is using positive strategies for coping with her losses and diabetes self-management.

Outcomes

As psychosocial behavioral interventions within DSME, coping strategies, utilizing techniques from cognitive therapy, and coping skills training may help individuals achieve and, more importantly, maintain diabetes self-management goals. These interventions may be particularly valuable given the multiple, and often stressful, competing demands of life.

Coping skills training for diabetes self-management has been tested in adults with type 2 diabetes.[79] Significant improvements in glycemic stability, quality of life, and self-efficacy and decreased diabetes-related emotional distress were demonstrated.

The report of the Psychosocial Therapies Working Group provides further rationale and evidence for the importance of assessing psychosocial factors and providing interventions that will ensure optimal psychosocial functioning for optimal health and quality of life.[80] Positive outcomes of stress moderation or elimination and modified stress response can result in restoration and maintenance of physiological and psychosocial well-being. The coping appraisal and strategies used in psychosocial interventions such as coping skills training and cognitive therapy techniques in the context of DSME are consistent with the AADE7 Self-Care Behaviors® and core outcomes and serve as a guide for the assessment, intervention, and evaluation of stress and coping in individuals with diabetes and their families.

Focus on Education

Teaching Strategies

Meet basic needs first. Understand that basic survival needs must be met before the process of identifying stressors and barriers can take place. This is key to problem solving and will affect motivation for higher order needs. For example, the basic needs for physical comfort and safety must be met, as well as the goal of stabilizing blood glucose, before introducing higher level problems to solve. This includes appreciating the family system, acknowledging the stage of development, and determining whether the person is experiencing depression.

Special circumstances related to the individual. Individual, cultural, spiritual/religious, and family traditions have an impact on beliefs and practices that shape future decision making. Before introducing problem-solving and coping skills, assist individuals with identifying stressors and treatment plans for optimal coping and illness adjustment based on individual, cultural, and religious influences.

Be aware of different focuses. It is critical for diabetes care and education specialists to understand the process that is typical for an individual person with diabetes or family and to do their best to work within the framework of that orientation. Whether they have a problem-focused orientation or are more emotionally focused, it is important for diabetes care and education specialists to be nonjudgmental in their approach. The overall goal is to achieve a working relationship that fosters a collaborative approach.

Support the individual's mental health. At each contact, promote good nutrition, regular physical activity, and proper sleep habits and offer problem solving to assist with engagement with the medication regimens.

Seek team collaboration. Maintaining ongoing communication with all members of the diabetes care team and mental health professionals is crucial for the appropriate care of individuals with mental health problems.

Regularly incorporate screening. Be familiar with screening tools and comfortable in initiating screening for symptoms of mental health problems during the education and care process. Be comfortable with the referral process and establish communication lines with mental health professionals.

Messages for People With Diabetes

Start a medical regimen. Begin testing the basic treatment plan and ask for assistance and clarification from the healthcare team. Frequent calls, e-mails, and clinic visits are expected in the first several weeks of a new plan while comfort with the plan is mastered.

Develop coping skills. Skills are developed through experience and information, trial and error. Learning coping skills is a process and can be encouraged by family, friends, and health professionals. An example of the process is problem solving: Define a problem or concern and discuss possible individualized solutions; consider the solutions and implement one plan; evaluate the plan and decide whether to modify, change, or adopt it; practice the plan. If it is working, develop a relapse prevention plan.

Discuss disorders openly. Individuals with diabetes may experience diabetes distress, depression, anxiety, or eating disorders. Talking about the possibility of this and creating awareness may offer quicker recognition and allow treatment opportunities to be scheduled sooner.

Consider mental health part of good diabetes management. Assessing diabetes distress and understanding how it can interfere with diabetes self-management and diabetes stability may help improve the provider-person with diabetes relationship and facilitate better care.

Referring to a mental healthcare practitioner shortly after receiving a diabetes diagnosis can help persons with diabetes build a relationship with a therapist, deal with initial issues, and improve outcomes when future problems arise. Periodic monitoring of mental health and feelings is also an important part of routine diabetes care.

Seek available help. Persons dealing with both diabetes and matters of mental health need to know they are not alone. Help and support are available. Ask your diabetes care and education specialist for handouts or Web site addresses with information on where to find additional support. Make an appointment with a mental health professional as the need arises.

Health Literacy

Health literacy and mental health. Health literacy includes the ability to recognize specific issues/disorders and seek mental health information; knowledge of risk factors and causes, and self-management and professional help available; and attitudes that promote recognition and appropriate help-seeking.[81]

Picture stories. Consider using a visual approach when screening for depression or other conditions. Picture storyboards can be used with individuals with low literacy skills or when language barriers are present. Picture stories are designed to be safe, impersonal prompts that allow individuals to discuss difficult topics, ask questions, and obtain information. For an example, see Picture Stories for Adult ESL Health Literacy (http://www.cal.org/caela/esl_resources/Health/healthindex.html#Depress).

References

1. Association of Diabetes Care and Education Specialists (ADCES). An effective model of diabetes care and education: revising the AADE7 self-care behaviors®. Published online ahead of print, Feb 2020. Diabetes Educ. doi: https://doi.org/10.1177/0145721719894903.
2. Walker JG, Jackson HJ, Littlejohn GO. Models of adjustment to chronic illness: using the example of rheumatoid arthritis. Clin Psychol Rev. 2004;24:461-88.
3. Kent D, Haas L, Randal D, et al. Healthy coping: issues and implications in diabetes education and care. Popul Health Manag. 2010 Oct;13(5):227-33.
4. Goebel-Fabbri AE. Detecting and treating eating disorders in young women with type 1 diabetes. In: Anderson BJ, Rubin RR, eds. Practical Psychology for Diabetes Clinicians. 2nd ed. Washington, D.C.: American Diabetes Association; 2002.
5. Lustman PJ, Clouse RE. Depression in diabetic patients: the relationship between mood and glycemic control. J Diabetes Complications. 2005;19(2):113-22.
6. Grigsby AB, Anderson RJ, Freedland KE, Clouse RE, Lustman PJ. Prevalence of anxiety in adults with diabetes: a systematic review. J Psychosom Res. 2002;53(6):1053-60.
7. LeBow, EB. Resolve ADHD to improve diabetes self-management. Endocrine Today. 2016;14(5):8-9.
8. Mazaika PK, Weinzimer SA, Mauras N, et al. Variations in brain volume and growth in young children with type 1 diabetes. Diabetes. 2016;65(2):476-85.
9. Cato A, Hershey T. Cognition and type 1 diabetes in children and adolescents. Diabetes Spectrum. 2016;29(4):197-202.
10. Nunley KA, Rosano C, Ryan CM, et al. Clinically relevant cognitive impairment in middle age adults with childhood onset type 1 diabetes. Diabetes Care. 2015;38(9):1768-76.
11. Moheet A, Mangia S, Seaquist ER. Impact of diabetes on cognitive function and brain structure. Annals of the New York Academy of Sciences. 2015;1353:60-71.
12. Munshi MN. Cognitive dysfunction in older adults with diabetes: what a clinician needs to know. Diabetes Care. 2017;40(4):461-7.
13. Devarajooh C, Chinna K. Depression, distress and self-efficacy: the impact on diabetes self-care practices. PLOS One 2017 (March 31):1-16.
14. LeBow EB. Addressing cognitive impact of hyperglycemia on diabetes self-management. Endocrine Today. February 2016;15(2):13.
15. Wolf MS, Curtis LM, Wilson EA, et al. Literacy, cognitive function, and health: results of the LitCog study. J Gen Intern Med. 2012;27(10):1300-7.
16. Department of Veterans Affairs http://medschool.slu.edu/agingsuccessfully/pdfsurveys/slumsexam_05.pdf Retrieved on July 21st, 2019.
17. Young-Hyman D, de Groot M, Hill-Briggs F, Gonzalez JS, Hood K, Peyrot M. Psychosocial care for people with diabetes: A position statement of the American Diabetes Association. Diabetes Care. 2016;39(12):2126-40.
18. Fisher L, Hessler D, Glasgow RE, et al. REDEEM: A pragmatic trial to reduce diabetes distress. Diabetes Care. 2013; 36(9):2551-8.
19. Berry E, Lockhart S, Davies M, Lindsay JR, Dempster M. Diabetes distress: understanding the hidden struggles of living with diabetes and exploring intervention strategies. Postgrad Med J. 2015;91(1075):278-83.
20. Nicolucci A, Kovas Burns K, Holt RI, et al; DAWN2 Study Group. Diabetes Attitudes, Wishes, and Needs second study (DAWN2™): cross-national benchmarking of diabetes-related psychosocial outcomes for people with diabetes. Diabet Med. 2013 Jul;30(7):767-77.
21. Berry E, Lockhart S, Davies M, Lindsay JR, Dempster M. Diabetes distress: understanding the hidden struggles of living with diabetes and exploring intervention strategies. Postgrad Med J. 2015;91(1075):278-83.
22. Hessler D, Fisher L, Polonsky WH, Johnson N. Understanding the areas and correlates of diabetes related distress in parents with type 1 diabetes. Journal of Pediatric Psychology. 2016,1-9.
23. Polonsky WH, Fisher L, Hessler D, Johnson N. Emotional distress in the partners of type 1 diabetes adults: worries about hypoglycemia and other key concerns. Diabetes Technology & Therapeutics. 2016;18(4).
24. Fisher L, Hessler DM, Polonsky WH, Mullan J. When is diabetes distress clinically meaningful? Establishing cut points for Diabetes Distress Scale. Diabetes Care. 2012;35(2):259-64.
25. Aikens JE.Prospective associations between emotional distress and poor outcomes in type 2 diabetes. Diabetes Care. 2012;35:2472-8.
26. Fisher, Lawrence, et al. When is diabetes distress cllinically meaningful? Diabetes Care. 2012;35:259-64.
27. Polonsky WF. Assessing psychological stress in diabetes: development of the Diabetes Distress Scale. Diabetes Care. 2005;28:626-31.
28. Behavioral Diabetes Institute. https://behavioraldiabetes.org/scales-and-measures/ Retrieved on July 21st, 2019.
29. Hou C, Carter B, Hewitt J, Francisa T, Mayor S. Do mobile phone applications improve glycemic control (HbA1c) in the self-management of diabetes? A systemic review, meta-analysis, and GRADE of 14 randomized trials. Diabetes Care. 2016;39:2089-95.
30. Golden SH, Lazo M, Carnethon M, et al. Examining a bidirectional association between depression symptoms and diabetes. JAMA. 2008;299(23):2751-9.
31. Pan A, Lucas M, Sun Q, et al. Bidirectional association between depression and type 2 diabetes mellitus in women. Arch Intern Med. 2010;170(21):1884-91.

32. Chen PC, Chan YT, Chen HF, Ko MC, Li CY. Population-based cohort analyses of the bidirectional relationship between type 2 diabetes and depression. Diabetes Care. 2013;36(2):376-82.

33. Roszler J, Rapaport WS. Approaches to Behavior. Alexandria, Va: American Diabetes Association; 2015.

34. Karimy M, Koohestani HR, Araban M. The association between attitude, self-efficacy and social support and adherence to diabetes self-care behavior. Diabetol Metab Syndr. 2018(10)86:1-6.

35. Ries A, Blackman LT, Page RA, Gizlice Z, Benedict S, Barnes K, Kelsey K, Carter-Edwards L. Goal setting for health behavior change: evidence from an obesity intervention for rural low-income women. Rural and Remote Health. 2014;14:2682.

36. Klinkner GE, Yaeger KM, Brenny Fitzpatrick MT, Vorderstrasse AA. Improving diabetes self-management support: goal setting across the continuum of care. Clinical Diabetes. 2017Dec;35(5):305-12.

37. Murawski ME, Milsom VA, Ross KM, Rickel KA, Debraganz N, Gibbons LM, Perri MG. Problem solving, treatment adherence, and weight loss outcome among women participating in lifestyle treatment for obesity. Eat Behav. 2009 August; 10(3):146-51.

38. National Institute of Mental Health. Washington, D.C.: National Institutes of Health; 2018 (cited July, 2018). On the Internet at: https://www.nimh.nih.gov/health/topics/anxiety-disorders/index.shtml.

39. Polonsky WF. Assessing psychological stress in diabetes: development of the Diabetes Distress Scale. Diabetes Care. 2005;28:626-31.

40. Polonsky WH, Anderson BJ, Lohrer PA. Assessment of diabetes-related distress. Diabetes Care.1995;18(6):754-60.

41. American Psychiatric Association. Diagnostic and Statistical Manual of Mental Disorders. 5th ed., text revision. Washington, D.C.: American Psychiatric Association; 2013.

42. Powers MA, Richter SA, Ackard DM, Craft C. Development and validation of the Screen for Early Eating Disorder Signs (SEEDS) in persons with type 1 diabetes. Eating Disord: J Treatment Prev. 2015.

43. Dimond M, Jones S. Chronic Illness Across the Lifespan. Norwalk, Conn: Appleton-Century-Crofts; 1983:165-76.

44. Leininger M. What is transcultural nursing and culturally competent care? J Transcult Nurs. 1999;10(1):9.

45. Melkus GD, Newlin K. Cultural considerations in diabetes care. In: Childs B, Cypress M, Spollett G, eds. Nursing Care of Persons With Diabetes. Alexandria, Va: American Diabetes Association; 2005:207-19.

46. Diller JV. Cultural Diversity. 3rd ed. Belmont, Calif: Brooks/Cole; 2007.

47. Miller R, Rollnick S. Meeting in the middle: motivational interviewing and self-determination theory. Int J Behav Nutr Phys Act. 2012;9(25):1.

48. Deci EL, Ryan RM. Self-determination theory in healthcare and its relation to motivational interviewing: a few comments. Int J Behav Nutr Phys Act. 2012;9:24.

49. Heisler M. Building Peer Support Programs to Manage Chronic Disease: Seven Models for Success. 2006; https://www.chcf.org/wp-content/uploads/2017/12/PDF-BuildingPeerSupportPrograms.pdf.

50. The final challenge: death and dying. In: Sigelman CK, Rider EA, eds. Life-Span Human Development, 6th ed. Belmont, Calif: Thomson Wadsworth Publishing; 2009:497-509.

51. Mbuagbaw L, Aronson R, Walker A, Brown RE, Orzech N. The LMC Skills, Confidence & Preparedness Index (SCPI): development and evaluation of a novel tool for assessing self-management in patients with diabetes. Health and Quality of Life Outcomes. (2017)15:27.

52. Aronson R, Brown RE, Jiandani D, Walker A, Orzech N, Mbuagbaw L. Assessment of self-management in patients with diabetes using the novel LMC Skills, Confidence and Preparedness Index (SCPI). Diabetes Research and Clinical Practice. 2018;137:128-36.

53. Ware JE, Kosinski M, Keller KD. A 12-item Short-Form Health Survey: construction of scales and preliminary tests of reliability and validity. Med Care 1996;34:220-33.

54. Shen W, Kotsanos JG, Huster WJ, Mathias SD, Andrejasich CM, Patrick DL. Development and validation of the diabetes quality of life clinical trial questionnaire. Med Care. 1999;37:45–66.

55. Nair R, Kachan P. Outcome tools for diabetes-specific quality of life. Canadian Family Physician Le Médecin de famille canadien. 2017:63.

56. Kroenke K, Spitzer RL, Williams JB. The PHQ-9: validity of a brief depression severity measure. J Gen Intern Med. 2001 Sep;16(9):606-13.

57. Tombaugh TN, McDowell I, Kristjansson B, Hubley AM. Mini-Mental State Examination (MMSE) and the Modified MMSE (3MS): a psychometric comparison and normative data. Psychological Assessment, 1996:8(1):48-59.

58. Skovlund SE, Peyrot M; for the DAWN International Advisory Panel. The Diabetes Attitudes, Wishes, and Needs (DAWN) program: a new approach to improving outcomes of diabetes care. Diabetes Spectr. 2005;18:136-42.

59. Dweck C. Mindset: The New Psychology of Success. New York: Ballantine Books; 2007.

60. Maciejewski PK, Prigerson HG, Mazure CM. Self-efficacy as a mediator between stressful life events and depressive symptoms: differences based on history of prior depression. Br J Psychiatry. 2000;176:373-8.

61. Jha S, Panda M, Kumar S, et al. Psychological insulin resistance in patients with type 2 diabetes. J Assoc Physicians India. 2015 Jul;63(7):33-9.

62. Wilkins C. Mindfulness and diabetes: working in tandem. On the Cutting Edge. 2015:35(6):4-6.

63. Kay AB. Yoga for type 2 diabetes and related comorbidities. On the Cutting Edge. 2015;35(6):7-9.

64. Trattner E, Stephens-Bogard K. Diabetes and traditional Chinese medicine: managing a modern epidemic with ancient medicine. On the Cutting Edge. 2015:35(6);24-7.

65. McCaffrey R, Zerwekh J, Keller K. Pain management: cognitive restructuring as a model for teaching nursing students. Nurse Educ. 2005;30(5);226-30.

66. Kanner S, Hamrin V, Grey M. Depression in adolescents with diabetes. J Child Adolesc Psychiatr Nurs. 2003;16(1):15-24.

67. National Institute of Mental Health. Major depression among adults. Washington, D.C.: National Institutes of Health; 2014 (cited 2016 May 23). On the Internet at: http://www.nimh.nih.gov/health/statistics/prevalence/major-depression-among-adults.shtml.

68. Dantzer C, Swendsen J, Maurice-Tison S, et al. Anxiety and depression in juvenile diabetes: a critical review. Clin Psychol Rev. 2003;23(6):787-800.

69. LeBow EB. Resolve ADHD to improve diabetes self-management. Endocr Today. 2016;14(5):8-9.

70. Vianna Paulo DL, Sanches Yassuda M. Elderly individuals with diabetes: adding cognitive training to psychoeducational intervention. Educ Gerontol. 2012;38(4):257-70.

71. Arvanitakis Z, Wilson RS, Bienias JL, et al. Diabetes mellitus and risk of Alzheimer disease and decline in cognitive function. Arch Neurol. 2004 May;61(5):661-6.

72. Taneilian T, ed. Invisible Wounds of War: Psychological and Cognitive Injuries, Their Consequences, and Services to Assist Recovery. Santa Monica, Calif: RAND Corporation; 2008.

73. Trief PM, Ouimette P, Wade M, Shanahan P, Weinstock RS. Post-traumatic stress disorder and diabetes: co-morbidity and outcomes in a male veterans sample. J Behav Med. 2006 Oct;29(5):411-8.

74. Tuffnell DJ, West J, Walkinshaw SA. Treatments for gestational diabetes and impaired glucose tolerance in pregnancy (review). Cochrane Database Syst Rev. 2003;(3):CD003395.

75. Daniells S, Grenyer BF, Davis WS, et al. Gestational diabetes mellitus: is a diagnosis associated with an increase in maternal anxiety and stress in the short and intermediate term? Diabetes Care. 2003;26:385-9.

76. Kozhimannil KB, Pereira MA, Harlow BL. Association between diabetes and perinatal depression among low-income mothers. JAMA. 2009;301(8):842-7.

77. Public Health Service. Mental health: culture, race, and ethnicity, a supplement to mental health: a report of the Surgeon General. Washington, D.C.: Department of Health and Human Services; 2001.

78. Kramer EJ, Guarnaccia P, Resendez C, Lu FG. No estoy loco/I'm not crazy. Understanding the stigma of mental illness in Latinos; 2009 (cited 2016 July 10). On the Internet at: https://ethnomed.org/clinical/mental-health/Facilitators%20Guide%20123108%20final%20_2_.pdf.

79. Surwit RS, van Tilburg MAL, McCaskill CC, et al. Stress management improves long-term glycemic control in type 2 diabetes. Diabetes Care. 2002;25(1):30-4.

80. Delamater AM, Jacobson AM, Anderson B, et al. Psychosocial therapies in diabetes: report of the Psychosocial Therapies Working Group. Diabetes Care. 2001;24(7):1286-92.

81. Provincial Health Services Authority. Towards Reducing Health Inequities: A Health System Approach to Chronic Disease Prevention. A Discussion Paper. Vancouver, BC: Population & Public Health, Provincial Health Services Authority; 2011.

CHAPTER 5

Healthy Eating

Cecilia Sauter, MS, RDN, CDCES, FADCES

Key Concepts

- Healthy eating is an effective, but challenging, self-care behavior that improves metabolic control and quality of life in persons with or at risk for diabetes.
- The diabetes care and education specialist should support healthy eating behaviors that are grounded in evidence-based research, such as the American Diabetes Association Clinical Practice Recommendations. Clinical recommendations can be translated into self-management education guided by the AADE7 Self-Care Behaviors®.
- Providers of diabetes self-management support (DSME/T and DSMS) should work with an interdisciplinary diabetes care team to tailor interventions to individual self-management education needs as well as to the stage of readiness to change behavior of persons with diabetes.
- To facilitate healthy eating, the DSME/T and DSMS provider assists the person with or at risk for diabetes in acquiring specific knowledge and skills by choosing the most appropriate meal-planning resource from the variety of approaches available. Key issues to address include, but are not limited to, portion sizes; food labels; meal planning, shopping, and cooking; modifying recipes; eating out; snacking; and special situations such as travel, alcohol, and parties/holidays.

Introduction

Healthy eating has a significant effect on the metabolic control of diabetes, including improvement in glycemic levels control and lipid profiles, maintenance of blood pressure in the target range, and weight loss or maintenance.[1] Many diabetes care and education specialists and clinicians consider healthy eating to be the most challenging of the AADE7 Self-Care Behaviors® to implement successfully.[2] Healthy eating involves basic behaviors and decisions such as when to eat, what to eat, and how much to eat. Influencing these decisions are complex factors such as habits, emotions, traditions, family and cultural eating patterns, health beliefs, food preferences, and food availability.[3,4] To help individuals with diabetes achieve effective behavior change to promote healthy eating, the diabetes care and education specialist's role encompasses the following:

- Providing the person with or at risk for diabetes with knowledge and skills training focused on healthy eating approaches grounded in evidence-based research
- Translating clinical recommendations into effective self-management education
- Facilitating successful behavior change by tailoring interventions to the individual's stage of readiness to embrace new behaviors
- Sharing practical information regarding meal-planning skills

Achieving successful self-management behaviors that are focused on making healthy food choices requires knowledge and skill on the part of the learner. This chapter focuses on the art of diabetes self-management education and training as well as diabetes self-management support (DSME/T and DSMS) and the areas that are important for the diabetes care and education specialist to teach, support, and promote to guide behavior change for healthy eating.

Promoting Healthy Eating: The Role of Medical Nutrition Therapy

Diabetes *medical nutrition therapy* (MNT) is the term for the specific nutrition diagnostic, therapy, and counseling services for the purpose of disease management furnished by a registered dietitian (RD)/registered dietitian nutritionist (RDN) or similarly qualified nutrition professional.[5,6,7] Successful MNT is grounded in evidence-based principles of nutrition for diabetes, which are then translated into self-management education for healthy eating behaviors. Although all diabetes care and education specialists must be able to apply the principles of MNT and use the same core set of behaviors to measure outcomes (see Table 5.1), the RD/RDN is the health professional with the greatest expertise in providing MNT.[7] The RD/RDN's effectiveness has been documented in research studies that have achieved positive outcomes. The Nutrition Therapy for Adults with Diabetes or Prediabetes[7] highlights a comprehensive review of the evidence for the effectiveness of MNT and healthy eating in diabetes management. The authors cite randomized controlled trials in which MNT was either implemented independently or delivered as part of an overall diabetes self-management training (DSMT) program. The studies demonstrated the following:

- Decreases in A1C: absolute decreases up to 1.9% (in type 1 diabetes) and up to 2.0% (in type 2 diabetes) at 3 to 6 months. These reductions are similar to or greater than what would be expected with treatment of currently available medications for diabetes. Ongoing support is helpful in maintaining glycemic improvement.
- With regards to cardiovascular risk factors evidence of positive effects of MNT is mixed.

TABLE 5.1 Outcomes for the AADE7 Self-Care Behavior® Healthy Eating

	*Immediate Outcome**			*Intermediate Outcome†*	
	Knowledge	*Skill*	*Barriers*	*Measures*	*Methods of Measurement*
Healthy Eating	• Effect of foods/beverages on metabolic parameters (including blood glucose, lipids, blood pressure, weight, etc) • Sources and distribution of nutrients (nutrient-dense carbohydrates, lean proteins, healthy fats) • Eating patterns (frequency of meals, timing, portions, etc.) • Resources to assist in food choices • Macronutrient composition (quality, quantity, combination, substitutions)	• Meal planning • Portion awareness and management • Planning Strategies (Carb counting, Exchanges, Plate Method, Mindful Eating) • Nutrition Facts Label comprehension • Special situations and problem solving (planning, shopping, meal delivery/kits, eating away from home at work/school/restaurants)	• Environmental factors • Cultural and family Influences • Food and health beliefs • Financial (food security) • Cognitive • Health literacy and numeracy • Emotional • Meal pattern sustainability	• Types of food choices • Amounts consumed • Timing of meals and snacks • Alcohol (with or without food, amount, frequency) • Fluids (adequate hydration) • Effect of food/beverages on metabolic parameters • Progress toward goal achievement	• Observation • Self-report (24-hour recall, typical day, food frequency, food diaries) • Monitoring tools with associated records • Goal setting

*Immediate outcomes are those that can be measured at the time of the intervention (eg, learning).

†Intermediate outcomes result over time (eg, behavior change) and require more than a single measurement.

Source: Adapted from Association of Diabetes Care and Education Specialists (ADCES). An effective model of diabetes care and education: revising the AADE7 self-care behaviors®. Published online ahead of print, Feb 2020. Diabetes Educ. doi: https://doi.org/10.1177/0145721719894903.

- Reductions in diabetes comorbidities and decreased use of medications led to a reduction in the use of health services and costs, indicating that MNT is also cost-effective.
- MNT improved overall quality of life.

The Diabetes Prevention Program (DPP) showed strong evidence that interventions such as intensive lifestyle modifications based on healthy eating habits and physical activity are effective in delaying or preventing the onset of type 2 diabetes by 58% to 71%.[8] The follow-up results from three large lifestyle interventional studies for diabetes prevention show sustained reduction of type 2 diabetes: Da Qing Diabetes Prevention study showed a 43% reduction at 20 years, the Finish Diabetes Prevention Study (DPS) showed a reduction of 43% at 7 years, and the original DPP study showed a 34% reduction in the rate of conversion to type 2 diabetes after 10 years and 27% reduction after 15 years.[9,10,11,12]

Registered Dietitian (RD)/Registered Dietitian Nutritionist (RDN)

The team member with the most academic preparation, training, skills, and demonstrated effectiveness in fostering healthy eating for diabetes is the RD/RDN. The initials RD or RDN after a dietitian's name ensure that he or she has met and maintains the standards of the Academy of Nutrition and Dietetics.

Goals of MNT for Prediabetes and Diabetes

The American Diabetes Association (ADA) outlines the following goals of MNT for prediabetes and diabetes:

- For individuals with prediabetes, the goal of MNT is to decrease the risk of diabetes and cardiovascular disease (CVD) by intensive lifestyle modification, specifically healthy food choices, and increased physical activity leading to moderate weight loss that is maintained.[13]
- For individuals with diabetes, the goals of MNT are the following:
  - —To promote and support healthful eating patterns, emphasizing a variety of nutrient-dense foods in appropriate portion sizes in order to improve overall health and specifically to
    - o Achieve and maintain body weight
    - o Attain individualized glycemic, blood pressure, and lipid goals. General recommended goals from the ADA for these markers are as follows:

      A1C <7% for non-pregnant adult (older adults: healthy <7.5%; complex/intermediate health <8.0%; very complex/poor health <8.5%)

      Blood pressure <140/90 mm Hg

      Triglycerides <150 mg/dL (1.69 mmol/L) and HDL cholesterol >40 mg/dL (1.04 mmol/L) for men and >50 mg/dL (1.30 mmol/L) for women. LDL goals need to be individualized.
    - o Delay or prevent complications of diabetes
  - —To address individual nutrition needs based on personal and cultural preferences, health literacy and numeracy, access to healthful food choices, and willingness and ability to make behavioral changes, as well as barriers to change
  - —To maintain the pleasure of eating by providing nonjudgmental messages about food choices
  - —To provide the individual with diabetes with practical tools for developing healthful eating patterns rather than focusing on individual macronutrients, micronutrients, or single foods[13]

Further information on the evidence-based research that supports these recommendations is provided in chapter 16, Nutrition Therapy.

MNT Considerations

Successful self-management for healthy eating requires DSME/T and DSMS that focuses on concerns that are specific to the person's medical condition. One size does not fit all when educating an individual. Focus areas for healthy eating for type 1 diabetes are quite different from those for gestational diabetes, for example. Below are highlights of specialized issues that must be considered during DSME/T and DSMS. Additional information on MNT can be found in chapter 16, Nutrition Therapy.

Nutrition Recommendations and Interventions for the Prevention of Diabetes

The prevalence of obesity continues to be high; more than one third of adults in the United States are obese.[14] Risk factors for developing type 2 diabetes include a first-degree relative with diabetes, habitual physical inactivity, certain ethnicities, history of gestational diabetes, hypertension, hyperlipidemia, polycystic ovarian syndrome, conditions associated with insulin resistance such as acanthosis nigricans (a thickening of the stratum corneum that becomes pigmented), history of cardiovascular disease, etc. Given that family history and overweight are strong risk factors for type 2 diabetes, healthy eating for the entire family is

Case: Healthy Eating Through DSME/T and DSMS

SM is a 30-year-old Caucasian female who has had type 1 diabetes since age 17. She is interested in preconception planning for her first pregnancy.

Assessment Data

- Height: 65 in (165 cm)
- Weight: 130 lb (58.5 kg)
- Body mass index (BMI): 21
- Blood pressure: 128/77 mm Hg

Most Recent Lab Values

- A1C: 8.5%
- Fasting blood glucose: 145 mg/dL (8.05 mmol/L)
- Total cholesterol: 226 mg/dL (5.85 mmol/L)
- Triglycerides: 128 mg/dL (1.45 mmol/L)
- High-density lipoprotein cholesterol (HDL-C): 42 mg/dL (1.09 mmol/L)
- Low-density lipoprotein cholesterol (LDL-C): 113 mg/dL (2.93 mmol/L)

SM lives with her husband and travels frequently for her pharmaceutical sales job. She has been instructed on basic carbohydrate counting, but she is not consistent with her intake. She often eats sporadically due to her hectic travel schedule. Breakfast during the workweek is typically a large bagel with low-fat cream cheese, a piece of fruit, and black coffee; on weekends at home she sleeps late and enjoys making a brunch of bacon, eggs, and fruit salad. On most days, lunch is a chef salad with low-fat ranch salad dressing, 2 packages of crackers, and a diet drink. SM often goes out for a late dinner with friends, choosing items such as pasta with tomato sauce or grilled chicken with salad and bread, and an occasional alcoholic beverage.

SM currently takes 10 units of a rapid-acting insulin analog with meals and 20 units of glargine (Lantus®, Sanofi-Aventis) at bedtime. She is not adjusting her mealtime insulin doses. She is interested in using an insulin pump. SM checks her fasting blood glucose daily and tries to check her blood glucose at least one more time each day. SM is taking cinnamon capsules because her hairdresser told her it was "good for blood sugar." She denies taking other medications.

Her physical activity program consists of running 3 miles per day on the weekends. Her activity level during the week is much less intense, although she tries to attend a step aerobics class twice a week. Otherwise, her activity level is rather sedentary, as she spends much of her day in the car, driving between physicians' clinics in her sales territory.

Questions to Consider

1. What are the key healthy eating issues you might address at this visit?
2. How can you use the steps of the Nutrition Care Process and Model (NCPM) during SM's visit? (The NCPM is discussed later in this chapter.)
3. What resources could you suggest to SM to assist her with carb counting?
4. What is 1 behavior-change goal that focuses on healthy eating that SM may set?
5. List 2 skills related to healthy eating that you will review with SM during this visit.

a critical factor in diabetes prevention. Results from the DPP confirm that lifestyle modification was nearly twice as effective as medication in preventing diabetes (58% versus 31% relative reductions, respectively).[8] The DPP Outcomes Study showed that after an average of 10 years' follow-up, intensive lifestyle changes reduced the rate of developing type 2 diabetes by 34%[12] and at 15 years showed a reduction of 27%.[11] Similar results were found in the Da Qing Diabetes Prevention Study, showing a 43% reduction at 20 years[9] and in the Finish Diabetes Prevention Study a 43% reduction at 7 years.[10] The greater benefit of weight loss and physical activity strongly suggests that lifestyle modification should be the first choice to prevent or delay diabetes. The following are recommended goals for diabetes prevention:[13]

- *Weight loss* of 7% of body weight
- *Increasing physical activity* to at least 150 minutes per week of moderate-intensity aerobic activity such as walking

Because this intervention not only has been shown to prevent or delay diabetes, but also has a variety of other benefits, healthcare providers should urge all overweight, obese, and sedentary individuals to adopt these lifestyle changes, and such recommendations should be made at every opportunity.

Healthy eating and physical activity strategies implemented in a community-based program can complement clinical preventive and treatment programs for those who are already obese. Studies have shown that either

DPP-modeled intensive lifestyle interventions based in the community or individualized MNT for prediabetes will assist individuals in achieving weight loss and have demonstrated to be cost-effective.[15,16,17,18]

Nutrition Recommendations for the Management of Diabetes

The Nutrition Therapy for Adults with Diabetes or Prediabetes consensus report[7] state that nutrition therapy is recommended for all people with type 1 diabetes or type 2 diabetes as an effective component of the overall treatment plan. There is no ideal percentage of calories from carbohydrate, protein, and fat for all people with diabetes, so the choice of a healthy eating approach should be based on an individualized assessment of current eating patterns, preferences, and metabolic goals. Nutrition therapy goals should be created in collaboration with the individual with diabetes; the nutrition counselor's role is to share strategies to support the behavior changes necessary to achieve those goals.

Type 1 Diabetes Individuals with type 1 diabetes require exogenous insulin, so their primary nutrition goal is to integrate insulin therapy into their preferred eating routine and physical activity pattern. The total and type of carbohydrate in meals and snacks directly affects blood glucose levels, so this is a main area of focus. Those individuals on a fixed insulin regimen should strive for consistency in the timing and amount of their carbohydrate intake. Those using a multiple daily injection plan or insulin pump should adjust their insulin based on the carbohydrate content of their meals and snacks and may benefit from using the carbohydrate-counting meal-planning approach. For those on fixed daily insulin doses, consistent carbohydrate intake can result in improved glycemic stability and reduced risk for hypoglycemia. Because hypoglycemia occurs more frequently in individuals with type 1 diabetes, reviewing the basics of hypoglycemia prevention and treatment is important. The diabetes care and education specialist needs to address the blood glucose lowering effect of physical activity, sharing strategies such as adjusting insulin dosage for planned exercise to prevent hypoglycemia and also carrying a source of carbohydrate to treat hypoglycemia if needed. Additional information on this topic can be found in chapter 6, which deals with physical activity.

Type 2 Diabetes For people with type 2 diabetes who are overweight and insulin resistant, the diabetes care and education specialist needs to emphasize healthy eating behaviors that result in a reduction of energy, saturated and *trans* fat, and cholesterol and sodium, and an increase in physical activity in an effort to improve glycemia, dyslipidemia, and blood pressure. As in type 1 diabetes, individuals on fixed daily insulin doses may benefit from consistent carbohydrate intake to improve glycemic levels and reduce risk for hypoglycemia.

- *Weight loss*—A single weight loss plan that is successful for all individuals with diabetes has yet to be created. Reducing energy intake while maintaining a healthful eating pattern is recommended to promote weight loss.
- *Physical activity*—Initial physical activity recommendations should be modest and based on the person's willingness and ability to change. Adults with diabetes should be advised to perform at least 150 minutes a week of moderate-intensity aerobic physical activity (50%-70% of maximum heart rate), spread over at least 3 days a week with no more than 2 consecutive days without exercise. In the absence of contraindications, adults with type 2 diabetes should be encouraged to perform resistance training at least twice per week.[13]
- *Behavior change*—Persons with diabetes who achieve behavior-change goals for weight loss will have better clinical outcomes and improved health status. Successful behavior-change strategies associated with weight loss and weight loss maintenance in addition to a reduced-energy/fat intake, included self-monitoring of weight and food intake; portion management and healthy food choices, simplified meal plans as well as a variety of eating patterns[19] and increased, sustained levels of physical activity. Some evidence suggests that lifestyle interventions targeting both dietary intake and physical activity are effective in reducing weight regain after the initial weight loss in obese adults within 12 months and up to 24 months after the initial weight loss. The evidence is very limited when looking beyond 24 months.[20]

Pregnancy and Lactation Data from the Hyperglycemia and Adverse Pregnancy Outcome study have led to changes in the recommended criteria for the diagnosis and classification of hyperglycemia in pregnancy.[13] However, the MNT goals for pregnancy with diabetes continue to focus on minimizing blood glucose excursions and maintaining glucose values within target goal ranges before and after meals; providing a calorie intake that is neither inadequate nor excessive and will achieve an appropriate gestational weight gain without maternal ketosis; and ensuring adequate, safe nutrients for maternal and fetal health.[21] Breastfeeding is encouraged in all women with diabetes, with an emphasis on education for the prevention and treatment of hypoglycemia for women who require insulin. Specific nutrition issues with preexisting diabetes and gestational diabetes mellitus are noted below.

- *Preexisting diabetes:* Whether type 1 or type 2 preexisting diabetes, a major goal is "stability before conception" because the risk of fetal anomalies is greater when blood glucose stability is poor during fetal organogenesis, which occurs early in pregnancy.[22] Pregnancy for a woman with *type 1 diabetes* is often a time for intensive diabetes management involving an insulin pump or multiple daily injections of insulin. Concepts such as insulin-to-carbohydrate ratio must be mastered. The diabetes care and education specialist also needs to emphasize issues relating to food and the response of blood glucose during pregnancy. Hypoglycemia occurs more commonly in the first trimester because insulin requirements decrease and morning sickness leads to decreased food intake. As the pregnancy progresses, insulin resistance increases due to weight gain and increased placental hormones, necessitating increased insulin dosages to maintain optimal blood glucose levels. Women with *type 2 diabetes* who become pregnant require much of the same information as women with type 1 diabetes. Often, a woman with type 2 diabetes is overweight or obese when she becomes pregnant. The diabetes care and education specialist should consider the pregravid BMI when setting gestational goals for weight gain, energy intake, and physical activity level. Additional information can be found in chapter 24, Pregnancy With Diabetes.
- *Gestational diabetes mellitus (GDM):* A healthy eating plan is the primary therapeutic strategy for managing GDM. Emphasis should be placed on maintaining normal blood glucose while consuming enough calories and carbohydrate to promote appropriate weight gain yet avoid maternal starvation ketosis. Dietary reference intakes are used to determine the estimated energy requirements in pregnancy. Because carbohydrate consumed affects postprandial blood glucose levels, the individualized eating plan for GDM should be based on the nutrition assessment and focuses on total amount, type, and distribution of carbohydrate.[21,23] Women who develop GDM should be made aware of the lifestyle changes they will need to adopt to delay or prevent their increased risk for developing type 2 diabetes later in life. Additionally, children who were born to mothers who had GDM may also be at increased risk for obesity and type 2 diabetes throughout their lives. Additional information on GDM can be found in chapter 24, Pregnancy With Diabetes.

Children and Adolescents With Diabetes Nutrition education to promote healthy eating for children and adolescents with diabetes should involve the entire family as well as caretakers and should be geared toward the appropriate developmental stage of the child.[24] Group sessions involving family members have been consistently associated with positive weight loss in children and adolescents. The overarching goal for children and adolescents with diabetes is to prescribe enough calories for normal growth and development. To determine normal growth and weight profiles, growth of children and adolescents should be monitored on a height-weight growth chart at a minimum of every 3 to 6 months. Food plans must be developed with both treatment goals and realistic lifestyle choices in mind. Consider these points for children with diabetes or at risk for type 2 diabetes when creating the healthy eating plan:

- Adjust the food plan to meet energy requirements for growth and activity.
- Focus on an intake of nutrient-dense foods (ie, fruits, vegetables, whole grains, and calcium-rich foods) versus nutrient-sparse foods (ie, excessive amounts of sweets or large amounts of juice and fruit drinks).
- Use the term *food plan* or *meal plan*, rather than *diet* to avoid furthering negative connotations regarding healthy eating.
- Engage the child or adolescent in development of the food plan as well as in shopping for and preparing healthy foods for the entire family.

Type 1 Diabetes In addition to the points mentioned above, nutrition education for children with type 1 diabetes revolves around achieving blood glucose goals without excessive hypoglycemia while promoting normal growth and development. The key concepts discussed earlier about type 1 diabetes in adults also apply to children with type 1 diabetes. Discussions of DSME/T and DSMS should address the following:

- Nutrition issues for school and day care, irregular schedules, sports activities, peer influences, and level of acceptance
- Effects of growth and hormonal changes on blood glucose

- Additional adjustments to be made in insulin administered at mealtime, for "picky" eaters

Type 2 Diabetes It is estimated that 2 out of every 5 Americans are expected to develop type 2 diabetes during their lifetime, and the numbers look even worse for some minority groups.[25] This is due, in part, to the increasing number of children who are medically classified as "pediatric overweight." In addition to the previously mentioned points, lifestyle considerations for children at risk for or diagnosed with type 2 diabetes should include the following:

- Managing portions by encouraging children to "eat to appetite" rather than "cleaning their plates" filled with adult-sized portions
- Slowing their rate of eating
- Striving for regular mealtimes and limiting distractions, such as eating while watching TV, working on the computer, or using a smartphone
- Promoting moderate physical activity of at least 60 minutes daily
- Limiting the amount of nonacademic "screen time" (TV watching, video games, or Internet or social media use) to less than 2 hours daily

Because of the strong genetic component of type 2 diabetes, the entire family often benefits from being involved in the lifestyle change program. Successful lifestyle change outcomes for children with type 2 diabetes are defined as follows:[26]

- Cessation of excessive weight gain with near-normal linear growth
- Near-normal fasting blood glucose and A1C values

The Academy of Nutrition and Dietetics' Pediatric Weight Management Evidence-Based Nutrition Practice Guidelines[27] provides updated recommendations that can be incorporated into the nutrition counseling of children with type 2 diabetes at the time of diagnosis and as part of ongoing management. It is important to let the child or adolescent choose what they would like to focus on to improve their overall health, instead of having the healthcare provider decide what would be the best change to make. Additional information on nutrition therapy for children and adolescents with diabetes can be found in chapter 16.

Older Adults With Diabetes Recommendations for making healthy food choices should be individualized regardless of a person's age, but the need for this is even more apparent when the numerous factors affecting the older adult are considered.

> **Older Adults**
>
> One-to-one sessions often eliminate visual and auditory barriers to learning. Family and caregivers can attend to offer additional support.

Older adults with diabetes vary widely in their physical and cognitive status; in the presence or absence of underlying chronic conditions and comorbidities; and in their cultural backgrounds, traditions, and beliefs. An older individual who is able and willing to undertake the responsibility for diabetes self-management should be encouraged to do so and should be treated using the previously stated metabolic goals for adults; for other older adults, glycemic goals may be reasonably relaxed.[28–31] The diabetes care and education specialist should provide meal-planning guidelines that incorporate cultural food favorites and meet calorie and nutrient needs, looking specifically at protein intake and micronutrients, while promoting glycemic stability control. Physical activity should also be encouraged as a regular part of the individual's daily routine educating on prevention of hypoglycemia if the older person with diabetes is on insulin or medications that potentially could cause a low blood sugar.[28] With the individual's permission, family and caregivers should be encouraged to attend the teaching sessions; one-to-one sessions may be preferable to group classes, in which visual and auditory barriers could arise. Healthy eating issues such as taste preferences, lifelong eating habits, finances, and food preparation ability are also important.[32] Additional information on nutrition therapy for older adults with diabetes can be found in chapter 16.

Eating Problems and Diabetes Eating problems (both disordered eating behavior and eating disorders) are more common in adolescents with type 1 diabetes compared with their peers without type 1 diabetes, and both eating problems and diabetes are associated with poorer glycemic stability.[33] Evidence also suggests an increasing trend in eating disorders for middle-aged women, as well as the trend of orthorexia nervosa, an unhealthful fixation about eating so-called healthful foods.[34] Types of eating disorders include the following:

- *Anorexia nervosa*, which centers on restricted energy intake relative to requirements, leading to a markedly low body weight; intense fear of gaining weight or becoming fat or persistent behavior to avoid weight gain, even though at a markedly low weight; disturbance in the way in which one's body weight or shape is experienced.

- *Bulimia nervosa*, which is characterized by recurrent episodes of binge eating with a sense of lack of control and inappropriate compensatory behavior; self-evaluation unduly influenced by body shape and weight; and not occurring exclusively during episodes of anorexia nervosa. Purging may occur with self-induced vomiting, laxatives, diuretics, insulin omission or reduction, fasting, severe diets, or vigorous exercise.
- *Binge eating disorder*, which is described as repeated episodes of overconsumption of food with a sense of a lack of control. While there may be no purging, there may be sporadic fasts or repetitive diets and often feelings of shame or distress after a binge.
- *Diabulimia,* reduction or omission of insulin doses, inducing hyperglycemia to lose glucose calories through the urine.

Disturbed eating can have a potentially life-threatening impact on individuals with diabetes. Early recognition of risk for an eating disorder may help with prevention. The diagnosis of eating disorder is usually confirmed by questionnaires specifically designed to evaluate unhealthy eating behaviors. There are a couple of tools that can be used to diagnose eating disorders: the revised Diabetes Eating Problem Survey includes 16 items and has excellent internal consistency and specificity; the Eating Disordered Inventory 3 has been modified to be used in persons with type 1 diabetes.[35] Diabetes care and education specialists should be alert to warning signs that may suggest the presence of an eating disorder, such as deterioration in psychosocial function, neglect of diabetes management (particularly insulin omission), erratic clinic attendance, significant weight gain/loss, poor body image/low self-esteem, and recurrent/frequent diabetic ketoacidosis. Because eating disorders may be well hidden, it's important for the diabetes care and education specialist to use sensitive, open-ended questions to encourage discussion about body weight and shape. If an eating disorder is suspected, early referral to a mental health professional with experience working with individuals with eating disorders is indicated.

A multidisciplinary team approach to treatment is considered the standard of care for both eating disorders and diabetes. Initially, treatment of an eating disorder involves establishing medical safety, while members of the treatment team work to establish a positive rapport with the patient. Cognitive behavioral therapy has proven successful in the treatment of binge eating behaviors, but its use in anorexia nervosa is challenging because disruptions in neurotransmitter secretions and functions limit a patient's response to treatment.[35] A focus on carbohydrate or calorie intake can lead to over-restrictive eating in an individual with diabetes, so the nutrition treatment plan for the eating disorder should emphasize flexible and non-depriving approaches to eating that can be adopted by the patient's entire family for overall health and wellness.[36] The total diet approach to healthy eating, which focuses on variety, moderation, and proportionality in the context of a healthy lifestyle, rather than targeting specific nutrients or foods,[37] may prove successful in the treatment of eating problems in individuals with diabetes.

Diabetes and the Gastrointestinal Tract *Celiac disease* and *gastroparesis* are 2 areas of concern relative to healthy eating, diabetes, and the gastrointestinal tract.

Celiac Disease Celiac disease (also known as gluten-sensitive enteropathy) is an immune-mediated disorder that occurs with increased frequency in persons with type 1 diabetes (1.6%-16.4% of individuals compared with 0.3%-1% in the general population).[13] Individuals with celiac disease sustain damage to their intestinal epithelium after ingestion of foods made from the gliadin fraction of wheat gluten and similar molecules from barley, rye, and possibly oats, most commonly causing abdominal pain, diarrhea, malabsorption, and failure to thrive. While many patients with celiac disease are asymptomatic, current practice recommends that healthcare providers consider screening children with type 1 diabetes for celiac disease soon after the diagnosis of diabetes. If the diagnosis of celiac disease is confirmed, patients should consult with an RD/RDN and begin a gluten-free eating plan to coordinate with their nutrition plan for diabetes management. In addition to strictly eliminating gluten-containing grains such as barley, bran, hydrolyzed wheat protein, oats, rye, wheat, wheat bran, wheat germ, and white, whole wheat, and graham flour, patients may require a multivitamin supplement daily to prevent deficiencies resulting from malabsorption.[38] Intensive education in label reading and identification of hidden sources of gluten is necessary. The FDA's 2013 gluten-free labeling rule is intended to help people with celiac disease to easily identify gluten-free foods. It also provides standardization of what the term "gluten-free" means on a food label. It is also important to share with the patients that have celiac disease information in how they can get different educational information such as pamphlets, books, and recipes,[39-341] although there is a need for more educational materials that address healthy eating for both celiac disease and diabetes.

Gastroparesis Gastroparesis is a form of autonomic neuropathy that delays the emptying of the stomach. Clinically, persons with diabetes and gastroparesis are at risk for erratic glycemic levels as a consequence of unpredictable nutrient delivery of food into the upper gut, where it is absorbed. Hypoglycemia has resulted when insulin has been administered and gastric emptying of nutrients did not follow. The management for the person with gastroparesis includes attempts in improving gastric emptying, relieving symptoms and improving glycemic and the nutritional state. The pharmacologic treatment options include anti-emetic and prokinetic medications, as well as the emerging option of gastric electrical stimulation. The first choice of treatment in patients with gastroparesis is often dietary advice. Most of the nutrition therapy interventions for gastroparesis are based on the knowledge of the pathophysiology and clinical judgement.[7] Currently, there is only one small randomized clinical trial that emphasizes that small particle size (<2 mm) foods may reduce the severity of gastrointestinal symptoms.[42] Some of the dietary recommendations for the treatment of gastroparesis may include the following:[7]

- Decrease volume of meals/eat smaller, more frequent meals throughout the day.
- Use more liquid calories—may need to switch to liquid calories over the course of the day as fullness worsens; if solids are not tolerated, consider a trial of a pureed/liquid diet.
- Chew foods well.
- Sit up for 1 to 2 hours after a meal.
- Decrease fiber in the diet, as it may delay gastric emptying and lead to bezoar formation.
- Evaluate fat intake—fat in liquid form is often tolerated; fat is a good source of calories and should only be limited after other measures have been exhausted or if intake of solid fat is excessive.
- Consider taking a daily multivitamin/mineral supplement if dietary intake is inadequate.

Because poor glycemic management and wide swings in blood glucose levels can exacerbate gastroparesis, it's important for people with diabetes to work toward improved blood glucose stability. A basal-bolus insulin regimen before meals and snacks is recommended to match insulin needs to carbohydrate intake and promote optimal glucose stability. The use of an insulin pump is an option for people with type 1 diabetes and insulin requiring people with type 2 diabetes. Frequent blood glucose monitoring is necessary to achieve improved glycemic stability.

In Summary: Which Approach to Healthy Eating for Diabetes Is the Most Effective?

Healthy eating for diabetes is a complex issue. At this time, no single, ideal approach to the amount of protein, fat, and carbohydrate in a diabetes meal plan has been established. An individualized assessment of a person with diabetes' current eating patterns, preferences, and metabolic goals can help determine macronutrient distribution. Emphasis should not be placed on individual micro- and macronutrients, but rather on *eating patterns*, a term used to describe combinations of different foods or food groups that characterize relationships between nutrition and health promotion and disease prevention. Framing nutrition recommendations in terms of eating patterns is consistent with the total diet approach suggested by the 2015 Dietary Guidelines for Americans, which consider the combinations of foods and beverages that provide energy and nutrients and constitute an individual's complete dietary intake, on average, over time.[44] Nutrition Therapy for Adults With Diabetes or Prediabetes: a Consensus Report[7] reviews the evidence base in support of several eating patterns to evaluate their impact on diabetes nutrition goals for type 1 diabetes or type 2 diabetes:

- The *Mediterranean-style* eating pattern leads to improved CVD risk factors in individuals with diabetes. When supplemented with mixed nuts or olive oil, the Mediterranean eating pattern lowered combined end points for cardiovascular events and stroke. Individuals following an energy-restricted Mediterranean-style eating pattern also achieved improvements in glycemic goals.
- *Vegetarian and vegan* eating patterns did not consistently improve glycemic stability or CVD risk in individuals with type 2 diabetes, except when energy intake was restricted and weight was lost.
- The *low-fat* eating pattern with reduced calories achieved moderate success for weight loss in the Look AHEAD trial, but in other cited research studies, lowering total fat intake didn't consistently improve glycemic stability or CVD risk factors. The benefit from a low-fat eating pattern is more likely when energy intake is also reduced and weight loss occurs.
- *Very low-fat: Ornish or Pritikin* eating pattern may improve glycemic stability, weight, blood pressure and HDL-C with a mixed effect on triglycerides.
- *Low-carbohydrate or very-low-carbohydrate* eating pattern, especially the very-low carbohydrate

eating pattern, have been shown to reduce A1C and the need for blood glucose lowering medications. Effects can be seen during the first 3 to 6 months but A1C benefits are lost at 12 and 24 months. More research is needed to better understand the effect of a very-low-carbohydrate eating pattern for people with chronic kidney disease, disordered eating patterns, and women who are pregnant. There also are no randomized control trials in people with type 2 diabetes where the type of fat used in the low and very-low-carbohydrate eating pattern is examined for its effect on glycemia, CVD risk factors, or clinical events.

- The *DASH (Dietary Approaches to Stop Hypertension)* eating pattern has been shown to stabilize blood pressure and reduce risk for CVD in people without diabetes. Limited evidence exists on the effects of the DASH eating plan in individuals with diabetes, but one would expect results similar to those of other studies using the DASH eating plan.
- *Paleo* eating pattern showed mixed effects on A1C, weight, and lipids.

Table 5.2 describes the key elements of each of these eating patterns and includes meal ideas to help translate these recommendations into a day's meals.

TABLE 5.2 Eating Patterns for Diabetes: Descriptions and Meal Ideas

Eating Pattern	*Description*	*Meal Ideas*
Mediterranean style	Includes plant-based food (fruits, vegetables, whole intact grains, beans, nuts, and seeds); fish and other seafood; olive oil as the principal source of dietary fat; dairy products (mainly cheese and yogurt) consumed in low to moderate amounts; fewer than 4 eggs per week; red meat consumed in low frequency and amounts; and wine consumption in low to moderate amounts; and concentrated sugars or honey rarely.	Breakfast—Greek yogurt topped with berries and walnuts, cubed cantaloupe Lunch—White bean soup, hummus and vegetables in a whole wheat pita Dinner—Grilled salmon stuffed with spinach and feta cheese, wheat berry salad (olive oil, vinaigrette, feta, parsley, and tomatoes), baked apples with cherries and almonds, glass of red wine Snacks—Nuts, whole grain crackers and cheese
Vegetarian and vegan	Vegan meal plans are devoid of all flesh foods and animal-derived products; vegetarian meal plans are devoid of all flesh foods but include egg (ovo) and/or dairy (lacto) products. These meal plans feature lower intakes of saturated fat and cholesterol and higher intakes of fruits, vegetables, whole grains, nuts, soy products, fiber, and phytochemicals.	Vegan meals: Breakfast—Whole grain cereal with soy milk, banana Lunch—Grilled vegetable sandwich (tomatoes, zucchini, peppers, onion, garlic, and beans), green spinach salad with vinaigrette dressing Dinner—Tofu stir-fry with sautéed vegetables such as broccoli, snow peas, baby corn, and water chestnuts, soy yogurt parfait Snacks—Fresh fruits and vegetables, soy almond milk fruit smoothie Vegetarian meals may include eggs and dairy products
Low fat	Emphasizes fiber-rich vegetables, beans, fruits, whole intact grains, starches (breads/crackers, pasta, starchy vegetables), lean protein, and low-fat dairy products. Defined as total fat intake <30% or total energy intake and saturated fat intake <10%	Breakfast—Whole grain English muffin with fat-free cream cheese, blueberries, skim milk Lunch—Chicken noodle soup, green salad with chicken and fat-free French salad dressing, fresh pineapple Dinner—Grilled shrimp skewers on brown rice, tossed salad with fat-free Caesar salad dressing, watermelon Snacks—Nonfat yogurt, low-fat cheese with whole wheat crackers

TABLE 5.2 Eating Patterns for Diabetes: Descriptions and Meal Ideas (continued)

Eating Pattern	*Description*	*Meal Ideas*
Very low-fat	Emphasizes fiber-rich vegetables, beans, fruits, whole intact grains, nonfat dairy, fish and egg whites and comprises 70%–77% carbohydrate (including 30–60 g fiber), 10% fat, 13%–20% protein	Breakfast—2 egg whites with vegetable scramble; blueberries, strawberries and raspberries, nonfat milk, whole grain bread Lunch—roasted tomato soup, asian noodle salad with grilled shrimp, whole-wheat peach griddle cake Dinner—wild salmon, butter salad, corn/black bean/tomato salad, bread pudding Snack—dark chocolate, apricots
Low carbohydrate/ Very low carbohydrate	Emphasizes vegetables low in carbohydrates (such as salad green, broccoli, cauliflower, cucumber, cabbage, and others) fat from animal foods, oils, butter, and avocado; and protein in the form of meat, poultry, fish, shellfish, eggs, cheese, nuts, and seeds. Some plans include fruit (eg, berries) and a greater array of nonstarchy vegetables. Avoids starchy and sugary foods such as pasta, rice, potatoes, bread, and sweets. Carbohydrate intake is between 26%–45% of total calories. The very low-carbohydrate pattern limits carbohydrate-containing foods even further and meals typically derive more than half of the calories from fat. Carbohydrates—no more than 20 to 50 g of non-fiber to induce nutritional ketosis. Carbohydrate intake <26%.	Breakfast—Eggs cooked in butter, Canadian bacon, fresh grapefruit Lunch—Sliced grilled chicken wrapped in lettuce with tomatoes and mayonnaise, Romaine lettuce salad with avocado slices and vinaigrette salad dressing Dinner—London Broil, mushrooms sautéed in oil, spinach salad with pecans and blue cheese dressing, sugar-free gelatin Snacks—Whole almonds, string cheese
DASH	Emphasizes fruits, vegetables, and low-fat dairy products, including whole grains, poultry, fish, and nuts; reduced in saturated fat, red meat, sweets, and sugar-containing beverages. The most effective DASH meal plan is also reduced in sodium.	Breakfast—Cooked oatmeal with low-fat milk, low-sodium vegetable juice, banana Lunch—Unsalted chicken salad on whole wheat bread with Dijon mustard, apple, low-fat milk Dinner—Baked turkey, broccoli, whole wheat roll with unsalted soft margarine, nonfat yogurt Snacks—Unsalted almonds or pretzels, fresh fruits and vegetables
Paleo	Emphasizes foods theoretically eaten regularly during early human evolution, such as lean meat, fish, shellfish, vegetables, eggs, nuts, and berries. Avoids grains, dairy, salt, refined fats, and sugar.	Breakfast—eggs with sausage and berries Lunch—shrimp bowl with zucchini Dinner—sweet potato chili with green chiles and ground bison or beef

Source: Adapted from AB Evert, M Denison, CD Gardner, et al; American Diabetes Association, "Nutrition therapy for adults with diabetes or prediabetes: a consensus report of the American Diabetes Association," *Diabetes Care* 42 (2019): 731-54.

Glycemic Index and Glycemic Load

Monitoring carbohydrate intake remains a key strategy in achieving glycemic stability. The *glycemic index* (GI) estimates the acute postprandial glycemic impact of a specified quantity of carbohydrate-containing foods and ranks these carbohydrates on a scale from 0 to 100 according to the extent to which they raise blood glucose levels after being consumed. Proponents of this often-controversial meal-planning approach explain GI by noting that foods with a high GI are those which are rapidly digested and absorbed and result in marked fluctuations in blood glucose levels; low-GI foods, by virtue of their slow digestion and absorption, produce gradual rises in blood glucose and insulin levels.[45] *Glycemic load* (GL) refers to the amount of carbohydrate found in a particular food eaten multiplied by the glycemic index.[46] The Human Nutrition Unit, School of Molecular Biosciences, University of Sydney (Australia) maintains a comprehensive database of foods that have been tested for the GI and glycemic load.[47] Research on the effects of using a GI meal-planning approach on glycemic stability and CVD risks factors is mixed; however, substituting low–glycemic load foods for high–glycemic load foods may modestly improve glycemic stability.[7] Implementing a GI meal-planning approach can be complex, but individuals with diabetes who choose to use the GI can begin by incorporating one lower GI food in each meal and snack and making simple changes such as substituting a grainy or sourdough bread for white bread, natural muesli for puffed grain cereal, lentils or beans for potatoes, and nuts for snacks such as pretzels.

Because the literature suggests that several approaches to healthy eating for diabetes may be effective in improving glycemic and/or CVD risk factors, the diabetes care and education specialist should offer a choice of eating patterns based on the individual's health goals, personal and cultural preferences, health literacy and numeracy, access to healthful choices, and readiness, willingness, and ability to change.[7] For a more in-depth discussion on the evidence base supporting healthy eating, see chapter 16, Nutrition Therapy.

Promoting Healthy Eating: The Role of DSME/T and DSMS

Diabetes education—also known as diabetes self-management training (DSMT), diabetes self-management support (DSMS), or diabetes self-management education (DSME)—is a collaborative process through which people with or at risk for diabetes gain the knowledge and skills needed to modify behavior and successfully self-manage the disease and its related conditions.[1] Using evidence-based clinical practice recommendations and taking into account the expected outcomes from MNT, diabetes care and education specialists translate clinical recommendations into self-management education. Registered dietitians/registered dietitian nutritionists are guided in this effort by 2 recommended tools, the Nutrition Care Process and Model and the Nutrition Practice Guidelines, both developed by the Academy of Nutrition and Dietetics.

The Nutrition Care Process and Model

The Nutrition Care Process and Model (NCPM)[48,49] outlines the consistent and specific steps to be used when delivering MNT and moves professionals beyond experience-based practice to evidence-based practice. Although the NCPM is intended for dietetics professionals, other healthcare professionals may find the process useful in providing quality care. Central to the effective provision of MNT is the relationship between the individual seeking care and the healthcare professional.

> **Four Steps in the NCPM**
>
> 1. Assessment
> 2. Diagnosis
> 3. Intervention
> 4. Monitoring and evaluation

Step 1: Nutrition Assessment

An RD/RDN who provides MNT and education on healthy eating should follow a systematic process that begins with a nutrition assessment. Nutrition assessment is a systematic approach to collect, record, and interpret relevant data from persons with diabetes, clients, family members, caregivers, and other individuals and groups. Nutrition assessment is an ongoing, dynamic process that involves initial data collection as well as continual reassessment and analysis of the individual's/client's status compared with specific criteria.[48,49] Other members of the diabetes healthcare team often provide information which makes the assessment more valuable. Types of data collected include the following:

- Food- and nutrition-related history
- Anthropometric measurements
- Biochemical data, medical tests, and procedures
- Nutrition-focused physical examination findings
- Client history

Conducting the assessment establishes rapport, which is particularly helpful as the process of DSME/T and DSMS continues. The diabetes care and education specialist must learn the following about the individual: level of knowledge and skills, attitude and motivation, and readiness to learn new behaviors and interest in changing old ones, if appropriate, as well as preferred ways of learning.

During the assessment phase, the diabetes care and education specialist can determine the individual's preference for learning. This enables the diabetes care and education specialist to present information in a style tailored to promote success. Some people prefer to learn by reading, others by listening, others by watching, and still others by a hands-on approach; at times, an individual may combine learning styles. Health literacy is particularly relevant for diabetes education. The assessment phase yields information related to the individualization of self-management education, which promotes consideration of each participant's educational concerns and priorities, recognizes the expertise and unique perspectives that each participant brings to the process of self-management education, incorporates psychosocial and behavioral aspects, and helps create collaborative partnerships between participants and diabetes care and education specialists that promote and sustain ongoing diabetes self-management.[48,49]

Health beliefs must be considered during the assessment. Food choices and why a person eats as he or she does are deeply embedded in the psyche and may be a result of strong cultural or ethnic traditions. The supportiveness of family members may not be obvious; further probing may be required. Visual status, disabilities, barriers to learning, and socioeconomic status are all important factors to determine in the assessment.

The Role of Ethnicity and Culture Because ethnic diversity continues to increase, and because the prevalence of diabetes in minority groups throughout the United States is extremely high, the diabetes care and education specialist must be prepared to tailor DSME/T and DSMS for healthy eating to fit a variety of cultural practices. The most effective diabetes care and education specialist are those who have a deep commitment to cultural sensitivity for the populations they serve.[51,52] Cultural competency is the ability to work effectively with people of different cultural backgrounds. Successful diabetes prevention and treatment in diverse ethnic populations require sensitivity to cultural differences in health beliefs and eating habits.

In cross-cultural counseling, as in other situations, the person who came for assistance should be involved in problem solving and in developing strategies for behavior change. Include family members who are involved in food preparation. Establish respect and trust by having a nonjudgmental attitude and accepting cultural differences. Include as many familiar foods as possible in the healthy eating plan and explore the person's use of special foods, beverages, or herbal therapies as folk remedies. Refer to chapter 21, on biological complementary therapies, for more information and a list of resources.

A variety of resources are available for learning more about a specific culture and are useful when providing MNT.[53–55] Existing educational materials may also be adapted to be culturally specific. Invite the individual with diabetes to teach the diabetes care and education specialist about the ingredients in and preparation of cultural and ethnic foods. Combining an individual's cultural expertise with the diabetes and nutrition knowledge of the diabetes care and education specialist allows for a true exchange of information that benefits both parties.

A comprehensive assessment is a crucial step in providing individualized diabetes medical nutrition therapy. The assessment requires adequate time to be performed thoroughly, but provides a wealth of information that allows the professional to tailor the intervention and the diabetes nutrition therapy to the individual. The RD/RDN cannot begin to develop a nutrition diagnosis or design a nutrition intervention without the sound basis of an assessment. A high-level assessment involves obtaining appropriate data as well as analyzing and interpreting the data in light of evidence-based standards.

Step 2: Nutrition Diagnosis

The nutrition diagnosis is the RD/RDN's identification and labeling of an existing nutrition problem that he or she is responsible for treating independently.[49] It determines the specific healthy eating behaviors that need to be modified. The nutrition diagnosis is not the same as the medical diagnosis, which is diabetes mellitus. Components of the nutrition diagnosis include a description of alterations in a patient's status, etiology of the problem, and signs/symptoms of the problem. While the individual may have a medical diagnosis of type 1 diabetes, after completing a nutrition assessment the RD/RDN establishes the nutrition diagnosis. A well-written nutrition diagnostic statement should be clear and concise, specific to a individual/client, limited to a single client problem, accurately related to one etiology, and based on signs/symptoms from the assessment data.[49] The following are examples of a nutrition diagnostic statement:

"Inconsistent carbohydrate intake"
"Overly large portion sizes"
"Excessive fat intake"

Determining a nutrition diagnosis will guide the diabetes care and education specialist and the person with or at risk for diabetes toward the appropriate selection of goals for behavior change and their desired outcomes.

Step 3: Nutrition Intervention

The third step of the NCPM, nutrition intervention, involves planning and implementing the activities that specifically facilitate or support the individual's healthy eating behavior. It consists of 2 interrelated components: planning and implementation. Steps in planning include prioritizing diagnoses, writing a nutrition prescription, collaborating with the person with diabetes to identify goals, selecting specific intervention strategies, and defining time/frequency of care, including intensity, duration, and follow-up. Implementing the plan involves collaborating with the person with diabetes to carry out the plan, communicating the plan, modifying the plan as needed, following up and verifying that the plan is being implemented, and revising strategies based on changes in condition or response to the intervention.[48]

Education, the process of providing accurate and timely information to the individual who has or is at risk for diabetes, is key at this step. However, the role of the diabetes care and education specialist goes beyond merely supplying facts. The diabetes care and education specialist is a counselor and a coach, whose role is to help the person understand the disease and cope with its implications. The diabetes care and education specialist is a partner in disease management, assisting individuals in making their own decisions about self-care and healthy eating while helping them discover how they may be motivated to change their behavior.

After the nutrition diagnosis is made and behavior goals and desired outcomes are established, the nutrition intervention begins and healthy eating skills can be taught. A number of healthy eating resources are available; several are described later in this chapter. No single meal-planning approach works for every individual. The initial meal-planning approach is chosen with the understanding that it may change as the person's understanding of the disease and motivation to self-manage evolve.

Step 4: Nutrition Monitoring and Evaluation

Nutrition monitoring and evaluation identifies the amount of progress made and whether goals are being met. This step includes 3 distinct and interrelated processes: monitor progress, measure outcomes, and evaluate outcomes.[49] Successful MNT involves the process of problem solving, adjustment, and readjustment. Food diaries and records, such as blood glucose readings, are reviewed, evaluated, and reassessed. Measurable goals help make evaluation a straightforward task. Helping the person with diabetes think in terms of a course correction, rather than a goal evaluation, makes this discussion less threatening. If initial goals are not met, they may need to be changed or renegotiated. If they have been met, new reasonable, attainable, and measurable goals should be designed.

Documentation is necessary at each stage of the NCPM. Documentation in the medical record aids in communication with other members of the healthcare team. Written documentation can be shared with the person with diabetes to demonstrate his or her progress and encourage further efforts.

Outline for a Well-Designed Diabetes Nutrition Education Encounter

- *Focus on the individual*—The encounter begins with the diabetes care and education specialist asking the individual what questions and concerns he or she has regarding their diabetes as it relates to healthy eating.
- *Assess, diagnose, plan*—The diabetes care and education specialist then completes the nutrition assessment, establishes a nutrition diagnosis, and works with the individual to set behavior-change goals and plan a nutrition intervention using an individualized healthy eating approach.
- *Wrap up for the individual's benefit*—The session ends with the diabetes care and education specialist answering remaining questions, asking the individual to summarize key points, and making a follow-up plan for the future.

The Nutrition Practice Guidelines

The Nutrition Practice Guidelines (NPGs) for type 1 diabetes and type 2 diabetes[56] and for GDM[21] have been developed to delineate the structure by which optimal care is provided. The NPGs are evidence-based protocols that, when used to deliver MNT, result in positive health outcomes. These guidelines outline both clinical outcomes and necessary lifestyle changes and suggest the frequency and length of contact with the RD/RDN as well as the amount of time between encounters, based on the specific situation of the person. For example, due to the time-sensitive nature of GDM, more frequent contact in a shorter period of time is generally required as compared with routine follow-up for an individual with long-standing type 2 diabetes. Together, the NCPM and NPGs form the framework for well-designed self-management education regarding healthy eating.

Promoting Healthy Eating: The Role of Behavior Change

Behavior change is the unique outcome measurement for DSME. For the individual who participates in self-management education focused on healthy eating, the goal is to improve overall health status by empowering him or her to do the following:

- Acquire knowledge (what to do)
- Acquire skills (how to do it)

- Develop confidence and motivation to perform the appropriate self-care behaviors (want to do it)
- Develop problem-solving and coping skills to overcome any barriers to self-care behavior (can do it)[57]

Outcomes

Measuring outcomes demonstrates the effectiveness of the diabetes care and education specialist and the unique contribution that he or she can make. For each of the AADE7 Self-Care Behaviors®, a continuum of outcomes related to diabetes education is expected[57]

- *Immediate outcomes:* Learning, knowledge, skill acquisition
- *Intermediate outcomes:* Behavior change
- *Post-intermediate outcomes:* Improved clinical indicators
- *Long-term outcomes:* Improved health status

Immediate Outcomes

Learning is the immediate outcome sought. After teaching a healthy eating behavior such as label reading, the diabetes care and education specialist can immediately ask the learner to demonstrate the new skill. The diabetes care and education specialist asks the learner, for example, to read a sample label for critical information, such as portion size or carbohydrate content. This enables the diabetes care and education specialist to determine whether the person learned the material that was taught.

Intermediate Outcomes

Behavior change, the intermediate outcome sought, is the unique outcome measurement for DSME/T and DSMS. Although the learner may have acquired important information regarding label reading, the desired outcome is that this person uses the information to change his or her behavior and make healthier food choices. Behaviors such as choosing the proper type and amount of food or dealing with special situations such as illness or travel can be measured by observation, self-report of food intake, and review of records of blood glucose readings. Feeling empowered about making positive, sustainable behavior changes leads to increased energy levels and improved monitoring results.

Post-Intermediate Outcomes

Improved clinical indicators, the desired post-intermediate outcome, can be measured via laboratory tests and clinical measurements such as A1C, blood pressure, and lipid levels.

Long-Term Outcomes

At the end of the continuum of outcomes are long-term outcomes such as improved health status. Long-term outcomes can be measured as improvement in quality of life, economic benefits from reduced healthcare costs, and increased productivity.

Behavior Change

Behavior-change theories and strategies are useful in planning effective counseling sessions on the topic of healthy eating. Using the Transtheoretical Model of Behavior Change,[58] the diabetes care and education specialist can match the nutrition intervention to the individual's stage of readiness to embrace new behaviors. In developing this model, Prochaska et al outlined the 5 stages of behavior change: precontemplation, contemplation, preparation, action, and maintenance. The stages are useful to consider when planning and implementing nutrition care. In making changes, people progress through these 5 stages, although not necessarily in a systematic manner. Being aware of the nature of this process can help the diabetes care and education specialist better understand and help the individual progress toward behavior changes that result in healthy eating. Recognizing that behavior change is a multistep process helps minimize unrealistic expectations. Table 5.3 illustrates the process.

The individual with diabetes and the diabetes care and education specialist work together to formulate goals and determine a plan of action. When establishing goals, the diabetes care and education specialist should distinguish not only between short-term goals for behavior change and long-term goals, but also between behavior-change outcomes that are the goals of the person seeking assistance and those that are the goals of the healthcare provider. Goals for both parties should be specific, reasonable, attainable, and measurable.[59] Examples of behavior-change goals for healthy eating are shown in Table 5.4. It is important to let the person with diabetes select a goal that he or she would like to work on—the diabetes care and education specialist will function as a guide to assist the person in making this goal more specific. Healthy eating goals evolve over time and need to be evaluated and renegotiated as circumstances change.

A brief counseling approach that can be integrated with other diabetes nutrition education and counseling resources is the 5As (Assess, Advise, Agree, Assist, Arrange), which has proven helpful in counseling for smoking cessation. Research has shown that when clinicians spend as little as 3 minutes talking about a new behavior, patients will consider and even adopt a behavior change.[60]

Additional information about outcomes, goal setting, and behavior change can be found in chapters 2 and 3.

TABLE 5.3 The Process of Behavior Change: Healthy Eating for Weight Loss

Stage of Change	*Characteristics*	*Common Comments That Can Indicate the Stage of Change*
Precontemplation	Unaware that change is needed or having no intention of changing	"I feel fine, even though I might be a few pounds overweight."
Contemplation	Intends to change in the next 6 months; aware of the benefits and costs of change	"I will try to lose some weight. It will help improve my blood glucose, but I don't know if I can give up my wife's down-home cooking."
Preparation	Ready to change in the next 30 days; tak' g steps to begin making a change	"I've looked at all the diets out there. I think I'll stick with the meal plan I learned about at my last diabetes clinic visit."
Action	Has been making changes over the past 6 months	"I've been following my meal plan and weighing myself every week for the past month."
Maintenance	Has successfully made a change for more than 6 months; making efforts to avoid slipping into past behaviors	"Since the holidays are coming up, I need to plan on sticking with my current strategies, so I won't gain weight again this year."

Source: P Geil, T Ross, *What Do I Eat Now? A Step-by-Step Guide for Eating Right With Type 2 Diabetes* (Alexandria, Va: American Diabetes Association, 2015).

TABLE 5.4 Sample Behavior-Change Goals for Healthy Eating

I will measure my food and beverage intake for 3 days, record the amounts, and bring the records to my next clinic appointment.
I will substitute diet soda or water for sweetened soda at lunchtime at least 3 days per week.
I will check and record my blood glucose levels 2 hours after each meal every day.
I will modify 3 favorite recipes into lower fat and lower carbohydrate versions before my next clinic appointment.
I will limit my carbohydrate intake to 60 g of carbohydrate at each of my 3 meals and 15 g of carbohydrate at each of my 2 snacks at least 5 days per week.

Source: P Geil, T Ross, *What Do I Eat Now? A Step-by-Step Guide for Eating Right With Type 2 Diabetes* (Alexandria, Va: American Diabetes Association, 2015).

Promoting Healthy Eating: Theory Into Practice

No single meal-planning approach works for every individual, and no single approach has been proven to be more effective than another. Positive behavior change for healthy eating depends greatly on readiness to learn and the individualized needs of the person with diabetes. For each phase of education, different educational resources may be needed. Key topics for nutrition education, including coordinating food with diabetes medications, are available in Nutrition Therapy for Adults With Diabetes or Prediabetes: a Consensus Report.[7]

Initial Education

Basic nutrition interventions are needed for beginning or "survival" education, while more in-depth tools may be needed as the counseling process continues. Basic or initial education provides the information needed at the time of diagnosis, when the treatment plan or person's lifestyle changes, or at the time of initial contact with a diabetes care and education specialist. Initial skill topics include the following:

- Information about basic nutrition guidelines
- Instruction on sources of carbohydrate, amount of carbohydrate to consume, portion sizes, and the need to space carbohydrates throughout the day to manage blood glucose
- Symptoms and treatment of hypoglycemia, if appropriate

More Advanced Topics

Continuing self-management training provides more advanced education and includes both management and lifestyle skills. Topics to cover are chosen based on the individual's situation, level of nutrition knowledge, and experience in planning, purchasing, and preparing food. Individuals with diabetes can be taught more in-depth topics such as making adjustments in food and medication for sick days, physical activity, travel, and eating away from home.

Meal-Planning Resources

A healthy eating plan for diabetes is individualized and should emphasize a variety of minimally processed nutrient-dense foods in appropriate portion sizes.[7] The following meal-planning resources are helpful in translating the evidence-based science behind current diabetes nutrition recommendations into a healthy meal plan for everyday use.

Because healthy eating for diabetes is not "one size fits all," preprinted diet sheets are ineffective and should not be used. A number of meal-planning approaches are available to teach basic diabetes nutrition guidelines as well as more in-depth nutrition interventions. The person with diabetes and the diabetes care and education specialist may begin with one meal-planning approach and then try other resources as the counseling process continues.

Dietary Guidelines 2015–2020[44] and the USDA Choose My Plate[61] (see Figure 5.1) can be used as an introduction to basic nutrition and to begin the process of changing eating behaviors. However, these resources do not address issues specific to diabetes; therefore, a diabetes-based resource such as the ADA's Create Your Plate[62] might prove more effective. These meal-planning approaches are especially useful for visual learners, those who do not speak English, persons with poor reading or math skills, and individuals with cognitive limitations.

Healthy Food Choices (English and Spanish)[63] is a pamphlet that illustrates the basics of good nutrition and includes food lists. It opens into a small poster that provides a general overview of what to eat and when. Space is provided to write in a detailed meal plan in any "meal-planning language" (ie, carbohydrate servings, food choice groups, or actual menu items).

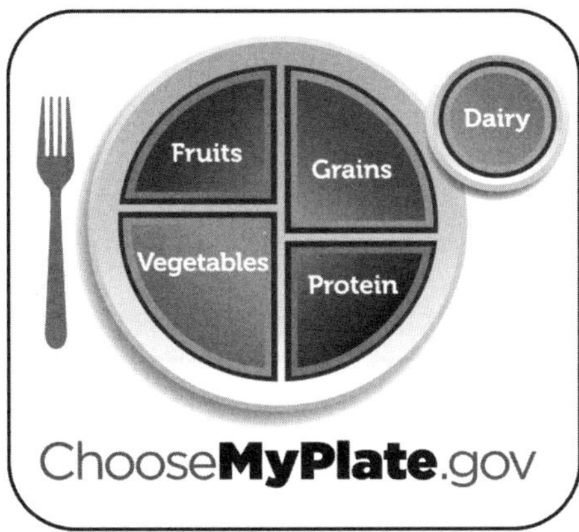

FIGURE 5.1 USDA Choose My Plate

Source: United States Department of Agriculture (USDA), "Choose my plate" (cited 2019 June 3), on the Internet at: http://www.choosemyplate.gov.

Individualized menus can be developed by the RD/RDN to provide a written description of exactly what and when to eat. Individualized, preplanned menus help people with diabetes achieve healthy eating by specifying the foods and amounts to be consumed for meals and snacks each day. Menu resources often include simple recipes to help people with diabetes prepare their food. Menus are useful for initial or simplified diabetes meal planning; for those who have little experience or interest in meal planning; and for individuals with poor reading and math skills, cognitive limitations, or difficulty using more structured approaches. The ADA has developed healthy menus that are available in the *Month of Meals™ Diabetes Meal Planner* book.[64]

Eating Healthy With Diabetes: Easy Reading Guide[65] is intended for persons with diabetes who have limited reading skills or impaired vision. The guide offers a large-print format, numerous photos, and very little text. Food lists are presented in the context of breakfast, lunch, dinner, and snack choices.

Choose Your Foods: Food Lists for Diabetes[66] (English and Spanish) lists groups of measured foods of approximately the same nutritional value. Foods in each list can be substituted or exchanged for other foods in the same list. This continues to be the most complete set of food lists on which all other diabetes nutrition resources are based. The food lists are used with an individualized meal plan that specifies when and how many choices from each group are to be eaten for meals and/or snacks.

Choose Your Foods: Plan Your Meals[67] (English and Spanish) is a colorful trifold poster that introduces meal planning for people newly diagnosed with diabetes. It includes tips for using a plate to plan breakfasts, lunches, dinners, and snacks and features a meal planner that can be personalized.

Carbohydrate Counting

Carbohydrate affects blood glucose more directly than protein or fat, the other 2 sources of energy/calories. Both the amount (grams) and the type of carbohydrate in a food influence the blood glucose level. Monitoring total grams of carbohydrate remains a key strategy in achieving glycemic stability. Using the carbohydrate-counting method, the person with diabetes counts the exact number of grams of carbohydrate in the foods eaten. Alternatively, each serving of starch, fruit, or milk and milk substitutes can be counted as 1 carbohydrate serving. Each carbohydrate serving has about 15 g of carbohydrate. An RD/RDN can help the person with diabetes determine the optimal number of carbohydrate servings or grams of carbohydrate to eat each day; the individual then follows this recommendation in planning meals. Food records and self-monitoring of blood glucose can be used to determine whether the amount of carbohydrate prescribed is appropriate. Carbohydrate counting can be effective for individuals with all types of diabetes. Meal-planning resources for carbohydrate counting are divided into 2 levels of instruction:

- *Count Your Carbs: Getting Started*[68] is a booklet that introduces basic concepts of carbohydrate counting and blood glucose management. It provides guidance on how much carbohydrate to eat, record keeping, and where to find carbohydrate information.
- *Advanced Carbohydrate Counting*[69] is a booklet that is designed to teach blood glucose and pattern management and how to use insulin-to-carbohydrate ratios. An advanced carbohydrate-counting vocabulary list, a list of needed skills, practice exercises, and questions and answers are included. This booklet is intended to be used in conjunction with the *Choose Your Foods: Food Lists for Diabetes* or other carbohydrate-counting nutrition references, as food lists are not included.

Meal-Planning Skills

In addition to mastering the basic concepts described in a selected meal-planning resource, individuals with diabetes need to learn practical healthy eating skills to apply in a variety of real-life situations. The individual's specific needs and learning priorities should guide the diabetes care and education specialist in teaching topics such as portion sizes; food label reading; planning, shopping, and cooking; eating out; and special situations.

Portion Sizes

Portion sizes served are often in excess of what's needed to satisfy hunger and meet carbohydrate goals for meals and snacks. Many individuals don't realize that portion size might vary from the standard serving size listed on food labels. The diabetes care and education specialist can advise the person with diabetes to take advantage of the "tools of the trade":

- Use a measuring cup to serve foods such as soup, casseroles, cereal, rice, and cut-up fruit.
- Use measuring spoons for salad dressing, margarine, and peanut butter to get a visual of food portions.
- When possible, measure out appropriate individual portions of food and try to remember how the portion looks for the next time.
- Portions for meats, poultry, and fish are based on cooked weight, so allow shrinkage from raw.
- Measure your drinking cups so you'll know how much you drink when you use that cup, and measure your bowls so you'll know how much cereal or soup you're eating.

Visualize Portion Size[59]

Knowing portion sizes is crucial to successful diabetes management. Use dietitian-approved plastic or similar food models to demonstrate portion sizes and foods that contain carbohydrates. Compare small portions of common foods such as a bunch of grapes, 8 oz plain yogurt, or whole grain crackers with the amount of carbohydrate in a 12-oz can of regular soft drink, gelatin, sweetened fruit yogurt, and other foods. Have the individual weigh and measure foods at home occasionally to improve portion-estimating abilities when eating away from home. Teach the following convenient guides to portion sizes:

- Thumb tip = 1 tsp
- Thumb = 2 Tb or 1 oz
- Fist = 1 c
- Palm = 3 oz of cooked meat
- Cupped handful = 1–2 oz or 1/4 c of snack food

Food Label Reading

Food labels provide valuable information for healthy eating, but individuals with diabetes may feel overwhelmed by the wealth of facts and figures, making them uncertain about which numbers are most important. Some tips to share with persons with diabetes about making the most of food label information are the following:

- *Take it from the top—size up the servings.* Compare the serving size recommended in diabetes meal-planning tools with the serving size listed on the food label and adjust the portion on your plate as needed.
- *How many servings are in there?* A quick check of the number of servings in the container is an easy portion tool.

- *Know your numbers—what's inside?* A quick way to determine whether the amount of a particular nutrient is high or low in a serving of food is to use the % Daily Value data on the label: 5% or less is low, 20% or more is high.
- *Make a smart choice—it's all about you!* The RD/RDN can provide additional individualized guidance if nutrients such as fat or sodium are of concern.
- Note: the updated US Food and Drug Administration (FDA) food labeling final rule of May 20, 2016, requires label compliance to start on January 2021. This change includes an updated nutrition facts panel format, updated serving sizes, and required nutrients and % Daily Values. For example, calories per serving will be prominent, potassium and Vitamin D will be required, and grams of added sugars will be listed beneath Total Sugars.[70,71]

If an individual with diabetes is still overwhelmed by label reading, he or she should be advised to go back to the basics and focus first on serving size and the amount of carbohydrate in the foods most commonly eaten.

Planning, Shopping, and Cooking

The heart of healthy eating is enjoying good food. With today's time crunch, cooking has become a lost art for many people. Encourage individuals with diabetes to take the time to plan meal and snack choices, shop economically, and begin cooking at home to improve their health and budget. Top tips include the following:

- Take the time to plan ahead for meals and snacks. Advance planning means healthier food choices, and using a list in the grocery store saves time and money.[72]
- Batch cooking (cooking once and serving twice) and planned-overs (key ingredients saved after a meal to use as part of another meal) help make the most of time in the kitchen.
- There's no need to give up favorite family recipes in order to eat healthfully for diabetes. Rethink recipes with an eye to reducing fat, sugar, and salt and increasing the fiber and flavor.

Eating Out

Individuals with diabetes often eat away from home. While dining out can make healthy eating a challenge, tips to share include the following:

- In a fast-food restaurant, keep it simple by choosing foods in their simplest forms, such as a grilled chicken sandwich rather than processed chicken nuggets.
- When dining in a restaurant, plan ahead. Think about when you'll eat, in order to time your medication correctly. Do some research on the menu prior to eating out, and identify choices at different restaurants that fit healthy eating needs so that ordering is simple.
- Don't hesitate to ask what's in a dish or to make special requests.
- Ask the host or server if nutrition information is available to review before ordering or check the restaurant's Web site ahead of time. Many chain restaurants currently provide this information.
- Note: The US FDA menu-labeling final rule that went into effect in 2017 requires all restaurants and food service businesses with 20 or more locations to post calorie information for standard menu items and provide additional nutrition information upon request. Smaller establishments can voluntarily comply.[73]

Smart Snacking

Snacks fuel the body, curb the appetite, head off hypoglycemia, and boost calorie intake. Not everyone with diabetes needs snacks, so the person with diabetes should discuss his or her specific situation with the diabetes care and education specialist to determine whether snacks are necessary to keep blood glucose and weight on target. While portion sizes for snacks are dependent on carbohydrate goals, some smart snack ideas include the following:

- Fresh fruit such as a medium-sized apple
- Frozen 100% fruit juice bar
- Air-popped or light microwave popcorn
- Fresh vegetable slices with salsa
- Lean turkey on whole grain crackers
- Celery sticks filled with peanut butter

Special Situations: Travel, Alcohol, Parties

Special situations are part of life. Individuals with diabetes need strategies for fitting them into their diabetes picture.

- Travel—Try to stay as close to your usual food and medication schedule as possible. Keep plenty of portable, ready-to-eat snacks on hand such as fresh fruit, small bags of high-fiber cereal, or

Case: Wrap-up

1. What are the key healthy eating issues you might address at this visit?
   - Improving glycemic stability prior to conception
   - Matching insulin to carbohydrate intake
   - Improving consistency of carbohydrate intake
   - Addressing the use of complementary therapy
2. How can you use the steps of the NCPM during SM's visit?
   - *Assessment*—Gather data, identify SM's goals and preferred learning style, establish rapport.
   - *Diagnosis*—Inconsistent carbohydrate intake.
   - *Intervention*—Choose the appropriate meal-planning resources. Begin with *Count Your Carbs: Getting Started* until SM achieves consistent carbohydrate intake and improved glycemic stability. Move to *Advanced Carbohydrate Counting* when she is ready to learn more about insulin-to-carbohydrate ratio.
   - *Monitoring and evaluation*—Review, evaluate, and reassess food and blood glucose records via telephone or on a return visit.
3. What resources could you suggest to SM to assist her with carb counting?
   - *Count Your Carbs: Getting Started* and *Advanced Carbohydrate Counting*
   - Choose Your Foods: Food Lists for Diabetes
   - Phone apps like MyFitnessPal, Calorie King, and SparkPeople
4. What is 1 behavior-change goal that focuses on healthy eating that SM might set?
   - "I will measure my food and beverage intake for 1 day, record the amounts, and bring the records to my next clinic appointment."
   - "I will keep my carbohydrate intake consistent by having 60 g of carbohydrate every breakfast and check my blood sugar 2 hours after breakfast to learn the effect of food on my blood sugar."
5. List 2 skill areas related to healthy eating that you will review with SM during this visit.
   - Portion management
   - Eating out
   - Special situations—travel, alcohol, parties

individually wrapped reduced-fat cheese in case of delays or when food is not available.

- Alcohol—adults with diabetes who consume alcohol should do so in moderation—the ADA recommends no more than 1 alcoholic drink per day for women and no more than 2 per day for men.[13] Alcohol consumption may place the person with diabetes at increased risk for hypoglycemia (up to 8 hours after consuming alcohol), especially if taking insulin or insulin secretagogues. It is important to provide education and awareness regarding the recognition and management of delayed hypoglycemia. Be aware of portion sizes of alcoholic drinks as they add many calories without added nutrition benefits.
- Parties—Focus on fun and fellowship rather than food. Eat a small snack before you leave home to curb your appetite. Take a look at the entire buffet table before filling your plate so you can make smart choices and plan the portions that best fit your carbohydrate goals.

Summary

Diabetes care and education specialists must be prepared to address healthy eating not only for diabetes itself but also for the many comorbidities that occur in individuals with diabetes. Behavior change, rather than content mastery, will continue to be the gold standard for outcomes of effective DSME/T and DSMS for healthy eating. Diabetes care and education specialists can contribute to conquering the challenge of healthy eating for individuals with diabetes by translating evidence-based research into effective self-management education and training.

In the future, there will be a continued and increased emphasis on prevention of diabetes and its complications. Individualized approaches to meal planning will require more in-depth assessment of an individual's health goals, personal and cultural preferences, and readiness to change. Methods of delivering education will rely more on electronic, online, and telemedicine approaches. Community-based programs will be used to deliver education alongside the traditional clinic-based programs.

Focus on Education

Teaching Strategies

Let the person with diabetes take the lead. Encourage the person with diabetes to select a topic of interest or set the agenda. Start DSME/T and DSMS sessions by asking the individual "what is the hardest for you in taking care of your diabetes?" Other open-ended question that can be used include: "What would you like to work on today?" If the individual is not sure what they would like to discuss you can display a list of nutrition-related topics and let the individual choose what seems most beneficial to learn. This technique encourages patient empowerment and relieves the diabetes care and education specialist of the unrealistic burden of trying to teach everything in a single session.

Engage the learner. Use menus from local restaurants or fast-food chains to help individuals plan a meal according to their healthy eating plan. Role-play so individuals can practice assertiveness skills by asking their "waiter" questions about ingredients, preparation, and presentation of food.

Recognize cultural, ethnic, and family traditions. Work to incorporate preferences or adapt recipes to include favorite foods and family traditions into meal planning to promote good health for the family. Ask persons with diabetes questions about foods that are omitted or included based on culture/religion and about the incorporation of practices such as fasting.

Stay current. Nutrition is ever-evolving. The knowledge that "sugar is not a poison" is just one example of how evidence-based research on dietary carbohydrate has guided the remarkable changes that have occurred in clinical practice recommendations for healthy eating in recent years.

Become familiar with diabetes apps. For those individuals with diabetes who appreciate new ways to manage their condition on the go, apps that track food intake, physical activity, and blood glucose levels are available for smartphones and tablets. Information on health apps, many of which are free, can be found on reliable diabetes Web sites such as those of the ADA (http://www.diabetes.org) and the Academy of Nutrition and Dietetics (http://www.eatright.org).

Messages for Persons With Diabetes

Be open to new information. Recognize that learning about making healthier food choices takes time, but the extra effort will help achieve goals for improved diabetes management and overall health. Also, remember that recommendations for diabetes nutrition change and evolve as more is learned. Learning about the most current guidelines is worthwhile.

Healthy eating is individualized. What works for your friend or neighbor may not be appropriate for you. For example, whether a person with diabetes includes snacks in his or her meal plan depends on that person's medication, activity level, blood glucose levels, nutrient needs, and personal preferences. Children with type 1 diabetes may require frequent snacks to maintain normal blood glucose levels, whereas adults with type 2 diabetes that are managed by lifestyle changes alone may not need the extra calories that snacks provide. A meal plan can be designed to meet your needs and work as part of your management plan.

Health Literacy

Individuals with low health literacy and numeracy may have difficulty translating information from traditional diabetes nutrition education programs and materials into effective self-management. The content of the material and its formatting should be designed to improve ease of use by adhering to a lower text-reading level, using illustrations for key concepts, and using color-coding and other modifications to guide persons with diabetes through instructions for healthy eating. *Eating Healthy With Diabetes: Easy Reading Guide*[65] is an example of a meal-planning resource that is effective when health literacy is of concern.

Consult additional resources on health literacy. The National Network of Libraries of Medicine provides an extensive resource on health literacy.[74]

Allow people with diabetes to experience healthy eating. Do food preparation demonstrations, supermarket tours, restaurant menu selections, and restaurant/dining clubs for people with diabetes. This provides people with hands-on skills in food preparation and healthy eating experiences that include social interaction.

Focus on what people can eat instead of what they can't eat. Examine what people eat for breakfast, lunch, dinner, and snacks in response to stress or special circumstances. Get an agreement from the person with diabetes on the alternative options. Write them down for easy reference.

Health literacy plays an important role in the adoption of healthy eating. Communication with the patient needs to focus on informed decision making within a typical environment and social economic circumstances. Each person with diabetes or specific population can be very different in seeking, interpreting, critically analyzing, and using information to make informed healthy eating decisions. Some persons with diabetes might interpret "An apple a day keeps the disease away" literally and think that the only healthy fruit is an apple. Others might exclude favorite foods like bananas and carrots from their diet with the assumption that "they have too much sugar."

Allow persons with diabetes to teach you about their healthy eating. Most people with diabetes know that they need to eat healthfully, but they might not be very good about it or do not really know what it means. Ask persons with diabetes to tell you what they think they need to eat in order to be healthy or achieve better blood glucose management. This will allow you to identify their misconceptions and adjust accordingly.

Focus on one meal at a time. People with low health literacy will find it more manageable to understand one behavior change at a time. Add a meal or a snack with the additional visits. Ask the person with diabetes to summarize the strategy for that meal; that way you can evaluate whether he or she recalls it accurately.

Focus on Practice

Invest in your physical environment. In your waiting room, use colorful displays of charts or test tubes showing the amounts of sugar or fat in common foods to stimulate discussions of healthy eating.

Make teaching creative and fun. Ask persons with diabetes to bring food labels from home and from the menu nutrition Web site of their favorite restaurant to teach carbohydrate awareness. Use the Nutrition Facts to point out the grams of carbohydrate, protein, fat, and number of calories per serving. Use the label to illustrate that the serving size may differ from the food list value; for example, a label for brown rice lists a serving size of 1 cup (cooked) while its serving size from the starch list is one-third cup (cooked). Use the Nutrition Facts package serving size and measuring tools to compare what is generally served at the restaurant.

Consider the financial implications. Diabetes self-management education and training for healthy eating should be part of the care plan of every individual with diabetes, regardless of his or her medication regimen. It is also part of diabetes prevention. Unfortunately, a large percentage of people with diabetes do not receive any structured diabetes education and/or nutrition therapy and may not be aware that these services are available to them. It is possible in this time of healthcare reform that DSME/T, DSMS, and MNT coverage will become more comprehensive and more accessible, given that healthy eating for diabetes helps improve quality of life and reduces healthcare costs.

References

1. Powers MA, Bardsley J, Cypress M, et al. Diabetes self-management education and support in type 2 diabetes—a joint position statement of the American Diabetes Association, the American Association of Diabetes Educators, and the Academy of Nutrition and Dietetics. Diabetes Educ. 2015;41(4):417-30.

2. Association of Diabetes Care and Education Specialists (ADCES). An effective model of diabetes care and education: revising the AADE7 self-care behaviors®. Published online ahead of print, Feb 2020. Diabetes Educ. doi: https://doi.org/10.1177/0145721719894903.

3. American Association of Diabetes Educators. Healthy eating: incorporating nutritional management into lifestyle. Diabetes Educ. 2012;38:124-8.

4. American Association of Diabetes Educators. Healthy eating. Practice synopsis. 2015 (cited 2019 May 30). On the Internet at: https://www.diabeteseducator.org/docs/default-source/default-document-library/practice-synopsis-final_healthy-eating.pdf?sfvrsn=0.

5. Institute of Medicine. The Role of Nutrition in Maintaining Health in the Nation's Elderly: Evaluating Coverage of Nutrition

Services for the Medicare Population. Washington, D.C.: National Academies Press; 2000.

6. Franz MJ, MacLeod J, et al; Academy of Nutrition and Dietetics Nutrition practice guideline for type 1 and type 2 diabetes in adults: systematic review of evidence for medical nutrition therapy effectiveness and recommendations for integration into the nutrition care process. J Acad Nutr Diet. 2017; 117(10):1659-79.
7. Evert AB, Dennison M, et al; Nutrition therapy for adults with diabetes or prediabetes: a consensus report. Diabetes Care. 2019;42:731-54.
8. Diabetes Prevention Program Research Group. Reduction in the incidence of type 2 diabetes with lifestyle intervention or metformin. N Engl J Med. 2002;346:393-403.
9. Li G, Zhang P, Wang J, et al; The long-term effect of lifestyle Interventions to prevent diabetes in the China Da Qing Diabetes Prevention Study: a 20-year follow-up study. Lancet. 2008;371:1783-89.
10. Lindström J, Ilanne-Parikka P, Peltonen M, et al; Finish Diabetes Prevention Study Group. Sustained reduction in the incidence of type 2 diabetes by lifestyle intervention: follow-up of the Finnish Diabetes Prevention Study. Lancet. 2006;368:1673-9.
11. Diabetes Prevention Program Research Group. Long-term effects of lifestyle intervention or metformin on diabetes development and microvascular complications over 15-year follow-up: The Diabetes Prevention Program Outcomes Study. Lancet Diabetes Endocrinol. 2015;3:866-75.
12. American Diabetes Association. Prevention or delay of type 2 diabetes. Sec. 3. In: Standards of medical care in diabetes—2019. Diabetes Care. 2019;42 Suppl 1:S29-33.
13. American Diabetes Association. Standards of medical care in diabetes—2020. Diabetes Care. 2020;43 Suppl 1:S1.
14. Centers for Disease Control and Prevention. NCHS data brief. Prevalence of obesity among adults: United States, 2015-2016. 2019 (cited 2019 May 30). On the Internet at: https://www.cdc.gov/nchs/data/databriefs/db288.pdf.
15. Jackson L. Translating the Diabetes Prevention Program into practice: a review of community interventions. Diabetes Educ. 2009;35:309-20.
16. Ritchie ND, Sauder KA, Fabbri S. Reach and effectiveness of the National Diabetes Prevention Program for Young Women. Am J Prev Med. 2017;53(5):714-8.
17. DiBenedetto JC, Blum NM, O'Brian CA, et al.; Achievement of weight loss and other requirements of the Diabetes Prevention and Recognition Program: a National Diabetes Prevention Program network based on nationally certified diabetes self-management education programs. Diabetes Educ. 2016;42:678-85.
18. Briggs Early K, Stanley K. Position of the Academy of Nutrition and Dietetics: the role of medical nutrition therapy and registered dietitian nutritionists in the prevention and treatment of prediabetes and type 2 diabetes. J Acad Nutr Diet. 2018;118:343-53.
19. Franz MJ, Boucher JL, Rutten-Ramos S, et al.; Lifestyle weight-loss intervention outcomes In overweight and obese adults with type 2 diabetes: a systematic review and meta-analysis of randomized clinical trials. J Acad Nutr Diet. 2015;115(9):1447-63.
20. Dombrowski SU, Knittle K, Avenell A, et al.; Long tern maintenance of weight loss with non-surgical Interventions in obese adults: systematic review and meta-analyses of randomized controlled trials. BMJ. 2014;348:g2646.
21. Duarte-Gardea MO, Gonzales-Pacheco DM, et al; Academy of Nutrition and Dietetics Gestational Diabetes Evidence Based Nutrition Practice Guideline. J Acad Nutr Diet. 2018; 118(9): 1719-42.
22. Kitzmiller JL, Block JM, Brown FM, et al. Managing preexisting diabetes for pregnancy. Diabetes Care. 2008;31:1060-79.
23. American Association of Diabetes Educators. Gestational diabetes mellitus. AADE practice paper. 2018 (cited 2019 May 30). On the Internet at: https://www.diabeteseducator.org/docs/default-source/practice/educator-tools/Gestational-Diabetes/gestational-diabetes-mellitus-practice-paper.pdf?sfvrsn=2.
24. Silverstein J, Klingensmith G, Copeland KC, et al; American Diabetes Association. Care of children and adolescents with type 1 diabetes: a statement of the American Diabetes Association. Diabetes Care. 2005;28:186-212.
25. Mayer-Davis EJ, Lawrence JM, et al; Incidence trends of type 1 and type 2 diabetes among youths, 2002-2012. N Engl J Med. 2017;376:1419-29.
26. Arslanian S, Bacha F, et al. Evaluation and management of youth onset type 2 diabetes: a position statement by the American Diabetes Association. Diabetes Care 2018;41:2648-2668. American Diabetes Association. ADA consensus statement: type 2 diabetes in children and adolescents. Diabetes Care. 2000;23:381-9.
27. Academy of Nutrition and Dietetics. Pediatric weight management evidence-based nutrition practice guideline. 2015 (cited 2019 May 30). On the Internet at: http://www.andeal.org/topic.cfm?menu=5296&cat=5632.
28. American Diabetes Association. Older adults. Sec 12. In: Standards of medical care in diabetes—2019. Diabetes Care. 2019;42 Suppl 1:S139-47.
29. Kirkman M, Briscoe VJ, Clark N, et al. Diabetes in older adults. Diabetes Care. 2012;35:2650-64.
30. Sesti G, Antonelli Incalzi R, Bonora E, et al. Management of diabetes in older adults. Nutr Met Card Disease. 2018; 28:206-18.
31. American Association of Diabetes Educators. Special considerations in the management and education of older persons with diabetes. AADE practice synopsis. 2016 (cited 2019 May 31). On the Internet at: https://www.diabeteseducator.org/docs/default-source/default-document-library/special-considerations-in-the-management-of-older-persons-with-diabetes.pdf?sfvrsn=0.

32. Stanley K. Nutrition considerations for the growing population of older adults with diabetes. Diabetes Spectrum. 2014;27(1):29-36.

33. Clery P, Stahl D, Ismail K, et al; Systematic review and meta analysis of the efficacy of interventions for people with type 1 diabetes mellitus and disordered eating. Diabet Med. 2017;34:1667-75.

34. American Dietetic Association. Position of the American Dietetic Association: nutrition intervention in the treatment of eating disorders. J Am Diet Assoc. 2011;111:1236-41.

35. Toni G, Giulia Berioli M, Cerquiglini L, et al; Eating disorders and disordered eating symptoms in adolescents with type 1 diabetes. Nutrients. 2017;906(9):1-11.

36. Goebel-Fabbri A, Uplinger N, Gerken S, et al. Outpatient management of eating disorders in type 1 diabetes. Diabetes Spectr. 2009;22:147-52.

37. Academy of Nutrition and Dietetics. Position of the Academy of Nutrition and Dietetics: total diet approach to healthy eating. J Acad Nutr Diet. 2013;113:307-17.

38. Jones AL. The Gluten-Free Diet: fad or necessity. Diabetes Spectr. 2017;30:118-23.

39. American Diabetes Association. Gluten-free diets. 2014 (cited 2019 May 31). On the Internet at: http://www.diabetes.org/food-and-fitness/food/planning-meals/gluten-free-diets/.

40. Academy of Nutrition and Dietetics. Gluten free diet: building the grocery list. 2018 (cited 2019 May 31). On the Internet at: https://www.eatright.org/health/diseases-and-conditions/celiac-disease/the-gluten-free-diet-building-the-grocery-list

41. Academy of Nutrition and Dietetics. Celiac disease: alleviating gastrointestinal symptoms. 2017 (cited 2019 May 31). On the Internet at: https://www.eatright.org/health/diseases-and-conditions/celiac-disease/celiac-disease-alleviating-gastrointestinal-symptoms.

42. Olausson EA, Storsrud S, Grundin H, et al. A small particle size diet reduces upper gastrointestinal symptoms in patients with diabetic gastroparesis: a randomized controlled trial. Am J Gastroenterol 2014; 109:375-85.

43. Camilleri M, Packman HP, Shafi MA, Abell TL, Gerson L. Clinical guideline: management of gastroparesis. Am J Gastroenterol. 2013;108:18-37.

44. US Department of Health and Human Services. Dietary guidelines 2015-2020 (cited 2019 May 31). On the Internet at: http://health.gov/dietaryguidelines/2015/guidelines/executive-summary/.

45. The University of Sydney. About glycemic index. 2017 (cited 2019 May 31). On the Internet at: http://www.glycemicindex.com/about.php.

46. Vega-Loez S, Venn BJ, Slavin JL. Relevance of the glycemic Index and glycemic load for body weight, diabetes and cardiovascular disease. Nutrients. 2018;10:E1361.

47. The University of Sydney. Search for the glycemic index. 2017 (cited 2019 May 31). On the Internet at: http://www.glycemicindex.com/foodSearch.php.

48. Academy of Nutrition and Dietetics. Nutrition Care Process and Model Update: Toward Realizing People-Centered Care and Outcomes Management. J Acad Nutr Diet.2017:117(12): 2003-14.

49. Academy of Nutrition and Dietetics. The nutrition care process. 2019 (cited 2019 May 23). On the internet at: https://www.ncpro.org/nutrition-care-process.

50. Kittler PG, Sucher KP. Diet counseling in a multicultural society. Diabetes Educ. 1990;16:127-34.

51. American Association of Diabetes Educators. Cultural sensitivity and diabetes education. Position statement. Diabetes Educ. 2012;38:137-41.

52. American Association of Diabetes Educators. Cultural considerations in diabetes education. AADE practice synopsis. 2015 (cited 2019 June 3). On the Internet at: https://www.diabeteseducator.org/docs/default-source/default-document-library/cultural-considerations-in-diabetes-management.pdf?sfvrsn=0.

53. Goody CM, Drago L, eds; Diabetes Care and Education Dietetic Practice Group. Cultural Food Practices. Chicago: American Dietetic Association; 2010.

54. Academy of Nutrition and Dietetics. Cultural competency for nutrition professionals. 2015 (cited 2019 June3). On the Internet at: http://www.eatrightstore.org/product/E2EBE1F2-A38E-49AB-B5B6-D1D432585F17.

55. National Diabetes Education Program. Approaches for specific populations. (cited 2019 June 3). On the Internet at: https://www.niddk.nih.gov/health-information/communication-programs/ndep/health-professionals/practice-transformation-physicians-health-care-teams/approaches-specific-populations.

56. MacLeod J, Franz MJ, Handu D, et al. Academy of Nutrition and Dietetics Nutrition Practice Guideline for type 1 and type 2 diabetes in adults: nutrition intervention evidence reviews and recommendations. J Acad Nutr Diet. 2017:117(10): 1637-58.

57. American Association of Diabetes Educators. Outcomes measurement. Position statement. 2011 (cited 2019 May 31). On the Internet at: https://www.diabeteseducator.org/docs/default-source/legacy-docs/_resources/pdf/research/outcomes_technical_review_2011.pdf?sfvrsn=2.

58. Prochaska J, Redding C, Evers K. The Transtheoretical Model and Stages of Change. 2nd ed. San Francisco: Jossey-Bass; 1997:60-84.

59. Geil P, Ross T. What Do I Eat Now? A Step-by-Step Guide for Eating Right With Type 2 Diabetes. Alexandria, Va: American Diabetes Association; 2015. Second edition.

60. Boucher J. Effective nutrition education and counseling. In: Franz MJ, Evert AB, eds. American Diabetes Association Guide to Nutrition Therapy for Diabetes. Alexandria, Va: American Diabetes Association; 2012:425-39.

61. US Department of Agriculture. Choose my plate. 2019 (cited 2019 May 31). On the Internet at: http://www.choosemyplate.gov.

62. American Diabetes Association. Create your plate. 2016 (cited 2019 May 31). On the Internet at: http://www.diabetes.org/food-and-fitness/food/planning-meals/create-your-plate/.

63. American Diabetes Association and Academy of Dietetics and Nutrition. Healthy Food Choices. Alexandria, Va, and Chicago: American Diabetes Association and Academy of Dietetics and Nutrition; 2014.

64. American Diabetes Association. Month of Meals™ Diabetes Meal Planner. Alexandria, Va: American Diabetes Association; 2010.

65. American Diabetes Association and Academy of Dietetics and Nutrition. Eating Healthy With Diabetes: Easy Reading Guide. Alexandria, Va, and Chicago: American Diabetes Association and Academy of Dietetics and Nutrition; 2014.

66. American Diabetes Association and Academy of Dietetics and Nutrition. Choose Your Foods: Food Lists for Diabetes. Alexandria, Va, and Chicago: American Diabetes Association and Academy of Dietetics and Nutrition; 2014.

67. American Diabetes Association and Academy of Dietetics and Nutrition. Choose Your Foods: Plan Your Meals. Alexandria, Va, and Chicago: American Diabetes Association and Academy of Dietetics and Nutrition; 2014.

68. American Diabetes Association and Academy of Dietetics and Nutrition. Count Your Carbs: Getting Started. Alexandria, Va, and Chicago: American Diabetes Association and Academy of Dietetics and Nutrition; 2014.

69. American Diabetes Association and Academy of Dietetics and Nutrition. Advanced Carbohydrate Counting. Alexandria, Va, and Chicago: American Diabetes Association and Academy of Dietetics and Nutrition; 2014.

70. Academy of Nutrition and Dietetics. Shop Smart–get the facts on the new food labels. 2018 (cited 2019 May 31). On the internet at: https://www.eatright.org/-/media/files/eatrightdocuments/nnm/shopsmartgetthefactsonfoodlabels.pdf?la=en&hash=573B14C8DB0198A7D2CE09C93F45BD8B9C726C39.

71. US Food and Drug Administration. New and Improved Nutrition Facts Label. 2019 (cited 201 May 31). On the Internet at: https://www.fda.gov/food/food-labeling-nutrition/nutrition-education-resources-materials.

72. Geil P, Ross T. Diabetes Meals on $7 a Day—or Less! Alexandria, Va: American Diabetes Association; 2007.

73. US Food and Drug Administration. Guidance for industry: a labeling guide for restaurants and retail establishments selling away-from-home foods—part II (menu labeling requirements in accordance with 21 CFR 101.11). 2018 (cited 2019 June 3). On the Internet at: http://www.fda.gov/Food/GuidanceRegulation/GuidanceDocumentsRegulatoryInformation/ucm461934.htm.

74. National Network of Libraries of Medicine. Health literacy. 2013 (cited 2019 June 3). On the Internet at: https://nnlm.gov/initiatives/topics/health-literacy.

CHAPTER 6

Being Active

Sheri R. Colberg, PhD, FACSM

Key Concepts

- Understand the role of physical activity and fitness in health and diabetes management.
- Distinguish among physical activity, exercise, and fitness in promoting the adoption of a physically active lifestyle.
- Understand assessment of the individual's readiness for physical activity participation, including medical evaluation and possible exercise stress testing.
- Implement the current recommendations for aerobic, resistance, and other structured exercise and physical activity for individuals with diabetes, along with daily lifestyle activity.
- Understand the physiological responses of blood glucose levels during physical activity, including the potential for hypoglycemia and hyperglycemia and how to manage both.
- Identify the individual's activity risks, particularly specific health complications, and apply clinical strategies to minimize those risks with exercise modifications and effective practices.
- Address concerns related to physical activity undertaken by specific populations, such as pregnant women, overweight/obese, youth, and older adults.
- Understand activity barriers and implement behavior change strategies effective in promoting self-care behaviors related to having a physically active lifestyle.
- Implement the use of technology-driven interactions and wearable devices to promote long-term adherence to physical activity.
- Use evidence-based strategies for self-directed fitness plans and goal setting, including SMART strategies and motivational interviewing.

Introduction

The Association of Diabetes Care and Education Specialists (ADCES) continues to provide an evidenced-based framework for assessment, intervention, and evaluation of individuals and populations living with diabetes and other cardiometabolic conditions to allow them to visualize and implement effective strategies for self-care management. The recently renewed and updated AADE7 Self-Care Behaviors® emphasize that even small changes in physical activity levels are considered beneficial.[1] The "being active" behavior is inclusive of all of types, durations, and intensities of daily physical movement, equating to prescribed bouts of aerobic or resistance exercise training (structured "exercise"), as well as unstructured activities. Diabetes care and education specialists and other healthcare facilitators have long been tasked with and continue to play an important role in assisting individuals with diabetes or prediabetes to become more physically active.

The benefits of regular physical activity on cardiometabolic health are widely recognized, even when activity is light or comprised of higher intensity intervals.[2–4] Increased physical activity is associated with a reduction in mortality from all causes and from cardiovascular disease (CVD) events,[5,6] and mortality is inversely related to cardiorespiratory fitness level.[7] In part, this inverse association is due to the favorable impact of physical activity on glycemic management, blood pressure, body mass index, and lipids. Given that insulin resistance is the root cause of type 2 diabetes, physical activity is a powerful and effective tool to improve insulin sensitivity. Leisure-time, vigorous, and lower intensity physical activity can all function as critical components of prediabetes and type 2 diabetes prevention through increased activity. Regular activity is a powerful and effective tool to improve insulin sensitivity and is important in both the prevention and the treatment of type 2 diabetes in particular, along with gestational diabetes and the health complications associated with any type of diabetes.[8–12]

Implementing and maintaining a health-related fitness program is regarded as a primary component of diabetes and health self-management, especially for individuals with type 2 diabetes or women with gestational diabetes who are attempting to reduce their levels of insulin resistance.[13] For individuals with type 1 diabetes, appropriate regimen changes are needed to effectively manage blood glucose levels with the addition of physical activity.[14] However, regular participation in physical activity can prevent an increase in insulin resistance that can lead to "double diabetes" (ie, insulin resistance more characteristic of type 2 diabetes in individuals with type 1) and greater exogenous insulin requirements if not managed effectively.[15]

In addition to improving insulin sensitivity, physical activity can lower blood glucose levels, improve body mass index (BMI), and reduce the risk factors for cardiovascular disease, which is at least doubled in people with diabetes. The risk for coronary death is significantly greater for women with diabetes than men. Insulin sensitivity may be related to the total exercise dose (expressed as average kilocalories expended per week) in a graded dose-response relationship, with exercise intensity being relatively more important than frequency.[16] Higher volumes of sedentary time alone may be associated with the onset of type 2 diabetes and other metabolic diseases, independent of physical activity and other factors,[17] and simply breaking up sedentary time with any activity may lower postprandial glucose and insulin levels.[18,19] Sedentary time has been associated not only with an increased risk of diabetes but also with cardiovascular disease and cardiovascular and all-cause mortality. Both high levels of sedentary time and low levels of moderate to vigorous physical activity are strong and independent predictors of early death from any cause in adults.[17,20]

Numerous barriers to being active exist for everyone, such as lack of time, physical pain, being overweight, and living in unsafe neighborhoods. In insulin users, fear of hypoglycemia can create an additional barrier.[21,22] However, most people with diabetes can undertake physical activity safely and manage their blood glucose levels effectively. Behavior-change strategies, coupled with a solid understanding of current recommendations for physical activity and exercise, can be powerful tools for helping individuals undertake regular physical activity. Diabetes care and education specialists must assist individuals in learning how to adjust variables within their treatment regimens, especially when insulin or select other medications are taken. When diabetes complications like neuropathy, nephropathy, and retinopathy exist, certain physical movements may pose challenges and safety issues. Learning to overcome barriers that interfere with a more physically active lifestyle is a large part of diabetes self-management education. Since not all individuals with diabetes are capable of participating or willing to participate in a fitness program, healthcare facilitators must introduce all options and alternatives available for the person with diabetes so that a safe, effective, and realistic fitness plan can be designed and successfully

Cases: Facilitating Self-Management of Physical Activity

Type 1 Diabetes

HW is a 48-year-old business manager who is married and a father of 2 boys. Athletic throughout his life, he often included sports or outdoor pursuits as part of his family time. Everyone was shocked when he was told at age 45 that he had diabetes, which was initially diagnosed and treated as type 2. Although the addition of medications helped at first, when his blood glucose levels did not improve on oral agents, his wife convinced him to see his healthcare provider. HW then had autoimmunity tests performed and was diagnosed with type 1 diabetes. He was somewhat relieved by this news as he had been working hard to manage his blood glucose—exercising to the best of his ability and eating almost no carbohydrates—but his blood glucose levels continued to rise steadily over time. As exercise became more physically difficult, he was ready to accept that hiking, camping, hunting, biking, kayaking, and ice hockey refereeing were all a thing of the past. The diagnosis of type 1 diabetes explained why his blood glucose levels had stayed so high despite his best efforts. He was started on insulin therapy and gained new hope that he may be able to resume the active lifestyle he and his family enjoyed.

Type 2 Diabetes

DK is a 62-year-old mother of 3 children. She was diagnosed with gestational diabetes mellitus during her third pregnancy. She learned then that her risk of developing type 2 diabetes would be higher, so she vowed to take off the 80 pounds that had accumulated over the 3 pregnancies. As the years went by, she found that her days were full working as a dental hygienist, being a wife, and raising her children. Instead of losing weight, she actually gained another 40 pounds. She was not surprised when she was diagnosed with type 2 diabetes 6 years ago when seeking treatment of recurrent vaginal yeast infections. She had lost 20 pounds over the previous year without any effort, and she suspected that her excessive thirst, fatigue, and blurry vision were not good signs. A blood glucose value of 370 mg/dL (20.6 mmol/L) confirmed her suspicion of having diabetes. She was immediately started on metformin.

implemented.[23] This chapter provides diabetes care and education specialists with tools and strategies for helping individuals with or at risk for diabetes make positive and lasting changes toward adopting a physically active lifestyle.

Defining Physical Activity, Exercise, and Fitness

Physical activity and *exercise* can be defined separately; however, these terms are used interchangeably in this chapter for simplicity. The use of the broader term "physical activity" in place of the narrower term "exercise" has caused some confusion, but many types of movement, including exercise, sports, leisure activities, dance, and more, have a positive impact on physical fitness and health.[24,25] This broader term may also be more acceptable to individuals who have a negative viewpoint of exercise *per se*. Structured exercise training programs for individuals with diabetes typically include activities to enhance cardiovascular capacity (aerobic fitness) and muscular fitness and strength in individuals of all ages, as well as flexibility and balance in older individuals.[26]

A related activity concept, *physical fitness* encompasses cardiorespiratory (aerobic) endurance, muscle endurance, strength and power, flexibility, balance, speed, reaction time (neuromotor), and body composition. More than one type of physical activity may be required to yield measurable improvements for its various components, and specific training may be necessary to adequately increase skill and coordination to perform well in sports.

What complicates physical fitness for the layperson is that there are many reasons to engage in a physically active lifestyle. Fitness is intended to be inclusive rather than athletic in nature when considering what affects an individual's ability to be active and health outcomes. However, most laypersons believe they need to possess skill-related talents, participate in sports, or work out at a fitness club to achieve physiological or health-related benefits. This misperception prevents many people from considering or engaging in a physically active lifestyle. A primary goal of the healthcare professional should be to encourage individuals to engage in appropriate physical activities of all types and at all levels.[25]

Defining Physical Activity, Exercise, and Fitness

- *Physical activity:* Bodily movement produced by the contraction of skeletal muscle that substantially increases energy expenditure
- *Exercise:* Subset of physical activity conducted with the intention of developing physical fitness, which includes cardiovascular, strength, balance, and flexibility training options
- *Physical Fitness:* Physical ability to carry out daily tasks with vigor and alertness, without undue fatigue and with ample energy to enjoy leisure-time pursuits and meet unforeseen emergencies

Preparing Individuals for Being Active

Most people with diabetes can safely begin physical activity that is no more vigorous than their usual activities of daily living without a medical checkup, which removes many barriers to their participation.[27] However, some may benefit from at least consulting a healthcare provider for assessment or obtaining medical clearance before beginning a structured physical fitness program, particularly if currently sedentary.[28] For those with diabetes and a higher cardiometabolic risk, obtaining medical clearance, and possibly even undergoing pre-participation exercise stress testing, may be recommended, particularly when planning to undertake vigorous physical activity to which they are unaccustomed.[26]

Pre-Activity Medical Exam and Assessment

For exercise that is more vigorous than brisk walking or that exceeds the demands of everyday living, sedentary and older individuals with diabetes may benefit from being assessed for conditions associated with cardiovascular disease or that may contraindicate certain types of exercise or predispose them to injuries, such as severe peripheral neuropathy, severe autonomic neuropathy, or preproliferative or proliferative retinopathy.[26] Before undertaking higher intensity physical activity, they should likely be advised to undergo a detailed medical evaluation and screening for blood glucose management, physical limitations, medications, and macrovascular and microvascular complications associated with the heart, blood vessels, eyes, kidneys, feet, and nerves. Comorbid health issues may require individualization of physical activity choices (eg, avoidance of weight-bearing physical activity with unhealed plantar ulcers), which serves as an opportunity for shared decision making and problem solving. Factoring in these and other relevant health considerations enhances the advice provided and can contribute to a safely designed exercise prescription. Table 6.1 lists the general categories to be considered during this examination.

TABLE 6.1 Components of the Pre-Participation Medical Exam
Measurement of
Body weight (body mass index [BMI], waist girth, body composition)
Apical pulse rate and rhythm
Resting blood pressure (seated, supine, standing)
Auscultation of
Lungs, with specific attention to uniformity of breath sounds in all areas (absence of rales, wheezes, and other breathing sounds)
Heart, with specific attention to murmurs, gallops, clicks, rubs
Carotid, abdominal, and femoral arteries
Palpitation of
Cardiac apical impulse, point of maximal impulse (PMI)
Carotid, abdominal, and femoral arteries
Inspection of lower extremities for edema and presence of arterial pulses
Evaluation of
Abdomen, for bowel sounds, masses, visceromegaly, and tenderness
Absence or presence of tendon xanthoma and skin xanthelasma
Tests of neurological function, including reflexes and cognition
Skin, especially lower extremity in persons with diabetes
Follow-up exam related to orthopedic or other medical conditions that would limit exercise

PAR-Q+ (Self-Assessment of Physical Activity Readiness)

Individuals may want to use a self-screening health tool before starting an exercise program, one known as the Physical Activity Readiness Questionnaire for Everyone, or the PAR-Q+ (accessible online at https://eparmedx.com). It begins with 7 basic questions about health, such as asking whether someone has a known heart condition, chest pain, dizziness, metabolic condition (like diabetes) and more. It is attempting to identify those unaccustomed to physical exertion who may experience an excessive stress on their cardiovascular system or risk having associated complications. If the answer to any of those questions is "yes," users are directed to a second questionnaire, the electronic Physical Activity Readiness Medical Examination (ePARmed-X+), available through the same Web site. These questionnaires will tell an individual whether it is likely necessary for him or her to seek further advice from a healthcare provider or a qualified exercise professional before becoming more physically active.

Pre-Exercise Stress Testing

For individuals who wish to participate in easy or moderate-intensity activities like walking, healthcare providers should use clinical judgment in deciding whether to recommend pre-exercise stress testing.[29] Conducting such testing prior to starting a walking program is not routinely necessary as a diagnostic tool for cardiovascular disease and requiring it may create barriers to participation. Current guidelines attempt to avoid automatic inclusion of lower risk individuals, in whom the risk of a false positive exercise stress test is higher and may outweigh the benefits of detection of cardiovascular abnormalities. Such testing is currently advised primarily for *previously sedentary* people with diabetes who want to undertake activity that is *more intense than brisk walking*.

Use of these criteria does not exclude the possibility of conducting electrocardiogram (ECG) stress testing on individuals with a low risk of coronary artery disease (CAD) or those planning to engage in less intense exercise, particularly if used to establish a fitness baseline and subsequent fitness goals. In the absence of contraindications to maximal stress testing, it can still be considered for anyone with diabetes.[29] The potential benefits should be weighed against the risks for each individual, based on criteria listed in Table 6.2.

Individuals who exhibit nonspecific ECG changes in response to exercise or who have nonspecific ST and

TABLE 6.2 Criteria for Conducting a Graded Exercise Stress Test
Age >40 years, with or without CVD risk factors other than diabetes
Age >30 years and any of the following: • Type 1 diabetes or type 2 diabetes of >10 years' duration • Hypertension • Cigarette smoking • Dyslipidemia • Proliferative or preproliferative retinopathy • Nephropathy, including microalbuminuria
Any of the following, regardless of age • Known or suspected CAD, cerebrovascular disease, and/or peripheral vascular disease • Autonomic neuropathy • Advanced nephropathy with renal failure

T wave changes on resting ECG may need follow-up testing. However, the cost-effectiveness and diagnostic value of more intensive testing remain in question.[29]

Controversy: The Graded Exercise Test

A controversial topic that healthcare facilitators often must address is whether a person should be recommended to undergo a graded exercise test with ECG monitoring prior to exercise participation. Diabetes is an independent risk factor for CVD. The established American Diabetes Association criteria give healthcare providers a broad referral base upon which to determine whether a graded exercise test is warranted. These criteria are more inclusive than exclusive. They can, therefore, be applied to most individuals seen in a diabetes practice. While this offers straightforward access, performing the test may not be the course of action required for each individual, depending on his or her physical activity and fitness goals. The risk of a false-positive result can overshadow the benefits an otherwise healthy individual receives from starting a fitness program. Likewise, a negative test result does not guarantee that the individual is protected from having a cardiovascular event. While careful consideration of the presence of such a disease is important, clinical judgment needs to be included when making the final determination on whether this test is necessary and in evaluating the individual's results.

Other Program-Design Considerations

Clinical status and health needs, as well as the individual's personal interests and past and present activity patterns, should be considered in program planning. Specific goals identified by the individual, whether related to diabetes management, health improvement, weight loss/maintenance, or increased energy, are the ultimate target. All exercise programs should to be designed to address intensity (how difficult), duration (how long), frequency (how often), and mode (type of activity), along with appropriate progression. Rates of progression will depend on an individual's functional capacity, medical and health status, age, activity preferences and goals, and tolerance for the current level of activity.

Promoting Greater Lifestyle Physical Activity

For individuals with diabetes, who are frequently deconditioned and sedentary, the first major challenge–and a good place to start–is to assist them in incorporating more physical activity into daily living. Engaging in unstructured or daily living activities has become a current focal point for improving health, lowering cardiometabolic risks, and enhancing quality of life in all adults.[30] Based on what is now known about sedentary behaviors, interventions may also benefit from simply attempting to decrease sitting time and periods of extended sedentary activity and promote more lifestyle physical activity. Simply taking more daily steps, standing more, and engaging in various forms of physical activity are all important to cardiometabolic health, as well as treatment and prevention of type 2 diabetes.[31–33] Also keep in mind that some individuals believe themselves as more active than they are when viewed in their own social context, such as relative to other assisted living residents.[34]

Promote an Active Lifestyle

Remaining physically active is an essential part of self-care for all persons with any type of diabetes. For individuals using insulin or certain oral medications that increase endogenous insulin release, additional regimen changes will likely be needed to balance blood glucose levels.

Many individuals may be classified as sedentary (see Table 6.3) while considering themselves more active than they really are. In almost all cases, significant health benefits, such as a reduction in coronary risk factors, can be obtained by incorporating frequent bouts of moderate-intensity activities on most, if not all, days of the week. While lifestyle physical activity does not entirely take the place of a traditionally structured exercise program, it can be highly effective in helping individuals increase their daily activity level, build a fitness base, and possibly improve glycemic management.[14] In addition, those who have successfully implemented more physical activity into their daily lifestyle may feel more confident and ready, as well as able, to initiate more structured forms of activity. Likewise, decreasing the amount of time spent sitting has also become a promising area of research for managing blood glucose levels, body weight, and functional fitness levels that allow for independent living.[35]

In particular, older adults may benefit from simply reducing their total sedentary time and avoiding prolonged periods of sitting by increasing the number of breaks during sedentary time.[12] The most advantageous frequency of these breaks (ranging from hourly to every 15 minutes) is unknown, but more frequent breaks appear to work better.[36,37] In addition, the best type of physical activity undertaken during such breaks

TABLE 6.3 Activity Classification Based on Steps per Day

Classification	*Daily Steps* (number)*	*Indications*
Sedentary	<5,000	Highly inactive and sitting too much, which raises health risks
Low Active	5,000-7,499	Typical of daily activity excluding sports/exercise; the average American walks 5,900 to 6,900 steps daily
Somewhat Active	7,500-9,999	Likely includes some exercise or walking (or a job with more walking)
Active	10,000-12,500	Taking 10,000 steps is the point used to classify most individuals as active enough; this is a good daily goal for healthy people striving to get enough daily activity
Highly Active	>12,500	Individuals in this category are getting more than the recommended amounts of physical activity, which may carry additional health benefits to some

* Measured, computed, or estimated using pedometers, other devices, or equivalent step counts.

Sources: C Tudor-Locke, CL Craig, WJ Brown, et al. "How many steps/day are enough? For adults." *Int J Behav Nutr Phys Act.* 2011;8:79.

C Tudor-Locke, CL Craig, JP Thyfault, JC Spence. "A step-defined sedentary lifestyle index: <5000 steps/day," *Appl Physiol Nutr Metab.* 2013;38(2):100-14.

(standing, walking, resistance activity, flexibility exercise), intensity (light vs. moderate), and duration (typically 3 to 5 minutes) remain to be fully elucidated.[19,38]

A visual tool, the Activity Pyramid can guide individuals on how to become more active (see Figure 6.1). It shows a variety of ways that physical activity, both structured and unstructured, can be included in daily life. Diabetes care and education specialists can use the Activity Pyramid to help individuals identify, plan, and progressively increase regular physical activity, including lifestyle components.

- Suggest individuals begin by focusing on undertaking more daily activities from the base of the pyramid, which includes various activities of daily living.
- Once the individual has established a solid activity base, encourage him or her to consider activities from other areas of the pyramid, starting and progressing slowly.
- Specific fitness areas can be enhanced by doing activities from a specific level of the pyramid:
  - —Activities from the base enhance overall health and well-being.
  - —Activities from the middle level focus on improving aerobic fitness, muscular strength and endurance, and balance and flexibility.
  - —The tip of the pyramid suggests ways to decrease sedentary activities.
- Advise individuals on ways to track their daily movement to promote adherence (see more on daily step counts and activity monitors later in this chapter).

Developing a Structured Physical Activity Program

A structured exercise program has several components, including how each training session is formatted, the actual plan for everyone (including activities to be prescribed), and specific about each activity selected (how much, how often, etc). It is important for diabetes care and education specialists to understand what should likely be prescribed and how to assist each person in formulating an individualized plan that meets his or her unique goals.

Exercise Training Session Format

Structured aerobic and resistance exercise sessions generally have 4 components:[39]

- Warm-up
- Conditioning
- Cool-down
- Stretching

Warm-up

The warm-up phase includes at least 5 to 10 minutes of a light or moderate intensity cardiorespiratory or muscular endurance activity. Warming up before moderate- or vigorous-intensity aerobic activity allows a gradual increase in heart rate and breathing at the start of the episode of activity.[40] It may also help reduce muscle injury and facilitate a safe transition from rest to exercise by stretching postural muscles, increasing blood flow, elevating body temperature, and increasing oxygen

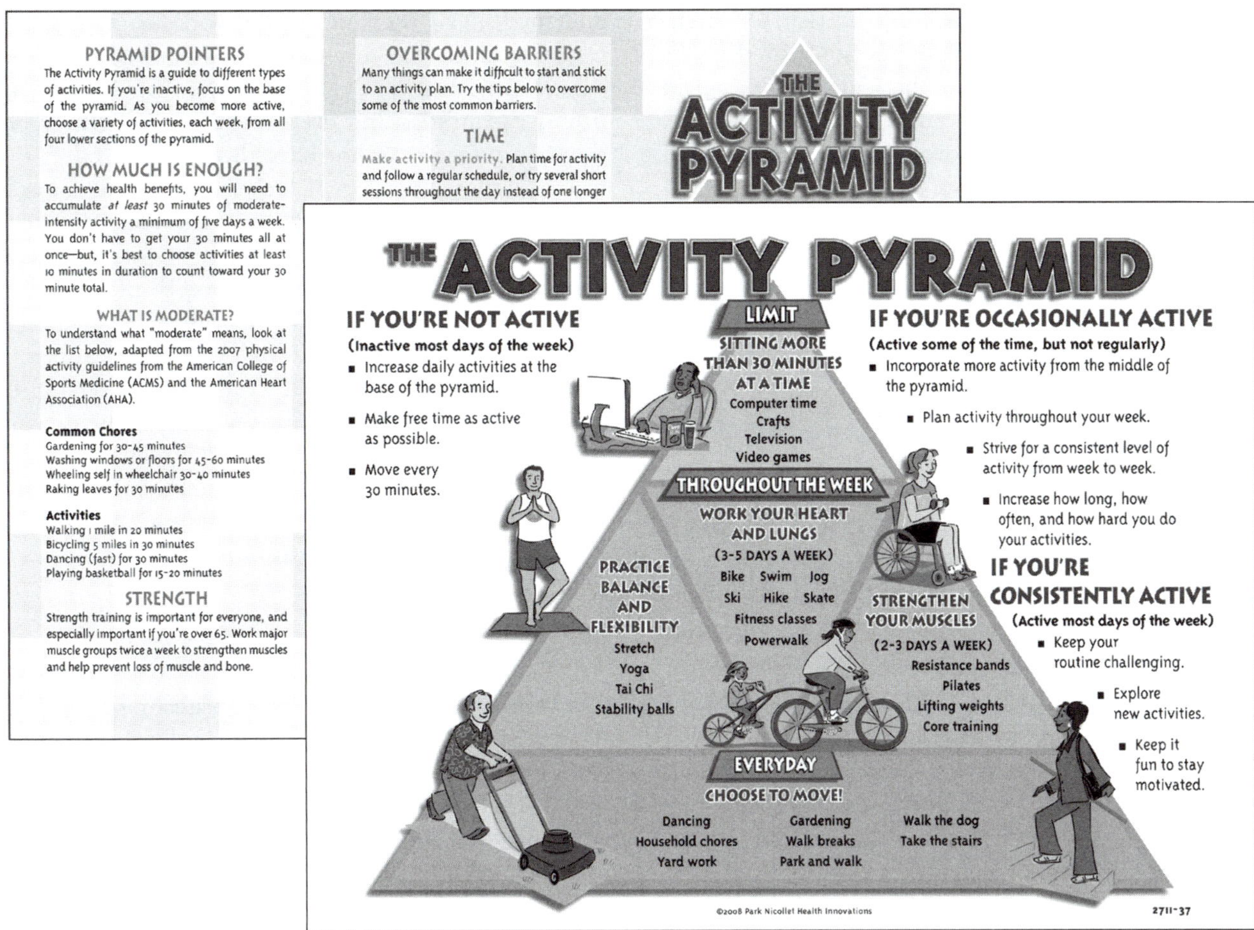

FIGURE 6.1 **The Activity Pyramid**

Source: From Type 2 Diabetes BASICS © 2010 International Diabetes Center. Adapted with permission from The Activity Pyramid © 2008 Park Nicollet HealthSource, Minneapolis, Minn.

availability and metabolic rate. Warming up for a muscle-strengthening activity commonly involves doing exercises with lighter weights to start.

Conditioning

The conditioning phase includes at least 20 to 60 minutes of aerobic, resistance, neuromotor, and/or sports activities that enhance cardiorespiratory fitness, muscle strength and endurance, or flexibility. Time spent warming up and cooling down may count toward meeting aerobic activity guidelines, but only if the activity is at least of moderate intensity (for example, walking briskly as a warm-up before jogging).[40]

Cool-down

The cool-down includes at least 5 to 10 minutes of a light or moderate intensity cardiorespiratory or muscular endurance activity to help the body gradually recover from the conditioning phase and safely transition back to a resting state. Doing so helps prevent blood from pooling in the arms and legs and removes metabolic by-products immediately after exercise.

Stretching

The stretching component includes at least 10 minutes of stretching exercises performed either after the initial warm-up phase or following the cool-down. This phase is distinct from the warm-up or cool-down and is best done when muscles are warmer and have a greater range of motion.

General Exercise Prescription

Simply put, the exercise prescription is *the plan the individual follows to achieve physical fitness or other exercise-related health goals.* In an ideal world, each person with diabetes would have access to an exercise physiologist (EP) for a well-designed exercise prescription. If your person with diabetes education team has no EP, then other educators can help the person with diabetes design a program that will meet his or her needs. Include the following components—often abbreviated as **FITT-VP**—into each person's written activity plan,[40] which includes an appropriate plan for progression once initial goals are met.

FITT-VP: The Basis for All Prescriptive Exercise

Frequency—How often

Intensity—How hard

Time—How long (duration)

Type of activity—Mode (or name)

Volume—Total amount of exercise (as a product of its frequency, intensity, and time)

Progression—How to increase exercise over time

With a few exceptions, recommendations for physical participation are similar for individuals with and without diabetes. Healthcare facilitators can access the recommended physical activity guidelines and prescription for adults and older adults through the American College of Sports Medicine (ACSM) (http://acsm.org) or the 2018 US federal guidelines (https://health.gov/paguidelines/second-edition). For a comprehensive, case study–based resource for exercise prescription that covers the gamut of diabetes types, complications, and other factors, readers are referred to *Exercise and Diabetes: A Clinician's Guide to Prescribing Physical Activity* (American Diabetes Association, 2013).

Frequency

Physical activity sessions can be performed in a variety of combinations of frequency and duration.[40] Most research concludes that physical activity should be performed 3 to 7 days per week to achieve significant health benefits. The latest federal guidelines from 2018[27] now state that adults will still derive benefits if they perform all of their weekly recommended physical activity on a single day rather than over the course of multiple days; however, adults with diabetes can better maintain higher levels of exercise-induced insulin sensitivity by allowing no more than 2 consecutive days to pass without engaging in some physical activity.[26,29]

Intensity

Determining the intensity of the physical activity takes the most care and attention for people with diabetes. This does not mean the harder the workout, the better the results in all cases. Rather, the intensity level of the physical activity must be matched to the individual's current fitness capabilities and exercise goals. An activity period that is too easy may not have the intended effect on the fitness level. Conversely, if the activity period is too hard, the individual will not be able to complete the workout or, worse yet, may become injured or discouraged from exercising. A greater emphasis should be placed on vigorous intensity aerobic exercise if fitness is a primary goal of exercise and not contraindicated by complications; both high-intensity interval and continuous exercise training are appropriate activities for most individuals with diabetes.[26] Appropriate measures of intensity, including the "talk test," ratings of perceived exertion (RPEs), and target heart rate based on the heart rate reserve (HRR) method, are detailed in the section that follows on aerobic exercise training.

Time

The time (duration) of the exercise session has been investigated as well. While 20 minutes had been the minimal recommendation to provide cardiovascular improvements, multiple shorter bouts of 10 minutes, repeated to equal 30 total minutes, have also resulted in measurable improvements.[40] Recently, federal guidelines backed away from recommending a minimum exercise time, taking the stance that activity of any length can be beneficial and better than none.[27] Generally, intensity and time are inversely related, and moderate exercise requires a longer duration than more intense exercise for individuals to gain the same cardiovascular benefits. Longer bouts of physical activity, lasting 60 minutes or more, may be necessary to achieve weight loss or to prevent weight regain in overweight or obese individuals while preserving muscle mass.[41] Each individual's needs, goals, and circumstances will vary; special considerations for children, teens, older adults, and pregnant women are discussed later in this chapter.

Type

The type of physical activity chosen by the individual is in many ways less crucial than other components of the exercise prescription. While aerobic, strength, and flexibility exercises are important to consider, any type of increased movement may initially improve an individual's fitness level.[40] Sedentary individuals who begin participating in almost any type of physical activity experience measurable results in their fitness levels. Accordingly, a wide range of physical activities can be explored and made part of the fitness plan. All opportunities that the individual identifies should be assessed and, if safe to perform, encouraged. The diabetes care and education specialist should ensure that the chosen activity is appropriate, considering the presence of any complications (eg, neuropathy, severe retinopathy, or heart disease). As the individual becomes more successful and confident, options can be expanded and other types of physical activities added or substituted, depending on individualized preferences and goals.

Volume

The volume of exercise performed is a product of its frequency, intensity, and time (FIT) undertaken. The total volume is important for reaching many health and fitness goals, particularly those related to body composition or weight loss/maintenance. It can be used to estimate gross energy expenditure for a specific activity or for an individual's exercise program in total, often expressed as calorie expenditure or metabolic equivalents (METs) per minute for a wide variety of physical activities to allow for calculation of accumulated expenditures.[39]

General Exercise Prescription by Diabetes Type

- *Type 1 diabetes:* For individuals of all ages with type 1 diabetes without complications, exercise recommendations are similar to those for individuals with no known health problems.[25,40]
- *Type 2 diabetes:* Recommendations for individuals with type 2 diabetes closely align with guidelines for sedentary adults and older adults[25,42] but also focus on duration to achieve expected levels of calorie expenditure, weight loss, or other health risk reduction goals.[20]
- *Gestational diabetes:* Women who develop diabetes during pregnancy are recommended to follow accepted pregnancy exercise guidelines,[43] although they will need to monitor blood glucose levels more similarly to those with pre-existing type 1 diabetes if their management regimen includes insulin use.

Progression

Many people lead sedentary lifestyles and do not think about spending, or even think it possible to spend, the recommended time each day doing any type of physical activity. Diabetes care and education specialists must, therefore, provide realistic instruction that includes both how to start a fitness program and what to reasonably expect in terms of progress (see Table 6.4). The individual must understand the type, quantity, and rate of progress. Over an average of at least 4 to 6 months, each individual moves through 3 distinct stages of a fitness plan:

Initial Stage
in which activity habits are established
↓
Improvement Stage
in which progress is seen, but habits may weaken
↓
Maintenance Stage
in which extensions are planned

Initial Stage Many people start structured exercise and never make it out of the critical initial stage before dropping out. They either attempt activities that are too difficult for their fitness level or develop unrealistic expectations of what they will be able to accomplish and when, leading them to quickly become discouraged. The real success from this stage comes from the individual beginning to form physical activity habits that can easily be integrated into his or her lifestyle while considering factors like initial fitness level, time availability, injury prevention, existing health complications, and motivation.

- Help the individual understand that measurable changes related to their exercise goals (fitness, weight loss, etc) may not occur during this period. Building an exercise habit takes at least 4 weeks and may take longer in individuals who start with very poor fitness levels.
- Sedentary individuals are more likely to form lasting exercise habits when the initial stage starts at a lower intensity and progresses very slowly over time, that is, "start low, go slow."

TABLE 6.4 Physical Activity Program Stages and Rates of Progression

Program Stage	*Week*	*Frequency (per week)*	*Intensity (% HRR)*	*Duration (minutes)*
Initial	1–4	3–4	30%–59%	15–30
Improvement	5–24	3–5	40%–89%	25–40
Maintenance	25+	3–5	40%–89%	20–60

- Persons with diabetes who are already active and have a foundational fitness base may be able to start at or progress more quickly to the second, improvement stage.

Habit Formation: The Initial Goal

In the first 4 weeks or so of a new fitness plan, the goal is not to achieve measurable changes in fitness but rather to establish habits and baseline levels of endurance that will make fitness progress possible.

Improvement Stage During the improvement stage, the focus shifts from developing habits to improving the fitness level and achieving other health goals. The individual now has improved stamina and endurance, can engage in physical activity for longer amounts of time, and can begin adding to the workload or intensity of the workout. Over the 3 or more months (or longer for deconditioned and older individuals) of this stage, measurable health benefits should start to be observed. However, individuals can interpret this initial success as permanent change, which may sabotage their efforts. The individual may allow other routine parts of everyday life to take priority again and start missing workout sessions.

- Identify and seek progress in fitness goals by aiming for a moderate (or higher) exercise intensity in this stage.
- Once improvements begin to be evident, help the person avoid becoming complacent or slacking off from seeking further improvement.
- Foster success beyond the first milestone and over the longer term.

Maintenance Stage Once an individual has successfully met the major goals originally defined, new goals and a new plan need to be developed (see SMART goal setting later in this chapter). The new goal may be as simple as "preventing weight regain" or as challenging as "training for a competitive event."

- Review goals routinely at medical and diabetes education visits.
- Reassess for medication changes, new diagnoses, or progression of existing diseases to ensure the fitness routine continues to be safe and effective.
- Develop new goals and plans once existing ones are achieved.
- Choose appropriate exercise goals with injury prevention and long-term participation in mind.

Benefits Gained Can Quickly Diminish

Beneficial effects of physical activity diminish quickly if activity does not occur regularly. Support persons with diabetes to ensure that both the activity and the benefits continue.

Aerobic Exercise Prescription

Cardiorespiratory or aerobic exercise is defined as continuous, dynamic exercise that uses large muscle groups and requires aerobic metabolic pathways to sustain the activity.[25,40] Examples include walking, jogging, biking, swimming, water aerobics, cycling, rollerblading, and cross-country skiing. Aerobic exercise has been the mode traditionally prescribed for diabetes management and prevention. Most of its benefits related to blood glucose stability are realized through acute and chronic improvements in insulin action. The acute effects of a recent bout of exercise account for most of the improvements in insulin action, but are short-lived, while regular exercise training generally results in a more lasting effect.[44] In addition, exercise mode, timing, intensity, and total volume potentially impact glycemic responses and cardiometabolic health in individuals with diabetes.[13,45–48]

Frequency of Aerobic Activity

Diverging from all prior recommendations, the latest (2018) federal guidelines state that the total recommended weekly activity can be performed in a single day (like a "weekend warrior" scenario), although stated that it is still considered more advantageous to spread activity out throughout the week.[27] However, for persons with diabetes it still is recommended not to let more than two days lapse between bouts of aerobic activity due to the transient nature of improvements in insulin sensitivity from such activity. Ideally, adults with diabetes of any type should be active at least 3 nonconsecutive days per week, but up to 7 weekly sessions of moderate activity will likely be even more beneficial to improving glycemic stability and cardiorespiratory endurance and achieving target caloric expenditure.[26] Exercise that is limited to 2 days per week generally does not result in significant improvements in cardiorespiratory endurance. In addition, to achieve sustained major weight loss, the optimal level of activity needed is typically greater than that needed to improve glycemic management.

Energy expenditure can also be used to guide exercise programming. The ACSM recommends a target range of 150 to 400 calories per day expended via physical activity.[40] This represents a minimum threshold of 1,000 calories a week, which is associated with a reduction in all-cause mortality risk. For previously sedentary individuals, educators should recommend the minimum threshold as the initial goal, but encourage progress toward the upper target range of expending 300 to 400 calories per day, or 2,000 calories per week, in physical activity to achieve maximal health benefits and weight loss. Energy expenditure in excess of 2,000 calories per week in physical activity has been associated with successful short- and long-term weight loss.

Intensity of Aerobic Activity

Moderate to vigorous physical activity is generally recommended for aerobic fitness and cardiometabolic improvements.[26,40] Lower intensity activities will expend calories and help with weight maintenance, but they may have a lesser acute impact on fitness and blood glucose levels.

Use of the "Talk Test" For individuals who cannot or prefer not to measure heart rate (HR) or use subjective ratings, they can gauge the upper limit of exercise intensity using the "talk test." This simply means that an individual should be able to carry on a conversation (but not sing) during aerobic activity without struggling to breathe while doing so. If an individual is breathing too heavily to talk, he or she is working above the ventilatory threshold and at an intensity that exceeds a moderate workload. Use of this test cannot as easily discern when exercise intensity is lower than desired, however.

Estimating Intensity The intensity of aerobic activity can be easily calculated based on measured or estimated maximal HR. The ACSM[40] recommends using heart rate reserve (HRR) rather than a percentage of maximal HR, with a recommended training intensity of 40% to 89% of HRR: moderate intensity is 40% to 59% HRR and vigorous is 60% to 89% HRR. Deconditioned individuals may need to start at even lower intensities (30%-39% of HRR), while individuals with greater fitness typically require a higher minimal threshold to progress with their cardiorespiratory fitness. The prescribed intensity range should be based on one's fitness level, individual fitness and health goals, duration of diabetes, and presence of complications.

Aerobic Exercise Target Intensity Ranges

Easy: 30%–39% HRR ***Moderate***: 40%–59% HRR
Vigorous: 60%–89% HRR

Determining Target HR Exercise intensity can be calculated most accurately using the results of a maximal exercise stress test. Based on the individual's maximum HR response to the exercise stress test, the following HRR formula, also known as the Karvonen formula, is the commonly accepted method to calculate target HR or HR range in beats per minute (bpm):

$$\text{Target HR} = [(\text{HRmax} - \text{HRrest}) \times \text{Desired percent intensity}] + \text{HRrest}$$

If the actual maximal HR is not known, the target HR range can be estimated using the following equation, although caution is required:

$$\text{Estimated HRmax} = 220 - \text{Age}$$

This equation should be used with caution due to the large standard deviation, which can cause the HR estimation to be off by 12 to 15 bpm. This procedure may also overestimate the maximal HR of some individuals with diabetes, particularly those taking medications like beta-blockers that lower maximal levels or anyone with autonomic neuropathy.[49] When cardiac autonomic neuropathy (CAN) is present, exercise intensity is better prescribed using the HRR method to approximate oxygen consumption during submaximal exercise with maximal HR dirctly measured, rather than estimated, for better accuracy.[50]

Due to the high prevalence of cardiovascular disease, caution should be used when applying standard HR formulas to an individual with diabetes. An alternate equation that utilizes 70% of age rather than full age may be more accurate for estimating maximal HR in an older population:

$$\text{Estimated HRmax} = 208 - (0.7 \times \text{Age})$$

Rating of Perceived Exertion The RPE is another useful guide for estimating exercise intensity (see Table 6.5). This is a subjective rating based on general fatigue and can be used along with target HR estimations or as a substitute to guide the intensity of activity. There are 2 RPE scales appropriate to use with adults, including those with diabetes:

- Original Category scale, which rates intensity from 6 to 20
- Category-Ratio scale, which rates intensity from 0 to 10+

When RPE scales are used, the individual is instructed to focus on full-body feelings of exertion and general

TABLE 6.5 Rating of Perceived Exertion

Category Scale	*Category-Ratio Scale*	*Perceived Exertion*
6	0 Nothing at all	No intensity
7 Extremely light	0.3–0.5 Extremely weak	Just noticeable
8	1 Very weak	
9 Very light	1.5	
10	2 Weak	Light
11 Light	2.5 Moderate	
12	3	
13 Somewhat hard	4	
14	5 Strong	Heavy
15 Hard (heavy)	6	
16	7 Very strong	
17 Very hard	8	
18	9	
19 Extremely hard	10 Extremely strong	Maximal intensity
20 Maximal exertion	11	
	Absolute maximum	Highest possible

fatigue. While performing the activity within his or her target exercise intensity, the individual is asked to identify feelings of exertion and fatigue. This elicits the recommended RPE range. Generally, a moderate-to-vigorous exercise intensity that corresponds to an RPE range of 12 to 16 ("somewhat hard" to "hard" using the 6-20 scale) or 3 to 7 (using the 0-10 scale) is recommended. A high correlation exists between a person's perceived exertion rating (6-20 scale) multiplied times 10 and the actual heart rate during physical activity (eg, RPE rating of 13 × 10 = HR of approximately 130 bpm), at least for younger individuals whose maximal heart rate is near 200 bpm. Therefore, perceived exertion may provide a fair estimate of actual HR during activity, and it is still valid to use when taking beta blockers or when HR is affected by autonomic neuropathy.[50]

Time of Aerobic Activity

The duration of exercise is directly related to caloric expenditure requirements and inversely related to the intensity of exercise required to achieve the same results. To gain maximum caloric and glycemic benefits, lower intensity exercise needs to be performed for longer periods of time compared to higher intensity exercise. The exercise duration required to meet the recommended weekly energy expenditure differs by which current guidelines are consulted.

Prior guidelines from the ACSM and the American Heart Association for adults and older adults[51,52] recommended 150 minutes of moderate activity (30 minutes, 5 days per week) or 60 minutes of vigorous physical activity (20 minutes on 3 days) for all adults, whereas the updated 2018 US federal guidelines now recommend 150 to 300 minutes of moderate or 75 to 150 minutes of vigorous activity, or an equivalent combination, with no specific guidelines on exercise frequency.[27] The updated guidelines for all Americans also state that additional health benefits may be gained from doing more than the recommended durations. The incidence of activity-related injuries does increase with duration,[53] however, and injury avoidance is a key for continued exercise participation.

Physical activity may be broken down into shorter sessions done throughout the day. Studies have shown that similar cardiorespiratory gains occur when physical activity is accumulated throughout the day in shorter bouts (3 bouts of 10 minutes) compared to a single prolonged activity session of similar duration and intensity (a 30-minute bout),[40] and glycemic benefits may be greater from the more frequent, shorter bouts of activity.[54] Structured exercise training of more than 150 minutes per week is associated with greater A1C declines than that of 150 minutes or less per week,[55] and total exercise volume matters most.[48] Severely deconditioned individuals may need to exercise in multiple sessions of short duration (5-10 minutes), begin at very low levels (30%-39% HRR) with brief rest intervals, and progress weekly to be able to sustain higher intensity exercise. Initially, sessions can be done for 10 to 15 minutes, increasing progressively over time to longer durations of continuous activity, and higher intensity intervals may be interspersed for greater fitness gains and glycemic benefits. The latest federal guidelines set no minimum duration for activities, taking the stand that doing anything for any length of time is better than not doing it.

Type of Aerobic Activity

The recommended types, or modes, of aerobic activity for diabetes are highly dependent on the individual's preferences and skill level. Health-related benefits of improved physical fitness do not appear to depend on the type of aerobic exercise done, and both continuous and interval training bestow health and glycemic benefits.[56,57] However, the safety and efficacy of low-volume, high-intensity interval training remain unclear for some adults with diabetes.[29–30] High-intensity intervals can vary by training protocol from just a few seconds to minutes undertaken at a higher (often near maximal) pace, interspersed among either periods of lesser work or rest. Those who wish to perform such intense training should be clinically stable, have been participating at least in regular moderate-intensity exercise, and likely be supervised at least initially.[58] The risks with advanced disease are unclear, and continuous, moderate-intensity exercise may be safer. Identifying activities that can safely and effectively improve cardiovascular endurance and maximize caloric expenditure is important.[42] Walking is the most common type of physical activity done by adults with diabetes and often the most convenient. However, other low-impact or non-weight-bearing types of activity, such as bicycling, swimming, and aquatic or chair exercises, may be more appropriate for those with complications or coexisting conditions like peripheral or autonomic neuropathy.[26]

Volume of Aerobic Activity

Exercise volume is the product of exercise frequency, intensity, and time, or the gross energy expenditure for a given week. An appropriate target aerobic exercise volume for most adults is ≥500 to 1,000 MET-min (MET equivalent of physical activity × number of minutes) per week, or approximately ~1,000 kcalories per week, which can be accumulated by engaging in ~150 minutes of moderate activity or compiling step counts of ≥5,400 to 7,900 steps per day. Some cardiovascular and glycemic benefits may be gained from lower exercise volumes (although a minimum dose has not been established), whereas additional benefits likely result from engaging in durations beyond recommended amounts and greater volumes may be needed for effective weight management in overweight/obese individuals.

To put this in context, an exercise volume of 500 to 1,000 MET-minutes per week can be achieved by doing 150 minutes per week of walking at 6.4 km/hour (4 mph; intensity of 5 METs) or 75 minutes of jogging at 9.7 km/hour (6 mph; 10 METs). Unfortunately, most individuals with type 2 diabetes and many older adults do not have sufficient aerobic capacity to jog for that duration, and they may have orthopedic or other limitations that would preclude them from doing so. The mean maximal aerobic capacity in individuals with diabetes has been reported to be only 22.4 ml/kg/min, or 6.4 METs.[59] Accordingly, 4.8 METs (~75% of maximal) is likely the highest sustainable intensity. Thus, most individuals with type 2 diabetes require at least 150 minutes of moderate to vigorous aerobic exercise per week to achieve optimal cardiovascular risk reduction.[29]

Individuals with higher aerobic capacities (>10 METs), such as many younger individuals with type 1 diabetes, may exercise at a higher absolute intensity for less time to achieve the same benefits. For all adults with diabetes of either type able to run steadily at 6 miles per hour (9.7 km/hour) for 25 minutes, 75 min/week of vigorous activity may provide similar cardioprotective and metabolic benefits.[26]

Aerobic Exercise Guidelines

- *Frequency:* 3 to 7 days per week, ideally with no more than 2 consecutive days without aerobic activity
- *Intensity:* moderate to vigorous (ie, 40%-89% of heart rate reserve, or rating of perceived exertion of 12-16 or 3-7, or "somewhat hard" to "hard")
- *Time:* a minimum of 150 to 300 minutes of moderate activity spread throughout the week, but a lower total time (75-150 minutes) is possible if done more intensely
- *Type:* Continuous exercise or high-intensity interval training, although the latter may not be appropriate or safe for all adults with diabetes
- *Volume:* ≥500 to 1,000 MET-min per week, ~1,000 kcal per week, ~150 minutes of moderate activity each week, or ≥5,400 to 7,900 steps per day

Progression Toward Aerobic Activity Goals

Recommend appropriate rates of progression to help individuals effectively and safely achieve aerobic exercise goals. Initially, focus on increasing frequency and duration of the exercise, rather than its intensity. This provides a safe level of activity that can be done with little effort and increases the likelihood of creating and sustaining an activity habit.[40] Alternatively, to increase intensity with a lower risk of injury or burnout, encourage individuals to intersperse faster intervals into any training session[4] and work on building foundational fitness first.

Aerobic Exercise Precautions

- Include proper warm-up and cool-down
- Use careful selection and progression of exercise program
- Make sure persons with diabetes are adequately educated about aerobic activity participation
- Monitor blood glucose before and after exercise, as well as during prolonged activities, especially when undertaken by insulin users
- Adjust medications and food intake to prevent hypoglycemia (or hyperglycemia) as needed
- Consult with healthcare personnel about regimen changes

Resistance Exercise Prescription

Resistance (strength) training improves musculoskeletal health, helps maintain independence in performing daily activities, and reduces the possibility of injury.[40,42] Properly designed resistance programs may improve indices of cardiovascular function, glucose tolerance, strength, and body composition. Higher-intensity resistance training may confer greater glycemic benefits.[60] Adding in resistance training early after a diagnosis of type 2 diabetes may result in the greatest glycemic benefit in previously sedentary adults.[61]

The term "muscular fitness" refers to aspects of both muscular strength and muscular endurance. Muscle strength is the ability of the muscle to exert force, while muscle endurance is the ability of the muscle to continue to perform without fatigue. For instance, muscular strength can be measured using a 1-repetition maximum and muscular endurance with the number of push-ups done in a minute. Muscular power, such as time to complete a 50-yard sprint, is a combination of the two. Resistance exercises can be tailored to improve all aspects of muscular fitness. Examples include the following:

- Weight lifting with free weights (dumbbells and barbells)
- Weight or resistance machines
- Resistance bands
- Isometric exercises
- Calisthenics using body weight as resistance (eg, push-ups)

Resistance Exercise Prescription Guidelines

Consider the following when helping individuals develop a resistance training program.

Exercise Selection Select at least 8 to 10 exercises that cover all the major muscle groups in the upper body, lower body, and core, which include the back, legs, hips, chest, shoulders, arms, and abdomen.[40] Exercise selection should be based on individual goals, preferences, and skill. Using different exercises to train the same muscle groups adds variety. Specific muscle groups may also be targeted to enhance other components of the activity program, such as biking or swimming.

Sequence Exercise large muscle groups before small muscle groups, doing chest and back exercises before specific arm exercises, for example. In addition, recommend performing exercises involving multiple joints before those for single joints, such as doing leg presses before leg extensions or leg curls. Doing exercises in this sequence helps ensure that adequate energy is available to effectively perform all exercises within a training session and lowers the potential for injury. Abdominal and core muscle exercises should always be performed at the end of the training session.

Amount of Resistance The resistance used is determined by the individual's 1-repetition maximum (1-RM), defined as the maximal amount of weight that an individual can successfully lift 1 time. Recommending training that is either moderate (50%-60% of 1-RM) or vigorous (75%-80% of 1-RM) in intensity allows for optimal gains in strength and insulin action.[60] No specific amount of time is recommended for muscle strengthening, but exercises should be performed to the point at which it would be difficult to do another repetition without help (ie, done to fatigue). Home-based resistance training is adequate for maintaining muscle mass and strength, but less effective than supervised, gym-based training for maintaining blood glucose levels as heavier weights or resistance may be needed to optimize insulin action.[62] Using resistance bands can increase strength, but likely has a lesser glycemic benefit.[63]

Frequency Recommend doing strength training exercises at least 2 times a week with a minimum of 48 hours of rest between sessions, but more ideally 3 nonconsecutive days per week, along with regular aerobic activities.[26]

Volume Each training session should involve completion of 10 to 15 repetitions to near fatigue per set on every exercise early in training, progressing over time to using heavier weights or resistance that allows for completion of only 8 to 12 repetitions.[40] Recommend doing a minimum of 1 set of repetitions to near fatigue to start, with a later goal of completing as many as 4 sets. The intensity of training and number of repetitions performed are inversely related, so the target number of repetitions may decrease as resistance increases.

Progression To avoid injury, progression of training should occur slowly. Recommend first undertaking increases in weight or resistance, and only when the target number of repetitions per set can consistently be exceeded, followed by a greater number of sets, and lastly by increased training frequency. Progression over 6 months or more to thrice-weekly sessions of up to 4 sets of 8 to 12 repetitions done at 75% to 80% of 1-RM on 8 to 10 exercises is an optimal goal for most individuals with diabetes.

Modifications For older or deconditioned individuals or anyone who needs to maintain a lower resistance program due to joint limitations or other health complications, recommend doing 1 set of exercises for all major muscle groups, starting with 10 to 15 repetitions at a very light or light intensity (40 to 50% of 1-RM) and progressing to 15 to 20 repetitions before adding additional sets.

Rest Adequate rest periods between sets are needed to successfully complete all sets on each exercise. Typically, lower intensity training requires 15 seconds to 1 minute of rest, while higher intensity training may necessitate up to 2 to 3 minutes of rest between sets. In addition, allow at least 48 hours between training sessions for optimal musculoskeletal recovery.

Resistance Exercise Guidelines

- *Frequency:* 2, but preferably 3, nonconsecutive days per week
- *Intensity:* moderate to vigorous; 50% to 80% of 1-RM, inclusive of 8 to 10 exercises that cover all the major muscle groups (ie, upper body, lower body, core)
- *Time:* 1 to 4 sets of each exercise; a minimum of 1 set of repetitions to near fatigue to start, with a later goal of completing as many as 4 sets, with rest intervals of 2 to 3 minutes between sets of any given exercise
- *Type:* Resistance machines, free weights, resistance bands, and/or body weight as resistance exercises
- *Volume:* 8 to 15 repetitions per set (eg, 1 set of 10-15 repetitions to fatigue initially, progressing to 8-12 harder repetitions, and finally to 4 or more sets of 8-12 repetitions)

Instruction and Supervision

Before starting a resistance exercise program, individuals must be instructed on proper weight lifting techniques to ensure that all exercises are performed safely and correctly. Recommend that a qualified exercise professional supervise the initial stages of the training program. Instruct individuals with the following recommendations:

- Breathe continually and avoid breath-holding during movements.
- Exhale during the exertion or lifting phase, and inhale while returning to starting position.
- Avoid sustained, tight gripping and static lifts that may cause hypertensive responses.
- Lift weights with slow, controlled movements.
- Emphasize using a complete range of motion around each joint.
- Maintain good form and keep the body properly aligned throughout the lift, especially when using free weights or resistance bands.
- Adjust the resistance equipment to fit the body frame.
- Stop exercising if warning signs or symptoms occur, such as dizziness, unusual shortness of breath, or chest pain.

Resistance Training Precautions

- Individuals with microvascular or macrovascular complications require program modifications to decrease strain on their cardiovascular system.
- Advise those with unstable proliferative retinopathy to avoid activities that dramatically elevate blood pressure, such as intense resistance training, as well as jumping, jarring, head-down, or breath-holding activities.[26]
- Before starting resistance training, individuals with diabetes and cardiovascular disease need to have an ejection fraction >45% and a cardiorespiratory fitness level of 7 METs, without ischemic ST segment depression hypotensive or hypertensive responses, serious ventricular arrhythmias, or symptoms of cardiovascular insufficiency.[64]
- Individuals with any complications that may be worsened by resistance training need to receive approval from their physician before starting a resistance program.

Flexibility Exercise Prescription

Flexibility is defined as the ability to move a joint through its complete range of motion and is considered an important part of physical fitness.[40,42] Some types of physical activity require more flexibility than others. Both dynamic and static stretching exercises are effective in increasing flexibility and thereby can allow individuals to more easily do activities that require greater movement around joints. For this reason, flexibility activities are an appropriate part of a physical activity program, even though it is unclear whether they reduce risk of injury. Flexibility exercises can be included as part of the warm-up or cool-down, but by themselves they are not counted toward meeting the aerobic or muscle-strengthening guidelines.[26]

Flexibility exercise, combined with resistance training, has been shown to increase joint range of motion in individuals with type 2 diabetes[50] and allow them to more easily engage in activities that require greater flexibility. For this reason, flexibility training may be included as part of a physical activity program, although it should not substitute for other training. Older adults are advised to undertake exercises that maintain or improve balance to prevent falls,[42,65] which may include flexibility training especially for many older individuals with type 2 diabetes or peripheral neuropathy who have a higher risk of falling.

Stretching should be considered an option to include in the fitness plan for individuals with diabetes. Traditional static and dynamic stretching, as well as exercises like yoga and tai chi, can provide fitness benefits.[66] However, it should not substitute for other recommended activities (ie, aerobic and resistance training), as flexibility training does not affect glucose stability, body composition or insulin action. Therefore, flexibility exercise recommendations should be based primarily on the individual's specific needs and interests but are recommended to be done at least 2 to 3 days per week to help maintain range of motion around joints.[26]

Balance and Other Training Prescription

Balance Exercise In addition to flexibility exercises, balance training is recommended for all adults to promote movement around joints and falls prevention, particularly for anyone over 40 years of age or with peripheral neuropathy, at least 2 to 3 times/week.[67,68] Many lower-body and core strengthening exercises concomitantly improve balance and may be included, along with other specific balance exercises, such as practice standing on one leg or a tandem stand. All exercises involving motor skills (eg, balance, agility, coordination, gait, proprioceptive) may be prescribed to enhance neuromotor function and lower risk of falls.

Yoga and Tai Chi Unconventional forms of physical activity, like yoga and tai chi, may benefit management of blood glucose, oxidative stress, flexibility, strength, balance, and more, but the results of studies investigating glycemic benefits have been mixed, and the inclusion of those activities as part of a weekly exercise program is not conclusively supported at this time.[69–71] Such exercises can be included according to individual preferences to increase flexibility, muscular strength, and balance, but their effects on aerobic fitness are lesser than other forms of training.

Flexibility and Balance Exercise Guidelines

- *Frequency:* Flexibility exercises at least 2 to 3 days per week (with daily being more effective), and balance exercises 2 to 3 or more days per week (especially for persons with diabetes over 40 or with neuropathy of any type)
- *Intensity:* Stretch to the point of feeling tightness or slight discomfort; for balance, an optimal intensity has not been determined
- *Time:* Total of 60 seconds per joint recommended for stretching; hold a single stretch for 10 to 30 seconds, 30 to 60 seconds more effective for older adults; for balance exercises, a minimum of 20 to 30 minutes per exercise session may be optimal
- *Type:* Static or dynamic stretching or yoga; balance, agility, coordination, gait, and proprioception exercise to enhance functional fitness and prevent falls; exercises using balance equipment, lower-body and core resistance exercises, tai chi, and practice standing on one leg
- *Volume:* A reasonable target for flexibility exercise is to perform 60 seconds of stretching during each flexibility exercise; older adults may benefit from frequent (daily) stretching and >60 minutes of weekly balance training, although the optimal volume is not known

Combined Aerobic and Resistance Training Including both aerobic and resistance exercise in a weekly exercise program is recommended. Combined aerobic and resistance training done thrice weekly in individuals with type 2 diabetes may be of greater benefit to blood glucose stability than either aerobic or resistance exercise alone.[72–74] However, in most studies, the total duration of exercise and caloric expenditure were greatest with combined training, and both were done on the same days during a single training session. One study that controlled for caloric expenditure reported that a group that performed a combination of aerobic and resistance training improved A1C levels in adults with type 2 diabetes compared with the nonexercise control group; this was not achieved by aerobic or resistance training alone.[75]

Exercise Order For individuals with type 1 diabetes, both the type and the order of activities undertaken during the same exercise session affects glycemic balance both during and following the combined activity. For example, performing resistance exercise before aerobic exercise improves glycemic stability throughout exercise and reduces the duration and severity of immediate postexercise hypoglycemia.[73,76] Although resistance exercise causes a lesser initial decline in blood glucose during the activity, it is associated with more prolonged reductions in postexercise glycemia than aerobic exercise.[76,77]

Exercise Energy Systems and Hormonal Effects

Blood glucose levels can change during and after physical activity, depending on the type, duration, intensity, frequency, and more. The underlying physiological responses associated with these changes are detailed in the following paragraphs. Most affect the fuels used by the body during the activity.

As Physical Activity Begins

Regardless of the fuel source, the release of phosphate from adenosine triphosphate (ATP) produces the direct energy for muscle contraction. Some stored energy is readily available in muscles for the first 10 seconds of activity (as depicted in Figure 6.2). Beyond that, muscles must use alternative energy systems to fuel physical activity, which is primarily accomplished via enzymatic pathways that initially break down carbohydrate and later fat and some protein. During the first few minutes of physical activity, most of the energy is derived from intramuscular glycogen, which is broken down without oxygen through rapid glycolysis. This anaerobic pathway provides only a limited amount of energy, peaks at about 30 seconds into an activity, and lasts a maximum of 2 minutes. When activity is intense, rapid glycolysis may result in acid byproducts that can cause muscular discomfort (a burning sensation) and a reduced exercise capacity. This energy pathway is particularly important at the onset of physical activity when aerobic conversion of energy is too slow to compensate or at any time during a workout when the exercise intensity is increased. As physical activity continues, an adequate supply of energy becomes available through the aerobic breakdown of carbohydrate, fat, and protein, although carbohydrate remains the body's preferred energy source for most activities.[78]

After 5 to 10 Minutes

During sustained movement, carbohydrate, fat, and protein are broken down to continuously provide energy to working muscles. For moderate and intense activity, the primary fuel remains carbohydrate, primarily muscle glycogen with a small amount of blood glucose. After 5 to 10 minutes, circulating glucose arising from glycogen breakdown in the liver (hepatic glycogenolysis) and glucose being synthesized there (hepatic gluconeogenesis) provide additional energy sources for working muscles.

Beyond 20 Minutes

As exercise continues beyond 20 to 30 minutes, muscle glycogen stores may start to become depleted.[79] The rate of glycogen utilization is highly dependent on exercise intensity and duration, with more being used at greater intensities and/or during longer durations. Whenever glycogen decreases, a shift in the fuel mix is required. During low to moderate exercise intensities, free fatty acids (FFAs) become an increasingly significant source of energy, in addition to blood glucose from hepatic sources. As physical exercise continues, hepatic gluconeogenesis becomes increasingly important for providing the required glucose. The main substrates for hepatic gluconeogenesis are lactate, amino acids (eg, alanine), and glycerol.

Longer Duration Activity

As exercise duration increases further, the contribution of FFA for fuel increases relative to glucose. Exercise of low to

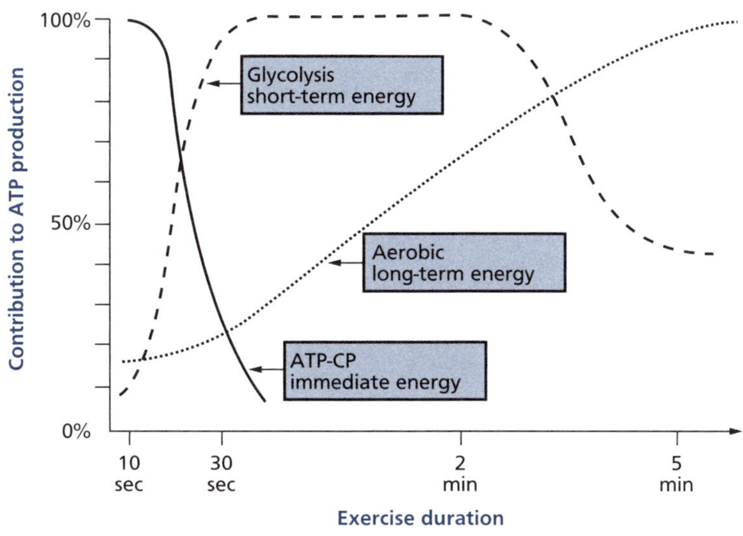

FIGURE 6.2 Energy Systems During Physical Activity

Reprinted with permission from SR Colberg, *The Athlete's Guide to Diabetes: Expert Advice for 165 Sports and Activities* (Champaign, IL: Human Kinetics, 2019), 29.

Cases—Part 2: Effects of Physical Activity on Blood Glucose

Type 1 Diabetes

HW was eager to take care of his diabetes and happy to get back into his fitness routine. He liked to work out in the evenings, the time of day he could most easily get to his fitness club or referee hockey games.

He read that hypoglycemia could be prevented by exercising after a meal. Since eating food increases blood glucose and exercise decreases it, he assumed everything would come out even. He took his usual premeal, rapid-acting insulin dose and ate dinner before going to his club one evening. Twenty-five minutes into his moderate aerobic workout, however, HW had to stop and treat a blood glucose of 57 mg/dL (3.2 mmol/L). This was not what he expected!

Type 2 Diabetes

When diagnosed with type 2 diabetes, DK decided to start exercising. She was motivated to lose a lot of weight, the faster the better. She used to be active and had enjoyed dancing, exercise classes, and playing games with her children. She was not sure how that person got lost, but she was determined to find herself again.

DK was cleared to exercise by her healthcare provider, who told her any weight loss would improve her hypertension and hyperlipidemia. A friend told her that a snack was important to eat before exercise to keep her blood glucose from going too low. She remembered that metformin did not cause low blood glucose levels, but she was not sure what to do for exercise.

To be safe, she ate a package of 4 peanut butter crackers before walking a mile around her neighborhood. She became frustrated when she figured out later that she had eaten 190 calories but walked off only 100. Also, her blood glucose readings were a little higher after her walk compared with before. This made no sense to her since she remembered being told that exercising should make her blood glucose go down, not up!

moderate intensity relies largely on circulating FFA as the oxidative fuel for muscle, although protein sources may provide up to 5% of the total energy during moderate duration activity and up to 15% during ultraendurance events. The oxidation of fat-derived substrates cannot completely replace carbohydrate use, given that there is a minimum amount of carbohydrate required for fat to be efficiently used as a fuel.[79] When carbohydrate sources are too limited, fat is not completely oxidized and ketone bodies are formed as a by-product of the incomplete combustion of fat. Ketones are not an efficient source of energy during exercise. Without an adequate supply of carbohydrate available, the exercise intensity cannot be maintained; this may explain exercisers "bonking" or runners "hitting the wall" during long-duration activities like marathons.

Role of Hormones in Exercise Blood Glucose Levels

Physical activity activates the release of the glucose-raising hormones, such as epinephrine and norepinephrine, which are released in an exaggerated fashion in response to intense exercise, and other hormones that significantly influence how the primary fuel substrates (carbohydrate, protein, and fat) are used for energy production (see Table 6.6).[80] Exercise-induced release of these hormones allows alternate fuels to be made available as energy sources while maintaining glucose homeostasis. Endogenous insulin secretion normally decreases during physical activity, and its suppression is an essential step in allowing hepatic glucose production to maintain the balance of glucose in the blood.

Glycogen stores in the liver and muscle need to be replenished following each bout of physical activity.[81,82] This demand is met by an increased rate of glucose uptake until the depleted glycogen stores are fully replaced. This activity may take 24 to 48 hours to complete.[82] This extended recovery period is also characterized by enhanced insulin sensitivity and improved fat oxidation.[83] There are many long-term adaptations to habitual physical activity that may alter carbohydrate use and storage and affect blood glucose management.[81,84]

Effect of Types of Physical Activity on Diabetes Management

Blood glucose levels related to being active can vary with the type of activity done, whether an individual is engaging in a single session or repeated bouts. Aerobic exercise, based on its frequency, intensity, and duration, may have a different effect than resistance training, balance exercise, or a combination of activities. The diabetes care and education specialist can play a role in educating individuals about expected outcomes to assist them in more effectively regulating their blood glucose levels around activities.

Aerobic Exercise

Regular aerobic exercise is an essential component of diabetes self-management behavior for most individuals with diabetes. Since the duration of glycemic improvement

TABLE 6.6 Normal Hormonal Responses and the Resultant Acute Metabolic Effects of Physical Activity

Hormone	*Response During Activity*	*Metabolic Effect of Hormonal Response*
Insulin	Decreases	Facilitates hepatic glucose production and free fatty acid (FFA) release from adipose tissues
Glucagon	Increases	Increases hepatic glucose production via glycogenolysis and gluconeogenesis, thereby increasing glucose supply available in the blood
Epinephrine	Increases	Stimulates muscle glycogen breakdown and FFA production, which provides glycerol as a substrate for gluconeogenesis; may enhance hepatic glucose production during exercise; decreases insulin secretion
Norepinephrine	Increases	Stimulates hepatic glucose production; reduces muscular glucose uptake during physical activity; decreases insulin secretion
Growth Hormone and Cortisol	Increase	Increase lipolysis; decrease insulin-stimulated glucose uptake (ie, heighten insulin resistance); increase supply of glycerol and amino acids to liver for new glucose production; result in primarily delayed effects that are important during prolonged activities

after an exercise session is usually greater than 2 hours but less than 72 hours, regular physical activity is needed to lower blood glucose. For those with type 2 diabetes, a sustained improvement in blood glucose management may be possible when a regular aerobic training program is maintained, although the impact of exercise and dietary intervention alone (without antihyperglycemic medications) is likely greater with shorter disease history and better glycemic management.[85] Postprandial exercise, especially following large meals, has been found to prevent or lower the rise in blood glucose levels at that time in adults with type 2 diabetes.[13]

Generally, aerobic exercise performed at low levels (<40% HRR) has less of an effect on glucose disposal than exercise performed at higher intensities, given that blood glucose disposal during exercise is roughly proportional to the total work performed (time × intensity). Total energy expenditure may be more important than the exercise intensity for overall glycemic balance, however. When matched for energy cost, low- to moderate-intensity aerobic training has been shown to be as effective as moderate- to high-intensity training in lowering A1C levels and increasing whole body and skeletal muscle oxidative capacity in obese individuals with type 2 diabetes.[86] Even a single bout of low-intensity, compared to high-intensity, exercise substantially reduces the prevalence of hyperglycemia throughout the subsequent 24-hour postexercise period.[87] As long as total exercise volume is equivalent, every other day training may have the same glycemic impact as daily exercise.[88] On the other hand, low-volume, high-intensity interval training may rapidly improve glucose management and induce adaptations in skeletal muscle that are linked to improved metabolic health in those with type 2 diabetes.[89]

For individuals taking insulin, being active on a daily basis may help balance caloric needs with insulin dosing, as well as maintain higher levels of insulin sensitivity to allow for reduced insulin dosing, but correcting managing food intake and insulin dosing is critical for maintaining glycemic target levels. Inconsistent A1C values may result with physical activity in this population, and care must be taken to achieve this goal when promoting blood glucose management as an expected outcome.[77] The glycemic response to aerobic exercise has some degree of reproducibility within an individual with type 1 diabetes, as long as many of the variables known to impact glucose homeostasis are held constant, such as the pre-exercise meal, the insulin dose, and the exercise task itself.[90] Intermittent high-intensity activities may be safer than continuous exercise because of lesser decline in blood glucose,[91] but vigorous exercise (>60% of HRR) may result in transient hyperglycemia.[89] To safely and successfully pursue a physically active lifestyle, the individual with type 1 diabetes needs to develop hypoglycemia prevention strategies, as do many individuals with type 2 diabetes using insulin or taking insulin secretagogues. Hypoglycemia prevention is discussed later in this chapter.

Resistance Exercise

Inclusive of both strength exercises and core conditioning, resistance training is an important means of preserving and increasing muscular strength, muscular endurance, power, and balance. Resistance exercise has been shown to improve glycemic levels, possibly even more so than aerobic training in persons with type 2 diabetes.[60,92,93] In adults with type 1 diabetes, the effects on A1C levels are less clear, but also likely beneficial to overall diabetes management.[92] Acute bouts of resistance exercise, sprints, and high-intensity intervals may all attenuate exercise-related declines in blood glucose both during and after exercise, although responses may vary based on age, sex, and fitness level.[94] Older adults receive the added advantage of preventing accidental falls and increased mobility with resistance work, even if peripheral neuropathy is present.[68] This can allow an elderly person to remain more independent and self-sufficient.

Flexibility and Balance Exercise

The benefits of alternative training like yoga and tai chi are less established, although yoga may promote improvement in glycemic management, lipid levels, body composition, and health-related quality of life in adults with type 2 diabetes.[69,70] Tai chi training may improve glycemic stability, balance, neuropathic symptoms, and some dimensions of quality of life in adults with diabetes and neuropathy.[71] Both of these modalities include basic stretching movements as part of the instruction, along with some elements of balance and strength. Flexibility exercise combined with resistance training can increase joint range-of-motion in individuals with diabetes[95] and allow them to more easily engage in activities that require flexibility. An older adult who engages in flexibility exercise has the added advantages of preventing accidental falls and increasing joint mobility during resistance work.[68] In addition, flexibility programs are easy to perform and may provide the perfect introduction to a more physically active lifestyle for deconditioned individuals.

Exercise Hypoglycemia Management

Being physically active is extremely beneficial to general health, important in the prevention of type 2 diabetes, and an essential health-management behavior for anyone with diabetes. Fear of hypoglycemia has been reported as a significant barrier, especially in those who use insulin or insulin secretagogues.[22] In collaboration with the healthcare team, people living with diabetes can develop strategies for avoidance of hypoglycemia, such as reductions in insulin or medication prior to physical activity, and inclusion of rapid-acting carbohydrate prior to and during activity. Due to distinctions in pathophysiology and treatment options, physical activity frequently affects blood glucose levels differently in people with type 1 diabetes or type 2 diabetes. Understanding these differences helps the diabetes care and education specialist identify and avoid common blood glucose concerns associated with physical activity.

Assessing Risk for Hypoglycemia

Particularly in individuals with type 1 diabetes, a number of factors can increase the risk for exercise-associated hypoglycemia, including the timing, duration, and intensity of the activity.[91,96,97] Engaging in a new or unfamiliar activity may also increase the risk, while endurance training may lower it.[98] Since hypoglycemia is one of the most common concerns associated with physical activity that people with diabetes have, the individual must understand whether the potential of this side effect exists with the medication regimen in use. Fear of hypoglycemia is the strongest reported barrier to regular physical activity in adults and youth with type 1 diabetes, highlighting the importance of information and support regarding hypoglycemia management for these individuals.[21,22]

> Assist individuals in understanding their individualized risk for hypoglycemia related to physical activity participation.

In addition, individuals with type 1 diabetes may have multiple impairments in their counterregulatory hormone response to hypoglycemia and exercise, placing them at high risk for severe hypoglycemia. Both antecedent hypoglycemia and exercise cause reduced neuroendocrine, metabolic, and symptom responses to subsequent hypoglycemia or exercise.[99] After the first few years of the onset of diabetes, the glucagon response to hypoglycemia is typically diminished or lost, although its response to exercise may still be intact.[100] Increases in epinephrine are also blunted during both exercise and hypoglycemia. Even if counterregulatory responses to hypoglycemia (and exercise) occur, excessive exogenous insulin dosing can blunt hepatic glucose production and increase peripheral glucose disposal, thereby resulting in rapid hypoglycemia. Other factors like inadequate carbohydrate intake, failure to monitor blood glucose levels, and exercising in the heat may also increase the risk of hypoglycemia. In older individuals with type 2 diabetes, a marked subjective unawareness of hypoglycemia has been reported that does not depend on altered neuroendocrine counterregulation and may contribute to the increased probability of severe hypoglycemia in these individuals.[101]

Medication Impact on Hypoglycemia Risk

Table 6.7 can be used to identify categories of diabetes medications that place the user at higher risk for exercise-related hypoglycemia. Most classes of newer medications

TABLE 6.7 Risk of Exercise-Related Hypoglycemia With Various Diabetes Medications

No or Minimal Risk	*Higher Risk*
Alpha-glucosidase inhibitors (eg, acarbose, miglitol)	Insulin (all types and delivery methods)
Biguanides (eg, metformin)	Meglitinides (eg, nateglinide and repaglinide)
Amylin mimetic (pramlintide)	Sulfonylureas (eg, glimepiride, glipizide) and combination pills containing sulfonyureas
DPP-4 inhibitors (eg, sitagliptin, vildagliptin, saxagliptin, linagliptin)	
Incretins and incretin mimetics (eg, dulaglutide, exenatide, liraglutide, semaglutide)	
SGLT2 inhibitors (eg, canagliflozin, dapagliflozin, empagliflozin, ertugliflozin)	
Thiazolidinediones (eg, pioglitazone, rosiglitizone)	

appear not to confer much risk. However, there are some anecdotal reports of hard-to-treat episodes of hypoglycemia related to physical activity undertaken when exenatide and pramlintide doses were taken close to initiation of activity.[102] Conversely, exenatide has also been shown to cause an exaggerated release of catecholamines and a rise in blood glucose during aerobic exercise in men without diabetes.[103]

Insulin—a part of medication treatment regimens for all individuals with type 1 diabetes and many with type 2 diabetes—is the medication that poses the greatest risk for hypoglycemia. Circulating levels of this hormone are normally reduced by the body naturally during exercise but injected (or pumped) insulin continues to be released from subcutaneous depots (and at a faster rate) during activity and, thus, cannot be regulated as effortlessly without pre-exercise planning.[104] In insulin users, hypoglycemia can occur during exercise, but also at varying times postexercise due to acutely increased insulin mobilization, enhanced insulin sensitivity, increased glucose utilization, replenishment of glycogen stores, and defective counterregulatory mechanisms.[83,105]

Administration of short- or rapid-acting human insulin or insulin analogs 2 to 3 hours before the onset of physical activity increases hypoglycemia risk,[97] particularly if doses are not adjusted downward in anticipation of being active, although 25%-75% reductions in doses (injected or pumped) may lower the risk.[106] Since exercise often occurs in a timeframe of 0 to 4 hours after insulin administration, persons taking regular or rapid-acting insulin analogs are typically exercising when circulating insulin levels are too high, relatively speaking, for low or moderate aerobic exercise. In these situations, corrections in insulin dosage and/or additional carbohydrates are typically needed.[107] The best indicator of risk is likely the individual's past experiences with repeated bouts of physical activity under similar conditions.

As an alternative or complement to carbohydrate intake, reductions in basal and/or bolus insulin dosing should be considered for exercise-induced hypoglycemia prevention. For example, basal insulin can be reduced by 20% in individuals with type 1 diabetes on multiple daily injections (MDI) both before and after exercise, but may not fully prevent hypoglycemia.[106] For individuals, using continuous subcutaneous insulin infusion (CSII, or an insulin pump) can reduce or suspend insulin delivery at the start of exercise.[108] Decreasing basal rates 30 to 60 minutes prior to the start of exercise may reduce hypoglycemia since CSII uses only rapid-acting insulin analogs for basal insulin delivery.[41] Frequent blood glucose checks are required when implementing insulin and carbohydrate adjustments. Basal insulin generally has a lesser acute impact on glycemic balance during most activities, but it may need to be adjusted prior to participation in long-duration events. Moreover, hypoglycemia risk may be higher with use of certain basal insulins.[109,110] Both insulin detemir and neutral protamine Hagedorn have been associated with less hypoglycemia than insulin glargine in people with relatively well managed type 1 diabetes during and after 30 minutes of exercise undertaken 5 hours after the last mealtime and basal insulin injection.

General Strategies to Prevent Exercise-Related Hypoglycemia

- Educate the person with diabetes about the possible causes of hypoglycemia.
- Reduce insulin doses (bolus and/or basal) as needed prior to, during, and following physical activity.
- Increase the amount of carbohydrate (and possibly protein and fat) consumed after physical activity.
- Make appropriate regimen changes to compensate for physical activity in proximity to bedtime (to prevent overnight hypoglycemia).
- Monitor blood glucose more frequently following physical activity.

By way of contrast, an individual with type 2 diabetes who is not prescribed any diabetes medications has a low risk of experiencing exercise-induced hypoglycemia. Even so, the degree of risk associated with hypoglycemia varies from person to person, based on medication regimen, food intake, and physical activity choices. For example, individuals with a low carbohydrate intake are more likely to deplete muscle glycogen stores rapidly during exercise and may increase their risk of exercise-associated hypoglycemia.[84] During assessment, the educator must identify other variables that may contribute to or protect the individual from hypoglycemia (ie, elevated versus near-normal A1C, usual timing of activity, type or duration of diabetes, and food preferences). At times, the best risk indicator for hypoglycemia is the individual's own personal experience. When the risk exists, strategies to prevent it during physical activity need to be reviewed.

Not all hypoglycemia associated with physical activity occurs during activity or even immediately afterward. Low blood glucose levels can be biphasic after exercise, occurring both immediately afterward and again 7 to 11 hours later, and occur for up to 24 or more hours after the exercise has stopped.[111,112] Later onset hypoglycemia becomes a greater concern when carbohydrate stores such as muscle and liver glycogen are depleted during an acute bout of exercise, usually one that is either higher intensity (aerobic or resistance training) or prolonged (usually aerobic). In particular, repeated interval workouts or intense resistance training can result in substantial depletion of muscle glycogen, thereby increasing the risk for later onset hypoglycemia particularly if supplemental insulin or longer lasting sulfonylureas or other insulin secretagogues are taken.[113,114] The consumption of moderate amounts of carbohydrates (5-30 grams, depending on the individual's postexercise blood glucose levels) during and within 30 minutes to 2 hours after exhaustive, glycogen-depleting exercise will lower hypoglycemia risk and allow for more efficient restoration of muscle glycogen.[115]

When the risk of hypoglycemia does not realistically exist, it is just as important to communicate this information to the person with diabetes and family members to eliminate a perceived barrier to a physically active lifestyle. The person with diabetes will no longer harbor fears or have concerns about what he or she has heard about physical activity and hypoglycemia and will better understand how to prevent unexpected and unwanted decreases in blood glucose levels associated with physical activity.

Other Medication Considerations

Certain diabetes medications must be considered when assessing risk of falls or other adverse outcomes potentially associated with physical activity. For example, a study assessed whether a link exists between metformin and falls in older persons with type 2 diabetes; while no direct connection was found, an indirect association caused by neuropathy secondary to vitamin B_{12} deficiency (resulting from metformin use) may be of concern.[116] In addition, insulin use has been demonstrated to increase the risk of falls related to hypoglycemia in the elderly, and thiazolidinediones increase fracture risk and thus may worsen fall-related outcomes.[117] When creating a physical activity plan, the risk of falls and fall-related complications associated with these medications should not be ignored in certain populations.

Steroids and beta-adrenergic blocking agents are two other classes of prescription medications that need to be considered when predicting or interpreting an individual's blood glucose response to physical activity. Steroids are likely to result in hyperglycemia, while beta-blockers can cause severe hypoglycemia due to the inhibition of glycogenolysis, as well as mask the usual adrenergic symptoms of hypoglycemia.[118] Moreover, beta-blockers also lower heart rate during submaximal and maximal exercise and may result in early fatigue.

Establishing Blood Glucose Targets for Exercise

Once the individual understands whether he or she is at risk for hypoglycemia, the next step is establishing reasonable blood glucose goals for physical activity. The diabetes care and education specialist must tailor the complexity of these steps to the individual's abilities. Additional complications or circumstances that may have an effect must also be considered. Complications like gastroparesis may already exist, making blood glucose levels erratic at times.[119] If the individual has hypoglycemia unawareness, taking additional blood glucose readings may be helpful.

Rapid changes in blood glucose can be directly measured with traditional fingerstick blood glucose monitoring, whereas continuous glucose monitoring (CGM) devices measure glucose in interstitial fluids rather than blood and their glucose readings may lag behind actual blood glucose levels during rapid changes in glycemia.[120] Many active individuals with type 1 diabetes have begun using these systems to track glucose trends in place of fingerstick readings. The accuracy of these latest devices has improved, even during exercise of varying intensities.[121,122] Advances in CGM and insulin delivery, integration of algorithms with other devices, and adaptive machine learning may together provide a feasible closed-loop system in the future that can better manage physical activities. Use of CGM has already been proven to increase time in range and lower severe hypoglycemia in people with type 1 diabetes,[123] and it may prove to be a useful technology to help people with type 1 diabetes improve metabolic stability around exercise. Specialists must be involved with persons with diabetes in learning the intricacies of new devices and helping the individuals using them to practice new skills, prioritize any data surplus, and overcome their technology phobias.

If more blood glucose readings cannot be performed due to finances or the individual's unwillingness to do so, other options should be explored to make sure any risks, including those associated with hypoglycemia, are minimized during and after participation in any physical activity. Modifications may, for example, capitalize on opportunities such as the following: exercising after meals when blood glucose levels may be higher; making bouts of physical activity shorter but more intense to keep glucose levels higher; exercising at the time of day when blood glucose levels are highest; or exercising in the presence of trained helpers or peers who can watch for symptoms of hypoglycemia.

The individual's personal history can help the diabetes care and education specialist establish reasonable blood glucose goals for physical activity. These guidelines are a good starting point:

- *Using insulin:* Keep blood glucose levels as close to normal as possible, but above 110 mg/dL (6.1 mmol/L) and under 250 mg/dL (13.9 mmol/L).
- *Using oral diabetes medication with potential for exercise hypoglycemia:* Keep blood glucose level above 90 mg/dL (5.0 mmol/L) during all physical activities.
- *Using oral agents that do not cause hypoglycemia or not on medication for diabetes:* No minimal blood glucose threshold is necessary.
- *With other complications or circumstances that predispose to hypoglycemia:* Keep blood glucose level above 120 mg/dL (6.7 mmol/L) and under 250 mg/dL (13.9 mmol/L).

Interpretation and Management of Hyperglycemia

In some circumstances, elevated blood glucose levels can be indicative of medical concerns like insulin deficiency. People with type 2 diabetes can experience hyperglycemia from a combination of insulin resistance and inadequate insulin secretion; in their case, extremely elevated glucose levels in combination with severe dehydration can result in hyperosmolar hyperglycemia, which may be aggravated by other extenuating health variables such as severe illness and infections.[124] These individuals typically do not produce ketones; if ketones do exist, they may be due to dietary restriction, as opposed to insulin deficiency. People with type 1 diabetes are more susceptible to insulin deficiency since they have almost no ability to produce any insulin; therefore, they need to receive instruction on why and when to check for ketones.[125] This is especially important if the individual is using an insulin pump. If ketones are present, then the higher blood glucose levels are a result of insulin deficiency, and corrective action should be taken immediately.

Most diabetes care and education specialists teach people with type 1 diabetes to check for ketones when their blood glucose levels are consistently above 300 mg/dL (16.7 mmol/L), but they should check whenever they have unexplained hyperglycemia (≥200 mg/dL, or 11.1 mmol/L) that persists more than a couple of hours. Exercise should be postponed or suspended if blood ketone levels are elevated (≥1.5 mmol/L or 8.7 mg/dL), equivalent to moderate to large urine ketones, since blood glucose and ketones may rise further with even mild activity.[14]

Insulin regimens paired with frequent blood glucose checks greatly diminish the chance of insulin deficiency developing, and significant levels of ketones are rarely found when performing blood or urine checks. In most circumstances, slightly elevated blood glucose levels should not interfere with exercise performance; however, some people report headaches, blurry vision, or lack of energy with even mild hyperglycemia, which may be reason enough to avoid physical activity until the glucose level improves. The healthcare facilitator must consider the ability of the individual to perform blood glucose and ketone testing and understand the complexity of the information.

In other situations, physical activity itself can raise normal blood glucose levels when performed at high intensity.[126] The catecholamine response to very intense activity results in an exaggerated hepatic production of glucose for fuel, and after the activity is stopped, the insulin need can double during the post-activity period. If not corrected with insulin dosing in insulin users, this hyperglycemia may last for several hours before drifting down, or it may not decrease without additional insulin.[127] Those using insulin pump therapy may bolus with a small amount of insulin to address this physiological need. If injecting insulin by syringe, an additional dose of short- or rapid-acting insulin can also be administered. The timing and amount of insulin given require careful consideration and monitoring to accomplish the desired blood glucose result. Individuals must consider any insulin remaining from their last injection or bolus in making subsequent adjustments to doses, as well as factor in the residual effects of the last bout of activity on blood glucose use (ie, postexercise enhanced insulin action).

Regardless of the delivery method, this additional insulin dose can result in hypoglycemia and may not be advisable in all cases.

Self-Management Strategies for Physical Activity

Determining the best routine to follow during periods of physical activity takes time, and the individual with diabetes must learn, practice, and problem solve. Often, information from multiple workout sessions is needed as well as frequent blood glucose monitoring and patience. To keep blood glucose levels above the target goal before, during, and after physical activity, many people–insulin users in particular–will need to adjust other aspects of the diabetes regimen. These adjustments are intended to either:

- *Raise the amount of glucose* available to active muscles with an adequate amount in the blood (through calorie intake), and/or
- *Lower the amount of insulin* in the blood during activity (with medication or timing adjustments).

Both strategies may result in the blood glucose level drifting higher for a short period of time. However, once the physical activity begins, increased glucose use by muscles will fuel some of the energy needs of the active muscles. While working out at higher intensities, some individuals may need to make adjustments that lower blood glucose levels instead if the release of glucose by hormones outpaces its use.

Questions for the Diabetes Specialist to Ask

Determining what people with diabetes know about their unique exercise responses and what they may have already tried is very helpful. Often, the individual understands basic concepts or recognizes patterns but has not implemented regimen adjustments correctly or may know to check blood glucose more often, eat a snack, or adjust the insulin dose, but still may not be seeing the desired blood glucose levels. Below are some appropriate questions to ask and points for discussion.

> Troubleshoot hypoglycemia with appropriate questions that allow individuals to prevent or treat it more effectively.

When Is Blood Glucose Being Checked? Frequently the blood glucose reported was checked hours before or after the physical activity was done. The person needs to check within minutes of starting and ending physical activity to determine its acute effect. Also, when later onset hypoglycemia is a concern, individuals may need to monitor more frequently and make adjustments for 8 or more hours afterward.[127]

Is Hypoglycemia During Activities a Possibility or Concern? If so, ask for an extra glucose check during the physical activity to establish usual patterns of response. Sometimes, higher blood glucose levels after the workout are caused by unrecognized hypoglycemia during the workout, which can lead to an excessive release of glucose-raising catecholamines. If this is the cause, discuss a plan to prevent the possibility of hypoglycemia during the activity.

Was a Snack Eaten? If so, was it appropriate (in both type and quantity), and was it eaten at the correct time? If not, should a snack be included in the future?

Would a Sports Drink With Carbohydrate Help With Both Hydration and Blood Glucose Stabilization During Exercise? If blood glucose is not a concern, plain water works equally well for hydration during most physical activities and avoids the intake of extra glucose and calories.

Why Was Blood Glucose Higher After Physical Activity? There are a few possibilities and responses:

- *How much did blood glucose increase?* Get specifics. If the level went from 105 mg/dL (5.8 mmol/L) to 117 mg/dL (6.5 mmol/L), that still reflects excellent results (and may be within the error of measurement). If the level went from 209 mg/dL (11.6 mmol/L) to 277 mg/dL (15.4 mmol/L), the person has an A1C of 11% and is trying to avoid insulin, adjustments need to be made so that physical activity can benefit diabetes management, not worsen it.
- *Could this be a normal response?* For some activities (such as intense ones), supply of blood glucose can exceed demand. This is usually short-lived and blood glucose tends to decrease within an hour or so postexercise but may be alarming to the individual or discouraging. One solution may be to exercise at a lower intensity or possibly at a different time of day. If someone is hyperglycemic and ketotic, though, exercise should be avoided until better metabolic stability is achieved.
- *What role did food have on the response?* Sometimes a meal or snack that was eaten before or during the activity can raise blood glucose during or afterward due to slower digestion while active. If this is the cause, the blood glucose is likely better than it would have been if the person had not

been physically active. This may not require any changes, only explanations, or food intake may need to be reduced around this activity.

- *Has this happened only once?* A single occurrence may not repeat itself. Consider potential confounding variables, such as environmental extremes, time of day that exercise was done, mental stress such as prerace anxiety, physical illness or infection, and hydration status.

Activity Glucose Monitoring

Glucose monitoring before and after a period of physical activity provides crucial feedback for the individual learning to adjust insulin and/or food intake. Levels at the start and end of the activity are the most common to monitor, but to identify trends it may be necessary to check within 15 minutes prior to exercise, during exercise, soon afterward, or periodically for a few hours after its completion.

Individuals using CGM devices may be able to more easily track blood glucose trends. These devices can provide useful information about blood glucose trends before, during, and after physical activity, but the individual should keep in mind that readings from CGM devices are somewhat time-delayed, may vary in accuracy with the type of activity done, and may not identify hypoglycemia during exercise before it occurs.[121,128] The interpretation of this information—particularly glucose trends during an activity—can lead to a better understanding of the insulin and food adjustments required to support exercise energy needs.

> Encourage frequent blood glucose monitoring for problem solving around physical activity.

Appropriate Snacking and Hydration

Snacking is the easiest adjustment for laypeople to understand and a strategy that those with diabetes often implement by themselves. Unfortunately, estimating the amount of food needed can be difficult. When the snack is insufficient or inappropriate, hypoglycemia can still happen. If a snack larger than necessary is eaten, some degree of hyperglycemia may result. When weight loss is a goal of the fitness plan, both circumstances can result in more total calories being consumed, and when too many extra calories are consumed, weight gain may result instead of weight loss.

Carbohydrate Snacks

Blood glucose readings taken at the *start, during,* and *end* of an exercise session allow the individual to gauge whether additional carbohydrates or another calorie source (that will be available later) are needed. For example, if the blood glucose usually drops 30 to 40 mg/dL (1.7 to 2.2 mmol/L) during a physical activity and the goal is to stay above 110 mg/dL (6.1 mmol/L), a pre-exercise snack should be eaten for readings below 130 mg/dL (7.2 mmol/L). For pre-exercise glucose levels between the target starting value and the goal, some—albeit a lesser amount—carbohydrate may still be needed.

A number of factors can influence actual intake needed, including intensity and duration of exercise, starting blood glucose level, circulating insulin levels, the medication regimen, recent food and caloric beverage consumption, and timing of exercise, just to name a few.[14] Even in individuals with type 2 diabetes not taking insulin, blood glucose levels are likely to decrease more during physical activity undertaken in the fed state (post-meal) compared with the fasted or premeal state at varying times of day.[129,130]

To prevent hypoglycemia in individuals with a relatively higher risk during exercise, a general guideline is that a snack containing 10 to 30 g of carbohydrate should be consumed for every 30 to 45 minutes of moderate aerobic physical activity. Requirements will vary with aerobic exercise intensity and duration as well as starting blood glucose levels, as shown in Table 6.8. Keep in mind that a lesser or no snack may be needed if insulin levels can be reduced enough with dosing changes. The actual need for carbohydrate will vary from person to person and even among activities done by one individual, making blood glucose monitoring critical for predicting snack requirements to optimize exercise performance and blood glucose management.

Composition of Snacks

The snack option must meet the fuel needs of the physical activity and the individual. Often, people with diabetes choose to consume juice or glucose tablets at the start of the physical activity because they know these options are used to treat hypoglycemic events and assume they are useful to prevent them as well. These choices work short-term but may not be the best for long-term prevention of hypoglycemia during extended exercise and afterward.

> Snacks to prevent hypoglycemia are not always the same as those used to treat it.

For *preventing* hypoglycemia during exercise, a pre-exercise snack with carbohydrates that are more slowly absorbed or with some protein may be a better match for exercise fuel requirements than a rapidly absorbed carbohydrate source like glucose tablets or regular soda (snacks

TABLE 6.8 Carbohydrate Increases for Aerobic Activities in Grams

Duration (min)	*Intensity*[a]	*Pre-Exercise Blood Glucose in mg/dL (mmol/L)*			
		<100 (5.6)	*100–150 (5.6-8.3)*	*150–200 (8.3–11.1)*	*>200 (11.1)*[b]
30	Easy	5–10 g[c]	0–10 g	0–5 g	None
	Moderate	10–20 g	10–20 g	5–15 g	0–10 g
	Vigorous	15–30 g	15–30 g	10–25 g	5–20 g
60	Easy	10–25 g	10–20 g	5–15 g	0–10 g
	Moderate	20–50 g	20–40 g	10–30 g	5–20 g
	Vigorous	30–75 g	30–60 g	15–45 g	10–30 g
>60	Easy	10 to 20 g of carbohydrate per additional hour			
	Moderate	20 to 40 g of carbohydrate per additional hour			
	Vigorous	30 to 60 g of carbohydrate per additional hour[d]			

[a] Easy activities are defined as less than 40%, moderate 40%–59%, and vigorous 60%–89% of heart rate reserve.

[b] For a starting blood glucose above 250 mg/dL with moderate or high ketones, individuals may need a dose of rapid-acting insulin to lower glucose during an activity, not any extra carbohydrate.

[c] Individuals should consume rapidly absorbed carbohydrates except possibly after the first hour when a mixture of carbohydrate sources or other foods may be helpful.

[d] Exercisers may need up to 75 grams per hour to prevent lows when they have higher insulin levels.

Used with permission from SR Colberg, *The Athlete's Guide to Diabetes: Expert Advice for 165 Sports and Activities* (Champaign, IL: Human Kinetics, 2019), 33.

used to *treat* hypoglycemia). People consume a variety of carbohydrate-based snacks during exercise, including sports bars, gels, and drinks, some of which contain protein (and fat) along with carbohydrate.[102] Carbohydrates that are more slowly absorbed can be found in whole grains, many whole fruits, yogurt, and many snack bars. The best option is based on the desired blood glucose level, the duration and intensity of the activity, the individual's unique glucose response to exercise and tolerance to foods, and personal preferences. Many are following lower carbohydrate food plans and prefer to snack on foods higher in protein and fat, even during activity.

Following physical activity, additional snacks may be needed to prevent later onset hypoglycemia. The first 30 to 60 minutes afterward is generally when muscles take up blood glucose to replace glycogen at the fastest rate and with the least insulin needed. Eating a small carbohydrate or protein snack within 30 to 120 minutes postexercise may prevent hypoglycemia during that time. The actual number of carbohydrates required will vary with the type of activity done, the regimen changes implemented for the activity (lower insulin and/or higher carbohydrate intake), and the individual's immediate postexercise blood glucose level.

Precautions may be needed to prevent late-onset hypoglycemia from occurring overnight during sleep.[106] The need for and composition of a bedtime snack depend on the blood glucose; for example, no snack may be necessary at levels >180 mg/dL (10 mmol/L), any snack may suffice at levels between 126 and 180 mg/dL (7 and 10 mmol/L), and a standard or protein snack may be needed for levels <126 mg/dL (7 mmol/L).[131] Postexercise and bedtime snacks used to prevent late-onset and nighttime hypoglycemia should likely contain some protein and fat (such as found in whole milk, soymilk, yogurt, peanut butter, etc), which are metabolized more slowly and keep blood glucose levels more stable over time than carbohydrate alone.[106,131] A higher fat dinner meal with the same carbohydrate and protein content as a lower fat one raises insulin resistance and insulin dosing requirements for individuals with type 1 diabetes.[132,133] Consumption of bedtime carbohydrates that are more slowly digested may also prevent nighttime hypoglycemia following exercise.

Timing of Snacks

The next consideration is when snacks should be eaten, if being used to prevent hypoglycemia during physical activity itself.

- *If the activity is soon after a meal or usual snack:* No extra food may be needed. If more food is required, the amount can be adjusted upward to achieve the desired blood glucose.

- *If the activity is being performed more than 2 hours after a meal:* A snack may be needed within 15 minutes of beginning the physical activity to give it sufficient time to be digested and to enter the bloodstream, making glucose available to active muscles.

Fluids and Electrolytes

Maintaining adequate hydration is important during physical activity. Replenishing fluids is especially important if the activity results in excessive perspiration or lasts longer than an hour, but excessive fluid intake (resulting in hyponatremia) should be avoided.[134]

If water is being consumed during the activity, additional carbohydrates can be introduced via a sports drink or other beverage. Drinks containing 6% to 8% carbohydrate (ie, 6-8 g carbohydrate per 100 ml of fluid) optimize gastric emptying.[135] However, drinks with a carbohydrate concentration greater than 10% should be avoided during exercise because their high osmolality not only delays gastric emptying but also favors fluid shifts into the gut. Fruit juices and most regular soft drinks contain approximately 12% carbohydrate and can lead to gastrointestinal upset, such as cramps, nausea, vomiting, diarrhea, or bloating and "sloshing" during exercise, if not diluted with water.

Since the carbohydrates in sports beverages are quickly absorbed, a few ounces must be consumed every 5 to 10 minutes to provide a consistent supply of fuel to prevent peaks and valleys in blood glucose levels. A 24-oz bottle of a typical sports drink contains about 42 g of carbohydrate, which satisfies the recommended hourly intake for most endurance workouts, along with supplying important electrolytes crucial for fluid and pH balance, neuronal and muscle function, and prevention of muscle cramps.

Medication Adjustments

As an alternate or in addition to snacking, the individual may be able to adjust medications to prevent hypoglycemia associated with being active. For those with type 2 diabetes, it depends on whether the medication is likely to cause hypoglycemia (the majority do not), whereas anyone with type 1 diabetes or any insulin user may need to consider dosing adjustments to maintain euglycemia with exercise.

Oral Agents

Meglitinides are the main class of oral antihyperglycemic agents that can be acutely adjusted for physical activity. Since both medications in this class (repaglinide and nateglinide) have a short duration of action, either one may be reduced or omitted if physical activity is undertaken a few hours after the meal. However, if physical activity is erratic or unpredictable, this may not be the best option.

The doses of select other oral medications that can increase the risk for exercise-associated hypoglycemia (ie, sulfonylureas) may need to be lowered once a physical activity routine that improves insulin action is established, but not in anticipation of a single exercise session. Longer-term adjustments may be needed for doses of sulfonylureas when exercise participation is regular.[113]

Cases—Part 3: Learning to Make Appropriate Adjustments

Type 1 Diabetes

Insulin Dose Adjustments

HW remembered being told that he may need to reduce his insulin dose before exercise. The next time he went to the health club, he took 1 unit less than his normal 10-unit dinner dose, thinking that a blood glucose of 154 mg/dL (8.6 mmol/L) before his aerobic workout was high enough. He hoped to see it go down during exercise and it did—but too fast: 15 minutes into his workout he had to stop and treat another low blood glucose, this time 63 mg/dL (3.5 mmol/L). After reducing his insulin by half the next time, he became alarmed when his blood glucose reading the next night was 287 mg/dL (15.9 mmol/L) before his workout. He remembered something about not exercising with a blood glucose over 250 mg/dL (13.9 mmol/L) and ketones. Since he did not have ketone strips to check, he skipped the workout and went home not knowing what to do.

Type 2 Diabetes

Snacks and Timing

DK thought about her pre-exercise snack and decided she did not need the peanut butter crackers before walking. However, she was still concerned about hypoglycemia and decided to walk only after she had eaten a meal. Sometimes this worked in her schedule, and sometimes it did not. When she was able to fit in a walk, DK noticed that her blood glucose levels had dropped by the time she finished. She was also glad she could skip all those extra calories. Yet she was sure she would have to walk a lot more to lose weight.

Insulin Adjustments

When engaging in physical activity, the individual using insulin must focus on the blood glucose level, which is affected by circulating levels of insulin and catecholamine release.

- If the circulating level of insulin is greater than physiological needs, hypoglycemia can occur.
- If the circulating level of insulin is insufficient, hyperglycemia can result.

The physiological decrease in circulating insulin levels, which is a typical response to physical activity, does not naturally occur in anyone treated with exogenous insulin. Reductions in the bolus insulin dose accompanying the meal before exercise or consumption of additional carbohydrate during exercise are typically needed to avoid hypoglycemia during prolonged exercise (>30 min). Individuals can reduce their rapid- or short-acting insulin dose administered within 1 to 2 hours by 20% to 30% prior to prolonged exercise of moderate intensity,[106–108] as outlined in Table 6.9. A dose administered within an hour after the activity ends may also need to be decreased to prevent postexercise hypoglycemia. Basal insulin doses may be reduced as well but are adjusted less frequently for shorter bouts of activity and more often for prolonged exercise or regular training; insulin pump users are able to change basal delivery more easily than individuals who take multiple daily injections.[136,137]

TABLE 6.9 General Bolus Insulin Reductions Before Aerobic Activities Based on Duration and Intensity

Duration (min)	*Intensity (%)*		
	Easy	*Moderate*	*Vigorous*
30	0–25	25–50	50–75*
60	25–50	50–75	50–100
120	25–75	50–100	75–100

Note: These premeal insulin changes assume that an individual is not eating extra food to compensate and that exercise starts within 1 to 2 hours after the bolus. Less or no insulin reduction may be needed if starting after that. For insulin pump users, basal rate reductions during an activity may be greater or less than these, whether done alone or with reduced boluses. Individuals may also need insulin reductions (bolus and basal) after activities to prevent later-onset lows.

* For intense, near-maximal exercise, individuals may need an increase in rapid-acting insulin (rather than a decrease) to counter the effects of glucose raising-hormones.

Used with permission from SR Colberg, *The Athlete's Guide to Diabetes: Expert Advice for 165 Sports and Activities* (Champaign, IL: Human Kinetics, 2019), 36.

For a more in-depth discussion on how to adjust insulin levels, refer to "Exercise management in type 1 diabetes: a consensus statement" (*Lancet Diabetes Endocrinol,* 2017).[14]

For specific, real-life athlete examples of regimen adjustments for 165 sports and activities, refer to *The Athlete's Guide to Diabetes* (Human Kinetics, 2019).[102]

With insulin pump therapy, basal rates and boluses can more easily be adjusted based on the timing, duration, intensity, and type of activity performed. Insulin pump users have these options to prevent hypoglycemia during periods of physical activity:

- Reduce the basal infusion rate (before, during, and/or after physical activity).
- Consume additional carbohydrates.
- Temporarily suspend pump or lower basal rates (before, during, and/or following activity).

Insulin should be injected into the subcutaneous fat layer as its intramuscular injection can lower blood glucose levels too rapidly when combined with muscular contractions during exercise. The absorption of all bolus insulins is accelerated somewhat by changes in cutaneous circulation during exercise,[138] and changing the subcutaneous injection site to a part of the body not involved in the activity does not reduce the risk of hypoglycemia. Any time the level of circulating insulin from exogenous sources is elevated during activities, hypoglycemia is more likely to occur.

Problem Solving

As discussed, many strategies can be used to assist individuals in maintaining euglycemia during and following physical activity. The diabetes care and education specialist must consider that the routine will vary from person to person. While one option may be preferred by an individual, there will be situations when a different strategy works better for achieving the desired blood glucose results. When problem solving after an unexpected blood glucose response, consider that each person's blood glucose response may differ due to any of the following:

- Type of diabetes
- Type of insulin taken and delivery method
- Effect of other medications (eg, insulin secretagogues, corticosteroids)
- Time of day exercise is undertaken

- Frequency, intensity, type, and total time of physical activity
- Fitness level of individual
- Blood glucose level at start of physical activity

Many other factors contribute to the blood glucose response to physical activity. As many of these factors can change over time, at each visit the educator needs to ensure that the prescribed exercise plan continues to fit the physiological needs of the person with diabetes. The following must also be regularly considered:

- Seasonal variations
- Weight loss or gain
- Changes in training state and fitness levels
- Impact of overtraining
- Altered medication dosing
- Sleep patterns
- Orthopedic limitations or injury
- Diabetes or other health complications
- Hormonal changes in women (monthly menstrual cycle, menopause)

In short, regimen changes should be tailored to each individual's specific response to physical activity (see Table 6.10). The choices depend on the individual's goals and may require using a combination of additional carbohydrate/food intake and insulin (or other medication) adjustments.

TABLE 6.10 Therapy Adjustments to Prevent Hypoglycemia Associated With Physical Activity
Adjust *insulin* (and insulin secretagogues) for:
Weight loss (may require less)
Improved blood glucose management (may require more or less)
Planned, regular physical activity (may require less overall)
Adjust with additional *carbohydrate* (or other macronutrients) for:
Pre-exercise blood glucose likely to result in hypoglycemia during activity
Long duration of physical activity
Spontaneous or erratic physical activity
No insulin adjustments made
Select oral diabetes medications (ie, sulfonylureas, meglitinides)

General Physical Activity Safety Considerations

- Teach all individuals with diabetes who are treated with insulin, sulfonylureas, or meglitinides to carry rapidly absorbed carbohydrates (eg, glucose tablets or gels) with them while performing physical activity so that they can treat hypoglycemia quickly.
- Teach individuals to monitor blood glucose, both before and after activity, to promote safety and understanding of the glycemic effects of exercise.
- Advise individuals to wear some form of diabetes and personal identification and carry a mobile phone that enables them to request assistance in case of emergency.
- Advise individuals to avoid exercising in extremely hot, humid, smoggy, or cold environments.
- Encourage individuals to wear clothing and shoes appropriate for the activity to reduce chance of injury, and check feet daily for signs of redness or trauma.
- Be aware that certain medications can impair exercise tolerance; for example, beta-adrenergic blocking agents lower the HR response to physical activity, as well as mask hypoglycemic symptoms and lessen counterregulatory responses.
- Advise individuals to stop the activity if symptoms like pain, lightheadedness, or shortness of breath occur.
- Since seasonal changes in A1C have been related to environmental temperature,[139] encourage individuals to find places to be active indoors when the weather is cold.

Modifying Exercise for Comorbid Health Issues

Individuals with health complications of diabetes or other comorbid health issues often do not undertake regular physical activity. Yet, being regularly active is especially useful for this group to improve or maintain functional capacity, strength, balance, and flexibility, even when diabetes and related conditions present additional challenges to participation. For instance, proliferative retinopathy may limit participation in activities that cause rapid blood pressure swings; cardiac autonomic neuropathy requires extensive warm-up and cool-down phases; peripheral neuropathy necessitates frequent foot inspections and possibly limiting weight-bearing activity; and peripheral vascular disease requires limiting intensity to a tolerable pain threshold.[26] Physical activity planning for specific groups of individuals, including those who are overweight or obese, pregnant, old, young, or underprivileged, needs to take their unique physical and/or emotional requirements into consideration. In addition, a lack of self-efficacy or self-esteem related to being active may be evident,[140] but individuals can participate in being active safely and effectively as long as certain precautions are taken.

Cardiovascular Disease and Hypertension

Cardiovascular disease is the major cause of morbidity and mortality for people with diabetes. As such, a careful cardiac assessment is warranted prior to initiating any moderate- to vigorous-intensity fitness program. The existence of any cardiac risk factors should be determined, and emphasis should be placed on their management to help prevent or slow the disease process. When a fitness program that exceeds the demands of everyday living (ie, more intense than brisk walking) is being considered for a previously sedentary individual, the ADA has established criteria[29] to help determine whether a graded exercise test is warranted (as shown previously in Table 6.2).

When working with individuals with cardiovascular (heart) disease, focus attention on blood pressure and heart rate responses to training. Advise these individuals to start resistance training with lighter resistances to help decrease the myocardial oxygen demand on the heart.[141,142] Heart rate and blood pressure need to be monitored during training and remain within the limits established by an exercise stress test, keeping in mind that myocardial perfusion will be similar or enhanced during resistance training at heart rate limits established during aerobic exercise testing. While cardiovascular disease is not a contraindication to any form of exercise, anyone with angina classified as moderate or high risk should preferably exercise in a supervised cardiac rehabilitation program, at least initially, and heart rate should be kept at least 10 bpm below the onset of exercise-induced angina (if present).

Since individuals with diabetes have an increased risk of cardiovascular disease, a comprehensive assessment is recommended for those meeting the pre-exercise screening criteria to determine the most appropriate physical activity options.

- For all individuals, assess risk with a physical activity history and/or an exercise test, to guide prescription.
- Recommend that high-risk individuals with established cardiovascular disease (eg, recent acute coronary syndrome or revascularization, heart failure) be supervised in a cardiac rehabilitation or other medically supervised program during exercise.
- Encourage 30 to 60 minutes of moderate-intensity aerobic activity, such as brisk walking, on most, preferably all, days of the week, supplemented by an increase in daily lifestyle activities (eg, walking breaks at work, gardening, household work).
- Recommend resistance training on at least 2 nonconsecutive days, but preferably 3, per week.
- Advise individuals to avoid activities that cause a hypertensive response (systolic blood pressure >260 mm Hg, diastolic blood pressure >125 mm Hg), including those that involve heavy lifting, straining, and Valsalva-like maneuvers.

Peripheral Artery Disease

Individuals with peripheral artery disease will experience ischemic pain in the lower extremities during physical activity due to an insufficient oxygen supply in those active muscles. A low-intensity walking program for intermittent claudication may improve collateral circulation and muscle metabolism and, in turn, decrease pain.[143] Generally, low- or moderate-intensity walking, arm ergometer, and leg ergometer are the preferred aerobic activities, but all other activities can be taken as pain permits. Lower-extremity resistance training also improves functional performance.[144]

- Advise individuals that daily physical activity sessions will maximize pain tolerance during movement.
- Help individuals determine the distance and duration for walking by a pain-limited threshold.
- Advise individuals to keep the intensity lower, as higher intensity demands a greater blood supply and will likely cause claudication pain.
- Encourage individuals to use conversation, music, and other elements to divert attention from the discomfort and pain.
- Stop activity when the discomfort or pain increases from moderate to intense and attention cannot be diverted from the pain.
- Recommend weight-bearing activities, although non-weight-bearing activities may be used if longer duration and higher intensity workouts are the goal.

Retinopathy, Visual Impairment, and Blindness

The presence of retinopathy (retinal eye disease) should be evaluated for all people with diabetes based on established clinical guidelines. People without diabetic retinopathy or who have only mild nonproliferative diabetic retinopathy (NPDR) do not have activity limitations. Those with moderate, severe, or very severe NPDR and those with

TABLE 6.11 Physical Activity With Retinopathy

Level of Retinopathy	*Physical Activity and Exercise Recommendations*
No diabetic retinopathy	No physical activity/exercise limitations
Mild nonproliferative	No physical activity/exercise limitations
Moderate nonproliferative	Avoid activities that dramatically elevate blood pressure (eg, power lifting)
Severe to very severe nonproliferative	Limit increase in systolic blood pressure (eg, Valsalva maneuver) and avoid activities that jar the head; heart rate should not exceed that which elicits a systolic blood pressure response greater than 170 mm Hg (boxing and intense competitive sports)
Proliferative	Avoid strenuous activity, high-impact activities, Valsalva maneuvers, and activities that jar the head (eg, weight lifting, jogging, high-impact aerobic dance, racquet sports, strenuous trumpet playing, and competitive sports) Encourage activities that are low impact and aerobic, and stress cardiovascular conditioning (eg, swimming without diving, walking, low-impact aerobic dance, stationary cycling, and endurance exercising)

proliferative diabetic retinopathy should be educated on the limitations during exercise and even routine physical activities. Macular edema and glaucoma should be evaluated by an ophthalmologist or optometrist and activity guidelines determined by the results of the examination. More specific information is provided in Table 6.11 for the different levels of retinopathy.

The level of retinopathy determines which activities are appropriate and which are better avoided. While background or preproliferative retinopathy requires no precautions, individuals with advanced proliferative retinopathy will have significant restrictions in their level of physical exertion and activity options. Visual impairment itself resulting from diabetes-related or other eye disease should not be considered a contraindication to exercise but may require precautions.

- Provide physical activity recommendations based on the severity and stage of diabetic retinopathy.
- Advise individuals with unstable proliferative diabetic retinopathy to seek clearance for exercise from their ophthalmologist due to risk of vitreous hemorrhage or traction retinal detachment.
- Advise individuals with unstable, advanced proliferative disease that activities producing large increases in blood pressure are not advised, such as high-intensity aerobic exercise, heavy resistance training, jumping or jarring activities, or exercises in a head-down position.[26]
- Recommend appropriate options for physical activity, such as swimming using lane guides, stationary cycling, treadmill walking, tandem cycling, and dancing, using a sighted person as a guide when appropriate for visual impairment.

Neuropathy

The main forms of diabetes-related neuropathy (nerve damage) are autonomic, gastroparesis, and peripheral.[145] Table 6.12 lists special considerations for physical activity that should accompany each of these forms. When progression of these symptoms presents safety issues, a clinically supervised exercise setting may be prudent. When this option is not available, self-monitoring is important; the person must be able to make appropriate decisions independently when engaging in physical activity.

Autonomic Neuropathy

For individuals with autonomic neuropathy, physical activity must be approached with caution because of the role that the autonomic nervous system plays in hormonal and cardiovascular regulation during exercise. The presence of cardiac autonomic neuropathy (CAN) doubles the risk of mortality and is associated with more frequent silent myocardial ischemia, orthostatic hypotension, and resting elevations in HR, leading to impaired exercise tolerance, low maximal HR, and slower HR recovery.[146] HR is also sluggish in responding to positional changes (eg, sitting to standing) and blunted during Valsalva maneuvers.[145] A blunting in heart rate variability increases an individual's chance of dying suddenly from cardiac arrest, possibly even during physical activities. Blood pressure responses may be abnormal when changing positions or performing isometric exercise, which may lead to orthostatic hypotension during activities, and an exaggerated rise in blood pressure is possible.[147] Dehydration is a greater concern, as is impaired thermoregulation during exercise, especially done in environmental extremes. Care must be taken with all components of the exercise prescription.

TABLE 6.12 Physical Activity Considerations With Neuropathy

Type of Neuropathy	*Safety Concern Associated With Type of Neuropathy*	*Action to Discuss*
Autonomic	Inability to recognize signs and symptoms of hypoglycemia	Monitor blood glucose during physical activity; set higher blood glucose goals
	Blunted heart rate response to physical activity (cardiac)	Monitor intensity with HRR, RPE, or "talk test"
	Erratic blood pressure response during exercise, increased risk of postural hypotension	Monitor blood pressure during physical activity; determine whether different positions (sitting, standing, reclining, supine) affect results
	Lack of effective thermoregulation for hot and cold environments	Monitor environment; drink fluids to prevent dehydration; wear proper clothing
Gastroparesis	Erratic emptying rate of stomach and digestion of food	Monitor blood glucose as needed; use foods absorbed in the mouth to treat hypoglycemia (eg, glucose tabs, glucose gels, and hard candies); delay injection of rapid-acting insulin until after activity
	Discomfort following consumption of a meal or specific type of food	Determine whether physical activity impedes or promotes food mobility; plan timing of physical activity as symptoms tolerate
Peripheral	Discomfort or pain with physical activity	Limit weight-bearing options based on level of tolerance
	Injury, infection, ulceration	Monitor feet daily for blisters, cuts, scrapes; teach proper hygiene techniques for foot and skin care; choose appropriate footwear (shoes and socks); consider need for orthotics or orthopedic shoes

Nonetheless, regular exercise participation is important for these individuals. Moderate-intensity aerobic training can improve autonomic function in individuals with and without CAN,[148] although anyone with CAN should have an exercise stress test and physician approval before commencing exercise. Exercise intensity may be accurately prescribed using the HRR method with maximal HR directly measured, rather than estimated, for better accuracy.[50]

- Advise individuals with autonomic neuropathy (particularly CAN) to avoid high-intensity physical activities unless they have been cleared by a physician to participate.
- Encourage individuals to avoid physical exertion in hot or cold environments since dehydration may be more likely to occur, or they may overheat due to faulty thermoregulation.
- Caution individuals that hypotension or hypertension may occur after vigorous activities or when making rapid positional changes during activities.
- Recommend recumbent cycling or water aerobics for individuals with orthostatic hypotension.
- For better accuracy, advise individuals to monitor exercise intensity using the HRR method, using a measured maximal HR rather than using an estimate, if possible.

Gastroparesis

A form of autonomic neuropathy, gastroparesis produces physically uncomfortable and potentially embarrassing episodes for the individual with this complication. Common complaints are nausea, vomiting, feeling overly full after eating, bloating, intestinal pain, alternating bouts of constipation and diarrhea, and lack of appetite.[119,149] Any of these can make physical activity difficult to perform. Medications and foods must be balanced as part of the exercise prescription to help minimize these symptoms.

- Encourage individuals to adopt eating practices that minimize problems, such as consuming only small portions and avoiding eating a large meal before exercise as doing so can delay gastric emptying.
- Advise individuals with gastroparesis that exercise-related hypoglycemia may be harder to treat quickly with food as its absorption may be slowed.
- Caution that to treat hypoglycemia, it may be necessary to consume some glucose tablets before blood glucose levels drop that low to prevent it from becoming severe.
- Recommend more frequent blood glucose monitoring, both before and after exercise when hypoglycemia is more likely to occur.

Peripheral Neuropathy, Ulcers, and Amputation

Peripheral neuropathy, with an associated decrease in sensation, carries with it an increased risk of injury as those with insensate feet may not have the pain sensation needed to recognize that an injury has occurred. A blister or repeated trauma to a bone may go unnoticed. Also, sensations connected to balance and strength can be diminished, and gait can be altered, contributing to development of orthopedic issues and a greater risk of falling. In fact, individuals with type 2 diabetes without overt peripheral neuropathy exhibit altered and less efficient gait patterns.[150] The individual may become fearful of falling and avoid physical activity. Walking, standing, or getting out of a chair can be difficult. In those with painful symptoms, greater discomfort may occur during physical activity, although that may not preclude participation.[151] Safety must be the prime consideration of the exercise prescription.

Physical activity cannot fully reverse the symptoms of peripheral neuropathy, but it can prevent further loss of muscle strength and flexibility commonly seen in individuals with sensory polyneuropathy. Prior recommendations stated that individuals with severe peripheral neuropathy should avoid weight-bearing activities to lower their risk of foot ulcerations; however, moderate-intensity walking does not appear to increase risk of foot ulcers or re-ulceration in those with peripheral neuropathy.[152,153] Moreover, mild to moderate exercise can actually prevent the onset of peripheral neuropathy itself.[154] Thus, individuals without acute foot ulcers can and likely should perform moderate weight-bearing exercise. All individuals should closely examine their feet on a daily basis to detect sores or ulcers early.

- Encourage individuals with any degree of peripheral neuropathy to wear shoes with silica gel or air midsoles (for optimal stability and shock absorption), along with wearing polyester or cotton-polyester blend socks to prevent blisters and keep feet dry during physical activities.
- Advise individuals without acute foot ulcers to engage in mild or moderate weight-bearing exercise to improve muscle tone, balance ability, and awareness of lower extremities.
- Recommend daily range-of-motion exercises to help minimize shortening of connective tissue surrounding lower extremity joints.
- Low-impact activities are viable options as well; recommended exercises include swimming, pool walking, water aerobics and other pool-based exercise, stationary bicycling, rowing, arm ergometer work, upper-body exercises, tai chi, qigong, yoga, seated aerobic and resistance exercises, and other non-weight-bearing activities.
- Recommend that individuals with a foot injury or open sore avoid weight-bearing activities because of an increased chance of soft tissue and joint injury; aquatic activities should be avoided when individuals have unhealed ulcers.
- Encourage individuals to wear proper footwear and inspect their feet after physical activity to prevent blisters and detect injuries.
- Advise individuals to avoid jogging, as it places a threefold increase in pressure on the foot compared with walking.
- Suggest chair or seated exercises for individuals with limited mobility or lower extremity amputations to improve fitness, flexibility, and strength.
- If present, amputation sites should be properly cared for daily; if amputation sites become irritated or traumatized due to weight-bearing activities, suggest switching to non-weight-bearing ones.

Diabetic Kidney Disease

Exercise does not accelerate progression of diabetic kidney disease, and greater participation in moderate-to-vigorous leisure time activity and higher physical activity levels may actually moderate the initiation and progression of diabetic nephropathy.[155,156] Although urinary albumin excretion rates can rise proportionally with increasing exercise intensity during the period following the activity, such changes should not be interpreted to mean that exercise is causing additional damage.[157]

The risk of developing specific comorbidities increases as nephropathy progresses. Often, the individual with overt nephropathy has diminished capacity for physical activity, causing a self-limitation of strenuous physical activity. Yet, people at all stages of nephropathy can benefit from staying physically active, and physical activity during dialysis sessions is possible and often recommended to increase functional capacity.[158] Table 6.13 provides information highlighting these considerations for the exercise prescription.

Cardiovascular disease is the leading cause of death within the chronic kidney disease population, with an inverse relationship between decreasing kidney function and increased prevalence of cardiovascular problems. In addition, individuals with diabetes kidney disease usually have low functional and aerobic capacity, particularly in the later stages of the disease. Aerobic activities are preferred, but the individual's degree of kidney impairment

TABLE 6.13 Physical Activity Considerations With Nephropathy

Increased Risk of	*Physical Activity*	*Points to Consider*
Bone disease	Strength training program	Promotes bone strength; improves balance and gait; reduces risk of falls and fractures
Hypertension or exaggerated blood pressure response to activity	Avoid or modify physical activities that cause extreme increases in systolic blood pressure	Blood pressure should be monitored; medications should be adjusted as needed to keep resting and exercise blood pressure in desired ranges
Edema	As tolerated	Instruction should be provided for dietary and fluid intake to minimize this condition; foot elevation or use of compression stockings may be useful
Anemia	As tolerated	Treat as needed to keep hematocrit levels between 33% and 36%
Loss of independence	Promote physically active lifestyle	Increases ability to maintain activities of daily living, which may limit dependence on others as disease progresses
Depression	Promote physically active lifestyle	Provides a level of protection from depression, hopelessness, and doom

dictates his or her ability to perform aerobic activity. Individuals who are weak can benefit from strength training interventions. Resistance and aerobic exercise programs should be initiated at relatively low intensity and progressed slowly as tolerated to avoid injury and discontinuation of exercise. Offering exercise programming during maintenance hemodialysis treatments may increase the likelihood of regular exercise participation, enhance quality of life, and lower symptoms of depression in those with end-stage renal disease.[159]

- Recommend that individuals begin aerobic activity at a low level, perhaps using interval work, followed by gradual increases in their activity plan.
- Advise individuals to progress over time to brisk walking, swimming, and cycling activities, as well as resistance training to improve strength.
- Encourage individuals on hemodialysis to incorporate exercise into the dialysis session to increase participation and tolerance but have them closely monitor blood electrolytes.

Cases—Part 4: Adjusting Workout Duration and Intensity

Type 1 Diabetes

Workout Intensity and Adjustments

HW decided to try another type of exercise with a reduced insulin dose, this time a heavy session of resistance (weight) training instead of an aerobic workout. Since his blood glucose had gone too high when he cut his predinner insulin in half, he reduced it by only 25% this time. About 30 minutes into his intense workout with heavy free weights, he started to feel funny so he pulled out his monitor and checked his blood glucose. He was shocked that his reading was even higher than before, this time at 318 mg/dL (17.7 mmol/L). He really had no idea why it had gone higher even with taking more insulin than the previous time, but he knew it was not supposed to get that high. He immediately stopped his workout and again went home not knowing what to do. He woke up in the middle of the night feeling shaky and sweating profusely with a blood glucose of 54 mg/dL (3.0 mmol/L), which was puzzling to him since he had not taken any extra insulin to bring down his high postworkout level and it had still been elevated (188 mg/dL [10.4 mmol/L]) at bedtime. Now he was really confused about how to handle his blood glucose and still engage in any type of exercise.

Type 2 Diabetes

Workout Duration and Progression

DK decided she would just have to walk longer to burn calories and improve her blood glucose level. She decided to walk 60 minutes each day on most days of the week. She was sure this would work—until she tried it. After the first 40 minutes on the first day, she was not even sure she would make it home. When she walked into her house, she felt very shaky and checked her blood glucose. It was 104 mg/dL (5.8 mmol/L), her lowest number yet. She immediately went to the freezer and pulled out the ice cream. To top off her woes, her right hip was in severe pain for days. She surely was not going to put herself through that again!

Overweight and Obese

Combined programs of physical activity, meal planning, and behavior change are effective for overweight and obese individuals. The introduction of several newer diabetes medications that induce satiety and reduce food intake or block reabsorption of blood glucose used alone or in conjunction with weight neutral medications provides therapeutic options to achieve glucose management without body weight gain. Physical activity combined with meal planning has been shown to be more effective for long-term weight loss than either done alone. Approaches that emphasize physical activity offer enhanced calorie expenditure and provide the benefits of improved fitness related to influencing blood lipids, blood glucose, blood pressure, mood, and attitude. Regular physical activity also helps maintain muscle mass while promoting fat loss during weight loss.[41,160] Visceral (ectopic) fat accumulation is also a concern in overweight and obese adults, and regular physical activity effectively reduces visceral and liver adipose tissue; therefore, being active should be a key feature of programs aimed at reducing visceral fat in obesity-related diabetes.[161,162]

The optimal volume of exercise needed to achieve sustained major weight loss is likely much larger than that needed to achieve improved blood glucose levels and cardiovascular health. Individuals who successfully maintain large weight loss over at least a year typically engage in about 7 hours per week of moderate- to vigorous-intensity exercise,[163] although greater exercise volumes (2,000 and 2,500 calories per week) produce greater and more sustained weight loss than smaller exercise volumes (1,000 calories per week). However, even simply engaging in more unstructured physical activity (eg, errands, household tasks, dog walking, gardening) increases daily energy expenditure and assists with weight management. Unstructured activity also reduces total daily sitting time. When working with obese individuals, use the following guidelines to increase their daily physical activity level:

- Encourage individuals to engage in more daily movement to further increase calorie expenditure and to reduce total sedentary time.
- Recommend moderate aerobic exercise that uses large muscle groups, with emphasis on increasing duration and frequency.
- Recommend walking as an effective choice for continuous aerobic exercise; alternative types of exercise include cycling and chair and water exercise.
- Encourage engaging in non-weight-bearing activities to reduce the risk of orthopedic injury; higher intensity weight-bearing activities like running and jogging are not recommended until body weight is reduced or for anyone with preexisting lower extremity joint issues.
- Recommend aiming for 45 to 60 minutes of activity 5 to 7 days per week.
- Recommend a target range of 300 to 400 calories of energy expenditure per day, or 2,000 calories per week in physical activity.
- Advise individuals to undertake recommended amounts of resistance training to build muscle strength and mass and retain muscle during periods of weight loss.
- If self-conscious about exercising with others due to body size, encourage overweight individuals to be active in more private settings (like at home) or by doing aquatic activities.

Pregnancy

Women with either gestational or preexisting diabetes during pregnancy are encouraged to engage in regular physical activity to help enhance insulin action and prevent excess weight gain. In fact, regular exercise may help prevent some cases of gestational diabetes.[164–167] Pregnant women with diabetes can generally follow recommendations made for all pregnant women by the American College of Obstetricians and Gynecologists.[43] Engaging in regular physical activity makes it easier for pregnant women with any type of diabetes to manage their blood glucose.[168] Exercise intensity should be mild or moderate and should be undertaken for up to 30 minutes at a time during most days of the week (eg, 150 minutes per week). Vigorous activities are generally not recommended during pregnancy unless women have been engaging in them prior to becoming pregnant.[169] Activities to undertake include moderate walking, indoor cycling, swimming and aquatic activities, low-impact aerobics, seated exercise routines, and mild or moderate resistance training.[170]

Safety concerns for pregnant women revolve around prevention of falls, blows to the abdomen, and reduced blood flow through the placenta. They should avoid contact sports, most racquet sports (requiring rapid movements and changes in direction), water and snow skiing, scuba diving, outdoor cycling (later in pregnancy), and running (unless the woman ran before becoming pregnant), as well as exercises done lying flat on the back (after the first trimester) or in environmental extremes. Precautions to avoid hypoglycemia or hyperglycemia resulting from exercise are similar for pregnant and nonpregnant women. Standing still for long periods of time should also be avoided. Women diagnosed with gestational diabetes mellitus are at substantially increased risk of developing type 2 diabetes later in life, and physical activity of all intensities may be considered a tool to prevent both Gestational Diabetes Mellitus (GDM) and possibly diabetes onset at a later date.

- Recommend engaging in 30 minutes of moderate exercise most days of the week, aiming for a total of 150 minutes; individuals who were sedentary pre-pregnancy should start out slowly.
- Recommend wearing comfortable clothing that will help individuals remain cool, along with a bra that fits well and gives adequate support.
- Encourage pregnant exercisers to drink plenty of water to avoid overheating and dehydrating.
- Recommend consuming enough daily calories to replace those used during exercise.
- Advise avoidance of exercise done in hot, humid weather or with a fever.
- Running, certain racquet sports, and vigorous resistance training can be continued by women doing these activities before becoming pregnant, but do not advise beginning them during pregnancy.
- Recommend that pregnant women avoid contact sports, downhill skiing, scuba diving, and sports requiring quick directional changes.
- Advise individuals to avoid doing any exercise lying flat on their back after the first trimester of pregnancy.
- Advise all pregnant women that they may safely engage in light to moderate resistance training throughout pregnancy.
- Advise pregnant women to stop exercising and call their healthcare team if they develop symptoms during activity, including vaginal bleeding, dizziness, increased shortness of breath, chest pain, headache, muscle weakness, calf pain or swelling, uterine contractions, decreased fetal movement, or fluid leaking from the vagina.

Older Adults

Older adults who have been primarily sedentary and may have physical limitations present a challenge for diabetes care and education specialists. Give special consideration to changes in body composition that may have occurred over the years (eg, declines in muscle mass and muscle strength, with resultant decreases in basal metabolic rate, activity level, and energy expenditure). Older adults who do any kind of physical activity can improve not only their blood glucose levels but also their muscle tone, bone health, flexibility, balance, and mental outlook. In fact, both high levels of sedentary time and low levels of moderate to vigorous physical activity are strong and independent predictors of early death from any cause in adults ages 50 years or older.[20] Brain health is also of increasing importance in an aging population, and being active has been shown to improve cognition, inclusive of executive function, attention memory, crystallized intelligence, processing speed.[42]

Table 6.14 summarizes the guidelines for aerobic exercise in older adults. Guidelines for adults ages 18 to 64 for aerobic exercise, resistance training, and flexibility also apply to older individuals, who should still adhere to the regimen prescribed for all adults, but they should also do multicomponent physical activity.[27] In particular, they should perform exercises that include lower extremity strength and balance training to reduce their risk of falls, and other special considerations may be needed. Osteoarthritis in lower extremity joints is common in older adults, particularly in those who are overweight or obese. However, participation in regular physical activity is possible and should be encouraged as moderate activity may improve joint symptoms and alleviate pain. Brisk walking, gardening, yard work, and housework are good examples of recommended

TABLE 6.14 Summary of Guidelines for Aerobic Exercise in Older Adults

Activity	Cycling, brisk walking, swimming, dancing, rowing
Duration	Intersperse initial activity sessions with brief rest periods until an activity can be performed for longer, and add 2–5 minutes per week until desired goal (30 minutes or more at a time) is met
Frequency	At least 3 nonconsecutive days per week, but ideally spread out over 5 or more days per week
Intensity	Base initial training intensity on the individual's graded exercise test, risk factors, and medical history: moderate to vigorous (ie, 40%–89% HRR), but starting at a lower level (ie, 30%–39% HRR), if sedentary and progressing slowly to a recommended intensity; determine level of effort relative to initial level of fitness
Volume	At least 150–300 minutes a week of moderate-intensity or 75–150 minutes a week of vigorous-intensity, or an equivalent combination of both, preferably spread throughout the week; if not attainable due to chronic conditions, be as physically active as abilities and conditions safely allow
Progression	Assess progress and reevaluate the individual's fitness plan every 4–6 weeks until minimal recommendations are met; avoid injuries due to overtraining or joint limitations

moderate-intensity activities. Adding resistance exercise can also promote stronger bone health, especially in women as they age.[171] Intensity is likely not as important as frequency of activity in this age group. Simply decreasing total sitting time and having active breaks during sedentary activities may also be a useful goal for all older adults.[172]

Safety concerns may preclude older adults from walking due to a high risk for falls and subsequent fracture. Osteoarthritis is also common in the lower extremity joints, particularly for older adults who are overweight or obese, and knee and hip pain may directly contribute to the progression of sarcopenia and increased falls risk in older adults, especially women.[173] Their participation in regular physical activity is possible and should be encouraged because moderate activity may improve joint symptoms and alleviate pain and lower falls risk. Activity options may include using a stationary cycle, lifting light or moderate weights, or exercising while seated. Exercise videos, classes, and routines that can be done from a chair, rather than standing, may be helpful in this population.

Aerobic Activity: Older Adults

- Highly recommend that adults have a thorough medical exam before starting an exercise program of moderate or higher intensity if they have been sedentary.
- Recommend that older adults do at least 150 to 300 minutes a week of moderate or 75 to 150 minutes of vigorous-intensity, or a combination of both, preferably spread throughout the week.
- Instruct individuals to increase exercise duration and frequency before intensity.
- Recommend a conservative approach when increasing exercise intensity, avoiding vigorous aerobic activity at first (except for possibly shorter intervals interspersed during an activity).
- Advise previously sedentary individuals to start at lower levels and gradually increase the duration and frequency to reach the desired fitness level.
- Advise older adults that if chronic conditions prevent reaching recommended activity goals, they should be as physically active as their abilities and conditions allow.
- Recommend aquatic or chair exercises and stationary cycling for individuals with less tolerance for weight-bearing activities, such as those with severe degenerative joint disease or osteoarthritis.
- Particularly if they have joint issues, recommend range of motion activities and light resistance exercise to increase strength of muscles surrounding affected joints.
- Advise avoidance of activities with high risk of joint trauma, such as contact sports and ones with rapid directional changes.
- Advise that no matter what its purpose—gardening, walking the dog, taking a dance or exercise class, or bicycling to the store—activity of all types counts toward meeting recommended levels.
- Recommend that all older adults break up sedentary time with frequent movement and avoid prolonged periods of uninterrupted sitting.

Resistance Training: Older Adults

- Recommend a minimum of 1 set of 8 to 10 exercises for each major muscle group 2 to 3 times a week, progressing up to 2 to 4 sets per exercise session.
- Recommend doing 10 to 15 repetitions, progressing slowly over time to 8 to 12 repetitions at a harder intensity.
- Recommend using a lower resistance for the first 8 weeks to accommodate changes in connective tissue and to prevent injury.
- Suggest using all means of muscle strengthening, including exercises using exercise bands, weight machines, hand-held weights, and using body weight as resistance; digging, lifting, and carrying as part of gardening; carrying groceries; some yoga exercises; and some tai chi exercises.
- Advise individuals with degenerative joint disease or osteoarthritis to avoid resistance training during active periods of joint inflammation or pain.

Flexibility and Balance Exercises: Older Adults

- Recommend a well-rounded stretching program to counteract decreases in flexibility and improve balance and agility.
- Advise doing exercises that maintain or improve balance (such as backward walking, sideways walking, heel walking, toe walking, and standing from a sitting position) 3 or more times a week.
- Let individuals know that doing any type of lower body and core resistance training also counts as balance training.
- For deconditioned individuals who are just beginning to be more active, recommend devoting a significant portion of the exercise session to improving flexibility.

Children and Adolescents

Although type 1 diabetes is most prevalent in youth, type 2 diabetes is being diagnosed in this population at increasing rates. While the causes for this looming epidemic are multiple, the decline in physical activity levels for children and adolescents in the United States is partially responsible. Physical activity has a direct impact on weight management, cardiovascular risk factors, bone development, and mental health over a lifetime. A sedentary lifestyle in young people is often seen to lead to negative health consequences in the near term and later in life. Federal guidelines continue to recommend that all youth ages 6 to 17 years engage in 60 min/day or more of moderate or vigorous-intensity aerobic activity, with equal portions of aerobic, muscle-strengthening and bone-strengthening activity spread throughout the week.[27] These guidelines additionally recommend that preschool-aged children (those between the ages of 3 and 5 years) should be physically active throughout the day. When working with children and adolescents, focus activity recommendations on enjoyable playtime activities, rather than structured exercise bouts. Encourage participation in school physical education classes, recreation leagues, school sports, and active family outings, as well as parental involvement in the planning and development of physical activity programs for children and adolescents.

For children with type 1 diabetes and those with type 2 diabetes taking insulin, careful review of insulin dosages, insulin peaks and durations of action, and timing of meals and snacks is critical if problems with widely variant blood glucose levels, related to physical activity, are to be avoided. Frequent self-monitoring of blood glucose (ie, before, during, and after exercise) will assist in guiding adjustments in insulin dosing that will help avoid the extremes of glycemia. Due to an increased uptake of glucose into skeletal muscle during exercise, children who have not had a regular pattern of activity or conditioning may be particularly susceptible to hypoglycemic episodes near the time of the exercise or hours later. To avoid problems, a decrease in circulating insulin during active periods and modifications in food intake may be needed.

A full discussion of insulin changes by regimen and activity in youth is beyond the scope of this chapter. For comprehensive coverage of insulin, food, and exercise regimen changes for youth with type 1 diabetes (and insulin users with type 2 diabetes), healthcare facilitators are referred to "Exercise management in type 1 diabetes: a consensus statement" (*Lancet Diabetes Endocrinol*, 2017)[14] and *The Athlete's Guide to Diabetes: Expert Advice for 165 Sports and Activities* (Human Kinetics, 2019).[102]

- Recommend that all youth ages 6 to 17 engage in 60 or more minutes of daily moderate or vigorous activity, most of which should be either moderate- or vigorous-intensity aerobic activity and should include vigorous-intensity physical activity on at least 3 days a week.
- Advise inclusion of both muscle-strengthening and bone-strengthening activities on at least 3 days per week as part of the 60 minutes of daily activity.
- Advise parents and caregivers that preschool-aged children (ages 3 through 5 years) should be physically active throughout the day to enhance growth and development, including active play of a variety of activity types.
- Encourage identification of safe and age-appropriate options for physical activity, which should evolve as youth undergo normal maturation in coordination, motor skills, social development, and personal interests.
- Advise parents that athletes with diabetes, especially youth who participate in sports year-round, may be prone to repetitive use, soft tissue injuries that can be avoided with a modified training schedule.
- Include clear assignment of blood glucose management responsibilities among parents and youth with diabetes and allow teenagers to begin to take on more of the responsibility and seek independence from parental supervision.
- Address the blood glucose changes that occur during physical activity to prevent hypoglycemia (and hyperglycemia) during sports and activities.
- Recommend beginning exercise at a target blood glucose level and consuming sufficient carbohydrate or lowering insulin levels to decrease the risk of hypoglycemia.
- Advise parents of young exercisers with diabetes not to overreact to postexercise hyperglycemia, which is usually only transient and may need reduced or no insulin to treat effectively for several hours afterward.
- Address the concern that disordered eating behaviors and compulsive exercise patterns are prevalent among teenagers and young adults with diabetes and advise parents to be vigilant for signs and symptoms of such behaviors.

Cultural and Socioeconomic Considerations

When assisting individuals in planning and preparing for physical activity, consideration must be given to their cultural practices and beliefs and how these may influence the adoption of physical activity behaviors.[174–177] Their ability to access and afford such behaviors must also be taken into consideration, particularly for adults of lower socioeconomic status who may have lesser access to planned physical activity for a variety of reasons.[178,179]

Understanding and being sensitive to beliefs and perceptions regarding physical activity, as well as accessibility, is crucial for successful planning of physical activity goals. Promote activities that do not offend or ignore the individual's cultural beliefs. Elicit information from individuals and provide culturally appropriate suggestions to help tailor suitable physical activity recommendations for their particular group. Consider cost when recommending that individuals with a lower socioeconomic status join an exercise facility and assist them in finding more affordable options if cost is an issue. Consider that their exercise resources may have a limited availability (eg, neighborhood unsafe for walking, lack of accessibility to green spaces and parks),[180–182] or time involvement may create barriers to participation (such as when economic pressures may necessitate working more than one job). Certain cultural traditions also downplay physical activity.

Dance and music are a vital part of tradition and celebration for many ethnically diverse groups, including Native, Hispanic, and African Americans. Asian and Middle Eastern groups may have other cultural traditions that can be brought into the fitness routine, such as yoga and tai chi. By reinforcing the regular inclusion of dance or other cultural physical activities as a healthy lifestyle choice, the diabetes care and education specialist can help individuals with diabetes (and their high-risk family members) make increased activity a regular part of the family routine. The activity helps strengthen families as well.

- Consider cultural practices and beliefs and socioeconomic barriers to regular adoption of a physically active lifestyle.
- Promote activities that are culturally acceptable to individuals, such as walking in groups or dancing for tradition or celebration, and tailor exercise prescription to fall within their beliefs.
- Address economic barriers and resources (eg, cost, availability, lack of childcare) to physical activity participation and assist them in finding viable options to overcome their unique barriers.
- Encourage the adoption of breaking up sedentary time and incorporating more daily movement to promote a more active lifestyle.
- Advise individuals to include family members and friends in their daily activities to create a supportive environment for continued participation.

Putting the Activity Program Into Action

Most diabetes care and education specialists are adept in interpreting and promoting recommendations for physical activity and exercise to individuals with diabetes. Specialists skilled in behavior-change strategies and able to effectively tailor exercise programs to an individual's goals, needs, and interests are better equipped to help individuals become and stay more active. Physical activity programs that are designed primarily by the individual are more likely to be sustained and choosing enjoyable and convenient activities makes it more likely that he or she will participate regularly.

Greater effort also needs to be focused on the promotion of regular exercise among individuals with or at risk for developing type 2 diabetes since lifestyle choices largely influence the onset of this condition. One of the most consistent predictors of greater levels of activity has been higher levels of self-efficacy, which reflect confidence in the ability to exercise. In individuals with type 2 diabetes, interventions should focus on enhancing self-efficacy, problem solving, and social-environmental support to improve self-management (which includes exercise, dietary, and medication behaviors).[183]

Adoption and Maintenance of Exercise by Persons With Diabetes

The following are central determining factors influencing activity across the life span in all individuals, with and without diabetes:

- Self-efficacy (ie, having confidence in one's ability to be active)
- Enjoyment of physical activity
- Lack of perceived barriers to being physically active
- Positive beliefs concerning the benefits of physical activity
- Support from others to continue exercising

Integrating Daily Activity Before Planned Exercise

Diabetes care and education specialists are charged with providing instruction related to the various components of physical fitness in the prevention and treatment of diabetes. As the individualized assessment is performed, the educator gathers information useful in addressing the role of physical activity in the self-management plan. Physical activity may not be one of the initial goals identified by the diabetes care and education specialist or the individual with diabetes to address. Many times, other skills or self-care concepts need to be covered first because they either are health priorities or are more interesting to the person with diabetes (who may already be struggling with the amount of information provided to master to manage blood glucose levels).

A place to start with all individuals may simply be to encourage more physical movement throughout the day. Stress the importance of standing, taking more daily steps, moving whenever possible, and taking frequent activity breaks during sedentary activities.[184–186] Encourage individuals, especially those with type 2 diabetes, to walk after meals to lower postprandial elevations in blood glucose levels.[187]

After briefly introducing the importance of eventually including planned exercise in diabetes management, the diabetes care and education specialist works with the individual to choose other goals on which to focus. However, when the time is right, the healthcare facilitator can redirect the person to goals involving planning, implementing, and assessing the impact of a personalized fitness program that goes beyond simply focusing on more daily activity. Specialists are encouraged to focus more on factors like choice and enjoyment in helping determine specifically how an individual would meet recommended participation.

Enhancing Self-Efficacy Related to Being Active

Beliefs about self-efficacy influence health behaviors. Individuals tend to pursue tasks they feel competent to perform and avoid those in which they feel incompetent.[188] Diabetes care and education specialists can help individuals enhance self-efficacy related to being physically active in the following ways:

- Help the individual develop realistic physical activity goals.
- Plan a gradual program with the individual that incorporates small, incremental steps.
- Encourage setting goals that the individual is likely to attain, to promote feelings of mastery.
- Provide suggestions or opportunities to observe others succeeding at being physically active, such as watching an exercise class.
- Rehearse or practice the intended exercise behavior with the individual.
- Provide regular, supportive feedback about physical activity participation.
- Identify the individual's perceived barriers or obstacles to being active (ie, fear of falling, hypoglycemia) and assist them in brainstorming ways to overcome them.

Identifying Activity Barriers and Finding Facilitators

Since frequent and consistent physical activity often requires sustained behavior change, combating potential barriers with appropriate strategies and goals is of significant importance.[23,188] For most adults, regular physical activity is most commonly discontinued due to a perceived lack of time, injuries, inappropriate starting

Cases—Part 5: Assessing Barriers to Physical Activity

Type 1 Diabetes

Lack of Understanding Leading to Creation of Self-Imposed Barriers

HW was frustrated by the large fluctuations in his blood glucose levels caused by his physical activity participation. His healthcare provider had told him he could be physically active, but it just wasn't working out for him. He wanted to call his educator the morning after his post-resistance training hypoglycemia since he desperately wanted to continue being active. Instead, he gave up, deciding that he would simply stop working out because it was just too hard to manage his blood glucose. He was worried about diabetes-related complications from hyperglycemia, though. That day he went to work depressed and had a hard time keeping his blood glucose levels low enough to get anywhere near his target level of 100 mg/dL (5.6 mmol/L) before meals.

Type 2 Diabetes

Identifying Medical Barriers Related to Prior Exercise

DK called her healthcare provider about the hip pain she had developed from walking. She was sure the type 2 diabetes was now causing some other problems and was afraid she was going to lose her leg. Once her healthcare provider reassured her that was not so, DK was scheduled to have a few medical tests. She learned that diabetes was not the reason for her hip pain; rather, she had some arthritis in her hips that was probably exacerbated by her excess body weight. She was told that while the arthritis would cause some discomfort, weight loss could help decrease the pain, as could regular moderate physical activity. Now exercise was more important for her than ever.

intensity, and a lack of enjoyment. Other barriers may relate to the environment (such as a lack of safe places for physical activity, availability of facilities, and pleasant places to walk),[180,181] social factors (a lack of social support for regular physical activity),[189] and work or home situations that lead to more sedentary behaviors.

Even though people may understand and acknowledge that physical activity is good for them, they may have specific barriers preventing them from making healthy choices. As important as it is to identify barriers to physical activity, it's just as important to consider the positives in each individual's situation (ie, facilitators). Looking deeper, individuals will likely find that there are more positives than they thought. Diabetes care and education specialists can work with individuals to identify their unique barriers and problem solve to come up with possible solutions to overcome those barriers.

Reality Scenario	*Problem Solving* *Possible Solutions/What Would You Do?*
Too out of shape	
It's been years since I did any real exercise. I feel flabby and out of shape. At this point, even walking up the stairs makes me tired.	Start with activities you can tolerate. Increase activity slowly over time.
Time constraints	
I work full time. I have young kids at home. Also, I'm involved with church and the PTA. It seems there is not enough time in the day to add one more thing.	Do an inventory of your time. Prioritize. Consider what else you can reasonably give up. Think of activities that you can do while watching TV. Get up earlier in the morning. Do things with the kids. Add in bits of activity throughout the day that count toward your goals.
Weather (too hot, too cold, rain or snow)	
I plan to go for a walk after dinner. But then it's too hot.	Do indoor activities. Get an exercise video or DVD. *Ask participants to share the name of any exercise DVDs or videos they use.* Go to the mall or large stores or retail centers to walk indoors.
Environment/lack of safe place	
I'd like to walk in my neighborhood, but there are [fill in the blank: mean dogs/gangs/heavy traffic/sidewalks with big cracks and potholes in them]. I'm afraid I might get hurt if I go out there.	Explore options for each barrier. Can you take a safer route to avoid dogs/people? Are there local resources like a Y or other community center? Is there a retail center (mall, large store) nearby? Can you consider another choice of activity, perhaps indoors?
Fear of low blood glucose	
One time I did an aerobics class at the gym after work. Afterward, I had a very low blood glucose level, and I nearly passed out in the locker room. Someone had to run for help. I was so embarrassed! I don't want that to ever happen again.	Monitor blood glucose levels before and after activity, and occasionally during. Be prepared with a carbohydrate snack, glucose tablets, juice, or regular soda. Plan to do activity after meals when your blood glucose is rising.
Self-conscious about body	
I feel like everyone is looking at me. Everybody else at the health club is lean and in great shape. I feel like a fat blob in my workout clothes.	Do indoor, solo activities. If active in a public area, wear loose clothes that don't emphasize your body shape. Find a gym that caters to people you feel comfortable being with. Try aquatic activities.
Boredom	
Exercise is just so boring! After a few days of the same old thing, I just want to quit.	Choose activities that you enjoy, even dancing. Having fun will help you stay motivated. Do different activities on different days or do a combination of activities on the same day. Get an exercise buddy, and make activity a social time, too. Listen to music during the activity to distract you.

(continued)

Reality Scenario	*Problem Solving* *Possible Solutions/What Would You Do?*
Lack of motivation	
I just don't have any motivation.	Focus on reasons for living and being more healthy, such as your children, your spouse, or accomplishing your long-term goals in life. Practice *positive affirmations*. These are statements that reflect who you want to be. If you want to be an active, motivated person, repeat to yourself several times a day: *"I am a motivated, active person."* Set small, realistic, and measurable (SMART) goals. Plan for a reward when you meet your goal. Get an activity *accountability partner*. This is someone who is counting on you to be active.
Unrealistic expectations	
I've been exercising for a week already, and I don't see any changes in my body. It's discouraging.	It takes time to see changes in your body. Focus on other positives that activity brings, like more energy, better glucose management, and just the fact that you're taking steps to improve your health. If you're exercising to lose weight, give it a month or more before you expect the scale to change since you may be gaining muscle mass. Use the "clothes test" (ie, do your clothes fit better?) instead of watching your scale weight.
Physical limitations	
Balance issues, joint problems, foot problems, obesity, etc. For example: "My bad knee won't let me go out and walk."	Choose activities that will not aggravate physical ailments. Consider doing stationary cycling, chair or other seated exercises, or water exercise. It is possible to do resistance exercises sitting down as well.

Common Facilitators

- Social support—activity buddy, family members, coworkers, friends and neighbors
- Community resources—accessible fitness center, local pool, community center, etc.
- Reminders and cues—notes, entry on calendar, reminder alarm
- Rewards—incentives to maintain motivation (preferably noncaloric ones)

Setting Practical Goals

When planning to increase physical activity levels by overcoming potential obstacles or problems, individuals should be encouraged to develop realistic and practical goals. Goals that are too vague, too ambitious, or too distant do not provide enough self-motivation to maintain long-term interest. Encourage individuals to write down and track their goals to help see their progress and identify barriers. The acronym SMART may be used to help individuals set appropriate physical activity goals. SMART stands for specific, measurable, attainable, realistic, and time-bound, as explained below:

- *Specific:* Encourage the individual to be as precise as possible when identifying details of frequency, duration, intensity, and type of activity.
- *Measurable:* Teach the person how to make goals that can be quantified so he or she can accurately track, measure, and identify progress.
- *Attainable:* Help the individual set goals that are challenging but reachable to increase confidence and the likelihood of setting even more challenging goals in the future.
- *Realistic:* Help the individual evaluate how likely he or she is to attain his or her chosen goals in a given situation.
- *Time-bound:* Encourage the individual to set short-term goals that provide more immediate feedback, such as setting goals for just the next week.

The participant sets an individual goal for physical activity. The educator and the participant schedule a date in which to evaluate progress with behavior change.

Providing Social-Environmental Support (In Person and Remotely)

Social support is associated with greater levels of physical activity, supporting the role of social networks in modifying behavior patterns.[23,189] Fortunately, the same social dynamics may be exploited to increase the effects of interventions beyond the target individual and can potentially help spread exercise behavior. Particularly in adults with chronic health conditions, social and cultural identities may have a greater impact on their willingness to exercise and how they perceive and value being active.[190] Having at least one supporter is likely to increase participation, and people who value the social and psychological benefits of attending group or supervised exercise are more likely to attend regularly. How individuals get their support can vary, however, particularly with the onslaught of digital and online options now available.

In-Person Counseling and Supervision

Counseling delivered directly by healthcare professionals has long been a meaningful source of support and an effective source for delivery.[191] Longer term behavioral intervention strategies (over several years) have resulted in a sustained increase in physical activity and decrease in sedentary time, at least in adults with type 2 diabetes.[192] Most exercise intervention studies showing the greatest impact on blood glucose stability have involved supervision of exercise sessions by qualified exercise trainers.[48,67,193,194] When supervision is removed, both engagement and glycemic management may suffer. Thus, individuals with diabetes engaging in supervised training gain benefits that exceed those of exercise counseling and increased physical activity undertaken alone.

Digital and Online Support

With the widespread adoption of mobile phones, digital health solutions that incorporate evidence-based, behaviorally designed interventions can also improve the reach of and access to diabetes self-management education and ongoing support.[195] Technology-enabled diabetes self-management improves overall glycemic management, especially when incorporating feedback loop components that connect individuals with diabetes with their healthcare team.[196] Digital diabetes care has demonstrated only modest HbA1c reduction in multiple studies and borderline cost-effectiveness, although satisfaction appears to be increased in persons with diabetes.[195] However, many different options are now available to persons with diabetes and their caregivers, all of which can benefit diabetes self-management.[197]

The technology used to support self-care now includes medical devices, digital therapeutics, wearable technology, insulin pumps, sensor augmented pumps, continuous glucose monitors, blood glucose meters, web-based programs and portals, mobile phone and smartphone applications, text messaging and electronic communications, and video conferencing. Technology tools have allowed for easier tracking, less time spent recordkeeping, and increased access to data. People with diabetes can receive healthcare services "virtually," outside of the clinic with use of the Internet and mobile devices, which eliminates barriers such as transportation or cost of travel.[198–200] Mobile phones (calls, texts), secure messaging, and web-based tools and education facilitate two-way communication, analysis of patient-generated health data, tailored education, and individualized feedback.

Using Wearable Activity Technologies

The latest trend is to improve engagement by assessing an individual's unique barriers to being more active and employing new and evolving technology like accelerometers and smartphone applications that track physical activity.[188] Others have benefited from use of newer technologies that monitor their heart rate, blood pressure, steps, sedentary time, exercise intensity, and other variables in real time. For instance, heart rate monitors are good for achieving and maintaining appropriate exercise intensity. Target heart rates, however, must be individualized based on health status and use of medication that may limit heart rate.

Many individuals with prediabetes or diabetes prefer walking as an aerobic activity, and pedometer- or accelerometer-based interventions can be effective for tracking and increasing such aerobic activity.[201,202] Pedometers (small monitors that record the number of steps taken), accelerometers (that monitor that record all movement, including variations in exercise intensity), and other activity-tracking devices can be useful tools for increasing lifestyle physical activity. Pedometers detect only walking-based activities and cannot detect changes in type, intensity, or pattern of activity, whereas accelerometers can measure activity patterns and intensity but have a low sensitivity to sedentary activities and are unable to register static exercise. Many cellular phones already have accelerometers incorporated in them that can be used to track daily movement.

Counting or estimating daily physical movement can be effective for motivating persons with diabetes to seek being active throughout the day, and not just during planned exercise times. A daily log of step counts can be used to show the correlation between physical activity and glucose management. Apps for tracking workout progress, analyzing glucose patterns related to different forms of exercise, can also supply needed feedback for making regimen adjustments in real time. As they are relatively inexpensive and easy to use, such technologies may be helpful to individuals in self-monitoring physical activity by providing immediate feedback, building confidence, and enhancing enjoyment.

For middle age or older adults, short-term (<6 months) weight loss interventions using wearable activity trackers has been shown to be a better option than following a standard weight loss program.[203] Similarly, wearable devices (pedometers, accelerometers, and other tracking devices) may positively impact physical health in clinical populations with cardiometabolic diseases.[204] People with type 2 diabetes, provided with an accelerometer or pedometer, substantially increase their free-living physical activity.[201] An important predictor of increased physical activity may be having a defined goal, such as to take a target number of steps per day. For instance, pedometer use in adults with type 2 diabetes increased their daily steps by 1,822 on average, but did not improve their overall glycemic stability, although using a daily steps goal (eg, 10,000 steps) led to increased participation, even when using self-selected step goals.[205] Specialists should encourage individuals to initially set feasible/achievable targets for steps per day before progressing toward higher goals.

Given that most individuals with type 2 diabetes have access to the Internet, technology-based support is appealing for extending clinical intervention reach. For adults with type 2 diabetes, Internet-delivered physical activity promotion interventions, including Fitbit and others, may be more effective than usual care.[206] Effective Internet-based programs included monitoring of physical activity, feedback, goal setting, and support from a coach via phone/email. Similarly, engaging and competing with peers around physical activity goals may also be effective. More evidence is needed regarding the use of social media approaches, given the importance of social and peer support in diabetes self-management.[207]

Tracking Daily Steps/Movement

Assist individuals in using tracking devices effectively. Pedometers must be worn correctly, usually attached to the waistband of pants and centered above the kneecap, or it can be placed on the small of the back for persons with a large abdomen. Other tracking devices like accelerometers may be worn on a wristband or attached to the waistband, depending on the device. Instruct individuals to follow these steps for the best outcomes:

- Establish an activity baseline by tracking steps or daily movement for a few days without intentionally increasing physical activity levels.
- Set appropriate step goals by progressively increasing steps or activity levels from baseline using small increases to start, such as setting a goal to take an extra 500 or 1,000 steps a day.
- Estimate step counts of time spent doing activities not recorded by the pedometer or other tracking device (refer to Table 6.15 for step equivalents).
- Alternately, use accelerometers to track both total movement and intensity of activity for extended periods of time.

Using Stage-Matched Interventions

The Transtheoretical Model of behavior change, which uses progressive stages of readiness for behavior change, can be used to tailor exercise interventions. Stage-matched interventions are widely accepted by healthcare practitioners in helping individuals make permanent lifestyle changes, including regular exercise.[192,193,208] (See more detail on these stages in Chapter 3.) The following stage-matched strategies can be used to specifically assist individuals in overcoming physical activity and exercise barriers.

Stages of Change for Exercise Behavior

1. *Precontemplation:* Not regularly active and has no intention of being active in the next 6 months
2. *Contemplation:* Not regularly active but thinking about starting in the next 6 months
3. *Preparation:* Doing some activity but not enough to meet current guidelines for regular physical activity
4. *Action:* Has become regularly physically active within the last 6 months
5. *Maintenance:* Has maintained regular physical activity for 6 months or more

Precontemplation

The goal at the precontemplation stage is for individuals to begin thinking about participating in more physical activity.

- Build trust with the individual and provide information as needed.
- Emphasize the individual's autonomy in decisions to be more active.
- Discuss pros and cons of physical activity.
- Encourage the individual to think about personally relevant benefits.
- Address the individual's specific barriers and encourage the individual to come up with possible solutions to these barriers.

TABLE 6.15 Equivalent Steps of Physical Activities for Adults (when not recorded by tracking device)

Activity	*Minute Step Count*	*15-Minute Step Count*	*30-Minute Step Count*
Aerobic dance	197	2,955	5,910
Ballroom dancing, slow to fast	91–167	1,365–2,505	2,730–5,010
Bowling	91	1,365	2,730
Canoeing	106	1,590	3,180
Circuit training	242	3,630	7,260
Climbing, rock or mountain	273	4,095	8,190
Gardening	121	1,815	3,630
Golf	136	2,040	4,080
Gymnastics	121	1,815	3,630
Health-club exercise, general	167	2,505	5,010
Hiking	182	2,730	5,460
Jogging	212	3,180	6,360
Jogging on mini-trampoline	136	2,040	4,080
Martial arts	303	4,545	9,090
Running, 5–8 mph	242–409	3,630–6,135	7,260–12,270
Shopping	70	1,050	2,100
Stationary cycling, moderate to vigorous	212–318	3,180–4,770	6,360–9,540
Step aerobics	273	4,095	8,190
Swimming laps, moderate to vigorous	212–303	3,180–4,545	6,360–9,090
Swimming leisurely	182	2,730	5,460
Water aerobics	121	1,815	3,630
Water jogging	242	3,630	7,260
Weight lifting, moderate to vigorous	121–182	1,815–2,730	3,630–5,460
Yoga and stretching	76	1,140	2,280

Based on metabolic equivalents (METs) of various physical activities.

Source: BE Ainsworth, WL Haskell, MC Whitt, et al, 2011. "Compendium of physical activities: a second update of codes and MET values," *Med Sci Sports Exerc* 2011;43: 1575-81.

- Use appropriate goal-setting activities focused on getting the individual to think about being more active, such as reading a pamphlet on the benefits of exercise.
- Suggest that the individual write down benefits of exercise, barriers to exercising, reasons to be active, and reasons not to be active.

Contemplation

The goal at the contemplation stage is for individuals to begin taking steps to be more active and to think about setting physical activity goals.

- Continue to use strategies from the precontemplation stage.
- Provide support and validation to the individual.
- Offer information on physical activity and exercise, emphasizing social, psychological, and general health benefits.
- Discuss the individual's personal preferences for physical activity.
- Encourage the individual to think about what has been successful in the past regarding physical activity or examples of family and friends who have been successful.
- Suggest that the individual use a reinforcement program that provides positive rewards when goals are achieved.
- Encourage the individual to identify other people to use for support.

Preparation

The goal at the preparation stage is for individuals to increase physical activity to recommended levels.

- Praise preparation taken to increase physical activity.
- Continue to use strategies from the precontemplation and contemplation stages.
- Assist the individual in setting goals to gradually increase physical activity levels.
- Encourage the individual to track progress with a physical activity log that details activity type, amount, duration, and frequency.
- Suggest the individual join an exercise class or club.

Action

The goal at the action stage is for individuals to begin making physical activity a regular part of their life.

- Praise all efforts of the individual.
- Work with the individual to develop a specific plan for tracking progress and setting short-term physical activity goals.
- Suggest the individual try new activities or train for an upcoming exercise event (such as walking or a bicycle race).
- Limit suggestions for additional changes to 1 or 2.
- Encourage the individual to begin to anticipate barriers.

Maintenance

The goal at the maintenance stage is for individuals to prepare for possible setbacks and find ways to continue to increase enjoyment with the personalized physical activity program.

- Praise all efforts of the individual.
- Use strategies from the action stage.
- Help the individual find ways to avoid boredom, such as varying exercise routines.
- Promote relapse-prevention strategies—distinguish between a lapse (slight slip) and a relapse (return to former behavior patterns) by having the individual identify potential high-risk situations and develop a plan to deal with them.
- Encourage the individual to reflect on the benefits achieved with regular physical activity.

Keep in mind that most people are not successful with their first attempt at increasing and maintaining new levels of physical activity. Some individuals may need 3 or 4 attempts before being active becomes a long-term habit. Individuals will progress through the stages as they learn from past attempts and successes and try different methods for increasing activity. The more an individual takes action to become more physically active, the better his or her chances of progressing forward. The role of the diabetes care and education specialist is to support the individual in all stages and apply appropriate intervention strategies as needed.

Using Motivational Interviewing

Motivational interviewing is an individual-centered directive method of communication for enhancing intrinsic motivation to change by exploring and resolving ambivalence. This technique can be used with individuals to help increase motivational readiness to make positive behavior changes in physical activity. Individuals with type 2 diabetes may be more receptive to motivational interviewing, given that its approach is more person-centered and empowering than traditional care,[209] although motivational interviewing may not be any more effective than usual care in some cases.[210]

Key strategies that diabetes care and education specialists can use with individuals experiencing ambivalence with physical activity participation include the following:

- Emphasize the individual's autonomy and freedom to choose not to be physically active.
- Encourage the individual's acceptance of responsibility for change and consequences of not changing activity habits.
- Use strategic feedback, reflections, and questions to help the individual develop internal discrepancies for remaining inactive.
- Use decisional balance scales to help the individual weigh being more active against remaining inactive or being less active.
- Obtain permission from the individual before providing information or offering advice.

A key tool of motivational interviewing is the use of rulers to explore importance and raise the individual's confidence regarding his or her exercise behaviors. Start by asking the individual to rate on a 10-point scale how important the exercise behavior is and how confident he or she is about the behavior, such as walking 3 times a week for 15 minutes. After the individual chooses a number, ask why that specific number was chosen, versus a higher number. See the sidebar for an example of how this technique is implemented.

Using Behavior-Change Rules

Importance Rulers

1. On a scale of 0 to 10, how *important* is it for you to begin walking 3 times a week for 15 minutes?

The answer given helps determine the individual's readiness to change physical activity patterns.

2. Why did you choose that number and not a lower one? (5 instead of 4, for example)

The individual's answer elicits conversation regarding behavior change.

Confidence Rulers

1. On a scale of 0 to 10, how *confident* are you that you could walk 3 times a week for 15 minutes?

The answer given helps determine the individual's confidence regarding increasing physical activity.

2. What would it take for you to move up just one number on the scale?

The answer given elicits conversation regarding the individual's ability to be more active.

Summary

This chapter reviews the current physical activity and exercise guidelines for individuals with diabetes and discusses a variety of strategies to assist both those with diabetes and those at risk for diabetes in adopting a more physically active lifestyle. Exercise prescription serves as a guide for safe and effective physical activity programs, even when complicated by the presence of diabetes-related and other health issues or when considering special populations (eg, obese, pregnancy, older adults, youth). The true art of program planning lies in the effective use of behavior-change strategies to tailor the program to each individual's health status, personal preferences, abilities, goals, and stage of readiness.

Case Wrap-Up: Education Aids Implementation of Exercise Prescription

Type 1 Diabetes

Data Interpretation and Support

HW went to his follow-up appointment with the diabetes care and education specialist. He was sure the educator was going to tell him he would have to stop being active. After all, trying to work out was making his blood glucose levels worse. The educator's response surprised him by not only explaining how his blood glucose numbers were affected by the type and intensity of training he did, but also encouraging him to keep trying different things until he found what worked best for him. They talked specifically about what he should try and what he should expect to see his blood glucose doing during both aerobic and resistance training activities. He agreed to check and record his blood glucose before and after exercise, along with the type and duration of exercise, to determine patterns. If he had a problem he could not solve on his own, he was to call the educator right away. He learned that figuring out the right balance of food, insulin, and exercise would take a little time but could be done. He also decided to join an online diabetes forum for athletic individuals to get more ideas on managing his exercise blood glucose levels.

Type 2 Diabetes

Identifying Activity Options

DK met with a diabetes care and education specialist. During her appointment, she learned more about her diabetes medication and how it does not place her at risk of exercise-induced hypoglycemia. She realized she could exercise whenever she could fit it into her day. The diabetes care and education specialist also talked about other exercise options. They decided she should add something besides walking because of the pain it caused with her hip. DK has a friend who does water aerobics—something she might consider trying. The diabetes care and education specialist also provided her with information about an exercise program for people with arthritis, and she decided to look into both of those options.

Working Systematically in Stages

The diabetes care and education specialist also helped DK chart a plan for how much time to spend exercising. DK then understood she would need to work on her fitness plan for a few months to get her fitness level to where it should be. She would start with a small amount of exercise and add more as she could tolerate it. She promised she would return to talk to the diabetes care and education specialist before she tried to add too much. After all that, DK felt she was finally getting her life back!

Focus on Education

Teaching Strategies

Perform a pre-exercise evaluation. Individuals who have or are at risk for vascular or cardiac complications likely need a pre-exercise evaluation to start activities more vigorous than daily living. Once the evaluation is completed, a tailored program can be developed. Aerobic activities may be a place to start, but goals should progress to include resistance training at some point.

Set goals using the SMART approach. Goals are set to achieve positive outcomes. Using the SMART approach (goals that are specific, measurable, attainable, realistic, and time-bound) encourages positive outcomes and helps establish lifelong habits. Encourage a plan for activity that is enjoyable, safe, and effective.

Use theory to guide interventions. Be familiar with theories to tailor and individualize interventions (eg, stage-matched strategies, goal setting, and motivational interviewing techniques).

Monitor progress and impact of exercise on metabolic management. Persons with diabetes can record and quantify daily physical activities and their impact on glycemic levels. Exercise can be a therapeutic strategy for daily glucose stability.

Help the individual who hates to exercise. Many people voice this opposition. When a person makes this statement, the diabetes care and education specialist or other provider has a huge opportunity to ask more questions. Digging deeper, the educator often finds the real root of the problem and can help prevent it from interfering again. Examples include the following:

- *Does not like to sweat.* Promote lighter types of activities such as stretching, pool activities, or easy walking. The individual may be surprised to find these are options in a fitness plan.
- *Had a bad experience.* Determine what went wrong and prepare a plan that will replace that experience with a positive one.
- *Feels self-conscious in front of others.* May be best to start with solo options, such as videos, home-based equipment, or a personal trainer. A group fitness class or specific fitness facility may provide support if the person feels he or she fits in with the other members.
- *Has always "failed" at fitness programs.* Help set reasonable goals, prescribe a fitness program that will meet those goals, and provide positive support to the person through each step whether the person experiences a success or a setback. Build in appropriate progression of exercise.

Help the individual who underestimates insulin adjustment needs. Many need reassurances that a large reduction in their insulin dose is the correct action to take. They are willing to take 1 or 2 units off a dose initially but hesitant to do more. With support, they can omit 20% to 50% or more of their dose for a given exercise session if needed to achieve acceptable glucose levels.

Help the person who delays or avoids snacks. Even when the blood glucose indicates a snack is needed, many individuals will wait to see if they really need a snack. This often results in either hypoglycemia and the need for a larger volume of food to treat the reaction or overtreatment. Pointing out that a smaller snack at the right time can help them avoid consuming a larger number of calories later to treat a reaction can help.

Identify support and assistance. Whether the individual is of school age, a working professional, a parent, or retired, support and assistance from others close to the individual are important. The person may need to ask someone to join him or her in a fitness program to promote consistency or ask someone to take over a chore or responsibility to free up time for recommended physical activity. Financial resources may also need to be allocated so that the individual can buy appropriate clothing and shoes or have access to exercise equipment.

Be a role model. Model a lifestyle incorporating physical activity and planned exercise to emphasize that physical activity is a lifestyle priority. Be a role model with your own activity plan, and wear and encourage use of a pedometer, accelerometer, or other activity tracker. Plan a group program such as a walking club or an exercise class; track activity and outcomes.

Help persons with diabetes establish a healthy relationship with fitness. Physical activity can be part of an eating disorder or just maladaptive functioning. Help individuals achieve a balance with how much they exercise and set reasonable SMART goals to better define their goals associated with being active.

Messages for Persons with Diabetes

Establish a routine for physical activity. Physical activity is a vital part of improved or continued diabetes management, and it has a positive effect on blood pressure and blood cholesterol and prevention of type 2 diabetes. Choose an activity you enjoy! Involve family or friends in a swim class, biking or hiking trip, or neighborhood street dance. Find ways to add extra activity in each day, such as walking around the parking lot before getting in the car, using the stairs when able, walking around the grocery store prior to picking up your first item, and frequenting safe places like malls to get in more daily steps. Simply taking frequent activity breaks during prolonged sitting time can help with blood glucose, body weight, and energy levels.

Identify health issues. Contact your healthcare provider for approval of an exercise plan if you have high blood pressure or any other complications (such as neuropathy or arthritis) that may impact your ability to be active safely and effectively.

Practice safety first. Wear diabetes identification. Check your blood glucose before and after activity, especially if you use insulin. Wear shoes and clothing that fit well and dress in layers so that you can easily adjust what you are wearing. Stop the activity if you are lightheaded or short of breath. If you are on medications for diabetes that can cause hypoglycemia with activity (eg, insulin, sulfonylureas, and meglitinides), be sure to carry a rapid-acting carbohydrate product to treat it if needed. Consider carrying fluids to stay hydrated during physical activity.

Establish an exercise support network. Create a network of friends and family who will support you, keep you accountable, partner with you, and motivate you to get going and keep the exercise habit. Make sure to talk to your healthcare professional team about your physical activity routine, any pain associated with it, any challenges, and the impact on your health.

Assess exercise relapse. Your usual physical activity routine can be interrupted for several days and consequently discontinued. Provide strategies for relapse prevention and its management. Also, reassess your physical activity routine and its impact annually.

Be prepared to troubleshoot your fitness plan. Determining the best routine to follow to safely and effectively engage in physical activity takes time (eg, frequent blood glucose checks and data from multiple physical activity sessions), patience, and problem solving. When in doubt, give another activity a try to see if it works better for you.

Monitor levels to gain valuable information. Recognize the need to measure blood glucose levels around exercise to facilitate good decision making in the future. Monitoring provides feedback on decisions about snacks, timing of exercise, and adjustments in medications. The interpretation of observed blood glucose patterns and effects of exercise can be reinforced with this information.

Time snacks appropriately to help keep calorie counts down. A smaller snack at the right time can help you avoid consuming a larger number of calories later to treat hypoglycemia. Also, never assume that snacks are needed for all exercise; determine first whether your diabetes medications place you at risk for a decrease in blood glucose levels during any activity.

Realize that insulin dose adjustments may be larger than you expect. A large reduction in your insulin dose may be the correct action to take. Encourage them to try omitting 25–50% or more of their dose for a given exercise session if needed to achieve their blood glucose targets.

Do not make spontaneous treatment judgments based on a single glucose reading. Determine whether this is a one-time-only situation or a pattern and adjust your therapy accordingly.

Establish a healthy attitude toward fitness. Your physical activity routine not only can help you keep glucose better managed but can improve overall well-being and empower you to do more.

Health Literacy

Low health literacy affects individuals' ability to locate proper health services, share personal information with providers, perform self-care behaviors, adopt healthy behaviors, make judgments, obtain tests, and follow up. Consider all these elements in developing realistic physical activity education. Your education approach needs to be so much more than just providing information on what to do and how to do it. Make it understandable and relatable for everyone.

Use or create low-literacy educational materials. It is recommended that health education material be written toward a sixth-grade level. However, most diabetes education materials are written at a ninth-grade level or above. Even college-level readers prefer materials written in easy-to-read formats. Use handouts with pictures that demonstrate each stage of the desired physical activity, its duration, and when to progress to the next stage. You can use a calendar with prompts to adjust the routine or to keep people motivated. The illustrations and text should focus on desired behavioral strategies rather than medical facts.

Use effective communication strategies with your persons with diabetes. Assume all your persons with diabetes have a low literacy level. Everyone, regardless of literacy level, deserves to be engaged in meaningful and strategic communication.

Focus on high-priority behaviors first, but make sure that they are as important to the person with diabetes as they are to you. Ask your persons with diabetes what matters most to them with regard to being active (eg, increased energy levels, better health, weight loss, blood glucose management) and then give them your input when it comes to prioritizing them to target some of the more high-priority ones first.

Use concrete examples of activities, places, and times. The more specific an individual can be when creating a fitness plan, the more likely it is that it can be followed and maintained. Instead of prompting them to exercise more, have them decide to walk at lunchtime with coworkers three days this week, for example.

Limit the number of topics covered in one session. It can be easy to overwhelm individuals by giving them too much information at one sitting, making it likely that they will retain very little of it. Limit the number of topics covered at one time to just a few core ones and build on those and add a few new ones at the next session.

Use the teach-back method to demonstrate adequate comprehension. To make certain that persons with diabetes truly grasp each concept, have them convey back to you their understanding of each one before moving on to the next. Give them a practice scenario and ask them to make a decision that reflects their level of comprehension.

Address health numeracy by having persons with diabetes identify methods of monitoring their physical activity with time, intensity, and duration. Also, health numeracy can affect a person's understanding of the impact of exercise on glucose readings and how to quantify its health benefits. One of the strategies used to understand the benefits is to have persons with diabetes check their blood glucose before and after physical activity. They can also use the "how do I feel" scale of 1 to 10 for days with exercise versus no exercise versus less exercise. Some persons with diabetes may not understand the difference between "set" and "repetition" in weight lifting.

Let the person with diabetes know that you will follow up by e-mail or with a phone call within the next few days to provide support and troubleshoot. With follow-up support guarantee, persons with diabetes will feel more empowered to try out activities, especially if they need help troubleshooting any problems that arise. Eventually, they will be empowered to exercise on their own and problem solve for themselves, but that initial support while they are establishing an exercise habit is critical.

Use analogies or stories to increase comprehension. You can relate that exercise works like medicine by showing a medication bottle with the name of the exercise, its benefits, and side effects. Share other people's stories on overcoming a challenge or demonstrating success. Normalize obstacles by sharing your own strategies and your daily routine.

Health Numeracy

Numbers can scare people and prevent them from exercising. You might think that pedometers or heart rate monitors are great, but they might be "scary" for persons with diabetes with low numeracy skills. Encourage their use but refrain from forcing anyone to use such devices.

Effective Behavior Change Strategies

Assess importance (why), confidence (how and what), and readiness (when).

- Explore importance by asking: Is it worthwhile? Why should I? How will I benefit? What will change? At what cost? Do I really want to? Will it make a difference?
- Explore confidence by asking: Can I? How will I do it? How will I cope with . . .? Will I succeed if . . .? What change . . .?
- Explore readiness by asking: Should I do it now? How about other priorities?

Challenge-based learning or situation problem solving. State a circumstance for a person with diabetes and have the person come up with the solution/strategy. For example: What will you do when you have hypoglycemia during exercise?

Focus on Practice

Pre-exercise needs. In the absence of known cardiovascular complications, requiring a pre-exercise evaluation may be a deterrent to physical activity and unnecessary prior to starting exercise programs involving only mild or moderate walking (ie, brisk walking or lower intensity exercise). Make sure you have access to proper footwear for weight-bearing activities like walking.

Socioeconomic barriers. A lower socioeconomic status may affect exercise opportunities because of cost (eg, joining an exercise facility), limited availability (neighborhood unsafe for walking), or time involvement (such as economic pressures necessitating working more than one job). Certain cultural traditions also downplay physical activity.

Community assets. Develop and maintain a referral list of appropriate exercise programs and other fitness resources available in your community that can be shared with persons with diabetes to facilitate their involvement. Online information about exercise recommendations and precautions is available at http://www.health.gov/paguidelines and other sources.

Physical inactivity is associated with an increased risk of chronic diseases. Various physical activity interventions should be part of any healthcare system. Physical activity interventions reduce disease incidence, are cost-effective, and offer good value for the money. Provide choices and variety in exercise programs and interventions.

Fitness facilities/structures and key community resources linked to health care. Formal partnerships and coalitions formed with community centers are needed to ensure continuity in care, along with a formal fitness referral system to community centers. Physical activity is a clinical intervention and should be treated as such.

Communities with access to various fitness channels. Advocate for healthy communities with sidewalks, bike trails, mall walking, yoga, tai chi, karate, parks, exercise clubs, and fitness centers. Give people choices and opportunities to choose what they like and change their strategies.

Medically supervised fitness facilities. Be part of a system providing evidence-based and medically supervised care. Such systems involve a network of healthcare professionals like physicians, psychologists, dietitians, exercise physiologists, and physical therapists, among others. Communicate with all the providers, exchange ideas, and advance the practice.

Population-based fitness. Focus on ensuring needed care to all members of a population rather than individual persons with diabetes (eg, use of registries). Fitness is part of a lifestyle. Quantify its impact.

References

1. American Association of Diabetes care and education specialists. Revision of the AADE7™ Self-Care Behaviors. The Diabetes care and education specialist 2019;45 (in press).
2. Ostman C, Jewiss D, King N, Smart NA. Clinical outcomes to exercise training in type 1 diabetes: a systematic review and meta-analysis. Diabetes Res Clin Pract. 2018;139:380-91.
3. Chastin SFM, De Craemer M, De Cocker K, et al. How does light-intensity physical activity associate with adult cardiometabolic health and mortality? Systematic review with meta-analysis of experimental and observational studies. Br J Sports Med. 2018;25:2017-097563.
4. Qiu S, Cai X, Sun Z, Zugel M, Steinacker JM, Schumann U. Aerobic interval training and cardiometabolic health in patients with type 2 diabetes: a meta-analysis. Front Physiol 2017;8:957.
5. Moholdt T, Lavie CJ, Nauman J. Sustained physical activity, not weight loss, associated with improved survival in coronary heart disease. J Am Coll Cardiol. 2018;71:1094-101.
6. Shin WY, Lee T, Jeon DH, Kim HC. Diabetes, frequency of exercise, and mortality over 12 years: analysis of the National Health Insurance Service-Health Screening (NHIS-HEALS) Database. J Korean Med Sci. 2018;33:e60.
7. Sadarangani KP, Hamer M, Mindell JS, Coombs NA, Stamatakis E. Physical activity and risk of all-cause and cardiovascular disease mortality in diabetic adults from Great Britain: pooled analysis of 10 population-based cohorts. Diabetes Care. 2014;37:1016-23.
8. Hamman RF, Wing RR, Edelstein SL, et al. Effect of weight loss with lifestyle intervention on risk of diabetes. Diabetes Care. 2006;29:2102-7.
9. Knowler WC, Barrett-Connor E, Fowler SE, et al. Reduction in the incidence of type 2 diabetes with lifestyle intervention or metformin. N Engl J Med. 2002;346:393-403.
10. Hoskin MA, Bray GA, Hattaway K, et al. Prevention of diabetes through the lifestyle intervention: lessons learned from the Diabetes Prevention Program and Outcomes Study and its translation to practice. Curr Nutr Rep. 2014;3:364-78.
11. Aune D, Sen A, Henriksen T, Saugstad OD, Tonstad S. Physical activity and the risk of gestational diabetes mellitus: a systematic review and dose-response meta-analysis of epidemiological studies. Eur J Epidemiol. 2016;31:967-97.
12. Aune D, Norat T, Leitzmann M, Tonstad S, Vatten LJ. Physical activity and the risk of type 2 diabetes: a systematic review and dose-response meta-analysis. Eur J Epidemiol. 2015;30:529-42.
13. Borror A, Zieff G, Battaglini C, Stoner L. The effects of postprandial exercise on glucose control in individuals with type 2 diabetes: a systemic review. Sports Med. 2018;2:018-0864.

14. Riddell MC, Gallen IW, Smart CE, et al. Exercise management in type 1 diabetes: a consensus statement. Lancet Diabetes Endocrinol. 2017;5:377-90.

15. Kilpatrick ES, Rigby AS, Atkin SL. Insulin resistance, the metabolic syndrome, and complication risk in type 1 diabetes: "double diabetes" in the Diabetes Control and Complications Trial. Diabetes Care. 2007;30:707-12.

16. Dube JJ, Allison KF, Rousson V, Goodpaster BH, Amati F. Exercise dose and insulin sensitivity: relevance for diabetes prevention. Med Sci Sports Exerc. 2012;44:793-9.

17. Wilmot EG, Edwardson CL, Achana FA, et al. Sedentary time in adults and the association with diabetes, cardiovascular disease and death: systematic review and meta-analysis. Diabetologia. 2012;55:2895-905.

18. Dempsey PC, Larsen RN, Sethi P, et al. Benefits for type 2 diabetes of interrupting prolonged sitting with brief bouts of light walking or simple resistance activities. Diabetes Care. 2016;39:964-72.

19. Dempsey PC, Sacre JW, Larsen RN, et al. Interrupting prolonged sitting with brief bouts of light walking or simple resistance activities reduces resting blood pressure and plasma noradrenaline in type 2 diabetes. J Hypertens. 2016;34:2376-82.

20. Schmid D, Ricci C, Leitzmann MF. Associations of objectively assessed physical activity and sedentary time with all-cause mortality in US adults: the NHANES study. PLoS One. 2015; 10:e0119591.

21. Jabbour G, Henderson M, Mathieu ME. Barriers to active lifestyles in children with type 1 diabetes. Can J Diabetes. 2016;40:170-2.

22. Brazeau AS, Rabasa-Lhoret R, Strychar I, Mircescu H. Barriers to physical activity among patients with type 1 diabetes. Diabetes Care. 2008;31:2108-9.

23. Avery L, Flynn D, Dombrowski SU, van Wersch A, Sniehotta FF, Trenell MI. Successful behavioural strategies to increase physical activity and improve glucose control in adults with type 2 diabetes. Diabet Med. 2015;32:1058-62.

24. Piercy KL, Troiano RP, Ballard RM, et al. The Physical Activity Guidelines for Americans. JAMA. 2018;320:2020-8.

25. Physical Activity Guidelines Advisory Committee. 2018 Physical Activity Guidelines Advisory Committee Scientific Report. In: Services USDoHaH, ed. Washington, D.C. 2018.

26. Colberg SR SR, Yardley JE, Riddell MC, Dunstan DW, Dempsey PC, Horton ES, Castorino K, Tate DF. Physical activity/exercise and diabetes: a position statement of the American Diabetes Association. Diabetes Care. 2016;39:2065-79.

27. Physical Activity Guidelines Advisory Committee. 2018 Physical Activity Guidelines Advisory Committee Scientific Report In: U.S. Department of Health and Human Services, ed. Washington, D.C. 2018.

28. Riebe D, Franklin BA, Thompson PD, et al. Updating ACSM's Recommendations for Exercise Preparticipation Health Screening. Med Sci Sports Exerc. 2015;47:2473-9.

29. Colberg SR, Sigal RJ, Fernhall B, et al. Exercise and type 2 diabetes: the American College of Sports Medicine and the American Diabetes Association: joint position statement executive summary. Diabetes Care. 2010;33:2692-6.

30. Tudor-Locke C, Craig CL, Thyfault JP, Spence JC. A step-defined sedentary lifestyle index: <5000 steps/day. Appl Physiol Nutr Metab. 2013;38:100-14.

31. Wolff-Hughes DL, Fitzhugh EC, Bassett DR, Churilla JR. Total activity counts and bouted minutes of moderate-to-vigorous physical activity: relationships with cardiometabolic biomarkers using 2003-2006 NHANES. J Phys Act Health. 2015;12:694-700.

32. Ponsonby AL, Sun C, Ukoumunne OC, et al. Objectively measured physical activity and the subsequent risk of incident dysglycemia: the Australian Diabetes, Obesity and Lifestyle Study (AusDiab). Diabetes Care. 2011;34:1497-502.

33. Yates T, Davies MJ, Haffner SM, et al. Physical activity as a determinant of fasting and 2-h post-challenge glucose: a prospective cohort analysis of the NAVIGATOR trial. Diabet Med. 2015;32:1090-6.

34. Costello E, Kafchinski M, Vrazel J, Sullivan P. Motivators, barriers, and beliefs regarding physical activity in an older adult population. J Geriatr Phys Ther. 2011;34:138-47.

35. Rejeski WJ, Ip EH, Bertoni AG, et al. Lifestyle change and mobility in obese adults with type 2 diabetes. N Engl J Med. 2012;366:1209-17.

36. Hawari NS, Al-Shayji I, Wilson J, Gill JM. Frequency of breaks in sedentary time and postprandial metabolic responses. Med. Sci Sports Exerc. 2016;48:2495-502.

37. Duvivier BM, Schaper NC, Hesselink MK, et al. Breaking sitting with light activities vs structured exercise: a randomised crossover study demonstrating benefits for glycaemic control and insulin sensitivity in type 2 diabetes. Diabetologia. 2017;60:490-8.

38. Benatti FB, Ried-Larsen M. The effects of breaking up prolonged sitting time: a review of experimental studies. Med Sci Sports Exerc. 2015;47:2053-61.

39. American College of Sports Medicine. *ACSM's Guidelines for Exercise Testing and Prescription*. 10th ed. Philadelphia: Wolters Kluwer; 2018.

40. Garber CE, Blissmer B, Deschenes MR, et al. American College of Sports Medicine position stand. Quantity and quality of exercise for developing and maintaining cardiorespiratory, musculoskeletal, and neuromotor fitness in apparently healthy adults: guidance for prescribing exercise. Med Sci Sports Exerc. 2011;43:1334-59.

41. Chomentowski P, Dube JJ, Amati F, et al. Moderate exercise attenuates the loss of skeletal muscle mass that occurs with intentional caloric restriction-induced weight loss in older, overweight to obese adults. J Gerontol A Biol Sci Med Sci. 2009;64:575-80.

42. Powell KE, King AC, Buchner DM, et al. The Scientific Foundation for the Physical Activity Guidelines for Americans, 2nd Edition. J Phys Act Health. 2018;17:1-11.

43. American College of Obstetrics and Gynecology. ACOG Committee Opinion No. 650: Physical activity and exercise during pregnancy and the postpartum period. Obstet Gynecol. 2015;126:e135-42.

44. Richter EA, Hargreaves M. Exercise, GLUT4, and skeletal muscle glucose uptake. Physiol Rev. 2013;93:993-1017.

45. Teo SYM, Kanaley JA, Guelfi KJ, et al. Exercise timing in type 2 diabetes mellitus: a systemic review. Med Sci Sports Exerc. 2018;50:2387-97.

46. Liubaoerjijin Y, Terada T, Fletcher K, Boule NG. Effect of aerobic exercise intensity on glycemic control in type 2 diabetes: a meta-analysis of head-to-head randomized trials. Acta Diabetol. 2016;53:769-81.

47. Batacan RB, Jr., Duncan MJ, Dalbo VJ, Tucker PS, Fenning AS. Effects of high-intensity interval training on cardiometabolic health: a systematic review and meta-analysis of intervention studies. Br J Sports Med. 2017;51:494-503.

48. Umpierre D, Ribeiro PA, Schaan BD, Ribeiro JP. Volume of supervised exercise training impacts glycaemic control in patients with type 2 diabetes: a systematic review with meta-regression analysis. Diabetologia. 2013;56:242-51.

49. Vinik AI, Casellini C, Parson HK, Colberg SR, Nevoret ML. Cardiac autonomic neuropathy in diabetes: a predictor of cardiometabolic events. Front Neurosci. 2018;12:591.

50. Colberg SR, Swain DP, Vinik AI. Use of heart rate reserve and rating of perceived exertion to prescribe exercise intensity in diabetic autonomic neuropathy. Diabetes Care. 2003;26: 986-90.

51. Haskell WL, Lee IM, Pate RR, et al. Physical activity and public health: updated recommendation for adults from the American College of Sports Medicine and the American Heart Association. Med Sci Sports Exerc. 2007;39:1423-34.

52. Nelson ME, Rejeski WJ, Blair SN, et al. Physical activity and public health in older adults: recommendation from the American College of Sports Medicine and the American Heart Association. Med Sci Sports Exerc. 2007;39:1435-45.

53. Tenforde AS, Sayres LC, McCurdy ML, Collado H, Sainani KL, Fredericson M. Overuse injuries in high school runners: lifetime prevalence and prevention strategies. PM&R. 2011;3:125-31.

54. Eriksen L, Dahl-Petersen I, Haugaard SB, Dela F. Comparison of the effect of multiple short-duration with single long-duration exercise sessions on glucose homeostasis in type 2 diabetes mellitus. Diabetologia. 2007;50:2245-53.

55. Umpierre D, Ribeiro PA, Kramer CK, et al. Physical activity advice only or structured exercise training and association with HbA1c levels in type 2 diabetes: a systematic review and meta-analysis. JAMA. 2011;305:1790-9.

56. Jelleyman C, Yates T, O'Donovan G, et al. The effects of high-intensity interval training on glucose regulation and insulin resistance: a meta-analysis. Obes Rev. 2015;16:942-61.

57. Tonoli C, Heyman E, Roelands B, et al. Effects of different types of acute and chronic (training) exercise on glycaemic control in type 1 diabetes mellitus: a meta-analysis. Sports Med. 2012;42:1059-80.

58. Levinger I, Shaw CS, Stepto NK, et al. What doesn't kill you makes you fitter: a systematic review of high-intensity interval exercise for patients with cardiovascular and metabolic diseases. Clin Med Insights Cardiol. 2015;9:53-63.

59. Boulé NG, Kenny GP, Haddad E, Wells GA, Sigal RJ. Meta-analysis of the effect of structured exercise training on cardiorespiratory fitness in type 2 diabetes mellitus. Diabetologia. 2003;46:1071-81.

60. Liu Y, Ye W, Chen Q, Zhang Y, Kuo CH, Korivi M. Resistance exercise intensity is correlated with attenuation of HbA1c and insulin in patients with type 2 diabetes: a systematic review and meta-analysis. Int J Environ Res Public Health. 2019;16(1). ijerph16010140.

61. Ishiguro H, Kodama S, Horikawa C, et al. In search of the ideal resistance training program to improve glycemic control and its indication for patients with type 2 diabetes mellitus: a systematic review and meta-analysis. Sports Med. 2016;46:67-77.

62. Willey KA, Singh MA. Battling insulin resistance in elderly obese people with type 2 diabetes: bring on the heavy weights. Diabetes Care. 2003;26:1580-8.

63. McGinley SK, Armstrong MJ, Boule NG, Sigal RJ. Effects of exercise training using resistance bands on glycaemic control and strength in type 2 diabetes mellitus: a meta-analysis of randomised controlled trials. Acta Diabetol. 2015;52:221-30.

64. Smith SC, Jr., Allen J, Blair SN, et al. AHA/ACC guidelines for secondary prevention for patients with coronary and other atherosclerotic vascular disease: 2006 update: endorsed by the National Heart, Lung, and Blood Institute. Circulation. 2006;113:2363-72.

65. Karlsson MK, Magnusson H, von Schewelov T, Rosengren BE. Prevention of falls in the elderly—a review. Osteoporos Int. 2013;24:747-62.

66. Behm DG, Blazevich AJ, Kay AD, McHugh M. Acute effects of muscle stretching on physical performance, range of motion, and injury incidence in healthy active individuals: a systematic review. Appl Physiol Nutr Metab. 2016;41:1-11.

67. Morrison S, Simmons R, Colberg SR, Parson HK, Vinik AI. Supervised balance training and Wii Fit–based exercises lower falls risk in older adults with type 2 diabetes. J Am Med Dir Assoc. 2018;19:185.e7-.e13.

68. Morrison S, Colberg SR, Mariano M, Parson HK, Vinik AI. Balance training reduces falls risk in older individuals with type 2 diabetes. Diabetes Care. 2010;33:748-50.

69. Innes KE, Selfe TK. Yoga for adults with type 2 diabetes: A systematic review of controlled trials. J Diabetes Res. 2016;2016:6979370.

70. Jayawardena R, Ranasinghe P, Chathuranga T, Atapattu PM, Misra A. The benefits of yoga practice compared to physical exercise in the management of type 2 Diabetes Mellitus: A systematic review and meta-analysis. Diabetes Metab Syndr. 2018;12:795-805.

71. Chao M, Wang C, Dong X, Ding M. The effects of tai chi on type 2 diabetes: a meta-analysis. J Diabetes Res. 2018;2018:7350567.

72. Yang P, Swardfager W, Fernandes D, et al. Finding the optimal volume and intensity of resistance training exercise for type 2 diabetes: the FORTE Study, a randomized trial. Diabetes Res Clin Pract. 2017;130:98-107.

73. Yardley JE, Kenny GP, Perkins BA, et al. Effects of performing resistance exercise before versus after aerobic exercise on glycemia in type 1 diabetes. Diabetes Care. 2012;35:669-75.

74. Sigal RJ, Kenny GP, Boule NG, et al. Effects of aerobic training, resistance training, or both on glycemic control in type 2 diabetes: a randomized trial. Ann Intern Med. 2007;147:357-69.

75. Church TS, Blair SN, Cocreham S, et al. Effects of aerobic and resistance training on hemoglobin A1c levels in patients with type 2 diabetes: a randomized controlled trial. JAMA. 2010;304:2253-62.

76. Yardley JE, Kenny GP, Perkins BA, et al. Resistance versus aerobic exercise: acute effects on glycemia in type 1 diabetes. Diabetes Care. 2013;36:537-42.

77. Yardley JE, Hay J, Abou-Setta AM, Marks SD, McGavock J. A systematic review and meta-analysis of exercise interventions in adults with type 1 diabetes. Diabetes Res Clin Pract. 2014; 106:393-400.

78. Burke LM, Ross ML, Garvican-Lewis LA, et al. Low carbohydrate, high fat diet impairs exercise economy and negates the performance benefit from intensified training in elite race walkers. J Physiol. 2017;595(9):2785-807.

79. Ørtenblad N, Westerblad H, Nielsen J. Muscle glycogen stores and fatigue. J Physiol. 2013;591:4405-13.

80. Adolfsson P, Nilsson S, Albertsson-Wikland K, Lindblad B. Hormonal response during physical exercise of different intensities in adolescents with type 1 diabetes and healthy controls. Pediatr Diabetes. 2012;13:587-96.

81. Volek JS, Freidenreich DJ, Saenz C, et al. Metabolic characteristics of keto-adapted ultra-endurance runners. Metabolism. 2016;65:100-10.

82. Jensen J, Rustad PI, Kolnes AJ, Lai YC. The role of skeletal muscle glycogen breakdown for regulation of insulin sensitivity by exercise. Front Physiol. 2011;2:112.

83. Roberts CK, Little JP, Thyfault JP. Modification of insulin sensitivity and glycemic control by activity and exercise. Med Sci Sports Exerc. 2013;45:1868-77.

84. Volek JS, Noakes T, Phinney SD. Rethinking fat as a fuel for endurance exercise. Eur J Sport Sci. 2015;15:13-20.

85. Gregg EW, Chen H, Wagenknecht LE, et al. Association of an intensive lifestyle intervention with remission of type 2 diabetes. JAMA. 2012;308:2489-96.

86. Hansen D, Dendale P, Jonkers RA, et al. Continuous low- to moderate-intensity exercise training is as effective as moderate- to high-intensity exercise training at lowering blood HbA(1c) in obese type 2 diabetes patients. Diabetologia. 2009;52: 1789-97.

87. Manders RJ, Van Dijk JW, van Loon LJ. Low-intensity exercise reduces the prevalence of hyperglycemia in type 2 diabetes. Med Sci Sports Exerc. 2010;42:219-25.

88. van Dijk JW, Tummers K, Stehouwer CD, Hartgens F, van Loon LJ. Exercise therapy in type 2 diabetes: is daily exercise required to optimize glycemic control? Diabetes Care. 2012;35:948-54.

89. Little JP, Gillen JB, Percival ME, et al. Low-volume high-intensity interval training reduces hyperglycemia and increases muscle mitochondrial capacity in patients with type 2 diabetes. J Appl Physiol. 2011;111:1554-60.

90. Garcia-Garcia F, Kumareswaran K, Hovorka R, Hernando ME. Quantifying the acute changes in glucose with exercise in type 1 diabetes: a systematic review and meta-analysis. Sports Med. 2015;45:587-99.

91. Hasan S, Shaw SM, Gelling LH, Kerr CJ, Meads CA. Exercise modes and their association with hypoglycemia episodes in adults with type 1 diabetes mellitus: a systematic review. BMJ Open Diabetes Res Care. 2018;6:e000578.

92. Reddy R, Wittenberg A, Castle JR, et al. Effect of aerobic and resistance exercise on glycemic control in adults with type 1 diabetes. Can J Diabetes. 2018;30:193.

93. Pan B, Ge L, Xun YQ, et al. Exercise training modalities in patients with type 2 diabetes mellitus: a systematic review and network meta-analysis. Int J Behav Nutr Phys Act. 2018;15:72.

94. Yardley JE, Sigal RJ. Exercise strategies for hypoglycemia prevention in individuals with type 1 diabetes. Diabetes Spectr. 2015;28:32-8.

95. Herriott MT, Colberg SR, Parson HK, Nunnold T, Vinik AI. Effects of 8 weeks of flexibility and resistance training in older adults with type 2 diabetes. Diabetes Care. 2004;27:2988-9.

96. Rempel M, Yardley JE, MacIntosh A, et al. Vigorous intervals and hypoglycemia in type 1 diabetes: a randomized cross-over trial. Sci Rep. 2018;8:15879.

97. Roy-Fleming A, Taleb N, Messier V, et al. Timing of insulin basal rate reduction to reduce hypoglycemia during late post-prandial exercise in adults with type 1 diabetes using insulin pump therapy: a randomized crossover trial. Diabetes Metab. 2018;27:30159-9.

98. Dube JJ, Broskey NT, Despines AA, et al. Muscle characteristics and substrate energetics in lifelong endurance athletes. Med Sci Sports Exerc. 2016;48:472-80.

99. Davis SN, Tate D, Hedrington MS. Mechanisms of hypoglycemia and exercise-associated autonomic dysfunction. Trans Am Clin Climatol Assoc. 2014;125:281-91.

100. Cryer PE. Hypoglycemia-associated autonomic failure in diabetes. Handb Clin Neurol. 2013;117:295-307.

101. Bremer JP, Jauch-Chara K, Hallschmid M, Schmid S, Schultes B. Hypoglycemia unawareness in older compared with middle-aged patients with type 2 diabetes. Diabetes Care. 2009;32:1513-7.

102. Colberg S. *The Athlete's Guide to Diabetes: Expert Advice for 165 Sports and Activities*. Champaign, IL: Human Kinetics; 2019.

103. Khoo EY, Wallis J, Tsintzas K, Macdonald IA, Mansell P. Effects of exenatide on circulating glucose, insulin, glucagon, cortisol and catecholamines in healthy volunteers during exercise. Diabetologia. 2010;53:139-43.

104. Frank S, Jbaily A, Hinshaw L, Basu R, Basu A, Szeri AJ. Modeling the acute effects of exercise on insulin kinetics in type 1 diabetes. J Pharmacokinet Pharmacodyn. 2018;3:018-9611.

105. Roberts CK, Hevener AL, Barnard RJ. Metabolic syndrome and insulin resistance: underlying causes and modification by exercise training. Compr Physiol. 2013;3:1-58.

106. Campbell MD, Walker M, Bracken RM, et al. Insulin therapy and dietary adjustments to normalize glycemia and prevent nocturnal hypoglycemia after evening exercise in type 1 diabetes: a randomized controlled trial. BMJ Open Diabetes Res Care. 2015;3:e000085.

107. Zaharieva DP, Riddell MC. Insulin management strategies for exercise in diabetes. Can J Diabetes. 2017;41:507-16.

108. Franc S, Daoudi A, Pochat A, et al. Insulin-based strategies to prevent hypoglycaemia during and after exercise in adult patients with type 1 diabetes on pump therapy: the DIABRASPORT randomized study. Diabetes Obes Metab. 2015;17:1150-7.

109. Yamamoto C, Miyoshi H, Fujiwara Y, et al. Degludec is superior to glargine in terms of daily glycemic variability in people with type 1 diabetes mellitus. Endocr J. 2016;63:53-60.

110. Heise T, Bain SC, Bracken RM, et al. Similar risk of exercise-related hypoglycaemia for insulin degludec to that for insulin glargine in patients with type 1 diabetes: a randomized crossover trial. Diabetes Obes Metab. 2016;18:196-9.

111. Davey RJ, Howe W, Paramalingam N, et al. The effect of midday moderate-intensity exercise on postexercise hypoglycemia risk in individuals with type 1 diabetes. J Clin Endocrinol Metab. 2013;98:2908-14.

112. McMahon SK, Ferreira LD, Ratnam N, et al. Glucose requirements to maintain euglycemia after moderate-intensity afternoon exercise in adolescents with type 1 diabetes are increased in a biphasic manner. J Clin Endocrinol Metab. 2007;92:963-8.

113. Joy NG, Tate DB, Davis SN. Counterregulatory responses to hypoglycemia differ between glimepiride and glyburide in non diabetic individuals. Metabolism. 2015;64:729-37.

114. Larsen JJ, Dela F, Madsbad S, Vibe-Petersen J, Galbo H. Interaction of sulfonylureas and exercise on glucose homeostasis in type 2 diabetic patients. Diabetes Care. 1999;22:1647-54.

115. Cermak NM, van Loon LJ. The use of carbohydrates during exercise as an ergogenic aid. Sports Med. 2013;43:1139-55.

116. Berlie HD, Garwood CL. Diabetes medications related to an increased risk of falls and fall-related morbidity in the elderly. Ann Pharmacother. 2010;44:712-7.

117. Khazai NB, Beck GR, Jr., Umpierrez GE. Diabetes and fractures: an overshadowed association. Curr Opin Endocrinol Diabetes Obes. 2009;16:435-45.

118. ter Braak EW, Appelman AM, van de Laak M, Stolk RP, van Haeften TW, Erkelens DW. Clinical characteristics of type 1 diabetic patients with and without severe hypoglycemia. Diabetes Care. 2000;23:1467-71.

119. Parkman HP, Fass R, Foxx-Orenstein AE. Treatment of patients with diabetic gastroparesis. Gastroenterol Hepatol (N Y). 2010;6:1-16.

120. Iscoe KE, Davey RJ, Fournier PA. Is the response of continuous glucose monitors to physiological changes in blood glucose levels affected by sensor life? Diabetes Technol Ther. 2012;14:135-42.

121. Bally L, Zueger T, Pasi N, Carlos C, Paganini D, Stettler C. Accuracy of continuous glucose monitoring during differing exercise conditions. Diabetes Res Clin Pract. 2016;112:1-5.

122. Yardley JE, Sigal RJ, Kenny GP, Riddell MC, Lovblom LE, Perkins BA. Point accuracy of interstitial continuous glucose monitoring during exercise in type 1 diabetes. Diabetes Technol Ther. 2013;15:46-9.

123. van Beers CA, DeVries JH, Kleijer SJ, et al. Continuous glucose monitoring for patients with type 1 diabetes and impaired awareness of hypoglycaemia (IN CONTROL): a randomised, open-label, crossover trial. Lancet Diabetes Endocrinol. 2016;4:893-902.

124. Umpierrez G, Korytkowski M. Diabetic emergencies—ketoacidosis, hyperglycaemic hyperosmolar state and hypoglycaemia. Nat Rev Endocrinol. 2016;12:222-32.

125. Kamata Y, Takano K, Kishihara E, Watanabe M, Ichikawa R, Shichiri M. Distinct clinical characteristics and therapeutic modalities for diabetic ketoacidosis in type 1 and type 2 diabetes mellitus. J Diabetes Complications. 2017;31:468-72.

126. Fahey AJ, Paramalingam N, Davey RJ, Davis EA, Jones TW, Fournier PA. The effect of a short sprint on postexercise whole-body glucose production and utilization rates in individuals with type 1 diabetes mellitus. J Clin Endocrinol Metab. 2012;97:4193-200.

127. Aronson R, Brown RE, Li A, Riddell MC. Optimal insulin correction factor in post-high-intensity exercise hyperglycemia in adults with type 1 diabetes: the FIT Study. Diabetes Care. 2019;42(1):10-16.

128. Biagi L, Bertachi A, Quiros C, et al. Accuracy of continuous glucose monitoring before, during, and after aerobic and anaerobic exercise in patients with type 1 diabetes mellitus. Biosensors (Basel). 2018;8(1).bios8010022.

129. Colberg SR, Zarrabi L, Bennington L, et al. Postprandial walking is better for lowering the glycemic effect of dinner than pre-dinner exercise in type 2 diabetic individuals. J Am Med Dir Assoc. 2009;10:394-7.

130. Gomez AM, Gomez C, Aschner P, et al. Effects of performing morning versus afternoon exercise on glycemic control and hypoglycemia frequency in type 1 diabetes patients on sensor-augmented insulin pump therapy. J Diabetes Sci Technol. 2015;9:619-24.

131. Kalergis M, Schiffrin A, Gougeon R, Jones PJ, Yale JF. Impact of bedtime snack composition on prevention of nocturnal hypoglycemia in adults with type 1 diabetes undergoing

intensive insulin management using lispro insulin before meals: a randomized, placebo-controlled, crossover trial. Diabetes Care. 2003;26:9-15.

132. Bell KJ, Smart CE, Steil GM, Brand-Miller JC, King B, Wolpert HA. Impact of fat, protein, and glycemic index on postprandial glucose control in type 1 diabetes: implications for intensive diabetes management in the continuous glucose monitoring era. Diabetes Care. 2015;38:1008-15.

133. Wolpert HA, Atakov-Castillo A, Smith SA, Steil GM. Dietary fat acutely increases glucose concentrations and insulin requirements in patients with type 1 diabetes: implications for carbohydrate-based bolus dose calculation and intensive diabetes management. Diabetes Care. 2013;36:810-6.

134. Hubing KA, Bassett JT, Quigg LR, Phillips MD, Barbee JJ, Mitchell JB. Exercise-associated hyponatremia: the influence of pre-exercise carbohydrate status combined with high volume fluid intake on sodium concentrations and fluid balance. Eur J Appl Physiol. 2011;111:797-807.

135. American College of Sports M, Sawka MN, Burke LM, et al. American College of Sports Medicine position stand. Exercise and fluid replacement. Med Sci Sports Exerc. 2007;39:377-90.

136. Zaharieva D, Yavelberg L, Jamnik V, Cinar A, Turksoy K, Riddell MC. The effects of basal insulin suspension at the start of exercise on blood glucose levels during continuous versus circuit based exercise in individuals with type 1 diabetes on continuous subcutaneous insulin infusion. Diabetes Technol Ther. 2017;19:370-8.

137. Garg S, Brazg RL, Bailey TS, et al. Reduction in duration of hypoglycemia by automatic suspension of insulin delivery: the in-clinic ASPIRE study. Diabetes Technol Ther. 2012;14:205-9.

138. Frank S, Jbaily A, Hinshaw L, Basu R, Basu A, Szeri AJ. Modeling the acute effects of exercise on insulin kinetics in type 1 diabetes. J Pharmacokinet Pharmacodyn. 2018;45:829-45.

139. Kang JH, Tseng SH, Jaw FS, Lai CH, Chen HC, Chen SC. Comparison of ultrasonographic findings of the rotator cuff between diabetic and nondiabetic patients with chronic shoulder pain: a retrospective study. Ultrasound Med Biol. 2010;36:1792-6.

140. Kaminsky LA, Dewey D. The association between body mass index and physical activity, and body image, self esteem and social support in adolescents with type 1 diabetes. Can J Diabetes. 2014;38:244-9.

141. Papataxiarchis E, Panagiotakos DB, Notara V, et al. Physical activity frequency on the 10-year acute coronary syndrome (ACS) prognosis; the interaction with cardiovascular disease history and diabetes mellitus: the GREECS Observational Study. J Aging Phys Act. 2016;24(4):624-32.

142. Piepoli MF, Corra U, Adamopoulos S, et al. Secondary prevention in the clinical management of patients with cardiovascular diseases. Core components, standards and outcome measures for referral and delivery: a policy statement from the cardiac rehabilitation section of the European Association for Cardiovascular Prevention & Rehabilitation. Endorsed by the Committee for Practice Guidelines of the European Society of Cardiology. Eur J Prev Cardiol. 2014;21:664-81.

143. Pena KE, Stopka CB, Barak S, Gertner HR, Jr., Carmeli E. Effects of low-intensity exercise on patients with peripheral artery disease. Phys Sportsmed. 2009;37:106-10.

144. McDermott MM, Ades P, Guralnik JM, et al. Treadmill exercise and resistance training in patients with peripheral arterial disease with and without intermittent claudication: a randomized controlled trial. JAMA. 2009;301:165-74.

145. Colberg SR, Vinik AI. Exercising with peripheral or autonomic neuropathy: what health care providers and diabetic patients need to know. Phys Sportsmed. 2014;42:15-23.

146. Vinik AI, Erbas T. Diabetic autonomic neuropathy. Handb Clin Neurol. 2013;117:279-94.

147. Weston KS, Sacre JW, Jellis CL, Coombes JS. Contribution of autonomic dysfunction to abnormal exercise blood pressure in type 2 diabetes mellitus. J Sci Med Sport. 2013;16:8-12.

148. Loimaala A, Huikuri HV, Koobi T, Rinne M, Nenonen A, Vuori I. Exercise training improves baroreflex sensitivity in type 2 diabetes. Diabetes. 2003;52:1837-42.

149. Tang M, Donaghue KC, Cho YH, Craig ME. Autonomic neuropathy in young people with type 1 diabetes: a systematic review. Pediatr Diabetes. 2013;14:239-48.

150. Ko SU, Stenholm S, Chia CW, Simonsick EM, Ferrucci L. Gait pattern alterations in older adults associated with type 2 diabetes in the absence of peripheral neuropathy–results from the Baltimore Longitudinal Study of Aging. Gait Posture. 2011;34:548-52.

151. Yoo M, D'Silva LJ, Martin K, et al. Pilot study of exercise therapy on painful diabetic peripheral neuropathy. Pain Med. 2015;16:1482-9.

152. Lemaster JW, Mueller MJ, Reiber GE, Mehr DR, Madsen RW, Conn VS. Effect of weight-bearing activity on foot ulcer incidence in people with diabetic peripheral neuropathy: feet first randomized controlled trial. Phys Ther. 2008;88:1385-98.

153. Lemaster JW, Reiber GE, Smith DG, Heagerty PJ, Wallace C. Daily weight-bearing activity does not increase the risk of diabetic foot ulcers. Med Sci Sports Exerc. 2003;35:1093-9.

154. Balducci S, Iacobellis G, Parisi L, et al. Exercise training can modify the natural history of diabetic peripheral neuropathy. J Diabetes Complications. 2006;20:216-23.

155. Waden J, Tikkanen HK, Forsblom C, et al. Leisure-time physical activity and development and progression of diabetic nephropathy in type 1 diabetes: the FinnDiane Study. Diabetologia. 2015;58:929-36.

156. Robinson-Cohen C, Littman AJ, Duncan GE, et al. Physical activity and change in estimated GFR among persons with CKD. J Am Soc Nephrol. 2014;25:399-406.

157. Kornhauser C, Malacara JM, Macias-Cervantes MH, Rivera-Cisneros AE. Effect of exercise intensity on albuminuria in adolescents with type 1 diabetes mellitus. Diabet Med. 2012;29:70-3.

158. Makhlough A, Ilali E, Mohseni R, Shahmohammadi S. Effect of intradialytic aerobic exercise on serum electrolytes levels in hemodialysis patients. Iran J Kidney Dis. 2012;6:119-23.

159. Lopes AA, Lantz B, Morgenstern H, et al. Associations of self-reported physical activity types and levels with quality of life, depression symptoms, and mortality in hemodialysis patients: the DOPPS. Clin J Am Soc Nephrol. 2014;9:1702-12.

160. Weiss EP, Jordan RC, Frese EM, Albert SG, Villareal DT. Effects of weight loss on lean mass, strength, bone, and aerobic capacity. Med Sci Sports Exerc. 2017;49(1):206-17.

161. Sabag A, Way KL, Keating SE, et al. Exercise and ectopic fat in type 2 diabetes: a systematic review and meta-analysis. Diabetes Metab. 2017;43:195-210.

162. Johnson NA, Sachinwalla T, Walton DW, et al. Aerobic exercise training reduces hepatic and visceral lipids in obese individuals without weight loss. Hepatology. 2009;50:1105-12.

163. Donnelly JE, Blair SN, Jakicic JM, Manore MM, Rankin JW, Smith BK. American College of Sports Medicine Position Stand. Appropriate physical activity intervention strategies for weight loss and prevention of weight regain for adults. Medicine & Science in Sports & Exercise. 2009;41:459-71.

164. Russo LM, Nobles C, Ertel KA, Chasan-Taber L, Whitcomb BW. Physical activity interventions in pregnancy and risk of gestational diabetes mellitus: a systematic review and meta-analysis. Obstet Gynecol. 2015;125:576-82.

165. Sanabria-Martinez G, Garcia-Hermoso A, Poyatos-Leon R, Alvarez-Bueno C, Sanchez-Lopez M, Martinez-Vizcaino V. Effectiveness of physical activity interventions on preventing gestational diabetes mellitus and excessive maternal weight gain: a meta-analysis. BJOG. 2015;122:1167-74.

166. Davenport MH, Ruchat SM, Poitras VJ, et al. Prenatal exercise for the prevention of gestational diabetes mellitus and hypertensive disorders of pregnancy: a systematic review and meta-analysis. Br J Sports Med. 2018;52:1367-75.

167. Ruchat SM, Mottola MF, Skow RJ, et al. Effectiveness of exercise interventions in the prevention of excessive gestational weight gain and postpartum weight retention: a systematic review and meta-analysis. Br J Sports Med. 2018;52:1347-56.

168. Davenport MH, Ruchat SM, Poitras VJ, et al. Glucose responses to acute and chronic exercise during pregnancy: a systematic review and meta-analysis. Br J Sports Med. 2018;52:1367-75.

169. Zavorsky GS, Longo LD. Exercise guidelines in pregnancy: new perspectives. Sports Med. 2011;41:345-60.

170. Zavorsky GS, Longo LD. Adding strength training, exercise intensity, and caloric expenditure to exercise guidelines in pregnancy. Obstet Gynecol. 2011;117:1399-402.

171. Watson SL, Weeks BK, Weis LJ, Harding AT, Horan SA, Beck BR. High-intensity resistance and impact training improves bone mineral density and physical function in postmenopausal women with osteopenia and osteoporosis: the LIFTMOR Randomized Controlled Trial. J Bone Miner Res. 2018;33:211-20.

172. Bankoski A, Harris TB, McClain JJ, et al. Sedentary activity associated with metabolic syndrome independent of physical activity. Diabetes Care. 2011;34:497-503.

173. Scott D, Blizzard L, Fell J, Jones G. Prospective study of self-reported pain, radiographic osteoarthritis, sarcopenia progression, and falls risk in community-dwelling older adults. Arthritis Care Res (Hoboken). 2012;64:30-7.

174. Cogbill SA, Thompson VL, Deshpande AD. Selected sociocultural correlates of physical activity among African-American adults. Ethn Health. 2011;16:625-41.

175. Lu Y, Dipierro M, Chen L, Chin R, Fava M, Yeung A. The evaluation of a culturally appropriate, community-based lifestyle intervention program for elderly Chinese immigrants with chronic diseases: a pilot study. J Public Health (Oxf). 2014;36:149-55.

176. Corsino L, Rocha-Goldberg MP, Batch BC, Ortiz-Melo DI, Bosworth HB, Svetkey LP. The Latino Health Project: pilot testing a culturally adapted behavioral weight loss intervention in obese and overweight Latino adults. Ethn Dis. 2012; 22:51-7.

177. Harley AE, Odoms-Young A, Beard B, Katz ML, Heaney CA. African American social and cultural contexts and physical activity: strategies for navigating challenges to participation. Women Health. 2009;49:84-100.

178. Laukkanen JA, Zaccardi F, Khan H, Kurl S, Jae SY, Rauramaa R. Long-term change in cardiorespiratory fitness and all-cause mortality: a population-based follow up study. Mayo Clin Proc. 2016;91:1183-8.

179. Cavalcante BR, Farah BQ, Barbosa JP, et al. Are the barriers for physical activity practice equal for all peripheral artery disease patients? Arch Phys Med Rehabil. 2015;96(2):248-52.

180. Karmeniemi M, Lankila T, Ikaheimo T, Koivumaa-Honkanen H, Korpelainen R. The built environment as a determinant of physical activity: a systematic review of longitudinal studies and natural experiments. Ann Behav Med. 2018;52:239-51.

181. den Braver NR, Lakerveld J, Rutters F, Schoonmade LJ, Brug J, Beulens JWJ. Built environmental characteristics and diabetes: a systematic review and meta-analysis. BMC Med. 2018;16:12.

182. Cerin E, Nathan A, van Cauwenberg J, Barnett DW, Barnett A. The neighbourhood physical environment and active travel in older adults: a systematic review and meta-analysis. Int J Behav Nutr Phys Act. 2017;14:15.

183. King DK, Glasgow RE, Toobert DJ, et al. Self-efficacy, problem solving, and social-environmental support are associated with diabetes self-management behaviors. Diabetes Care. 2010;33:751-3.

184. Climie RE, Grace MS, Larsen RL, et al. Regular brief interruptions to sitting after a high-energy evening meal attenuate glycemic excursions in overweight/obese adults. Nutr Metab Cardiovasc Dis. 2018;28:909-16.

185. Thorp AA, Kingwell BA, English C, et al. Alternating sitting and standing increases the workplace energy expenditure of overweight adults. J Phys Act Health. 2016;13:24-9.

186. Sardinha LB, Santos DA, Silva AM, Baptista F, Owen N. Breaking-up sedentary time is associated with physical function in older adults. J Gerontol A Biol Sci Med Sci. 2015;70:119-24.

187. Reynolds AN, Mann JI, Williams S, Venn BJ. Advice to walk after meals is more effective for lowering postprandial glycaemia in type 2 diabetes mellitus than advice that does not specify timing: a randomised crossover study. Diabetologia. 2016;59:2572-8.

188. Sallis R, Franklin B, Joy L, Ross R, Sabgir D, Stone J. Strategies for promoting physical activity in clinical practice. Prog Cardiovasc Dis. 2015;57:375-86.

189. Lindsay Smith G, Banting L, Eime R, O'Sullivan G, van Uffelen JGZ. The association between social support and physical activity in older adults: a systematic review. Int J Behav Nutr Phys Act. 2017;14:56.

190. Pentecost C, Taket A. Understanding exercise uptake and adherence for people with chronic conditions: a new model demonstrating the importance of exercise identity, benefits of attending and support. Health Educ Res. 2011;26:908-22.

191. Armit CM, Brown WJ, Marshall AL, et al. Randomized trial of three strategies to promote physical activity in general practice. Preventive Medicine. 2009;48:156-63.

192. Balducci S, D'Errico V, Haxhi J, et al. Effect of a behavioral intervention strategy on sustained change in physical activity and sedentary behavior in patients with type 2 diabetes: the IDES_2 Randomized Clinical Trial. JAMA. 2019;321:880-90.

193. Balducci S, D'Errico V, Haxhi J, et al. Effect of a behavioral intervention strategy for adoption and maintenance of a physically active lifestyle: The Italian Diabetes and Exercise Study 2 (IDES_2): A Randomized Controlled Trial. Diabetes Care. 2017;40:1444-52.

194. Bgeginski R, Ribeiro PAB, Mottola MF, Ramos JGL. Effects of weekly supervised exercise or physical activity counseling on fasting blood glucose in women diagnosed with gestational diabetes mellitus: A systematic review and meta-analysis of randomized trials. J Diabetes. 2017;9:1023-32.

195. Cahn A, Akirov A, Raz I. Digital health technology and diabetes management. J Diabetes. 2018;10:10-7.

196. Greenwood DA, Gee PM, Fatkin KJ, Peeples M. A systemic review of reviews evaluating technology-enabled diabetes self-management education and support. J Diabetes Sci Technol. 2017;11:1015-27.

197. Rollo ME, Aguiar EJ, Williams RL, et al. eHealth technologies to support nutrition and physical activity behaviors in diabetes self-management. Diabetes Metab Syndr Obes. 2016;9:381-90.

198. Deacon AJ, Edirippulige S. Using mobile technology to motivate adolescents with type 1 diabetes mellitus: A systematic review of recent literature. J Telemed Telecare. 2015;21:431-8.

199. Nakhasi A, Shen AX, Passarella RJ, Appel LJ, Anderson CA. Online social networks that connect users to physical activity partners: a review and descriptive analysis. J Med Internet Res. 2014;16:e153.

200. Kohl LF, Crutzen R, de Vries NK. Online prevention aimed at lifestyle behaviors: a systematic review of reviews. J Med Internet Res. 2013;15:e146.

201. Baskerville R, Ricci-Cabello I, Roberts N, Farmer A. Impact of accelerometer and pedometer use on physical activity and glycaemic control in people with type 2 diabetes: a systematic review and meta-analysis. Diabet Med. 2017;34:612-20.

202. Funk M, Taylor EL. Pedometer-based walking interventions for free-living adults with type 2 diabetes: a systematic review. Curr Diabetes Rev. 2013;9:462-71.

203. Cheatham SW, Stull KR, Fantigrassi M, Motel I. The efficacy of wearable activity tracking technology as part of a weight loss program: a systematic review. J Sports Med Phys Fitness. 2018;58:534-48.

204. Kirk MA, Amiri M, Pirbaglou M, Ritvo P. Wearable technology and physical activity behavior change in adults with chronic cardiometabolic disease: a systematic review and meta-analysis. Am J Health Promot. 2018;26:0890117118816278.

205. Qiu S, Cai X, Chen X, Yang B, Sun Z. Step counter use in type 2 diabetes: a meta-analysis of randomized controlled trials. BMC Med. 2014;12:36.

206. Connelly J, Kirk A, Masthoff J, MacRury S. The use of technology to promote physical activity in type 2 diabetes management: a systematic review. Diabet Med. 2013;30:1420-32.

207. Merolli M, Gray K, Martin-Sanchez F. Health outcomes and related effects of using social media in chronic disease management: a literature review and analysis of affordances. J Biomed Inform. 2013;46:957-69.

208. Duff OM, Walsh DM, Furlong BA, O'Connor NE, Moran KA, Woods CB. Behavior change techniques in physical activity eHealth interventions for people with cardiovascular disease: systematic review. J Med Internet Res. 2017;19:e281.

209. Dellasega C, Anel-Tiangco RM, Gabbay RA. How patients with type 2 diabetes mellitus respond to motivational interviewing. Diabetes Res Clin Pract. 2012;95:37-41.

210. Ekong G, Kavookjian J. Motivational interviewing and outcomes in adults with type 2 diabetes: a systematic review. Patient Educ Couns. 2016;99(6):944-52.

CHAPTER 7

Taking Medication

Devra K. Dang, PharmD, BCPS, CDCES, FNAP

Key Concepts

- Self-care behaviors related to taking medication are important to develop, evaluate, and enhance engagement. The diabetes care and education specialist plays an important role in this.
- The diabetes care and education specialist must have the ability to recognize potential barriers that could interfere with an individual's engagement with his or her medication regimen. An important part of the diabetes care and education specialist's job is to assist the person with diabetes in identifying and addressing these barriers.
- The diabetes care and education specialist must be well versed in medication-taking considerations (eg, administration technique, dosing, frequency, potential adverse reactions, possible drug interactions) for each type of prescription diabetes medication and be able to convey this information clearly to the person living with diabetes.
- The diabetes care and education specialist should also be familiar with basic concepts for common categories of nonprescription medications and dietary supplements that persons with diabetes may use.

Introduction

Taking medication is a crucial self-care behavior that contributes to optimal diabetes management. In this chapter, considerations related to medication use in persons living with diabetes are discussed. Special focus is on the diabetes care and education specialist's role and opportunities to reinforce self-care behaviors related to taking diabetes medications. The chapter begins by examining what enhances the individual's ability to follow the regimen and what enhances the actual administration of the medication. Risk factors and warning signs for the diabetes care and education specialist to recognize are summarized. This section describes the following:

- Promoting the use of medication administration aids that enhance the individual's ability to follow the medication plan
- Choosing medication delivery methods and treatment regimens appropriate to the individual
- Addressing cost (affordability)

Strategies to improve individuals' ability to follow their medication regimens and derive the intended benefit of the medications are also discussed.

Next, the chapter describes clinical considerations relevant to specific medications used in glycemic management, with an emphasis on education strategies for the person with diabetes. In regard to this, each of the following is discussed separately:

- Alpha-glucosidase inhibitors
- Amylin analog
- Biguanides
- Bile acid sequestrants
- Dipeptidyl peptidase-4 inhibitors
- Dopamine receptor agonists
- Glucagon-like peptide-1 agonists
- Insulin
- Sodium-glucose co-transporter 2 inhibitors
- Sulfonylureas and meglitinides
- Thiazolidinediones

The discussion of insulin includes consideration of delivery method options and regimen choices. An outline of basic and advanced education topics is presented, along with a summary of teaching topics regarding insulin use. Strategies to overcome barriers of injection and fears related to taking insulin are presented to promote better medication-taking behaviors.

Other drugs that the individual with diabetes may be taking are considered next. Drug interactions and use of the following nonprescription medications and products are addressed:

- Alcohol- and sugar-free products
- Cough and cold products
- Pain and fever products
- Products for gastrointestinal ailments
- Dietary supplements
- Topical and dermatologic products
- Products for oral hygiene and dental care
- Ophthalmologic products

The chapter also provides an overview of the unique needs of children, adolescents, and the elderly with regard to medication taking.

Case—Part 1

You are a diabetes care and education specialist working at a primary care clinic. AB is a 53-year-old African-American woman diagnosed with type 2 diabetes 15 years ago. She has also been diagnosed with hypertension and hyperlipidemia. She is currently prescribed glyburide twice daily, metformin three times daily with meals, pioglitazone once-daily, lisinopril once-daily, hydrochlorothiazide once-daily, amlodipine once-daily, and atorvastatin once-daily. AB's A1C readings in the past year have ranged from 8.5% to 9.5%, and AB's primary care provider is interested in initiating insulin therapy. However, he is concerned that she may not be taking the medications as prescribed. You meet AB, and she immediately states that she is very reluctant to start insulin because within 2 years after her father was initiated on insulin, he became blind and was also started on dialysis. AB wants to know if there is another "pill" she can take to manage her diabetes instead.

Medication Taking in Diabetes

Following a prescribed medication program is integral to the success of most medical treatment plans, and in the management of a chronic condition such as diabetes, following the medication regimen is crucial self-care behavior. Following the medication plan includes not only taking prescribed medications but also taking them on time, at the right time to get the best effects, and at the correct frequency, and utilizing appropriate medication administration techniques. Long-term engagement with taking oral glucose-lowering agents has been reported as ranging from 36% to 93%, with insulin engagement in persons with type 2 diabetes ranging from 62% to 80%.[1,2] The Diabetes Attitudes, Wishes, and Needs study found that a third of those with diabetes reported feeling tired of following their medication regimen.[1] Poor medication nonadherence has been shown to correlate with worse glycemic and lipid stability.[2,3] Although medication nonadherence is typically viewed as not taking medication, or not taking enough doses, it is important to remember that medication nonadherence also encompasses taking too much medication.

Risk Factors for, and Warning Signs of, Poor Medication-Taking Behavior

Awareness of the risk factors for, and warning signs of, poor medication-taking engagement is the first step in resolving this problem. Warning signs of an individual's poor engagement with the medication and treatment plans include the following:[3]

- Poorly managed diabetes
- Erratic fluctuations in blood glucose
- Lack of engagement with office visits and/or recommended clinical testing
- Lack of engagement with self-monitoring of blood glucose or with reporting these results

Asking the person with diabetes to bring in their prescription bottles or reviewing the refill history can also provide clues to medication-taking engagement. For example, if an individual is refilling medications too early, he or she may be taking more medication than prescribed due to elevations in blood glucose. Although the medication refill history pattern can be quite helpful in assessing medication-taking engagement, this record does not always accurately reflect medication-taking behavior. Many community pharmacies offer an automatic refill service whereby prescriptions are automatically refilled on the day they are due based on the day supply of the original prescription, thereby making it appear that the person is perfectly engaged with their medication regimen. A multifaceted approach to assessing medication-taking behavior should be utilized. Risk factors for poor medication-taking behavior include the following:[2,4–6]

- Age—the elderly and adolescents are at the highest risk
- Medication dosing frequency and complexity of the regimen
- Number of medications the person with diabetes is taking
- Presence of other concurrent medical conditions

TABLE 7.1 Medication-Taking Barriers to Diabetes Mellitus Medication Use

Person with Diabetes Factor	*Medication Factor*	*Provider or System Factor*
Fears: disease worsening, hypoglycemia, needles, social stigma, weight gain Knowledge, understanding, and skill: education Self-efficacy Health beliefs Depression Lack of confidence in immediate or future benefits of the medication Remembering doses and refills	Complexity of regimen (eg, more than 1 diabetes medication or other drugs, splitting tablets, drawing up insulin) Frequency of dosing (2 or more times daily results in poorer medication taking) Cost Adverse effects	Fear that person with diabetes will not be able to use therapy Knowledge: medications, use of insulin, monitoring, diabetes treatment Skill: able to demonstrate proper use of devices Inadequate educational support Inadequate follow-up resources Clinical inertia

Source: Adapted from PS Odegard, K Capoccia. "Medication taking and diabetes: a systematic review of the literature," *Diabetes Educ* 2007; 33:1014–29; discussion 1030–1.

- Presence of depression or other psychiatric disorders
- The individual's understanding of the treatment regimen and its potential benefits and side effects
- Perception of the severity of the disease
- Socioeconomic status
- Health insurance status
- Cost of medications
- Poor family dynamics or lack of social support
- Poor relationship with prescriber
- Duration of diabetes

There are also medication-related and provider- or system-related barriers to medication taking. Table 7.1 summarizes the person with diabetes-, medication-, and provider- or system-related barriers to medication taking in the management of diabetes.[7] Health literacy is another significant barrier to medication taking and is discussed in the Focus on Education section at the end of this chapter.

Strategies to Improve Medication-Taking Behavior

An interprofessional approach is crucial in the management of diabetes. The entire team of physicians, nurses, pharmacists, dietitians, physician assistants, social workers, and others can share information to increase the likelihood of positive clinical outcomes. Collaboration with the pharmacist can optimize both identification and resolution of medication-related problems, including but not limited to, medication-taking engagement barriers. Consultation with the pharmacist regarding medication formulations, frequency, pharmacology, pharmacogenomic factors, and cost can optimize efficacy and minimize adverse drug reactions and drug interactions, leading to improved medication taking and clinical outcomes.

Relationship and Communication

Establishing a trusting, nonjudgmental relationship between the healthcare professional and the person with diabetes is a crucial component in enhancing the individual's engagement with medication taking and the treatment plan. The person with diabetes should feel that he or she has a level of control over treatment decisions, including medication therapy, and that his or her wishes are viewed as important. He or she should feel comfortable expressing any concerns about medication therapy. It can be easy for healthcare professionals to forget that persons living with diabetes don't always share the same view and understanding of the efficacy and necessity of medications that they do.

The diabetes care and education specialist should explain to the person with diabetes the expected benefits and rationale of the medication and treatment plans. The educator should help the person understand the natural course of diabetes, how the prescribed medications work to prevent complications of diabetes, and why frequent monitoring and intensification of therapy are needed to prevent these complications. It can also be helpful to explain the predicted target dose and titration schedule at initiation of therapy so that the person with diabetes does not feel discouraged every time the dose is increased. For example, metformin is often initiated at 500 mg once or twice daily with a goal of titrating to a total daily dose of 2,000 mg/day over the course of several weeks. Not having this background therapeutic knowledge, the person with diabetes may become frustrated and discouraged if they see the metformin dose increased at every visit (to the planned target dose) even though they have been working hard at medication-taking engagement and therapeutic lifestyle changes.

The diabetes care and education specialist should also acknowledge the potential for adverse drug reactions and discuss the expected likelihood that these may occur, ways that the individual can minimize or avoid these reactions, what the healthcare team is doing to monitor for these reactions, and how the individual can actively participate in this via self-monitoring. When applicable, the educator should also explain why more than 1 drug is often needed in order to address the multiple pathophysiologic processes of diabetes and associated complications. Cultural and religious beliefs and socioeconomic factors should also be taken into consideration when communicating about the treatment plan.

Regimen Changes and Adjustments

Some simple strategies specific to medication formulation that can enhance an individual's ability to follow the medication plan include the following:

- Decreasing the frequency of medication administration—by using once-daily medications whenever possible
- Decreasing pill burden—by using combination tablets

Combination tablets are available for glucose-lowering drugs (see Table 7.2) and many antihypertensive drugs, including various combinations of an angiotensin-converting enzyme (ACE) inhibitor or angiotensin II receptor blocker (ARB) plus the diuretic hydrochlorothiazide. Combinations of a calcium channel blocker and ACE inhibitor, such as amlodipine plus benazepril (Lotrel®, Novartis; generics), or a calcium channel blocker and a 3-hydroxy-3-methylglutaryl-coenzyme A reductase inhibitor, such as amlodipine plus atorvastatin (Caduet®, Pfizer; generics), are also available. It is important to recognize that cost may be a barrier, as some combination tablets are available as brand only or are at a higher co-pay tier on insurance formularies. Two fixed-ratio combinations that incorporate a once-daily glucagon-like peptide-1 agonist and a basal insulin into a single pen are also available.

TABLE 7.2 Combination Oral Glucose-Lowering Medications

Generic Name	*Trade Name*
Alogliptin-metformin	Kazano®
Alogliptin-pioglitazone	Oseni®
Canagliflozin-metformin	Invokamet®, Invokamet® XR
Dapagliflozin-metformin XR	Xigduo XR®
Dapagliflozin-saxagliptin	Qtern®
Dapagliflozin-saxagliptin-metformin XR	Qternmet® XR
Empagliflozin-metformin	Synjardy®, Synjardy® XR
Empagliflozin-linagliptin	Glyxambi®
Empagliflozin-linagliptin-metformin XR	Trijardy™
Ertugliflozin-metformin	Segluromet™
Ertulgliflozin-sitagliptin	Steglujan™
Glipizide-metformin	Available as generic only
Glyburide-metformin	Available as generic only
Linagliptin-metformin	Jentadueto®, Jentadueto XR®
Pioglitazone-metformin	ACTOplus met®, generics
Pioglitazone + glimepiride	Duetact®, generics
Sitagliptin-metformin	Janumet® and Janumet XR®
Saxagliptin-metformin XR	Kombiglyze™ XR

Product Aids

A variety of medication administration aids are available from pharmacies, via online Web sites, and directly from manufacturers. Administration aids may help the individual follow the medication plan and include the following:

- Pill organizers
- Medication reminders, including alarms and mobile apps
- Medication calendars
- Blister packaging
- Insulin injection aids

One study found that 80% of adults with diabetes use at least 1 form of a medication-use aid, including use of a pill organizer in 50% of persons with diabetes.[8] The diabetes care and education specialist should be aware of the different types of administration aids available in order to help persons with diabetes select the most appropriate product.

Addressing Medication Cost

No matter how effective a medication's clinical effects may be, those who cannot afford to have the prescription filled cannot benefit from it. In a study in adults with diabetes, 19% of those surveyed reported decreasing medication use due to cost, and 28% reported going without food or other essentials in order to afford medications.[9]

Strategies to Reduce Cost

Occasionally, the use of more expensive medications is necessary due to factors such as intolerable adverse drug reactions or the need to obtain clinical benefit, and less expensive medications may be less desirable. However, there is typically an array of medications available and different strategies to decrease cost. For those who have health insurance, selecting a medication that is not only on the insurance plan's formulary but also at the lowest co-pay tier (eg, generics) is one option. For medications that are still branded, there is often one medication within the drug class that is considered "preferred." Therefore selecting or switching to that medication within the drug class can result in a lower copay. Drug manufacturers often have coupons or savings program for branded medications, especially newly marketed ones. A simple check of the Web site for each medication should reveal this. For those without medication insurance, various national and local pharmacy chains run discount programs whereby generic medications can be purchased for approximately $4 to $16 for 30 to 100 tablets/capsules. At least one of the national community pharmacy chains also offers selected nonprescription medications through the same discount plan. Some community pharmacy chains also advertise that they provide metformin, second-generation sulfonylureas, lancets, and insulin syringes at no cost. Prescription savings cards that enable the holder to receive a discount at participating pharmacies are also available to those who belong to various organizations (eg, the American Automobile Association's Prescription Savings program, AARP's Prescription Discounts program). If a person with diabetes chooses to use more than one pharmacy to obtain medications due to cost considerations, the diabetes care and education specialist should educate the person that the complete list of medications should be provided to both the healthcare team and the community pharmacists to ensure that there are no duplicate or interacting medications.

Individuals who are uninsured and meet income qualifications can overcome the cost barrier by using manufacturer-sponsored medication assistance programs. A listing of such programs is available at medicationassistance tool.org, a search engine sponsored by the Pharmaceutical Research and Manufacturers of America, and the non-profit NeedyMeds (www.needymeds.org). Both Web sites allow the user to enter the name of their medication(s), which results in a list of matching manufacturer assistance programs, coupons/rebates, savings card, and other potential resources for each medication. The American Diabetes Association has a web page dedicated to prescription assistance resources insulinhelp.org. Other resources include some local and state health departments, which carry a limited formulary of medications for lower income individuals, and free clinics, where medical care and medications are provided free or at a minimal cost (usually on a sliding scale based on income).

Older adults and others who qualify for Medicare are able to purchase prescription drug coverage insurance through Medicare Part D; these individuals should be encouraged to sign up as soon as they are eligible as there is a late-enrollment penalty (https://www.medicare.gov/find-a-plan/questions/home.aspx). They should review their Part D plan once a year to determine whether the particular plan selected the previous year still provides adequate coverage and at an acceptable co-pay level for their current medication regimen, especially if they were initiated on new medications during the year. The Medicare Prescription Drug Plan Web site contains a section where the individual can compare prescription medication plans available in his or her zip code (medicare.gov/plan-compare).

It is important for diabetes care and education specialists to remember that most Medicare Part D plans have a period during which out-of-pocket medication costs are increased, which may greatly affect engagement with medication taking. This coverage gap (also referred to as the "donut hole") may vary each year. In 2019, once the individual and the plan have spent $3,820 in covered medications, the individual is in the donut hole. During this time, the individual will pay up to 25% of the Part D plan's cost of covered brand-name prescription medications. A different coinsurance rule is applied for generic medications. The individual is out of the donut hole upon reaching $5,100 in medication expenses, after which he or she will pay only a small medication copayment for the rest of the year. There are slightly different rules starting in 2020. The donut hole is typically reached during the latter part of the year, and the diabetes care and education specialist should be aware of this, especially in individuals who are prescribed multiple brand-name medications. More information about the Medicare Part D donut hole is available at https://www.medicare.gov/drug-coverage-part-d/costs-for-medicare-drug-coverage/costs-in-the-coverage-gap. Due to potential changes in healthcare reform regulations, it is important to check the www.medicare.gov Web site for the latest information.

Education and Basic Clinical Considerations for Diabetes Medications

The diabetes care and education specialist should be well versed in the potential efficacy and adverse drug reactions, and education points for all medications prescribed for hyperglycemia management. A review of education points specific to optimizing medication-taking behavior is provided below. More detailed information on the pharmacology, efficacy, adverse reactions, and other factors for each drug and drug class is provided in chapter 17, on pharmacotherapy for glucose management.

Alpha-Glucosidase Inhibitors

Alpha-glucosidase inhibitors work by delaying the absorption of carbohydrates from the intestinal tract, which reduces the rise of postprandial blood glucose. Products available are acarbose (Precose®, Bayer) and miglitol (Glyset®, Pharmacia and Upjohn). Normally, hypoglycemia is not a risk with monotherapy of these medications. However, when hypoglycemia does occur due to concomitant administration with other glucose-lowering drugs, the person needs to understand that only glucose tablets can be used for treatment, due to the mechanism of action of these drugs. See also the more detailed discussion on alpha-glucosidase inhibitors in chapter 17, on pharmacotherapy for glucose management.

Amylin Analog

Pramlintide (Symlin®, Amylin) can be used in the management of both type 1 and type 2 diabetes who use mealtime insulin. The diabetes care and education specialist should explain the difference between this medication and insulin, including how it works and the difference in dosing units compared with insulin. Pramlintide is taken before meals that contain at least 250 calories or at least 30 g of carbohydrates and should be skipped if a meal is skipped or if the person is experiencing hypoglycemia. Persons taking pramlintide should also know that the mealtime insulin doses will need to be decreased by 50% initially. Education about the potential for hypoglycemia, recognition of hypoglycemic symptoms, and specific corrective actions that can be taken if it occurs should be provided. In addition, the potential for drug-induced nausea and vomiting should also be acknowledged. Persons taking pramlintide should be educated that pramlintide can delay absorption of certain oral medications, and these may need to be administered at least 1 hour before or 2 hours after pramlintide injection.[10] See also the discussions on pramlintide in chapter 17, on pharmacotherapy for glucose management.

Biguanides

The only medication currently available in the biguanide drug class is metformin. Metformin (Glucophage® and Glucophage® XR, Bristol-Myers Squibb, generics; Glumetza®, Santarus Inc, generics; Riomet® and Riomet ER™ (Sun Pharma)) is the first-line agent for the treatment of type 2 diabetes in most persons with diabetes, and it has several advantages over the other oral medications for hyperglycemia (does not cause weight gain, has no risk of hypoglycemia in most persons when used as monotherapy, allows for lower doses of insulin, comes in combination tablets with most other oral medications). Thus, every therapeutically appropriate effort should be made to maintain metformin as a viable treatment option in treating persons with type 2 diabetes.

In clinical practice, an oft-cited reason for discontinuation of metformin is intolerance to the gastrointestinal side effects. In many cases, these side effects are likely due to titrating the dose too quickly. Metformin should be initiated at the lowest dose (500 mg once or twice daily) and titrated slowly (eg, by 500 mg per week) to decrease the risk of gastrointestinal side effects such as diarrhea, nausea, vomiting, and abdominal discomfort. Taking metformin with meals also minimizes the risk of these side effects. In most persons, gastrointestinal side effects, if they occur, are mild and typically abate with time. However, if a person is taking the full daily dose of metformin and stops taking it for more than several days, the medication should be re-titrated when it is restarted. Another reason for "intolerance" and/or lack of engagement with metformin therapy is the very large tablet size, especially for the 1,000-mg strength. Also, some formulations of metformin tablets emit a very strong odor that has been likened to "old locker-room sweat socks" or "fishy" and that in itself may lead to nausea and self-discontinuation of the drug.[11] Both of these barriers can be overcome by using liquid metformin (Riomet®, Mikart Inc.), which is available as a 500-mg/5-ml oral solution with a non-offensive cherry or strawberry flavor and odor. One drawback to the liquid form is that a person cannot rely on a pill organizer as medication-use aid. Using the film-coated, extended-release formulation can decrease the offensive odor while still allowing the person to place the tablets in a pill organizer, but it does not overcome the concern about tablet size. Some manufacturers of immediate-release metformin advertise that their formulation of metformin does not have an offensive odor. The diabetes care and education specialist can consult a pharmacist for recommendations on the formulation and manufacturer. Persons taking any formulation of metformin should be advised to report the use of this medication to all of their healthcare providers, as its use is contraindicated when receiving intra-arterial iodinated contrast and in other conditions that predispose the individual to the risk of renal failure or lactic acidosis, such as dehydration, heart failure, or liver disease and alcoholism. See also the more detailed discussion of metformin in chapter 17, on pharmacotherapy for glucose management.

Bile Acid Sequestrants

The main use of bile acid sequestrants is in the management of hyperlipidemia, but colesevelam (Welchol®; generics, Daiichi Sankyo) has an additional FDA-approved indication for the management of type 2 diabetes as an adjunct to lifestyle changes. Bloating, nausea, and constipation are the main adverse reactions with this class of medication, and they can interfere with absorption of other medications the person with diabetes is taking and the fat-soluble vitamins (A, D, E, and K). Therefore, these affected medications should be taken at least 4 hours prior to colesevelam administration, which can adversely affect medication taking in those juggling multiple medications. Another factor that may affect engagement with administration is that colesevelam tablets are large, and a dose is 6 tablets once-daily or 3 tablets twice daily with a meal. The large tablets may cause dysphagia or esophageal obstruction, and the medication should be taken with food and liquid. An oral powder for suspension formulation (to be mixed with water, juice, or diet beverages) and a chewable bar are available.[12] See also the more detailed discussion of colesevelam in chapter 20, on pharmacotherapy for dyslipidemia and hypertension.

Dipeptidyl Peptidase-4 Inhibitors

Medications in the dipeptidyl peptidase-4 (DPP-4) inhibitors class currently available in the United States are alogliptin (Nesina®, Takeda Pharmaceuticals America, Inc.), linagliptin (Tradjenta®, Boehringer Ingelheim), saxagliptin (Onglyza™, AstraZeneca), and sitagliptin (Januvia®, Merck), with various others currently in development. Persons taking one of these medications should be advised to monitor for symptoms of pancreatitis and seek medical attention immediately should these occur. They are also associated with severe arthralgia. An increased risk of hospitalization for heart failure has been observed with alogliptin and saxasgliptin. See also the more detailed discussion of DPP-4 inhibitors in chapter 17, on pharmacotherapy for glucose management.

Dopamine Receptor Agonists

Bromocriptine (Cycloset®, VeroScience) is the only medication in the dopamine receptor agonists drug class that has been approved by the US Food and Drug Administration (FDA) at the time of writing. Bromocriptine should be taken with food within 2 hours of waking in the morning. A potential adverse reaction is orthostatic hypotension and syncope and may be especially problematic in those who take concomitant antihypertensives. This medication can also cause somnolence. The medication's labeling advises caution while operating heavy machinery.[13] See also the discussion of bromocriptine in chapter 17, on pharmacotherapy for glucose management.

Glucagon-Like Peptide-1 Receptor Agonists

The glucagon-like peptide-1 (GLP-1) receptor agonists available at the time of writing are dulaglutide (Trulicity®, Eli Lilly), exenatide (Byetta®, Bydureon®, Amylin), liraglutide (Victoza®, Novo Nordisk), lixisenatide (Adlyxin®, Sanofi-Aventis), and semaglutide (Ozempic®, Novo Nordisk). These are all injectable medications, though an oral formulation of semaglutide recently received FDA approval in September 2019. Liraglutide and lixisenatide are also available in combination (in the same pen) with insulin degludec and insulin glargine, respectively. Persons using these medications should understand that they are not a substitute for insulin in those who require insulin for glycemic management, as they may mistakenly think they are trading one type of injectable medication for another. The fact that these medications are associated with weight loss may be especially appealing for those individuals with diabetes who are overweight/obese and insulin resistant.

Those who are prescribed these injectable therapies should be carefully taught how to administer them, including differences in dosing units compared with insulin. They should be advised to monitor for symptoms of pancreatitis and seek medical attention immediately should these occur. Nausea and vomiting are potential common side effects. Those prescribed the once-weekly GLP-1 receptor agonists (dulaglutide, exenatide LAR, semaglutide) should clearly understand the very specific instructions for what to do if a dose is missed, as they can be confusing to some. See also the discussions on these medications in chapter 17, on pharmacotherapy for glucose management.

Sodium-Glucose Co-Transporter 2 Inhibitors

Sodium-glucose co-transporter 2 (SGLT2) inhibitors are the most recently-introduced class of oral glucose-lowering medications available for the management of type 2 diabetes. Canagliflozin (Invokana®, Janssen Pharmaceuticals, Inc.), dapagliflozin (Farxiga®, AstraZeneca), empagliflozin (Jardiance®, Boehringer Ingelheim), and ertugliflozin (Steglatro™, Merck & Co.) are available in the United States in this drug class at the time of writing. A number of potential adverse drug reactions have been described with these agents and should be discussed with the person with diabetes. In particular, genital mycotic infections in both sexes, urinary tract infection, increased urination, and hypotension are potential adverse drug reactions that may be quite distressing to the individual prescribed this medication and lead to lack of engagement. A potential benefit is weight loss and a slight reducion in blood pressure. For additional education points on monitoring for potential adverse drug reactions, see the more detailed discussion of SGLT2 inhibitors in chapter 17, on pharmacotherapy for glucose management.

Sulfonylureas and Meglitinides

Only second-generation sulfonylureas should be used, due to the lower potency and higher risk for hypoglycemia with first-generation sulfonylureas. The second-generation sulfonylureas are glipizide (Glucotrol® and Glucotrol XL®, Pfizer; generics), glyburide (Diabeta®, Sanofi Aventis; Glynase®, Pharmacia and Upjohn; generics), and glimepiride (Amaryl®, Sanofi Aventis; generics). All of the second-generation sulfonylureas are dosed once or twice daily. The XL version of glipizide should not be cut in half, because doing so may cause the medication to be released faster than intended and increase the risk of hypoglycemia. Sulfonylureas achieve their maximum glucose-lowering effect at half the maximum daily dose.[14] Nonsulfonylurea secretagogues—repaglinide (generics) and nateglinide (Starlix®, Novartis; generics)—are given immediately prior to meals to specifically lower postmeal glucose elevations. Unlike sulfonylureas, which can be given once or twice daily, meglitinides must be given up to 3 (nateglinide) or 4 (repaglinide) times a day (before each meal) due to their short half-life, which may adversely affect medication taking. However, this property is an advantage in persons who have an erratic meal schedule, as they can skip the dose if the meal is not eaten or delay the dose if the meal is delayed. Discussion of the risks of hypoglycemia and weight gain should be provided to persons taking either drug class. See also the more detailed discussions on these medications in chapter 17, on pharmacotherapy for glucose management.

Thiazolidinediones

Persons prescribed a thiazolidinedione (TZD) should understand that the maximum glucose-lowering effect of this medication may not be apparent until after 8 to 12 weeks of use. Products available are pioglitazone (Actos®, Takeda; generics) and rosiglitazone (Avandia®, SB Pharmco; generics). Those starting one of these medications need to be encouraged to keep taking it until a full effect can be determined. Persons taking TZDs should be educated about the risks of fluid retention (including precipitation and exacerbation of heart failure symptoms) and weight gain and how to self-monitor for these adverse events. See also the more detailed discussion of TZDs in chapter 17, on pharmacotherapy for glucose management.

Insulin

Insulin is essential for treatment of type 1 diabetes and is also used in persons with type 2 diabetes, especially in those with glucose toxicity or ineffective beta cell function. Insulin can be used at any time during the lifespan of type 2 diabetes and should not be considered a "last resort" option. Insulin is available in formulations that differ in their onset, peak and length of action, and source. In addition to therapeutic considerations, the choice of which insulin regimen to use should be individualized based on the person's daily schedule, willingness to check blood glucose levels, and the number of daily insulin injections the individual is willing to receive or administer.

The most physiologic insulin regimen is the so-called basal-bolus regimen, which uses a long-acting insulin as the basal dose and a rapid-acting insulin as the bolus dose given at meals. Advantages of this regimen include a lower risk of hypoglycemia and the ability to adjust the dose of the rapid-acting insulin according to meal content and timing.

Premixed insulins may be chosen over a basal-bolus regimen due to the individual's preference for no more than twice-daily insulin injections, the individual's inability to remember >2 doses of insulins throughout the day, or financial constraints. However, premixed insulins have a number of disadvantages compared to the basal-bolus regimen, including inability to separately adjust the dose of the 2 components and increased risk of hypoglycemia.

Whether subcutaneously-administered insulin is given via a syringe, pen device, pump, or needle-free jet injector is determined by the individual's personal choice, physical limitations, insurance coverage, educational level, and/or financial resources. A prandial version of insulin is also available as an inhaled formulation, which can reduce injection burden but requires appropriate selection and monitoring given the potential for respiratory adverse drug reactions. See also the more detailed discussion on insulin in chapter 17, on pharmacotherapy for glucose management.

Fears of Insulin

Taking insulin can be a particularly challenging self-care behavior for people with diabetes. Resistance to taking insulin (to initiation of insulin therapy, engagement with current insulin therapy, or both) due to fears and other beliefs has been described extensively in the literature. This "psychological insulin resistance" is a significant barrier to treatment and may be due to many factors—fear of needles and injections, fear of an adverse reaction (hypoglycemia, weight gain), concern about alterations in lifestyle/schedule, concerns about ability to self-manage the demands of an insulin regimen, misconceptions about insulin including lack of efficacy, and perceived failure of self-management of diabetes are but a few examples.[1,15] Fear of insulin and misconceptions about insulin are fairly common in clinical practice, but these beliefs are not always shared with the healthcare team. The diabetes care and education specialist needs to be able to elicit concerns about insulin from the person with diabetes and assist the healthcare team in addressing these beliefs. One way to do this is through the establishment of a trusting relationship and open communication, as discussed earlier, as well as the use of motivational interviewing techniques. A thorough discussion of motivational interviewing is beyond the scope of this chapter. Welch et al provide a good review of motivational interviewing in diabetes.[16] In brief, motivational interviewing "instructs us to appreciate the limits of a direct-persuasion, advice-giving model of clinician influence, guides toward a strong appreciation of the role of ambivalence in behavior change and the value of eliciting change talk from the person with diabetes, and models the use of effective listening skills to build rapport, engage, understand, and facilitate behavior change."[16(p10)]

Explanations of the benefits of insulin and its crucial role for glycemic management, and hence potential prevention of long-term complications of diabetes, need to be carefully communicated. Some prescribers inadvertently communicate the need for insulin therapy to persons with diabetes as a "have to" medication (eg, "If you are not able to managed your diabetes with diet, exercise, and the oral pills, I will have to put you on insulin"). The diabetes care and education specialist should strive to avoid any type of tone and wording that impart a negative connotation to the use of insulin.

Fear of hypoglycemia can be a particularly strong barrier to initiation of, and engagement with, insulin therapy. The fear of hypoglycemia because of past experiences with insulin (by the person or by a close friend or relative) may be ingrained in a person's mind. The educator should make such persons aware of the availability of insulin analogs that, compared with the older insulins, more closely mimic the body's natural release of insulin and have been shown to decrease the incidence and severity of hypoglycemia. Detailed education regarding steps to avoid hypoglycemia, recognition of signs and symptoms of hypoglycemia, and corrective actions to take should it occur should always be provided to those prescribed insulin. Some people associate insulin initiation with the development of long-term complications of diabetes, such as nephropathy and dialysis. The diabetes care and education specialist should explain that the complication was most likely present before the insulin was initiated and may have been avoided if insulin initiation to improve glucose levels had not been delayed.

Showing the person the different options for administration (which may, as appropriate, include short needles, an insulin pen device, a needle-free jet injector, or the inhaled insulin) may help alleviate some of the fears about injections and allow the person to make some choices in how to improve individual outcomes. Some people associate injections, especially with syringes, with drug abuse. The use of insulin pens may be more acceptable to those with this belief. Again, the diabetes care and education specialist should thoroughly discuss insulin administration and its crucial role in diabetes management with the individual.

Education Topics for Persons Taking Insulin

Minimal skills to be taught to those on insulin therapy are the following:

- Proper storage of insulin
- Preparation of dose
- Correct administration, including site selection, injection site rotation, and gently rolling the vials or inverting the pens for suspended insulin formulations prior to administration
- Priming insulin pens before each injection
- The maximum number of unit that can be dialed for each insulin pen, including when the pen cartridge can only be dialed up to the amount of insulin remaining in the cartridge
- Removing the pen needle from the pen cartridge after each administration
- Strategies to avoid inadvertent needlesticks
- Safe disposal of syringes or needles
- Recognition of hypoglycemia signs and symptoms and corrective actions to take
- Hypoglycemia prevention
- Timing of prandial insulin in relation to meals
- Correct administration of the inhaled insulin

To minimize potential adverse events, the individual's understanding of and ability to perform these skills should be assessed before the medication is prescribed.

The following are more advanced skills that are also important to teach. However, not all persons with diabetes will be able to learn and manage all of these skills:

- Mixing 2 insulins in the same syringe
- Pattern management
- Insulin adjustments for physical activity, sick days, and differing amounts of carbohydrate intake

The diabetes care and education specialist must individualize the educational strategies and message to each person's educational and coping levels. A number of chapters in this book address these topics individually (see index). See also the sections on hypoglycemia and insulin in chapter 17, on pharmacotherapy for glucose management.

Overcoming Insulin Administration Problems

As with other aspects of diabetes management, matching the insulin delivery device to the unique needs of the individual with diabetes is important. Any mismatch will increase the likelihood that the device or equipment will not be used as prescribed and the individual may be at increased risk for hypoglycemia or hyperglycemia. Chapters 17 and 19 describe insulin delivery devices: syringes, insulin pumps, jet injectors, and pen devices.

Individuals with dexterity problems or visual impairment may have difficulty drawing up a dose of insulin. The use of different injection aids (eg, syringe magnifying guide) or devices that are easier to use, such as an insulin pen, may be helpful for some. A list of insulin injection aids for those using the syringe and vial is published annually in the *Consumer Guide* of the American Diabetes Association's *Diabetes Forecast* magazine.

Persons with diabetes may be pleasantly surprised to learn that needle length and diameter are much smaller than they may have anticipated. The length of needles for insulin injection typically ranges from 4 mm (for pen needles) or 6 mm (for syringes) to 12.7 mm (for both pen needles and syringes). Shorter needles are often more acceptable to most individuals with diabetes, but healthcare providers may not be aware of the existence of these shorter pen and syringe needle lengths. In particular, providers have traditionally prescribed the longer needle lengths (8 mm and 12.7 mm) for obese individuals to ensure that the insulin delivered reaches the subcutaneous fat. However, while the thickness of the subcutaneous tissue varies significantly by body mass index, body site, and sex, it has been demonstrated among adults with diabetes that the average skin thickness at the 4 common insulin injection sites (abdomen, thigh, buttock, and arm) varies by only 0.5 mm between the thinnest (thigh) and the thickest (buttock) sites.[17] Furthermore, the difference in skin thickness is not clinically different among those with different body mass index, race, or age.[17] The average thickness of the skin at the thickest site (buttock) in the study was 2.4 mm; therefore, a needle as short as 4 mm is adequate to reach past the epidermis and dermis into the subcutaneous fat layer, while at the same time minimizing risk of intramuscular administration. Recent studies have demonstrated equivalent glycemic stability and less pain with the shorter needles compared with the longer needles.[18–21]

The international Third Injection Technique Workshop in Athens (TITAN)—a conference consisting of 127 physicians, nurses, diabetes care and education specialists, and psychologists from 27 countries who provide evidence-based consensus recommendations on injection techniques for insulin and glucagon-like peptide-1 agonists—recommended that children, adolescents, and adults with diabetes use a 4-, 5-, or 6-mm needle and concluded that "there is no medical reason" for recommending needles longer than 8 mm.[22] Table 7.3 provides recommendations for insulin injection with different needle lengths.[23]

The gauge of the needle is also important for comfort. Most insulin syringes are available in the smaller 30 or 31 gauge, which may make the injection less painful. The unit markings on the side of the syringe differ, depending on whether the syringe holds 30 units (3/10 cc), 50 units (1/2 cc), or 100 units (1 cc). Individual markings may be in 1/2-unit, 1-unit, or 2-unit increments. If a person is injecting less than 30 units for a dose, using a syringe that closely matches the dose—in this case a 3/10 cc syringe—will allow the person to see the units easier than using a 1-cc syringe. However, the risk for error in administration may be increased if the insulin dose is increased and the person is prescribed a different syringe size with a different unit increment but not given education regarding this. Insulin pens are typically easier to use and more discreet, and the unit markings may be easier to read than the markings on a vial and syringe; thus, they can provide greater accuracy and are usually preferred by persons on insulin therapy.[24] The thinnest pen needle available at the time of writing is 32 gauge.

TABLE 7.3 Tips for Angle of Injection and for Pinching a Skinfold Prior to Injection

1. Most needles should be inserted at a 90° angle; however, a 45° angle is advised for frail elderly or cachexic adults or children.
2. Persons with diabetes using 6-, 8-, or 12.7-mm needles do need to pinch a skinfold for the medication to reach its intended absorption site.
3. Four- or five-millimeter needles may be used by any person with diabetes, including lean or obese children and adults. Persons with diabetes do not need to pinch a skinfold when using 4- or 5-mm needles. *Exception:* Children and adults with lesser amounts of subcutaneous fat who use their arms or thighs for injection sites are advised to pinch a skinfold when using 4- or 5-mm needles.

Source: Reprinted with permission from R Saltiel-Berzin, M Cypress, M Gibney. "Translating the research in insulin injection technique: implications for practice." *Diabetes Educ* 2012; 38:635-43.

Key Points on Insulin Use: What to Review With Persons With Diabetes

- Determine what barriers to, and misconceptions of, insulin therapy exist. These may include fears of injection, complications, and hypoglycemia; fear that insulin initiation signals that the diabetes is end-stage; social concerns; cost; and weight gain.
- Show the person when and how the insulin is working to lower blood glucose levels and discuss with him or her the proven clinical benefits of insulin therapy. Printed educational materials and information from the insulin manufacturer's Web site, the American Diabetes Association (ADA), and the Association of Diabetes Care and Education Specialists (ADCES) may be beneficial.
- Explain how to properly administer the insulin, including proper mixing and resuspension (if appropriate), appropriate injection sites, site rotation, and storage.
- Educate the person about the potential for hypoglycemia, recognition of hypoglycemic symptoms, and specific corrective actions that can be taken if it occurs. Discuss risk factors for hypoglycemia, including missed or irregular meals, and hypoglycemia after exercise or physical activity. Discuss how to minimize or prevent the occurrence of hypoglycemic episodes. Educate the individual and family members and any caregivers about hypoglycemia unawareness and the use of a glucagon emergency kit for treating severe hypoglycemia. Educate family members and caregivers about how to recognize signs and symptoms of hypoglycemia.
- Properly match the amount and timing of food to the type and dose of insulin to minimize hypoglycemic events. If the person is able to perform carbohydrate counting, carbohydrate-to-insulin ratios should be developed with persons using basal-bolus regimens.
- Educate the person about what to do when engaging in exercise or sports.
- Educate the person about what to do when eating out or traveling.
- Discuss the disposal of syringes, pen needles, and testing supplies. This varies by city, county, and state.
- Discuss methods to avoid accidental needlesticks. One practice that is universal is to teach people not to recap syringes and pen needles after use.
- Discuss reusing syringes and pen needles and whether this is recommended. This should normally be avoided in most persons. Discuss that refrigerating the syringes for reuse later and wiping the needle off with alcohol are not recommended. Reusing needles dulls the needle tip and removes the lubricated coating, making the injection more painful. Discuss sick-day management and development of a sick-day plan (see chapter 23).
- Avoid potential medication prescribing and dispensing errors by educating all persons taking insulin products on both the brand and generic names for their insulins; those taking insulin mixes should know the generic names of both insulin components. Also explain the differences in the relevant concentrations of insulin (insulin regular in U-100 and U-500 formulations, insulin lispro in U-100 and U-200 formulations, insulin glargine in U-100 and U-300 formulations, and insulin degludec in U-100 and U-200 formulations) if the person is switched from one concentration to another.

Fixed Ratio Combination of GLP-1 Receptor Agonists and Basal Insulin

An increasingly common treatment strategy for persons with type 2 diabetes who have not achieved glycemic stability with basal insulin or a GLP-1 receptor agonist is to use the combination. This method has several advantages over the basal-bolus regimen, including lower risk of hypoglycemia and potential weight reduction. It also enables few injections: 8 injections per week (if using a once-weekly GLP-1 receptor agonist and a once-daily basal insulin) or 14 injections per week (with a once-daily GLP-1 receptor agonist and a once-daily basal insulin combination pen) compared to 28 injections a week (once-daily basal insulin plus 3 times daily prandial insulin). At the time of writing, 2 products that combine a once-daily GLP-1 receptor agonist with a basal insulin in the same pen are available in the U.S.: insulin degludec/liraglutide 100/3.6 (Xultophy® 100/3.6) and insulin glargine/lixisenatide (Soliqua® 100/33). These may potentially enhance engagement with medication taking by decreasing the number of injections to 7 per week. Because of the unique dosing and titration schema of these products, the diabetes care and education specialist should carefully explain to persons taking these products the amount of basal insulin and GLP-1 receptor agonist present in each dose. Other education points regarding medication administration such as dialing to the correct dose, storage, injection, disposal, etc should also be provided. Additionally, some

Case—Part 2

You acknowledge AB's fears about insulin initiation and help her realize that it was most likely the delay in insulin initiation that led to the retinopathy and nephropathy he experienced. You also help AB understand the risks of both short-term and long-term hyperglycemia and inform her that insulin is the most effective medication currently available to treat hyperglycemia. You educate AB, in lay language, that insulin is not a strange or foreign substance but a natural hormone made by all living persons to maintain glucose homeostasis, and that the pancreas of persons with diabetes either does not make any insulin or does not make enough to manage the hyperglycemia. You also help AB recognize that insulin can resolve the symptoms of hyperglycemia (excessive thirst, polyuria, blurry vision) that she is experiencing. These explanations seem to help AB feel more comfortable with initiating insulin, and she states that she is willing to try it. However, she is concerned about remembering to take "so many" different medications and admits to not remembering to take all of her medications each day. You consult with the pharmacist team member and AB's primary care provider and recommend several ways to decrease pill burden:

1. A combination tablet of pioglitazone and a different sulfonylurea, glimepiride (Duetact®, Takeda Pharmaceuticals, generic), is available. Glimepiride is also associated with a lower risk of hypoglycemia than glyburide.
2. Switching AB to extended-release metformin will allow her to take the full dose just once-daily.
3. A combination tablet for lisinopril and hydrochlorothiazide is also available; although if AB is currently taking the usual doses of 40 mg of lisinopril and 25 mg of hydrocholorthiazide, she will still need to take 2 tablets, as the combination only comes as lisinopril-hydrocholorthiazide 20 mg-12.5 mg or 20-25 mg.
4. A combination tablet of amlodipine and atorvastatin is available (Caduet®, Pfizer; generics).
5. Alternatively, a combination tablet of amlodipine and an ARB (either valsartan, telmistartan, or olmesartan) is also available.
6. Another alternative is to switch the ACE inhibitor to valsartan and combine it with the amlodipine and hydrochlorothiazide into the triple combination tablet (Exforge HCT®, Novartis; generics).
7. The sulfonylurea can be discontinued once the optimal dose of insulin is reached. You also advise AB to purchase a pill organizer to help her remember which doses have already been taken for the day and to associate the medication taking with a regular daily activity such as eating breakfast.
8. If appropriate and after a discussion with AB's primary care provider, you can educate AB about the benefits of GLP-1 receptor agonists and/or SGLT2 inhibitors as potentially better therapeutic options than the TZD.

AB is especially interested in taking "natural herbal products" to manage hyperglycemia. What should you tell her?

differences exist between the 2 products regarding administration: the insulin glargine/lixisenatide product should be administered with 1 hour of the first meal while the insulin degludec/liraglutide product can be administered without regards to meals; the maximum of basal insulin units in a single injection is 60 units of insulin glargine compared to 50 units of insulin degludec. See also the discussions on these medications in chapter 17, on pharmacotherapy for glucose management.

Drug Interactions

Persons living with diabetes often take a number of medications concurrently for comorbid conditions such as hypertension, hyperlipidemia, coronary artery disease, and heart failure. They may also take medications to treat long-term complications of diabetes such as peripheral neuropathy. Thus, the diabetes care and education specialist should be aware of the potential for drug interactions and increased adverse drug reactions and help the person with diabetes and the healthcare team monitor for these. A complete discussion of the many potential drug interactions and medication-related problems that may occur is beyond the scope of this chapter. A brief discussion of medications that can adversely affect glycemic levels is included in the paragraphs that follow. Chapter 17 also briefly discusses drug-drug, drug-disease, and drug-food interactions of concern when using medications for diabetes management. Consultation with a pharmacist and/or inclusion of a pharmacist into the healthcare team helps reduce the potential for medication misadventures.

Many medications have the potential to induce hyperglycemia and worsen glycemic levels. Commonly prescribed medications in this category include glucocorticoids, protease inhibitors, atypical antipsychotics, thiazide diuretics, beta-adrenergic blocking agents (beta-blockers), and niacin. Worsening of preexisting diabetes, new-onset diabetes, impaired fasting glucose, and impaired glucose tolerance have all been reported with these medications. Proposed mechanisms for hyperglycemia vary by drug class but include decreased peripheral insulin sensitivity, decreased insulin secretion, and increased gluconeogenesis. Atypical antipsychotics can also cause weight gain and dyslipidemia. Protease inhibitors can cause dyslipidemia and lipodystrophy. The risk of hyperglycemia may vary among drugs within a class. For example, clozapine (Clozaril®, Heritage Life; generics) and olanzapine (Zyprexa®, Eli Lilly; generics) appear to have the highest association with hyperglycemia, although any of the atypical antipsychotics may adversely affect blood glucose levels. The risk of hyperglycemia is also dependent on other factors such as the dose administered (as with glucocorticoids and niacin) and the route of administration (eg, lower risk with inhaled and topical formulations of glucocorticoids compared with oral and intravenous formulations).[25]

Use of Nonprescription Medications

In the United States, nonprescription medications, also known as over-the-counter (OTC) drugs, are reviewed by the FDA.[26] There are more than 300,000 marketed OTC drug products on the market; the FDA reviews the active ingredients and the labeling of the 80+ therapeutic categories of drugs only, not each individual OTC product.[26] Some of the more frequent ailments that are treated with nonprescription products include cough, cold and flu, pain and fever, allergy and sinus complaints, dermatologic conditions, gastrointestinal distress, and musculoskeletal pain. People with diabetes may want to treat a common ailment but may take something that adversely affects their blood glucose or blood pressure. The labeling of the product should always be checked prior to administration, as nonprescription products are frequently reformulated and ingredients may change. Diabetes care and education specialists need to be knowledgeable about the ingredients in these products in order to assist in selecting appropriate self-care therapies. Due to the complexity involved (eg, multitude of drug ingredients and formulations, adverse drug reactions, contraindications to self-care, and the potential for drug-drug, drug-disease, and drug-food interactions), consultation with a pharmacist prior to commencing use is especially important.

Alcohol-Free and Sugar-Free Products

Whether a person with diabetes needs to exclusively use alcohol-free and sugar-free products depends on the person's glycemic stability, medications, and comorbid medical conditions. Individuals taking insulin or insulin secretagogues should be advised against using products with alcohol. If a product contains carbohydrates, the carbohydrate count needs to be added into the number of grams of carbohydrates the person consumes. The dosage of these products varies by product; therefore, just as with foods, labels have to be read carefully to prevent hyperglycemia or hypoglycemia. The amount of carbohydrate in some products may be so small that the potential increase in blood glucose is minimal. The illness being treated with the OTC product itself may also increase blood glucose levels, so this needs to be considered. Information on the carbohydrate content of products may be found on each product's Web site or by calling the consumer toll-free phone number listed on the package. The alcohol content of many nonprescription products can also be found this way and is also given in the ingredients list on the product's label (listed as an inactive ingredient).

Cough and Cold Products

One common mistake people make when self-treating with OTC products is taking a multi-symptom remedy when only a single symptom needs to be treated. For example, a person attempting to self-treat nasal congestion may purchase a product that has both a decongestant and a cough suppressant. Most OTC products marketed to treat cough and cold symptoms contain more than 1 active ingredient. They also may contain ingredients that adversely affect blood glucose and blood pressure. This effect varies by product and formulation. Selecting a product that treats only the symptom(s) present, and being cognizant of the carbohydrate and alcohol content (especially with liquid formulations), allows individuals with diabetes to better select products for self-care. In most cases, tablet and gelcap formulations to treat cough and cold symptoms do not contain any, or contain only a limited amount of, carbohydrate and alcohol. Nasal sprays used to treat nasal congestion and allergies should have limited systemic effects if used according to the directions on the label and with proper administration techniques. Oral decongestants such as pseudoephedrine or phenylephrine should be used with caution and under medical supervision, mainly due to their effects on increasing blood pressure and heart rate. Two of the major contraindications for the use of these medications are in those with coronary artery disease and those with arrhythmia. The labeling for oral and nasal decongestant products includes a warning against use in persons with diabetes, unless with medical supervision, because these sympathomimetic agents may increase blood glucose.

Pain and Fever Products

Pain and fever are commonly treated with nonprescription medications. Examples include acetaminophen and nonsteroidal anti-inflammatory drugs (NSAIDs) such as ibuprofen and naproxen. The person with diabetes should be aware that, unless directed otherwise by a healthcare professional, NSAID use should be avoided in those with renal impairment, hypertension, heart failure, or gastrointestinal ulcer. Some OTC pain reliever products contain large quantities of sodium and should be avoided in persons with hypertension and heart failure. For example, at the time of writing, Alka-Seltzer® Original (Bayer) contains 567 mg of sodium per tablet, along with 325 mg of aspirin, and the directions instruct adults to take 2 tablets per dose for a maximum of 8 tablets in a 24-hour period.[27] Aspirin may increase the risk of hypoglycemia when taken with sulfonylureas due to displacement of the sulfonylurea from plasma protein-binding sites. Aspirin also appears to possess hypoglycemic actions (proposed mechanisms include increasing pancreatic insulin secretion and insulin sensitivity and decreasing gluconeogenesis). However, these effects are usually only clinically relevant at higher (anti-inflammatory) doses.[25]

Products for Gastrointestinal Ailments

The diabetes care and education specialist should inquire about use of nonprescription products for gastrointestinal ailments, as this may be a sign that the person with diabetes is experiencing gastrointestinal autonomic neuropathy. Many nonprescription products for the treatment of gas, heartburn, constipation, and diarrhea do not contain noticeable amounts of carbohydrate or alcohol and do not possess any mechanisms of action that would adversely affect blood glucose levels. Most antacids contain magnesium, aluminum, a combination of the 2, or calcium carbonate. Products containing aluminum should be avoided in persons with impaired renal function or those at risk for constipation. Calcium antacids (and supplements), as well as products containing iron, may also cause constipation.

Nonprescription agents for treating constipation include bulk-forming laxatives (methylcellulose, polycarbophil, psyllium), osmotic agents (eg, glycerin, polyethylene glycol 3350), stimulant laxatives (bisacodyl, senna, castor oil), lubricant laxatives (mineral oil), saline laxatives (magnesium citrate or hydroxide, sodium phosphate, magnesium sulfate [Epsom salt]), and stool softeners (docusate).[28] Differences in these products include the onset of action, potential adverse drug reactions, and drug interactions. These products do not affect blood glucose, but the stimulant, osmotic, and saline laxatives may lead to electrolyte imbalances, especially with overuse. Sodium phosphate laxatives dosed at higher than the recommended amount have been reported to cause a number of cases of life-threatening and fatal dehydration, electrolyte disturbances, acute kidney injury, and gastrointestinal and cardiac sequelae.[29] It is important to remember that constipation may be a symptom of an underlying medical condition, including diabetic gastroparesis. Because of the availability of a number of self-treatment options for constipation, the person living with diabetes may not discuss this symptom with their healthcare provider until it becomes truly bothersome and recurrent many weeks to months later. All OTC products for constipation should not be used for more than 1 week.[29] The diabetes care and education specialist can help identify persons engaging in self-treatment and advise them to seek medical guidance promptly. A number of laxatives can decrease the absorption and therefore bioavailability of oral prescription medications; administration of these medications should be separated by at least 2 hours from the laxative.[28] Consultation with a pharmacist or prescriber to evaluate for potential drug interactions is recommended.

The nonprescription agents approved by the FDA for the treatment of diarrhea include loperamide (eg, Imodium® A-D, Johnson and Johnson; generics) and bismuth subsalicylate (eg, Pepto-Bismol®, Procter and Gamble; generics). These do not adversely affect blood glucose levels. Products containing bismuth subsalicylate may interact with other medications that persons with diabetes take, such as aspirin and other antiplatelet drugs, NSAIDs, and anticoagulants, but generally do not adversely affect blood glucose levels in recommended nonprescription doses. As with all nonprescription products, the ingredients list should be carefully reviewed each time an OTC product is purchased, even if the person believes he or she is buying the same product because its name is the same. Due to frequent reformulations of OTC products, the risk of adverse events or lack of efficacy is increased if the person takes an OTC product with an ingredient or ingredients that are inappropriate for his or her current medication regimen or medical condition(s). For example, in the first decade of the 21st century, the Kaopectate product that used to contain attapulgite, an ingredient to treat diarrhea, was reformulated so that Kaopectate® Anti-Diarrheal (Pfizer Consumer Healthcare) contained bismuth subsalicylate. However, Kaopectate® Stool Softener (Pfizer Consumer Healthcare) actually contained docusate. Adverse effects are likely to occur if the person buying the product to self-treat an episode of diarrhea inadvertently selects Kaopectate® Stool Softener (due to paying attention only to the brand name of the product and not reading the actual ingredients list) instead of the Kaopectate® Anti-Diarrheal. At the time of writing, all Kaopectate® products contain bismuth subsalicylate.

In the 2000s, 2 prescription proton pump inhibitors (omeprazole [Prilosec® OTC, AstraZeneca] and lansoprazole [Prevacid® 24 Hour, Novartis]), along with all of the prescription histamine-2 receptor blockers, became available as OTC medications. In 2014, the prescription proton pump inhibitor esomeprazole (Nexium 24 Hour) also became available OTC. The medications are indicated for the self-treatment of heartburn. The OTC proton pump inhibitors are indicated for self-treatment for no more than a 14-day course, and each course may be repeated no more frequently than every 4 months, unless directed differently by a healthcare provider. There is not a maximum time limit on the labeling for the OTC histamine-2 receptor blockers, although there is a warning to ask a physician before use if heartburn symptoms have been present for over 3 months. The diabetes care and education specialist should help the person with diabetes who is using these products understand how to monitor his or her symptoms and when to seek medical attention, as gastrointestinal symptoms may be a sign of underlying gastrointestinal autonomic neuropathy. All of these medications are substrates and/or inhibitors of the cytochrome P450 (CYP450) enzyme system that metabolizes many prescription medications; consultation with a pharmacist is advised if the person is also taking other medications. Especially problematic among the OTC histamine-2 receptor blockers is cimetidine, which inhibits most of the CYP450 isoenzymes, increasing the risk for drug interactions and adverse drug reactions.

Products for Common Genitourinary Conditions

Persons with diabetes arc in general, more susceptible to microbial infections, and urinary tract infection and genital yeast infection (in both men and women) are potential side effects of SGLT2 inhibitors. Antifungal products for treating vaginal yeast infections are available as creams, ointments, and suppositories and vary by the number of days (1-7) required for treatment. Self-treatment of vaginal yeast infections can be recommended only if the person has symptoms consistent with those of an episode previously diagnosed by a healthcare professional, if the person has had fewer than 4 infections per year, and if the current episode is at least 2 months after the previous.[30] However, commonalities in symptom presentation exist among the 3 most common vaginal infections—vulvovaginal candidiasis (commonly known as vaginal yeast infection), bacterial vaginosis, and trichomoniasis—and therefore correct self-diagnosis can be quite difficult. Only mild-to-moderate vulvovaginal candidiasis can be treated with an OTC antifungal product; the other 2 conditions require a medical evaluation and prescription for an antibiotic. The diabetes care and education specialist should advise persons with diabetes who wish to self-treat for a vaginal yeast infection to obtain medical supervision especially if they have taking other medications. The OTC antifungals may have significant drug-drug interactions, including with warfarin, and a dose adjustment of the prescription medication may be needed.[30] Any person who is concerned about experiencing symptoms of an urinary tract infection should seek medical evaluation as the treatment can vary from a few days of antibiotic to hospitalization, depending on severity and clinical characteristics of the person with diabetes.

Dietary Supplements

It is important that diabetes care and education specialists be aware of alternative remedies persons with diabetes may be using and how those therapies interact with recommended or prescribed treatments.

Dietary supplements may include herbs, vitamins, minerals, and nutritional supplements. Unlike prescription products, dietary supplements are not regulated by the FDA, and product quality may vary among manufacturers or even among lots of the same product. Some manufacturers have voluntarily submitted to testing and verification by the US Pharmacopeia (USP; https://www.quality-supplements.org/), the organization responsible for setting standards and quality control for all FDA-approved prescription and nonprescription medications. Evidence-based information about dietary supplements can be found via the Natural Medicines databases (https://naturalmedicines.therapeuticresearch.com/) and the National Center for Complementary Medicine and Integrative Health (https://nccih.nih.gov).

Persons with diabetes who wish to use an herbal product to help with glycemic levels should be educated that the scientific evidence for effectiveness of these agents is equivocal and that these products cannot substitute for FDA-approved glucose-lowering medications. If a person still wishes to use these products, a careful check for potential drug interactions and adverse drug reactions should be completed. The diabetes care and education specialist should advise the person to use only USP-verified products, as noted above. Chapter 21, on biological complementary therapies, provides more information to assist educators and those with diabetes in evaluating complementary products.

Topical and Dermatologic Products

Persons with poorly managed diabetes are at risk for fungal infections, dry skin, and possible skin ulcerations. Trauma to the skin from wearing ill-fitting shoes can lead to blisters. Education regarding proper foot care, discussed in chapters 9, and 28 (on reducing risks and diabetic neuropathies), should be provided.

Tinea pedis, or "athlete's foot," is common in many persons with diabetes. Nonprescription antifungal products may take up to 4 weeks of continuous treatment to resolve the problem. Many people do not use these products long enough, which leads to recurrent or unresolved tinea infections. Therefore, education regarding engagement with medication taking for the duration of therapy is key. If there is not significant improvement, systemic antifungal prescription medications may be needed. Fungal infections of the nails (onychomycosis), especially toenails, are also a frequent condition in those with diabetes. A number of nonprescription products are advertised for this condition, but persons affected by this condition should be educated that onychomycosis can be effectively treated only with prescription medications.

Autonomic neuropathy and polyuria caused by hyperglycemia may lead to dry skin. Various moisturizers containing glycerin, mineral oil, and lanolin are available to prevent and treat dry skin. Those containing alcohol should be avoided, as the alcohol promotes drying of the skin.

Nonprescription products marketed for the removal of corns and calluses should not be used and are required by the FDA to be labeled with "do not use if you are diabetic or if you have poor blood circulation." Using these products without medical supervision and misapplying them can lead to inflammation and ulcer formation,[31] The person with diabetes should be referred to a podiatrist for the evaluation and treatment of foot disorders.

Products for Oral Hygiene and Dental Care

Gum disease and dental caries may occur more frequently in people with inadequately managed blood glucose. Proper brushing, flossing, and regular dental appointments as well as achieving and maintaining good glycemic stability will minimize the risk of gum disease and dental caries in most people. Many mouth rinses contain large amounts of alcohol and should be avoided, even if the rinse is not swallowed, since they can lead to dry mouth, which can promote dental caries. Many people have problems with ill-fitting dentures if they have gingivitis. Oral candidiasis may occur in persons with poorly managed blood glucose and may be prevented with adequate blood glucose management and removal of dentures at bedtime. Dentures should be cleaned as directed and rinsed thoroughly to prevent contact irritation. See also the discussion on oral care in chapter 9, on reducing risks.

Ophthalmologic Products

The use of nonprescription moisturizing eyedrops containing only lubricants is usually safe. As with all nonprescription medications, labels should be read carefully, as some products may contain more than 1 drug. Ophthalmic decongestants such as phenylephrine, naphazoline, oxymetazoline, and tetrahydrozoline are vasoconstrictors and are contraindicated in persons with angle-closure glaucoma. Medical supervision is advised when using these products, as incorrect administration or overuse may lead to appreciable systemic absorption and subsequent increases in blood pressure, heart rate, or blood glucose. Some ophthalmic decongestants are coformulated with ophthalmic antihistamines (eg, pheniramine) for the treatment of allergic conjunctivitis. Ophthalmic antihistamines are also contraindicated in angle-closure glaucoma.[30] The labeling for ophthalmic products containing an antihistamine also recommends consultation with a prescriber before taking if the person has difficulty urinating due to an enlarged prostate.

Case—Part 3

Utilizing motivational interviewing techniques, you discuss with AB how she thinks herbal supplements would be helpful to her. You share with AB that the herbal products marketed for diabetes have not been adequately studied for both efficacy and safety. In addition, these products are not regulated by the FDA, and the contents of the products are not guaranteed to be manufactured under the stringent conditions that prescription medications are subject to. You also advise AB that some of these herbal products may interact with the medications she is currently prescribed, which could put her at risk for hypoglycemia. You discuss with AB that if she still feels strongly about taking an herbal product, or any OTC products, she should check with a pharmacist or other healthcare professional before purchasing the product.

Considerations in Children, Adolescents, and Older Adults

Children and Adolescents

Medication administration for children can be challenging, with different challenges at different ages—when children are young, when they are of school age, and when they become adolescents. Medication administration away from home can affect young children in day care as well as school-aged children and can sometimes still be a factor in the teen years. Psychosocial challenges related to medication taking must also be considered.

Appropriate Insulin Type

The availability of rapid-acting insulin analogs has allowed parents of young children who are fussy eaters to be able to both give insulin after the child decides to eat and adjust the dose based on the amount of carbohydrates the child actually ate. Prior to the availability of these insulins, a dose of short-acting insulin was prepared based on the child's blood glucose and the amount of carbohydrate for the meal. Since this type of insulin had to be administered 30 minutes before the meal, the risk of hypoglycemia was present if the child decided not to eat or did not consume the entire meal.

Medication Administration by Others

Some medications, including some regimens of insulin, may require administration at school and in care settings away from home. Education of school, day care, and camp staff is key to successful management. Another potential challenge is that different insulin schedules may be used on different days, depending on the level of physical activity typical for that day. Children who usually take a mixed dose of neutral protamine Hagedorn (NPH) and a rapid-acting analog insulin may, on occasion, be advised to use a premixed insulin, such as Humalog® Mix 75/25™ (lispro protamine suspension/lispro, Eli Lilly), to allow for simpler administration (not requiring mixing) away from home. Some children may be prescribed premixed insulin to allow for administration to occur only at home. This may not provide the child with optimal blood glucose stability, but it may be a way to ensure that the insulin is given and given correctly. In all children taking glucose-lowering medications, both the child and personnel at school, day care, and camps need to be able to recognize the signs and symptoms of hypoglycemia and perform the necessary corrective actions. Parents and personnel at school, day care, and camps also need to be educated on when to use glucagon to treat hypoglycemia. Teachers may try to administer this to conscious children, causing unnecessary fear and anxiety. Chapter 14, on type 1 diabetes, discusses information relevant to challenges that children with diabetes face when they are at school, when they are away from home at other care settings, and when they are physically active, such as when participating in sports.

Adolescent Considerations

The combination of having diabetes and managing it well during adolescence can be challenging for a child with diabetes, the family, and others involved in the individual's care and well-being. This period of growth, with its hormonal changes, poses a challenge to even those teens and parents who are firmly committed to managing diabetes well. Unfortunately, adolescents with chronic medical conditions, including diabetes, have been reported to exhibit poor engagement with treatment plans.[2,32] Teenagers need to be educated about the dangers of omitting their insulin doses. Some teenagers may feel that their parents are too protective and may become rebellious and seek attention through hospitalization. Teenagers trying to lose weight may purposely omit their insulin to improve their self-image. Teenagers also need to be educated on the detrimental effects of alcohol or illicit drug use on their medical condition and medications. Severe hypoglycemia may occur if they binge drink and pass out from intoxication. Referral to a psychologist or family counselor may be necessary for some families. Health-care providers should be aware that insulin requirements will increase during puberty. See chapters 12 and 14 for more information on topics in adolescence relevant to taking medication. See chapter 4 for psychological and mental health issues, such as eating disorders and depression, which may also have a bearing on medication-taking behavior.

Insulin Administration

The advent of 4-mm and 5-mm insulin pen needles allows some children to inject their insulin at a 90° (instead of a 45°) angle; these shorter needles are also less intimidating (see Table 7.3). Insulin pens may be a better option for children who have a fear of syringes as well as trouble operating the syringe and vial. Insulin injection aids (a list is published in the annual *Consumer Guide* of the American Diabetes Association's *Diabetes Forecast* magazine) can help those who need to inject via a syringe and vial. Various products for hiding the needle of the syringe and decreasing the injection sensation are available. Insulin pens allow for more discreet insulin delivery than the vial and syringe method. For children using an insulin pump, a variety of insertion sets with variable lengths of needles and cannulas are available to match individual preference for comfort and to promote best insulin absorption. The child with diabetes, the parents of the child, caregivers, and school/day care/camp personnel need to be educated on how to address problems that may occur with pump use. No matter which delivery devices and injection aids are used, careful education and monitoring of insulin administration must always be provided.

Type 2 Diabetes in Children and Adolescents

For many years, the assumption was that the only type of diabetes that children could develop was type 1 diabetes, and terminology such as *juvenile-onset diabetes* was used. It is now commonly known that children may develop both type 1 diabetes and type 2 diabetes. At the time of writing, the only oral glucose-lowering agent approved by the FDA for children 10 years of age and older with type 2 diabetes is immediate-release metformin.[32] These children may not need to have medication administered at school, since this medication can be given twice daily. Similarly, the GLP-1 receptor agonist liraglutide, recently approved by the FDA for children 10 years and older with type 2 diabetes, can be given once-daily at home.

In teenagers with type 2 diabetes treated with metformin, the risk of lactic acidosis and binge drinking needs to be discussed. Insulin is required for some children with type 2 diabetes, and the potential challenges with medication taking and administration discussed earlier should be taken into consideration.

Coping Skills for the Child/Adolescent With Diabetes

Social support and education about coping skills should be provided to the child and his or her family members. The diabetes care and education specialist should also recognize psychosocial risk factors for poor diabetes management, which include the presence of other medical conditions, poor school attendance, learning disabilities, and emotional and behavioral disorders in the child. Family-related risk factors include a single-parent home, chronic physical or mental health problems in close relatives, a recent major life change for the parent, lack of adequate health insurance, complex child-care arrangements, health/cultural/religious beliefs affecting engagement with treatment plans, and having a parent with diabetes.[33] Additionally, the transition from adolescent to adulthood, with its multitude of changes in psychosocial factors and increasing responsibility for self-care, is another period in which decreased medication taking, worsened glycemic stability, and diabetic complications may occur and a strong transition care plan and support should be developed.[34,35]

Healthcare professionals should understand the effect of these factors on self-management of diabetes and help children with diabetes and their families overcome these barriers. Resources such as support groups and summer camps are available in some communities, but finding one that is age-appropriate, meets the needs of the family, and is within an acceptable geographic location may be a barrier. See chapter 4 for more on healthy coping.

Older Adults

Older individuals with diabetes who are living at home are at increased risk for medication-related adverse events due to multiple factors, including polymedication, multiple comorbidities, cost, dietary intake including dental considerations, and psychosocial barriers. Medication-use aids (such as medication planners and schedulers and pill organizers) and administration aids (such as insulin pens and injection guides) can help older people remember to take their medications and to administer them correctly. However, medication administration may still prove to be difficult due to decreased manual dexterity, decreased vision and mobility, or cognitive impairment. In addition, if inadequately or improperly trained, family members and other caregivers may give medication at the wrong time or in the wrong dosage. Involving them in the education session or discussing by phone can be critical in preventing errors from occurring. The use of combination tablets, of both oral glucose-lowering medications and cardiovascular medications, can decrease the pill burden in those taking multiple medications. However, the cost of the combination product (some of which may still be branded) compared to the individual (generic) components should be kept in mind.

The risk of falls should always be assessed in all older persons, and those living with diabetes may be at an even higher risk. Many factors, such as visual impairment, gait instability from arthritis, or peripheral neuropathy, play a role. Another important contributing factor to the risk of falling in older persons with diabetes is medication side effects. Older persons with diabetes may have to contend with hypoglycemic symptoms from glucose-lowering agents, dizziness from antihypertensive medications and medications acting on the central nervous system (CNS), sedation and confusion from CNS-acting agents and psychotropics, and blurred vision from a variety of medications. The diabetes care and education specialist can remind the prescriber to assess for fall risk and assist in the discussion of fall prevention with both the person living with diabetes and any family member or caregiver. The diabetes care and education specialist should have an open discussion with these same parties about any concerns regarding the risk of falling due to side effects of prescribed medications that may lead to lack of engagement with the regimen. The diabetes care and education specialist can also initiate a referral to a pharmacist or prescriber for evaluation of the entire medication regimen and potential simplification. An important consideration is whether the therapeutic goals are still appropriate as the person ages and the life expectancy changes. The ADA Standards of Medical Care in Diabetes provides guidelines on A1c, fasting and preprandial blood glucose, bedtime glucose, blood pressure, and lipid targets in older persons depending on health status and life expectancy. It also provides an algorithm for simplifying complex insulin regimen in older adults with type 2 diabetes.[36]

Community-dwelling older persons with diabetes are more likely to be admitted to a long-term care facility than their counterparts without diabetes. Although this may present a difficult situation for the person with diabetes to accept, it provides an opportunity for members of the healthcare team to collaborate and work closely with the resident, family, and long-term care staff, so problems with medication taking can be avoided.

Older adults and people residing in assisted-living facilities may also have impaired liver and kidney function. They may be taking multiple medications that increase the risk of drug-drug interactions. Defects in the metabolism and excretion of medications can lead to episodes of hypoglycemia and hyperglycemia. Sulfonylureas and meglitinides are metabolized in the liver and excreted in the urine. People with hepatic or renal impairment have an increased risk of hypoglycemia, especially if the individual has irregular eating habits. If a sulfonylurea is chosen, glimepiride or glipizide is the drug of choice due to minimally active or inactive metabolites, respectively. On the other hand, given that the mechanism of action of both sulfonylureas and meglitinides is to stimulate insulin release from functioning pancreatic beta cells, older persons with long-standing diabetes may find that they no longer receive any benefit from these medications. Metformin is excreted by the kidneys, and renal function should be monitored before therapy is started and periodically, especially in the elderly and in those with known mild renal impairment. In persons with renal insufficiency prescribed insulin, the insulin dose will usually need to be adjusted downward as renal function worsens. The dose of sitagliptin, saxagliptin, and alogliptin should be adjusted based on the degree of renal insufficiency. Caution is advised with the use of GLP-1 receptor agonists and SGLT2 inhibitors in those with renal impairment and use is contraindicated in moderate or severe renal impairment, depending on the drug. Thiazolidinediones can precipitate new-onset heart failure or worsen existing heart failure and may also precipitate or worsen diabetic macular edema. Sudden weight gain, edema, and difficulty in breathing should be brought immediately to the healthcare provider's attention. Body weight should be closely monitored in those receiving these medications. Use of TZDs may also lead to increased bone fracture risk. (See chapter 20 for more details on renal and hepatic considerations with diabetes medications.) Finally, decreased thirst and hunger mechanisms in the elderly increase the risk for dehydration, malnutrition, and swings in blood glucose levels, including the risk for a hyperosmolar hyperglycemic state. (Chapter 23, on hyperglycemia, describes a case study with an elderly adult in a hyperosmolar hyperglycemic state of care and provides more information). For a detailed review of overall diabetes management considerations in older adults, see the annual update of the Older Adults section in the ADA Standards of Medical Care for Diabetes.

Summary

There are many ways to ensure that optimal clinical outcomes are achieved with minimization of significant adverse effects when people who have diabetes and other conditions take prescription and nonprescription products. The person with diabetes, family members, caregivers, and healthcare professionals all need to contribute to the process. The diabetes care and education specialist should assess medication-taking behaviors for each agent, prescribed and OTC, in all persons living with diabetes and assist them in developing strategies to overcome identified barriers in order to take their medications safely. Using an interprofessional team-based approach to identify and correct barriers to therapy can also increase the likelihood of optimal clinical success. Most importantly, persons living with diabetes should be active participants in their own care and be included in all healthcare decisions.

Focus on Education

Teaching Strategies

Show and tell/demonstrate and discuss. Construct the information/presentation by function/category of drug, relating the information to how the drug affects the body and blood glucose (sensitizers, secretagogues, and so on). Pictures of how the medications are used in the body and what they look like are useful. A poster board display of actual pills helps identify actual dosing and aids in recognition but is typically best for medications that are still branded. Involve family and others to assist with learning drug names (brand and generic), dosing, frequency of administration, potential side effects (including how to monitor for them and what to do if they occur), and other important information.

Assess medications prescribed and barriers to taking them. Have the person bring all medications to the appointment to determine the date of each prescription, dose, prescriber, pharmacy used, and other pertinent details. Ask the person to also bring nonprescription medications and alternative medicines. Have the person describe how he or she takes each medication and if there are any concerns and/or challenges with taking prescribed medications. Work with the pharmacist to check for trade and generic duplication, outdated medicines, formulation availability, contraindicated medications, and other medication-related problems. Pharmacists can create a medication care plan to address both medication-related problems (eg, drug interactions, dosing, adverse effects) and medication taking.

Messages for Persons with Diabetes

Safety. Establish one local pharmacy or mail-order pharmacy for consistency in medication refills. Ask if there is any lab work to be done once you have started taking a medication (to monitor for both therapeutic effects and potential side effects). Keep an up-to-date listing of all medications including OTC vitamins, minerals, dietary supplements, and other products, and bring this list to all healthcare appointments, including specialist appointments, hospital visits, or procedures for review by the healthcare provider at each visit. Nonprescription products and dietary supplements may interact with your prescription medications or your conditions. Before taking any of these products, check with the prescriber or pharmacist.

Side effects. All medications, including OTC medications as well as herbals and alternative medicine products, have the potential for a side effect. Follow the prescription. Do not add medications on your own, including taking medications prescribed to others. Remind the prescriber of current medications you are taking, including any OTC medications, vitamins, and herbal supplements. When a new medication is prescribed, ask how the medicine will work with any current medicines you are taking, exactly how the medicine should be taken (such as before or after meals, at bedtime), and how to monitor for any potential side effects. Also ask what happens if illness occurs or if a procedure is scheduled that requires fasting overnight—ask whether you should take the medication or skip the dose and when to restart the drug. When in doubt, contact your healthcare team for instructions.

Family and caregiver involvement and education. Have a key member of your family, significant other, roommate, or close friend attend healthcare visits or classes with you to learn about the medications you take. Give this person a list of medications, side effects, treatment, and healthcare phone numbers in case of an emergency. Have the person demonstrate use of blood glucose testing equipment, discuss use of glucagon, and describe the number of glucose tablets used in case of low blood glucose.

Health Literacy

Assessment. Be vigilant for signs that the person may have low literacy and low health literacy. Some signs that the person may not be able to read, and therefore not able to correctly follow the directions on the label of the medication bottle, include the following: If the person does not know the names of the medications and what the directions say when asked but instead opens the bottle and relies on recognizing the shape and color of the medication in order to provide this information, or if the person is not able to read education handouts or fill out forms because he or she "forgot to bring my glasses" to healthcare appointments. Inspection of the medication bottles may show that the labels have symbols and other markings that indicate how to take the medications. When the dose is changed but a new prescription does not need to be provided at the appointment (such as when the dose is decreased from 2 tablets to 1 tablet), the person unable to read or write may ask the healthcare professional to make a mark on the medication bottle instead of writing the actual directions on the label. The problem of low literacy also extends to those who are able to read and write but at a level inadequate for optimal engagement with the medication and treatment plans. The diabetes care and education specialist should assess how well the person understands the messages being delivered by all members of the diabetes care team, including those delivered by both oral and written communications. Several health literacy assessment tools are available at http://www.ahrq.gov/professionals/quality-patient-safety/quality-resources/tools/literacy/index.html.

Strategies to overcome health literacy problems relevant to medication taking. In persons unable to read, the use of symbols, colors, and pictures can assist with correct administration of medications. United States Pharmacopeia has a library of pictograms related to medication taking that can be downloaded from usp.org/health-quality-safety/usp-pictograms. Be certain to clearly explain the meaning of the pictogram to avoid any misinterpretation. In persons with low health literacy, avoiding the use of technical jargon is crucial in effectively conveying the educational message. Using the "teach-back" method is key in the education of all persons living with diabetes and doubly so both in those who are unable to read or write and in those with low health literacy. Involvement of caregivers and family members, including accompanying the person to healthcare appointments, should also be encouraged.

References

1. Skovlund SE, Peyrot M. DAWN International Advisory Panel. The Diabetes Attitudes, Wishes, and Needs (DAWN) program: a new approach to improving outcomes of diabetes care. Diabetes Spectr. 2005;18:136-42.
2. Cramer JA. A systematic review of adherence with medications for diabetes. Diabetes Care. 2004;27:1218-24.
3. Pladevall M, Williams LK, Potts LA, Divine G, Xi H, Lafata JE. Clinical outcomes and adherence to medications measured by claims data in patients with diabetes. Diabetes Care. 2004;27:2800-5.
4. Leichter SB. Making outpatient care of diabetes more efficient: analyzing noncompliance. Clin Diabetes. 2015;23:187-90.
5. Lin EH, Katon W, Von Korff M, et al. Relationship of depression and diabetes self-care, medication adherence, and preventive care. Diabetes Care. 2004;27:2154-60.
6. Rubin RR. Adherence to pharmacologic therapy in patients with type 2 diabetes mellitus. Am J Med. 2005; 118 Suppl 5A:27S-34S.
7. Odegard PS, Capoccia K. Medication taking and diabetes: a systematic review of the literature. Diabetes Educ. 2007; 33:1014-29; discussion 1030-1.
8. Littenberg B, MacLean CD, Hurowitz L. The use of adherence aids by adults with diabetes: a cross-sectional survey. BMC Fam Pract. 2006;7:1-5.
9. Piette JD, Heisler M, Wagner TH. Problems paying out-of-pocket medication costs among older adults with diabetes. Diabetes Care. 2004;27:384-91.
10. Symlin [package insert]. AstraZeneca Pharmaceuticals LP, Wilmington DE; 2015.
11. Pelletier AL, Butler AM, Gillies RA, May JR. Metformin stinks, literally. Ann Intern Med. 2010;152:267-8.
12. Welchol [package insert]. Basking Ridge, NJ; 2019.
13. Cycloset [package insert]. Tiverton, RI: VeroScience; 2016.
14. Inzucchi SE. Oral antihyperglycemic therapy for type 2 diabetes: scientific review. JAMA 2002;287:360-72.
15. Polonsky W. Psychological insulin resistance: the patient perspective. Diabetes Educ. 2007;33 Suppl 7:241S-4S.
16. Welch G, Rose G, Ernst D. Motivational interviewing and diabetes: what is it, how is it used, and does it work? Diabetes Spectr. 2006;19:5-11.
17. Gibney MA, Arce CH, Byron KJ, Hirsch LJ. Skin and subcutaneous adipose layer thickness in adults with diabetes at sites used for insulin injections: implications for needle length recommendations. Curr Med Res Opin. 2010;26:1519-30.
18. Hirsch LJ, Gibney MA, Albanese J, et al. Comparative glycemic control, safety and patient ratings for a new 4 mm × 32G insulin pen needle in adults with diabetes. Curr Med Res Opin. 2010;26:1531-41.
19. Hirsch LJ, Gibney MA, Li L, Bérubé J. Glycemic control, reported pain and leakage with a 4 mm 32 G pen needle in obese and non-obese adults with diabetes: a post hoc analysis Curr Med Res Opin. 2012;28:1305-11.
20. Kreugel G, Keers JC, Kerstens MN, Wolffenbuttel BH. Randomized trial on the influence of the length of two insulin pen needles on glycemic control and patient preference in obese patients with diabetes. Diabetes Technol Ther. 2011;13:737-41.
21. Schwartz S, Hassman D, Shelmet J, et al. A multicenter, open-label, randomized, two-period crossover trial comparing glycemic control, satisfaction, and preference achieved with a 31 gauge x 6 mm needle versus a 29 gauge x 12.7 mm needle in obese patients with diabetes mellitus. Clin Ther. 2004;26:1663-78.
22. Frid A, Hirsch L, Gaspar R, et al. New injection recommendations for patients with diabetes. Diabetes Metab. 2010;36 Suppl 2:S3-18.
23. Saltiel-Berzin R, Cypress M, Gibney M. Translating the research in insulin injection technique: implications for practice. Diabetes Educ. 2012;38:635-43.
24. Pearson TL. Practical aspects of insulin pen devices. J Diabetes Sci Technol. 2010;4:522-31.
25. Dang DK, Pucino F, Ponte CD, Calis KA. Drug-induced glucose and insulin dysregulation. In: Tisdale JE, Miller DA, eds. *Drug-Induced Diseases: Prevention, Detection, and Management*, Third Edition. Bethesda, MD: American Society of Health Systems Pharmacists; 2018:679-96.
26. US Food and Drug administration, US Department of Health and Human Services. Drug applications for OTC (Nonprescription) drugs. Last updated 2015 Jan 7 (cited 2019 June 3). https://www.fda.gov/drugs/types-applications/drug-applications-over-counter-otc-drugs.
27. Bayer HealthCare. Alka-Seltzer Original [product information]. 2014 (cited 2019 June 3). On the Internet at: http://labeling.bayercare.com/omr/online/alka-seltzer-original.pdf.
28. Weitzel KR, Goode JVKR. Constipation. In: Krinsky DL, Ferreri SP, Hemstreet B, et al, eds. *Handbook of Nonprescription Drugs: an Interactive Approach to Self-Care.* Washington, DC: American Pharmacists Association;2018:265-85.
29. US Food and Drug Administration. FDA Drug Safety Communication: FDA warns of possible harm from exceeding recommended dose of over-the-counter sodium phosphate products to treat constipation. 2014 Jan 8 (cited 2019 June 3). On the Internet at: http://www.fda.gov/Drugs/DrugSafety/ucm380757.htm.
30. Lodise NM. Vaginal and vulvovaginal disorders. In: Krinsky DL, Ferreri SP, Hemstreet B, et al, eds. Handbook of Nonprescription Drugs: an Interactive Approach to Self-Care. Washington, DC: American Pharmacists Association;2018:131-46.
31. Coffey CW, Srivastava SB. Minor foot disorders. In: Krinsky DL, Ferreri SP, Hemstreet B, et al, eds. Handbook of Nonprescription Drugs: an Interactive Approach to Self-Care. Washington, DC: American Pharmacists Association;2018:821-39.
32. Datye KA, Moore DJ, Russell WE, Jaser SS. A review of adolescent adherence in type 1 diabetes and the untapped potential of diabetes providers to improve outcomes. Curr Diab Rep. 2015; 15:51.

33. Silverstein J, Klingensmith G, Copeland K, et al. Care of children and adolescents with type 1 diabetes: a statement of the American Diabetes Association. Diabetes Care. 2005; 28:186-212.

34. Children and Adolescents: Standards of Medical Care in Diabetes-2019. Diabetes Care. 2019;42:S148-64.

35. Chiang JL, Maahs DM, Garvey KC, et al. Type 1 Diabetes in children and adolescents: a position statement by the American Diabetes Association. Diabetes Care. 2018;41:2026-44.

36. Older Adults: Standards of Medical Care in Diabetes-2019. Diabetes Care. 2019;42:S139-47.

CHAPTER 8

Monitoring

Molly McElwee-Malloy, CDCES, RN

Key Concepts

- Monitoring is the self-care behavior that acts as a springboard into the other six self-care behaviors. Monitoring generates data, and understanding how to use these data supports change.
- Monitoring is a tool for prevention and early diagnosis and to delay progression of the related complications and comorbidities that result in disabilities that may compromise effective self-management and reduce quality of life.
- Diabetes care and education specialists need to be aware of both technological and clinical skill set requirements of continuous glucose monitoring, blood glucose and ketone monitoring, medication tracking, blood pressure testing, weight measurement, routine lab visits, and the operational and interpretive aspects of each.
- It is equally important to teach persons with diabetes how to understand the data being monitored and when they may need to alert their healthcare provider for additional assistance.

Introduction

Monitoring is one of the AADE7 Self-Care Behaviors® and is recognized as an important component of the treatment plan for persons with diabetes. With the advancement of technology, the monitoring behavior encircles many aspects of diabetes management, including healthy eating, being active, taking medications and healthy coping.[1] Today, monitoring has expanded beyond self-monitoring of blood glucose to include monitoring of blood pressure, activity, nutritional intake, weight, medication, feet/skin, mood, sleep, symptoms like shortness of breath, and other aspects of self-care.[1] Although monitoring can still include the use of paper and pencil to record data, new methods of data collection are available that enable individuals to more easily record data.[2] Although diabetes is mostly a self-managed disease, the persons with diabetes still rely on healthcare professionals for monitoring, advice, and support as life changes and health needs change.[3] Healthcare professionals need to understand the parameters that require monitoring, as well as what can be monitored by different technologies, with knowledge of the difference of what should be monitored by them and those that are or can be self-monitored by the person with diabetes.[4] This chapter focuses on monitoring clinical, microvascular, macrovascular, diabetes self-management education and support (DSMES), medical nutrition therapy (MNT), acute complications, and psychosocial parameters related to diabetes. Chapter 18 focuses exclusively on glucose monitoring, from self-monitoring of blood glucose (SMBG) through continuous glucose monitoring (CGM).

When monitoring diabetes, it is important to start with a baseline evaluation. This includes a comprehensive medical and medication history, physical exam, and standard lab tests. Key information includes the age of the person and characteristics of the onset of diabetes (eg, diabetic ketoacidosis [DKA], asymptomatic laboratory finding), the type of diabetes the person has, and the person's understanding of his or her diabetes. Lifestyle habits must also be assessed, including eating patterns, physical activity, nutritional status, and weight history (such as weight gain or weight loss). In addition, the growth and development of children and adolescents with diabetes should be reviewed.

A thorough review of the person's diabetes education history should include a review of previous treatment regimens and the person's response to that therapy (A1C records as well as self-report). The healthcare professional needs to obtain the person's current treatment plan, including medications and medication regimen participation, meal plan and food patterns, physical activity patterns, CGM and/or SMBG patterns and readings (including how the person uses the data). Obtaining these data are made easier through the use of apps and other self-monitoring options offered through most smartphones today.[4]

Next, a review of the person's history of diabetes-related complications should be obtained. The healthcare professional needs to review the person's history of acute and chronic complications for how often the person experiences DKA (including the severity and cause) and for microvascular complications such as retinopathy, nephropathy, and neuropathy (sensory [including history of foot lesions] and autonomic [including sexual dysfunction and gastroparesis]), as well as monitoring for glycemic variability.[5] The healthcare professional also needs to assess the person's history of macrovascular complications, such as chronic heart disease, cerebrovascular disease, and peripheral artery disease. Finally, any additional chronic complications should be discussed, such as depression, psychosocial problems (to include diabetes distress in appendix), and dental disease.

A complete lab evaluation should be done to establish a baseline of the person's lab parameters. This includes an A1C; fasting lipid profile with low-density lipoprotein (LDL), high-density lipoprotein (HDL), and triglycerides; liver function tests; serum creatinine and calculated glomerular filtration rate (GFR); and thyroid-stimulating hormone in persons with type 1 diabetes or dyslipidemia, or in women over 50.

Children with type 1 diabetes, and adults who are symptomatic, should be screened for celiac disease, since there is a genetic link between type 1 diabetes and celiac disease.[6] Additional parameters that need to be monitored or assessed periodically are often completed by medical specialists. These include an annual dilated eye exam, family planning for women of reproductive age, MNT from a registered dietitian, DSMES from a recognized or accredited education program, a dental examination, and, if needed, referral to a mental health professional.

Monitoring checklists can be helpful to the healthcare professional and the person with diabetes. See Tables 8.1 and 8.2.

Monitoring of all these parameters is valuable, and with connected devices and other technologies, remote patient monitoring and virtual collaborative care and telehealth are possible.[2] Assisting persons with diabetes in using technology to monitor behaviors and issues related to appropriate and useful monitoring is an area of diabetes care that clearly combines the diabetes care and education specialist's skills of management and education.[1]

TABLE 8.1 Monitoring Checklist for Healthcare Professionals

Clinical	• A1C • Lipids • Blood pressure
Microvascular	• Neuropathy • Nephropathy • Retinopathy • Reducing glycemic variability
Macrovascular	• Smoking • Antiplatelet
DSMES	• Nutrition (related apps) • Activity (related apps) • Support (peer support and social media) • SMBG/CGM • Medication taking/ tracking (apps)
Acute complications	• Hypoglycemia • DKA • Hyperosmolar hyperglycemic state
Psychosocial	• Depression • Preconception planning • Transitional care • Diabetes Distress Scale

TABLE 8.2 Self-Monitoring Checklist for Persons With Diabetes

- SMBG or CGM
- Blood pressure
- Daily foot exam
- Daily dental care
- Acute complications, ie, hypoglycemia or hyperglycemia
- Ketones
- Chronic complications, ie, kidney function, neuropathy, eye health
- Meal plan/food intake
- Stress/emotional health

SGLT2 Inhibitors and Risk of Euglycemic Diabetic Ketoacidosis[7–10]

There are known benefits for individuals using SGLT-2 inhibitors for weight loss, cardiovascular health, and increased glycemic stability. However, an individual taking insulin and SGLT-2 is at an increased risk of experiencing DKA, possibly without high blood glucose.[8] The risk for DKA is known for persons with diabetes on insulin. Traditional episodes of DKA present with high blood glucose, in addition to all other associated symptoms. However, an individual taking an SGLT-2 inhibitor on insulin therapy may experience euglycemic values and still be diagnosed with DKA. With high blood glucose symptoms absent, the individual and the provider may not be considering the possibility of ketoacidosis occurring. Individuals on SGLT-2 and insulin should regularly monitor for blood ketones to help alert to possible episodes of ketoacidosis early to their healthcare provider.[7,9]

Euglycemic DKA with SGLT-2 inhibitors has an increased risk of occurring in individuals who have excessive alcohol intake, who may be dehydrated, may be on a very low carbohydrate diet, and have extensive and extended exercise, or reduction or omission of insulin dosing.[10] Individuals on SGLT-2 inhibitors and insulin therapy who experience an increase in ketones should discontinue SGLT-2 therapy and follow up with their healthcare provider.

Monitoring: A Comprehensive Approach to Person-Centered Care Beyond Glycemic Management

Daily SMBG or CGM use provides persons with diabetes the information they need to assess how food, physical activity, and medications affect their glucose levels and guide decisions to improve glycemic stability, if needed. The needs of people with diabetes, however, are not limited solely to adequate glycemic stability; they also include learning to identify and prevent the related complications that result in disability and reduced quality of life. In keeping with these expanding needs of the person with diabetes, the role of the diabetes care and education specialist has evolved to address the global aspects of chronic disease management. Diabetes education should include both monitoring for the comorbidities and complications that frequently accompany diabetes and supporting person-centered self-management education and training in those areas.

Diabetes education should include helping persons with diabetes understand how to prevent complications as well as the risks for and the benefits of the identification and treatment of the complications of diabetes. Monitoring parameters of the various accompanying disease states should include common signs and symptoms, timing and frequency of testing, target values and goals, instruction on self-monitoring and devices, and interpretation and use of information and results. Today's diabetes care and education specialist is charged with knowing what information is needed, how this information can be collected and analyzed, how often it should be evaluated, and how best to help support positive self-management behaviors in all areas of monitoring. This aspect of self-care is as crucial as glycemic management in improving outcomes in individual with diabetes.

Complications and Comorbidities

The importance of protecting the body from the effects of hyperglycemia cannot be overstated. The direct and indirect effects on the vasculature are the major sources of morbidity and mortality in both type 1 diabetes and type 2 diabetes. Typically, the injurious effects of diabetes are identified as either microvascular or macrovascular complications and include diabetes nephropathy, retinopathy, neuropathy, coronary artery disease, peripheral arterial disease, and stroke. There are, however, several other complications and disease states that have been associated with diabetes and should be included in risk assessment and routine monitoring: periodontal disease, thyroid disorders, mental health and depression, osteoporosis, sleep apnea, and ensuring immunization schedules are met. Monitoring parameters for common complications and comorbidities will be discussed as they relate to the role of the diabetes care and education specialist in assessment, follow-up, and individual self-management skills.

Initial Assessment

When monitoring people with diabetes, it is important to start with a baseline evaluation. This should include a comprehensive medical and medication history, physical exam, and standard lab tests.

The physical exam should include height, weight, and body mass index (BMI) as well as blood pressure (including orthostatic measurements when indicated), fundoscopic examination, thyroid palpation, skin examination, and comprehensive foot exam.

A complete lab panel should also be performed that includes A1C, fasting lipid profile, liver function tests, serum creatinine, and calculated GFR. Measurement of thyroid-stimulating hormone (TSH) should be included in persons with type 1 diabetes or dyslipidemia and in women over 50 years of age. Children with type 1 diabetes and symptomatic adults should be screened for celiac disease, since there is a genetic link between type 1 diabetes and celiac disease.

The initial assessment and lab profile will be important points of reference for the healthcare provider when evaluating disease progression, assessing lifestyle and therapeutic interventions, and making future recommendations. It is important to ensure that the individual's type of diabetes is being treated correctly. Persons with LADA are often misdiagnosed as having type 2 diabetes,[11] while up to 5% of all diabetes cases are neither type 1 or type 2 and rather fall into another etiologic category.[11,12]

Macrovascular

Persons with diabetes should be regularly assessed for cardiovascular risk factors and the presence of macrovascular disease. The assessment should include an inquiry about symptoms of macrovascular disease, follow-up on recommended testing and monitoring parameters, an evaluation of goals, and education and support. Persons with high glycemic variability are at greater risk for macrovascular (as well as microvascular) complications.[13]

Blood Pressure

All persons with diabetes should be monitored for hypertension and educated on reducing risks of cardiovascular disease. Hypertension is a common comorbidity among persons with type 2 diabetes, which magnifies the risk of diabetes-related complications. The aggressive treatment of high blood pressure decreases the incidence of CVD as well as microvascular complications.[14,15] Today, there are numerous apps and other mobile health technology that can assist healthcare providers and persons with diabetes in monitoring cardiovascular health.[16]

According to the ADA, blood pressure should be measured routinely to a goal of <140/80 mm Hg for most people with diabetes. A lower systolic target of <130 mm Hg may be appropriate for certain individuals, such as younger people with diabetes, if this can be achieved without undue treatment burden.[17] Because hypertension often presents without symptoms, the accurate measurement of blood pressure is fundamental to both the diagnosis and effective management of the disease. In light of this, specific procedures have been developed that describe the proper method for obtaining the most accurate blood pressure reading possible. These procedures, as outlined in Table 8.3, should be followed for both in-office and home blood pressure measurement.

The most common error in blood pressure measurement is the use of an inappropriately sized cuff. Considerable overestimation of readings can occur if the cuff is too small. To determine the correct cuff size, use a cloth measuring tape to measure the circumference of the arm that will most often be used for blood pressure measurements. Place the tape around the upper arm, midway between the elbow and the shoulder. Refer to the chart in Table 8.4 for appropriate sizing.

In-office blood pressure measurements are subject to a high degree of variability[18]; therefore, readings should be performed by trained individuals, using validated equipment to ensure consistency in measurements. With rare exceptions, blood pressure machines found in supermarkets and pharmacies are usually not properly maintained and should not be used. For home blood pressure monitoring, the American Heart Association recommends using an automatic cuff-style upper-arm monitor.[19] Wrist and finger monitors are not recommended, because they yield less-reliable readings.[19] Electronic home monitors are easy to use, are cost-effective, and may have integration into smartphone technology making therapeutic

TABLE 8.3 Blood Pressure Tips and Procedures

- The individual sits quietly for at least 5 minutes before the blood pressure is taken.
- Caffeine, smoking, and exercise are avoided for at least 30 minutes before the reading.
- Individual sits with back supported and both feet on the floor, legs uncrossed.
- The arm is supported at heart level.
- Outer garments are removed; avoid rolling sleeves if this will cause constriction.
- Talking is avoided during the reading.
- Place the lower edge of the cuff about 1 inch above the bend of the elbow.
- Record the reading and which arm was used for the reading.
- Take another reading and record the second reading.

TABLE 8.4 Sizing Blood Pressure Cuffs

Distance Around the Arm	*Blood Pressure Cuff Size*
7–9 inches	Small adult cuff
9–13 inches	Standard adult cuff
13–17 inches	Large adult cuff

participation easier. Additionally, home blood pressure monitoring may help identify individuals with nocturnal hypertension, white-coat hypertension, or masked hypertension. Persons with diabetes should be prescribed devices that have been tested, validated, and approved by the Association for the Advancement of Medical Instrumentation, the British Hypertension Society, and the International Protocol for the Validation of Automated BP Measuring Devices. A list of validated monitors is available on the Dabl Educational Trust Web site (http://www.dableducational.org).

At home, blood pressure is typically measured twice daily—once in the morning before taking any medications, and once in the evening. Two or three readings taken 1 minute apart should be taken at the same time each day and all of the results recorded. Blood pressure may vary throughout the day and is typically higher in the morning. *Orthostatic hypotension* may be identified by lightheadedness when standing, or if the blood pressure falls by >20 mm Hg systolic or >10 mm Hg diastolic from baseline upon standing.

Review of in-office and home blood pressure readings will provide information to help assess treatment goals, therapies, and the individual's options. The diagnosis of hypertension, as well as changes in therapy, will usually require confirmation of elevated blood pressure readings on a separate day or visit. Persons with diabetes should understand their blood pressure numbers and the importance of blood pressure management to reduce complications and maximize quality of life. Diabetes self-management education should include discussions around medications and engagement with the medication regimen, critical blood pressure values, and development of a plan for identifying and managing hypertensive crisis.

Cholesterol: Lipids

Diabetes is correlated with a high risk for CVD. Management of the dyslipidemia of diabetes is a key element in the multifactorial approach to preventing CVD in persons with type 2 diabetes. The most typical lipoprotein pattern in type 2 diabetes consists of a moderate elevation in triglyceride levels, low HDL cholesterol values, and increased small, dense LDL particles. This pattern has been associated with insulin resistance and may present even before the onset of type 2 diabetes.

An annual fasting lipid profile is recommended for most adults with diabetes.[17] However, individuals with low-risk lipid values (LDL-C <100 mg/dL, HDL-C >50 mg/dL, and triglycerides <150 mg/dL) may be eligible for screenings every 2 years.[17] More frequent monitoring may be indicated after initiation or intensification of lipid-lowering therapies.[20,21]

In the absence of severe hypertriglyceridemia, lowering LDL-C to target is the first priority for most people with diabetes. The recommended treatment goal is LDL-C <100 mg/dL for individuals without overt CVD and <70 mg/dL for individuals with overt CVD. For individuals on high-dose statin therapy who are unable to achieve the LDL-C goal, a 30% to 40% reduction in LDL-C from baseline is an acceptable alternate target.[17] Lipid panel consisting of total cholesterol (TC), HDL-C, LDL-C, and triglycerides is most accurate if performed after a 9- to 12-hour fast, and if alcohol is avoided for 24 hours before the test. Concurrent conditions such as nephrotic syndrome[17] and hypothyroidism may cause elevated TC and/or LDL-C, while the presence of infection or inflammation results in lower HDL-C values and/or increased triglycerides.[22] Additionally, lipid levels may be altered after an acute myocardial infarction, making a lipid panel vital within the first 24 hours after the infarct.[23]

Healthcare providers should be monitoring to ensure the required lipid panels and follow-up are completed. Assessment should include a review of goals, therapeutic engagement, barriers to regimen participation, and the importance of risk reduction. For persons with diabetes not at goal, consider lifestyle modifications and initiation or intensification of medications. When intensification of statin therapy is warranted to reach the LDL-C goal, a doubling of the current dose generally achieves a modest, incremental reduction in the LDL-C of 5% to 6%,[24] a pattern that should be considered when escalating statin therapy to get to goal. Those individuals on statins or fibrates should be monitored for possible medication side effects and counseled on the signs and symptoms of myositis and rhabdomyolysis.

Antiplatelet Therapy

The ADA recommends the use of low-dose aspirin, 75 to 162 mg per day, as a primary prevention strategy in most persons with type 1 diabetes or type 2 diabetes at increased risk for CVD. Randomized control trials show that the dose should be person-specific and consider for bleeding risks.[25]

At each visit, the educator should monitor for all of the following: participation in the antiplatelet therapy, signs and symptoms of gastrointestinal (GI) bleed, and concomitant therapies that may increase the risk of bleed. Symptoms of upper GI bleeding can include bright red blood, dark clots, coffee-ground-like emesis, and black, tar-like stools. Symptoms of lower GI bleeding may include passing bright red or maroon blood alone or mixed in the stool. The use of enteric-coated aspirin may help alleviate stomach irritation but does not decrease the risk of GI bleed.

Smoking Cessation

Smoking cessation is associated with substantial health benefits.[26] Screening all persons with diabetes at every visit for tobacco use and providing those who do smoke with behavioral counseling and advice on pharmacologic interventions as well as wellness apps and technology are valuable preventive strategies. While the benefits of smoking cessation far outweigh the risks, the healthcare provider should be prepared to discuss the possible symptoms of nicotine withdrawal in order to maximize the likelihood that the individual will succeed. These include insomnia, anxiety, weight gain, depression, restlessness, and poor concentration. The most effective way to promote smoking cessation is to combine pharmacologic and behavioral interventions with ongoing support from the trained staff available through quit lines/programs. An example of such a program can be found at https://smokefree.gov (a free app), which provides online support 24/7 to help quit smoking.

Microvascular

Hyperglycemia as an important risk factor for the development of microvascular disease in people with diabetes.[27] Intensive glycemic management can reduce the risk of microvascular complications including progression of nephropathy, manifestation and progression of retinopathy, and retinal photocoagulation. The educator should be aware that persons with diagnosed retinopathy with extensive hyperglycemia can experience a worsening of retinopathy with sudden intensive glucose management. An attempt to gradually and methodically stabilize glucose levels is advised.[28]

Retinopathy

Diabetic retinopathy is the most common ophthalmic complication of poorly managed glucose and blood pressure and can eventually lead to blindness.[29] It occurs when blood vessels in the retina swell and leak fluid or become completely blocked. In some cases, abnormal new blood vessels grow on the surface of the retina. These ocular manifestations of diabetes affect up to 80% of all people who have had diabetes for 10 years or more.[29] Despite these intimidating statistics, research indicates that at least 90% of these new cases could be reduced through proper and vigilant treatment and monitoring of the eyes.[30] Early detection and treatment are critical because the risk of developing eye problems increases with the amount of time an individual has diabetes.[31] An initial dilated and comprehensive eye examination by an optometrist or ophthalmologist is recommended in persons with type 1 diabetes within 5 years of diagnosis. In people with type 2 diabetes, the eye exam should be performed shortly after diagnosis because this population is more likely to have retinopathy at diagnosis.[32] Annual comprehensive follow-up exams are recommended after the initial evaluation; however, more frequent follow-up may be required if retinopathy is progressing. Less-frequent exams (every 2 to 3 years) may be considered following 1 or more normal eye exams.[32] Retinal fundus photography may serve as a screening tool for retinopathy, but it is not a substitute for a comprehensive eye exam.

TABLE 8.5 Risk Factors for Development of Diabetic Retinopathy

- Duration of diabetes
- High blood pressure
- Hyperlipidemia
- Pregnancy
- Use of tobacco products

Women with preexisting diabetes who are pregnant or are planning pregnancy should have a comprehensive eye examination and should be counseled on the risk of development and/or progression of diabetic retinopathy. The eye examination should occur in the first trimester with close follow-up throughout pregnancy and for 1-year postpartum.[31] Risk factors for the development of diabetic retinopathy are shown in Table 8.5.

There are 4 stages of retinopathy progression: mild non-proliferative, moderate non-proliferative, severe non-proliferative, and the advanced stage, proliferative retinopathy. The early stages of the disease are often symptom-free; however, monitoring for blurred vision, blocked vision, floaters, or bleeding in the eyes should be done at each visit. Persons with diabetes with or at high risk for retinopathy should be counseled to avoid heavy lifting and jarring exercise that could lead to microvascular retinal bleeding and possible retinal detachment.[33] Educational and behavioral interventions should focus on reducing risks and participation in regular eye examinations.

Nephropathy

In healthy individuals, protein (albumin) is typically not found in the urine, because the spaces in the glomerular membrane of the kidney are too small to allow protein molecules to escape. If the membrane is damaged, however, these molecules can leak through into the urine. People with diabetes are at significant risk of kidney damage leading to increased albumin in the urine and possible progression to diabetic nephropathy (DN). Reduced renal blood flow and the presence of albumin in the urine make the body retain excess amounts of water and salt, which may manifest in symptoms such as weight gain, ankle swelling, fatigue, and loss of appetite.

Diabetic nephropathy affects approximately 38% of people with diabetes.[34] It is the leading cause of end-stage renal disease (ESRD) in the United States,[35] and people at all stages of DN have a significantly increased risk of heart disease.[36] There are usually no symptoms in the early stages of DN, so the only sign of kidney damage may be small amounts of protein in the urine, referred to as microalbuminuria, or moderately increased albuminuria.

Screening for DN is done by measuring the albumin-to-creatinine ratio on a spot urine specimen or total urinary albumin in a 24-hour collection. The spot urine test is the most practical method to assess the albumin-to-creatinine ratio because it is easy to perform and collection errors occur less frequently. The 24-hour urine collection can be burdensome and adds little predictive value or accuracy to the results.[37,38] Measurement of a spot urine for albumin only, without measuring urine creatinine, is somewhat less expensive but is more susceptible to yielding false-negative and false-positive results. Falsely elevated urine protein levels may be produced by conditions such as urinary tract infections, exercise, and hematuria. Abnormalities of albumin excretion are defined in Table 8.6.

Because of variability in urinary albumin excretion (UAE), 2 of 3 specimens collected within a 3- to 6-month period should be abnormal before considering an individual to have crossed 1 of these diagnostic thresholds. Exercise within 24 hours, infection, fever, congestive heart failure, marked hyperglycemia, and marked hypertension may elevate UAE over baseline values. False positives can also result from an improperly collected or stored specimen.

Microalbuminuria rarely develops in persons with type 1 diabetes during the first few years of the disease. For this reason the ADA recommends an annual test to assess UAE that begins 5 years after diagnosis.[31,39] Persons with type 2 diabetes are more likely to have albuminuria at diagnosis because of the long duration of abnormal glucose metabolism that often precedes diagnosis. Thus, persons with type 2 diabetes should begin an annual UAE at the time of diagnosis.[31,40] Serum creatinine should be measured at least annually in all adults with diabetes regardless of the degree of UAE. The serum creatinine should be used to estimate GFR and stage the level of chronic kidney disease (CKD) if present.[31,41]

Treatment is rigorous glycemic management combined with blood pressure management. An angiotensin-converting enzyme (ACE) inhibitor, an angiotensin II receptor blocker (ARB), or both should be used to treat hypertension at the earliest sign of microalbuminuria or even before, because these drugs lower intraglomerular blood pressure and thus have renal protective effects. Diabetes self-management education and support should focus on routine assessment to include monitoring for symptoms, regular testing, follow-up, and referral to a specialist as needed as well as ongoing education and support in line with the individual's needs and goals.

TABLE 8.6 Abnormalities of Albumin Excretion

Category	*Spot Collection (μg/mg creatinine)*
Normal	<30
Microalbuminuria or moderately increased albuminuria (early diabetic nephropathy)	30–299
Macroalbuminuria or severely increased albuminuria	≥300

Neuropathy

Neuropathies are the most common complication of diabetes, characterized by a progressive loss of nerve fiber function. People with diabetes can, over time, develop nerve damage throughout the body, to which the clinical manifestations will depend on what nerves are affected, sensory or autonomic. Diabetic neuropathy can result in significant disability that may impair daily self-management activities, lower quality of life, and increase the risk of death.[42]

The prevalence of neuropathy increases with the duration of diabetes and severity of hyperglycemia, and while it is considered a progressive disease, individuals may present without symptoms. For this reason, comprehensive screening for both distal symmetric polyneuropathy and diabetic autonomic neuropathy should take place annually beginning 5 years after diagnosis for people with type 1 diabetes and at diagnosis for people with type 2 diabetes.[31]

Management of diabetic neuropathy has 2 approaches: therapies that help relieve symptoms and therapies that may slow progression of the disease. Of all the available treatments, optimal glycemic stability is probably the most important for slowing the progression of neuropathy.

Peripheral Neuropathy It is estimated that approximately half of the people with diabetes will develop neuropathy during their lifetime.[43] Diabetic peripheral neuropathy (DPN) is the most common form of neuropathy in this population, with the most common presentation being distal symmetrical polyneuropathy, a stocking-and-glove pattern of numbness, pain, tingling, or weakness.

All people with diabetes should receive routine visual inspection of their feet at each diabetes-related visit with their healthcare provider and an annual comprehensive foot exam.[31] The routine visual foot inspection is used to detect the presence of acute problems as well as reinforce the importance of preventive strategies and self-care behaviors for foot health. The exam should include all areas indicated in Table 8.7.

Beyond the routine visual inspection, an annual comprehensive foot exam should be performed[3] to assess risk status and disease progression and to determine the need for referral and prescription footwear. The annual exam should include both visual inspection of the feet and the use of some simple, in-office tests that assist in revealing decreased sensation to vibration, pressure, and superficial pain.[31]

A simple vibratory sensation exam consists of a 128-Hz tuning fork placed on the bony prominence at the dorsum of the great toe using the following steps:

1. Strike the tuning fork to initiate vibration.
2. Touch the tuning fork to the medial aspect of the great toe (avoid callused areas).
3. Ask the individual to state when he or she first feels the vibration and when it stops. If the individual indicates the vibration has stopped before the vibration has stopped in the examiner's hand, the test is abnormal (–).
4. Document the results as (+) for normal or (–) for abnormal.

TABLE 8.7 Routine Visual Foot Inspection

- Inspect feet, heels, and between the toes.
- Check for signs of compromised blood flow such as thin and shiny skin, bluish-colored skin, or lack of hair.
- Check for wounds, calluses, blisters, ulcers, or deformities.
- Inspect nails for thickening, appropriate length, and signs of fungal or bacterial infection, and look for any ingrown nails.
- Check socks for discharge or blood.
- Check shoes for wear and for foreign objects.
- Check footwear for appropriate materials and support.
- Educate individuals about daily foot inspections and self-care of the feet.
- Refer individuals to healthcare provider or specialist as needed.

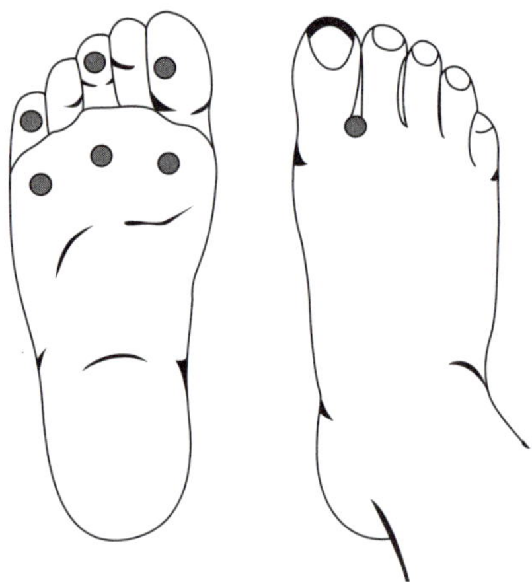

FIGURE 8.1 Performing the Semmes-Weinstein Monofilament Exam

Pressure sensation can be assessed using a simple clinical test such as the Semmes-Weinstein monofilament exam. (See Figure 8.1.) The Semmes-Weinstein 5.07 monofilament nylon wire exerts 10 g of force when bowed into a C shape against the skin for 1 second. Individuals are asked if they detect the sensation. Individuals who can't reliably detect application of the monofilament to designated sites on the plantar surface of their feet are considered to have lost protective pressure sensation. When performing this exam, the healthcare provider should follow these guidelines:

1. Place the individual in either a supine or sitting position with shoes and socks removed.
2. Touch the monofilament wire to the individual's skin on the arm or hand to demonstrate what the touch feels like.
3. Have the individual close his or her eyes and keep toes pointed straight upward during the exam.
4. Have the individual say "yes" or "now" each time he or she feels the pressure of the monofilament on the foot during the exam.
5. Hold the monofilament perpendicular to the individual's foot and press it against the foot, increasing the pressure until the monofilament bends into a C shape. (The individual should sense the monofilament by the time it bows.)
6. Hold the monofilament in place for about 1 second.
7. Repeat 2 to 3 times and then move to the next spot.
8. Test both feet on the locations according to the diagram. Avoid callused areas.
9. Record responses on a foot screening form with "+" for yes and "–" for no.

Neuropathy usually starts in the first and third toes and progresses to the first and third metatarsal heads. These areas will likely be the first to have negative results with the Semmes-Weinstein monofilament exam. For more information on monofilament exams, see Figure 28.1 in Chapter 28.

Superficial pain sensation is tested with a pinprick. The test is performed with a pin or needle gently applied to an area of skin that the subject cannot observe. The application of the pin is alternated with the pressing of a dull object against the skin, and the individual is asked to report pain.

Monofilament examination, vibration testing with a tuning fork, and superficial pain sensation testing have similar efficacy in detecting neuropathy.[44] The mobility, gait, and balance of a person with diabetes also should be assessed because individuals with DPN and balance problems have a two- to threefold increased risk of fall.[45]

Foot examinations can assist the healthcare provider with identification of risk factors and early detection and treatment, as well as provide an opportunity to reinforce healthy self-management behaviors. Self-management education should include encouraging individuals to perform daily foot inspections and to contact their healthcare provider with any concerns. For example, look for cracks in skin, calluses, blisters, change in color, ingrown toenails, and reddened areas. Use of a mirror or a support person can help in visual self-examination. The routine, in-office inspection offers the educator the opportunity to discuss appropriate footwear and foot care, and to reinforce the importance of glycemic management. People who receive foot self-management education and have a foot examination performed by a healthcare provider are significantly more likely to regularly check their feet than people who do not receive such services.[46]

Autonomic Neuropathy Diabetic autonomic neuropathy (DAN) is a form of polyneuropathy affecting the nonvoluntary, non-sensory nerves, leading to damage mostly to the internal organs such as the bladder, cardiovascular system, digestive tract, and genital organs. Risk factors include duration of diabetes, increasing age, female sex, and higher BMI.[47]

The diagnosis of DAN is difficult given that it does not usually present with overt pain. In addition, the number of organs that can be affected and the similarity of symptoms with other medical conditions can make this diagnosis more difficult. Clinical symptoms generally do not develop until many years after the onset of diabetes, so clinicians must rely on quantitative functional testing to help identify DAN. Healthcare providers should include assessment of risk as well as routine screening for symptoms associated with these complications. Some common clinical manifestations and symptoms of DAN may include those listed in Table 8.8.

Hypoglycemic unawareness can pose a serious threat to the person with diabetes. Persons with autonomic neuropathy may not experience the typical symptoms of low blood glucose, such as shakiness, making detection of hypoglycemia more difficult.

Persons showing symptoms of DAN should be referred to the primary care provider or specialist for a complete physical assessment and follow-up. Diagnostic tests that evaluate autonomic function include tests that measure heart rate variability, response of heart rate and blood pressure to breathing exercises such as the Valsalva maneuver, and the tilt-table test. Additional assessment tools include gastric-emptying evaluation, thermoregulatory sweat test, urinalysis, ultrasound, and bladder function testing.

When DAN is undiagnosed or left untreated, the impact can be serious, resulting in complications ranging from discomfort and pain to heart attack and death. Identification of persons at risk for neuropathy in conjunction with routine monitoring for possible signs and symptoms is critical to preventing the onset of the disease and slowing disease progression. Strict glycemic management can slow the onset of DAN and sometimes reverse it.

Peripheral Arterial Disease

Peripheral arterial disease (PAD) is a narrowing of the arteries resulting in reduced blood flow to the extremities. People with diabetes are at an increased risk of developing this disease as well as develop it faster than the average population.[48] Hyperglycemia, hypertension, dyslipidemia, and tobacco use are known risk factors for PAD. Screening for PAD should be done at diagnosis and then annually, and should include the individual's history of claudication as well as assessment of pedal pulses.

Early signs of PAD in persons with diabetes are the onset of lower extremity pain associated with walking and cold feet. It is notable that a person with PAD may not experience physical symptoms that would indicate PAD screening or follow-up is necessary, particularly in type 1 diabetes.[49] A physical exam may reveal the presence of muscle atrophy, bruits, cool skin, thickened toenails, and possibly ulcers and gangrene. The ankle-brachial index (ABI) provides a simple, reliable, and noninvasive means for screening and diagnosing PAD. It is recommended that the ABI be performed on any person with diabetes

TABLE 8.8 Common Clinical Manifestations and Symptoms of Diabetic Autonomic Neuropathy (DAN)

Site	*Monitoring/Assessment*	*Symptoms*
Cardiovascular	Blood pressure	• Persistent or resting tachycardia (>100 beats per minute) • Orthostatic hypotension (a drop in systolic blood pressure of >20 mm Hg upon standing) • Syncope/light-headedness
	Heart rate	• Exercise intolerance where heart rate remains unchanged in response to changing activity levels
Gastrointestinal	Gastrointestinal function	• Constipation (may lead to bloating and esophageal reflux) • Diarrhea • Abdominal pain • Nausea or vomiting • Loss of appetite
	Swallow evaluation	• Difficulty in swallowing
	Gastric emptying	• Gastroparesis (delayed gastric emptying)
Genitourinary	Bladder function	• Urinary incontinence • Difficulty starting urination • Frequent urinary tract infections
	Sexual dysfunction	• Female sexual dysfunction • Vaginal dryness • Erectile dysfunction
Sudomotor	Perspiration	• Heat intolerance • Heavy sweating • Absence of perspiration • Gustatory sweating
	Skin hydration	• Dry or cracked skin • Skin infections
Pupillary	Vision problems	• Pupil response to light (difficult to adjust to changes in light/brightness) • Problems driving at night

Sources: American Diabetes Association. Adapted with permission from AJ Boulton, A Vinik, J Arezzo, et al, "Diabetic neuropathies (position statement)," *Diabetes Care* 28, no. 4 (2005): 956-62.

over the age of 50 or who has positive risk factors that include the following:

- Duration of diabetes >10 years
- Tobacco use
- High blood pressure
- Hyperlipidemia

The ABI is the ratio of systolic blood pressure in the ankle to systolic blood pressure in the arm using a hand-held Doppler and a blood pressure cuff. A normal ABI value is from 0.9 to 1.2. Any value less than 0.9 is indicative of PAD.[49]

Additional Areas to Monitor

Depression/Cognitive Assessment

Depression is an comorbid condition in persons with diabetes with nearly a threefold increase in type 1 diabetes and approximately 2 times higher in type 2 diabetes than the rest of the population.[50] It is important for healthcare providers to monitor for signs of depression in persons with diabetes. Signs of depression may include poor glycemic stability despite ongoing adjustments, insomnia or hypersomnia, changes in weight by more than 5% within the last month, general malaise, and episodes of crying or tearfulness.

According to the ADA, it is reasonable to include psychological and social assessments of the individual as part of diabetes management. Screening and follow-up may include attitudes about diabetes, management expectations, mood, quality of life, and financial, social, and emotional resources, as well as psychiatric history. In the presence of poor self-management, monitoring for depression, anxiety, eating disorders, and cognitive impairment is recommended.[51]

Many validated tools for screening for depression are available; however, obstacles, including length, cost, and degree of expertise required for use and interpretation, preclude inclusion in routine assessments. The Patient Health Questionnaire-2, or PHQ-2, and PHQ-9 are 2 tools proven to be effective in identifying individuals who might benefit from a more complete evaluation for depression.[52] This PHQ-2 is a quick assessment tool that can easily be incorporated into the diabetes care and education specialist's routine follow-up as it consists of only 2 questions:

> Over the past 2 weeks, have you often been bothered by:
>
> 1. Little interest or pleasure in doing things?
> 2. Feeling down, depressed, or hopeless?

An affirmative answer to *either* question is a provisional positive screen and does not establish a final diagnosis or determine depression severity and signals that the PHQ-9 should be administered.

For an individual with a positive screening, the healthcare provider

- May ask the individual to complete a more robust screening tool
- Should report the findings to the referring primary care provider
- Should provide a list of resources available for referral to a mental health professional

Depression and cognitive impairment screening and treatment should become routine components of diabetes care. Integrating simple screening tools for depression into DSMES is likely to be the most effective means for ensuring their routine use. Diabetes care and education specialists are in a key position to monitor for depression in adults with diabetes, and can help ensure appropriate referral, coordinate follow-up care, and develop goals aimed at optimizing individuals' self-care of both their depression and diabetes.

The Diabetes Distress Scale is an important validated tool used to measure the psychosocial and emotional distress attributed to having and managing diabetes.[53] Diabetes Distress is distinctly different than clinical depression, with a link to elevated A1C, poor self-care even when controlling for depression. Glycemic management and A1C are not always associated with poor clinical depression; however, with diabetes distress there often is a link.[54]

Weight

In persons with diabetes, managed weight loss using nutritional interventions and increased physical activity is associated with many beneficial effects. For persons with insulin dependent diabetes, weight loss has been linked to reductions in insulin resistance and subsequent insulin levels. Conversely, high insulin resistance and obesity have been associated with higher insulin levels. Since insulin is anabolic and promotes fat storage, reductions in insulin levels may augment weight loss.

While intentional weight loss in persons with diabetes is usually safe, unintentional weight loss may be associated with unmanaged glucose levels or other underlying conditions. Factors that could be attributed to weight loss include hyperglycemia, dehydration, thyroid disease, and cancer. Causes of weight gain should also be explored to include medication use or nonuse, thyroid disease, and nutritional sources.

The educator should be alerted if an individual suddenly develops significant involuntary weight loss, especially if it is accompanied by pronounced thirst or an increased need to urinate. Individuals should be encouraged to weigh themselves once or twice a week and record these values in a log or smartphone app for comparison. Diabetes self-management education should include identification of the individual's weight goals and education around the safe and appropriate loss of body mass as well as weight loss programs, support, and surgical options.

Thyroid

People with diabetes have a higher prevalence of thyroid disorders than the general population. Up to one third of women with type 1 diabetes have some form of autoimmune thyroid disease, and postpartum thyroiditis is 3 times more common in women with type 1 diabetes.[55,56] A number of reports have indicated a higher occurrence of thyroid diseases, particularly hypothyroidism, among people with type 2 diabetes. There is a particular increase in thyroid dysfunction for persons with A1C above 8%.[57]

Abnormal thyroid function may have profound effects on blood glucose stability. Hyperthyroidism is typically associated with worsening glucose levels and increased insulin requirements. The rapid heart rate resulting from excessive thyroid stimulation can worsen heart problems, and prolonged, untreated hyperthyroidism can exacerbate osteoporosis and risk of bone fractures. Hypothyroidism may be linked to insulin resistance in type 2 diabetes and should be routinely screened.[58] Low thyroid function may result in lipid abnormalities, including elevated triglyceride and LDL-C levels—changes that can further increase the risk of CVD.

In people with diabetes, the diagnosis of abnormal thyroid function based solely on clinical manifestations is difficult. Routine screening for thyroid function abnormalities in all persons with diabetes allows for early detection and treatment. Measurement of anti-thyroid peroxidase (anti-TPO) antibodies may detect subclinical hypothyroidism because those who are antibody positive have a higher risk of developing overt thyroid disease.[59] For persons with type 1 diabetes, it is recommended to test for anti-TPO antibodies at diagnosis. If anti-TPO antibodies are present, it is recommended that clinicians perform annual TSH screenings. In persons with type 2 diabetes, it is recommended that clinicians measure TSH at diagnosis of diabetes and every 5 years thereafter.[60] The AACE recommends TSH screening in women of childbearing age before pregnancy or during the first trimester.[14] The educator plays an important role in ensuring routine testing and follow-up of thyroid function as well as monitoring for symptoms of thyroid dysfunction. The signs and symptoms of hypothyroidism tend to be more subtle than those of hyperthyroidism and include dry skin, cold sensitivity, fatigue, muscle cramps, weight gain, and constipation. Symptoms commonly associated with hyperthyroidism include rapid heart rate, sweating, weight loss, shortness of breath, skin thickening on knees and elbows, and in women, changes in menstruation.

Treatment goals include initiating levothyroxine therapy when applicable, ongoing diabetes education and support, and improving glycemic stability.

Given the low therapeutic index for thyroid medications and the diversity of available products, it is recommended that individuals be maintained on the same brand of levothyroxine throughout the course of their therapy. In the event they are switched to another brand or generic product, measurement of serum TSH in 6 weeks to make adjustments is indicated.

Vitamin D

Vitamin D and its active metabolite, calcitriol, are important regulators of serum calcium and bone health. Vitamin D deficiency is present in a large portion of the population, and there have been several suggested links between vitamin D status and diabetes.[61] For persons with type 1 diabetes, this relationship is mediated by the effects of vitamin D on the immune system; in type 2 diabetes, vitamin D has been associated with improved beta cell activity as well as insulin sensitivity.[62] However, evidence from clinical studies evaluating vitamin D supplementation to improve glycemic stability in people with diabetes is conflicting.[63,64] Dialysis patients, many of whom have diabetes, are especially at risk for vitamin D abnormalities.

The most accurate way to determine vitamin D status is to measure a 25-hydroxy vitamin D level, with the optimal range typically between 25 and 80 ng/ml. Although vitamin D deficiency is prevalent, routine measurement of serum 25(OH)D levels is expensive. Therefore, it has been suggested that healthcare providers routinely monitor for vitamin D deficiency only in those individuals at risk for severe deficiency. This would include individuals with musculoskeletal symptoms such as bone pain or myalgia, those who have low bone mineral density (BMD) or prior fracture, those at risk for falls, and individuals with CKD.[65,66]

The diabetes care and education specialist should assess individuals who may be at high risk for vitamin D deficiency and recommend follow-up monitoring with the primary care provider or specialist for diagnostic testing if applicable.

The diabetes care and education specialist can play an important role in helping individuals select an appropriate vitamin D supplement, encouraging mealtime dosing of supplements, and recommending dietary sources of vitamin D.

Osteoporosis

Osteoporosis is a condition in which bone loses density and becomes fragile and more likely to fracture. There is growing evidence that people with diabetes are at increased risk of nontraumatic fracture and that poor glycemic management may contribute to deterioration of bone health.[67] People with type 1 diabetes typically have lower BMD, resulting in an increased risk of fractures, while vision problems, nerve damage, and hypoglycemic events heighten the propensity for falls. People with type 2 diabetes and complications were once thought to be protected from osteoporosis because of their higher BMD, but they may actually be at higher risk of fracture.[67] This may be attributable to the high rate of obesity and sedentary lifestyles in this population.

The routine care of people with diabetes should include an assessment of bone health. Specialized tests known as BMD tests measure bone density in various body parts. These tests not only detect existing osteoporosis but also predict risk for a future fracture. The most widely recognized BMD test is the dual-energy X-ray absorptiometry (DEXA or DXA) test, which measures bone density at the hip or spine.[68] It is a noninvasive test that typically takes less than 15 minutes and is repeated every 1 to 2 years. The results are reported as a T-score, and risk assessment is based on this value. The lower the T-score, the lower the bone density, as indicated in Table 8.9.

Although there is no cure for osteoporosis, treatment options are available. Treatment includes a balanced diet rich in calcium and vitamin D, an exercise plan and healthy lifestyle, and prescription therapies. Osteoporotic medications are divided into 2 categories: anti-resorptive medications and bone-forming medications. The anti-resorptive class includes the bisphosphonates, calcitonin, and the selective estrogen receptor modulators. There is presently only 1 bone-forming medication marketed as a synthetic version of parathyroid hormone.

The diabetes care and education specialist is afforded opportunities within the traditional assessment to evaluate the person's risk for osteoporosis and fracture and provide appropriate intervention and referral. A comprehensive assessment should include key indicators that can help identify those at greatest risk (see Table 8.10).[69] The diabetes care and education specialist should work with the individual to achieve optimal glycemic stability, improve nutritional status, make lifestyle changes, and create an exercise program to help improve bone health and decrease the chance of falls and fracture. Referral to specialists may include endocrinologists, bone specialists, podiatrists, ophthalmologists, occupational and physical therapists, and home care providers.

TABLE 8.9 T-Score Risk Assessment

+1 to −1	Indicates normal bone density
−1 to −2.5	Indicates low bone mineral density (osteopenia)
−2.5	Indicates osteoporosis

TABLE 8.10 Risk Factors for Falls and Osteoporotic Fracture

Nonmodifiable risk factors for osteoporotic fracture
Age
Female gender
Race: Caucasian and Asian at greater risk than African American
Weight: less than 127 lb
Bone structure: small framed
Early menopause (natural or surgical) and amenorrhea
Family and personal history of fracture as an adult
Medications (glucocorticoids, excessive thyroid hormone, anticonvulsants, gonadotropin-releasing hormones, methotrexate, cyclosporine A, heparin, and cholestyramine)
Diseases: type 1 diabetes, gastrointestinal and malabsorption
Modifiable risk factors for osteoporotic fracture
Cigarette smoking
Excessive caffeine intake
Excessive alcohol use
Inadequate intake for weight maintenance and bone health
Inadequate calcium or vitamin D
Disordered eating and low body weight
Insufficient weight-bearing exercise
Risk factors for falls more common with diabetes
Hypoglycemia
Hyperglycemia causing polyuria (nocturnal frequency when balance is impaired)

Immunizations

People with diabetes may have abnormalities in immune functions, putting them at risk for increased morbidity and mortality from infection. Therefore, immunization against influenza and pneumococcal disease is an important part of preventive services. An annual influenza vaccine should be recommended beginning on September 2 of each year for persons with diabetes 6 months of age or older.[70] Given that the influenza virus can be transmitted from person to person, vaccination of healthcare workers and family members of persons with diabetes may be justified. The flu vaccine does not contain a live virus, so the most frequent side effect is mild soreness at the injection site. Caution should be used for individuals with a chicken egg allergy.

Persons with diabetes are also susceptible to pneumococcal infections and are at increased risk for bacteremia from this organism.[70] Additional risk is associated with individuals 65 years of age or older who have chronic cardiovascular, pulmonary, and renal disease. Pneumococcal vaccination is recommended for persons with diabetes aged ≥2 years. A onetime revaccination is encouraged in individuals over 64 years of age if they were previously immunized at an age of <65 years, and if it has been more than 5 years since their last pneumococcal dose. Repeat vaccination is also encouraged in individuals with nephrotic syndrome, chronic renal disease, or other immune-compromised states. Common side effects include mild flu-like symptoms lasting less than 48 hours.

Hepatitis B vaccination should be administered to all infants, children, and unvaccinated adults with or without diabetes and considered in unvaccinated adults ≥60 years old.[71] Tetanus boosters should be repeated every 10 years.

Effective immunization strategies should include targeting the persons with diabetes *and* their family members. The diabetes care and education specialist's visit should include monitoring and updating the individual's vaccination records, as well as education on the importance of immunizations. Finding community resources that provide immunizations and that are both accessible and affordable remains an important intervention.

Sleep Apnea

Sleep apnea is a common, yet potentially serious sleep disorder in which breathing repeatedly stops and starts. Obstructive sleep apnea (OSA), the most common form, occurs from relaxation of the throat muscles. Breathing pauses can last from a few seconds to minutes and may occur in excess of 30 times per hour. Typically, normal breathing restarts with a loud snort or choking sound. This chronic condition disrupts normal sleep patterns, resulting in poor quality of sleep and subsequent excessive daytime sleepiness. Risk factors for OSA are listed in Table 8.11. Type 2 diabetes and OSA share several clinical findings—obesity, hypertension, and impaired glucose tolerance—and OSA may be an under-recognized comorbidity of diabetes mellitus.[72] The possibility of OSA should be considered in the assessment of all persons with type 2 diabetes and the metabolic syndrome. Monitoring for symptoms associated with sleep apnea can easily be incorporated into routine assessments and follow-up visits. Symptoms may include the following:

- Excessive daytime sleepiness (hypersomnia)*
- Loud snoring, which is usually more prominent in OSA
- Episodes of breathing cessation during sleep witnessed by another person
- Awakening with a dry mouth or sore throat
- Abrupt awakenings accompanied by shortness of breath, which more likely indicates central sleep apnea
- Difficulty staying asleep (insomnia)
- Morning headache
- Attention problems

* Although daytime sleepiness is the top associated symptom of OSA, there are a significant number of individuals with sleep apnea, particularly women, who do not exhibit this symptom. There is an increasing amount of the population that is diagnosed with OSA, but research suggests that it's the ability to diagnose more readily as the reason.

TABLE 8.11 Risk Factors for OSA
Excess weight
Large neck circumference
Being male—males have twice the risk of OSA than females
Age >60 years
Family history
Ethnicity—in persons <35 years, African Americans are at increased risk
Use of alcohol or sedatives
Smoking—smokers are 3 times more likely to have OSA than nonsmokers
Nasal congestion or allergies

Source: K Diaz, P Faverio, A Hospenthal, MI Restrepo, ME Amuan, MV Pugh, "Obstructive sleep apnea is associated with higher healthcare utilization in elderly patients," *Ann Thorac Med* 9 (2014): 92-8.

One available screening tool that could easily be applied in the primary care setting as a means of identifying persons with type 2 diabetes mellitus who are likely to have sleep apnea is the STOP-Bang questionnaire.[73] It can serve as a valuable screening instrument to help recognize individuals at increased risk of OSA who may benefit from further diagnostic studies and treatment. Considering the serious adverse health and quality-of-life consequences of OSA, efforts to expedite diagnosis and treatment are needed. The diabetes care and education specialist can play a critical role in improving screening for, and early diagnosis and treatment of, this potentially disabling condition.

Peridontal Disease

People with diabetes are at increased risk for periodontal (gum) disease, an infection of the gum and dental bone that hold the teeth in place. Periodontal disease can often lead to mouth pain, difficulty chewing, and possible loss of teeth. People with diabetes may also experience decreased flow of saliva and increased glucose in the saliva and the fluid between the teeth and gums, which can lead to increased plaque formation and contribute to a higher risk for caries. Xerostomia or dry mouth can contribute to the development of candidiasis, which may necessitate the use of antifungal agents for management. The management of oral burning symptoms can include maintaining adequate oral hydration and restricting intake of caffeine and alcohol. Diabetes care and education specialists must be aware of the symptoms of thrush or candidiasis in the mouth as a reflection of the individual's glucose levels, ability to heal, and potential for additional periodontal disease.[74]

Preventive measures for infection and delayed wound healing need to be monitored and reinforced by the diabetes care and education specialist. Preventive measures include daily brushing and flossing, regular dental visits, good glucose management, and the avoidance of compounding risk factors such as smoking. People with poor blood glucose levels get gum disease more often and more severely than people whose diabetes is well managed.[75] Just as the diabetes care and education specialist will closely monitor persons with diabetes for glucose management, regimen participation, and overall systemic health, he or she will do the same for oral health, because periodontal disease can be monitored and managed with careful attention to home care and regular visits to the dentist.

Summary

The management of diabetes is multifaceted. Successful diabetes management requires monitoring multiple aspects of the disease, in addition to glucose management, in order to reduce complications of the disease and improve quality of life.

The success of glucose management is dependent on SMBG or CGM data and its utilization by individuals and their healthcare providers in taking action to improve glucose stability. This requires that the educator teach not only the operational skills of monitoring glucose but also the interpretive skills, and that the glucose monitoring be personalized and embedded in a diabetes management plan.

Diabetes self-management education should include self-monitoring beyond the single focus of glycemic management. Diabetes care and education specialists can teach individuals to approach all monitoring data as information which they can use to reinforce their active role in the self-management of their disease. Monitoring provides a comprehensive approach to the prevention, recognition, and management of the comorbidities and complications that frequently accompany this disease. Table 8.12 provides a comprehensive monitoring checklist.

TABLE 8.12 Monitoring Checklist

Monitoring Parameter	*Goals*	*How Often*	*Patient Monitoring Behaviors*	*Professional Monitoring Parameters*
Macrovascular				
Blood pressure (BP)	• <140/80 mm Hg • <130/80 mm Hg may be appropriate in some patients	Each visit	• Home BP check • Once to twice daily • Validated home BP monitoring • Upper arm measurement • Goals	• Office BP every visit • Check for orthostatic hypertension • Check home BP machine • Medication adherence • Self-management education
Lipids	Low risk • LDL <100 mg/dL • HDL >50 mg/dL • TG <150 mg/dL Overt CVD • LDL <70 mg/dL	Annually	• Lifestyle changes and healthy eating habits • Monitor for muscle pain, soreness, or weakness if on statin	Annual lipid panel • Repeat more frequently if not at goal or to assess treatment regimen • Low-risk patients may repeat every 2 years For statin/fibrates, monitor: • Lipid function tests at baseline and as needed • Creatine kinase (myositis)

(continued)

TABLE 8.12 Monitoring Checklist (continued)

Monitoring Parameter	*Goals*	*How Often*	*Patient Monitoring Behaviors*	*Professional Monitoring Parameters*
Antiplatelet	Reduce CV risk: • 75–162 mg per day low-dose aspirin primary prevention in at-risk type 1 diabetes mellitus (T1DM) and type 2 diabetes mellitus (T2DM)	Each visit	• Recognize and report symptoms of GI bleed	• Patient criteria for use • Therapy adherence • Bleeding
Smoking cessation	• Avoid smoking and all tobacco products	Each visit	• Smoking cessation counseling, treatment, and support	• Advise not to smoke • Assess readiness to quit • Discuss therapeutic options • Encourage use of quit lines
		Microvascular		
Retinopathy	• Early detection/slow progression • Avoid permanent vision loss	Each visit Annually	• Glycemic control: avoid glycemic excursions	• Monitor at each visit for vision changes/disturbances • Support risk reduction strategies • Pregnancy and postpartum exams • Referral to specialist • Comprehensive eye exam • Referral as needed
Nephropathy	• Albumin: creatinine level <30	Each visit Annually	• Control BP • Good glycemic control	• Monitor weight gain, peripheral edema, fatigue, loss of appetite • Treatment adherence: ACE-I or ARB • UAE ratio, serum creatinine, and calculated GFR
Neuropathy: Peripheral	• Avoid infection, complications, and loss of sensation • Slow progression	Each visit Annually	• Daily visual foot inspection • Appropriate footwear selection • Sensory changes • Glycemic control	• Visual foot inspection • Check footwear • Sensation testing • Assess gait, balance, and motor skills • Self-management support • Referral if needed • Comprehensive foot exam • Referral if needed
Neuropathy: Autonomic	• Prevention, early identification, and treatment	Each visit	Monitor for various symptoms	• Risk assessment • Identification of symptoms • Support glycemic control: DSMES • Referral for quantitative testing and treatment

Focus on Education: Pearls for Practice

Teaching Strategies

Appreciate a global definition of monitoring. Monitoring in diabetes care includes monitoring of glucose, activities related to metabolic stability and health maintenance, as well as the chronic complications associated with diabetes.

Demonstrate empathy when asking an individual living with a chronic condition to add to their workload of taking care of themselves. Monitoring the many aspects of diabetes management can be an overwhelming task, even for the most dedicated and goal-directed individuals with diabetes. Ensure that the monitoring being done is being used to inform or achieve a goal specific to the individual. At clinic appointments, outpatient visits, and phone calls, recognize and acknowledge the work that those you are serving have done in performing monitoring activities.

Teach not just how but why. The diabetes care and education specialist's job is to teach those with diabetes not only the how of using a blood glucose meter but also the why so individuals with the disease are empowered to use the knowledge gained to make healthy, informed choices in their food intake, exercise, medication adjustments, and sick-day and stress management.

Be aware of the words used to describe monitoring. *Testing* may be interpreted as passing or failing. Terms such as *monitor*, *check*, or *measure* are value neutral and may be more acceptable to individuals. *Good* or *bad* data points may subconsciously be viewed as personal value judgments. Instead, consider using *above or below target* or *above or below range* for glucose and other monitoring activities.

Use appreciative inquiry techniques when questioning individuals about their monitoring habits. The goal is to ask questions in a positive way (see Table 18.15).

Facilitate goal setting. Consider what data will best serve the individual in making informed decisions about diabetes management and obtaining a specific, yet big-picture view of his or her glycemic stability.

Messages for Persons With Diabetes

Make the data work for you. Monitoring, in all its forms, puts valuable information in your hands. Take advantage of the technology available and the support of your diabetes care and education specialist to make informed decisions and improve your tools for diabetes management.

Try something different. Use an app to log meals with glucose values to see if you can find any patterns. Try counting your steps using your smartphone to see if increasing your activity affects your ability to more easily manage your diabetes.

Know your numbers. Diabetes care involves more than just glucose numbers. Discuss with your healthcare team other data points that will give you and your healthcare team the information needed to best manage your diabetes.

Monitor progress. Keep track of your laboratory values, your exercise activity, or other goals you are working towards achieving. Observing progress or trends will give you and your healthcare team the information needed to know what types of strategies work best for your diabetes management.

Health Literacy

Research indicates that individuals with limited health literacy can achieve similar or better improvement in self-management behaviors through the use of DSME.[76]

Self-monitoring is not just about numbers. Numeracy is defined as the ability to understand and use numbers and math skills in daily life. Individuals might not understand the meaning of the numbers if they are not familiar with quantitative description terms such as the following: *small*, *decrease*, *weight*, *reduce*, and *chance*.[77]

Everyone can benefit from low health literacy education methods. Everyone appreciates when information is simple, practical, and usable. When providing education, consider the following strategies for low literacy:

Introduce one concept at a time. Use one strategy per sentence. Make sure the concept is comprehended and then add additional applications. Instead of "If you have hypoglycemia, which is classified when your glucose is 70 mg/dL or below, have 2 to 5 glucose tablets, half a cup (4 oz) of fruit juice, or half a cup of a regular soft drink to raise your blood glucose," say, "Your blood glucose is considered too low when it is lower than 70 mg/dL." Then pause and ask, "What would you do if your blood glucose got that low?" Add additional concepts, one step at a time. Evaluate comprehension and actual applications of the information.

Demonstrate/illustrate the information. You can draw a picture, use analogies, show physical representations of quantity, encourage persons with diabetes to create their own images, use vivid language, and teach with stories. Even drawing images on the white board when you explain the concepts can provide more time to think through the process and its applications (this is much more effective than briefly showing them complex pictures of complex processes).

Focus on Practice

Self-monitoring considered a therapeutic intervention only when the results are interpreted and appropriate interventions adjusted. Create opportunities to work with persons with diabetes to review all monitoring results and provide specific feedback and recommendations. Evaluate the effectiveness of the corresponding recommendations/adjustments.

Since monitoring encompasses such a large volume of behaviors and data that can be collected, continuing education is necessary to understand the best tools to collect and interpret information from individuals. Often times this collection of information is done via an app, smartphone, or medical device. Since these technologies are always evolving, it's important to evaluate your knowledge and comfort level in using technology to give you and the persons with diabetes the best tools with the least amount of effort to gain progress toward a goal.

Clinical information systems need to work together. The systems that help integrate data from a wide range of systems will allow for healthcare professionals to offer efficient services. Healthcare professionals need to be able to access and share information quickly in order to work more efficiently and make better decisions.

References

1. Association of Diabetes Care and Education Specialists (ADCES). An effective model of diabetes care and education: revising the AADE7 self-care behaviors®. Published online ahead of print, Feb 2020. Diabetes Educ. doi: https://doi.org/10.1177/0145721719894903.

2. American Diabetes Association. Comprehensive medical evaluation and assessment of comorbidities: standards of medical care in diabetes—2019. Diabetes Care. 2019;42(suppl 1):S34-45.

3. Powers MA, Bardsley J, Cypress M, et al. Diabetes self-management education and support in type 2 diabetes: a joint position statement of the American Diabetes Association, the American Association of Diabetes Educators, and the Academy of Nutrition and Dietetics. Diabetes Educ. 2015;41(4):417-30.

4. Akturk H, Garg S. Technological advances shaping diabetes care. Current Opinion in Endocr Diabetes Obes. 2019;26(2): 84-9.

5. McEwan P, Foos V, Palmer J, et al. Validation of the IMS CORE diabetes mode. Value in Health. 2014;17(6):661-756.

6. Vajravelu ME, Keren R, Weber DR, et al. Incidence and risk of celiac disease after type 1 diabetes: a population-based cohort study using the health improvement network database. Pediatr Diabetes. 2018 Sept:19(8):1422-8.

7. Patel NS, Van Name MA, Cengiz E, et al. Altered patterns of early metabolic decompensation 1 diabetes during with a SGLT2 inhibitor: an insulin pump suspension study. Diabetes Technol Ther. 2017;19(11):618-22.

8. Goldenberg RM, Bernard LD, Cheng AYY, et al. SGLT2 inhibitor–associated diabetic ketoacidosis: clinical review and recommendations for prevention and diagnosis. Clin Ther. 2016;38(12):P2654-64.

9. Wolfsdorf, JI, Ratner RE. SGLT inhibitors for type 1 diabetes: proceed with extreme caution. Diabetes Care. 2019;42(6):991-3.

10. Dorcely B, Nitis J, Schwartzbard A, et al. A case report: euglycemic diabetic ketoacidosis presenting as chest pain in a patient on a low carbohydrate diet. Curr Diabetes Rev. 10.2174/1573399816666200316112709. [Epub ahead of print Mar 2020]

11. Chatzianagnostou K, Iervasi G, Vassalle C. Challenges of LADA diagnosis and treatment: Lessons from 2 case reports. American J Ther. 2016;23(5):e1270-4(5).

12. Ducloux R, Safraou M, Altman J. Etiologic diagnosis of diabetes mellitus in adults: questions to ask, tests to request. Int J Diabetes Dev Ctries. 2015;35, 604-11. doi:10.1007/s13410-015-0336-x.

13. Bergenstal RM, Glycemic Variability and Diabetes Complications: does it matter? Simply put, there are better glycemic markers! Diabetes Care. 2015;38(8):1615-21.

14. American Association of Clinical Endocrinologists. Medical Guidelines for Clinical Practice for Developing a Diabetes Comprehensive Care Plan. Endocr Pract. 2015;21 Suppl 1:1-87.

15. Mechanick JI, Pessah-Pollack R, Camacho P, et al. American Association of Clinical Endocrinologists and American College of Endocrinology. Protocol for standardized production of clinical practice guidelines, algorithms, and checklists—2017 Update. Endocr Pract. 2017;23(8):1006-21.

16. Hoang H, Nguyen Silva JNA. Use of smartphone technology in cardiology. Trends Cardiovasc Med. 2016;26(4):376-86.

17. American Diabetes Association. Cardiovascular disease and risk management: *standards of medical care in diabetes—2020.* Diabetes Care. 2020;43(Suppl 1):S111-134.

18. Wang J, Zgibor J, Matthews J, et al. Self-monitoring of blood glucose is associated with problem-solving skills in hyperglycemia and hypoglycemia. Diabetes Educ. 2012;38(2):207-14.

19. American Heart Association. Monitoring Your Blood Pressure at Home. On the Internet at: https://www.heart.org/en/health-topics/high-blood-pressure/understanding-blood-pressure-readings/monitoring-your-blood-pressure-at-home. Last accessed: 24 March 2020.

20. Jellinger PS, Handelsman Y, Rosenblit PD, et al. American Association of Clinical Endocrinologists and American College of Endocrinology Guidelines for Management of Dyslipidemia and Prevention of Cardiovascular Disease. Endocr Pract. 2017; 23(Suppl 2):1-87.

21. Mark PB, Winocour P, Day C. Management of lipids in adults with diabetes mellitus and nephropathy and/or chronic kidney disease: summary of joint guidance from the Association of British Clinical Diabetologists (ABCD) and the Renal Association (RA). Br J Diabetes. 2017(2):64-72.

22. Alvarez C, Ramos A. Lipids, lipoproteins and apolipoproteins in serum during infection. Clin Chem. 1986;32:142-5.

23. Ryder RE, Hayes TM, Mulligan JP, et al. How soon after myocardial infarction should plasma lipid values be assessed? BMJ. 1984;289:1651-3.

24. Srikanth, S., Deedwania, P. Management of dyslipidemia in patients with hypertension, diabetes, and metabolic syndrome. Curr Hypertens Rep. 2016;18, 76. https://doi.org/10.1007/s11906-016-0683-0.

25. Seidu, S, Kunutsor, SK, Sesso, HD, et al. Aspirin has potential benefits for primary prevention of cardiovascular outcomes in diabetes: updated literature-based and individual participant data meta-analyses of randomized controlled trials. Cardiovasc Diabetol. 2019;18, 70. doi:10.1186/s12933-019-0875-4.

26. American Diabetes Association. Standards of medical care of diabetes—2020. Diabetes Care. 2020;43(Suppl 1): S32-6. S60.

27. Gudla S, Tenneti D, Pande M, et al. Diabetic retinopathy: pathogenesis, treatment, and complications. In: Patel R, Sutariya V, Kanwar J, Pahak Y, eds. Drug Delivery for the Retina and Posterior Segment Disease. Springer, Cham, Switzerland: Springer;2018:83-94.

28. Bain SC, Klufas MA, Ho, A, et al. Worsening of diabetic retinopathy with rapid improvement in systemic glucose control: a review. Diabetes, Obes Metab. 2019;21(3):454-66.

29. Whitehead M, Wickremasinghe S, Osborne A, et al. Diabetic retinopathy: a complex pathophysiology requiring novel therapeutic strategies. Exp Op Biol Ther. 2018;18(12):1257-70.

30. Tapp RJ, Shaw JE, Harper CA, et al. The prevalence of and factors associated with diabetic retinopathy in the Australian population. Diabetes Care. 2003;26(6):1731-7.

31. American Diabetes Association. Microvascular complications and foot care: *Standards of Medical Care in Diabetes–2020.* Diabetes Care. 2020;43(Supplement 1):S135-51.

32. Solomon SD, Chew E, Duh, EJ, et al. Diabetic Retinopathy: A Position Statement by the American Diabetes Association. Diabetes Care. 2017;40(3):412-18.

33. Stewart M. (2010) Pathophysiology of diabetic retinopathy. In: Browning D., ed. Diabetic Retinopathy. New York: Springer. 2010. 1-30.

34. Centers for Disease Control and Prevention. Chronic Kidney Disease in the United States, 2019. Atlanta, GA: US Department of Health and Human Services, Centers for Disease Control and Prevention; 2019.

35. Saran R, Robinson B, Abbott KC, et al. US Renal Data System 2017 annual data report: epidemiology of kidney disease in the United States [published correction appears in Am J Kidney Dis. 2018 Apr;71(4):501]. Am J Kidney Dis. 2018;71(3 Suppl 1):A7.

36. Digsu N, Koye DJ, Magliano RG, et al. The global epidemiology of diabetes and kidney disease. Adv Chronic Kid Disease. 2019;25(3):121-32.

37. Tziomalos K, Athyros VG. Diabetic neuropathy: New Risk Factors and Improvements in Diagnosis. *Rev Diabet Stud.* 2015;12(1-2):110-18. doi:10.1900/RDS.2015.12.110.

38. Vassalotti JA, Centor R, Turner BJ, et al. Practical approach to detection and management of chronic kidney disease for the primary care clinician. Am J Med. 2016;129(2):153-62.e7.

39. Alleyn CR, Volkening LK, Wolfson J, Rodriguez-Ventura A, Wood JR, Laffel LM. Occurrence of microalbuminuria in young people with type 1 diabetes: importance of age and diabetes duration. Diabet Med. 2010;27(5):532-7. doi:10.1111/j.1464-5491.2010.02983.x.

40. Roett MA, Liegl S, Jabbarpour Y. Diabetic nephropathy—the family physician's role. Am Fam Physician. 2012;85(9):883-9.

41. Molitch ME, DeFronzo RA, Franz MJ, et al. Nephropathy in diabetes. Diabetes Care. 2004;27 Suppl 1:S79-83.

42. Schreiber AK, Nones CF, Reis RC, et al. Diabetic neuropathic pain: Physiopathology and treatment. World J Diabetes. 2015;6(3):432-44. doi:10.4239/wjd.v6.i3.432.

43. Perkins BA, Olaleye D, Zinman B, Bril V. Simple screening tests for peripheral neuropathy in the diabetes clinic. Diabetes Care. 2001;24:250-6.

44. Maser RE, Steenkiste AR, Dorman JS, Nielsen VK, Bass EB, Manjoo Q, Drash AL, Becker DJ, Kuller LH, Greene DA, et al. Epidemiological correlates of diabetic neuropathy. Report from Pittsburgh Epidemiology of Diabetes Complications Study. Diabetes. 1989;38(11):1456-61.

45. Agrawal Y, Carey JP, Della Santina CC, Schubert MC, Minor LB. Diabetes, vestibular dysfunction, and falls: analyses from the National Health and Nutrition Examination Survey. Otol Neurotol. 2010;31:1445-50.

46. De Berardis G, Pellegrini F, Franciosi M, et al; QuED Study Group—Quality of Care and Outcomes in Type 2 Diabetes. Are type 2 diabetic patients offered adequate foot care? The role of physician and patient characteristics. J Diabetes Complications. 2005;19(6):319-27.

47. Azmi S, Petropoulos IN, Ferdousi M, Ponirakis G, Alam U, Malik RA. An update on the diagnosis and treatment of diabetic somatic and autonomic neuropathy. *F1000Res*. 2019;8:F1000 Faculty Rev-186. Published 2019 Feb 15. doi:10.12688/f1000research.17118.1

48. Thiruvoipati T, Kielhorn CE, Armstrong EJ. Peripheral artery disease in patients with diabetes: epidemiology, mechanisms, and outcomes. World J Diabetes. 2015;6(7):961-9. doi:10.4239/wjd.v6.i7.961.

49. Thompson AT, Pillay S, Aldous C. The use of ABI in screening for diabetes-related lower limb peripheral arterial disease in IDF middle- and low-income countries: a scoping review. Int J Diabetes Dev Ctries. (2019). https://doi.org/10.1007/s13410-019-00753-y.

50. Bădescu SV, Tătaru C, Kobylinska L, et al. The association between diabetes mellitus and depression. J Med Life. 2016;9(2):120-5.

51. American Diabetes Association. Facilitating behavior change and well-being to improve health outcomes: standards of medical care in diabetes—*2020*. Diabetes Care. 2020 Jan; 43(Suppl 1):S48-S65.

52. New York State Dept of Health, Office of Mental Health. Administering the Patient Health Questionnaires 2 and 9 (PHQ2 and 9) in Integrated Care Settings. July 2016. Pages 1-5. On the Internet at: https://health.ny.gov/health_care/medicaid/redesign/dsrip/docs/2016-07-01_phq_2_and_9_clean.pdf. Last accessed 24 March 2020.

53. Polonsky WH, Fisher L, Earles J, et al. Assessing psychosocial distress in diabetes: development of the Diabetes Stress Scale. Diabetes Care. 2005;28(3):626-31.

54. Fisher, L, Hessler, DM, Polonsky WH, et al. When is diabetes distress clinically meaningful? Establishing cut points for the Diabetes Distress Scale. Diabetes Care. 2012;35(2):259-64.

55. Kadiyala R, Peter R, Okosieme OE. Thyroid dysfunction in patients with diabetes: clinical implications and screening strategies. Int J Clin Pract. 2010;64(8):1130-9.

56. Pearce EN. Thyroid disorders during pregnancy and postpartum. Best Pract Res Clin Obst Gyn. 2015;29(5):700-6.

57. Elgazar EH, Esheba NE, Shalaby SA, et al. Thyroid dysfunction prevalence and relation to glycemic control in patients with type 2 diabetes mellitus. Diabetes Metab Synd: Clin Res Rev. 2019;13(4):2513-17.

58. DeVito P, Candelotti E, Ahmed, G, et al. Role of thyroid hormones in insulin resistance and diabetes in immunology, endocrine & metabolic agents in medicinal chemistry (Formerly current medicinal chemistry - immunology, endocrine and metabolic agents), Vol. 15, Number 1, 2015, 86-93(8).

59. Hossein GR, Tuttle M, Baskin HJ, Fish LH, Singer PA, McDermot MT. Subclinical thyroid dysfunction: a joint statement on management from the American Association of Clinical Endocrinologists, the American Thyroid Association, and the Endocrine Society. J Clin Endocrinol Metab. 2005;90(1):581-5.

60. Sawka AM, Carty SE, Haugen BR. American Thyroid Association guidelines and statements: past, present, and future. Thyroid. 2018;28(6):692-706.

61. Takiish T, Gysemans C, Bouillon R, Mathieu C. Vitamin D and diabetes. Endocrinol Metab Clin North Am. 2010;39:419.

62. Mathieu C, Gysemans C, Guilietti A, et al. Vitamin D and diabetes. Diabetologia. 2005;48:1247.

63. Jorde R, Figenschau Y. Supplementation with cholecalciferol does not improve glycaemic control in diabetic subjects with normal serum 25-hydroxyvitamin D levels. Eur J Nutr. 2009;48:349-54.

64. Soric MM, Renner ET, Smith SR. Effect of daily vitamin D supplementation on HbA1c in patients with uncontrolled type 2 diabetes mellitus: a pilot study. J Diabetes. 2012;4:104-5.

65. Chapuy MC, Arlot ME, Duboeuf F, et al. Vitamin D_3 and calcium to prevent hip fractures in elderly women. N Engl J Med. 1992;327:1637-42.

66. Bischoff-Ferrari HA, Willett WC, Wong JB, et al. Fracture prevention with vitamin D supplementation: a meta-analysis of randomized controlled trials. JAMA. 2005;293:2257-64.

67. Kothari S, Chadha M., Chapter 53: Osteoporosis: an underappreciated complication of diabetes. In: Chawla R, Jaggi S, eds. RSSDI Diabetes Update 2018. New Dehli: Jaypee Brothers Medical Publishers, 2019;262-7.

68. Siddapur PR, Patil AB, Borde VS. Comparison of bone mineral density, t-scores and serum zinc between diabetic and non-diabetic postmenopausal women with osteoporosis. J Lab Physicians. 2015;7(1):43-8. doi:10.4103/0974-2727.151681.

69. Kemmis K, Stuber D. Diabetes and osteoporotic fractures: the role of the diabetes educator. Diabetes Educ. 2005;31:187-96.

70. Grohskopf LA, Sokolow LZ, Olsen SJ, Bresee JS, Broder KR, Karron RA. Prevention and control of influenza with vaccines: recommendations of the Advisory Committee on Immunization Practices, United States, 2015-16 Influenza Season. MMWR

Morb Mortal Wkly Rep. 2015;64(30):818-25. doi:10.15585/mmwr.mm6430a3.

71. Centers for Disease Control and Prevention, Division of Viral Hepatitis, National Center for HIV/AIDS, Viral Hepatitis, STD, and TB Prevention. Hepatitis B questions and answers for health professionals. On the Internet at: https://www.cdc.gov/hepatitis/hbv/hbvfaq.htm. Page last reviewed: March 16, 2020.

72. Cass AR, Alonso WJ, Islam J, et al. Risk of obstructive sleep apnea in patients with type 2 diabetes mellitus. Fam Med. 2013;45(7):492-500.

73. Nagappa M, Liao, P, Wong, J, et al. Validation of the STOP-Bang Questionnaire as a Screening Tool for Obstructive Sleep Apnea Among Different Populations: A Systematic Review and Meta-Analysis. PLoS One. 2015 Dec 14;10(12):e0143697. doi:10.1371/journal.pone.0143697.

74. Rodrigues CF, Rodrigues ME, Henriques M. *Candida* sp. Infections in patients with diabetes mellitus. J Clin Med. 2019;8(1):76.

75. Preshaw, P, Bissett, S. Periodontitis and diabetes. Br Dent J. 2019;227, 577-84.

76. Kim S, Love F, Quistberg DA, et al. Association of health literacy with self-management behavior in patients with diabetes. Diabetes Care. 2004;27:2980-2.

77. Cavanaugh K, Huizinga MM, Wallston KA, et al. Association of numeracy and diabetes control. Ann Intern Med. 2008;148:737-46.

CHAPTER 9

Reducing Risks

Kimberly Coy DeCoste, RN, MSN, CDCES, MLDE, FADCES
David K. Miller, RN, MSEd, BSN, CDCES, LDE, FADCES

Key Concepts

- All people with diabetes should be knowledgeable about the tests, exams, and interventions contained within the Standards of Care, including the frequency with which they are to be performed. Inclusion and monitoring of these can help reduce risks for diabetes complications.
- Targeted, therapeutic goals are recommended for people with diabetes to reduce risks of complications. To best meet an individual's needs and to optimize health, these goals need to be personalized; this is especially critical for vulnerable populations.
- People with diabetes should receive preventive healthcare services to maximize their health.
- To reduce risks for diabetes complications, people with diabetes must learn and acquire skills that will help them develop and maintain healthy behaviors. Ongoing support is essential for maintenance of the behavior change.
- Assist the person with diabetes to identify barriers and facilitate interventions to help remove identified barriers.
- Identifying and linking to other health system, community-based, or technology-driven programs or resources, especially for ongoing behavior-change support, may also assist the person with risk reduction.

Introduction

Reducing risks, as contained in the AADE7 Self-Care Behaviors®, refers to identifying risks and implementing behaviors to minimize and/or prevent complications or adverse outcomes.[1] These include acute complications like hypoglycemia, hyperglycemia, DKA, and HHS and chronic complications like retinopathy, kidney disease, neuropathy, and cardiovascular disease. Although both are important to the person with diabetes this chapter will focus on the chronic complications. Important to risk reduction is early identification of prediabetes and/or diabetes. Ongoing self-management education and support for the person with diabetes is critical to preventing acute complications and reducing the risk of long-term complications.[2] Those involved in diabetes education assist the person with diabetes to recognize the importance of risk reduction, acquire the appropriate skills, identify and overcome barriers to implementation, and adopt preventative behaviors. In addition, linking people with diabetes to other sources of support and services including new technologies and working to ensure that other services are available may help reduce the risk of developing complications.[3]

This chapter discusses knowledge content areas, skills, and barriers to be addressed when guiding people with diabetes through behavior changes that reduce their risk for complications and maximize their heath. The focus is on the modifiable risk factors. Due to the interconnectedness of reducing risk to the other behaviors, references are often made to other chapters in the book where specific risks and approaches to reducing them are discussed in more detail.

Knowledge Content Areas

Being knowledgeable about the Standards of Medical Care in Diabetes, clinical practice guidelines for recommended tests and exams, preventive care services, and understanding personal/individualized therapeutic goals is important for people with diabetes as they engage in behaviors that minimize their risk of developing complications. Quality diabetes self-management education and support (DSMES) facilitates the acquisition of knowledge and skills necessary to self-manage diabetes and prevent or delay complications. Evidence supports a person-centered approach for presenting the information and engaging the learner. Sensitivity to learning preferences, culture, language and health literacy are important. New technological platforms and systems, as well as other self-management support services, provide more options for the person to engage in effective self-management of their diabetes.

Standards of Care: Diabetes

The Standards of Medical Care in Diabetes[2] provide a comprehensive list of preventive-care practices (eg, assessments, physical examinations, laboratory tests, interventions) and describe how frequently each should be recommended to all people with diabetes. The American Diabetes Association (ADA) is the primary organization responsible for developing the Standards of Medical Care in Diabetes and publishes them annually. However, important updates will be included online if new evidence or regulatory changes come available. These are formulated from a thorough review of the literature and rating of the scientific evidence currently available and include screening, diagnostic and therapeutic actions that are known or believed to positively affect health outcomes of the person with diabetes.[4] They also include recommendations for special populations like children and adolescents, pregnant women and older adults. Table 9.1 summarizes the Standards of Care relevant to risk reduction.

TABLE 9.1 Summary of Standards of Care*

Test/Exam/Service	*Frequency*
Psychosocial assessment	At diagnosis and at least annually: Screen for depression, anxiety, and disordered eating. May require referral for further assessment or intervention. Consider assessment for cognitive impairment. Identify existing social supports.
Comorbid conditions	Ensure regular assessment for depression and health distress. Assess need to screen for other psychosocial issues, fatty liver disease, obstructive sleep apnea, cancer, fracture risk, cognitive changes, hearing impairments, and in men, low testosterone levels. Specifically, people with type 1 diabetes may need to be screened for autoimmune thyroid disease and celiac disease soon after diagnosis.
Self-monitoring of blood glucose (SMBG)	Evaluate frequency at each visit. Those using multiple insulin injections or insulin pump therapy usually test 6 to 10 times per day. For those using basal insulin, fasting glucose supports informed dose adjustments results in lower A1C. Those using less frequent insulin injections or noninsulin therapies: As needed to meet treatment goals. Evidence is insufficient on frequency.
Technology Use	Use of apps, online education, patient portals, etc at initial visit and annually. Glucose monitoring results and data use at every visit. For those using insulin pumps, review settings and use at every visit.
A1C	At least twice per year if meeting glycemic targets. Quarterly if treatment changes or not meeting glycemic targets. Note: More timely changes in treatment can occur when point-of-care testing is employed.
Renal status	At least annually, assess urinary albumin (spot urinary albumin-to-creatinine ratio) estimated glomerular filtration rate in persons with type 1 diabetes for ≥5 years and in all persons with type 2 diabetes regardless of treatment. Persons with urinary albumin >30 mg/g creatinine and/or an eGFR <60 mL/min/1.73 m^2 should be monitored twice annually.
Weight (BMI)	Each regular diabetes visit
Blood pressure	Every routine visit
Lipids	Lipid profile at initial visit and every 5 years thereafter if under the age of 40, obtain lipid profile at initiation of statins, 4 to 12 weeks after initiation, or a change of dose, and annually thereafter.

TABLE 9.1 Summary of Standards of Care* (continued)

Test/Exam/Service	*Frequency*
Dilated eye exam	At diagnosis for those with type 2 diabetes and after 5 years for those with type 1 diabetes, and then annually. If there is no evidence of retinopathy for 1 or more annual eye exams and glycemic targets are met, then every 2–3 years may be considered (more frequent exams needed if retinopathy is progressing).
Comprehensive foot exam	At least annually. Those with sensory loss or history of ulceration should have feet inspected at every visit.
Skin examination	At initial visit and annually (acanthosis nigricans, insulin injection or insertion sites).
Neuropathy	Assess for peripheral neuropathy starting at diagnosis for person with type 2 and 5 years after diagnosis for type 1, then annually. Assess for autonomic neuropathies in those with microvascular and neuropathic complications.
Medical nutrition therapy (MNT)	Refer at diagnosis and as needed throughout the lifespan and during times of changing health status to achieve treatment goals.
Diabetes self-management education (DSMES) and support	Four critical times to evaluate the need for DSMES: At diagnosis, annually, when complicating factors arise, and when transitions of care occur. Note: DSMES should be delivered according to National Standards for DSMES
Physical activity plan	Assess at least annually
Immunizations	Influenza vaccination annually for those ≥6 months of age. Vaccination against pneumococcal disease, including pneumococcal pneumonia, with 13-valent pneumococcal conjugate vaccine (PCV13) is recommended for all children before age 2 years. People with diabetes ages 2 to 64 should also receive 23-valent pneumococcal polysaccharide vaccine (PPSV23). At age ≥65 year, regardless of vaccination history, additional PPSV23 is needed. Depending on the vaccine, administer a 2- or 3-dose series of hepatitis B vaccine. Consider administering a 3-dose series to those aged 60 years and older. Provide routinely recommended vaccinations by age for children and adults with diabetes
Dental care	At least annually, more often as recommended by dentist.
Tobacco use status	At initial visit and at least annually
Pregnancy Planning	For women of childbearing capacity, preconception counseling and contraceptive needs at every visit.

*Standards listed are for adults with diabetes; some standards are different for children or pregnant women living with diabetes.

Source: Adapted from American Diabetes Association, "Standards of medical care in diabetes—2020," *Diabetes Care* 43,Suppl1(2019).

Glycemic Targets

It is recommended in The Use of Language in Diabetes Care and Education[5] that the term "control" not be used. To correctly report evidence from several studies demonstrating the strong association of A1C to delaying or preventing several complications and the current standards of care, the term "control" is used.

The results of the Diabetes Control and Complications Trial (DCCT)[6] and the UK Prospective Diabetes Study (UKPDS)[7] have demonstrated that intensive glycemic control is associated with decreased rates of retinopathy, nephropathy, and neuropathy. Follow-up of DCCT and UKPDS participants has shown that those who were in the intensive glycemic therapy arms of the studies continued to have lower rates of microvascular complications even though their glycemic control returned to that of the standard treated group; this is known as the "legacy effect."[8,9] In addition, for those with type 1 diabetes, the positive effects of early blood glucose control have been shown to last for decades and have even been associated with a slightly lower rate of all-cause mortality.[10] Randomized controlled trials of intensive versus standard glycemic control did not show a significant reduction in cardiovascular disease (CVD) during the initial trial, but long-term follow-up from the DCCT and UKPDS suggests that A1C targets around 7% or below in years soon after diagnosis are associated with a long-term reduction in risk of macrovascular disease.[11,12] The results of 3 additional large trials (ADVANCE, ACCORD, and VADT)[13] in those with long-term type 2 diabetes (10-15 years) and either a history of a CVD event or a significant CVD risk suggested no significant reduction in CVD events with intensive glycemic control. Findings from the studies suggest that caution should be taken when treating diabetes aggressively, toward near near-normal A1C goals, and that higher glycemic goals be considered for those who have had diabetes for many years, have a history of severe hypoglycemia, suffer from significant atherosclerosis, or have a limited life expectancy. In addition, the person with diabetes' individual preferences, resources, and support may also influence glycemic goals. However, in cooperation with their physician/provider, persons with long life expectancy and little co-morbidity may aim for more intensive targets if they can achieve them safely and without undue burden. The standards offer guidance on determining individualized A1C targets based on disease factors.[14] Recommendations for assessment of A1C are to perform the test at least two times a year in persons who are meeting their treatment goals and have stable glycemic control and quarterly in persons whose therapy has changed or they are not meeting glycemic targets.[15,16] The A1C test has a strong predictive value for diabetes complications.[15,16]

Though glycemic management is primarily assessed with the A1C test, many people utilize results from self-monitoring of blood glucose (SMBG) to help achieve glucose targets. In recent years, newer technology like continuous glucose monitoring (CGM) has proven very helpful in assessing blood glucose levels. SMBG and CGM are especially important to persons intensively managed with insulin and can be very useful in determining an individual's response to a therapy or change in treatment. Evidence shows that when A1C levels are closer to target range the postprandial glucose level has the greatest effect. Conversely, the farther away from A1C target, the fasting glucose has the greatest impact.[17,18]

Self-monitoring of blood glucose is most useful when individuals with diabetes learn how to use the monitoring information to assist with diabetes management. It can help the individual determine if glucose targets are being safely achieved and can help guide personal decision-making surrounding nutrition, activity, medication adjustment, hypoglycemia treatment, and other risk-reducing behaviors. To reinforce this important self-management behavior, include individuals in a review of the results and show them how the results can be used in an effective and timely way to make self-management decisions. The frequency and timing of SMBG are based on the needs and goals of the individual and are decided in collaboration with their provider. Both SMBG and CGM results are reliant upon correct user technique. It is important that the user be well trained and their technique be reviewed at regular intervals. (See chapter 18 on Monitoring Glucose.)

Reducing Risks for Chronic Complications

This section discusses recommendations for diabetes care and education specialists to use as they support the person with diabetes to successfully increase risk-reduction behaviors and preventive practices. Important knowledge, skills, measures, and behaviors related to the following chronic complications are discussed. The importance of individualizing therapeutic goals is emphasized. It is important to acknowledge the importance of the other AADE7® behaviors in reducing risks related to these specific complications, though those will not be discussed in detail in this chapter:

- Cardiovascular disease
- Retinopathy
- Diabetic kidney disease
- Neuropathy
- Foot care

Preventive services of importance in diabetes care, specifically for the following, are also discussed:

- Immunizations for influenza, pneumonia, and hepatitis B
- Dental care
- Pre-pregnancy counseling

Cardiovascular Disease

Cardiovascular disease (CVD) is the leading cause of death for people with diabetes and is a major contributor to healthcare costs related to diabetes. The prevalence of overall heart disease is higher among adults with diabetes than adults without diabetes. Numerous studies have demonstrated the benefits of managing CVD risk factors in people with diabetes. Implementation of evidence-based interventions has likely contributed to the significant reductions in CVD events and mortality seen in people with diabetes in recent decades.[19] People with type 1 diabetes are also at high risk of CVD, particularly after several decades of the disease. The following modifiable CVD risk factors are topics for diabetes education:

- Hypertension
- Dyslipidemia
- Smoking
- Increased platelet adherence

Blood Pressure: There are different definitions of hypertension depending on the organization. The American Academy of Pediatrics, American Heart Association, and the ADA define hypertension differently. It is important to know which recommendations your institution follows so the person with diabetes does not get confused or frustrated. Hypertension, defined as a sustained blood pressure, ≥140/90 mmHg by the ADA, is a major risk factor for cardiovascular and cerebrovascular disease as well as for microvascular complications including diabetic nephropathy and retinopathy. Studies show that blood pressure higher than 115/75 mmHg is associated with progressive increases in CVD events and mortality in people with diabetes.[19] The Seventh Report of the Joint National Committee on Prevention, Detection, Evaluation and Treatment of High Blood Pressure (JNC7)[20] provides evidence-based guidelines for diagnosing and classifying people with hypertension. See Table 9.2.

The diabetes care and education specialist should place emphasis on ensuring that people with diabetes know their blood pressure values and how to use MNT, physical activity, and, when necessary, medication to keep blood pressure values at their therapeutic goals. The Standards of Care recommend that blood pressure be measured at every routine diabetes visit and that elevated levels be confirmed on a separate day. All hypertensive persons with diabetes should be encouraged to monitor their blood pressure at home. Goals should be individualized and discussed between the person with diabetes and the healthcare team. Goals of therapy for people with diabetes and hypertension, according to the ADA, are the following:

Adults. Treat systolic blood pressure to less than 140 mmHg and diastolic pressure to less than 90 mmHg. Lower systolic (less than 130) and diastolic (under 80) blood pressure may be appropriate for some. Additional medications should not be used in older adults to achieve blood pressure levels below 130/70, as this may lead to increased mortality and has not been shown to improve cardiovascular health.[19]

- In pregnant women with diabetes and preexisting hypertension who are treated with antihypertensive therapy, blood pressure targets of <135/85 mmHg[21] are suggested in the interest of optimizing long-term maternal health and minimizing impaired fetal growth.
- Children and adolescents. Hypertension in childhood is defined as an average systolic or diastolic blood pressure greater than or equal to the 95th percentile for age, sex, and height.[22] "High-normal" blood pressure is defined as average systolic or diastolic blood pressure greater than or equal to the 90th percentile but less than the 95th percentile for age, sex, and height. Children found to have hypertension or "high normal" should have elevated blood pressure confirmed on three separate days.[22]
    - Blood pressure levels for age, sex, and height are available at nhlbi.nih.gov/files/docs/resources/heart/hbp_ped.pdf.

TABLE 9.2: Classification of Hypertension in Adults[20]

Classification of Hypertension in Adults		
Stage	*Systolic Pressure (mmHg)*	*Diastolic Pressure (mmHg)*
Normal	<120 and	<80
Prehypertension	120–139 or	80–89
Stage 1 hypertension	140–159 or	90–99
Stage 2 hypertension	≥160 or	≥100

Source: AV Chobanian, GL Bakris, HR Black, et al, "The Seventh Report of the Joint National Committee on Prevention, Detection, Evaluation, and Treatment of High Blood Pressure: the JNC 7 report," JAMA. 289(2003);2560-72.

Both the ADA and the AACE have developed recommended therapeutic goals for A1C, preprandial and postprandial plasma blood glucose, blood pressure, and lipids. See Table 9.3.

Adults: Lifestyle management is an important component of hypertension treatment because it lowers blood pressure and enhances the effectiveness of some antihypertensive medications. Lifestyle therapy consists of reducing excess body weight through caloric restriction, restricting sodium intake (<2,300 mg/day), increasing consumption of fruits and vegetables (8-10 servings per day), and low-fat dairy products (2-3 servings per day), avoiding excessive alcohol consumption (no more than 2 servings per day in men and no more than 1 serving per day in women) and increasing activity levels.

Children and Adolescents: Initial treatment of high normal blood pressure includes dietary modification and increased exercise, if appropriate, aimed at weight management. If target blood pressure is not reached within 3 to 6 months of initiating lifestyle intervention, pharmacological

TABLE 9.3 Therapeutic Goals for Nonpregnant Adults

	American Diabetes Association	*American Association of Clinical Endocrinologists*
A1C	<7.0%*	≤6.5% or lower for most*
Preprandial capillary plasma glucose	80–130 mg/dL (4.44–7.21 mmol/L)	<110 mg/dL (6.10 mmol/L) (fasting)
Peak postprandial capillary plasma glucose	<180 mg/dL (9.99 mmol/L) (1–2 hours after the beginning of a meal)	<140 mg/dL (7.77 mmol/L) (2 hours postprandial)
Blood pressure Systolic Diastolic	<140 mmHg† <80 mmHg†	<130 mmHg† <80 mmHg†
Lipids LDL-C	<100 mg/dL (5.55 mmol/L)‡	<100 mg/dL (5.55 mmol/L) (high risk) <70 mg/dL (3.88 mmol/L) (very high risk)
HDL-C	*Men:* >40 mg/dL (2.22 mmol/L) *Women:* >50 mg/dL (2.77 mmol/L)	No recommendation
Triglycerides	<150 mg/dL (8.32 mmol/L)	<150 mg/dL (8.32 mmol/L)
Non HDL-C	No recommendation	<160 mg/dL (moderate risk) <130 mg/dL (high risk)
TC/HDL-C ratio	No recommendation	<3.5 (moderate risk) <3 (high risk)

*Goal adjusted based on individual factors.

†Lower systolic and/or diastolic blood pressure appropriate for some.

‡If the maximum dose of a statin that a patient can tolerate fails to lower LDL cholesterol more by than 30%, there is no convincing evidence to add an additional agent.

Sources: American Diabetes Association, "Standards of medical care in diabetes—2020," *Diabetes Care* 43, Suppl 1(2020): S111-S134; American Association of Clinical Endocrinologists, Consensus Statement by the American Association of Clinical Endocrinologists and American College of Endocrinology on the Comprehensive Type 2 Diabetes Management Algorithm – 2020 Executive Summary." *Endocr Pract.* 26, No. 1(2020):107-129.

treatment should be considered. Pharmacological treatment should be considered and lifestyle modifications implemented as soon as hypertension is identified.[23]

Angiotensin converting enzyme (ACE) inhibitors and angiotensin receptor blockers (ARBs) have traditionally[19] been recommended as first-line therapy in people with diabetes, due to their known kidney protection effects. Multiple-drug therapy may be necessary to achieve optimal blood pressure targets. It is important that the diabetes care and education specialist help the person with diabetes understand multiple-drug therapy for more effective management of blood pressure. Initial therapy should begin with blood pressure between 140/90 and 159/99 mmHg. In persons with diabetes whose blood pressure is >160/100mm Hg, two anti-hypertensive medications are recommended in order to more effectively achieve adequate blood pressure levels.[21]

Lipids. Lipid abnormalities are more common in people with type 2 diabetes than in those with type 1 diabetes or those without diabetes. People with type 2 diabetes commonly have elevated triglycerides, reduced HDL-C, and same levels of LDL-C than those without diabetes. Lipid management should target lowering LDL-C, raising HDL-C, and lowering triglycerides. The Standards of Care recommend that statin therapy not only be initiated in all people with diabetes, who have overt heart disease, but also be considered for those over the age of 40, regardless of cardiovascular disease status.[19]

The Standards of Care recommend the following[21]:

- **Adults.** Adults with diabetes should be tested for lipid disorders both at diagnosis and at their first medical evaluation. In adults with low-risk lipid values (LDL-C less than 100 mg/dL[5.55 mmol/L], HDL-C greater than 50 mg/dL [2.77 mmol/L], and triglycerides less than 105 mg/dL[8.32 mmol/L]), lipid assessment may be done every 5 years. Obtain panel prior to the start of statin or other lipid-lowering therapy, 4-12 weeks after the start or change of dose, and annually thereafter.

- **Children and adolescents.** Obtain a fasting lipid profile in children ≥10 years of age soon after the diagnosis of diabetes (after glucose stability has been established). If LDL cholesterol values are within the accepted risk level (<100 mg/dL [2.6 mmol/L]), a lipid profile repeated every 3 to 5 years is reasonable. After the age of 10, if lifestyle interventions including nutrition therapy have not lowered the LDL (<160 mg/dl or <130 mg/dl with one additional CV risk factor) a statin may be considered. Treatment guidelines are the same as for children with type 1 diabetes.[23]

Lifestyle modifications are indicated for people with diabetes. These modifications include reducing the intake of saturated fat, trans fat, and cholesterol, and increasing omega-3 fatting acids, fiber, and plant stanols/sterols. Other interventions include increasing physical activity and weight reduction if needed, and statin therapy as indicated. The two statin dosing intensities that are recommended for use in clinical practice: high-intensity statin therapy will achieve approximately a 50% reduction in LDL cholesterol, and moderate-intensity statin regimens achieve 30% to 50% reductions in LDL cholesterol.[19]

Smoking Cessation. Cigarette smoking is the most important modifiable cause of premature death for those with and without diabetes. Studies of people with diabetes have repeatedly found an increased risk of morbidity and premature death associated with the development of macrovascular complications among smokers.[2] Smoking is also related to earlier development of microvascular complications.[2]

Smoking cessation counseling has been shown to be efficacious and cost-effective in reducing tobacco use.[19] The Standards of Care recommend advising all people with diabetes not to smoke or use other tobacco products, including e-cigarettes. This counseling should be used as a regular part of care.

The diabetes care and education specialist should address the issue of smoking cessation in a non-judgmental and supportive way. There are many programs (eg, telephone help lines for counseling) and tools (eg, gum, patches, and other pharmacologic agents) available to assist with cessation efforts. Special consideration should be given to assessing the level of nicotine dependence, which is associated with the difficulty of quitting and relapse. Several attempts at stopping are often required for success with cessation.[19]

Obstructive Sleep Apnea (OSA). Sleep disordered breathing conditions like obstructive sleep apnea (OSA) have been associated with insulin resistance and glucose intolerance. OSA is typically characterized by loud snoring and pauses in breathing while sleeping. Excess weight is often considered the cause of OSA because fat deposits around the upper airways obstruct breathing. Obesity has been identified as a significant risk factor for OSA as well as diabetes. Also, diabetes itself is a major risk factor and complication of OSA. In addition to causing poor sleep quality and daytime sleepiness, OSA has other important clinical consequences, including an increased risk of hypertension and cardiovascular disease (CVD).[24]

OSA is commonly found in people with type 2 diabetes. Diabetes care and education specialists need to ask individuals about daytime drowsiness, snoring, and impaired sleep symptoms in order to identify the problem. Lifestyle changes are among the most important treatments for mild cases of OSA, but other therapies are more effective for moderate-to-severe cases. These include continuous positive airways pressure (CPAP) devices, oral appliances, and surgery.[25]

Antiplatelet Therapy. Aspirin therapy has been shown to be effective in reducing cardiovascular morbidity and mortality in people with diabetes and previous stroke or myocardial infarction (secondary prevention) (reference). However, studies have not found a clear benefit of low-dose aspirin for primary prevention. The Standards of Care for the use of aspirin therapy include:

- **Secondary prevention:** Use aspirin therapy (75-162 mg per day) in those with diabetes who have a history of CVD as a secondary prevention tactic.
- **Primary prevention:** Aspirin therapy (75-162 mg per day) may be considered as a primary prevention strategy in those with type 1 diabetes or type 2 diabetes at increased cardiovascular risk. This includes most men >50 years of age or women >60 years of age who have at least 1 additional major risk factor (family history of CVD, hypertension, smoking, dyslipidemia, or albuminurea).
- **Contraindications:** Other antiplatelet agents should be considered in those with aspirin contraindications.
- **Younger adults and children:** Aspirin therapy is not recommended for those under 21 years of age, as it is linked to an increased risk of Reye's Syndrome.[19]

Diabetic Retinopathy

Diabetic retinopathy is a microvascular complication of both type 1 and type 2 diabetes. The duration of diabetes and level of glycemic stability strongly affect the prevalence. Diabetic retinopathy is the leading cause of new cases of blindness in working adults.[26] Glaucoma, cataracts, and other disorders of the eye are more common in people with diabetes. Nephropathy, hypertension, and dyslipidemia have also been associated with a higher risk of developing retinopathy. Optimal glycemic and blood pressure management can reduce the risk, or slow the progression, of retinopathy.

The Standards of Care regarding eye care for the person with diabetes include the following:[27]

- Adults with type 1 diabetes should have an initial dilated and comprehensive eye examination by an ophthalmologist or optometrist within 5 years after the onset of diabetes.
- Persons with type 2 diabetes should have an initial dilated and comprehensive eye examination by an ophthalmologist or optometrist at the time of the diabetes diagnosis.
- If there is no evidence of retinopathy for one or more annual eye exams and glycemia is well managed, then exams every 1 to 2 years may be considered. If any level of diabetic retinopathy is present, subsequent dilated retinal examinations should be repeated at least annually by an ophthalmologist or optometrist. If retinopathy is progressing or sight-threatening, then examinations will be required more frequently.
- Telemedicine programs that use validated retinal photography with remote reading by an ophthalmologist or optometrist and timely referral for a comprehensive eye examination when indicated can be an appropriate screening strategy for diabetic retinopathy.

Persons with diabetes experiencing any level of macular edema, severe nonproliferative diabetic retinopathy (a precursor of proliferative diabetic retinopathy), or any proliferative diabetic retinopathy should be referred to an ophthalmologist who is knowledgeable and experienced in the management of diabetic retinopathy.

The traditional treatment, laser photocoagulation therapy, is indicated to reduce the risk of vision loss in persons with high-risk proliferative diabetic retinopathy and, in some cases, severe nonproliferative diabetic retinopathy. Intravitreous injections of anti–vascular endothelial growth factor ranibizumab is also indicated to reduce the risk of vision loss in persons with proliferative diabetic retinopathy.[27]

Women with preexisting type 1 or type 2 diabetes who are planning pregnancy or who have become pregnant should be counseled on the risk of development and/or progression of diabetic retinopathy. A comprehensive eye exam should be performed prior to becoming pregnant or in the first trimester of pregnancy. Monitoring should occur at each trimester and for 1 year postpartum as indicated by the degree of retinopathy.[27]

The role of the diabetes care and education specialist is to prepare the person with diabetes for the eye exam. Explaining what to expect when the eyes are dilated is important. These exams can be uncomfortable and may cause some people to not follow through with the exam. They may not believe they have any eye concerns because they have not experienced any vision changes.

Diabetic Kidney Disease

Chronic kidney disease (CKD) attributed to diabetes (diabetic kidney disease or DKD) is the leading cause of end-stage renal disease (ESRD).[28] Ethnic and racial minorities have a higher prevalence of ESRD but are increasingly reporting lower mortality rates on dialysis then non-Hispanic whites.[29] Intensive glucose management has been shown to delay or reduce the onset and progression of DKD in people with type 1 or type 2 diabetes. Optimal blood pressure management is also recommended to reduce the risk or slow progression of CKD. Diabetic kidney disease is also associated with an increased risk of cardiovascular disease in people with type 1 or type 2 diabetes. In addition to glycemic and blood pressure management, Medical Nutrition Therapy (MNT) may be recommended to assist with nutrition needs related to desirable protein (0.8 kg/day) and dietary sodium and potassium levels for individuals with CKD who are not on dialysis. For persons with CKD and type 2 diabetes, use of SGLT2 inhibitor or GLP1 receptor agonist should be considered to reduce the risk of CKD progression and cardiovascular events. Among non-pregnant adults with diabetes and hypertension, angiotensin converting enzymes or angiotensin receptor blockers are recommended for a modestly elevated urinary albumin-to-creatinine ratio and estimated glomerular filtration rate. See chapter 28, Diabetes Kidney Diabetes.

Normal UACR <30 mg/g Cr
Normal eGFR >60 mL/min/1.73 m

Education related to DKD should include the importance of glucose and blood pressure management as well as the importance of annual screening of kidney function. Assessment of tobacco use and encouragement and support in smoking cessation are important.[2] People at all stages of kidney disease can benefit from staying physically active.

Physical activity plans are individualized to fit the needs of the person with diabetes. Since people are asymptomatic throughout the early stages of DKD, the diabetes care and education specialist plays a key role in helping persons with diabetes understand the importance of routine tests to assess kidney function. Recommendations from the standards are annual screening for urinary albumin (eg, spot urinary albumin-to-creatinine ratio) and estimated glomerular filtration rate in people with type 1 diabetes diagnosed for 5 or more years and in all people with type 2 diabetes and with comorbid hypertension. Education about urine albumin testing should include information about the transient elevations that may occur related to marked hyperglycemia, exercise within 24 hours of test, infection or fever, marked hypertension, heart failure, and menstruation. A positive test is to be repeated. Two to 3 tests within the next 3 to 6 months must be positive before a person is considered to have microalbuminuria. The importance of taking prescribed medications and an individualized nutrition plan along with the need for additional testing or treatment based on DKD stage should be stressed by the diabetes care and education specialist. It is recommended that persons with an eGFR <30 mL/min/1.73 m^2 be referred to a nephrologist.[21,27] ESRD treatments and considerations like medication, dialysis, and transplants are part of the education plan.

Neuropathy

A multitude of neuropathies may occur in people living with diabetes. Prevention focuses on early intervention with lifestyle modification and glucose management. In persons with type 1 diabetes near-normal glycemia greatly reduces the risk of distal symmetric polyneuropathy, often called diabetic peripheral neuropathy and cardiac autonomic neuropathy and can slow their progression in persons with type 2.[27] Up to 50% of diabetic peripheral neuropathies may be asymptomatic. If this is not recognized and preventive foot care put in place, the person will be at high risk of injuries to their insensate feet. Autonomic neuropathies may affect every system in the body and may result in hypoglycemic unawareness, constipation, diarrhea, gastroparesis, urinary problems, erectile dysfunction, female sexual dysfunction, orthostatic hypotension, resting tachycardia, and difficulty regulating sweating. Cardiac autonomic neuropathy is associated with increased morbidity and mortality. Educating individuals about the importance of early recognition of neuropathies, glucose management, and the availability of treatment options should be included in the diabetes education plan. Lifestyle modifications and preventive behaviors like self-foot exams are very important for improving symptoms and reducing complications like foot ulcerations. Currently there are no available treatment options targeting the pathogenesis of diabetic neuropathy. Therefore, it is important that the diabetes care and education specialist work with the individual to support them as they implement behaviors and therapies to help manage their symptoms and reduce secondary complications. Educate the individual on what to expect and the importance of the simple clinical tests used in screening for diabetic neuropathy. Ask about neuropathic pain or other symptoms of neuropathy that may interfere in the individual's daily activities and their motivation to engage in their self-management plan. Recognition of the impact that neuropathic complications may have on quality of life is important. A growing body of evidence indicates the diabetic neuropathy is a risk factor for depression. There is also evidence that depression and self–foot care play a role in the incidence of developing a first foot ulcer.[30] Compared to persons with diabetes without depression, persons with diabetes and major depressive disorder have a twofold increase in the risk of developing a foot ulcer.[31] Working collaboratively, the person with diabetes and the diabetes care team will implement a plan to promote risk-reduction strategies that help maintain or improve quality of life.[32a]

Neuropathy Assessment

- Assess for diabetic peripheral neuropathy starting at diagnosis of type 2 diabetes and 5 years after diagnosis of type 1, then at least annually.
    - To identify feet at high risk for ulceration and amputation, clinical tests like annual 10-g monofilament testing pinprick sensation, vibration perception with a tuning fork, and ankle reflexes are used in assessment.

        Consider assessing gait and balance to evaluate the risk of falls as evidence indicates and increased risk of falls among older adults with diabetes.[32b]
- Diabetic neuropathy is a diagnosis of exclusion. Nondiabetic neuropathies may occur in persons with diabetes and may be treatable. In persons with peripheral neuropathy, assess for B12 and other vitamin deficiencies, alcohol use disorder, hypothyroidism, and exposure to heavy metal or toxins.
- Signs and symptoms of autonomic neuropathy should be assessed in individuals with evidence of microvascular complications. It is suggested that screening for cardiac cardiomyopathy be done in persons with hypoglycemia unawareness. This includes assessment of signs such as resting tachycardia, exercise intolerance, and orthostatic hypotension.[33]

Foot Care

Diabetes is a leading cause of non-traumatic lower limb amputations. Foot ulceration and amputation caused by peripheral neuropathy and peripheral arterial disease (PAD) are common and are major causes of morbidity and mortality in persons with diabetes.[3] Early detection, treatment, and management of loss of protective sensation (LOPS) and PAD are key to delaying and preventing adverse outcomes. All persons with diabetes, especially those with high-risk foot conditions, should receive education on risk factors and how to care for their feet to prevent complications. Education includes how to care for the feet, selecting proper socks and shoes (including footwear behavior at home), and identifying foot problems, and when to report problems to the healthcare provider.

Also key to preventing foot problems are the comprehensive foot exam, performed at least annually by the health professional and the daily self-foot exam performed by the person with diabetes or their caretaker. The Lower Extremity Amputation Prevention Program (LEAP), utilized since 1992, uses a Five Step Model.[34] Steps are: 1. Annual Foot Screening using 10-gram monofilament testing to identify LOPS. Persons identified as "at-risk" should be seen at least 4 times a year to check feet and shoes. 2. Patient Education: Teaching simple self-management skills, assisting the person with diabetes to become a full partner with their healthcare team in preventing foot problems. 3. Daily Self-Inspection: Studies have shown that daily self-inspection is the single most effective way to protect feet with LOPS. Early detection of foot injuries like blisters, redness or swelling, callus or toe nail problems is important for preventing more serious problems. Some problems will be reported immediately and others may be self-managed. 4. Footwear Selection: Persons who have LOPS can develop problems from wearing poorly designed or improperly fitting shoes. They should never walk barefoot around the house. 5. Management of Simple Foot Problems: In addition to LOPs, neuropathy can also cause autonomic nerve changes that affect the feet. These include decreased perspiration and increased bone reabsorption. The decreased perspiration and lead to dry cracked skin increasing the likelihood of foot injuries. LEAP emphasizes the importance of reporting all foot injuries to the healthcare provider.

Standards of Care for Foot Care Include:[35]

- A comprehensive foot evaluation at least annually to identify risk factors for ulcers and amputations. Persons with evidence of sensory loss or a history of ulceration or amputation should have their feet inspected at every visit.
- Obtain prior history of ulceration, amputation, Charcot foot, angioplasty or vascular surgery, cigarette smoking, retinopathy, and renal disease, current symptoms of neuropathy (pain, numbness, burning), and vascular disease (leg fatigue, claudication).
- The comprehensive evaluation includes visual inspection of the skin, assessment of foot deformities, neurological assessment for loss of protective sensation (10-g monofilament testing with at least one other assessment: vibration using 128-Hz tuning fork, pinprick sensation, ankle reflexes, or vibration, temperature, or pinprick sensations) (testing of hot and cold thermal changes is also recommended by AACE). Vascular assessment should include pulses in the legs and feet.
- For individuals with diminished or absent pedal pulses or signs of claudication, further vascular assessment and ankle brachial index are indicated.
- Smokers or those with previous lower-extremity complications or other risk factors like LOPS, structural abnormalities, or PAD should be referred to foot care specialists for ongoing preventive care and surveillance.
- In children, consider comprehensive foot exams starting at puberty or ≥10 years (whichever is earlier), once the youth has had diabetes for at least 5 years.

Persons who smoke or who have history of lower extremity complications, loss of protective sensation, structural abnormalities, or PAD should be referred to a foot specialist for on-going care.[34]

- o The use of specialized therapeutic footwear is recommended for persons who are high risk for foot complications.

Many diabetes care and education specialists are responsible for performing foot exams. The diabetes care and education specialist must be appropriately trained to perform foot exams and refer individuals to foot care specialists when appropriate. LEAP offers free on-line training for health professionals, Comprehensive Management of the Neuropathic Foot (https://www.hrsa.gov/hansens-disease/training.html#leap-online). Diabetes care and education specialists are also key in demonstrating and reinforcing desirable foot self-care practices. This may include assessing the person with diabetes ability to perform self-foot exams and assisting those who have difficulty with a plan for daily care.

Barriers related to visual impairment, cognitive ability and physical constraints must be considered and assistance with adaptations like long-handled mirrors or a support person to perform the exam should be put in place.

Sensory Impairment

Though not widely recognized as a chronic complication of diabetes, over two thirds of adults with diabetes are affected with some level of hearing impairment. This is about twice as high as persons without diabetes. Adults with prediabetes have a 30% higher rate of hearing loss.[36] It is believed that this hearing is caused by damage to nerves and blood vessels in the inner ear. Consider assessing for hearing loss. The Hearing Handicap Inventory for the Elderly Screening (HHIE-S) tool is a 5-minute, 10-item questionnaire that can be used with persons of all ages (see Table 9.4). It is used to assess how an individual perceives the social and emotional effects of hearing loss. Those who perceive their hearing loss to be a problem are

TABLE 9.4 Hearing Handicap Inventory for the Elderly -Screening (HHIE-S)

ITEM	*YES* (4 points)	*SOMETIMES* (2 points)	*NO* (0 points)
Does a hearing problem cause you to feel embarrassed when you meet new people?			
Does a hearing problem cause you to feel frustrated when talking to members of your family?			
Do you have difficulty hearing when someone speaks in a whisper?			
Do you feel handicapped by a hearing problem?			
Does a hearing problem cause you difficulty when visiting friends, relatives, or neighbors?			
Does a hearing problem cause you to attend religious services less often than you would like?			
Does a hearing problem cause you to have arguments with family members?			
Does a hearing problem cause you difficulty when listening to TV or radio?			
Do you feel that any difficulty with your hearing limits or hampers your personal or social life?			
Does a hearing problem cause you difficulty when in a restaurant with relatives and friends?			
RAW SCORE ____________ (sum of the points assigned each of the items)			
INTERPRETING THE RAW SCORE 0 to 8 = 13% probability of hearing impairment (no handicap/no referral) 10 to 24 = 50% probability of hearing impairment (mild-moderate handicap/refer) 26 to 40 = 84% probability of hearing impairment (severe handicap/refer)			

Source: I Ventry, B Weinstein, "Identification of elderly people with hearing problems," ©*American Speech-Language-Hearing Association*, July (1983), 37-42. Reprinted with permission.

Note: The American Speech-Language-Hearing Association allows copies of this tool to be made and used with patients.

more likely to have further testing and accept the need for a hearing aid. The higher the HHIE-S score, the greater the handicapping effect of a hearing impairment. Referral for further testing is recommended for individuals scoring 10 or higher on the inventory. Hearing loss can be a barrier to diabetes care and education. It is important that accommodations be made for the individual with hearing impairment when receiving diabetes education in an individual or group setting. Minimize background noise and make sure the individual has an unobstructed view of the speaker. Asking the person for return demonstrations or to rephrase information that has been shared can help the diabetes care and education specialist evaluate if the message has been received.[37]

It has also been noted that impairment in smell has been reported in people with diabetes.[38]

Resources to Aid in Implementing Standards of Care

The National Diabetes Education Program Web site (https://www.cdc.gov/diabetes/ndep/index.html) contains a variety of educational resources and tools that the busy diabetes care and education specialist may find helpful. The Association of Diabetes Care and Education Specialists (ADCES) and the American Diabetes Association (ADA) also have many tools aimed at supporting individuals in their risk-reduction behaviors. Many industry partners also offer unbranded educational resources for persons with diabetes and for healthcare professionals. You may also find diabetes data and resources through the Centers for Disease Control (CDC) or the agency in your state that addresses public health concerns.

Preventive Care Services

In addition to the tests, exams, and interventions that are important for reducing risks for microvascular and macrovascular complications, there are other preventive care services that people with diabetes should receive to improve their health:

- Influenza, pneumococcal, and hepatitis B immunizations
- Dental care
- Prepregnancy counseling

Immunizations

People with diabetes are at higher risk of serious complications from certain diseases like influenza and pneumonia that are mostly preventable with vaccines. Both flu and pneumonia are associated with high morbidity and mortality rates among certain populations. In addition to diabetes, other health and age-related risk factors include heart disease, obesity (body mass index >40), adults 65 or older, children younger than 2 years, pregnant women, American Indians and Alaska Natives, and people living in nursing homes or other long-term care facilities. It is estimated that persons with diabetes have a three-times higher death rate from pneumonia than persons without diabetes.[39]

In addition, hepatitis B virus (HBV) vaccinations are now recommended as part of preventive care for many previously unvaccinated adults with diabetes. Among the general population over age 23, HBV is 2 times more common in those living with diabetes, and multiple HBV outbreaks have occurred in long-term care facilities and hospitals among people with diabetes. Hepatitis B virus is stable for long periods of time on lancing devices and glucose meters; receiving assistance with testing glucose in a location where others are also being tested increases the likelihood of spreading HBV.[40]

Immunization Recommendations:

- Provide recommended vaccines per age for adults and children with diabetes.
  - https://www.cdc.gov/vaccines/schedules/index.html
- Provide an annual influenza vaccine to all people with diabetes 6 months of age and older.
- Vaccination against pneumococcal disease, including pneumococcal pneumonia, with 13-valent pneumococcal conjugate vaccine (PCV13) is recommended for all children before age 2 years. People with diabetes ages 2–64 should also receive 23-valent pneumococcal polysaccharide vaccine (PPSV23). At age ≥65 year, regardless of vaccination history, additional PPSV23 is needed.
- A 2- or 3-dose (depending on the vaccine) series of hepatitis B vaccine should be given to adults with diabetes ages 18–59 years. Consider giving a 3-dose series of hepatitis B vaccine to unvaccinated adults with diabetes ≥60.

Individuals may express a belief that the flu shot gave them the flu in the past and that it is something they do not really need. The diabetes care and education specialist must address these concerns and explain the benefits of getting immunizations as recommended (a helpful resource from the CDC is at http://www.cdc.gov/flu/diabetes/). The influenza nasal spray vaccinations are currently not recommended for people with diabetes.[41]

Even persons who have well-managed diabetes are at an increased risk for flu and pneumonia. Having flu or pneumonia can cause glucose levels to increase and can make managing diabetes very difficult. (See sick day recommendations in chapter 23.) Confirming that the person does not have any contraindications for receiving the vaccine is also important. Best practice guidelines for evaluating contraindications to vaccines are found at https://www.cdc.gov/vaccines/hcp/acip-recs/general-recs/contraindications.html.

Dental Care

Periodontal disease may occur more frequently in people with diabetes, and it tends to be more severe. Evidence points to a bidirectional relationship. Diabetes worsens periodontal disease, and periodontal disease can make diabetes management more difficult. In general, people with type 2 diabetes and periodontitis have higher levels of A1C. Insufficient evidence is available for an association for people with type 1.[42,43] In addition, they interact in a manner that increases the risk of all-cause cardiovascular mortality. Evidence also points to a higher rate of other chronic complications in persons with periodontal disease. Regular dental care and improved managing blood glucose to targets may reduce the risk of periodontal disease.

The ADA does not provide specific guidance on how often a person with diabetes should see a dentist. However, Healthy People 2020[44] has a goal to increase the number of people with diabetes who see a dentist at least once a year and the Consensus report[43] and guidelines of the joint workshop on periodontal diseases and diabetes by the International Diabetes Federation and the European Federation of Periodontology provides the following recommendations.

- Oral health education should be provided to all persons with diabetes as part of their overall educational program.
- Individuals with all forms of diabetes should be told that periodontal disease risk is increased, and if untreated, the periodontitis has a negative impact on glucose management and may also increase the risk of complications such as cardiovascular and kidney disease.
- Individuals should be advised that successful periodontal therapy may have a positive impact upon their glucose management and diabetes complications.
- For people with diabetes, physicians should ask about a prior diagnosis of periodontal disease. If a positive diagnosis has been made, the physician should seek to ascertain that periodontal care and maintenance are being provided.
- Investigating the presence of periodontal disease should be an integral part of a diabetes care visit. People with diabetes should be asked about any signs and symptoms of periodontitis, including bleeding gums during brushing or eating, loose teeth, spacing or spreading of the teeth, oral malodor, and/or abscesses in the gums or gingival suppuration.
- If a positive history is elicited, then a prompt periodontal evaluation should be recommended before their scheduled annual check-up.
- In the case of a negative history, people with diabetes should be advised to check for the above symptoms, and if a positive sign appears, they should visit their dentist.
- For all people with newly diagnosed diabetes mellitus, referral for a periodontal examination should occur as part of their ongoing management of diabetes. Even if no periodontitis is diagnosed initially, annual periodontal review is recommended.
- For children and adolescents diagnosed with diabetes, annual oral screening is recommended through referral to a dental professional.
- Individuals with diabetes who have extensive tooth loss should be encouraged to pursue dental rehabilitation to restore adequate mastication for proper nutrition.
- Persons with diabetes should be advised that other oral conditions such as dry mouth and burning mouth may occur, and if so, they should seek advice from their dental practitioner. Also, persons with diabetes are at increased risk of oral fungal infections and experience poorer wound healing than those who do not have diabetes.
- The physician should consult with the dentist over diabetes management prior to the oral intervention and/or surgery to avoid hypoglycemia and to consider its potential impact on the person's ability to eat.

The diabetes care and education specialist should include dental care practices in their diabetes education assessment and education plan. Ask the person with diabetes about signs of gum disease like red, swollen or bleeding gums or loose teeth and refer as appropriate. Educate the person on the association of periodontitis and difficult-to-manage blood glucose and the association with cardiovascular disease and other complications. Encourage regular visits to the dentist along with routine self-care, including brushing teeth and gums twice daily and flossing each day.

Prepregnancy Counseling

Preconception care has been shown to reduce the risk of congenital malformations. Several nonrandomized studies have compared rates of malformations in infants between women who participated in preconception diabetes care and women who initiated intensive diabetes management after they were already pregnant.[45-49] The preconception care programs were multidisciplinary and trained participants in diabetes self-management with MNT, intensified insulin therapy, and SMBG. In all studies, the incidence of major congenital malformations in infants was much lower in those who participated in preconception care than in those who did not participate.

Standard care for all women with diabetes in their reproductive years with childbearing potential should include the following:[50]

- Starting in puberty, incorporate preconception counseling into the routine diabetes care visit.
- Discuss the importance of near normal blood glucose (under 6.5%), as long as it can be achieved safely, for women planning to become pregnant.
- Counsel women on the importance of family planning and prescribe an effective contraceptive until they are ready to have a child.
- Share risks of retinopathy development and progression with women who may become pregnant, and stress the importance of eye exams prior to pregnancy or in the first trimester of pregnancy and then every trimester and 1 year postpartum.
- Evaluate medications in those who are or may become pregnant, as some medications used to treat women with diabetes are not recommended during pregnancy (ie, statins, ARBs, ACE inhibitors, and most noninsulin glucose-lowering medications).

Women contemplating pregnancy should undergo specific diabetes preconception testing and counseling, which includes:

- A1C testing, which should be close to 6.5% without excessive hypoglycemia
- Review of medication list to change meds that may be harmful during pregnancy, such as ACE inhibitors and statins
- Thyroid stimulating hormone testing
- Identifying, evaluating, and treating long-term complications of diabetes (retinopathy, neuropathy, nephropathy, and CVD)

Blood glucose stability is critical in women with diabetes who become pregnant or those who develop gestational diabetes. Please refer to chapter 24 for detailed coverage of pregnancy in those with preexisting diabetes or gestational diabetes.

Skills

To practice behaviors that minimize the risk of developing complications, people with diabetes must master skills that include SMBG, self-monitoring of blood pressure, self-examination, and maintaining a personal care record. A key component to possessing skills is problem solving. People with diabetes must be taught how to use this information to make treatment decisions regarding food, medication, and physical activity.

Self-Monitoring of Blood Glucose and Continuous Glucose Monitoring

As discussed earlier in this chapter and in chapter 18, most persons with diabetes monitor their blood glucose utilizing SMBG or CGM. To help receive the most benefit out of these two self-management tools, the diabetes care and education specialist will assist the individual with mastering proper techniques for use of the equipment, including proper storage and other variables that may affect meter accuracy. Technique and understanding of SMBG or CGM should be reviewed by the diabetes care and education specialist at regular frequency. This will include assessing the individual's understanding of results and ability to interpret them correctly to use in self-management of their diabetes to make treatment decisions related to food, medication, physical activity, and various stressors.

Self-Monitoring of Blood Pressure

In addition to blood pressure monitoring by a healthcare professional during each diabetes visit, some individuals may benefit from self-monitoring their blood pressure. While this issue has not been specifically studied in people with diabetes, a meta-analysis found that home monitoring, or self-monitoring, of blood pressure improved blood pressure in those with essential hypertension (reference). If the healthcare profession and the person with diabetes determine that this level of monitoring is important, the individual may choose to use a home blood-pressure monitor.

The diabetes care and education specialist should have the person with diabetes bring the home blood-pressure monitor to a diabetes care appointment to be sure that he or she understands how to use it. It is also valuable to note the differences in readings between the home monitor and the office equipment. Having the person demonstrate use of the monitor is a good way to assess the individual's skills and provide feedback and support. The diabetes care and education specialist must also assess the size of the cuff and technique (measurement in the seated position, with feet on the floor and arm supported at heart level, after 5 min of rest. Cuff size should be appropriate for the upper-arm circumference.[19]

Self-Examination of Feet and Foot Care

Careful foot care and proper education have been shown to reduce the amputation rate associated with diabetes.[51] Daily foot inspection is the single most effective way to protect feet in the person who has lost protective sensation and is unable to feel pain.[34]

During the annual comprehensive foot exam, the importance of the individual's foot care and self-examination can be stressed. Additionally, this is a time when the diabetes care and education specialist can assess an individual's vision and mobility to determine whether they will pose difficulties in performing self-exams. If the person with diabetes has poor vision, a manual palpation may be substituted for the visual inspection. If mobility is impaired, making it difficult to reach the feet, a regular or magnifying hand mirror or long-handled mirror can be used to help visualize the plantar surface and other areas of the feet. When both vision and mobility are severely impaired, another individual may need to assist with foot inspections.

Before teaching foot exam and foot care skills, the diabetes care and education specialist needs to assess the person's present knowledge, behaviors, beliefs, and abilities by finding out what the individual is currently doing for foot care and self-examination. The following foot exam and foot care skills should be taught to all persons with diabetes. Close inspection is important for all but is critical for those who have LOPS that puts them at higher risk for developing foot problems: It is encouraged that people choose a specific time of day that they will check their feet.

- Look at both feet (top, bottom, and sides) and between the toes daily. This can be done when putting on or taking off socks and shoes. Look for cuts, calluses, blisters, thick or ingrown toenails, and signs of infection such as redness, swelling, or pus. Seek prompt medical attention for any problems.
- Wash and dry feet thoroughly, especially between the toes. Avoid routine foot soaks. To avoid hot water burns, test the temperature of bath and shower water with an elbow before stepping in.
- Moisturize dry skin (not between the toes) with an emollient such as lanolin or a hand or body lotion. Avoid using lotions that contain alcohol, as this can dry the skin. Talcum powder may be used between the toes, if desired.
- Cut toenails straight across and file the sharp corners to match the contour of the toe (this is best done after a bath or shower).
- Do not use chemicals on or cut corns and calluses.
- Inspect shoes daily by feeling the insides for torn linings, cracks, pebbles, nails, or other irregularities that may irritate the skin. Get in the habit of shaking out shoes before putting them on. Changing shoes during the day can limit repetitive local pressure.
- Avoid going barefoot or sock-footed. Wear appropriate footwear at the pool or beach and apply sunscreen to avoid burns.
- Avoid using hot water bottles or heating pads if your feet are cold.
- Wear lightly padded clean socks and shoes that fit well.

Having the person with diabetes perform a self-examination of the feet is important. This will allow the diabetes care and education specialist to provide positive reinforcement for those aspects that have been successfully done and to point out areas needing additional attention. Education on the importance of appropriate footwear should be provided to the individual along with tips like buying shoes later in the day when the feet may start to swell and breaking new shoes in gradually. For individuals with high-risk feet, it will be important to encourage them to discuss availability of special inserts or shoes that may be covered by insurance. It is widely accepted that educating the individual with diabetes and their family on self-foot care will lead to improved knowledge, self-care behaviors, and reduction of foot complications.[52,53]

Personal Care Record

A personal care record is a valuable tool for people with diabetes to keep track of their therapeutic goals and the tests and exams that are recommended in the Standards of Care. These records come in various formats and sizes, and individuals should select a type according to their personal preferences. Some may prefer a pocket-sized paper tool while others may use a smartphone app or a web-based record to monitor and record care. Self-monitoring of blood glucose may be done several times per day, and thus a separate log for SMBG is usually more practical. In addition, many blood glucose meters come with software that allows results to be downloaded to personal computers or personal digital assistants.

The personal care record is a great way to teach people with diabetes about the Standards of Care. It provides a concise listing of the necessary tests, exams, and interventions that should include places for the person to record his or her measured values. Diabetes care and education specialists can assist people with diabetes in keeping their personal care record up to date and using it to help them determine whether they are getting all the necessary Standards of Care and meeting treatment goals. Reviewing the personal care record is a useful way to guide this discussion in a logical and complete manner.

Barriers and Other Factors That Influence Self-Management

People with diabetes face many challenges that influence their self-management. These challenges can be placed into three areas. These areas are physical limitations, psychosocial, and social factors. The person with diabetes is most vulnerable at diagnosis and whenever medical status changes (eg, intensification of treatment or when complications are diagnosed).[54] Other factors include diagnosis of additional health conditions and when medications are added. The diabetes care and education specialist is key in assisting in identification and overcoming these barriers.

Physical barriers include visual impairment, dexterity issues, and physical activity restrictions. The diabetes care and education specialist can help persons with diabetes to manage these limitations through education and support resources. For example, magnifiers for insulin syringes and talking meters for those with visual impairments.

Social factors include difficulty paying for food, medication, medical supplies, and housing. When persons with diabetes struggle with meeting basic living needs, diabetes self-management becomes more difficult. They often chose between paying the rent, buying food, and medications. Persons with diabetes will often "stretch" their insulin or other medications. Other social factors include lack of insurance, high deductible plans, underinsured, and lack of access to DSMES services or healthcare providers.

Psychosocial and emotional factors include depression, anxiety, and diabetes-related distress. The DAWN (Diabetes Attitudes, Wishes, and Needs) study indicated that more than 4 out of 5 people living with diabetes are not engaging with prescribed treatments. In addition, at diagnosis and 15 years after diagnosis, the majority of people with diabetes were still experiencing distress linked to living with diabetes. Even if individuals are equipped with accurate knowledge and sufficient skills to reduce their risk, the ability to carry out healthy behaviors can be significantly impacted by their psychological and social state.[55] In the DAWN2 study, 45% of participants voiced they had diabetes distress. However, fewer than one fourth said their healthcare team asked them how diabetes was impacting their lives.[55] Diabetes-related distress has a greater impact on behavioral and metabolic outcomes than does depression. Diabetes-related distress is responsive to DSMES and focused attention.[55]

Another barrier to consider is clinical inertia. Many people with diabetes fail to achieve glycemic stability promptly after diagnosis and do not receive timely treatment intensification. This may be in part due to clinical inertia, defined as the failure of healthcare providers to initiate or intensify therapy when indicated. Physician-, person with diabetes, and healthcare-system-related factors all contribute to clinical inertia. Delay in treatment intensification can happen at all stages of treatment for people with diabetes, including prescription of lifestyle changes after diagnosis, introduction of pharmacological therapy, use of combination therapy where needed, and initiation of insulin. Clinical inertia may contribute to people with diabetes living with suboptimal glycemic stability for many years, with dramatic consequences for the person with diabetes in terms of quality of life, morbidity, and mortality.[56]

The diabetes care and education specialist should include psychological and social situation as part of ongoing diabetes management. The diabetes care and education specialist should conduct a thorough psychosocial screening with follow-up for issues like affect/mood, quality of life, expected medical management outcomes, perception of illness, psychiatric history, and resources (emotional, social, and financial). Regular screening for diabetes distress, depression, anxiety, eating disorders, and cognitive impairments should also be screened. If any of these factors are present during DSMES the diabetes care and education specialist should address them immediately and arrange for additional resources.[54]

Disparities in Chronic Complications and Risk-Reduction Behaviors

It is well known that there are disparities in the prevalence of diabetes among certain race/ethnic populations.[57] The same is true with the long-term complications of diabetes. Minority populations are more likely to be affected by retinopathy and nephropathy.[58] Data is conflicting on neuropathy, but studies show that there are disparities in amputations, especially those related to peripheral vascular disease or diabetes.[59] Despite the increased risk for retinopathy and nephropathy among non-Hispanic blacks and Mexican-Americans, these groups have a lower prevalence for hearing impairment when compared with other minority groups or non-Hispanic whites.

Disparities among risk-reduction behaviors are also well documented; for example lower rates of leisure time physical activity among Native Americans and

Mexican-Americans and higher rates of smoking among Native Americans.[60,61] In spite of being aware of the risk of eye complications, screening for diabetes retinopathy is underutilized among low-income minority populations.[62] Different barriers were noted among African American versus Hispanic populations.[62] Understanding the disparities and recognizing barriers that may be common among certain populations is very important for the diabetes care and education specialist as they collaborate with the person with diabetes to help remove barriers, helping support risk-reduction behaviors, decreasing the risk of complications.

Children and Adolescents

The management of diabetes in children and adolescents cannot be the same as care routinely provided to adults with diabetes. The diabetes care team must consider epidemiology, pathophysiology, developmental considerations, and response to therapy in pediatric-onset diabetes are different from adult diabetes. There are also differences in recommended care for children and adolescents with type 1 as opposed to type 2 diabetes. Due to the nature of clinical research in children, the recommendations for children and adolescents with diabetes are less likely to be based on clinical trial evidence. Most recommendations are based on professional opinion. This section will look at the different recommendations for children and adolescents with type 1 diabetes and for children and adolescents with type 2 diabetes.

Glycemic stability in children and adolescence with type 1 diabetes must consider the risk of hypoglycemia. Most children younger than 6 or 7 years of age have immature counterregulatory mechanisms, which result in a form of hypoglycemia unawareness. In addition, young children do not have the cognitive capacity to recognize and respond to hypoglycemia.[23] The A1C level attained in the "intensive" adolescent cohort in the DCCT was 1% above that achieved by adult participants (DCCT). The therapeutic goals for plasma blood glucose premeal and bedtime/overnight as well as A1C are listed for youth in Table 9.5.

Transitioning from pediatric to adult care is also important for youth with diabetes. The Standards of Care recommend that both adult and child healthcare providers provide support for teens with diabetes. The general consensus is that providers and parents should prepare youth for the change to adult care at least 1 year before they make the change.

The National Diabetes Education program has materials to help families and children with diabetes make the transition from a pediatrician to an adult provider (available online at http://ndep.nih.gov/transitions). Another tool, developed by the Endocrine Society in concert with the ADA and other partners, can be found online at http://www.endo-society.org/clinicalpractice/transition_of_care.cfm.

TABLE 9.5 Blood Glucose and A1C Goals for Children With Type 1 Diabetes

Plasma blood glucose goal range		
Before meals	*Bedtime/overnight*	*A1C*
90–130 mg/dL (5.0–7.2 mmol/L)	90–150 mg/dL (5.0–8.3 mmol/L)	<7%*

Key concepts in setting glycemic goals:

Targets should be individualized and lower targets may be reasonable based on a benefit-risk assessment.

Blood glucose targets should be modified in children with frequent hypoglycemia or hypoglycemia unawareness.

Postprandial blood glucose values should be measured when there is a discrepancy between preprandial blood glucose values and A1C levels and to assess preprandial insulin doses in those on basal-bolus or pump regimens.

A goal of <7% is appropriate for many children. Less-stringent A1C goals (such as <7.5% may be appropriate for individuals who cannot articulate symptoms of hypoglycemia; have hypoglycemia unawareness; lack access to analog insulins, advanced insulin delivery technology, and/or continuous glucose monitors; cannot check blood glucose regularly; or have nonglycemic factors that increase A1C (e.g., high glycators).

Source: Reproduced with permission for the American Diabetes Association, "Standards of medical care in diabetes–2020." *Diabetes Care* 43, Suppl 1(2020): S163-182.

Technology

Diabetes technology is the term used to describe the hardware, devices, and software that people with diabetes use to help manage their disease. Diabetes technology can also consist of digital therapeutics, wearable technology, insulin pumps, sensor augmented pumps, continuous glucose monitoring, meters, mobile apps, portals, text messaging, electronic communication, and video conferencing.[1] The use of continuous glucose monitoring has made it possible to see what person's glucose level is at any point during the day. Consequently, a new endpoint for glycemic stability has come into popularity: time in range, which is the percentage of time a person's glucose level is within a range of 70 to 180 mg/dL. In some studies CGM has shown an increase in time in range as well as reducing severe hypoglycemia in persons with type 1 as compared to SMBG.[63] More research is needed to see the effects of technology monotherapy (pump or CGM) and technology dual therapy (sensor augmented insulin pump). Although the advancement of technologies provide more options for effective self-management, complications are still prevalent.[64]

Mobile applications for self-management of diabetes is an emerging portion of technology. Apps, as they are generally called, are developed for both type 1 and type 2 diabetes. The apps, common features include setting reminders, tracking blood glucose, A1C, medication use, physical activity, and weight. Limited evidence suggests the use of commercially available apps, combined with support from a healthcare provider, improves at least one outcome, most often A1C.[65] The long-term impact of apps is unclear and more research is needed.

The use of electronic health records may show an improvement in clinical outcomes as well as engagement by the person with diabetes. Diabetes technology remains a promising area of innovation that can drastically improve the lives of people with diabetes. By reducing the need for constant finger sticking or insulin injections, technology can make glucose monitoring, drug delivery, and health decision-making more efficient. This gives person with diabetes and caregivers more time to dedicate to other aspects of their lives, such as relationships and careers. Diabetes technology also promotes mindfulness in making daily life decisions, the discipline for self-management and self-care, and the formation of health habits. Not only can this help prevent or reduce the progression of diabetes and its complications, but it also can help reduce the costs of diabetes treatment and management.[66] By collaborating with a diabetes care and education specialist, people can learn how to use these technological tools effectively to improve their clinical and quality of life outcomes.[67]

Summary

Reducing risks is multifaceted and influenced by family, friends, cultural background, community, and societal pressures. Reducing risks involves identifying risks and implementing behaviors to minimize and/or prevent complications or adverse outcomes. Diabetes care and education specialists help people with diabetes gain knowledge and understanding about the necessary tests, exams, interventions, and achievement of therapeutic goals that can help them reduce their likelihood of developing complications of diabetes. In addition, those living with diabetes must acquire self-care skills and develop strategies that will maximize their level of health and quality of life.

Reducing risks can be a challenging aspect of self-care behavior to address. The individual must be encouraged to address potential problems, yet practicing preventive behaviors may not always be a priority in the face of current life demands. The delicate balance the diabetes care and education specialist must strike falls between helping people with diabetes gain an understanding of and appreciation for the future benefits linked to preventive behaviors and employing methods that do not undermine self-efficacy. The evidence is strong that following the Standards of Care and achieving therapeutic goals greatly reduce the likelihood of diabetes complications. The diabetes care and education specialist plays a vital role in partnering with the person with diabetes, family members, and the other members of the healthcare team to translate the evidence supporting risk-reduction behaviors into practice.

Focus on Education

Teaching Strategies

Establish the importance. Help people with diabetes gain an appreciation for the importance of risk-reduction behaviors by partnering with them to make these behaviors personal and meaningful. Tailor information to appeal to the individuals, learning preferences, beliefs, culture, language, and educational level.

Deliver Risk Information

Use as much interactive teaching as possible, such as asking the person with diabetes to suggest specific actions he or she will take to reduce personal risk for complications and poor health. Ask individuals to demonstrate skills related to diabetes management to be sure they are performed correctly. Directly and specifically address feelings and concerns in addition to knowledge and skills acquisition. Use phrases like "What might stop you (hold you back) from trying this?"

Achieve targets. Though there may be differences in therapeutic goals recommended by various associations and groups, targets should be individualized based on assessment of co-morbidities, life expectancy, cognitive function, willingness to participate in treatments, and quality of life. These variables should be included when planning education to increase knowledge and improve skills to support risk-reduction behaviors.

Keep records. Personal care records are a valuable tool for engaging people with diabetes in risk-reducing self-care behaviors. They provide a list of the recommended tests, exams, and interventions based on the Standards of Care and help people with diabetes track their results. Encourage individuals to use a record-keeping tool that includes reminders for visits, follow-up lab testing, and immunizations and to consider keeping it in their purse or billfold for quick reference or use a smartphone or web-based tool.

Messages for Persons With Diabetes

Learn the skills

Realize that it's a lot of work! Diabetes management is a lot of work, but you and your health are worth it! Take advantage of the knowledge and recent advances in diabetes research and technology to help keep yourself healthy and reduce your risk for complications.

You can be a healthy person living with diabetes. There is no better time than the present to begin taking steps toward living a healthier life and reducing. Every day that your blood glucose, blood pressure and blood cholesterol levels are closer to your target range, you are building a healthier future.

Keep records. Work closely with your diabetes team to track blood glucose levels, blood pressure, and blood lipids. Make time for the recommended visits to associated healthcare providers and for suggested exams and immunizations. Keep a record of the results of your diabetes tests and exams and your medications (and changes). Bring this information to each clinic visit, educational class, and urgent care visit.

Health Literacy

Health literacy can negatively impact the interactions and the relationship between persons with diabetes and healthcare providers. Communicating meaningfully with persons with diabetes with low health literacy levels will maximize concordance. Persons with low literacy often are viewed as not engaging with their self-care regimen. Learning more about ways to effectively communicate with those who may have low health literacy can improve the ability of persons with diabetes to make lifestyle changes and engage with their medical treatment. All persons with diabetes should be assessed for literacy issues, including the use of numbers.

Low health literacy affects what happens during healthcare appointments, after the visit, and in potential future concordance. Existing miscommunications and, consequently, inaccurate perceptions about self-care among persons with diabetes can prevent adequate future risk-reduction behaviors. Some persons with diabetes may be intimidated by the overwhelming amount of information it takes to manage the new diagnosis of diabetes and may be resistant to preventive care. Craft your messages with empowered but realistic expectations of what it really takes to manage diabetes effectively at each stage. Use supplemental tools like videos, pictures, and models to assist with teaching. In addition, be certain to use demonstration and the teach-back method to ensure the person with diabetes understands the information.

Choose words that people understand. The main purpose of self-management education is to help the person with diabetes own the information so that they can improve their health. Choose words that the person can relate to and translate into action. For example, instead of asking, "What are your goals?" ask, "What will you do differently till the next time I see you?"

Teach people with diabetes what questions to ask their healthcare providers. What is my main problem? What do I need to do about it? And why is it important for me to do it?

Consider the needs of people whose primary language is not English. People whose primary language is not English are at high risk for having difficulty with health literacy. Providing a translator and material in their primary language may be needed. Additionally, using culturally sensitive care is important.

Online courses are available to help individual clinicians or health systems improve their dealings with those living with low literacy levels. Examples include the following:

- Health literacy tools and information are available through the Health Resources and Services Administration at http://www.hrsa.gov/publichealth/healthliteracy/.
- Centers for Disease Control and Prevention health literacy resources at http://www.cdc.gov/healthliteracy/.

Focus on Practice

Understand the standards of medical care for diabetes and incorporate them into practice. The diabetes care and education specialist should collaborate with the healthcare team and the person with diabetes to make sure the person is aware of recommended tests and exams and their frequency. Utilize the patient assessment to help identify gaps and barriers to care.

Integrate the clinical preventive services. Integrate the clinical preventive services and chronic disease management through the delivery of usual care among doctors, physician assistants, nurse practitioners, nurses, and administrators at their practice sites. Every clinical encounter creates an opportunity to inspire, support, and encourage the person with diabetes in preventive care and management. Use of brief, targeted messages through verbal communication, visuals, or media can bring up important issues at the right time and the right place for those who are ready to receive them.

Create an environment that supports health and wellness. A community that supports risk-reduction behaviors is important for an individual's health and well-being and for the health of the population. Healthy behaviors need to become part of the culture and a way of life. Community interventions to create safe places for physical activity, mitigating food insecurity, increasing access to quality medical care and creating opportunities for people to interact with other healthy people are all important to create a culture where healthy behaviors are a priority.

References

1. Association of Diabetes Care and Education Specialists (ADCES). An effective model of diabetes care and education: revising the AADE7 self-care behaviors®. Published online ahead of print, Feb 2020. Diabetes Educ. doi: https://doi.org/10.1177/0145721719894903.
2. American Diabetes Association. Facilitating Behavior Change and Well-being to Improve Health Outcomes: Standards of medical care in diabetes—2020. Diabetes Care. 2020;43(Suppl 1):S48-65.
3. Stange KC, Nutting PA, Miller WI, et al. Defining and measuring the patient-centered medical home. J Gen Intern Med. 2010 (cited 2019 December 4):25 (60):601-12. On the internet at: https://www.ncbi.nlm.nih.gov/pubmed/20467909.
4. American Diabetes Association. Improving care and promoting health in populations: standards of medical care in diabetes—2020. Diabetes Care. 2020;43(Suppl 1):S7-13.
5. Dickinson, JK, Guzman, SJ, Maryniuk, MD, et. al. The use of language in diabetes care and education. Diabetes Care. 2017; 40:1790-99.
6. Diabetes Control and Complication Trial. The effect of intensive treatment of diabetes on the development and progression of long term complications in insulin dependent diabetes. NEJM. 1993;329:977-86.
7. UK Prospective Diabetes Study (UKPDS) Group. Effect of intensive blood glucose control with metformin on complications in overweight patients with type 2 diabetes (UKPDS34). Lancet. 1998;352:854-65.
8. Martin CL, Albers J, Herman WH, et al: DCCT/EDIC Research Group. Neuropathy among the diabetes control and complications trial cohort 8 years after trial completion. Diabetes Care. 2006;29:340-4.
9. Holman RR, Paul SK, Bethel MA, Mathews DR, Neil HA. 10 year follow up of intensive glucose control in type 2 diabetes. N Engl J Med. 2008;359:1577-89.
10. Orchard TJ, Nathan DM, Zinman B et al. Writing Group for the DCCT/EDIC Research Group. Association between 7 years of intensive treatment of type 1 diabetes and long-term mortality. JAMA. 2015;313:45-53.
11. Duckworth W, Abraira C, Moritz T, et al; VADT Investigators. Glucose control and vascular complications om veterans with type 2 diabetes. N Engl J Med. 2009;360:129-39.
12. Nathan DM, Cleary PA, Backlund JY, et al; Diabetes Control and Complications Trial/Epidemiology of Diabetes Interventions and Complications (DCCT/EDIC) Study Research Group. Intensive diabetes treatment and cardiovascular disease in patients with type 1 diabetes. N Engl J Med. 2005;353:2643-53.
13. Skyler JS, Bergenstal R, Bonow RO, et al. Intensive Glycemic Control and the Prevention of Cardiovascular Events: Implications of the ACCORD, ADVANCE, and VA Diabetes Trials. A position statement of the American Diabetes Association and a scientific statement of the American College of Cardiology Foundation and the American Heart Association. Diabetes Care. 2009;32(1):187–92. doi: 10.2337/dc08-9026.
14. American Diabetes Association. Glycemic Targets: Standards of medical care in diabetes—2020. Diabetes Care. 2020;43 (Suppl 1):S71.
15. American Diabetes Association. Glycemic Targets: Standards of medical care in diabetes—2020. Diabetes Care. 2020;43 (Suppl 1):S66-76.
16. Stratton IM, Alder AI, Andrew NH, et al. 2000. Association of glycaemia with macrovascular and microvascular complications

of type 2 diabetes (UKPDS 35): prospective observational study. BMJ. 2000;321:405-12. doi: https://doi.org/10.1136/bmj.321.7258.405.

17. Little RR, Rohlfing C, Sacks DB. The National Glycohemoglobin Standardization Program: Over 20 Years of Improving Hemoglobin A_{1c} Measurement. Clin Chem. 2019;65(7):839-48.

18. Monnier L, Lapinski H, Colette C. Contributions of fasting and postprandial plasma glucose increments to the overall diurnal hyperglycemia of type 2 diabetic patients. Diabetes Care. 2003;26(3):881-85. https://doi.org/10.2337/diacare.26.3.881.

19. American Diabetes Association. Cardiovascular disease and risk management: standards of medical care in diabetes—2019. Diabetes Care. 2019;42(Suppl 1):S103-23.

20. Chobanian, AV, Bakris GL, Black HR, et al. "The Seventh Report of the Joint National Committee on Prevention, Detection, Evaluation, and Treatment of High Blood Pressure: the JNC 7 report. JAMA. 2003;289:2560-72.

21. American Diabetes Association. Cardiovascular disease and risk management: standards of medical care in diabetes—2020. Diabetes Care. 2020;43(Suppl 1):S111-34.

22. American Academy of Pediatrics. Clinical practice guideline for screening and management of high blood pressure in children and adolescents Pediatrics. 2017;140(3).

23. American Diabetes Association. Children and adolescents: standards of medical care in diabetes—2020. Diabetes Care. 2020;43(Suppl 1):S163-182.

24. Doumit J, Prasad B. Sleep apnea in type 2 diabetes. Diabetes Spectrum. 2016;29(1):14-19.

25. Medical Evaluation and Assessment of Comorbidities. Standards of medical care in diabetes—2019. Diabetes Care. 2019;42 (Suppl 1):S34-45.

26. National Diabetes Education Program. *Guiding Principles for the Care of People with or at Risk for Diabetes.* Atlanta, GA: National Diabetes Education Program, US Department of Health and Human Services' National Institutes of Health and Centers for Disease Control and Prevention; 2018.

27. American Diabetes Association. Microvascular complications and foot care: standards of medical care in diabetes—2020. Diabetes Care. 2020;43(Suppl 1)S135-51.

28. Centers for Disease Control and Prevention. *Chronic Kidney Disease Fact Sheet 2017.* Atlanta, GA: Centers for Disease Control and Prevention. 2017. (Cited 20 Jan 2020) On the Internet at: https://www.cdc.gov/diabetes/pubs/pdf/kidney_factsheet.pdf.

29. Spanikas E, Golden S. Race/Ethnic Difference in Diabetes and Diabetic Complications. Curr Diabetes Rep. 2013(6).

30. Vileikyte L, Gonzalez J. Recognition and management of psychosocial in diabetic neuropathy. Handbook of Clinical Neurology. 2014;126:195-209. https://doi.org/10.1016/B978-0-444-53480-4.00013-8.

31. Williams LH, Rutter CM, Katon WJ, et al. Depression and Incident diabetic foot ulcer. Am J Med. 2010;123(8):748-54.

32a. Pop-Busui R, Boulton AJ, Feldman EL, et al. Diabetic Neuropathy: A position statement by the American Diabetes Association. Diabetes Care. 2017; 40(1):136-54. doi: 10.2337/dc16-2042.

32b. Xang Y, Xinhua H, Quiang Z, Zou R. Diabetes mellitus and risk of falls in older adults: a systematic review and metaanalysis. Age and Ageing. 2016;45(6):761-67. https://doi.org/10.1093/ageing/afw140.

33. American Association of Clinical Endocrinologists. *Type 2 Diabetes Management Goals.* Jacksonville, FL: American Association of Clinical Endocrinologists AACE (Cited 19 Jun 2019) On the Internet: https://www.aace.com/disease-state-resources/diabetes/depth-information/type-2-diabetes-glucose-management-goals.

34. Health Resources & Services Administration. *Lower Extremity Amputation Program (LEAP).* Rockville, MD: Health Resources & Services Administration (Cited 25 Jun 2019). On the Internet at: https://www.hrsa.gov/hansens-disease/training.html#leap-online.

35. American Diabetes Association: 11 Microvascular complications and foot care: Standards of Medical Care in Diabetes–2020. Diabetes Care. 2020;43(Suppl 1):S135-151.

36. Bainbridge KE, Hoffman HJ, Cowie CC. Diabetes and hearing impairment in the US: audiometric evidence from the NHANES, 1999-2004. Ann Intern Med. 2008;149:1-10.

37. McLellan M. Hearing *Loss and Diabetes: Does Your Patient Her Your Clearly?* (Cited 20 Jan 2020). On the Internet at: http://dbcms.s3.amazonaws.com/media/files/ef419745-09a7-48e6-a0bf-d81e74b9c27d/McLellan_OTCE_Winter_2012.pdf.

38. Rassmussen VF, Vestergaard ET, Heijlesen O, et al, Prevalence of test and smell impairment in adults with diabetes: a cross-sectional analysis of data from the National Health and Nutrition Examination Survey (NHANES), Prim Care Diabetes. 2018;12:453-9.

39. Kesavadev S, Misra A, Das AK, et al. Suggested use of vacines in diabetes. Indian J of Endocrinol Metab. 2012; 16(6):886-93.

40. Centers for Disease Control and Prevention. Use of hepatitis B vaccination for adults with diabetes mellitus: recommendations of the Advisory Committee on Immunization Practices (ACOP), MMWR Morv. Mortal Wkly Rep. 2012;60: 1709-11.

41. Centers for Disease Control and Prevention. Seasonal influenza (cited 26 Jan 2020). On the Internet at: https://www.cdc.gov/flu/prevent/nasalspray.htm.

42. Casanova L, Hughes FJ, Preshaw PM. Diabetes and periodontal disease: a two-way relationship. Br Dent J. 2014;217(8):433-7. doi: 10.1038/sj.bdj.2014.907.

43. Sanz M, Ceriello A, Buysschaert M, et al. Scientific evidence on the links between periodonaltal diseases and diabetes: consensus report and guidelines of the joint workshop on periodontal diseases and diabetes by the International Diabetes Federation and the European Federation of Periodontology. Diabetes Research and Clinical Practice. 2018:137:231-41.

44. Office of Disease Prevention and Health Promotion. Healthy People 2020: Diabetes. Washington, DC: Office of Disease Prevention and Health Promotion. (Cited 20 Jan 2020) On the Internet at: https://www.healthypeople.gov/2020/topics-objectives/topic/diabetes/objectives.

45. Kitzmiller JL, Gavin LA, Gin GD, Jovanovic-Peterson L, Main EK, Zigrang WD. Preconception care of diabetes: glycemic control prevents excess congenital malformations. JAMA. 1991;265:731-6.

46. Goldman JA, Dicker D, Feldberg D, Yeshaya A, Samuel N, Karp M. Pregnancy outcome in patients with insulin-dependent diabetes mellitus with preconception diabetic control: a comparative study. Am J Obstet Gynecol. 1986;155:293-7.

47. Rosenn B, Miodovnik M, Combs CA, Khoury J, Siddiqi TA. Pre-conception management of insulin-dependent diabetes: improvement of pregnancy outcome. Obstet Gynecol. 1991;77:846-9.

48. Tchobroutsky C, Vray MM, Altman JJ. Risk/benefit ratio of changing late obstetrical strategies in the management of insulin-dependent diabetic pregnancies. Diabete Metab.1991;17:287-94.

49. Willhoite MB, Bennert HW Jr, Palomaki GE, Zaremba MM, Herman WH, Williams JR, Spear NH. The impact of preconception counseling on pregnancy outcomes. Diabetes Care. 1993;16:450-5.

50. American Diabetes Association. Management of diabetes in pregnancy: Standards of medical care in diabetes–2020. Diabetes Care. 2020;43(Suppl 1):S183-92.

51. Boutlton AJ, Armstrong DG, Albeer SF, et al. American Diabetes Association, American Association of Clinical Endocrinologists. Comprehensive foot examination and risk assessment: a report of the task force of the foot care interest group of the American Diabetes Association with endorsement by the American Association of Clinical Endocrinologists. Diabetes Care. 2008:31:1679-85.

52. Bonner T, Foster M, Spears-Lanoix E. Type 2 diabetes-related foot care knowledge and foot self-care practice interventions in the United States: a systematic review of the literature. Diabet Foot Ankle. 2016;7:29758. doi: 10.3402/dfa.v7.29758. eCollection 2016.

53. Bonner T, Foster M, Spears-Lanoix E. Type 2 diabetes–related foot care knowledge and foot self-care practice interventions in the United States: a systematic review of the literature. Diabetic Foot & Ankle. 2016;7:1, 29758, DOI: 10.3402/dfa.v7.29758.

54. Powers MA, Bardsley J, Cypress M, et al. Diabetes self-management education and support in type 2 diabetes. The Diabetes Educator: 2015;41(6):417-30.

55. Funnell MM, Bootle S, Stuckey HL. The diabetes attitudes, wishes and needs second study. Clinical Diabetes. 2015;33:32-36.

56. Strain WD, Blüher M, Paldánius P. Clinical inertia in individualising care for diabetes: is there time to do more in type 2 diabetes? Diabetes Ther. 2014;5(2):347-54. doi: 10.1007/s13300-014-0077-8. Epub 2014 Aug 12.

57. Centers for Disease Control and Prevention. *Prevalence of Diagnosed Diabetes*. Atlanta, GA: Centers for Disease Control and Prevention; 2018. (Cited 20 Jan 2020) On the Internet at: https://www.cdc.gov/diabetes/data/statistics-report/diagnosed.html.

58. Elias EK, Golden SH. Race/ethnic difference in diabetes and diabetic complications. Curr. Diabetes Report, 2013; (13)6:814-23.

59. Lefebvre KM, Lavery LA. Disparities in amputations in minorities. Clin Orthop Relat Res. 2011;469(7):1941-50.

60. Golden SH, Brown A, Cauley JA, et al. Health disparities in endocrine disorders: biological, clinical, and nonclinical factors–an Endocrine Society scientific statement. J Clin Endocrinol Metab. 2012;97(9):E1579–E1639. doi:10.1210/jc.2012-2043.

61. Kurin AK, Cardarelli KM. Racial and ethnic differences in cardiovascular disease risk factors: a systemic review. Ethnicity & Disease. 2007;17(1):143-52.

62. Yang, L, Sepra L, Genter P, et al. Disparities in diabetic retinopathy screening rates within minority populations: differences in reported screening rates among african american and hispanic patients. Diabetes Care. 2016;39(3):e31-2. https://doi.org/10.2337/dc15-2198.

63. Van Beers CA, Devries JH, Kleijer SJ, et al. Continuous glucose monitoring for patients with type 1 diabetes and impaired awareness of hypoglycemia (IN CONTROL): a randomized open0lable, crossover trial. Lancet Diabetes Endocrinol. 2016;4(11):893-902.

64. Centers for Disease Control and Prevention. *National Diabetes Statistics Report, 2017*. Atlanta, GA: Centers for Disease Control and Prevention, U.S. Dept of Health and Human Services; 2017.

65. Veazie S, Winchell K, Gilbert J, et al. Rapid evidence review of mobile applications for self-management of diabetes. J Gen Intern Med. 2018 Jul;33(7):1167-76. doi: 10.1007/s11606-018-4410-1.

66. Davies N. Smart Technology for Diabetes Self-Care. Diabetes Self-Management: 2016, June. (Cited 20 Jan 2020) On the Internet at: https://www.diabetesselfmanagement.com/diabetes-resources/tools-tech/smart-technology-diabetes-self-care/.

67. Greenwood DA, Gee PM, Fatkin, KJ, et al. A systematic review of reviews evaluating technology-enabled diabetes self-management education and support. J of Diabetes Sci Technol. 2017;11(5),1015-27.

CHAPTER 10

Problem Solving

Carolé Mensing, RN, MA, CDCES, FADCES

Key Concepts

- Problem solving is a core outcome of diabetes self-management education and support (DSMES) and one of the core AADE7 Self-Care Behaviors®. Problem-solving skills are challenging skills to teach and also difficult skills to learn.
- Diabetes care and education specialists use both direct instruction and problem-solving skill building when identifying and assessing problematic situations and barriers that impact diabetes self-management.
- The problems that affect diabetes self-management occur on 3 levels: (1) clinical issues and emergencies, (2) self-management behaviors that could be problematic, and (3) problematic situations affecting self-management decisions.
- Diabetes care and education specialists can identify potential stages in diabetes management that support educational interventions: at diagnosis, annual health visits, emergence of new complicating conditions, and transitions in care.
- The assessment can identify possible problem situations and potential barriers affecting an individual's behavior.
- The diabetes care and education specialist can assist the individual in choosing approaches for future problem solving and identify individualized, effective methods tailored to each person.
- Technology offers new resources and skills for individuals to support their self-management
- When working in a group setting, the diabetes care and education specialist can offer to help select appropriate problem-solving strategies based on an assessment of the individuals or the specific characteristics of the group.

Introduction

Problem solving is an essential tool for diabetes self-management and for facilitating behavior change.[1] As one of the AADE7 Self-Care Behaviors®, problem solving can be applied to the other 6 behaviors: healthy eating, being active, taking medication, monitoring, healthy coping, and reducing risks. Problem solving is a skill that can be learned and applied to all diabetes self-care behaviors. However, problem-solving skills can be the most challenging for the diabetes care and education specialist to teach and for the person with diabetes to learn.[2]

Problem solving is not a onetime event. It is a complex, fluid process that involves active engagement from both the person with diabetes (which may include family, friends, others) and the diabetes care and education specialist. What makes problem solving a unique behavior is that it cuts across all AADE7 Self-Care Behaviors, which is why it is such an important skill for people to master in order to better manage their diabetes. Unlike the other six self-care behaviors, a foundation of knowledge and skills in the other six behaviors is helpful for first effective problem solving in diabetes self-management.[1]

This chapter discusses the application of problem-solving education by a diabetes care and education specialist so that individuals with diabetes can learn about effective problem-solving skills, recognition of situations or potential problems, and apply them to their own diabetes self-management.

What Is Problem Solving?

Problem solving is a core outcome of diabetes self-management education and support (DSMES) and is defined as follows:

> A learned behavior that includes generating a set of potential strategies for problem resolution,

selecting the most appropriate strategy, and evaluating the effectiveness of the strategy[3] and determining a broader variety of techniques.[4]

Theoretical Model

Theories and models provide the building blocks for teaching and practicing problem-solving techniques with individuals and groups. Problem solving is often conceptualized as a process involving these steps:

1. Identify the problem or situation.
2. Develop alternative solutions.
3. Select, implement, and evaluate the solution.

However, the ability of the person with diabetes to effectively execute these steps is affected by a number of environmental components, as described in Table 10.1.

The problem-solving components described in Table 10.1 exist within a specific setting and context within which the situation occurs. This includes the individual's social and physical environment and the observed characteristics of the situation (potential problem) itself.

As part of the assessment process, the diabetes care and education specialist can use the environmental observation, theory components, timing of diagnosis, treatment change, and observed behaviors as a guide for determining how best to begin working with the individual to introduce new skills or improve his or her existing problem-solving abilities.

Anticipated Situational Problem-Solving Opportunities

Powers et al identified critical times to assess for and provide DSMES: at diagnosis, at annual health and follow-up visits, when medical conditions change or become complicated, and when there is a transition in the person's care environment.[5]

The diabetes care and education specialist's awareness of these times in clinical care, follow-up encounters, class settings, phone discussions, etc, offers opportunities to introduce new skills or improve problem-solving abilities by identifying other possible solutions.

Using Problem Solving in Diabetes Self-Management

While knowledge is necessary, it is insufficient for effective and maintained self-management. Problem solving requires more than just knowledge or skill acquisition.[3] The diabetes care and education specialist must determine whether an individual's issue requires direct knowledge/instruction or support in seeking additional solutions.

Direct Knowledge Through Instruction Versus Problem Solving

Direct instruction refers to specific directions for a person with diabetes to follow. This can be used when there is a specific course of action to follow and it would be too great a risk for the person with diabetes to consider alternatives. For example, if there is only one way to use a specific device, like a blood glucose meter or continuous glucose monitor (CGM), then there is no need to generate alternative solutions. Following the instructions, practicing the skills, ensures appropriate and accurate usage of the device.

Direct instruction is recommended for situations meeting the following criteria. The identified situational problem:

- Is well defined and straightforward[6]
- Has a single best strategy for resolution[6]

TABLE 10.1 Components of Problem Solving

	Component	*Effective Behaviors for Problem Solving*	*Ineffective Behaviors for Problem Solving*
Environment The setting and context within which the problem occurs	Approach to problem solving	Rational, logical	Impulsive, careless, avoidant
	Motivation toward managing problems	Positive attitude	Negative attitude
	Ability to learn from prior experience and apply that learning to new situations	Able to learn from experiences and transfer this learning to new situations in an appropriate manner	Unable to learn from experiences and transfers this learning to new situations in an inappropriate manner
	Knowledge base	Sufficient, accurate, and applicable	Insufficient, inaccurate, and not applicable

Source: F Hill-Briggs, "Problem solving in diabetes self-management: a model of chronic illness self-management behavior," *Ann Behav Med* 25, no. 3 (2003): 182-93.

- Has a known, specific course of action that the individual with diabetes could utilize for situational problem resolution
- Could be detrimental or life threatening if using the trial-and-error approach

Two common examples are the following:

- Selection of a blood glucose site for self-monitoring—such as an ear lobe, fingertip, or forearm
- Selection of a CGM site such as the abdomen, back of arm
- Using trial and error for treatment of risky acute hypoglycemia or hyperglycemia, and acute illness

Issue: Detecting Hypoglycemia and Hyperglycemia

- *Direct instruction.* This includes education about the symptoms of hypoglycemia and hyperglycemia, how to monitor one's blood glucose using appropriate sites, technology (CGM), and when to check ketone levels, as well as being able to state the blood glucose levels that indicate hypoglycemia or hyperglycemia (ketones present) for that person with diabetes.
- *Problem solving.* This includes identifying specific and reliable symptoms the individual experiences during hypoglycemia or hyperglycemia, identifying any barriers to detection such as blood glucose unawareness, determining barriers to monitoring with appropriate frequency and sites, and problem solving how these data can be used to act quickly, appropriately, and adjust one's regimen with regard to medication, eating, and/or activity.

Preventing Hypoglycemia and Hyperglycemia

In the case of quick recognition and prevention of hypoglycemia and hyperglycemia, problem solving is a particularly important strategy to employ. Selecting the most appropriate and effective strategies for a given individual to integrate and maintain in their lifestyle will result from effective problem solving.

Problem solving can focus on identifying the unique situations that tend to lead to these acute complications in the individual's life, devising tailored strategies for prevention, developing strategies to address both daily and long-term resolution of barriers to effective self-management, and planning for ongoing adjustment or maintenance of self-management behaviors.

Identifying and Assessing Potential Problems and Barriers

Recognizing the emotional effect of diabetes, an individual's coping skill is included in an opening assessment. Then, initial step in situational problem solving is identifying the potential problems and possible barriers (situations that disrupt usual action) preventing the person with diabetes from solving or managing the situation.

Types of Problems

Problem identification occurs on 3 levels:

Level 1: Clinical markers and emergencies
Examples: Suboptimal blood glucose management, acute complications (including illness), ER visits

Level 2: Problematic self-management behaviors
Examples: Unhealthy meal or snack choices, sedentary lifestyle, medication misuse or omission due to medical appointments, procedures, travel time changes, severe weather

Level 3: Problems impacting self-management
Examples: Lack of self-management knowledge and skills, environment changes, personal issues, and interpersonal issues

Management examples include:

- When a person is referred for consultation due to difficulties with disease management (a level 1 problem).
- When assessment is needed to determine the individual's use of self-management behaviors, gaps in information, new technology opportunities (level 2). (See chapter 2 for more on assessment.)
- When providing education and counseling to identify gaps or improve these behaviors, level 3 factors must be determined. Once the level 3 problems are identified, they become prime times for problem-solving education or counseling.

Whether a problem exists on levels 1, 2, or 3, it becomes essential to both identify and manage the situation and/or barriers to addressing the problem. A quick reference summary is seen in the Association of Diabetes Care and Education Specialists paper, "An effective model of diabetes care and education: revising the AADE7 self-care behaviors."[1]

Types of Barriers

In working to better understand the variety of barriers the person may be facing when trying to resolve his or her self-management problems, it can be helpful to think of barriers in 3 broad categories:

1. Personal: Emotional well-being and depression,[7,8] physical disabilities, poor coping styles, cultural

or unusual health beliefs, and poor health literacy and numeracy skills

2. Interpersonal: Conflict with family or significant other, lack of rapport with diabetes care and education specialist or others on the healthcare team
3. Environmental: Financial barriers for middle-aged and older adults[9,10]; social pressures for children and adolescents; socioeconomic, language, and knowledge barriers for minorities[10,11,12]

For the healthcare educator, assessing and understanding these barriers is essential for ensuring that the problem-solving intervention is appropriate for the unique barrier the individual is experiencing. Barriers to problem solving must be identified in order to provide culturally sensitive care and to make sustainable change.

Each state, Washington, D.C., and the US territories have a diabetes prevention and control program (also known as the DPP) available to help diabetes care and education specialists identify community resources. The diabetes care and education specialist should be aware of local resources, including referral to the appropriate agencies and professionals. Conduct an Internet search on "Diabetes Prevention and Control Program & Your State/DC/territory" to find a local Web site.

Common Problem Areas, Associated Barriers, and Potential Approaches

People Self-management decisions can be influenced in both positive and negative ways by people in the person's life. This includes their family, friends, employer, healthcare team, and others who can have an impact on the person's behavior. For example, a diabetes care and education specialist might discover that what appears to be a person's unwillingness to adjust their eating habits stems from their perception that such a change could be an inconvenience to others in the family. Sometimes the problem may be family members who are not supportive, or it may be healthcare professionals who give incorrect information. Diabetes care and education specialists need to work with the person to identify the real issue and how others in their life may also be involved.

Resources Determine what type of resources the person may need to manage their diabetes. Do they have access to these resources? Are there local volunteer groups or support organizations in the area? Is the diabetes care and education specialist knowledgeable about the resources available within the person's community or healthcare team? Recent publications document the advantages of

TABLE 10.2 Who Is on the Healthcare Team?
The following are some of the people who can be on the healthcare team of the person with diabetes. All should be considered as resources when problem solving with your person with diabetes.
Person with diabetes and his or her family
Primary care provider (eg, physician, nurse-practitioner, advanced nurse practitioner)
Board-Certified-Advanced Diabetes Management (BC-ADM)
Certified Diabetes Care and Education Specialist® (CDCES)
Master Certified Health Education Specialist® (MCHES)
Nurse educator
Registered dietitian
Pharmacist
Eye doctor
Foot doctor
Dentist
Social worker
Psychologist
Psychiatrist
Marriage/family therapist
Exercise physiologist
Physical therapist
Trained healthcare worker/paraprofessional
Case manager
Health educator
Peer Counselor

Source: Adapted with permission from G Kanzer-Lewis, *10 Steps to Better Living With Diabetes* (Alexandria, Va: American Diabetes Association, 2007), 17.

American Association of Diabetes Educators, The Role and Value of Ongoing and Peer Support in Diabetes Care and Education. 2019 (cited 28 Jan 2020), on the Internet at: https://journals.sagepub.com/doi/epub/10.1177/0145721719882007.

American Association of Diabetes Educators, *Community Health Workers' Role DSMES and Prediabetes.* 2019 (cited 28 Jan 2020), on the Internet at: https://www.diabeteseducator.org/docs/default-source/practice/practice-resources/comp003.pdf.

including trained healthcare workers (paraprofessionals).[13] Table 10.2 identifies a number of the resources.

Financial Diabetes technology, equipment, and supplies can be expensive. Can the person with diabetes afford them? Does the person have insurance? If yes, does the person's insurance cover the equipment and supplies? Is the diabetes care and education specialist aware of agencies or resources that can provide assistance?

Scheduling Are appointments and classes available at appropriate times when people can attend them? Are weekend and evening appointments and classes available? Are they located near public transportation? How does the diabetes care and education specialist resolve scheduling problems?

Choice of Action Problems can arise when the person does not want to follow a specific course of action that may be of help to him or her. Could the person benefit from learning about other meal planning choices using the plate method or carbohydrate counting? Or, for example, is the person unwilling to change from oral meds to injections? Would a change in timing of the medication make a difference? Will the person agree to try a new injectable medication or medication injection device? Is a continuous infusion device such as an insulin pump an appropriate change? Would a different monitoring device be useful, less of a burden? Could a short-term loan or lease of a CGM offer more-detailed information? A diabetes care and education specialist can help the person assess options by creating a decision tree. Decision trees are discussed later in this chapter.

Strategy Based on Assessment Does this person need individual teaching or group session? Will the person be able to adjust to changes in their life? How can the diabetes care and education specialist help and support the person to make that happen?

Communication/Comprehension Each person is an individual with his or her own history and beliefs. How does the diabetes care and education specialist explain issues in a way in which they may better understand *and* learn methods to solve their situation and problems?

Constraints Are there other issues that prevent the problem from being solved? Does the person have language, budget, insurance, literacy, or numeracy issues that affect his or her ability to manage the medication regimen? Perhaps the person has physical conditions that will not allow him or her to inject his or her own insulin. See the following example.

AM is a married woman with a number of adult children who were very supportive of their mother's need to manage her diabetes. The whole family attended every class and physician visit. AM was injecting her own insulin and doing well, but she had a stroke and is unable to use her right hand to inject her insulin. The diabetes care and education specialist decided she could teach AM to use an insulin pen with her left hand. However, her family was adamant that her culture and religion did not allow her to use the "dirty hand" for administering medication.{ In her culture the right hand is for eating and for "clean tasks" such as brushing teeth and taking medication, and the left hand is the "dirty" hand for toileting. }

Initially, the diabetes care and education specialist was concerned that the family was setting rules that AM did not understand, but she spoke to AM and asked what she wanted to do. AM agreed with her family.

When working with individuals, the goal is to find a suitable solution, not to try to convince the person to do what the diabetes care and education specialist determines is best. Work with the family and the individual to solicit ideas and approaches that fit with their cultural beliefs. This helps everyone problem solve the situation together.

Identifying and Assessing Problems and Barriers: Gather the Facts

- What is the *real* problem? Sometimes the actual issue is hidden within many smaller problems.
- Who is affected? Aside from the person with diabetes, are others affected by the problem? Are they a barrier, or can they be part of the solution?
- Who should be involved in the decisions? Does the diabetes care and education specialist need to discuss the inclusion of family members, others in the discussion?

Table 10.3 provides examples of the barriers and strategies for addressing 4 self-care behaviors.

Create an Environment That Encourages Problem Solving

The diabetes care and education specialist can support problem-solving skills by creating an environment in which the person is comfortable in practicing new skills and honestly discussing the concerns, barriers faced in trying to self-manage their diabetes.

TABLE 10.3 Barriers to Diabetes Self-Management Behaviors

AADE7 Self-Care Behaviors®	*Barriers*	*Strategies for Addressing Barriers*
Healthy Eating	*Personal: "Health food tastes bad"*	Explore what health food means to them and ask what foods they have already tried.
	Interpersonal: "My mother cooks true to our culture and she won't change her cooking style for me"	Listen, seek clarification about what the person with diabetes eats (along with portion size), discuss family's willingness to change, and suggest a family discussion
	Environmental: "My school doesn't offer healthy options in the cafeteria"	Appreciate the challenge, create list of alternatives
Being Active	*Personal: "I'm not athletic"*	Promote discussion of the person with diabetes's perception of being active versus being an athlete
	Interpersonal: "I am committed to taking care of my family and don't have time to exercise"	Explore the person with diabetes's ambivalence about caring for self and commitment to caring for others, and discuss solutions. Also discuss the perception difference of "exercise" and "activity"
	Environmental: "I don't live in a safe neighborhood so I can't exercise outside"	Explore the perception of being active and help the person with diabetes create alternatives
Taking Medication	*Personal: "My grandmother died after taking insulin, so insulin will hurt me, not help me"*	Cognitive Behavior Therapy to assist in new cognitions
	Interpersonal: "My family will think I'm weak if I take medication"	Discuss and examine beliefs about family perceptions in a family meeting
	Environmental: "I don't own a car, so I can't drive to the pharmacy to pick up my medications"	Identify alternatives and assist in choosing solutions to obtain medication
Monitoring	*Personal: "I can just feel what my glucose is. I don't need to poke myself again"*	Seek understanding of why person with diabetes does this, and challenge with an actual blood glucose check to compare the actual number with the person with diabetes's guesstimate
	Interpersonal: "My wife gets woozy at the sight of blood, so for her sake I don't check my blood glucose"	Acknowledge concern for spouse, challenge the excuse, and help find alternative locations to check blood glucose
	Environmental: "I'm not allowed breaks at work to check my blood glucose"	Identify and role-play discussion points to be had with supervisor

- *Give permission to ask questions.* People may avoid asking questions unless they are encouraged to ask them. Diabetes care and education specialists can encourage persons with diabetes to keep a list of things they want to know about their diabetes and to bring the list with them to appointments. Remember to provide adequate detail, encourage additional questions, and request feedback to ensure they understand the meaning.
- *Offer a non-judgmental environment for checking skills; observing injection, BGM techniques, meal portion selection. Remember to remain neutral while performing their technique. Once completed, offer alternative suggestions, "Have you thought about . . . ?"*
- *Collaboration, not confrontation.* People may withhold information or lie to healthcare providers either because they fear they will be criticized or lectured by the diabetes care and education specialist or because they are concerned that they will disappoint their diabetes care and education specialist.[14] By establishing an environment that recognizes that the person will have setbacks and challenges, the diabetes care and education specialist and the person can be honest with each other and focus on collaborative problem solving rather than confrontation.
- *Confirm understanding.* The diabetes care and education specialist should be aware that the person

may not understand the language of diabetes and health care in the same way that the diabetes care and education specialist does.

For example, what does "fasting" mean? Does it mean no meat on Friday or no water or food for 8, 10, or 24 hours? Does it mean don't take your pills before the test, or take only your blood pressure pills and not your blood glucose pills? Telling someone that their blood lab work is better or worse is meaningless if they are just asked what their A1C is. People need to know and understand the significance of the values for them personally. Ask the person what their last blood work numbers were compared with the newest labs. Showing a trending graph of a lab value, for example, A1C each time is up or down, yet over time, it has continued to rise. To quote Fred R. Barnard, in 1927, "A picture is worth a (10,000) words."

- *Ask, don't tell.* If the diabetes care and education specialist **tells** a person what to do without asking what he or she is **willing** to do, the diabetes care and education specialist may inadvertently place themselves in conflict with the person's beliefs. The result is that the person is not open to the suggestion or now learning what is important information for self-managing their diabetes.
- *Prioritize.* Once situations, problems, or barriers have been identified, consider assisting the person to prioritize the problem(s) that need to be addressed first based on importance for both the person and their family and the diabetes care and education specialist. Willingness to change is increased when all are able to agree and to collaborate on the goals.

In prioritizing. It is important to consider the person's readiness for change and to be clear about the process and the goal. Recognition of how this situation fits into the hierarchy of needs; ie, safety, comfort, etc. is as important.[15] Some situational problems and barriers require personal actions, several may require action by the diabetes care and education specialist, and others require collaboration. See the following section for more information on determining when a problem could be solved by the diabetes care and education specialist, by the person and the diabetes care and education specialist together, or by the person and their family or caregiver.[15]

Applying Problem Solving in Diabetes Education

There are different ways that problem solving might be used within an education or counseling session:

1. Clinical problem solving by the diabetes care and education specialist
2. Personal observation or partial partner to problem solving primarily by the diabetes care and education specialist
3. Person as problem solver facilitated by the diabetes care and education specialist
4. Person and diabetes care and education specialist as collaborators, sharing in the decision making[16]

Clinical Problem Solving by the Diabetes Care Education Specialist

In this type of scenario, the diabetes care and education specialist, often the nurse or team leader, is the only problem solver.[17] This diabetes care and education specialist assesses the problem, plans a course of action or treatment with the team, and evaluates the effectiveness, eg, hospitalization for severe hypoglycemia, ketosis, etc.

Observer or Partial Partner Contributor to Problem Solving

In this scenario, the person may provide some input, but the diabetes care and education specialist takes the active role as the problem solver.[17] This approach should be used carefully and only under special circumstances, such as when time or other constraints of the education session necessitate a more directive role by the diabetes care and education specialist,[3,6,17] or when the person with diabetes is not able or prefers not to assume an autonomous role in decision making (see the section on special considerations later in this chapter). For example, some elderly persons with diabetes may need and prefer clear directions on how to manage a situation due to declining cognitive abilities such as memory, eg, living conditions, urgent transition to a new plan of care.

Facilitated Problem Solving by Diabetes Care and Education Specialist

In this scenario, the person with diabetes is the problem solver.[3,6,18] Notice that the diabetes care and education specialist, through skillful person-centered questions and responses, guides the person in using a problem-solving process to come up with his or her own solution(s)[18] or uses instructional methods to train the person in problem solving to resolve problems independently.[18] This person-centered approach is illustrated in the following example:

PWD: I've been having a hard time remembering to take my blood glucose and then my long-acting insulin at bedtime, and I end up high in the morning and feel terrible.
DE: What do you think gets in your way of remembering?
Pt: I don't know, it gets late and I want to go to bed and just forget. My mom used to remind me, but now that I'm on my own I don't have that reminder.
DE: How do you remember to get up in the morning, or go to class, or work?
Pt: I just set the alarm on my cell. I suppose I could give that a try for reminding myself to take my insulin. *[Available phone technology—apps, alarms—supports this approach.]*

Collaboration

Once a person receives their initial diabetes education, the collaborative approach between the person and the diabetes care and education specialist is preferred in helping the person feel engaged in the treatment and in follow-up planning. This team approach, where the health professional has the ideal diabetes information and the person has the self-knowledge of whether it can be implemented, facilitates clarity and a feeling of equalizing power. They are joining each other in a common direction, as shown in the following outpatient encounter example:

Diabetes care and education specialist (DCES): I see your A1C has been a bit high lately.
Person with diabetes (PWD): Yes, after I went to college I vowed I wouldn't have any more lows. So I've been running it high; it's safer.
DCES: So, how are you feeling?
PWD: A bit crabby, not too sharp, but I'm not having lows.
DCES: You know, there might be some other ways to not run so high and still stay safe. Do you know what I'm talking about?
PWD: You mean like test more?
DCES: That is one way, or take a little more insulin, wear a pump, watch your carbs a bit closer. Are you open to any of these? *[This approach uses the wording "test" instead of "check" and then gives the person with diabetes only a "yes or no" response option—limiting choices, and potentially stifling problem solving, and setting up the following strong response.]*
PWD: I'm not doing the pump! Or a CGM!
DCES: I'm not saying those are the only choices; I'm offering you a number of choices, based on what you're OK with. I know lows are unpleasant, and being in college you need to stay safe, but a high A1C isn't safe either. Let's work together to come up with a plan. *[This diabetes care and education specialist modifies the response, opens the option for discussion and seeking alternatives, and states empathy for how hypoglycemia is affecting this person's life.]*
An alternative approach might be to offer working together to figure out if the team has this person on the best treatment plan now that life has changed. The diabetes care and education specialist uses the approach that the person is not wrong, it may be the treatment plan. "Let's be detectives together and see if we can figure this out."

Therapeutic Relationship Through a Problem-Solving Approach

Maintaining a therapeutic rapport is essential throughout all stages of self-management education and counseling. The way in which problem solving is used can be a source of conflict between the individual and the diabetes care and education specialist. One study of such conflict described the perspectives of diabetes care and education specialists and individuals regarding different approaches to problem solving.[17] In this study, when the diabetes care and education specialist rather than the individual was in the role of problem solver, individuals viewed professionals as not understanding their difficulties and as unable to help them resolve problems. In contrast, a preferred model involves both the professional and the individual. They agree that the individual ought to take the problem-solver role, fostering both support and a planned action by the individual. A previously published model of problem-solving conflict is shown in Table 10.4.

Use of communication methods from empowerment,[19,20] shared decision making,[16] and solution-focused therapy approaches[16] also facilitate maintenance of a therapeutic relationship in which persons with diabetes feel valued, supported, and autonomous, becoming more whole "person (person with diabetes) centered" in the community of care planning.[21] To learn more about

TABLE 10.4 Conflict Between Person With Diabetes and Diabetes Specialist: Influence of Problem-Solving Approaches

Problem-Solving Approach	*Professional's Perception of the Person With Diabetes*	*Person With Diabetes' Perception of the Professional*
Failure-expecting approach Conflict deadlocked	"Person with diabetes is a problem"	"My diabetes care and education specialist has tried to help but has not been able to do so"
Compliance-expecting approach Conflict unchanged	"Person with diabetes has a problem that we can solve"	"My diabetes care and education specialist has decided how I should manage my diabetes but she has no idea how hard it is for me"
Mutuality-expecting approach Conflict resolved; situational reflection takes advantage of a potential for change in different points of view	"Person with diabetes is a problem solver"	"My diabetes care and education specialist understands how difficult it is for me to manage diabetes and has helped me problem solve how I can manage my blood glucose levels"

Source: Adapted with permission from Sage Publications Inc. V Zoffman, M Kirkevold, "Life versus disease in difficult diabetes care," *Qual Health Res* 15, no. 6 (2005): 758.

empowerment and solution-focused approaches, see chapter 3, on motivational interviewing and empowerment models.

Empowering the Person With Diabetes as Problem Solver

Planning for Problem-Solving Training and Intervention

The planning process for designing any training or intervention begins with assessing a person's needs and assets, which should include an assessment of his or her knowledge, skills, and beliefs. Understanding an individual's problem-solving skills is integral to designing problem-solving training and selecting intervention techniques.

Formalized Problem-Solving Assessment Strategies and Measures

Assessing problem solving in the context of self-management education provides useful information regarding the problem-solving skills or styles of the individual. This information helps guide the problem-solving training or education. In practice, interviewing (discussed in chapter 2, on assessment) is often used by the diabetes care and education specialist to determine an individual's intervention needs or priorities; however, formal measures are also valuable. Formal measures have the advantage of standardizing the problem-solving assessment while quantifying the person's problem-solving ability. Problem-solving assessment also allows for outcomes measurement to determine the impact of the intervention on an individual's problem-solving ability.[22]

Healthcare educators who have the resources may wish to conduct a large-scale self-management intervention and may consider using diabetes-specific or generic measures in evaluating their educational program. This could offer a variety of alternative problem-solving paths to choose from. It might also assist newer staff in problem-solving alternatives. However, the majority of healthcare educators intervene on an individual or small group basis and rely solely on regular clinical measures (A1C, body mass index [BMI], blood pressure, blood lipids, etc) and self-administered questionnaires to assess impact and outcomes which may limit useful data. Cardiometabolic indicators are more actively being assessed and offer additional educational opportunities for the diabetes care and education specialist and care options for the person affected by all aspects of diabetes.

Diabetes-Specific Measures

A majority of studies examining associations between problem solving and diabetes self-management behaviors or blood glucose management have used diabetes-specific measures.[11,22,6-25] These measures were administered in different formats (interviews, questionnaires), include various response formats (multiple choice, open-ended, Likert scales), and address different content (diabetes-specific knowledge-based problem solving, specific problem-solving style or ability).

Diabetes-Specific Problem-Solving Skill Training

Research studies have used a variety of methods to train individuals in diabetes-specific problem-solving skills and techniques. Some of these techniques include the use of visual media,[26] computer-based education, discussion group formats,[27] new technologies, and applications.[28] Interventions have also been conducted in a variety of different settings that include routine DSMES classes,[29,30] diabetes summer camps,[26] and primary care offices, support groups, senior centers, YMCA's, etc. Some studies have incorporated problem solving as part of a more comprehensive intervention approach,[30,31] while others have focused on problem-solving skills training, alternative approaches, or problem resolution as the core intervention. The ADCES has developed a tool for accessing, reviewing, and assessing new technologies to use in care practices. This Web-based technology resource, Danatech, can be accessed via the ADCES Web site.

Problem Solving: Individual Options

Self-directed learning has become a popular method to support the interested individual in building information, skills, decision making, and situational problem solving by use of media resources. Web-based independent learning modules with topic-specific information are available on a variety of subjects (eg, meal planning, weight loss, exercise). Smartphone applications ("there's an app for that") and skill-building tutorials (such as use of devices for blood glucose monitoring and CGM, specific device functions, and troubleshooting) are located on the manufacturer's Web pages. Social media and E-tivity opportunities, eg, communities of inquiry, blogs, e-learning classes, offer another resource opportunity.[32,33] The National Center for Telehealth & Technology (http://t2health.dcoe.mil) portfolio lists a number of self-directed problem-solving mobile apps.

While these media resources have increased in number, variety of topics, and popularity, there is ongoing debate regarding their utilization and effectiveness. Each of these resources offers information and self-directed learning. Diabetes care and education specialists will want to follow up with persons with diabetes who are utilizing these resources for their own problem-solving. Diabetes care and education specialists are advised to assess for accuracy, relevancy, and timeliness of this information, as it may impact the individual's treatment plan. Literature is supporting the use of social media and care management technology for increased successful engagement in self-care, improved outcomes, and the use of alternative documentation options.[28,34,35] This technology has appeal for a variety of age groups, lifestyles, comorbidities, and interests.

Problem Solving in Group Settings

In many ways the characteristics of working with a group are similar to the characteristics of working with individuals: The diabetes care and education specialist builds rapport, answers questions, and helps the person with diabetes develop and implement goals. But in a group setting, the person, the diabetes care and education specialist, and the group help identify, develop, and evaluate the goals.

In some cases, the group setting may be the first time the diabetes care and education specialist meets the person with diabetes; however, optimally, an individual assessment could still be completed. This can be done before the class starts or in a telephone conversation before or after the group class; the individual could also complete an assessment form and bring it to class. New technology offers onsite form completion on iPads, with direct uploading to a data system of immediate classroom use. The diabetes care and education specialist benefits from having baseline information about each person attending a session and can therefore individualize the group class content and meet the needs of all participants.[36] Using an exercise, such as in the examples below, at the beginning of the group program can be an effective tool for determining diabetes knowledge gaps among the group members. This method helps to surface potential misinformation, personal care concerns, or problems.

Example 1: Jeopardy!® Game Identifies Knowledge Deficit

At the beginning of the class, play a game similar to Jeopardy!® with the group members. The members answer questions about diabetes and receive a score. At the end of the class or course the game is repeated and the scores are compared as an outcome measurement tool. The diabetes care and education specialist can then identify, on the assessment tool, the lack or gain in cognitive knowledge. This type of group "quiz" game allows the entire group to identify similar situational problems and then work to solve them. In addition, the diabetes care and education specialist can develop exercises or activities to learn things about the group members and then revise the teaching plans accordingly for that individual or group.

Remember—any test or quiz only measures knowledge, not skills or attitudes.

Example 2: Problem-Solving Scenario—Delayed Appointment

MM is 49 years old, and insulin requiring. She has taken a Blood Glucose reading (in range), administered her insulin, and is in the waiting room for her routine NP clinical visit at 11:00 am.

By 11:45 she is still in the waiting room; her appointment is delayed due to a patient emergency. Her usual lunch meal time is 12:30 pm.

Have the participants discuss what things to prepare for in the following categories:

- Monitoring
- Meal
- Medication
- Activity

Discussion Points:

Monitoring—bring equipment to the appointment, re-check at usual time

Meal—bring a small snack, and treatment for hypoglycemia if needed

Medication—pack noon medication and carry with her to the appointment

Activity—check BG before driving, or leaving the clinic (in range, or as close as possible, or take precautions as needed)

Monitoring—bring equipment to the appointment, re-check at usual time

Meal—bring a small snack, and treatment for hypoglycemia if needed

Medication—pack noon medication and carry with her to the appointment

Activity—check BG before driving, or leaving the clinic (in range, or as close as possible, or take precautions as needed)

Example 3: True or False (Or Not a Clue)

Post flip chart paper around the room with True of False Statements written on them.

Provide participants with 3 colors of Stickies (Green for True, Red/Pink for False, Yellow for Not a Clue)

Participants place a sticky on the flip chart paper, indicating their choice.

Once everyone participates, the educator leads a discussion, observing the color of the answers, allowing for information discussion and "correct" answers to evolve. "How have you handled illness in the past?" allows for discussion and alternatives to be revealed.

Tip: some statements might be situational, both True and False. Example statements, "Alcohol raises Blood Glucose," or "If ill, withhold food as your glucose is already elevated."

Group participation and interaction for the adult learner add interest to the learning experience and may help the participant's comfort level. Opening activities allows for the participants to socialize, and may increase their group comfort level. This method allows for teachable moments to occur. It also helps the diabetes care and education specialist assess the audience's base knowledge, experience level, and determine priorities for content to be reviewed. These activities are sometimes referred to as icebreakers.

An interactive automated response system makes answers to a question anonymous and thus more objective and less personal. A hand clicker is used to group the answers and display them in the aggregate. Answers may be discussed and alternatives described. This interactive teaching tool is useful for both persons with diabetes and professional audiences.

Another potential skill-building tool that can be effective in one-on-one settings as well as in group settings is a decision tree. A decision tree is a graphical representation of all possible outcomes of a decision that one can think of related to the situation. The purpose of the decision tree is to show how the user's initial decision could impact later outcomes.

In the example in Figure 10.1, the person with diabetes doesn't want to take his medications. Rather than telling him why he needs to take the medications, the diabetes care and education specialist creates a decision tree with him so he can see, step by step, the consequences of a decision not to take his medications. The decision tree in Figure 10.1 starts with the question "Should I take meds?"

In Figure 10.2, the diabetes care and education specialist is using the decision tree tool to work with a person who does not want to monitor her blood glucose.

Special Considerations for Problem Solving

One reason situational problem solving is considered to be among the most difficult skills to teach and learn is

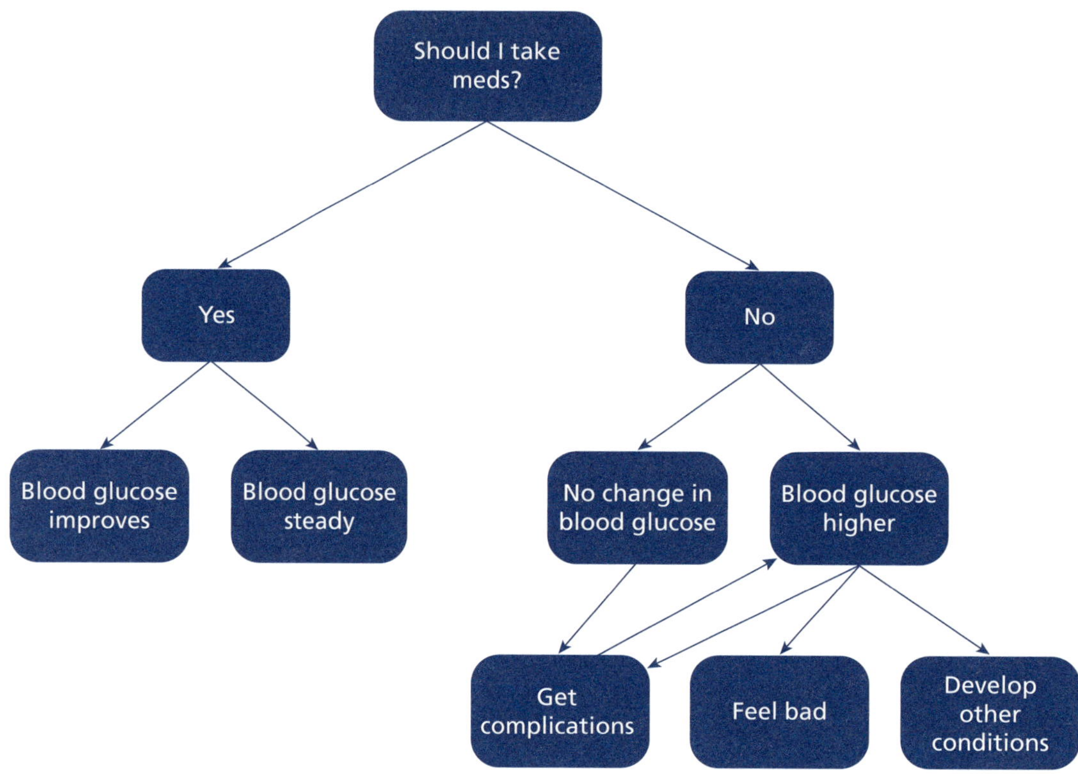

FIGURE 10.1 **Decision Tree: Should I Take Meds?**

that it is influenced by a number of factors. These factors are to be considered when planning or implementing problem-solving-based education.

Factors That Influence Problem Solving

1. Cognitive impairment: Because problem solving is a cognitive skill involving knowledge, some individuals may not understand enough to solve problems independently. These people may require the diabetes care and education specialist or their support structure to develop solutions to their problems.
2. Younger age: Children and adolescents solve problems differently, and problem-solving efforts should be aligned with the maturity level and cognitive development of each individual. There is no one right answer for each age group. The diabetes care and education specialist should work with the child, family, and support structure and healthcare team to decide what will work best for each child.
3. Older age: Older adults may have multiple physical conditions and psychosocial conditions to manage, in addition to diabetes, which may further complicate their lives. This may make problem solving more difficult and sometimes frightening. End-stage-of-life issues may result in family conflicts and confusion. People with diabetes should always be made aware and have input into decisions involving their care, even if they cannot participate fully.
4. Education: A higher level of educational attainment or literacy and numeracy does not necessarily mean the person has good problem-solving skills. It is important to evaluate each individual's ability to comprehend knowledge about their diabetes as well as their willingness and ability to address the problems and issues involved.
5. Cultural issues: To date, neither the diabetes scale nor intervention studies have examined whether diabetes-related problem-solving differences are related to ethnicity or culture. The diabetes care and education specialist should remember that factors including cultural appropriateness, education, and literacy should guide selection of strategies and materials for best outcomes.
6. Intellectual capacity: Individuals with depression, dementia, or other compromised cognitive

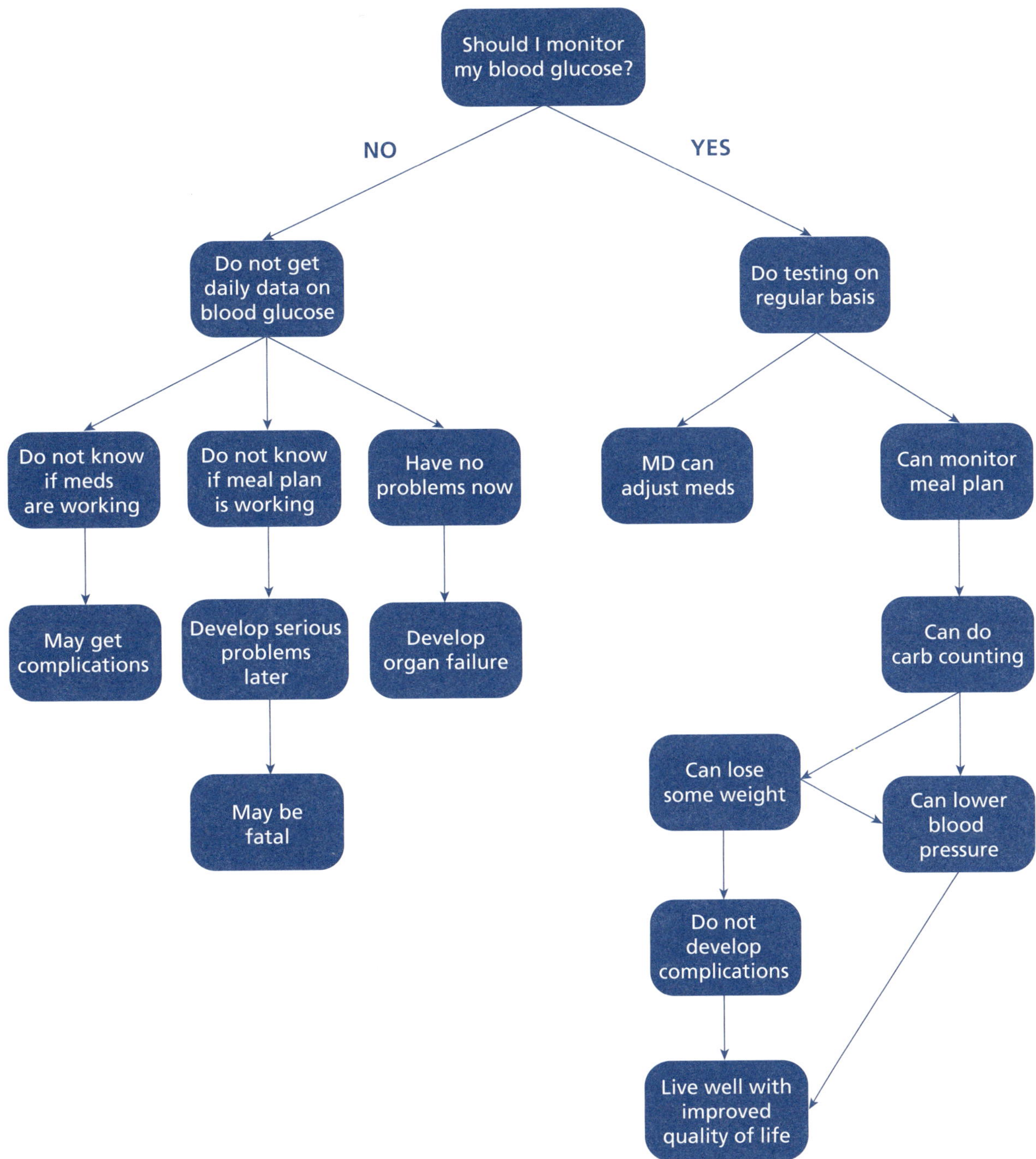
Should I monitor my blood glucose?
NO
YES
Do not get daily data on blood glucose
Do testing on regular basis
Do not know if meds are working
Do not know if meal plan is working
Have no problems now
MD can adjust meds
Can monitor meal plan
May get complications
Develop serious problems later
Develop organ failure
Can do carb counting
May be fatal
Can lose some weight
Can lower blood pressure
Do not develop complications
Live well with improved quality of life

FIGURE 10.2 **Decision Tree: Should I Monitor My Blood Glucose?**

executive functioning abilities are more challenging. Families, caregivers, and friends become an important part of the assessment, problem-solving, and planning process.

7. Fear of change: Change disrupts routine and may require new skills or new decisions. It may also involve money, technology, and altering relationships. The "unknown" is seen as exciting by some, and "scary" by others. Guidance from family, friends, and the diabetes care and education specialist offer a support system and safety net.

Case: Beliefs About Medicine

RC is a 68-year-old African-American man who was diagnosed with type 2 diabetes 3 years earlier. He was prescribed medications for diabetes and for hypertension at that time. RC stopped taking all the medications over 2 years ago because, "they make me sick." He added, "Pills cost money, and they don't work, anyway."

Progress:

Since the time he stopped taking his medications, RC has not returned to see the internist who was treating his diabetes. A cardiologist referred RC for counseling and education due to his poorly managed diabetes and hypertension and because of his refusal to take his diabetes and antihypertensive medications. RC was treated surgically by the cardiologist 6 years earlier for congestive heart failure stemming from a congenital heart defect.

RC feels he has done a good job of taking care of himself independently by making wise food choices, watching his weight, and taking vitamins.

Physical Assessment Results:

- Height: 68 in
- Weight: 182 lb
- BMI: 27.7
- Blood pressure: 161/81 mm Hg
- Does not smoke, quit 6 yrs ago

Lab Results:

- A1C: 9.7%
- Fasting blood glucose: 199 mg/dL
- LDL-C: 102 mg/dL
- HDL-C: 44 mg/dL

Home Life:

- Divorced, lives with his son
- Steelworker, 10th-grade education
- Sixth-grade reading level (Wide Range Achievement Test—WRAT-3), uses large print

RC reports that when he was diagnosed with diabetes, his internist prescribed oral medications for him. He was not sure what the medications were, but "the names were long" and he had difficulty finding out information about them. He reported that the medications made him feel sick, so he stopped taking them. When he told his internist about how the medications made him feel, the internist reminded him of the importance of continuing to take the medications. RC then decided that he would not return for follow-up visits, since he was not planning to take the medications anyway.

He reports a family history of diabetes. Both parents had diabetes. RC's father suffered a stroke and his mother suffered a heart attack. Both are deceased. He said his father always told him to be careful about medications because they "do more harm than good." RC believes strongly, as his father taught him, that medications are designed to help pharmaceutical companies make a profit and that the properties of medication and the side effects are harmful and should be avoided. RC does not believe that medications are good for the human body.

RC states that he manages his diabetes and blood pressure through healthy foods, herbs, vitamins, and other natural supplements. He reports that he does not add salt to foods. He shops for low-salt versions of foods like crackers and snacks. For breads, he relies on wheat and whole grains. RC does the cooking in his household. He often cooks large meals for his son and for neighbors, but he does not eat them "because I'm not supposed to have all that fried food." He often makes himself his favorite meal, spaghetti and meat sauce. He cooks with olive oil, prepares spaghetti sauce from a jar, and usually uses ground turkey instead of ground beef. He doesn't eat fresh fruits and vegetables, but buys canned vegetables that he cooks with seasoning salt for flavor, and often consumes frozen foods, processed meats, and cheeses. He eats canned fruits in light syrup. His weakness is candy bars, which he craves in the evenings. He states that he generally is able to resist his craving, but he keeps a few bars in his nightstand drawer in case he needs extra energy.

RC quit smoking 6 years earlier when he was diagnosed with congestive heart failure. He has arthritis that limits his ability to do rigorous exercise, but he does get physical activity through routine walking. He doesn't own a car, so getting from one point to another always involves some walking—either to and from the bus or to and from the destination itself. He feels confident that with his healthy eating and his walking he can manage his health without medication. He says, "What I can't do, I will turn over to God."

RC feels very confident that he is on the right track. He is hopeful about his ability to take charge of his health. He states that he plans to live to see his 100th birthday. The cardiologist wants to see RC learn more about behavioral methods for managing his blood glucose and blood pressure. He also hopes RC will return to see an internist, who will resume medications if RC's metabolic management has not shown any improvement in 3 to 6 months' time.

Case: Beliefs About Medicine (continued)

Questions for Consideration

1. RC appears disengaged from a problem-solving process because he feels he is already on the right track and doing a good job. Moreover, although his diabetes care and education specialist considers his refusal to take medication a problem, RC does not. Using components of the problem-solving model, how might you select ways to re-engage him?

Assess Diabetes-Specific Knowledge

RC's level of management does not match his stated understanding of diabetes and health behaviors—or his goal of seeing his 100th birthday. The discrepancy is an opportunity to establish that there is a problem to be worked on. What can be done?

First is to acknowledge the actions he has taken, giving credit for his efforts, building some trust with the diabetes care and education specialist. To help him evaluate whether he is fully on the right track and identify goals to work on, review target numbers for A1C, blood pressure, and BMI. Have him compare his current results with those targets. Ask if he knows why it is important for his numbers to be close to target. Share the connection between being in the target range and diabetes outcomes/complications; emphasize the importance of diabetes and blood pressure management for his heart. Provide information on how—and what—medications can help. Keep in mind that factors such as reduced literacy and difficulty seeing may have impeded his understanding of health information he received previously. Make sure wording and materials are at or below a sixth-grade reading level and in large-print format. Continue to acknowledge his participation, any progress made, and achievements, however small.

Assess Situational Problem-Solving Skills

Problem solving can be introduced as a self-management tool that will help RC figure out what's going on and what he can potentially change. What can be done? Help RC look at his current approach to dealing with his diabetes self-management (rational/logical, impulsive, careless, or avoidant). Reinforce that taking a logical, step-by-step approach will help him make the best decisions regarding his health and self-management behaviors.

Assess Problem-Solving Motivation

Connect managing his diabetes and blood pressure to his goal of living to see his 100th birthday. What can be done? Reinforce his approaches and emphasizing that problem solving is an opportunity for him to use new tools and work on skills for managing his diabetes—ones that could give him a potential chance at reaching his goal.

Discuss Transfer of Past Experience/Learning

RC has learned quite a bit about diabetes and managing diabetes from his parents and from his experiences. What he has learned may not achieve optimal self-management. This is an opportunity for RC to look at what he has learned from his parents' situations and what happened to them. What can be done? Encourage him to learn from both his parents' experiences and his own experiences so that his outcome will be different from theirs. Encourage him to think about modifying those things that have not been working as well as he thought.

2. Identifying possible situations, potential problems, and where to begin to make changes could be clarified by breaking his situation down into level 1, level 2, and level 3 problems. Here are some potential, immediate situational problems at each level.

Level 1: Clinical

- Suboptimal blood glucose levels, elevated blood pressure, complications

Level 2: Behaviors

- Desire not to take medication
- Suboptimal medical follow-up
- Some unhealthy eating patterns
- Experiences with delayed appointments, restaurant meals served late, Illnesses

Level 3: Environment

- Identify differences regarding the issue of medication taking.
- Although RC has stopped adding table salt to foods, he continues to have a high sodium intake through canned and jarred foods and seasonings.
- He is consuming more carbohydrate from canned fruit than he was aware of and keeps candy bars readily available for when he has cravings.

Barriers

- Personal: Beliefs about taking medications and about sodium in canned foods; likes candy bars
- Interpersonal: Cooks for others and they like fried foods; lack of communication or follow-up with internist

(continued)

Case: Beliefs About Medicine (continued)

- Environmental: Support people don't focus on his needs. The diabetes care and education specialist needs to include family in DSME classes.

3. Considering the 3 levels of problems can help clarify goals to be set. Level 1 goals were stated in the referral (improvement in blood glucose levels and blood pressure in 3 to 6 months). Level 2 has several areas for goals (medication taking, appointment keeping, healthy eating, increasing activity, monitoring). How might you help RC set level 2 goals?
   - Have him choose which level 2 problem he is willing to work on first.
   - Help him set a goal for the problem that is specific, easily measured, and realistic. (See chapter 2 for more on goal setting.) Give information about label reading and discuss the sodium content of canned food as opposed to frozen or fresh food.
4. Discuss with RC what he might want to alter to meet his goal of living a long life.
   - Help him identify what would give him the biggest payoff and motivate him to keep going.
   - Have him review his previous approaches, solutions for Insite Into success, and ones not useful.
   - Help him consider what he is most confident about being able to do.
   - Discuss his choices to help meet his overall goal, and let him identify what he can do given new facts about food and medications.
   - Determine his commitment to new skills, choices.
5. How might you help RC generate alternative solutions?
   - Have him brainstorm as many ideas as possible, without worrying about whether they will work, and then add additional ideas he might not have thought of. Then ask him what worked/did not work before.
6. How might you help RC select an alternative to try?
   - Have him consider what is most likely to work (stress desired outcomes while minimizing undesired outcomes) and to have the biggest payoff for his efforts.
   - Have him consider what is most doable and what he feels most confident about trying.
7. How would you help RC evaluate progress/achievements toward his goals?
   - Ask him what would be a sign that he was achieving some success with his goals and what would be a sign that he was not achieving his goals.
   - Have him keep a record of what he is trying and the outcomes; use worksheets to help RC commit to his chosen action plan and then evaluate whether it worked as he had planned and discuss what changes happened.
8. How would you plan a follow-up for RC?
   - See him for follow-up appointment(s) preferably throughout his progress toward completion of all identified goals, but at least identify progress of the first identified goal. Ideally, follow-up visits would extend over the 3- to 6-month time frame stated in the referral.
   - Use the time between follow-up visits to make check-in phone calls for him to report on progress or reevaluation. Suggest he keep some worksheets that document what he is working on and the outcomes of those efforts.

Summary

In this chapter, you learned that problem solving is defined as "a learned behavior that includes generating a set of potential strategies for situational problem resolution, assisting in the selection of the most appropriate strategy, applying the strategy, and evaluating the effectiveness of the strategy."[3]

Problem-solving techniques can be used to overcome problems and barriers encountered in day-to-day self-management situations, especially those that may have several possible solutions. However, direct instruction rather than trial and error is recommended for problems where the individual is at risk, such as hypoglycemia. The diabetes care and education specialist may choose to have a conversation with the individual in order to assess what he or she is doing well and what situations, concerns, problems, and barriers are affecting his or her self-management. Offering technology options helps to engage learners and may open clearer communication channels to surface concerns and situational problems, though there is evidence that adolescents may use technology in a reactive rather than preventive manner.

However, technology could facilitate some decision-making skills.[28,34,35]

Problems fall into 1 of 3 levels: clinical markers and emergencies, problematic self-care behaviors, and problems impacting self-management. It is essential to identify and understand the problems in order to better comprehend the nature of the individual's self-care problems. Barriers fall into 1 of 3 broad categories: personal, interpersonal, and environmental.

Another approach to problem solving is to utilize the decision tree. This may be useful and can be more engaging and fun to do with persons with diabetes. It is also a skill that may help the diabetes care and education specialists make decisions about their own diabetes education program, job, and indeed their own life.

Once problems and barriers are identified, people with diabetes and providers collaborate to prioritize them based on importance and readiness to change. Identified problems require action by the person, action by the provider, or collaborative action by both.

Information gathered from the individual (eg, personal, interpersonal, and environmental) can be used to design a tailored, solution-focused approach to problem solving. It may be helpful to use a motivational interviewing style in counseling individuals in developing problem-solving skills.

Many diabetes care and education specialists work with their clients in group settings. It can be challenging to work with several people at once; however, by establishing rapport with the group and effectively facilitating discussion, groups can feel empowered by having the opportunity to share experiences and offer their own expert experiences. As an individual presents a problem, other group participants can weigh in and learn to find their own answers/solutions.

In addition to group participation, technology options such as e-learning, mobile apps, and software programs are readily available and offer record-keeping, skill-building, feedback, and community support options. Danatech offers additional technology resources.

In order to provide effective care for either individuals or groups, it is important to take into account several factors that affect the cognitive process of problem solving, such as cognitive impairment, age, education, cultural issues, and urgent situations. Being aware of these factors will help the healthcare educator plan the most effective problem-solving counseling interventions.

The emerging role of the skilled community health worker (paraprofessional) expands the individual contacts and support options available in the community.

Problem solving and self-management situations are not a onetime event. They are a complex, fluid process that involves active engagement from the person with diabetes, family, caregivers, and the diabetes care and education specialist. What makes problem solving a unique behavior is that it cuts across all AADE7 Self-Care Behaviors®, which is why it is such an important skill for individuals to master in order to better manage their diabetes.[1]

Focus on Education

Teaching Strategies

When to use situational problem solving? Problem solving is best used when there are a variety of situations to review and options or courses of action from which to choose and learn from. People with diabetes will appreciate a collaborative approach that fits with their preferences, lifestyle, and goals. Remember, it is their life and they are responsible for managing their own care.

Interviewing techniques. Use a variety of interviewing techniques and skills to identify situations, problems, and barriers that will be the focus of problem solving. Identify the problem-solving ability of the individual—for example, by role-playing or discussing alternatives to real-life situations. Trying new techniques like games and exercises as an assessment strategy instead of formal interviewing sessions can be more interesting for you as well as the individual. It can be useful in assessing your own classes and teaching techniques as well as knowledge levels of your participants.

Techniques for empowerment. Work with the person's goals, not just the diabetes care and education specialist's goals. Assist with identifying what is most important to each person and setting realistic goals that fit with their priorities. Make sure you know how to create and set goals that are measurable, realistic, sustainable, and clear. Goals should be attainable and meaningful; avoid setting goals that are impossible to reach. Empower the person by building on successes, progression toward achievement.

Avoid using words with negative connotations (eg, "bad" numbers, unmotivated, noncompliant). Instead, use words focused on the positive (*making progress, looking at the treatment plan for any gaps*, etc). Focus on the appropriateness of the care plan as well as the person's approaches. Use positive terms ("situation" more often than "problem," "person with diabetes" more often than "patient").

Tailored approaches to problem solving. Approaches need to fit the capability and preference of the individual. Using motivational interviewing styles and skills can help the person feel more empowered and competent. An individual who believes that the diabetes care and education specialist is supportive and truly understands him or her is more apt to work to identify situations and solve problems. Shared decision making and selection of a variety of approaches support this strategy.

Utilizing technology resources, e-learning, and other social media or Web-based media may offer additional sources of information. This information should be evaluated for timeliness, accuracy, and relevancy and individualized for appropriateness to the person's treatment plan. More research is needed to support a better understanding of the nature of technology and its utilization in situational problem solving for all ages, extenuating situations, and all stages of the disease process. The Association of Diabetes Care & Education Specialists', Danatech, is a reliable online technology resource.

Focused on the person. Each person knows the diabetes care and education specialist cares about him or her, and sometimes, in an effort to please, the person will not always tell the truth. If the individual does not achieve the goals that were set or continue the activities he or she was taught, the goals can be reevaluated, rewritten, or placed on hold. People may need to be reminded that they are in charge of their lives and that the diabetes care and education specialist's job is to provide them all the information they need to make decisions that work for them in order to succeed in their diabetes self-management.

Messages for Persons With Diabetes

Problem solving is a learned skill. By identifying potential risk situations, discussing alternatives, and brainstorming solutions, you can develop effective problem-solving skills.

Identifying potential situations, possible problems, and the variety of possible solutions takes time. To broaden possible solutions, discuss, role-play, and consider the experiences of others (eg, friends with diabetes, caregivers) and the different approaches they may offer. This collaboration will strengthen problem-solving skills when unusual situations are present, such as traveling, rotating work schedules, snowstorms, illness, and other situations that alter the daily routine.

"Situations" are the day-to-day events that just happen, or could happen; "problems" are those which interfere with desired outcomes, and "problem-solving" is the learned skill to prepare for these events.

Health Literacy and Fluency

Early in the assessment, determine the person's health literacy ability. Even the most well-educated individual who is fluent in many skills, may not be well-versed in the language of health care and available resources. Literacy includes fluency in language vocabulary and healthcare resources.[37]

Individual "person with diabetes"-focused education versus content-driven teaching. People with diabetes need to learn new information and skills by a method that allows them to retain the content and apply it in practice. "Person with diabetes"-focused methodology allows people with diabetes to interpret the content/information in their own way. They may need to internalize the information and come up with their own strategies to implement it. In order to internalize the information, people need to have the opportunity to hear it, think about it, and verbalize their understanding of the information.

What can people with diabetes teach diabetes care and education specialists? A person who is not engaged with his or her diabetes regimen often has misinformation or mistaken understanding, or sometimes knows why he or she was not able to implement or do what he or she should be doing. It is counterproductive for the diabetes care and education specialist to keep on teaching the same information in the same way while knowing that it does not work. (The same information will continue to bring about the same results.) The diabetes care and education specialist could ask the following questions: What do you think you can do to . . . ? What might you have done differently to . . . ? What are you going to do about this challenge? How will you know if this made a difference? Asking these kind of open-ended questions or statements asking for conversation are useful. Asking questions with a "yes" or "no" response does not encourage participant conversation or participants to think about their answers.

Educating versus facilitating. Diabetes care and education specialists are dedicated and determined to teach persons with diabetes information that they need to know in order to manage their diabetes. As facilitators, diabetes care and education specialists assist in altering the learning process. They navigate the teaching process, focus on the person's individualized agenda, and give him or her an opportunity to process the content. It is not about diabetes care and education specialist and what they know, but about the person with diabetes and what they know and whether they are open to new opportunities to learn.

Education is all about retention and application of information. Explore all the information by answering the 5 Ws and 1 H questions (who, what, where, when, why, and how). People learn best when they practice, perform, and work with new knowledge, skills, and attitudes. Self-reflection is also an important part of learning. A follow-up visit allows individuals to verbalize what they have discovered, what they have tried to do, how they feel about it, and what their strategy is to keep the momentum.

Focus on Practice

The diabetes education delivery systems are encouraged to align with the assumption of andragogy, or the art and science of helping adults learn[38]

- *Changes in self-concept:* As people develop with age, so does their perception on life and self-care. People with diabetes need to be given continuous opportunities to self-reflect on existing circumstances and how diabetes fits within them.
- *The role of experience:* As people mature, they define who they are by their environment at that time. They may be influenced by their coworkers, church, children, or financial status, as well as factors such as well-being, health, and pain management.
- *Readiness to learn:* As people mature, their perspective on learning progresses from "other directed"—what they "ought to" learn because of their biological and academic development—to what they "need to" learn to problem solve (situational problem solving) because of the development phases they are approaching in their roles as workers, spouses, parents, leaders, leisure time users, and so forth.
- *Orientation to learning:* Most of the learning among children is subject-centered, whereas among adults it is problem-centered.

References

1. Association of Diabetes Care and Education Specialists (ADCES). An effective model of diabetes care and education: revising the AADE7 self-care behaviors®. Published online ahead of print, Feb 2020. Diabetes Educ. doi: https://doi.org/10.1177/0145721719894903.
2. Bonnet C, Gagnayre R, d'Ivernois JF. Difficulties of diabetic person with diabetess learning about their illness. Person with diabetes Educ Couns. 2001;42(2):159-64.
3. Mulcahy K, Maryniuk M, Peeples M, et al. Diabetes self-management education core outcomes measures. Diabetes Educ. 2003;29(5):790-1.
4. Marriott J, Davies N, Gibson L. Teaching, learning and assessing statistical problem solving. J Stat Educ. 2009;17(1):790-1.
5. Powers M, Bardsley J, Cypress M, et al. Diabetes self-management education and support in type 2 diabetes—a joint position statement of the American Diabetes Association, the American Association of Diabetes Educators, and the Academy of Nutrition and Dietetics. Clin Diabetes. 2016;34(2):70-80.
6. King EB, Schlundt DG, Pichert JW, Kinzer CK, Backer BA. Improving the skills of health professionals in engaging person with diabetess in diabetes-related problem solving. J Contin Educ Health Prof. 2002;22(2):94-102.
7. Hill-Briggs F, Cooper DC, Loman K, Brancati FL, Cooper LA. A qualitative study of problem solving and diabetes control in type 2 diabetes self-management. Diabetes Educ. 2003;29(6):1018-28.
8. Ciechanowski PS, Katon WJ, Russo JE. Depression and diabetes: impact of depressive symptoms on adherence, function, and costs. Arch Intern Med. 2000;160(21):3278-85.
9. Hill-Briggs F, Gary TL, Hill MN, Bone LR, Brancati FL. Health-related quality of life in urban African Americans with type 2 diabetes. J Gen Intern Med. 2002;17(6):412-9.
10. Schoenberg NE, Drungle SC. Barriers to non-insulin dependent diabetes mellitus (NIDDM) self-care practices among older women. J Aging Health. 2001;13(4):443-66.
11. Lawton J, Ahmad N, Hanna L, Douglas M, Hallowell N. "I can't do any serious exercise": barriers to physical activity amongst people of Pakistani and Indian origin with type 2 diabetes. Health Educ Res. 2006;21(1):43-54.
12. Samuel-Hodge CD, Headen SW, Skelly AH, et al. Influences on day-to-day self-management of type 2 diabetes among African-American women: spirituality, the multi-caregiver role, and other social context factors. Diabetes Care. 2000;23(7):928-33.

13. American Association of Diabetes Educators. Community health workers in diabetes management and prevention. AADE practice synopsis. 2015 Jun (cited 2016 Jul). On the Internet at: https://www.diabeteseducator.org/docs/default-source/default-document-library/community-health-workers-in-diabetes-management-and-prevention.pdf?sfvrsn=0.

14. Kanzer-Lewis G. Ten Steps to Better Living With Diabetes. Alexandria, Va: American Diabetes Association; 2008:18.

15. Cherry K. Maslow The five levels of Maslows Heirarchy of needs, How Maslow's famous heirarchy of needs, explains human motivation. Theories. Behv Psych. 2018.

16. Tamhane S, Rodriguez-Gutierrez R, Hargraves I, Montori VM. Shared decision making in diabetes care. Curr Diab Rep. 2015;15(12):112.

17. Zoffmann V, Kirkevold M. Life versus disease in difficult diabetes care: conflicting perspectives disempower person with diabetess and professionals in problem solving. Qual Health Res. 2005;15(6):750-65.

18. Bodenheimer T, Lorig K, Holman H, Grumbach K. Patient self-management of chronic disease in primary care. JAMA. 2002; 288(19);2469-75.

19. Anderson RM, Funnell MM, Barr PA, Dedrick RF, Davis WK. Learning to empower person with diabetess: results of professional education program for diabetes educators. Diabetes Care. 1991;14(7):584-90.

20. Anderson B, Funnell MM. The Art of Empowerment: Stories and Strategies for Diabetes Educators. Alexandria, Va: American Diabetes Association; 2000.

21. GSI Health.com; Value-Based Care, the Future of Health Care, 2016. White paper.

22. Glasgow RE, Toobert DJ, Barrera M Jr, Strycker LA. Assessment of problem-solving: a key to successful diabetes self-management. J Behav Med. 2004;27(5):477-90.

23. Cook S, Aikens JE, Berry CA, McNabb WL. Development of the diabetes problem-solving measure for adolescents. Diabetes Educ. 2001;27(6):865-74.

24. Hill-Briggs F, Yeh HC, Brancati FL. Development of the diabetes problem-solving scale. Ann Behav Med. 2005;30 Suppl:S-091.

25. Hill-Briggs F, Gary TL, Yeh HC, Batts-Turner M, Brancati FL. Validity of a novel diabetes problem-solving scale. Diabetes. 2005;54 Suppl 1:A471.

26. Schlundt DG, Flannery ME, Davis DL, Kinzer CK, Pichert JW. Evaluation of a multicomponent, behaviorally oriented, problem-based "summer school" program for adolescents with diabetes. Behav Modif. 1999;23(1):79-105.

27. Cook S, Herold K, Edidin DV, Briars R. Increasing problem solving in adolescents with type 1 diabetes: the choices diabetes program. Diabetes Educ. 2002;28(1):115-24.

28. Greenwood, DA, Gee PM, Fatkin KJ, Peoples M, A systematic review of reviews evaluating technology enabled diabetes self-management education and support. J Diabetes Sci Technol. 2017;11(5):1015-27.

29. Rubin RR, Peyrot M, Saudek CD. Effect of diabetes education on self-care, metabolic control, and emotional well-being. Diabetes Care. 1989;12(10):673-9.

30. Wysocki T, Harris MA, Greco P, et al. Randomized, controlled trial of behavior therapy for families of adolescents with insulin-dependent diabetes mellitus. J Pediatr Psychol. 2000;25(1):23-33.

31. Grey M, Boland EA, Davidson M, Li J, Tamborlane WV. Coping skills training for youth with diabetes mellitus has long-lasting effects on metabolic control and quality of life. J Pediatr. 2000;137(1):107-13.

32. Wright P. "E-tivities from the front line": a community of inquiry case study analysis of educators' blog posts on the topic of designing and delivering online learning. Educ Sci. 2014;4(2):172-92.

33. TKI. Beyond the classroom. 2016 Jul. On the Internet at: http://elearning.tki.org.nz/Beyond-the-classroom.

34. Kumah-Crystal YA, Ho K, Ho YX, et al. Technology for diabetes problem solving in adolescents with type 1 diabetes: relationship to glycemic control. Diabetes Technol Ther. 2015;17(7):449-54.

35. Markowitz JT, Harrington KR, Laffel LM. Technology to optimize pediatric diabetes management and outcomes. Curr Diabetes Rep. 2013;13:877-85.

36. Beck J, Greenwood DA, et al. 2017 National standards for diabetes self-management education and support. The Diabetes Educator. 2018;44(1):35-50.

37. Osbourne H. Health Literacy from A to Z: Practical Ways to Communicate Your Health Message. 2nd ed. Burlington, Mass: Jones & Bartlett Learning; 2011.

38. Knowles M, Holton EF, Swanson RA. The Adult Learner: The Definitive Class in Adult Education and Human Development. 7th ed. Oxford, UK: Butterworth-Heinemann; 2011:138, 140.

CHAPTER 11

Diabetes Education Program Management

Mary Jean Christian, MA, MBA, RD, CDCES

Key Concepts

- Diabetes care and education specialists have opportunities to establish and manage diabetes self-management education and support (DSMES) programs, that may also include diabetes prevention programs (DPP), but they may need to augment their skill set to manage the operational and business aspects of these programs.
- The process of establishing and managing a DSMES program is similar to the 5-step process of DSMES:
  1. assessment
  2. goal setting
  3. planning
  4. implementation
  5. evaluation/monitoring/documentation.
- Whether starting a new DSMES program or managing an existing program, the business skills required include program financial management, strategic planning, human resource management, integration of technology, marketing, quality improvement, and outcomes management.
- Because managing an education program usually involves completing an application for accreditation from the Association of Diabetes Care and Education Specialists (ADCES) or recognition from the American Diabetes Association (ADA), awareness of critical components in this process is helpful for program managers for appropriate resource allocation.

Introduction

Access to quality, formal diabetes education should be a right of all Americans with diabetes. The government-sponsored initiative Healthy People 2020 continues to have as one of its key objectives, "to increase the proportion of persons with diagnosed diabetes who receive formal diabetes education." Currently, only 57% of adults with diabetes reported ever receiving some sort of formal diabetes education.[1] Recent data reveal that insurance coverage is not a barrier, as only 6.8% of individuals with newly diagnosed type 2 diabetes with private insurance[2] and only 5% of Medicare participants[3] received diabetes self-management education and support (DSMES) within 12 months of diagnosis.[2] Although insurance coverage for DSMES has improved, beneficiaries are often faced with large co-pays for this service and defer enrollment. However the medical nutrition therapy (MNT) benefit is exempt from deductibles/co-pays and a registered dietitian diabetes care and education specialist can be employed to provide services to bridge the gap until deductibles have been met and the co-pay for DSMES is less.

Thus, there is an opportunity for diabetes care and education specialists to establish, operate, and manage effective and efficient quality DSMES/DPP programs. While diabetes care and education specialists are experts in the subject of diabetes, they may be less comfortable with their skills as a program manager when it comes to the overall management and business operations of a program. The purpose of this chapter is to highlight the essentials of program operations. It is intended to be relevant for the diabetes care and education specialists who find themselves starting a new program or who are being asked to manage an existing program. In this chapter, the term *program* is used broadly to include DSME in all delivery models, ranging from a small service provided by one diabetes care and education specialist in a physician office, to a large multidisciplinary comprehensive program delivered in an academic medical center, and everything in between, including diabetes education delivered in retail pharmacies, local health clinics, and independent practices. The term *program manager* is used to describe the diabetes care and education specialists with program management responsibilities. This term applies to both diabetes care and education specialists for whom program management is a full-time job and diabetes care and education specialists who are solo practitioners filling all roles, including counseling persons with diabetes on all relevant topic areas as well as overseeing the operations of the program. Diabetes care and education specialists in the role of program manager have the opportunity to drive integration in chronic disease management incorporating diabetes prevention program and diabetes self-management education and support into population health models of care.

The process of starting and running a diabetes education program is very similar to the 5-step process of DSME as described in the *AADE Scope of Practice, Standards of Practice, and Standards of Professional Performance for Diabetes Educators*.[4] The steps for providing DSMES are as follows:

1. Assessment
2. Goal setting
3. Planning
4. Implementation
5. Evaluation/monitoring/documentation

Keeping these steps in mind will help organize the process for the program manager. This chapter is organized into 3 sections. It first addresses the steps involved in starting a DSMES program (assessment, goal setting, and planning). Then it moves into operating and maintaining a program (implementation) and concludes with program evaluation, monitoring, and documentation. These same steps can be used to incorporate a DPP into the DSMES services.

As access to education services increases and more people with diabetes are able to take advantage of diabetes education programs, the nation will come closer to not only meeting but exceeding the Healthy People 2020 goals.

Starting a Diabetes Self-Management Education and Support Program

Assessment

As part of good person with diabetes care, the diabetes care and education specialist understands the importance of a thorough assessment to design the best education intervention for the person with diabetes. Similarly, to design a successful diabetes education program, the diabetes care and education specialist in the role of program manager must also do a thorough assessment. Questions such as the following will need to be answered as part of the assessment:

What are the expectations for the program? (to improve diabetes outcomes? to bring in more persons with diabetes to the hospital system? to reach into underserved populations? to incorporate DPP?)

What resources exist? (staff? budget? educational materials?)

Who is the target population and what are their needs? (existing persons with diabetes? new persons with diabetes? Or is the target to serve large groups of primary care physicians who could be bringing other business to a hospital system?)

Are there similar programs in the region, and how might this program be similar or different? (hospital based? private practice? programs within provider offices?)

Assess Expectations and Guidelines

If the program is part of a larger organization or business (such as a hospital, pharmacy, or medical office), it is important to make sure that the expectations of the administrators are understood. Does the senior leadership expect a program that will reach a certain target population? Break even in terms of expenses? Contribute revenue to other departments? It is critical for the program manager to understand as fully as possible what expectations are held by the executive team. If expectations are not realistic, the program manager needs to discuss with the leaders what may actually be possible, instead of focusing on what is *not* likely to happen.

A thorough understanding of the National Standards for Diabetes Self-Management Education and Support (NSDSMES) is essential to starting and running a quality diabetes education program.[5] The National Standards are guidelines designed to define quality DSMES and to assist diabetes care and education specialists who work in a variety of settings to provide evidence-based diabetes education. The most recent review and revisions acknowledge the importance of ongoing support for sustaining behavior change, and thus the name of the standards was revised to emphasize this. Table 11.1 provides a summary of the 10 standards. To receive Medicare reimbursement for services, the program manager must demonstrate that every standard has been met.

TABLE 11.1 National Standards for Diabetes Self-Management Education and Support (NSDSMES)

Standard 1: Internal structure	The provider(s) of DSMES will define and document a mission statement and goals. The DSMES services are incorporated within the organization—large, small, or independently operated.
Standard 2: Stakeholder input	The provider(s) of DSMES will seek ongoing input from valued stakeholders and experts to promote quality and enhance participant utilization.
Standard 3: Evaluation of Population Served	The provider(s) of DSMES will evaluate the communities they serve to determine the resources, design, and delivery methods that will align with the population's need for DSMES services.
Standard 4: Quality Coordinator Overseeing DSMES Services	A quality coordinator will be designated to ensure implementation of the Standards and oversee the DSMES services. The quality coordinator is responsible for all components of DSMES, including evidence-based practice, service design, evaluation, and continuous quality improvement.
Standard 5: DSMES Team	At least 1 of the team members responsible for facilitating DSMES services will be a registered nurse, registered dietitian nutritionist, or pharmacist with training and experience pertinent to DSMES, or be another healthcare professional holding certification as a diabetes care and education specialist (CDCES) or Board Certification in Advanced Diabetes Management (BC-ADM). Other healthcare workers or diabetes paraprofessionals may contribute to DSMES services with appropriate training in DSMES and with supervision and support by at least one of the team members listed above.
Standard 6: Curriculum	A written curriculum reflecting current evidence and practice guidelines, with criteria for evaluating outcomes, will serve as the framework for the provision of DSMES. The needs of the individual participant will determine which elements of the curriculum are required.
Standard 7: Individualization	The DSMES needs will be identified and led by the participant with assessment and support by one or more DSMES team members. Together, the participant and DSMES team member(s) will develop an individualized DSMES plan.
Standard 8: Ongoing support	The participant will be made aware of options and resources available for ongoing support of their initial education, and will select option(s) that will best maintain their self-management needs.
Standard 9: Participant progress	The provider(s) of DSMS services will monitor and communicate whether participants are achieving their personal diabetes self-management goals and other outcome(s) to evaluate the effectiveness of the educational intervention(s), using appropriate measurement techniques.
Standard 10: Quality improvement	The DSMES services quality coordinator will measure the impact and effectiveness of the DSMES services and identify areas for improvement by conducting systematic evaluation of process and outcome data.

Source: J Beck, D Greenwood, et al, "2017 National Standards for Diabetes Self-Management Education and Support," The Diabetes Educator. 2017; 43(5):449-64.

Assess Available Resources

As part of the assessment process, the program manager must determine what is available in terms of existing resources and what needs to be acquired (purchased) or developed. As a first step, the program manager may assess his or her own competencies, skills, and experience and compare them with those outlined in the ADCES *Competencies for Diabetes Care and Education Specialists*. Within that resource, a series of objectives for both program and business management provides the newly appointed program manager with specific guidance for skills and knowledge he or she may need to acquire in order to be successful in the role.

Look for ways to develop and launch a program that makes the most efficient use of resources as possible. Ask questions that assess the program's finances: Has a budget been allocated for the program? Will the program manager be able to control the budget and plan for allocation of resources for staff, materials, continuing education training, marketing, materials development, etc? The most expensive resource is staff. It may sound ideal to have a full-time nurse educator, a full-time dietitian, and a full-time secretary, but can the volume of persons with diabetes you are projecting justify the staff desired? It is better to start small with part-time staff and ramp up as needed. Likewise, it may be ideal to have your own classroom or your own equipment (such as a projector), but this can also be costly. Can space and equipment be shared with other departments or programs? Ensure the resources necessary to meet the program expectations of senior leadership are available. For example, if the leaders requesting a DSMES program are expecting to review clinical outcomes on the entire population of persons with diabetes getting DSMES, an electronic health or education record of some sort will be a necessary investment.

It may be helpful to keep your scope of services narrow at first, so the program does not have to acquire too many resources or stretch the staff too thinly. For example, the logical place to start may be to serve a population of adults with diabetes, with a focus on the major minority group in your community that has a high incidence of diabetes. Adding services for pediatrics or gestational diabetes, or adding other languages, may have to wait until the program is well established. It may be to the program's advantage financially to have a registered dietitian on the team who can also bill for medical nutrition therapy (MNT), as that allows for another set of services to be offered.

Assess Community Needs

When a diabetes care and education specialist conducts an assessment of the needs of the person with diabetes in order to understand the person's diabetes skills and knowledge of diabetes education, the diabetes care and education specialist does the best he or she can given the limited time frame. The diabetes care and education specialist does not go live in the home of the person with diabetes and follow him or her around. Likewise, understanding the needs of the community where the program will be based is essential, but it can be done in a practical manner. Many program managers make the mistake of over-interpreting the NSDSMES and turn what was intended to be a quality guideline into something far too complex and unnecessary. For example, Standard 3 of the NSDSMES states that "the provider(s) of DSMES services will evaluate the communities they serve to determine the resources, design, and delivery methods that will align with the population's need for DSMES services."[5] It does not say that a 10-item survey needs to be designed, validated, and mailed to all residents with diabetes in a 20-mile radius for a scientific analysis. Getting input from several potential referring providers in the community about the kinds of persons with diabetes they see and the barriers in skills/knowledge/behaviors they hope a diabetes program will address will fill this requirement quite adequately. County Departments of Health can also be valuable resources for assessing the health care needs of the community, having data on prevalence of chronic diseases and the demographics of the community you aim to serve.

In addition to assessing the needs of the persons with diabetes in a community, it is equally valuable to assess the needs of the providers (physicians and nurse practitioners) who will be referring persons with diabetes to the program. Ask if they currently refer persons with diabetes for diabetes education services and if not, why not. What would make them more likely to refer? How do they want to receive communication from the diabetes education program? How much involvement would they like you to have in terms of adjusting medications? The success of a diabetes education program is largely based on the satisfaction of referring providers (and the subsequent volume of persons with diabetes they refer), so aim to keep them happy.

Finally, a program manager will be well served by taking time to assess the competition. What other programs are in the area? Whom do they serve? What features do they have? Don't be deterred from building a diabetes education program just because there may already be one in the community. When you consider the size of the population that may have diabetes, there are usually plenty of potential clients, even in small communities. Chances are, by learning about the competition, you can find ways to collaborate with and complement each other rather than compete with each other.

Assess Resources for Ongoing Support

DSME is more effective when coupled with some sort of ongoing diabetes self-management support (DSMS) to help reinforce behavior change. Diabetes self-management support is part of the minimum quality standards (see Table 11.1, Standard 8) and can be behavioral, educational, psychosocial, or clinical.[5] While the DSMES program does not need to provide formal support, it does need to be familiar with resources that could serve this function. Diabetes self-management support can be provided through one-on-one interaction such as with a trained peer counselor or community health worker, or via a telephone call with a nurse case manager or lifestyle coach that is part of the person with diabetes' insurance plan. A growing number of online healthy living programs and apps include some kind of ongoing support and encouragement to stick with new behaviors and assist with goal setting. Persons with diabetes can also receive ongoing support through their own primary care team, something that has become possible with the organization of person-centered medical homes in many practices. Diabetes self-management support can involve joining a community-based program such as a mall walking group, weight management program, or the local fitness group at a senior center. It might even involve strengthening an existing relationship with a community pharmacist who can chat with the person with diabetes about his or her goals and progress. But no matter the method of ongoing support, the DSME instructor and person with diabetes must agree on a plan together, which is communicated back to the referring provider in writing at the end of the formal education program.

Goal Setting

Goal setting for DSMES requires knowing the plans of the referring provider and balancing them with the person with diabetes' own goals. It is important that goal setting be collaborative among the provider, the person with diabetes, and the diabetes care and education specialist. The same applies to the goal-setting process for program management. Begin with defining the program mission (and ensure there is agreement on the mission from all stakeholders) and then define more specific, measurable program goals. Just as with participant education, make sure the goals that are set are realistic and are clearly agreed upon by all parties (eg, institutional administrators, advisory board, and program staff). The business plan for a program is like the education plan for a person with diabetes in that it must describe what is expected to be done for the upcoming year of operations. All goal-setting activities should be assessed annually and revised as needed.

Define the Program Mission

The development and adoption of a mission statement is something a program manager can draft and present to the advisory group for discussion. A good mission statement may be short and state the obvious, but it helps focus the direction and clarifies the purpose of your program. Mission statements should be reviewed annually and edited as needed to ensure they remain relevant. Two sample mission statements that could serve as a starter for your advisory group to review and refine are as follows:

- The mission of ABC Diabetes Program is to provide comprehensive diabetes medical care and self-management education to individuals with diabetes and prediabetes.
- The mission of ABC Pediatric Diabetes Program is to provide the highest-quality diabetes education services to children with diabetes seen at XYZ Health Clinic and their families and thus help them better manage their disease and reduce their risks of complications.

Define the Program Goals

Establishing program goals is a good way for the program manager to stay accountable to the mission and help measure success. Written program goals are part of an annual program plan and should be reviewed annually both to assess progress on the previous year's goals and to modify the upcoming year's goals accordingly. Ensure goals have input from all stakeholders (such as institutional administrators) and are well understood by the instructional staff. The following are examples of first-year goals:

- To provide diabetes education services to persons with diabetes from at least ____ different referring providers (or to increase the number of referring providers by ____ percent)
- To deliver services that meet the needs of persons with diabetes by having at least ____ percent of persons with diabetes complete the program
- To demonstrate success in moving persons with diabetes toward achieving behavioral goals by at least ____ percent of persons with diabetes showing progress toward the goal
- To operate a financially responsible program by showing a break-even budget at the end of the first operating year

Write a Business Plan

A written business plan and pro forma statements including budgets help establish clear expectations for the diabetes program. The business plan should be aligned with the program mission and goals. The term *pro forma* means "as a matter of form" and is applied to the process of presenting financial projections for a specific period in a standardized format. Pro forma statements are used for decision making, program management, and plans for expected expenses and revenues by which the program can be managed and evaluated. Essential to the development of a useful business plan is having a set of realistic assumptions in terms of expenses (salary, educational materials, and other operating supplies) and revenues (number of persons with diabetes expected to be seen, expected revenues based on reimbursement rates, etc).

In addition to financial projections, the business plan may include the marketing plan as well as a plan for annual educational activities—or these may all be separate documents. Table 11.2 outlines key elements to think about in a business plan, including the following:

1. Defining the program overview
2. Describing program activities and timeline
3. Preparing the budget
4. Identifying marketing plans
5. Planning for program evaluation

TABLE 11.2 Sample Business Plan for a Diabetes Education Program

A business plan is a written document that helps you chart your course and follow it. Use this template as a guide to help you think about the steps involved in launching a successful diabetes education program.

Program Overview	Organizational structure: • Reporting relationships • Sponsoring organization Mission/Goals: What is the purpose of the program?
	Target Audience (both persons with diabetes and referring providers): • Who is the program aimed at reaching? Will you be providing gestational diabetes education, prediabetes education, insulin pump training, and continuous glucose monitoring system training in addition to general education for individuals with type 1 diabetes or type 2 diabetes? • What are the needs as expressed by potential referring providers? • Will you have resources to address the culturally and socioeconomically diverse needs of your target population, including resources needed by individuals with varying literacy levels and language needs?
	Staff/Team: • Who is on your planning/support team? • Who will deliver services? • Who is on the advisory board? • Who else do you need to connect with to build support? • Can you afford the staff size that you think is ideal? If not, what compromises might need to be made? What staff-to-participant ratios are reasonable and justify staff time?
	Resource Needs and Accessing Local Specialists/Community Resources: What resources are needed? (instructional, AV aids, etc) Program evaluation and continuous quality improvement: • Proposed dates for key activities (eg, advisory group meetings, large community events, continuing education programs) If you need to refer to others, do you know where to find a: • Podiatrist • Registered dietitian who offers MNT • Mall walking group • Reduced-cost exercise program • Weight management program • Mental health provider with expertise in chronic disease or diabetes
	Location/Space: • Where will the program be held? • What preprogram preparation is needed? • Is the classroom large enough to handle the numbers of registrants needed to meet your budget, as well as provide space for guests or interactive activities? • How often will you offer group classes, and how long will they be? Will you offer any support groups?
Program Activities and Timeline	• What program activities and materials need to be developed? Examples include: – Curriculum – Documentation and referral forms

TABLE 11.2 Sample Business Plan for a Diabetes Education Program (continued)	
Program Activities and Timeline (continued)	– Participant handouts and resources – Plan for continuous quality improvement • When do the program activities need to be completed? • How soon can you submit to an accreditation/recognition program for review?
Program Budget	**Overview:** • Do you plan to have the program make a profit, break even, or operate at a loss? • How will persons with diabetes be charged? • How will you get paid? • What are the expectations of the senior administrators for the program budget (are your expectations aligned? realistic?) • What is the landscape of the insurance companies in the region regarding covering diabetes education services? Is there a state mandate to cover diabetes education? Income: (see Table 11.3) Expenses: (see Table 11.3)
Marketing	**Building an Audience:** How do you plan to market the program? What are free/low-cost sources of spreading the word?
Evaluation	How will you know if the program is successful?

Planning

Develop a Budget Based on Expected Income and Expenses

An important way to measure the financial success of the diabetes education program is to track the direct expenses of the program that are related to participant care and the revenue associated with those activities. In the case of diabetes education programs, salaries are the largest expense. Revenue is defined as cash you are entitled to receive once any contract discounts you have agreed on are taken into consideration. Dividing revenue by expenses gives you an indicator that is referred to as your return on investment (ROI), which helps determine whether expenses are being covered and, ideally, returning something to the hospital or larger organization or yourself. This overage can be used to cover expenses such as rent, or it can be reinvested in improving the operations. For your program to be financially viable, covering direct expenses, it should produce an ROI of at least 1.

As part of the process of developing the budget, explore the following questions:

- What are the expectations of administrators for the program?
- Does there need to be a break-even budget or one that yields a profit, or will the program be partially subsidized by the hospital or physician's office as a service to persons with diabetes?
- In addition to billing for person with diabetes visits (group and one-on-one), are there additional opportunities to generate revenue through conducting professional education programs, charging fees for diabetes care and education specialist's speaking engagements, selling books or educational resources, or billing for lab tests such as point-of-care A1C in the education office?
- If your center offers both medical and educational services, would a program of shared medical visits provide both a participant support benefit and clinical and financial benefits?

Use the budget planning worksheet in Table 11.3 to help think about sources of income and expenses. Plan for the practice to build over time. While breaking even in the first year may be difficult, a budget can be designed to show increasing revenues over the first several years, until a break-even point or profit is realized in the second or third year.

How the money will be collected needs to be determined. You can capture more revenue if you consistently collect co-pays up front. In addition, you can maximize revenue if you operate a cash-only program and have persons with diabetes submit a bill to their insurance company on their own.

TABLE 11.3 Diabetes Education Budget Planning Worksheet

Use this worksheet as a guide to help you think about expenses you might have. Look for ways to decrease expenses or increase income by sharing expenses and seeking donations in the form of goods (AV equipment and participant education material from pharmaceutical companies) or services (volunteer time to help organize participant packets).

Projected expenses: ______________________

Item	*Considerations*	*Dollar Amount*
Staff	This is your largest expense: • Do you need to include only salary, or benefits as well? • Can any of the staff be part-time?	
Space/Overhead	• Do you need to pay for the space, or will it be donated by the sponsoring organization (hospital or physician's office)? Keep in mind that space cannot be "free" or donated to the program if Medicare is being billed for the education services, or it will violate kickback laws. • How will services such as electricity, heat, telephone, and postal services be covered? • You may need to pay for coding/billing support in your overhead expenses.	
Program materials	• This includes curricula, handouts, and teaching materials as well as AV aids (such as an LCD projector or flipcharts). See if you can share resources or seek donations from pharmaceutical companies for some items.	
Marketing	• This not only includes activities to promote your program, such as placing ads and mailing flyers, but also includes costs of printing things like stationery and brochures. • Plan time to make referral development visits to provider offices to describe your services and leave behind referral pads and/or other helpful information.	
Professional fees	• Do you need to generate enough revenue to cover expenses like continuing education unit credit hours and meeting attendance, professional association membership, and journal subscription? • Budget for application fees for ADCES accreditation or ADA recognition.	

Projected income: ______________________

Source	*Considerations*	*Dollar Amount*
Participant revenue	• Will you bill the participant directly and have him or her submit to insurance? • If you will accept insurance, which plans cover DSME and MNT and at what reimbursement rate? • What participant volume will you need to see to meet your expenses? • What percentage is billable time? • What percentage is scheduled time? • How will you account for no-shows and what no-show rate do you anticipate?	
Sales of books/ educational materials	• Will you sell any books and educational materials at a break-even cost or at a profit?	
Special events	• Fees can be charged for special events such as a continuing education program for healthcare providers or diabetes prevention and awareness classes and/or classes for grandparents or caregivers (as they are not billable to insurance).	

Establish an Advisory Group

The NSDSMES require that the advisory group include valued stakeholders and experts to promote quality and enhance participant utilization. It is important to give careful thought to members and include not only obvious program supporters (such as a local endocrinologist) but also people who might be somewhat resistant to the program and would be advantageous to win over (such as a doctor from a group practice where a medical assistant who has diabetes herself is doing all the teaching). Advisory group members found to be helpful include:

1. People who have an "in" with marketing opportunities (staff member of a local newspaper)
2. People who may be potential sources of referrals (local podiatrists, a retail pharmacist from the corner drugstore, or a representative from the community health clinic)
3. Individuals who might have knowledge of competitive programs in the area (pharmaceutical industry representatives)
4. Community leaders who can influence persons with diabetes and providers to use your service

The standards are intentionally vague on how often an advisory group should meet, and the review criteria require, at a minimum, only annual input from the group. There is no requirement that the meeting be conducted face-to-face. However, it has been the experience of many program managers that well-planned meetings that tap into the ideas and expertise of advisors can really help shape the program and identify possible problems and barriers to growth before they arise.

Adopt, Adapt, or Create a Curriculum

The NSDSMES require that a program have a defined curriculum that is reviewed and updated annually and covers all required content areas (see Table 11.4). A curriculum includes learning objectives, methods of delivery, and criteria for evaluating learning for the populations served. It is not a set of slides and handouts sorted by topic area. The curriculum must define teaching approaches that are interactive and tailored to individual needs. Is the curriculum age appropriate? Does it address both literacy and health literacy? Literacy is an individual's ability to read and write. Health literacy is an individual's ability to obtain, read, understand, and use healthcare information to make appropriate health decisions and follow instructions for treatment.

Evaluate whether it is more cost-effective for the program to build or buy. In other words, is it better to create everything, including learning objectives, teaching materials, and participant handouts, or purchase a complete program and tailor it to fit your needs? While commercial comprehensive curricula such as Healthy Interactions Conversation Maps can be useful, time must be allowed to annually review and update the objectives, content outlines, and support materials as needed and make any needed adaptations to fit the target population. Take care to identify resources that can meet a variety of literacy needs.

TABLE 11.4 DSMES Curriculum Content Areas Required by the NSDSMES

1. Diabetes pathophysiology and treatment options
2. Healthy eating
3. Physical activity
4. Medication usage
5. Monitoring and using patient generated health data (PGHD)
6. Preventing, detecting and treating acute and chronic complications
7. Healthy coping with psychosocial issues and concerns
8. Problem-solving

Source: J Beck, D Greenwood, et al., "2017 National Standards for Diabetes Self-Management Education and Support," The Diabetes Educator. 2017;43(5):449-64.

Determine Realistic Space Needs

In addition to traditional space options in hospital outpatient clinics and physician offices, explore other locations, including community centers, public library meeting rooms, senior centers, and shopping mall conference rooms. Think about accessibility issues, parking, and safety factors. If you have access to a classroom in a medical clinic, share it with other groups to minimize costs. Keep in mind that if you plan to bill for services and you use another health facility or physician office not owned by your institution, you will need to pay fair market value for use of the space to avoid violating kickback laws.

Identify Instructional and Support Staff

A common problem is overstaffing and not maximizing the use of group education. Having both a nurse and a dietitian work in a center may be ideal but not financially realistic. If only one education discipline is represented, consider identifying diabetes care and education specialists from other disciplines who might contribute to your advisory board, accept referrals, and deliver programs such as a special topics lecture. Hiring support staff may be desired, but it may not always be feasible. Tap into the hospital volunteer network or consider using former persons with diabetes as volunteers who can help with mailings or preparing class materials. Maintain a written list of specialists and resources available within the community for referrals as needed, such as experienced mental health providers, exercise physiologists, and specialty medical providers (eg, endocrinologists, podiatrists, and psychiatrists). Identify community pharmacists who have a special interest in diabetes and might be able to help with medication therapy management. In addition, maintain a list of support services that may be suggested to program participants, such as weight management programs, fitness or mall walking groups, diabetes support groups, and healthy cooking classes.

To best ensure program sustainability, program managers should ensure all staff are working at the top of their license. With training and mentoring from experienced diabetes care and education specialists, primary care offices can involve other office staff in education programs, including medical assistants and licensed practical nurses.[7] Many programs have found that involving community health workers or trained peer support counselors can be very valuable, especially with patient populations that represent diverse ethnic and cultural backgrounds.[8] When well trained and managed, these individuals can effectively work closely with the diabetes care and education specialists to deliver elements of the diabetes education classes, provide real-world examples to facilitate behavior change within unique community settings, and take leadership roles in programs offering ongoing support.

While having diabetes care and education specialists with additional certifications such as CDCES (certified diabetes care and education specialist) or BC-ADM (board certified–advanced diabetes manager) may be ideal, it is not required for billing or reimbursement purposes. Obtaining such certifications has other benefits, however; individuals who hold either of these credentials do not need to provide detailed documentation of continuing education hours. Two significant changes have been made to broaden eligibility to apply for the CDCES credential: (1) a new group of professionals, masters certified health education specialists, may now sit for a CDCES exam, and (2) volunteer hours working in DSMES may now count toward the total 1,000 practice hours needed before applying for the credential.[9]

Determine Information Technology Needs

Technology is a powerful tool, and program managers need to be aware of how it can be used within their programs. Evaluating information technology (IT) needs, available resources, and the kinds of data that program leaders are expected to analyze will help the program manager decide what kinds of IT resources need to be built and/or purchased.

Program managers are responsible for reporting participant and program outcomes and identifying methods for collecting individual and population-based data. Useful IT systems include the following:

- Electronic medical records
- Personal health records
- Diabetes data management systems and external large-scale Web programs through diabetes organizations, the government, and/or insurers

Information technology capabilities to aggregate, analyze, and report robust data need to be taken into consideration along with participant information security.

Implementation: Operating and Maintaining a DSMES Program

Once all the assessment, goal-setting, and planning activities have been completed, the next step is program implementation. Like the fourth step in the DSMES process for education of persons with diabetes, the implementation process for a diabetes program involves many components. The program manager oversees all operations related to the diabetes program, but turns to the advisory group whenever possible as a sounding board or for advice and recommendations. As part of day-to-day program operations, a review of key roles and responsibilities in the following 6 areas will help both new and experienced program managers improve the implementation process for their programs:

1. Managing staff
2. Communications
3. Front-end operations
4. Metrics and data
5. Marketing
6. Meeting the NSDSMES

These roles and responsibilities need to be reviewed regardless of program size, as they apply to both one-person operations and large multidisciplinary specialty centers. Program management of a diabetes center can sometimes feel like a lonely job (you don't have others in your institution who do that same job), but know that there are others across the country who are often happy to network and share ideas.

Managing Staff: The Most Important Resource for Overall Program Success

Staff development is a critical role for successful program coordinators. Whether the staff is just a team of 2 or a large team including diabetes care and education specialists and support staff, part of the coordinator's job is to keep the team members motivated, aligned in their goals, and competent in their overall roles and responsibilities. Program staff is the most important resource from the standpoint of the budget as well as from program delivery. Care must be taken to select the right person for the job and to make sure that tasks are clearly assigned (see Clear Communication section below) and that all employees are used to their maximum capacity (see Metrics and Data section below). Clear and frequent feedback to employees (including lots of praise when things are going well) helps shape appropriate behaviors. The program coordinator will be aware of where staff need further development, for both job satisfaction and job performance, and will identify ways to help each employee obtain those additional skills for growth and continuous quality improvement (CQI). Finally, the program coordinator will likely be the individual to maintain necessary records of updated clinical licenses, registration, CDCES credential status (if appropriate), and records of continuing education for all clinical employees.

Clear Communication: Enhances Overall Program Operations

The importance of documentation and clear communication as a basis for a well-functioning program is emphasized within the NSDSMES. Policies and procedures that are understood by the team and reviewed with the advisory board are an integral part of a quality process. Referrals to the education program from the medical care provider need to be documented in the medical record, as does communication back to the referring provider reporting on achievement toward goals and plans for ongoing support. The diabetes care and education specialist will need to document that the needs for self-management education have been assessed in all content areas, and that those areas found lacking are addressed in the education plan. Responsibilities and expectations for care must be clarified between the diabetes care and education specialist and the referring provider. For example, diabetes care and education specialists should assume only those roles within their scope of practice related to medication adjustment if operating under clear orders or guidelines from the referring provider. The referring provider should not expect the diabetes care and education specialist to handle routine phone follow-up unless it has been built into the budget. Discussing roles and clarifying expectations are an important part of accepting referrals and developing a collaborative care model with the person with diabetes.

In addition to clear communications within the team regarding clinical care, the program manager needs to ensure that all team members understand their productivity goals. Keep in mind that if the job can't be done in a cost-effective manner, it may not be done at all. Thus, to help ensure employment security (and to reach the maximum number of persons with diabetes in a timely fashion), each healthcare provider should know what is expected of him or her in terms of numbers of persons with diabetes to be seen in order to generate revenue to meet the program budget.

Although the NSDSMES require that an advisory group convene only once a year, most experienced program managers will agree that regular communication with members of this group can greatly enhance program operations. Advisory group members should be selected based on their connections with the wider community and ability to represent different points of view. Advisory group members bring the most value when they are kept in the loop regarding program activities and periodically asked for input or advice. Maximize the use of the advisory group members and the program will benefit.

Programs that are larger than a one-person operation will benefit by creating written policies or guidelines on a variety of topics to ensure clear communications. The program manager will want to guide the implementation and annual review of policies and procedures on clinical care topics such as the handling of medical emergencies (eg, hypoglycemia) and medication adjustment guidelines. Operational policies are also needed, such as when and how to refer to other diabetes care and education specialists (especially if the program is only offered by a single diabetes care and educations specialist or representing one discipline, such as nutrition) and how to handle persons with diabetes who miss appointments, along with policies related to billing and collection.

Finally, remember to keep the widest audience in mind when evaluating ways to enhance communication and keep everyone informed. In larger multidisciplinary programs, formal communication is all too often only between the healthcare providers, and the front/back office team is left out of the loop. Look for ways to obtain feedback from persons with diabetes as well as from other customer groups (such as referring providers) to assess satisfaction with program services and operations. Clear and effective communications will help ensure effective program operations. Take the time to assess whether all systems are working as well as they can be or if there is room for improvement.

In addition to communicating with the team and referral sources, the program manager is responsible for communicating with the regional Centers for Medicare and Medicaid Services (CMS) and other government insurers, such as Tricare, to provide copies of accreditation/recognition certificates as soon as the program is approved. In addition, the program manager is responsible for ensuring that these agencies have NPI (national provider identifier) numbers for any dietitian instructors, especially if they plan on billing for MNT. It would be prudent for the program manager to find out who his or her contact is at these agencies and keep communication lines open.

Front-End Operations: An Integral Part of the Overall Program

Even though many diabetes care and education specialists prefer to steer clear of anything related to the business operations of a diabetes program, it has to be recognized that good business is good medicine. The program manager must stay abreast of all operational aspects of the program, including the following:

- Scheduling
  - Are schedules filled tightly and efficiently?
  - Is a waiting list maintained in the event of a cancellation?
- Registration and participant data collection
  - Are new persons with diabetes asked how they were referred to the center?
  - Are names of referring providers analyzed to assess impact of marketing efforts?
  - Are pre-authorizations obtained if required?
  - Is accurate insurance information collected?
  - Are persons with diabetes expected to verify coverage or is that done by staff?
  - Are co-pays consistently collected at the time of visit?
  - Are reports summarizing collection rates being run?

Regardless of whether the front-end operations are handled within the diabetes education program or by employees who are off-site (or within another department as part of hospital operations), the program manager should do his or her best to communicate and collaborate with these essential team members so they fully understand their role in the overall diabetes education program.

Individuals who are the "voice" of the program on the phone should have a very thorough understanding of the diabetes education program. Ideally, invite them to go through one or more of the classes. Help them understand the high value of diabetes education services. Offer a written script for training so receptionists can accurately articulate the services, benefits, and expectations for a new participant appointment.

The program manager is responsible for understanding all aspects of accurate billing and coding for the services provided, including diabetes self-management education/training(DSME/T) and MNT. Even if these services are handled by another department within the institution, it is important that the program manager oversee what is happening to help maximize revenue opportunities. The program manager should establish good working relationships with the billing department to review denial reports and identify systemic billing problems.

Metrics and Data: Assess Program Operations and Impact

Ensuring clinical quality in a diabetes education program should be obvious. The NSDSMES require continuous quality improvement (CQI), so program managers will review performance metrics to demonstrate improvement in clinical and/or behavioral outcomes. However, while not required for a quality DSMES program, operational metrics such as monthly participant visits (new and follow-up) and analysis of number of referrals by providers are essential to track in order to continuously improve program operations, thus ensuring its survival. In addition, the program manager often is responsible for budget planning and a monthly review of revenue and expense reports. If careful projections are not done for developing budgets, managing expenses, and increasing revenue streams, there will be no program.

To keep a diabetes program operating, there have to be clear expectations and accountability for revenue and expenses. Schedules for participant visits need to be built to maximize productivity and meet revenue goals. At Joslin Diabetes Center (and all of its affiliated programs), the standard has been set for 2 metrics. Joslin productivity data evaluate "outpatient hours billed as a percent of paid time" as well as "percent of time spent treating billable outpatients" (also known as face-to-face time). The goal for diabetes care and education specialists is to achieve 100% each month for the first metric and 60% for the second. For example, consider Chris, a CDCES who in 1 week saw 20 hours of one-to-one appointments and conducted 2 2-hour classes, each with 6 participants (resulting in 24 billable hours). Chris kept that same schedule for the whole month (4 weeks), resulting in 80 billable one-to-one hours plus 96 group hours for a total of 176 billable participant care hours during the 4-week period. If that number is divided by the standard number of working hours in a month (160), Chris is considered to be very productive by this standard, as she is billing for 101% of her time.

Using the same figures, how much time is Chris actually face-to-face with persons with diabetes? This calculation provides an estimate of resource efficiency and productivity. The goal is for 60% of a diabetes care and education specialists' time to be face-to-face with persons with diabetes, either one-to-one or in a group. Using the figures above, in a typical week, Chris sees persons with diabetes for 24 hours (or 96 hours in a month). This calculates to 60% face-to-face time, which meets the goal of time spent face-to-face with persons with diabetes. It is clear that by seeing persons with diabetes in groups, diabetes care and education specialists can be more productive.

One way to assess and improve productivity is to have staff complete a time study.[10] Ask diabetes care and educations specialists to document for at least 2 weeks exactly how much time is spent in the following activities: billable participant care (group versus one-to-one), charting, phone calls, meetings, and other (be specific). By tracking exactly how time is spent, the program manager can assess whether the highest and best use is made of the resources. Are diabetes care and education specialists doing tasks that could be handled by the medical assistant or receptionist? How much time is spent on nonbillable participant care activities—and can that be reduced? The results are often surprising, as most are always very "busy" but not necessarily doing valuable billable activities. An analysis of diabetes care and education specialist productivity in 22 sites demonstrated that, on average, diabetes care and education specialists were billing 0.55 hours of education (one-to-one or group) for each hour of salary they were paid (range 0.19-1.21) but spent only 25% of their time on billable activities (range 11%-46%).[11] Findings such as this do not justify the types of salaries that diabetes care and education specialists are paid. Thus, diabetes care and education specialists not only need to be clear on what their productivity goals are for participant visits, but also need to participate in systems improvements to make sure they can meet or exceed those expectations. Be aware of other "billable" participant care time in chronic disease management such as non-face-to-face time billing codes and telemedicine care opportunities.

Marketing: Ensuring Ongoing Program Growth

A large part of what most program managers do is related to ensuring a consistent flow of new persons with diabetes into the education program and helping retain them for ongoing care and follow-up. Marketing activities do not necessarily mean that high-priced ads need to be placed in regional newspapers or magazines or heard over the radio, although that does help. Many things should be done on an ongoing basis to keep the participant schedules filled. A few tips are discussed below.

Focus Attention on Referring Provider

Referring providers are the most reliable source of persons with diabetes and well worth the time it takes to make personal visits to primary care providers or endocrine groups to ensure they know about the diabetes education services offered. In addition to explaining the services of the diabetes education program and asking for referrals, it may be appreciated if you offer some services to the office staff, such as providing handouts on treating hypoglycemia or foot care guidelines, or conducting a lunchtime diabetes education program. Educating the office staff about diabetes will usually result in more referrals as they begin to understand that the disease is more complex than they first realized.

Implement the Algorithm

Ensure that your staff as well as referring providers recognize the 4 critical times to refer for diabetes education as described in the ADA-ADCES-AND Joint Position Statement and Education Algorithm.[12–15] The 4 times are as follows: at diagnosis, annually, when complicating factors influence self-management, and when transitions occur. Marketing activities could include sharing copies of the figures contained within the algorithm (see chapter 2, Figures 2.1 and 2.2) with referring providers and providing a short inservice to enhance their understanding of the referral times and how this can benefit their persons with diabetes.

Don't Overlook the Obvious

Often diabetes education programs are part of a larger institution such as a hospital or multispecialty outpatient medical practice. These days, everyone knows someone with diabetes, so make sure all employees know about the diabetes program. Offer an annual open house for staff, conduct diabetes awareness activities in March and November in the employee cafeteria, and see where posters or brochures promoting program activities can be distributed. Consider having persons with diabetes who complete the education program mail a preprinted "thank you for referring me" postcard to their healthcare provider and share a flyer with a friend. A happy customer is a great source of referrals.

Keep Existing Persons with Diabetes in the System

All too often, persons with diabetes come for a comprehensive class series or a set of one-to-one counseling visits but return only in the event of a crisis. As part of the initial education program, help persons with diabetes understand that because diabetes is a chronic disease, education also should be ongoing. The assistance a diabetes care and education specialist offers over time becomes even more valuable as it moves from providing vital survival-skills information that is part of the initial diagnosis to providing more complex problem-solving skills and ongoing DSMS. Take advantage of the Medicare reimbursement benefit that allows for up to 2 hours of education annually for DSME (after the initial 10 hours in the first year) and 2 hours of MNT (after the initial 3 hours in the first year). This can also be incorporated into a system of providing DSMS and thus keeping the person with diabetes engaged and supported over time.

No matter what strategies are used to market the program, keep all team members informed of the different initiatives so that they can help track the results and evaluate the effectiveness of the activity. For example, if spending a day at a health fair resulted in only 1 new person with diabetes, it may not be worth repeating that activity next year. On the other hand, if the front desk receptionists handling new callers are aware that the program manager has been working to build a relationship with the new internal medicine practice in town, they can provide reports on the numbers of persons with diabetes coming from the practice and the program manager can respond with timely "thank you" acknowledgments for the referrals. Once again, communication is key.

Meet the Standards (NSDSMES/DPP)

There are 2 organizations that accredit or recognize diabetes education programs that meet quality standards as outlined by the NSDSMES.[16] The ADCES and the ADA offer accreditation or recognition status to programs meeting established criteria. The Centers for Disease and Control (CDC) offer certification for diabetes prevention programs. The Joint Commission provides accreditation for inpatient diabetes management. Ensuring that a diabetes education program meets minimum standards as outlined by the NSDSMES is important for 3 reasons:

1. It helps ensure a high level of quality.
2. It protects consumers with diabetes by helping them identify programs that meet the standards.
3. It is required in order for a program to be eligible for Medicare reimbursement.

Despite the detailed instructions prepared by each organization regarding the program guidelines and application process, there are many misunderstandings.

Table 11.5 outlines some of the common myths and reports the facts for each topic.

ADCES: Diabetes Education Accreditation Program (DEAP): http://www.diabeteseducator.org
ADA: Education Recognition Program (ERP): http://professional.diabetes.org
CDC: Diabetes Prevention Program certification (DPP) http://www.cdc.gov

Evaluation, Monitoring, and Documentation

Evaluation is defined in the broad sense as a method of determining the significance or value of something by careful appraisal and study. An essential and ongoing step in

TABLE 11.5 Myths Versus Facts About Program Accreditation and Recognition

Myth	*Fact*
All 8 content areas must be documented as taught in order for a participant to have completed the program.	It is true that there must be documentation to assess the participant's skills, knowledge, and behavior in all 8 content areas, but the participant only needs to be taught in areas that the assessment deems necessary.
At least 1 CDCES needs to be on staff for a program to be accredited or recognized.	Having a CDCES on staff is not required. However, an advantage to having a CDCES or BC-ADM on staff is that he or she does not have to maintain documentation of all continuing education hours.
Accreditation or recognition will automatically guarantee reimbursement.	Accreditation or recognition is required for Medicare reimbursement of the G codes for diabetes self-management training (DSMT). Accreditation or recognition does not, however, guarantee reimbursement. Although most payers require that a DSME/T program have accreditation or recognition, reimbursement criteria vary.
A comprehensive education program should take about 10 hours.	Do not confuse what Medicare has agreed to cover in terms of diabetes education (up to 10 hours in the first year) with how long a program "should" be.

the process of providing quality DSMES is for the program manager to evaluate his or her programs on an individual (person with diabetes) level, a program level, and a system level. The terms frequently referred to in DSME programs are *outcome measurement*, *evaluation*, and *continuous quality improvement*. To ensure that all of the evidence-based standards and program requirements have a mechanism for evaluation, it would be wise to use and refer to each standard in the NSDSMES. The standards direct baseline and repeated measurements to assess the impact of DSMES for individuals as well as programs or populations. The design of DSMES programs varies widely, and reliance on the standards and respective measures provides a framework for evaluating practice consistently. In this chapter, evaluation will be addressed from the program level.

Program-Level Evaluation

Evaluation helps determine which interventions are most appropriate and will produce the best outcomes for the population served by the DSMES program. Just as education is not considered complete until outcomes are reviewed and evaluated, a program cannot be considered comprehensive if the overall clinical effectiveness and operational metrics are not routinely assessed. Regardless of whether the DSMES service is provided by a single discipline diabetes care and education specialist or a multidisciplinary team, the need for program evaluation remains. The standards that address program structure and processes also require attention to evaluation.

Ongoing Quality Improvement

Program evaluation and monitoring activities should look not only at the program and participants but also at the diabetes care and education specialists involved in teaching and conducting the program. Ensure that expectations for teaching and counseling skills are clearly communicated and offer regular mentoring and feedback for performance improvement to ensure that diabetes care and education specialists are communicating in an effective, interactive, and person-centered manner. Invite team members to participate in program assessment activities. Table 11.6 is the AIDE tool (areas to improve in diabetes education). It is used within Joslin Affiliated Programs to stimulate program improvement, trigger discussion among diabetes care and education specialists and program staff, and identify specific steps toward improvement activities. Much like with education, when staff are involved in identifying the gaps and suggesting solutions, it is more likely that specific small-step behavior changes toward improvement will occur.

Organizational Structure

Standard 1 requires that the DSMES entity have documentation of its mission statement and goals.[5] The mission statement sets the stage for the program and should be articulated, understood, and supported by the larger organization's stakeholders, administrators, staff, persons with diabetes, volunteers, and community members. The DSMES staff should review the mission statement annually with the advisory group or board to ensure its relevance and make modifications as necessary.

In accomplishing the mission, program goals and objectives first need to be identified and then monitored. The objectives can include statements regarding the target audience as well as metrics related to the reach and volume of persons with diabetes to be seen. A review of the program goals and objectives should be conducted annually with the program's advisory board. It is essential to obtain an understanding of the program goals of the various program stakeholders. For example, don't assume that hospital administrators are only interested in program goals that demonstrate clinical excellence. They may be looking at goals that establish financial return or increased outreach to community providers. Take the time to understand the kinds of goals that are important to each of your stakeholders. Three sample program goals are as follows:

- To increase the percentage of patients discharged from the hospital who receive follow-up care in the diabetes program from 20% to 40%
- To increase the number of women with gestational diabetes seen at the center by 10%
- To increase the number of referring providers by 50%

Careful measurement and documentation of these goals is critical in meeting the program's mission.

Standard 2 mandates that the DSMES entity appoint an advisory board to include broad participation of organization(s) and community stakeholders, including health professionals, people with diabetes, consumers, and other community groups.[5] The advisory board members are responsible for the development, ongoing planning, and outcomes evaluation process for the program.

It is the program manager's responsibility to reassess the makeup of the board and participation of the members. Measures can include attendance records, member satisfaction surveys, and a review of meeting minutes to ensure active involvement. Focus groups led by a trained investigator also provide a unique opportunity to collect qualitative information about the community needs and program services. Advisory board members should be

TABLE 11.6 Areas to Improve in Diabetes Education (AIDE)

Instructions: Which of the following diabetes issues are currently a problem for your diabetes education program? Circle the number that gives the best answer for you. Please provide an answer for each question.

	Not a Problem	*Minor Problem*	*Moderate Problem*	*Somewhat Serious Problem*	*Serious Problem*
1. Not getting as many patients (class or 1:1) as planned?	0	1	2	3	4
2. Having trouble retaining patients for subsequent sessions and follow-up?	0	1	2	3	4
3. Having less than ideal outcomes on patient satisfaction surveys?	0	1	2	3	4
4. Hearing feedback that educators are not enjoying teaching classes?	0	1	2	3	4
5. Internal healthcare providers not referring as per protocol?	0	1	2	3	4
6. External primary care providers in the community not referring as much as possible?	0	1	2	3	4
7. Feeling your marketing material may be lacking some pizazz?	0	1	2	3	4
8. Not getting as many referrals from former class members as you'd planned?	0	1	2	3	4
9. Not able to demonstrate behavioral improvements in DSMES?	0	1	2	3	4
10. Front office staff lacks clarity about the program and/or conviction as to its importance for scheduling?	0	1	2	3	4
11. Each class minimizes "lectures" and maximizes interactions and opportunities for application?	0	1	2	3	4
12. Each attendee feels the information in the class has been made personally relevant for them?	0	1	2	3	4
13. Diabetes educators engage in personal CQI activities to continuously improve presentation skills?	0	1	2	3	4
14. Systems are in place to trigger automatic reminders when patients may be up for an annual refresher class/visit?	0	1	2	3	4
15. Too much time spent on nonbillable activities such as documentation/paperwork/phone calls?	0	1	2	3	4

Source: Copyright © 2016 by Joslin Diabetes Center, Inc. (Boston), reprinted with permission.

routinely polled to determine their preferences for meetings and communications (e-mail, face-to-face meetings, timing of meetings, etc).

Standard 3 refers to the identification of the diabetes education needs of the target population(s).[5] Thus, it is the responsibility of the diabetes care and education specialist to carefully assess the target population and determine its self-management education needs. The assessment process should identify the educational needs of all persons with diabetes, not just those who routinely attend clinical appointments. Demographic variables, such as ethnic background, age, formal education level, and reading ability, and barriers to participation in education must be considered to maximize the effectiveness of DSMES for the target population. Diabetes care and education specialists can assess this information using a variety of methods, including interviewing other providers in the target area, talking with the persons with diabetes, and evaluating their own participant data, as well as reviewing epidemiological data available on federal and state Web sites. Surveys such as the Behavioral Risk Factor Surveillance System (http://www.cdc.gov/brfss/) and the National Health and Nutrition Examination Survey (NHANES) (http://www.cdc.gov/nchs/nhanes.htm) provide useful, reliable large-scale data.

Identification of access issues is an essential part of the assessment process. Although DSMES is considered to be a critical component of diabetes care, the majority of individuals with diabetes do not receive DSMES. It is the program manager's responsibility to understand the barriers within the community. A thorough program evaluation process will help ensure that the education program reaches a wide audience.

1. How are the services being marketed?
2. How are programs being deployed?
3. What is the effectiveness of the different marketing interventions?

Tracking and evaluating the results of each type of marketing intervention can help assess its overall effectiveness in reaching the target audience and ideally result in increased visits.

Measuring participant satisfaction provides important insights from the population served. When evaluating satisfaction, it is helpful to have a core group of basic assessment questions as well as several questions that may be specific to a particular time period or need. For example, the standard evaluation assessment tool might always ask persons with diabetes to respond on a scale from 1 to 5 how satisfied they were with the following:

- Diabetes care overall
- Ease of reaching someone in an emergency
- Lab tests reviewed and explained
- Concern, courtesy, respect, and sensitivity of the provider you saw
- Would you recommend your diabetes care provider if a family member or friend needed diabetes care?

Questions asked on a consistent basis are valuable for benchmarking progress over time. Many commercial participant satisfaction survey businesses benchmark results against similar institutions or programs that are also their customers. Optional questions that could be varied based on need might address issues related to parking, time of day for classes, interest in different kinds of support groups, or satisfaction with new educational materials being offered. It is valuable to regularly review your satisfaction survey and ensure you are obtaining information that can truly help effect program improvement and change as needed.

Remember that persons with diabetes are not the only group that needs to be satisfied. Think about other consumers who influence the business of the diabetes program. Consider surveying referring providers to determine whether the education services are meeting their needs. It can also serve as a good marketing tool and reminder to the referring providers of the diabetes education program services. Other customer groups might include inpatient unit managers or hospital staff nurses and medical office assistants. Do they know of the diabetes consultation service? Are there improvements that could be made? Are there ways to improve their diabetes knowledge, skills, or awareness of services?

Standards 4 and 5 attend to program staff.[5] A quality coordinator is designated to oversee the planning, implementation, and evaluation, while instructors are responsible for providing DSMES. Careful evaluation of the credentials and skills of these individuals is critically important, and a mechanism must be in place to ensure that the participants' needs are met if those needs are outside the instructors' scope of practice and expertise. In addition to registered nurses, dietitians, and pharmacists, other health professionals (eg, physicians, behaviorists, exercise physiologists, ophthalmologists, optometrists, and podiatrists) and, more recently, lay health and community workers and peers provide information, behavioral support, and links with the healthcare system as part of DSMES.

By assessing various operational metrics regularly, the program manager can determine whether personnel and other resources are used efficiently. Without adequate operational data, it is difficult to justify the addition of new staff members or the expense of equipment such as practice management software and computers. An in-depth study of how diabetes care and education specialist's time is used can guide the program administrator to ensure that the diabetes care and education specialists' time is put toward person-centered, billable activities and that nonbillable or nonclinical tasks are delegated to others. Ultimately, the goal is to use the right person for the right task. Table 11.7 offers a tool that program managers and diabetes care and education specialists may use for setting goals, measuring baseline productivity, and tracking improvement.[16]

Standards 6 and 7 require a written evidence-based curriculum and an assessment tool.[5]

The content and questions within a standardized curriculum and assessment tool provide the foundation for direct evaluation measures. For example, if the curriculum content addresses nutrition strategies for women with gestational diabetes, specific questions should be

TABLE 11.7 Diabetes Care and Education Specialist Productivity Metrics

Category	*Definition*	*Your Program Goals*	*Month 1 Actual Results*	*Month 2 Actual Results*	*Month 3 Actual Results*	*Quarterly Actual Results*
Diabetes Care and Education Specialist paid hours	Total hours paid including hours worked and paid time off					
Billed 1:1 hours	DSMT and MNT provided ONLY if billed and ONLY for time billed					
Billed group hours	Total number of group hours times the number of participants in the group					
Total billed hours	Total billed 1:1 hours and total billed group hours					
% paid hours billed	Divide the number of total billed hours by diabetes care and education specialist paid hours					
Group face time	Number of hours spent teaching billable group classes					
Total face time hours	Number of hours spent in billable interventions in front of persons with diabetes. Total billed 1:1 hours and group face time					
% face time	Total face time hours divided by diabetes care and education specialist paid hours					

developed regarding nutrition habits in the persons with diabetes educated about gestational diabetes. If the assessment tool includes questions regarding cultural themes, a companion evaluation tool should include questions regarding the program's attention to culture and ethnicity. The use of evidence-based tools and outcome measures has been adopted by organizations and initiatives such as CMS, the National Committee for Quality Assurance, the Diabetes Quality Improvement Project, the Healthcare Effectiveness Data and Information Set, the Veterans Health Administration, and the Joint Commission.

The standards emphasize the importance of employing clear communication principles, avoiding jargon, making information culturally relevant, and using language- and literacy-appropriate education materials.

Health literacy is defined as the degree to which an individual can obtain, process, and understand basic health information and services needed to make appropriate health decisions. This involves both reading words and using numbers (numeracy).[17] It is estimated that 14% of adults have below basic literacy, and an additional 22% have only basic literacy.[18] Limitations in literacy are most common in older adults, those with lower education levels, immigrants, and racial/ethnic minorities. Two questions which have been validated as effective as a basic literacy screen are the following:[17]

How often do you have someone help you read hospital materials?

Answers: always, often, sometimes, rarely, never (answers other than "never" may indicate a literacy concern)

How confident are you filling out medical forms by yourself?

Answers: extremely, quite a bit, somewhat, a little bit, not at all (answers other than "extremely" or "quite a bit" may indicate a literacy concern)

It has been shown that persons with diabetes need ongoing DSMS to sustain behavior. Standard 8 refers to the development of a personalized DSMS follow-up plan.[5] A variety of innovative strategies are being made available for providing DSMS both within and outside the DSMES entity. For example, nurse case managers, disease-management programs, trained peers and community health workers, community-based programs, use of technology, ongoing education and support groups, and MNT are providing this key service. Although many of these programs are expected to be effective, evaluation is crucial to informing healthcare practices and ultimately policy change and reimbursement. Program managers and diabetes care and education specialists would be wise to document follow-up processes, their frequency, and methods for delivery. Currently, it is not known which methodology is most effective in supporting DSMES and in which environment.

The need to measure attainment of person with diabetes-defined goals and outcomes at regular intervals is the basis of Standard 9.[5] Measuring behavior change is the unique domain for DSMES.[19] The AADE7 Self-Care Behaviors® determine the effectiveness of diabetes education at the individual and group levels. Evaluation measures should be made at baseline and at regular intervals after the education program. Although systems to measure behavior change should be built into the education documentation systems and forms, program managers and diabetes care and education specialists may also consider tracking software that can help identify trends and progress.

Finally, Standard 10 states that the DSMES program will use a CQI process to evaluate the effectiveness of the education experience provided, and determine opportunities for improvement.[5] Continuous quality improvement is a methodology used to evaluate how businesses and organizations deliver quality to customers. The first step toward providing a quality DSME program is reflected in these questions:

- Are your participants (persons with diabetes) receiving the information/services they want?
- Are the methods used to provide these services effective and efficient?

A quality DSME program will evaluate its effectiveness (quality) on several levels:

- Process evaluation, which examines the degree to which recommended steps of care are currently being delivered
- Outcomes evaluation, which follows the impact of care on clinical indicators (A1C, lipids, blood pressure) and on the general health and well-being of participants served
- Utilization review, which determines whether persons with diabetes are receiving appropriate care and treatment

Not only is CQI a mechanism to ensure the delivery of quality clinical and education services, it also is a valuable way to evaluate and improve a program's operational success and thus leads to an improved financial bottom line. Table 11.8 offers 2 sample CQI projects that are written following the ADCES suggested format,[10] although there are several different formal processes for writing a CQI plan that may be used.

TABLE 11.8 CQI Case Examples

CQI Case #1 Determining whether behaviors actually change as a result of DSME	
1. Identify the problem	When the CDCES manager was asked, "How effective is your program in changing behaviors?," she realized she did not have concrete data on which to base her reply. She decided to see if the team could get a better understanding of how often people actually do meet their behavioral goals by doing a chart review and phone survey.
2. Collect and analyze data	Charts were pulled from 20 participants who had completed the DSME program 3 to 6 months earlier (so there would have been time for a change to be assessed or documented in a behavioral goal). Two behaviors were chosen to study: 1. Increasing activity 2. Using a meal plan Data were available on 6 participants, either through an education follow-up visit documented in the medical record or via a follow-up phone call. Results showed 2 participants maintained or increased their activity level and 3 participants reported using a meal plan >75% of the time.

(continued)

TABLE 11.8 CQI Case Examples (continued)	
2. Collect and analyze data (continued)	The analysis revealed the following additional problems: • The percentage of participants available for follow-up analysis was lower than expected. • Education records were not well designed to capture behavioral outcomes, and it took a long time to search for them. • Some participants' goals were unrealistic and needed better oversight before they were documented in the chart.
3. Consider possible solutions	The diabetes care and education specialists were disappointed in the results and brainstormed the following solutions: 1. Familiarize the staff with motivational interviewing and/or empowerment techniques to promote person-generated realistic goals. 2. Hire more staff just to do follow-up. 3. Redesign education documentation tools to be easier to assess outcomes. 4. Ask participants to provide a phone number where they can be reached in 3 months for a follow-up phone call (instead of using home numbers in the chart). 5. Conduct an additional class on writing measurable goals. 6. Ask participants to self-address 2 reminder postcards to themselves. One would be sent about 6 weeks post program with an upbeat message of support. The other would be sent a week before the follow-up call to remind them that the call is coming and that if they are not available, they should call in. 7. Use an outcomes charting tool. 8. Use a follow-up assessment form to re-measure behaviors.
4. Make recommendations	The CQI team narrowed the list down to choose 3, 6, and 7, as they appeared to be lower cost options (time and money).
5. Implement	The CQI team (including all staff) designed and printed the postcards and discussed exactly how the follow-up assessment tool would be used. (Participants would complete at last class and then again at follow-up, even if it was over the phone.) The CDCESs were much more vigilant in reviewing participants' behavioral goal choices and suggesting modifications if the goals were too ambitious.
6. Evaluate	After 2 comprehensive programs, the new methods had been implemented with 20 participants. Eighty-five percent of the participants were reached at follow-up by phone or by clinic appointment. Of those, 80% met or exceeded their meal plan and exercise goal. The program could now say that at baseline, participants walked an average of 30 minutes a week and at follow-up they walked an average of 60 minutes a week. In addition, 80% of participants say they follow their meal plan >75% of the time, an increase from 20% saying they use a meal plan at baseline.
7. Have a maintenance plan	Participants reported liking the postcard reminders. The clinic found that address labels could be easily printed, so the participants only needed to affix the label to their cards. Goal sheets are kept on file but may be moved to a computerized record.
CQI Case #2 Improving appointment scheduling at diabetes class	
1. Identify the problem	Although participants were encouraged as part of a group class to schedule a 1:1 follow-up appointment, they were leaving class before scheduling an appointment.
2. Collect and analyze data	At the monthly comprehensive class attended by 10 participants, the team determined that only 1 person made a follow-up appointment after class, and 1 more called before the next scheduled class. At the next class, each person was asked individually the reason an appointment was not made. Five of the 8 said "forgot" or "didn't understand that I was supposed to do it."
3. Consider possible solutions	The team brainstormed the following solutions: 1. Ask the secretary to come to class to schedule appointments.

TABLE 11.8 CQI Case Examples (continued)

3. Consider possible solutions (continued)	2. CDCESs will call participants to schedule appointments. 3. CDCESs will write possible class dates on the board and each participant will select a date and turn it in. 4. Mount a large piece of paper in front of the class listing date options for the follow-up class and invite participants to write their name next to the class they will attend.
4. Make recommendations	The fourth choice above was selected since it not only requires the least amount of time but also empowers the person with diabetes to take the action and potentially join a class that a classmate/friend has signed up for.
5. Implement	For the next 2 series of classes, a large piece of poster paper was mounted in the front of the class with options for 3 different follow-up classes. The CDCESs and scheduling staff met to discuss implementation. CDCESs introduced the follow-up class sign-up at the beginning of the class and again at the end.
6. Evaluate	After the first class series, 7 out of 10 participants signed up for class, and 6 actually attended. After the second series, 9 out of 11 signed up and 8 attended.
7. Have a maintenance plan	The solution demonstrated an excellent improvement, without the staff needing to commit extra time. When participants sign up for a follow-up class, they are given the choice of 2 different kinds of classes, at 2 different times. They can also complete and take home a reminder card.

Source: Adapted with permission from "Diabetes Education Programs and the CQI Process: Recommendations for Joslin Education Programs," in *Education Program Planning Manual* (Boston: Joslin Diabetes Center, 2015).

Summary

As the epidemic of diabetes continues to escalate, the need for diabetes education programs remains high. However, in order to survive, programs must operate at a high level of efficiency. This means that the program manager not only needs to understand diabetes and chronic disease, but also needs to be skilled in business operations. A successful DSMES/DPP program can be measured against the quadruple aim of quality care that is cost effective and meets the needs of the participant and the provider.

This chapter offered specific resources and suggestions to help program managers build and strengthen skills in program management and operations. The process of successful program management that was outlined follows the same 5 steps defined for DSMES: (1) assessment, (2) goal setting, (3) planning, (4) implementation, and (5) evaluation/monitoring. Keeping these steps in mind will help organize the process for the program manager.

Focus on Education

Teaching Strategies

DSME programs that produce good results share common qualities. These include culturally relevant clinical approaches; adequate contact time; and treatment goals that are based on collaboration between the person with diabetes and the provider, involve competent diabetes care and education professionals, are group based, and have a strong foundation of collaboration between diabetes care and education specialists and physicians.

Developing a learner-centered curriculum should be an ongoing process.

- Use program evaluations to determine whether the content and delivery of diabetes education meet the needs of each participant. Adjust accordingly.
- Make sure that the curriculum is evidence based, with both teaching content and education methods.
- Align the curriculum with your teaching philosophy.
- Know which theories underpin your curriculum (eg, Common Sense/Health Belief Model, Social Learning/Self-Efficacy, Dual Processing Theory).
- Assess how your teaching style works with the curriculum.
- Audit participant feedback and adjust the curriculum as needed.

Design your teaching facility to bring out the best of the learning experience. Create comfortable counseling and classroom spaces that are roomy enough for family members to join, have space for small group practice activities, and yet feel private enough for intimate, personal conversations. To make waiting rooms more comfortable, consider adjusting the lighting and adding chairs for people of different sizes. Flowers and relaxing art are also a nice addition.

Messages for People With Diabetes

Diabetes self-management education programs are designed to assist you in managing your diabetes. Diabetes care and education specialists are skilled in teaching you about diabetes and how to incorporate diabetes self-management skills into your daily routine.

Education is ongoing. Diabetes education is not just a onetime event. Take as much time as you need to understand your options and make choices. As your life changes, so will your diabetes self-management. Your body changes, your diabetes changes, and your perspectives and ability to take care of your diabetes change. Adjust your diabetes self-management therapies accordingly.

You are in charge of your diabetes. You have the right and responsibility to ask questions, seek clarification, and make changes in managing your diabetes and overall health. You have a right to know all of your options and alternatives and the potential outcomes of your choices. You have the right to a second opinion, to ask your family or others for advice, and to take as much time as needed. And you have the right to receive information in a way that best matches your learning style, literacy level, and needs.

You can learn about and manage your diabetes well regardless of your health literacy level. *Education is the kindling of a flame, not the filling of a vessel—Socrates.* Socrates never told people what the correct answer was, but rather he engaged them in a conversation, asking questions that were designed to make them aware of their own beliefs and judge for themselves whether they were based on mistaken information or contradictions. Explore your own diabetes and solutions to your diabetes care.

Focus on Practice

The NSDSMES set a foundation for developing and implementing a quality diabetes education program. To receive Medicare reimbursement for services, a program manager must be able to demonstrate that every standard is implemented.

There are 10 standards in the NSDSMES: (1) organizational mission statement, and goals; (2) stakeholder input; (3) population(s) served; (4) a quality coordinator; (5) DSMES team; (6) curriculum; (7) individualization of DSME participant plan; (8) ongoing support; (9 participant progress; (10) quality improvement.

There are 8 content areas of DSMES: (1) diabetes pathophysiology and treatment options, (2) healthy eating, (3) physical activity, (4) medication usage, (5) monitoring and using patient-generated health data, (6) acute complications and chronic complications, (7) healthy coping, (8) problem-solving.

There are 4 critical times for DSMES: (1) at diagnosis, (2) at an annual assessment of educational, nutritional, and emotional needs by the primary care provider with a particular emphasis on times when a referral for more education and support is recommended, (3) when complicating factors arise that affect diabetes management, and (4) when transitions in care occur.

Before you establish your DSMES program, carefully assess the needs of all parties. This includes persons with diabetes, the community, providers, and financial stakeholders. Examine all existing available resources to either complement the existing services or provide a competitive edge. Set program expectations by defining program goals, its mission, and a business plan. Outline a strategy with a budget, advisory group, curriculum, office space, staffing, and IT needs.

Effective implementation of a DSMES program involves several factors: ongoing marketing, clear operational communication, metrics collection, and meeting desirable accreditation standards, as well as a good understanding of coding and reimbursement for the services offered.

Put a system in place in which providers are given consistent feedback on performance. Feedback should be both quantitative (eg, A1C) and qualitative (eg, observations with persons with diabetes) by the healthcare system and/or respected colleagues.

Ask what the DSMES program will do and how it will do what it is meant to do. How will it improve participant care outcomes? How will it improve the delivery of care? How will it help the person with diabetes? How will it help the clinician?

Review the requirements for accreditation/recognition of programs early in your planning so that you know what you will need to report and put in place to get your program approved in order to bill CMS.

References

1. Department of Health and Human Services. Healthy People 2020 topics and objectives (cited 2016 Jun 16). On the Internet at: https://www.healthypeople.gov/2020/topics-objectives/topic/diabetes/objectives.

2. Li R, Shrestha SS, Lipman R, et al. Diabetes self-management education and training among privately insured persons with newly diagnosed diabetes—United States 2011-2012. MMWR Morb Mortal Wkly Rep. 2014 Nov 21;63(46):1045-9.

3. Strawbridge LM, Lloyd JT, Meadow A, et al. Use of Medicare's diabetes self-management training benefit. Health Educ Behav. 2015 Aug;42(4):530-8.

4. American Association of Diabetes Educators. The scope of practice, standards of practice, and standards of professional performance for diabetes educators. Chicago: American Association of Diabetes Educators; 2010.

5. Beck J, Greenwood, D, et al. 2017 National Standards for Diabetes Self-Management Education and Support. The Diabetes Educator. 2017; 43(5):449-64.

6. Association of Diabetes Care and Education Specialists (ADCES). Competencies for diabetes care and education specialists. (forthcoming).

7. Maryniuk MD, Mensing C, Imershein S, Gregory A, Jackson R. Enhancing the role of medical office staff in diabetes care and education. Clin Diabetes. 2013;31:116-22.

8. Tang TS, Funnell MM, Oh M. Lasting effects of a 2-year diabetes self-management support intervention: outcomes at 1-year follow-up. Prev Chronic Dis. 2012;9:E109. Epub 2012 Jun 7.

9. National Certification Board for Diabetes Educators (NCBDE) (cited 2013 Aug 6). On the Internet at: http://www.ncbde.org/ncbde-announces-changes-regarding-initial-certification-effective-2014/.

10. Sullivan E, Goodwin J. Where does your time go? In: AADE in Practice. Chicago: American Association of Diabetes Educators; Spring 2008.

11. Maryniuk MD, Moore T, Weinger K, et al. Diabetes educator productivity: an outpatient time study of daily activities. Diabetes. 2001;50 Suppl 2:A75.

12. Powers MA, Bardsley J, Cypress M, et al. Diabetes self-management education and support in type 2 diabetes: a joint position statement of the American Diabetes Association, the American Association of Diabetes Educators, and the Academy of Nutrition and Dietetics. Diabetes Care. 2015;38:1372-82.

13. Powers MA, Bardsley J, Cypress M, et al. Diabetes self-management education and support in type 2 diabetes: a joint position statement of the American Diabetes Association, the American Association of Diabetes Educators, and the Academy of Nutrition and Dietetics. Diabetes Educ. 2015;41(4):417-30.

14. Powers MA, Bardsley J, Cypress M, et al. Diabetes self-management education and support in type 2 diabetes: a joint position statement of the American Diabetes Association, the American Association of Diabetes Educators, and the Academy of Nutrition and Dietetics. J Acad Nutr Diet. 2015;115(8):1323-34.

15. Powers MA, Bardsley J, Cypress M, et al. Diabetes self-management education and support in type 2 diabetes: a joint position statement of the American Diabetes Association, the American Association of Diabetes Educators, and the Academy of Nutrition and Dietetics. Diabetes Educ. 2015;41(4):417-30.

16. American Association of Diabetes Educators. CQI: A Step-by-Step Guide for Quality Improvement in Diabetes Education. 3rd ed. Chicago: American Association of Diabetes Educators; 2015.

17. Powers BJ, Trinh JV, Bosworth HB. Can this patient read and understand written health information? JAMA. 2010;304(1):76-84.

18. Chew LD, Bradley KA, Boyko EJ. Brief questions to identify patients with inadequate health literacy. Fam Med. 2004 Sept;36(8):588-94.

19. Mulcahy K, Maryniuk M, Peeples M, et al. AADE position statement: standards for outcomes measurement of diabetes self-management education. Diabetes Educ. 2003;29:804-16.

CHAPTER 12

Transitional Care

Amy Hess Fischl, MS, RDN, LDN, BC-ADM, CDCES
Christie A. Schumacher, PharmD, BCPS, BCACP, BC-ADM, CDCES

Key Concepts

- Transitional care occurs throughout the life span, is continuously evolving, and must be tailored to each individual.
- There are important differences between children/adolescents/young adults and adults in regard to diabetes education and management. Focusing on the methods of communication, teaching tools, setting, and goals that meet the needs and pace of each individual is key to successful transition.
- Education in the hospital can play an important role in diabetes management and should begin upon admission and continue through discharge.
- Self-care and engagement should be encouraged through disease state education. Barriers to inpatient and outpatient care should be identified early in the education process.
- The patient's knowledge should be assessed and continually reassessed throughout the transition period to maintain an appropriate knowledge base and confirm important concepts.
- An individualized plan that promotes self-care should be developed for each person with diabetes.
- Communication among the person with diabetes, his or her family, and the healthcare team is a vital component of diabetes care. Confirm that everyone involved in the person's care understands the goals and the individualized care plan at every stage of transition.

Introduction

Transitional care has become an essential component of patient care within the inpatient and outpatient settings and at all ages and stages of life. Transitions for persons with diabetes are multifaceted throughout the life span since responsibilities are closely tied to age and maturity. The transition from pediatric to adult care has also become an integral element within diabetes education. The competing demands of relationships and careers, as well as the psychological and physical changes, make this a challenging time.[1] A successful path for good diabetes self-management is founded on a collaborative approach, with the healthcare team and the individual actively involved in the process from the beginning.

"Transitional care" is a diverse term. It includes the care of diabetes across the life span and transitions between different institutions and settings, all of which are an important part of patient care. It has been shown that one half of hospitalized patients experience at least one medical error in medication management, diagnostic workup, or follow-up testing as they change between healthcare settings. The majority of errors and adverse drug events can be attributed to lack of communication between healthcare providers at the different settings.[2,3] This is an important area for diabetes care and education specialists as they are in a position to facilitate communication between settings while encouraging self-care and engagement.

Infancy Through Young Adulthood

While children at different ages will be able to accomplish tasks and accept responsibilities at different ages and stages, diabetes is a family condition. During this time, it is important not to expect more from children than they are able to do and be certain that the family understands this as well. Age does not always equal maturity, and increasing diabetes responsibility must be individualized. Table 14.3 in chapter 14 lists the normal developmental tasks for the developmental stages from infancy through age 19.

Pediatric Care: Infant to Age 3

Tips for managing diabetes in an infant include the following:[4,5]

- Adjust insulin program around eating patterns.
- Use small lancets and small needles for blood glucose testing and injections.
- Try an auto-injector and numbing cream to help minimize the fear and pain of injections.
- Have supplies ready before blood tests and injections to minimize stress.
- Avoid glucose testing or injections in the child's bed (keep the bed a "safe" place).
- Use play as a teaching tool.
- Use the toes or heels for blood glucose testing. If using continuous glucose monitoring, insert in the hips or upper buttocks or the back of the arms (off-label use), away from the child's line of eye sight.
- Distract the child with a game or song so that he or she is not focused on the task at hand.
- Speak in soothing tones so the infant or child is not frightened.

During this time of rapid growth and development, key motor and brain maturity is taking place:[4,5]

- Sitting—age 6 to 8 months
- Crawling—age 6 to 12 months
- Walking—age 12 to 18 months
- Language development

Diabetes tasks are essential components of healthy growth and development. Parents and caregivers must attempt to remove emotion from the equation while completing these tasks. Infants and toddlers can identify emotional cues from their caregivers. Most outbursts regarding diabetes care are due to an interruption in the child's activity rather than true pain. Infants and toddlers develop trust during this time, so it is important to provide diabetes care with love and affection while making it part of the routine. The child may then accept it more readily. Since the child cannot independently perform self-care activities at this age, diabetes care is the responsibility of the parent. As the toddler demonstrates increased interest in participation, this interest should be fostered. It is important to reassure the parents that age-related responsibilities are merely a guideline, not a blueprint set in stone. Each child will progress along different timelines.

Once mobility begins, blood glucose levels will likely be affected due to increased energy expenditure. At this age, hypoglycemia unawareness is more common. Parents and caregivers need to be alert to outward symptoms as they may not be evident to the child. It will be important to test blood glucose levels more frequently as well as adjust insulin doses or add more carbohydrate snacks to reduce the risk of hypoglycemia.[4,5] With increased use of continuous glucose monitors, this could ease the burden of the parents to more proactively reduce the risk of hypoglycemia and frequent glycemic variability in toddlers by identifying rate of change and direction in glucose values.[6]

Tips for managing diabetes in the toddler include the following:[4,5]

- Align foods in blocks of time.
- Limit choices for food, injection sites, and blood test times to minimize stress.
- Have the child help with blood tests and injections, perhaps by placing the test strip in the blood glucose meter or placing the lancet in the lancing device.
- Have supplies ready before blood tests and injections to minimize stress; for example, Buzzy® devices assist children with pain management (https://buzzyhelps.com/).
- Use stories, books, and games as teaching tools.

School—Early and Middle School

Table 12.1 lists the average age for mastery of specific diabetes-related skills.

Tips for managing diabetes in the preschooler include the following:[7–9]

- Reassure the child that diabetes is no one's fault.
- Allow the child to do his or her own blood glucose tests and push the plunger on the syringe.
- If using continuous glucose monitoring, involve the child by having them inform an adult when the CGM receiver or phone app alarms or alerts.
- Use reward systems, such as a sticker chart, to help with involvement.
- Avoid labeling blood glucose test results as good or bad.
- Help the child identify feelings of low blood glucose.
- Involve the child in meal plan decisions.
- Use stories, books, and games as teaching tools.

The school-age child is beginning to have expanded cognitive, athletic, and social skills and more refined motor skills. While school-age children continue to fear a loss of control, they also have an intense fear of failure or not measuring up to others' expectations. To reduce these concerns, it is essential to create flexible diabetes self-management tasks. When working with the school staff, it would be helpful to review the following table of skills for school-age children:

Skills a school-age child may perform[10]	
Diabetes tasks a school-age child CAN do	Diabetes tasks a school-age child SHOULD NOT do
• Help check their own blood sugar • Help count carbohydrates • When ready, give their own insulin injection • Tell an adult when they feel like they have a low blood sugar • Start to learn their insulin doses • Help by doing the math problem when calculating an insulin dose • Check ketones, with help of a caregiver	• Be responsible for always understanding when to check blood sugar • Be expected to count carbs independently at all times • Give injection without supervision • Always know how to anticipate or prevent a low blood sugar • Know when and how to make insulin dose changes • Always be expected to calculate insulin doses • Be left alone or know what to do when sick

TABLE 12.1 Average Ages for Diabetes-Related Skills

Skill	*Average Age of Mastery (Years)*
Hypoglycemia management	
• Recognizes and reports	7–10
• Able to treat	10–12
• Anticipates/prevents	14–16
Hyperglycemia management	
• Recognizes and reports	After age 7
• Understanding cause and effect	Not well developed until after adolescence
• Anticipates/prevents	Not well developed until after adolescence
Blood glucose testing	8–10 may be able to perform fingerstick by 4–5 y of age Ability to interpret results not typical until school-age years
Insulin injection	
• Gives to self (at least sometimes)	8–12
• Able to adjust doses	14–16 Able to anticipate dose change needs by mid-adolescence (typically after age 16)
Meal planning	
• Can identify appropriate pre-exercise snack	10–12 Skills needed to evaluate impact of exercise on glycemic levels, medications, and meal intake are not well developed until after age 16
• States role of meal planning	14–16
• Able to alter food intake in relation to blood glucose level	14–16
• Emergency management	After age 16

Source: T Wysocki, P Meinhold, DJ Cox, WL Clarke, "Survey of diabetes professionals regarding developmental changes in diabetes self-care," *Diabetes Care* 13, no. 1 (1990): 65. LK Scott, "Developmental mastery of diabetes-related tasks in children," *Nurs Clin N Am*. 2013;48:329-42.

Tips for managing diabetes in the school-aged child include the following:[7–10]

- Incorporate school lunches, parties, and special events into the meal plan.
- Plan meal, exercise, and insulin schedules around usual activities.
- Make sure the school understands and provides for the child's needs.
- Monitor school attendance and performance.
- Ask the school to provide accommodations for blood glucose testing and/or use of continuous glucose monitoring and/or insulin pump therapy.

Adolescence

There are several differences in behavior and development between early, middle, and late adolescence, the time between 12 and 21 years of age. Characteristics of each of these stages are highlighted in Table 14.4 in chapter 14. Adolescence is a period of rapid growth and increasing physical, cognitive, and emotional maturity. These changes may occur slowly or rapidly and are determined by genetic familial factors, the economy, nutrition, health, and the environment.[8] Diabetes affects normal adolescent development, but identity and self-image concerns can revolve around diabetes concerns such as the appearance of the injection site or self-identification as being different. Normal independence issues may be impeded as a result of parental protectiveness or the teen's failure to assume responsibility for self-care. Adolescents with diabetes can become particularly concerned about their growth and sexual maturation. Metabolic management tends to deteriorate in adolescence due to a multitude of factors. Attitudes of experimentation and rebellion in addition to risk-taking behaviors can affect diabetes issues such as taking insulin regularly, monitoring, and the quality and quantity of food consumption.[7] It is highly probable that adolescents with type 1 diabetes may experience reduced quality of life. Adolescents who must self-manage their diabetes care not only face the pressures of diabetes but also the same biological, cognitive, hormonal, and physical changes as their peers. Most adolescents with type 1 diabetes experience challenges related to pursuing their own identities, being apprehensive about being seen as different from their peers, and feeling pressure (real or imagined) to independently manage their diabetes. This may lead some adolescents to mismanage their conditions, such as eliminating blood glucose monitoring, omitting insulin doses, following unreliable meal planning methods and engaging in high-risk behaviors that may reduce quality of life. Diabetes self-management education is identified as the best existing intervention program to help those with type 1 diabetes understand self-management options and make informed decisions about their care and improve quality of life.[8]

Tips for helping the early adolescent with diabetes management include the following:[7–10]

- Personal meaning of diabetes.
- Who and when to tell about diabetes.
- Determining roles and responsibilities in care.
- Incorporate both direct (eg, SMBG and insulin administration) AND indirect behavioral skills (stress reduction, coping strategies, conflict resolution, goal setting)
- Incorporate a hectic lifestyle into the diabetes plan.
- Begin to work on problem-solving skills and work up to independence.
- Discuss treatment options (multiple daily injections [MDIs], insulin pump therapy, meal planning, and continuous glucose monitoring) and benefits and barriers to each based on the individuals' needs and preferences.
- Allow independent visits with the healthcare team.
- Include sex education as part of diabetes education.
- Monitor school attendance and performance.
- Allow independence in problem solving.
- Be nonjudgmental (eg, there is no such thing as a "bad" blood glucose reading).
- Keep social issues separate from diabetes.
- Help establish realistic goals.
- Watch for risk-taking behaviors, such as not taking insulin or substance use.

Transitional Care (Adolescence to Young Adulthood)

According to Blum et al, "Transition is a purposeful, planned movement of adolescents and young adults with chronic physical and medical conditions from child-centered to adult-orientated health care systems."[11(p570)]

But, it is critical to understand that transition covers the lifespan, while transfer is the singular action of moving from one healthcare process to another. When transition care is described in the context of young adulthood, many mistakenly focus on the transfer component instead of the more critical long-spanning process of transition.[12] In 2018, the American Academy of Pediatrics, the American Academy of Family Physicians, and the American College of Physicians updated a clinical report on healthcare transition from adolescence to adulthood in the medical home.[13] It was updated to include the new research and international statements on the topic of healthcare transition. While the original 2011 report included the critical first steps for successful transitional care, these steps have not changed and are as follows:

- Identify an adult healthcare professional who can meet the individual's needs and provide uninterrupted, comprehensive, and accessible care.
- Identify the core knowledge and skills needed for successful transition and make them a required knowledge skill for primary care professionals in practice.
- Create a detailed medical summary of the individual.
- Create a written transition plan for the individual by age 14.
- Apply the same guidelines to all individuals and identify resources needed for those with special healthcare needs.
- Ensure affordable and continuous healthcare coverage.[13]

This update also focuses on the Six Core Elements of Health Care Transition, which is a structured process for use within healthcare practices to meet with needs of the adolescent into young adulthood. The elements include:

- Transition policy discussion—between ages 12 to 14
- Transition tracking and monitoring progress—between ages 14 to 18
- Transition readiness to assess skills—between ages 14 to 18
- Transition planning—between ages 14 to 18
- Transfer and/or integration into adult-centered care—between ages 18 to 21
- Transition completion and ongoing care with adult clinician—between ages 18 to 26
- Complete resources for the Six Core Elements can be found at https://www.gottransition.org/resources/index.cfm##six.

To encourage safe and successful diabetes management into adulthood, transitional care from the pediatric setting to the adult setting is essential. Typically, most pediatric practices transition the young person to adult care after age 18. However, some pediatric practices allow the person to remain until postsecondary education is completed. At this point, there are no established long-term guidelines in place that fits the global need, but rather multiple recommendations based on expert opinion.[15,16] Several studies have highlighted key components to successful transition care within their respective countries. In Canada, researchers found that transition support requires intensive and structured intervention, which led to increased clinic attendance, improved satisfaction with care and decreased diabetes-related distress, but these benefits were not sustained 12 months after completing the intervention.[17] Survey data from Ontario also illustrated that there was variation in transition processes, but challenges included transition preparation, communication with adult teams, adult programs' abilities to meet the needs of young adults and loss to follow-up.[18] It is clear that healthcare professionals throughout the world understand the need for transitional care, and researchers around the world are searching for the one true method that will meet the needs of the young adult and will be implemented effectively. Many position statements and recommendations have been developed globally in order to create continuity in the transition process, but each is typically focusing on an individual country's healthcare models.[19–21]

Additional research has shown that young adults who have gone through transition mention the following issues with the process: (1) the mean age for adult referral was 17, not allowing sufficient time for transition to an adult provider at age 18, (2) transition was too abrupt, (3) very little accessibility to adult healthcare providers when transferring to adult care, as compared with communication received in pediatric care, (4) lack of coordination for the transfer, (5) unexpected differences between pediatric and adult healthcare systems, and (6) delays greater than 6 months in establishing adult diabetes care. When young adults receive appropriate and effective transition care throughout their childhood into young adulthood, they did tend to have less diabetes-related distress and higher engagement with their regimen. Key factors that tend to influence effective communication with healthcare providers include interaction style, consistency, support for autonomy, parental involvement in medical care, and the young adult's comfort with disclosure.[22–24] A discussion with adolescents and young adults identified that in the development of a smooth transition, a patient would ideally feel as though nothing has changed and that any transition was a "natural" process.[26] Adolescents have also described unique barriers to and facilitators of self-care behaviors in their diabetes management. They found that situational influences included biological factors such as hunger, cravings, hypoglycemia, fatigue, and time of day; psychological factors such as knowledge, affect, cognition, motivation, and life goals; and environmental factors such as school, competing priorities, and peer relations. System influences include the health system, which refers to the type and quality of healthcare and diabetes education. They felt that diabetes care and education specialists assisted them in acquiring the knowledge and skills they need to manage their diabetes, and high-quality diabetes care and education specialists can have positive influences on self-care behaviors. But, it is important to understand that goal setting with the patient and working toward their specific goals can be a vital motivating factor.[27] Good outcomes have been achieved when clinics have implemented models in which there is a gradual and well planned move away from joint consultations, where the young person has the opportunity to have independent sessions with clinicians and where there is a specific service to meet the needs of parents.[28] It is crucial that healthcare providers, particularly diabetes care and education specialists, since they may have more allotted time to meet with the teen, initiate conversations about engagement in risky behaviors and transition to adult medical care as well as ensure teens have time without their parents to discuss these topics unencumbered. Recent research has found that instead of a focus on blood glucose target levels, the focus should be redirected to psychosocial support much earlier and more often. It was found that diabetes self-care confidence and perception of diabetes as a problem could be an indication of follow-up appointment attendance after transition.[29]

Also, once transition occurs and the individual leaves pediatric care, an increasing number of individuals become lost to follow-up or are dissatisfied with their care from adult endocrinologists.[24] Recent studies have shown that a structured transition program that included the use of joint appointments (including members from both pediatric and adult teams) and a transition coordinator as well as coordinated care between pediatric and adult providers can improve participation with follow-up after transition.[30,31] While studies have focused on transition clinics and many have found some success, this option is not realistic for the majority of the United States, and the entire globe, for that matter, due to lack of resources and locations of services. Transition clinics work well in large university settings due to the plethora of staff and monetary resources available to them. However, the majority of diabetes self-management education is conducted far from those services. It is crucial that transition guidelines and resources are applicable and available for the majority who are interacting with this age group.

A meta-summary discussed patient perspectives of transition as well as factors or "conditions" that can successfully facilitate transition to adult care. The first condition refers to the *meaning* given to transition by the individual and his or her family. It is important that the discussion reiterate that transition is normal and is not a punishment or form of abandonment by the pediatric healthcare providers. *Transition* should have a positive connotation. The second condition is related to the individual's *expectations* regarding transition. The goal of preparing for transition is to reduce the stress involved. Assessing the individual's thoughts regarding the process can help move the individual in the right direction and make this a positive experience with realistic expectations. The third condition is the individual's level of *knowledge and skills* before the transfer. Empowerment is key to diabetes care. The earlier this can be fostered, the less likely this process will need to be a "cram session" prior to transition. The fourth condition encompasses the actual *planning* itself. While timing of the transfer may vary depending on maturation and individual goals, it is essential that planning begin early and be embedded in the conversation at every office visit. The final condition includes the *environment* and the resources necessary for continued success.[32] It has been found that various transition interventions may improve outcomes, but it is crucial to understand the audience and their needs in order to facilitate success. In a recent review, several common themes were found across all interventions that improved transition: 1) continuity – strategies that facilitate contact between young adults and diabetes services; 2) support – strategies for addressing the psychosocial and diabetes-specific needs of the young adult; 3) education – strategies for informing young adults regarding diabetes management; and 4) tailored to young adults – strategies for delivering appropriate and acceptable interventions.[13] It is obvious young adults do want to be involved in their care, but on their terms. The role of the diabetes care and education specialist is to weave these themes within the context of diabetes self-management education and support. Another review also posited that an underappreciated component of the transition process is the responsibility of adult providers to actively participate in the stewardship of young adults. While it is well documented that young adults found issues with the timing and method of transfer, additional structured support in the adult care setting is necessary to continue and enhance the ongoing diabetes self-management skills. Key recommendations for adult providers include: 1) Communicate with pediatric colleagues during transition to coordinate care and minimize gaps; 2) Objective assessment of knowledge and skills levels can help the adult provider capitalize on strengths and identify needs for intervention; 3) Focus on establishing a relationship, not just perfecting A1C; 4) Develop a strategy to routinely identify and address psychosocial needs; and 5) A team-based approach can help young adults stay engaged.[20]

Effective transition is essential for continued quality care and successful long-term follow-up for the individual as well as the healthcare provider involved after transition. Several articles have summarized transition experiences, barriers, and needs from both healthcare providers and young adults themselves. A 2014 survey of adult endocrinologists used to assess current transition experiences, resources, and barriers found that only 11% reported receiving summaries for transitioning young adults although they felt it was important for patient care. The respondents reported easy access to diabetes care and education specialists and dietitians, but fewer reported access to mental health professionals, which led to barriers to diabetes management for young adults with depression, substance abuse problems, and eating disorders.[34] A 2015 survey of pediatric endocrinologists found that there is wide variation in transition care with regards to the transfer process. Barriers found to affect transfer of care included having to end long relationships with their patients, lack of transition protocols, and perceived deficiencies in adult care.[35] The earlier the conversation begins, the more prepared the individual and family can become. Regardless of the individual's age at transfer, it is important to include the individual in the decision-making process.[36] Table 12.2 provides age-specific decision points for diabetes self-care and management.

Recommendations and guidelines for transition from around the world are summarized in Table 12.3.

The National Alliance to Advance Adolescent Health created the Web site Got Transition to help improve transitional care. Numerous resources, assessment tools, and checklists are available for download at http://www.gottransition.org/resources/index.cfm. Of particular importance within these resources are the transition readiness checklists for both the patient and parent. If psychological support is available, this is an ideal tool for their use in assessing readiness. However, if that is not available, this tool can easily be used by the diabetes care and education specialist to assess the patient's individual needs to begin their transition journey. They can be accessed at https://www.gottransition.org/resourceGet.cfm?id=224 for youth and https://www.gottransition.org/resourceGet.cfm?id=225 for parents and caregivers. The Endocrine Society spearheaded an initiative that included the Hormone Health Network, American Academy of Pediatrics,

TABLE 12.2 Examples of Teaching Points for Transitions—the goal is to review all previous concepts as the individual transitions to the next age range

Ages 8–10:

- Begin to answer questions in clinic
- Why it is important to attend clinic every 3 months
- The importance of A1C values and target goals
- What it means to have diabetes
- Why some people have diabetes and others do not
- Importance of testing blood sugar and learning to test blood sugar (if not already)
- If using CGM, what should I do if the low and high BG alarms go off
- How to administer insulin (if not already)
- How the body uses food
- Identify carbohydrates
- How to make healthy food choices using MyPlate (USDA; http://www.choosemyplate.gov)
- The causes and symptoms of hypoglycemia and its treatment
- The role of insulin during sick-day management
- Identification of insulin types
- The effect of the school day and scheduling on blood sugar levels
- How sports, outside play, and other types of physical activity affect blood sugar levels and insulin doses
- Introduce the concept of transition
- Medical identification

Ages 11–12:

- Assume responsibility to check blood sugars on your own at specific times of the day
- Define healthy eating and how it fits into your meal plan Discuss ways to make healthy choices at school, when eating out with friends, and at other special occasions. Also discuss how to incorporate "occasional" foods.
- Begin to understand how an illness like a cold or the flu can affect your body and blood sugar
- What are urine or blood ketones, what do they signify, and how to test for them
- Begin to name insulin types taken, their actions, reasons for taking them, and the proper doses
- How sports (especially practices versus games), play, and other exercise (including gym class) affect your blood sugar levels and insulin doses
- How diabetes affects your school day
- Introduction to drinking, smoking, peer pressure, and diabetes
- Effects of growth, puberty, and sexual development on diabetes

(continued)

TABLE 12.2 Examples of Teaching Points for Transitions—the goal is to review all previous concepts as the individual transitions to the next age range (continued)

Ages 13–15:

- Answer questions independently in clinic and meet alone with the certified diabetes care and education specialists for part of the visit
- Inject insulin/change insulin pump with minimal reminders
- Parents review blood sugar logs and help you think through and double-check insulin doses
- Let parents know when you need medications or supplies
- The significance of A1C, how the choices you make affect it, and how you can change it
- The role of diabetes distress on diabetes care
- Screen for depression at every visit
- Discuss the blood tests that are completed each year and why
- Effects of growth, puberty and sexual development, sexual activity, and reproduction on diabetes
- Females only: discuss impact of menstrual cycle on diabetes self-management
- Understand reproductive choices and the impact on your diabetes and overall health – discuss contraception options
- The impact of diabetes on driving and the importance of checking blood sugar levels prior to driving
- Discuss the differences between pediatric and adult care
- Introduce the concept of confidentiality between patient, parent, and provider
- Begin shared responsibility between young adult and family for:
  - Making appointments
  - Calling the healthcare provider with questions or problems

Ages 16–17:

- Independent with monitoring and recording blood sugars
- Independent with all insulin doses without parents reminding you
- Begin to call/e-mail the diabetes team and speak directly with staff if there are changes in your health
- The impact of diabetes on driving, the importance of checking blood sugar levels prior to driving, and steps to take if blood sugar is low prior to getting behind the wheel
- Discuss the effect of smoking, drugs and alcohol on diabetes
- Know your health history including major illnesses, surgeries, allergies, and healthcare providers (dentist, eye doctor, psychologist)
- The impact of college, work, and career choices on diabetes management
- Effects of growth, puberty and sexual development, sexual activity, and reproduction on diabetes
- Females only: discuss impact of menstrual cycle on diabetes self-management
- Understand reproductive choices and the impact on your diabetes and overall health – discuss contraception options

Ages 18–21:

- Routinely call the diabetes team and speak directly with staff if there are changes in your health
- Understand reproductive choices and the impact on your diabetes and overall health
- Discuss long-term complications of diabetes, the need for routine follow-up and tests, and the importance of glucose management into adulthood
- Establish care with a primary care health professional and with an adult diabetes team
- Review the American Diabetes Association guidelines versus the American Association of Clinical Endocrinologists guidelines (http://www.aace.com/files/dm-guidelines-ccp.pdf) and the International Diabetes Federation guidelines (http://www.idf.org/diabetesatlas) for managing diabetes
- HIPAA—parents need permission from the young adult to be in the exam room, see test results, discuss any part of care with healthcare providers; document to be completed and signed by patient for chart authorizing parents to participate
- Review resources available for transition care
- Suggest annual review with a diabetes care and education specialist regarding updates and new technology

Source: Curriculum created by A Hess Fischl for the University of Chicago Kovler Diabetes Center, 2006; updated 05 Jan 2019 and available at http://www.kovlerdiabetescenter.org.

TABLE 12.3 Key Global Transition Recommendations/Guidelines

International Society for Pediatric and Adolescent Diabetes (ISPAD)[1]

- Appropriate age of transfer varies according to location and type of healthcare delivery system, maturity of adolescent, local practices and resources, patient and family preferences, national policies, and availability of appropriate services
- Transition preparation should include counseling on diabetes self-management, healthcare navigation, diabetes complications, and differences between pediatric and adult care systems
- A joint pediatric and adult clinic working together to facilitate the transition process or a liaison between pediatric and adult services
- Discussion of transition well in advance of transfer will allow the adolescent and family to choose the appropriate time based on their own preference and readiness as well as availability of services and healthcare insurance requirements
- Formal clinic-specific transition policies and clear communication between all services providing care for the transitioning patients

American Diabetes Association Transitions Work Group[2]

- Preparation of at least 1 year prior to transfer
- Preparation should focus on self-management skills with a gradual transfer of care from the parent to the teen
- Information regarding the differences between pediatric and adult care should be included in the preparation for transition
- Written summary of transfer needed for adult provider and patient

National Institute for Health and Clinical Excellence (NICE)[3,4]

- Should be allowed sufficient time to become familiar with the practicalities of transition from pediatric care to adult care in order to improve clinic attendance
- Planning should begin by age 13 or 14 at the latest
- Age of transfer should depend on the individual's physical and emotional development and maturity
- Transition planning should be developmentally appropriate and take into account the young person's capabilities, needs, and hopes for the future
- Transition should occur at a time of relative stability in the individual's health and should be coordinated with other life transitions
- Young people with type 1 diabetes who are preparing for transition to adult services should be informed that some aspects of diabetes care will change at transition

National Health Service England[5]

- Services for young people with diabetes aged up to 25 will require engagement with both pediatric and adult diabetes services
- Themes to be considered in the development of good transition services:
  - person centered and responsive
  - access and engagement
  - partnerships and coordination/integrated services
  - independence and autonomy
  - staged and timely
  - structures and systems
  - psychological support
  - clinical standards
  - continuing care and assessment
- Early preparation and planning are essential for managing expectations, promoting understanding and involvement in the wider process, and ensuring that the young adult is well informed and empowered.
- Planning must be based on the young person's physical development, emotional maturity, and local circumstances.
- Diabetes care for those aged 19–25 may be best provided in dedicated clinics, with the same staff from adult diabetes services that contribute to transitional diabetes clinics.

(continued)

TABLE 12.3 Key Global Transition Recommendations/Guidelines (continued)
Australasian Paediatric Endocrine Group and the Australian Diabetes Society[6] • Flexible timing of transfer • Flexibility in provision of health services • A "transition case manager" for each individual • Preparation period • Choice of adult provider • Coordinated transfer • Joint consultations • Accessible medical documentation • Maintaining contact after transfer • Psychosocial support • Education needs while preparing for transition must include: –Skills training, including diabetes self-management, self-advocacy, and the ability to independently negotiate services and to actively participate in a medical consultation –Education about general adolescent health issues, such as drug taking, alcohol use, and mental and sexual health issues –Educational and vocational issues, particularly career, work experience, and disclosure
Diabetes Care Program of Nova Scotia[7] Preparation Phase • Age 13 (or at age of diagnosis if >13): Initiate transition process, knowledge, and skills assessment • Ages 15–17: Continue completion of skills and education review and reinforcement, initiate education on complications of diabetes Transition Phase • Ages 17–18: Assess readiness for transition, fill knowledge gaps, begin transition but have pediatric continue with follow-up; pediatric and adult "designate" (case manager) collaborate for transition Integration Phase • Ages 18–19: Appointment with adult team and adult designate; communication between pediatric and adult designate • Additional resources including transition flow sheets and knowledge and skills checklists for ages 13–16 and 17–18 available on their Web site (below).

Sources:

1. FJ Cameron, K Garvey, KK Hood et al., "ISPAD Clinical Practice Consensus Guidelines 2018: Diabetes in Adolescence," *Pediatr Diabetes*. 2018;19 (Suppl 27):250-61.
2. A Peters, L Laffel; the American Diabetes Association Transitions Work Group, "Diabetes care for emerging adults: recommendations for transition from pediatric to adult diabetes care systems," *Diabetes Care*. 2011;34:2477-85.
3. National Institute for Health and Clinical Excellence. Diagnosis and Management of Type 1 Diabetes in Children, Young People, and Adults. London: NICE; 2004. On the Internet at: http://www.nice.org.uk/guidance/cg15.
4. National Institute for Health and Clinical Excellence. Transition from children's to adults' services for young people using health or social care services. London: NICE; 2016. On the Internet at: http://www.nice.org.uk/guidance/ng43.
5. National Health Service England. Diabetes Transition Service Specification. January 2016. Located at: https://www.england.nhs.uk/wp-content/uploads/2016/01/diabetes-transition-service-specification.pdf
6. GME Craig, SM Twigg, KC Donaghue, et al for the Australian Type 1 Diabetes Guidelines Expert Advisory Group, National evidence-based clinical care guidelines for type 1 diabetes in children, adolescents and adults. Australian Government Department of Health and Ageing. Canberra; 2011.
7. Diabetes Care Program of Nova Scotia. Moving on . . . with diabetes: adolescent transition resources. 2019 Mar. Located at:http://diabetescare.nshealth.ca/guidelines-resources/youth-transition.

American Diabetes Association, Pediatric Endocrine Society, American College of Physicians, Juvenile Diabetes Research Foundation, International Society for Pediatric and Adolescent Diabetes, and the Association of Diabetes Care and Education Specialist (formerly the American Association of Diabetes Educators) to develop transitional care resources for people with type 1 diabetes. The resources include a provider assessment of a patient's skill set and a patient assessment of worries, concerns, and burdens related to diabetes. These assessments and other resources can be found at https://www.endocrine.org/education-and-practice-management/quality-improvement-resources/clinical-practice-resources/transition-of-care or https://www.acponline.org/system/files/documents/clinical_information/high_value_care/clinician_resources/pediatric_adult_care_transitions/endo_type_1_diabetes_transitions_tools.pdf. Several other resources have emerged over the years to aid individuals in navigating the teen years and transitioning to college. In 2011, the American Diabetes Association created Going to College with Diabetes: A Self Advocacy Guide for Students. It is available for download at http://main.diabetes.org/dorg/PDFs/Advocacy/Discrimination/going-to-college-with-diabetes.pdf. The Juvenile Diabetes Research Foundation also has a Teen T1D toolkit through their Web site for free by request at https://www.jdrf.org/t1d-resources/living-with-t1d/toolkits/request-toolkit-teen/. Founded in 2009, the College Diabetes Network is a non-profit organization enhancing peer relationships among young adults with type 1 diabetes on college campuses. To date, there are over 200 chapters on college campuses with over 3,000 members. Their Web site, https://collegediabetesnetwork.org, includes various resources, including the Off to College booklets available for free of charge by request on their site.

Transitional Care and Technology Use

The technology landscape has evolved drastically over the last decade, for emerging adults and for children and adolescents with diabetes. Based on a recent survey, 95% of teens have smartphone access, up from 73% in 2014, regardless of gender, race, ethnicity, and socioeconomic status. Depending upon household income and parental education level, computer access ranges from 75% to 95%. Regardless of computer or phone use, 45% of teens describe their Internet use as near-constant.[37] Based on this information, diabetes self-management education and support options can include a variety of methods in conjunction with face-to-face meetings. In one survey of teens with type 1 diabetes, it was found the five most commonly used and available technologies for diabetes include social networking, diabetes Web sites, mobile diabetes apps, text messaging, and blood glucose meter/insulin pump software.[38] Telemedicine services that utilize videoconferencing services, apps and Internet to complement diabetes self-management education is becoming more popular and more readily available as a reimbursable service. While few studies have focused on use of telemedicine in young adults, those who have included teens found the use of services tend to decrease with time.[39] A small pilot study of 10- to 17-year-olds focused on the use of text messaging and its impact on behavior change. Twenty teenagers received five text messages per week related to their goal, and two times per week they were asked to rate their progress. The users found the process easy and the text facts and reminders useful.[40] A small Australian study also highlighted the possible benefit of using multiple methods for diabetes care. Finding alternate methods to deliver messages several ways could improve self-care and these teen subjects valued relevant and real-time information delivered online through mobile health systems along with allowing opportunities for peer support through web-based platforms.[41] Since teens and young adults with diabetes find it difficult to manage their care due to competing priorities, having multiple options to increase their engagement may aid in a more successful transition into adulthood. Using technology to assess psychosocial barriers to care could also be a very useful option within the context of usual care. Given that many pediatric offices or diabetes centers may not have a psychologist on staff, implementing methods to screen for depression, distress and anxiety in the teen and the parent, problem solving skills and resilience/positive coping factors would prove to be instrumental in successful transition.[42] The diabetes care and education speciaist should stay up to date with web-based options that may be useful for their transitioning teens.

Diabetes devices continue to evolve and become more enhanced as each year passes. Given that there has been a significant increase in insulin pump and continuous glucose monitor use in the diabetes community, it has still been found that teens and young adults continue to have the lowest use of these technologies. Typical barriers include the hassle of wearing the devices and disliking devices on their bodies.[43] Despite the data collected, it is still important for the diabetes care and education specialist to continue to introduce new diabetes devices to their patients and families as well as discuss possible methods to utilize them within the context of their patients' needs. For example, teenagers may not agree to wear a continuous glucose monitor 24/7, but suggesting a more flexible schedule such as using it monthly or every 6 weeks may be more reasonable for them. While it may not be the ideal method of use, it can still aid in problem-solving insulin doses, effect of different types of meals, physical activity, and impact of alcohol use.

Case: Transition to Young Adulthood

CT is a female who was diagnosed with diabetes at age 3. What are the expectations for self-care?

At the time of diagnosis, her parents were responsible for all her diabetes care. At this age she was not able to identify hypoglycemia, so her parents needed to test her blood glucose levels more than usual since typical outbursts of a 3-year-old and the symptoms of hypoglycemia may be similar.

There were times when CT was not cooperative with her diabetes care. Her parents and caregivers made sure to incorporate the care into her usual routine so there was no disruption in her daily life or increased episodes of acting out.

CT's parents encouraged her to participate in her care by allowing her to choose which finger to poke for blood glucose testing as well as which arm to use for her insulin injection.

As CT grew older, more diabetes tasks were transferred to her, depending on her maturity level. At age 7, she was very willing to check her blood glucose on her own as well as give her own injections. While her mother in particular was worried about having CT begin injecting on her own, it was important to foster this independence. However, setting guidelines was important to maintain safety. She did not inject her own insulin doses until she discussed the dosage with an adult.

At age 15, CT enrolled in driver's education. Discussing the importance of blood glucose monitoring prior to driving was cornerstone to her current care. She learned that in the event her blood glucose is under 80 mg/dL (4.4 mmol/L), she must wait 30 to 60 minutes before driving. While most teenagers would not comply with this recommendation due to time constraints, it was important to set realistic expectations and suggest that she check her blood glucose at least an hour before driving so that she could safely increase it if needed. At this time, to foster independence, all questions were directed to CT during her quarterly diabetes visits.

Eventually, CT prepared for college. In the years leading up to fall enrollment, conversations regarding drinking, smoking, drugs, and sex were typical during each visit with the diabetes care and education specialist. While the conversations were not an invitation to engage in these behaviors, they were an essential component of diabetes care and education to help her understand what can occur in these situations and how to stay safe. At this time, CT feels mentally prepared to begin using a continuous glucose monitor. She feels that having a device that will alert her when her blood glucose levels are low or high would be extremely helpful during college. She is willing to connect her CGM data to the office web-based program and communicate with the diabetes care and education specialist at least every 2 to 4 weeks to review the glucose readings and assess if changes to insulin doses are needed. She does not want to begin insulin pump therapy but is willing to use one of the new smart insulin pens that she can use with a mobile app to calculate her doses and keep track of when she gives her meal-time insulin.

CT has been enjoying her time in college and has joined an intramural soccer team. Unfortunately, she tore her ACL during one of the games and spent the night in the hospital undergoing surgery to repair it. She will be discharged tomorrow afternoon and will resume her typical diabetes self-management plan. The nurse reviewing CT's chart notices that CT has diabetes. At a minimum, what should the nurse make sure CT is educated on before she leaves the hospital?

Case Wrap-Up

CT should be able to perform basic survival skills upon discharge from the hospital. CT's medication regimen should be confirmed to make sure that she is taking each medication correctly, and she should be notified of any changes in her home regimen during her hospital stay. It should be confirmed that CT is capable of checking her blood glucose and able to recognize the signs and symptoms of hypoglycemia and know how to treat it. CT should receive information regarding a follow-up appointment for her diabetes management. It is important that she schedule a follow-up appointment since her activity level will change, along with her food and insulin requirements. It is also important to provide CT with contact information for a member of the healthcare team whom she can call with questions.

After being discharged from the hospital, CT will return to college and will be receiving physical therapy three days per week. What education should be provided to CT to assist her in managing her diabetes during physical therapy?

CT should receive education on checking her blood glucose before and 15 minutes after exercise and should be educated to record and understand the relationship between her physical therapy exercises and her blood glucose. She should inform the staff at physical therapy that she has diabetes as well as check her blood glucose before exercising and have a modified exercise plan or consume a 15-g carbohydrate snack for a value of less than 100 mg/dL (5.5 mmol/L). If CT experiences hypoglycemia during physical therapy, she should target a higher blood glucose before exercise or consider reducing insulin. CT should be advised to keep carbohydrate snacks with her during exercise in case she develops hypoglycemia during physical therapy. It is important to educate patients on the importance of meal planning around exercise to prevent excess caloric intake and weight gain.

Children in Foster Care/Residential Settings

There continues to be limited research regarding children with diabetes in foster care and residential settings, and several reviews of literature have highlighted that the accountability for healthcare access and quality in these groups is limited.[44,45]

A 2012 case study reviewing foster care in the Bronx revealed poor glycemic management and suboptimal social outcomes for children with type 1 diabetes.[46] In 2015, the American Academy of Pediatric declared all children in foster care as children with special healthcare needs due to the high rate of medical and mental health needs as well as their poor healthcare access. While this change is warranted, it does cause difficulty in distinguishing between those with higher medical complexity, like diabetes. Medical foster care is typically the most expensive foster placement in terms of daily rates provided to foster parents, although pay incentives have not increased the number of medical foster parents to meet the current demand.[47] It was also identified that children with a healthcare need are at higher risk of remaining in foster care for a prolonged period of time.[48] However, there are methods to optimize health outcomes in these situations. Improving the well-being of children with medical complexity in foster care requires intentional collaborations between the healthcare and child welfare systems to direct resources to those children who need them the most. For any children or young adults with diabetes who are in foster care or residential settings, it is important to incorporate the following strategies:

- Work with a social worker and maintain communication in between health visits.
- Create and utilize a care plan to be followed by all adults involved in the care of the individual.
- Require the foster family to be involved in all health visits.
- Provide access to health data, especially if the individual is frequently moved to different foster homes.[49]

Transition continues throughout the life span. While transition of diabetes care from one age to another can encounter difficulties, transitions to and from acute and long-term care also present challenges and obstacles. Since transition between healthcare settings includes unique variables, collaboration with multiple healthcare professionals is key to successful transition from admission to discharge, and all components in between.

Transition Into the Hospital

Upon admission to the hospital, it is important to collect information regarding the individual's outpatient diabetes management and home regimen (see Table 12.4). Reviewing admission laboratory values, especially the glycosylated hemoglobin (A1C) and blood glucose, is useful to gain a better understanding of the efficacy of the individual's home regimen. It is recommended that all persons with diabetes or hyperglycemia admitted to the hospital have an A1C performed, if one has not been performed in the previous 3 months.[9] An A1C upon admission will help guide inpatient medication use and education delivery in the hospital as well as facilitate the decision to initiate, intensify, or de-escalate the outpatient regimen upon discharge.[9,50] It should be noted that there are instances when the A1C is not accurate, such as patients with anemias, renal or liver failure, heavy bleeding, in patients that are pregnant, or those who receive blood transfusions.[9]

On admission, determine the efficacy of the medication regimen and the individual's knowledge of and satisfaction with his or her diabetes care. Diabetes self-management knowledge and behaviors should be assessed on admission, and a plan for diabetes self-management education should be created and provided throughout the entire hospital stay.[9] Patients may or may not bring in their medication bottles. The process of obtaining a medication history involves integration of information from several sources, including patient and caregiver recollections, a patient-provided medication list, prescription bottles, outpatient medical records, and prescription refill

TABLE 12.4 Assessment of A1C and Blood Glucose on Admission

A1C	*Blood Glucose*	*Explanation*
↑	↑	Inadequate management to meet glycemic goals or prolonged reversible cause of hyperglycemia
↑	↔	Improved management of diabetes mellitus Possible recent medication change
↔	↑	Good management of diabetes mellitus with recent lack of engagement with regimen or stress hyperglycemia

TABLE 12.5 Assessment at Admission

Important Questions to Ask the Patient on Admission	*Explanation*
Do you have prescriptions from more than 1 physician?	Patient may be receiving duplicate therapy from multiple providers.
Do you take medications that are not tablets or capsules, such as patches or inhalers?	It is important to include all medication delivery systems in medication reconciliation.
Can you tell me how you take your medications?	To assess medication use.
How long have you been taking the medication and when was the last dose administered?	To determine when it would be appropriate to administer next dose in the hospital.
Do you use any over-the-counter products and/or herbal or vitamin supplements?	Over-the-counter supplements and products may contribute to drug-drug, drug-supplement, or drug-disease interactions.
Which vaccines have you received?	Hospital admissions are an important time to assess vaccination status and administer appropriate vaccinations.
Do you have any medication allergies or intolerances?	To determine whether patient can tolerate recommended therapy and improve medication use.
How many times last week did you miss your medications?	It is important to assess medication use upon admission, so barriers can be addressed before discharge.

Source: S Kripalani, A Jackson, J Schnipper, E Coleman, "Promoting effective transitions of care at hospital discharge: a review of key issues for hospitalists," *J Hosp Med* 2, no. 5 (2007): 314-23.

information from community pharmacies. Prescriptions are often updated, and the patient may be taking the medication differently than instructed on the prescription; this is most commonly seen with insulin therapy. Always ask the patient or caregiver to confirm the dose he or she is taking, as they are the most important source of information regarding how medication is taken. It is important to ask the patient about a typical day and have him or her clarify which medications are taken at what time of day. Any discrepancies should be resolved with the patient and the caregiver upon admission, and all medications and dose instructions should be put on a list and saved for comparison at discharge (see Table 12.5). It is also important to identify any medication taking issues upon admission so that barriers to care can be appropriately assessed and addressed upon discharge. Home blood glucose monitoring values are important as well as the frequency of hypoglycemic events. If the patient is admitted from a nursing home setting, the institution should be contacted for confirmation of medication and medical history.[51]

A thorough medication review and disease management assessment is also important upon admission because any delay in home medication therapy may lead to missed doses of diabetes medications and subsequently hyperglycemia. It is important to confirm when patients last took their noninsulin and insulin medications, as missing a dose of insulin in a ketosis prone patient may lead to severe hyperglycemia and potentially diabetic ketoacidosis (DKA). On the flip-side, if a patient recently took their medications before coming to the hospital, an additional dose of insulin upon admission may result in hypoglycemia. It is important to determine the patient's regimen and previous dosing schedule prior to arrival to ensure optimal blood glucose management throughout their stay.[50]

Case Study 2: Hospital Admission

HK is a 75-year-old female who was recently admitted to the hospital for a complicated urinary tract infection. Upon further workup, it is found that HK has new-onset type 2 diabetes, with an A1C of 8.1% and a fasting plasma glucose of 235 mg/dL (13 mmol/L). HK receives long-acting basal insulin in the hospital to manage her blood glucose; however, her physician would like to start her on metformin (Glucophage®, Bristol-Myers Squibb Company) 500 mg twice daily to take at home. When should HK start taking metformin, and what should she be educated on during her hospital stay?

Medication Use in the Hospital

It is recommended that insulin therapy be used to treat hyperglycemia in hospitalized patients.[52] In certain situations, oral medications may be continued (e.g., stable patients admitted with good glycemic management, consistent diet, and anticipated short hospital stay); however, in acute illness, insulin therapy is the preferred method of treatment.[53] When evaluating the use of noninsulin medications in the inpatient setting several factors should be considered. Hospitalized patients may be at an increased risk for changes in fluid, electrolyte, and renal status; therefore, medications such as metformin may be discontinued if the eGFR decreases below 30 ml/min/1.73 m^2 and the dose should be decreased to a maximum dose of 1,000 mg daily or discontinuation should be considered in those patients with an eGFR <45 ml/min/1.73 m^2 during the hospital stay to minimize the risk of lactic acidosis. In addition, metformin should be discontinued if the patient is likely to receive radiocontrast media or other nephrotoxic medications. Sulfonylureas are not commonly used in the hospital setting, as patients are often at risk for worsening renal function, which may decrease the clearance of the medication and increase the risk of hypoglycemia. Many hospitalized patients also have reduced oral intake, which can increase the risk of hypoglycemia with sulfonylureas. Thiazolidinediones (TZDs) have the potential to cause fluid retention and are typically held in the hospital setting. Sodium-glucose co-transporter-2 (SGLT-2) inhibitors are generally avoided in the hospital setting due to the increased risk of euglycemic diabetic ketoacidosis (euDKA), which is precipitated by changes in insulin regimens, decreased food and fluid intake, dehydration, acute renal failure, surgical interventions, and stress.[54,55] If continued in the hospital setting, SGLT-2 inhibitors should be discontinued 2 to 3 days prior to surgery. The dipeptidyl peptidase-4 (DPP-4) inhibitors may have a role in the inpatient setting with recent literature supporting their use in combination with basal insulin demonstrating a reduction in glycemic variability and insulin requirements compared with a basal-bolus insulin regimen.[56,57] Sitagliptin or linagliptin would be preferred agents for an inpatient formulary based on their demonstrated safety in recent cardiovascular outcomes trials compared to saxagliptin or alogliptin, which had signals for increased risk of heart failure.[9] When considering the use of a glucagon-like peptide-1 receptor agonists (GLP-1-RA), other disease states and treatment adverse effects should be considered as gastrointestinal related adverse effects, such as nausea, vomiting, decreased appetite may be undesirable.[9]

Patients presenting to the hospital who were previously treated with insulin should have their clinical status assessed and dose modified to prevent hypoglycemia and hyperglycemia during their hospital stay.[52] It is also important to review the patient's basal and bolus insulin prescriptions and make sure the patient is appropriately converted to hospital-specific formulary agents with similar pharmacodynamic parameters, as many hospitals only have one rapid-acting insulin on formulary and may not carry all basal and premixed insulin products.[50,58] Patients started on insulin in the hospital who were well managed on noninsulin medications at home will need an insulin dose calculated that is based on their weight, age, and kidney function. The first step is to determine the patient's total daily dose.[59,60] This is illustrated in Table 12.6. Once insulin therapy is initiated, a target glucose range of 140 to 180 mg/dL is recommended.[9]

For noncritically ill patients who have poor oral intake or are taking nothing by mouth, the preferred regimen is a basal plus bolus correction insulin regimen. Patients with good nutritional intake should be started on an insulin regimen which includes a basal, prandial, and correction component. These patients should receive a total daily dose of insulin which is divided into 50% basal and 50% bolus components to match their carbohydrate intake.[9] An additional correction dose of insulin should be utilized to cover elevations in the patient's blood glucose. The use of sliding scale regimens provides suboptimal blood glucose management and is no longer recommended and strongly discouraged.[9] Patients who present to the hospital on mixed insulin regimens should be converted to basal plus bolus regimens in the hospital.[9] A study of mixed insulin versus basal-bolus therapy showed comparable glycemic management; however, the frequency of hypoglycemic episodes was significantly increased in the mixed insulin group.[61] Patients who were well managed on noninsulin agents at home can be transitioned back to these agents at discharge as long as they are clinically stable. The use of insulin in the hospital does not suggest that the patient be transitioned to a home insulin regimen. If oral medication therapy was held during the hospital stay, it should be reinitiated at discharge.[9] Patients who present on insulin pumps may continue to use their pump, provided they have the mental and physical capacity to do so, and should be monitored according to a uniform hospital policy to ensure safety.[9,53,60]

The use of continuous subcutaneous insulin infusion (CSII) devices has increased dramatically and recent guidelines suggest that they can be continued in the hospital setting in patients who are able to self-manage their insulin.[9] While continuing CSII may be appealing to patients and the healthcare team, there are limitations to their use. Many clinicians are not familiar with all of the available devices, which is compounded by the lack of standardized components and complexity of software. In addition, there is potential for medication errors when the patient does not inform the nursing staff of self-administered doses, or if the patient chooses to omit one of their scheduled doses.[50] Hospitals should have specific policies and procedures in place for continuing CSII therapy. Included in the policy should be recommendations for implementing processes to identify appropriate candidates to continue CSII

TABLE 12.6 Determining Patient's Total Daily Dose of Insulin

Patient Characteristics (Insulin Naïve)	*Recommendation for Initiation of Subcutaneous Insulin*
Patients aged ≥70 years and/or glomerular filtration rate less than 60 mL/min/1.73 m^2	0.2 to 0.3 units/kg/day
Patients with normal body weight and kidney function who have blood glucose concentrations of 140–200 mg/dL (7.8–11.1 mmol/L)	0.4 units/kg/day
Patients with obesity, a glomerular filtration rate greater than 60 mL/min/1.73 m^2, and/or a blood glucose concentration of 201–400 mg/dL (11.2–22.2 mmol/L)	0.5 units/kg/day
Patient Characteristics (Insulin Prior to Hospitalization)	*Recommendation for Initiation of Subcutaneous Insulin*
Patients with basal and bolus insulin regimen	Continue home insulin regimen; consider reducing the dose by 20% unless home blood glucose is always high • Greater reduction needed for patients with type 2 diabetes who will be NPO or whose dose of basal insulin is >50% of their total daily dose of insulin
Patients with pre-mixed insulin regimen	Order 50%–60% of patients total daily insulin dose as basal insulin and other 40%–50% as premeal insulin, divided into 3 premeal doses which can be held if patient is made NPO
Patients with basal insulin (with or without noninsulin agents) regimen	Order 60%–80% of home basal insulin dose plus correction insulin. Consider initiation of rapid-acting insulin if required.

Source: GE Umpierrez, R Hellman, MT Korytkowski, et al, "Management of hyperglycemia in hospitalized patients in non-critical care setting: an endocrine society practice guideline," *J Clin Endocrinol Metab.* 97, no. 1 (2012): 16-38.

AC Donihi, JM Moorman, A Abla, R Hanania, D Carneal, HW MacMaster, "Pharmacists' role in glycemic management in the inpatient setting: an opinion of the endocrine and metabolism practice and research network of the American College of Clinical Pharmacy," *J Am Coll Clin Pharm.* 2019;2:167-76.

CCL Wang, B Draznin, "Insulin use in hospitalized patients with diabetes: navigate with care," *Diabetes Spectr.* 2013;26(2):124-30.

self-management, development of a specific order set for insulin pump use in the hospital, patient responsibilities for self-management, and a process for documenting blood glucose measurements and insulin doses administered.[62]

Real-time continuous glucose monitoring (CGM) may also have an advantage in hospitalized patients as it is able to reduce the incidence of hypoglycemia in the hospital setting.[63,64] Studies on CGM use in the hospital setting have shown that use did not improve glycemic management; however, it was able to detect a larger number of hypoglycemic events than point-of-care testing. While data are promising, a recent review has recommended against the use of CGMs in adults in the hospital setting until more safety and efficacy data are available.[65]

In the critical care setting, continuous insulin infusion has been shown to be the best method for achieving glycemic targets.[9] When starting a patient on a continuous insulin infusion, the calculated total daily dose (Table 12.6 for patients new to insulin) can be divided over a 24-hour period. The transition from intravenous (IV) insulin therapy to subcutaneous (SC) insulin therapy can be more challenging, requiring a 20% decrease in the total daily dose.[66,67] An example case of how to convert IV to SC insulin therapy is described below.

Example: Transitioning From IV Insulin Drip to SC Insulin Injections[66–68]

The SC total daily dose (TDD) is 80% of the 24-hour insulin requirement.

Calculate an SC dose for a patient who received 5 units/hour of rapid-acting insulin IV over the previous 24 hours.

Step 1: 80% of (5 units/hour × 24) = 96 units

Step 2: Basal dose is 50% of SC TDD: 96 units × 50% = 48 units of long-acting insulin

Step 3: Bolus total dose is the other 50% divided among meals: 48 units/3 meals daily = ~16 units with each meal

SC insulin should be given before the drip is discontinued in order to allow an overlap that takes into consideration the onset of action. The first dose of basal insulin should be given 1 to 2 hours *before* the insulin infusion is discontinued.

Discharge Planning: Transition to Outpatient Care

Hospitalizations are an important time to initiate education with patients to prevent complications and readmissions. An adverse event after discharge occurs in about 20% of adult patients and is most commonly caused by an adverse drug event.[68] An increase in communication between the hospital team and the patient or the primary care physician can reduce the risk of an adverse event.[3,51,69]

The patient should be assessed upon admission to determine his or her baseline disease state knowledge. Patient education should commence during admission and continue throughout the entire stay. The patient's level of education should be assessed throughout the stay, and the education plan should be modified accordingly to meet the patient's needs.[9] Diabetes self-management education should include skills needed after discharge, such as appropriate use of antihyperglycemic medications, glucose monitoring and interpretation, and signs and symptoms of hypoglycemia and how to treat.[9]

Disease state education and proper medication therapy management can improve long-term diabetes care. Patients are more likely to retain the information if it is divided over the entire stay. It is also important to include family members if they will be assisting in the patient's care. Inpatient diabetes education focuses on basic skills and knowledge base. It should serve as a bridge to ongoing outpatient education centered on the AADE7 Self-Care Behaviors®.[70] Table 12.7 lists things to consider when a person with diabetes is transitioning from inpatient to outpatient care.

TABLE 12.7 Transitioning From Inpatient to Outpatient Care

Consideration	*Comments*
Goal of this patient's diabetes care	Care should be individualized and based on cognitive and physical ability. Also, the diabetes care and education specialist should assess the patient's readiness to learn at the beginning of the educational sessions and should inquire about his or her preferred learning style.
Past history of diabetes mellitus	Does the patient have a past history of diabetes mellitus, and are the A1C and blood glucose readings at diagnosis within target range? The patient's previous medical history and disease state management should play a role in his or her discharge education and home regimen. Newly diagnosed patients will require more discharge education, and previously diagnosed patients who are not meeting glycemic targets will need to be assessed for barriers to medication use and, if needed, an intensification in medication therapy.
Hypoglycemia risk factors	If the patient has declining physical ability and/or cognitive impairment and is living at home, consider a simplified regimen with low risk for treatment errors and hypoglycemia.
Patient's medication history	The patient's home medication regimen should be evaluated upon admission, and the medication summary should include: • Medications the patient was taking before hospitalization • Medications started during hospitalization • New medications to be taken upon discharge • Medications discontinued/continued It is important to highlight changes in the regimen and make sure the patient understands why the changes were made. Most confusion occurs when the patient is unable to distinguish which medications were discontinued prior to discharge and which medications he or she should take when at home. (Consider asking the patient what a typical day is like and when he or she takes his or her medications, to assess medication use and accuracy of medication administration.)
Patient's knowledge of diabetes and treatment recommendations	Always assess patient thoroughly and tailor education appropriately to match learning style. The focus of newly diagnosed patients should be "survival skills" with referral for outpatient follow-up.

(continued)

TABLE 12.7 Transitioning From Inpatient to Outpatient Care (continued)

Consideration	*Comments*
Financial stability	Is the patient able to pay for the recommended and prescribed blood glucose monitoring supplies, medications, and healthy food choices?
Access to healthcare services	Does the patient have established care with a primary care physician and health insurance to pay for medications and follow-up appointments? Consider transportation issues and make sure the patient has transportation for the first follow-up appointment.
Available support	Consider the patient's home support system. Does the patient have family and friends who can offer support?
Lifestyle	Ability to perform self-care activities: • What is the patient's current level of self-care? Physical/cognitive barriers: • Does the patient have any physical limitations, such as diminished vision or neuropathies, and what is his or her anticipated activity level? • Assess mobility, visual acuity, hearing loss, and dexterity. –Will the patient be able to check his or her blood glucose, draw up insulin from a syringe, or use an insulin pen? • Will the patient be able to remember to take the medications as instructed? –Will the patient need a pill box or a log to record information to assist with medication use? Psychological/social barriers: • Does the patient have social support at home? • Is the patient capable of adhering to the care plan, or does the plan need to be simplified? • Does the patient feel comfortable injecting insulin or checking his or her blood glucose in front of others? –Will he or she skip doses with variations in his or her work or social schedule? –Identify and address barriers to using insulin or checking blood glucose when not at home.
Culture	Ask the patient about diet restrictions and, if needed, assist him or her in planning for days of fasting.
Health literacy	Will the patient be able to comprehend the educational materials? The education provided should not exceed a fourth- or fifth-grade reading level.

Sources: C O'Malley, M Emanuele, L Halasyamani, A Amin, "Bridge over troubled waters: safe and effective transitions of the inpatient with hyperglycemia," *J Hosp Med* 3, Suppl 5 (2008): 55-65; S Rogers, "Inpatient care coordination for patients with diabetes," *Diabetes Spectr.* 21, no. 4 (2008): 272-5; A Nettles, "Patient education in the hospital," *Diabetes Spectr.* 18, no. 1 (2005): 44-8; A Brown, C Mangione, D Saliba, et al, "Guidelines for improving the care of the older person with diabetes mellitus," *J Am Geriatr Soc.* May, 51 Suppl 5 (2003): S265-80; A Migdal, SS Yarandi, D Smiley, GE Umpierrez, "Update on diabetes in the elderly and nursing home residents," *J Am Med Dir Assoc* 12 (2011): 627-32; American Diabetes Association, "Standards of medical care in diabetes—2019," *Diabetes Care.* 42 (2019): Suppl 1:S1-193.

Discharge Counseling

The main focus of discharge counseling should be survival skills. At a minimum, the patient should have knowledge of the following:[70,71]

- The diabetes disease state and treatments available
- How to take each medication (eg, drawing up and administering insulin)
- Any changes in the medication regimen from admission
- How to check blood glucose and record in logbook
  - Patients should be educated to check relative to meals
- Signs and symptoms of hypoglycemia and how to treat
- Basic meal planning with an emphasis on eating consistently
- Sick-day management

TABLE 12.8 Agency for Healthcare Research and Quality (AHRQ) Recommendations for Hospital Discharge

Consideration	*Comments*
Medication reconciliation	• The patient's medications must be checked to make sure chronic medications are continued and to ensure safety of new medications with previous home medications. • New and modified medications should be filled and reviewed with the patient and family members at or before discharge.
Structured discharge communication	• Information on medication changes, pending tests, and follow-up needs should be accurately and promptly communicated to the patient's primary care physician and care team. • The patient's discharge summary should be provided to the primary care physician as soon as possible. • The patient should have an appointment scheduled with an outpatient physician for follow-up prior to discharge to improve engagement with outpatient appointments.
Areas of knowledge to review and address prior to hospital discharge	• Identify the healthcare provider who will provide diabetes care after discharge • Level of understanding related to the diabetes diagnosis, self-monitoring of blood glucose, home blood glucose goals, and when to call the provider • Definition, recognition, treatment, and prevention of hyperglycemia and hypoglycemia • Information on making healthy food choices at home and referral to an outpatient registered dietitian nutritionist to guide individualization of meal plan, if needed • When and how to take blood glucose-lowering medications, including insulin administration, if applicable • Sick-day management • Proper use and disposal of needles and syringes

Source: American Diabetes Association, "Standards of medical care in diabetes—2019," *Diabetes Care.* 42 (2019): Suppl 1:S1-93.

- Contact information for follow-up appointments and education
- When to call a member of the healthcare team and who to call with questions

The Agency for Healthcare Research and Quality has also created similar recommendations regarding discharge planning, which are listed in Table 12.8. Educational sessions should be short and should be structured to optimize learning and utilize active learning techniques.[70,71] Education should be divided over the length of the hospital stay to be less overwhelming for patients, to reinforce previously taught concepts, and to spread the responsibility to more providers.[9,66]

Always ask the patient if he or she foresees any barriers or reasons why he or she would not be able to follow through with the recommended plan. An assessment of potential barriers should be conducted to identify any potential issues.

Common barriers that may prevent a patient from following the recommended insulin regimen include the following:[72]

- Association of needles and injections with pain
- Weight gain
- Fear of complications of diabetes
- Inconvenience
- Complex, time-consuming regimen
- Cost

The diabetes care and education specialist should provide written information in addition to verbal instruction because patients are unlikely to remember all verbal instructions at discharge. Written instructions for patients and family members are a useful tool to reinforce important self-care instructions. These materials should be written at a fourth- to fifth-grade reading level and should be written in patient-friendly language. The "teach-back" method should be used to confirm understanding. Through this method, the diabetes care and education specialist asks patients to repeat back what they understood from the discharge instructions and education.[51,52] Patients should be asked to demonstrate any new self-care tasks that they will be required to carry out at home, such as administering a subcutaneous injection. Open-ended questions should be utilized to confirm understanding and to allow the patient and family members to voice questions and concerns; avoid questions with "yes" or "no" responses.

When creating a home medication list for the patient, avoid stating "continue home medications" or "resume all medications." Patients should be provided with a complete list of all their medications, including correct dosages and indications to be taken at home, highlighting new medications and home medications taken prior to admission that have been changed. To improve engagement to the recommended regimen, patients should understand why medications have been added or discontinued. The medication list should also include specific instructions for administration, including the times of day. It is also important to make sure the patient has prescriptions for blood glucose testing supplies and insulin pen needles or syringes (if applicable) so that he or she has all the supplies necessary to carry out the discharge plan.[51,52]

Transitioning to an Outpatient Care Provider

An outpatient follow-up visit with the primary care provider, endocrinologist, or diabetes care and education is recommended within 1 month for all persons with diabetes having hyperglycemia in the hospital.[9] Patients are more likely to engage with their post-hospital follow-up appointments if they are given a set appointment that is reviewed before or at discharge.[51] If glycemic medications are changed or glucose levels are not optimal at discharge an earlier appointment in 1 to 2 weeks is preferred, and more frequent contact may be needed to avoid hyper- or hypoglycemia. Another method to improve participation with the discharge regimen is to conduct a telephone follow-up 2 to 3 days after discharge.[9,51] The additional telephone follow-up allows persons with diabetes to inquire about any new medication issues and to ask any questions that they may not have thought to ask during hospitalization. The call also provides an opportunity for the diabetes care and education specialist to assess medication-taking issues with the home regimen and determine whether there are any barriers to the prescribed regimen. Evidence shows that follow-up telephone calls improve patient satisfaction, medication use, and decrease preventable adverse drug events and the number of emergency room visits and hospital readmissions.[51] Additional considerations for improving transitions in persons with physical limitations are listed in Table 12.9.

Electronic health record (EHR) systems have demonstrated value in care transitions by reducing fragmented care and by improving care coordination. EHRs have the potential to integrate and organize patient health information and distribute information in a timely manner to all authorized providers involved in a patient's care. It is important to make sure all of the education provided, patient concerns and barriers to care, and medication changes and rationale are effectively documented in the EHR. Clear communication with outpatient providers either directly or via printed and electronic hospital discharge summaries facilitates safe transitions to outpatient care.[73]

Medication Use at Discharge

Newly diagnosed patients should receive appropriate treatment based on the current guidelines.[9] Patients with a previous diagnosis of diabetes mellitus who were meeting their

TABLE 12.9 Improving Transitions for Persons with Diabetes With Physical Limitations

Consideration	*Comments*
Age-related changes	• Decreases in the olfactory system and subsequent loss of taste may result in loss of appetite and malnutrition. • Malnutrition can also result from poor dentition. Persons with diabetes may no longer be able to eat solid foods as easily and may start substituting with meal replacement drinks. • There is an increased risk of dehydration, which can lead to hyperglycemic hyperosmolar state (HHS) as the kidneys are no longer able to concentrate urine in response to fluid deficit. • Cognitive changes such as confusion, depression, and social isolation may also lead to an inability to provide adequate self-care.
Diabetic neuropathies	• Persons with diabetes may not want to check their blood glucose because they fear additional pain in their hands or may have tremors that make them unable to check their blood glucose or draw up insulin.
Visual deficits and retinopathy	• Visual deficits and retinopathy can also present a barrier to person with diabetes self-care. Patients with visual deficits may miss taking certain medications or draw up an inaccurate dose of insulin.

Source: C O'Reilly, "Managing the care of patients with diabetes in the home care setting," *Diabetes Spectr.* 12, no. 3 (2005): 162-6.

glycemic targets prior to hospitalization can be discharged on their home regimen. Treatment should be intensified if the patient is not meeting appropriate glycemic targets; however, changes in lifestyle and stressors in the hospital which may have influenced glycemic levels, such as illness, decreased food intake, or glucocorticoid use, should be taken into consideration. Before reinitiating medications, check the patient's electrolytes, renal function, liver function, cardiac stability, and nutritional status to reduce the risk of complications.[68,74,75] In addition, an evaluation of the patient's disease state goals should be addressed. While a glycemic goal of less than 7% may be appropriate for younger patients, glycemic goals should be modified based on the patient's life expectancy, cognitive function, functional status, and comorbid conditions. Older adults with few chronic illnesses and intact cognitive function may still benefit from a glycemic goal of less than 7.5%, while elderly patients with limited life expectancy or those with multiple chronic Illnesses and cognitive impairment have a less stringent glycemic goal of less than 8% or 8.5%.[9] Medications with a low risk of hypoglycemia are preferred in the elderly population and deintensification should be considered for patients with complex regimens to reduce the risk of hypoglycemia and to ease disease state burden.[9]

Recent literature recommends that patients admitted with an A1C below their glycemic target can be discharged on the same preadmission diabetes regimen, including oral agent or insulin, while patients with an A1C above their glycemic target should have their therapy intensified.[76] It is important for diabetes care and education specialists to review the patient's diabetes management at discharge to prevent clinical inertia, which is defined as failure to initiate or intensify therapy when clinically indicated.[76] Insulin regimens and blood glucose levels during hospitalization should be taken into consideration in patients that require insulin at discharge. It is also important to recognize that the hospital formulary may differ from the patient's prescription insurance formulary and cost of new products that differ from the pre-admission medication list should be confirmed.[50] Despite guidance with regard to the importance of intensification of a patient's regimen at discharge, barriers still exist. It is important to recognize barriers such as fear of hypoglycemia, lack of provider confidence to effectively address these therapies at discharge, lack of effective transitions of care processes, and patient-specific factors, such as fear or refusal to initiate insulin, mental or physical disabilities, or financial and social barriers to prevent clinical inertia.[76]

For patients discharged on oral agents, discontinue basal insulin before discharge and use bolus insulin when starting oral agents if extra coverage is needed.[66,68] Consider the onset and duration of each medication. Sulfonylureas, meglitinides, metformin, DPP-4 inhibitors, SGLT2 inhibitors, and daily GLP-1 receptor agonists will begin to work shortly after administration; however, pioglitazone (Actos™, Takeda Pharmaceuticals U.S.A.) has a delayed onset of 4 weeks, and full effect may not be seen until 12 weeks. Weekly GLP-1 receptor agonists may have a delayed onset of action as well, which should be taken into consideration in patients with significant hyperglycemia in the hospital. Other important considerations when choosing a medication regimen include the setting in which the patient is being treated (home, skilled nursing facility, rehabilitation facility, etc), physical and cognitive ability, and family and social support. To prevent hypoglycemia and improve medication taking, a basic medication therapy regimen may be required for an elderly patient with declining physical and/or cognitive ability who lives alone.[68]

Hospitalizations can also serve as an important time to assess preventive care measures to reduce the risk of micro- and macrovascular complications. Vaccination history should be reviewed and persons with diabetes should receive indicated vaccinations, if not previously received.

Case Wrap-Up

HK should discontinue basal insulin 12 to 24 hours before discharge. She may start metformin 500 mg twice daily with breakfast and dinner if her kidney function and electrolytes are stable. Metformin will begin to work within 1 to 3 hours after the first dose and can be taken concomitantly with insulin to achieve euglycemia in the hospital. Metformin is cost-effective, so cost should not be a barrier for HK; however, she may need a pillbox to help with medication use.

The main focus of discharge counseling should be on survival skills. Since HK is newly diagnosed, she should be educated on the diabetes disease state and treatments available. HK should also be educated on how to take her medication and what to do if she misses a dose. She should learn how to check her blood glucose, confirmed though the teach-back method, and the diabetes care and education specialist should ensure that HK has the proper prescriptions for a glucometer, strips, and lancets to check her blood glucose at home. HK should know the signs and symptoms of hypoglycemia and how to treat and basic meal planning skills. She should receive contact information for follow-up appointments and educational sessions and should be given contact information for a member of the healthcare team whom she can call with questions. HK's physical and cognitive ability should be assessed as well as family and social support. It may be beneficial for HK to have a family member or friend present when reviewing survival skills, as the initial education process may be overwhelming, especially if she is learning additional information related to other co-morbid conditions during her hospital stay.

Transitioning to a Skilled Nursing Facility or Other Acute Care Hospital

Discharge education and procedures for patients transitioning to skilled nursing facilities or long-term care institutions should include education and medication reconciliation similar to that given to the patient and caretaker when the patient is going home. Many nursing home facilities do not have an algorithm for managing patients with diabetes or have a blood glucose monitoring policy; therefore, it is important that patients going to another institution receive the same education as a patient going home.[74] In long-term care facilities, medical providers are not required to evaluate patients daily. Assessments are conducted at a minimum of every 30 days for the first 90 days, followed by every 60 days thereafter.[74,77] Patients may be seen more frequently; however, patients are not managed daily and may have large glycemic variability without nursing home providers being notified. Patients should be educated to contact their provider or diabetes care and education specialist if they notice large changes in blood glucose levels, if they are ill and cannot keep food down, or if they notice changes in appetite.[9]

The variability in living arrangements in the long-term care population creates a challenge for the management of patients with diabetes. Some adults live independently, while others receive partial support or full supervision for medical management.[77] It is important for the diabetes care and education specialist to evaluate the formulary, processes, and staffing to determine whether the facility is similar to a hospital versus the patient's home. Hypoglycemic events are common and reported in up to 48% of nursing home residents; it should not be assumed that patients receive full diabetes care in the nursing home.[66,69,78,79]

Patients residing in skilled nursing or long-term care facilities may have impaired food intake, difficulty swallowing, and/or decreased appetite, leading to unpredictable meal consumption. Meal planning should be tailored to the patient's food preferences and culture to increase quality of life and nutritional status.[9] Meal planning, including carbohydrate counseling and diet education, is an important educational component in the elderly population. For patients who have a poor nutritional status, the focus should be on medication management and lifestyle rather than diet restriction. In addition, the risk of hypoglycemic events with intensive glucose management may precipitate complications, such as falls and cardiovascular events that are more harmful to the elderly population than hyperglycemia.[74] Because of this risk, diabetes medications should be simplified and initiated at the lowest possible dose that will allow residents to meet their glycemic goals, and sliding-scale insulin regimens should be avoided.[77] Glycemic goals should be based on cognitive and physical status.[80] All of these factors should be considered when assessing an elderly patient at discharge.

The diabetes care and education care should provide patients with hypoglycemia education, including signs and symptoms and how to treat to prevent complications of hypoglycemia. Care transitions may result in changes in carbohydrate intake and activity levels, stress, or illness. Lifestyle changes, in addition to medication therapy changes, can increase the risk for hypoglycemia or hyperglycemia in the outpatient setting. A resident who is being transferred should check his or her blood glucose 2 to 4 times daily until glycemic levels are stabilized.[80] In addition, it is important to convey to the long-term care facility staff any medication changes made in the hospital. Medications may be changed due to formulary issues, and all changes should be conveyed to staff at the new setting.[80]

The transition between facilities can be challenging because there is no standard transition of care document with all of the necessary information for diabetes management. It is recommended that the facility request information on the patient's meal plan, activity levels, self-care education, laboratory tests, hydration status, blood glucose readings, and ability to detect and treat hypoglycemia.[77] Discharge summaries often do not include diagnostic test results, treatment received during hospital course, discharge medications, test results pending at discharge, and follow-up plans. This leads to duplicate testing and potential continuation of incorrect medication regimens.

Transition to a Correctional Institution

Correctional institutions have policies and procedures in place for the management of persons with diabetes, and trained staff available; however, the transition to prison can be a new challenge for a person with diabetes, as he or she will have to learn how to manage diabetes mellitus with access to fewer resources.[81] The transition to a correctional institution will require additional considerations in meal planning and medication use, as people with diabetes may not be able to test their blood glucose as frequently and will have to learn how to count carbohydrates effectively to prevent hypoglycemia or hyperglycemia during times when food is not available.

The patient's medical history should be conveyed to the correctional institution as early as possible to prevent hypoglycemia or hyperglycemia and complications of diabetes. Not all persons are screened for diabetes mellitus upon arrival at a correctional institution, as screening for diabetes mellitus is not required, so it is important that persons with diabetes inform personnel at screening and check-in that they have diabetes mellitus to receive appropriate care. Other information that is important for the correctional institution to receive includes the following:[81]

- Type and duration of diabetes
- List of current therapy and date and time of last medication administration
- Identified barriers to self-care
- Presence of complications and concurrent illnesses
- Family history
- History of alcohol and drug use
- Behavioral health issues, such as depression, distress, and suicidal ideation
- Information regarding follow-up if patient needs transportation to a provider outside the facility
- Name and contact information of provider at transfer institution who can provide additional information to correctional facility if needed

Each correctional institution has its own formulary, which will not include all insulin preparations and medications.[82] The diabetes care and education specialist should call the institution to determine which medications on the formulary would best fit the patient's care plan. Rapid-acting insulin should be avoided in most circumstances and is not typically included on the formulary due to the inability to coordinate administration with the timing of food. If a person requires meal time insulin, short-acting insulin is preferred.[81]

Insulin pumps may not be allowed in the correctional institution, so the individual with diabetes may need to change insulin delivery methods. Glucometers should be provided, and persons with diabetes will be allowed to use them in accordance with regulatory guidance that addresses security, logistical, and infection control issues. Individuals with diabetes should be well educated about carbohydrate counting because they may not have access to resources for rapid correction of low or high blood glucose. They may encounter situations where they have to self-detect hypoglycemia because frequent blood glucose monitoring is unavailable. Meal planning and signs and symptoms of hypoglycemia should be an important focus of disease state education when transitioning to correctional facilities. Encourage persons with diabetes to buy extra food from the canteen to have with them in the event of hypoglycemia.[81,82]

Individuals with diabetes in correctional institutions should also be counseled on the signs and symptoms of hyperglycemia and diabetic ketoacidosis (DKA). When counseling persons with diabetes transitioning to correctional facilities, it is important to focus on self-care and problem-solving skills. Peer and family support will not be available, and resources are limited. Staff members should be adequately trained; however, not all are comfortable, nor do they understand the consequences of improper diabetes management. The Federal Bureau of Prisons has produced a 2017 clinical guidance resource for the management of diabetes which can be provided to institutions needing additional resources and education.[81]

For people with diabetes transferring out of correctional facilities it is important to reinforce that information from the correctional institution medical record should be taken to their next provider. Most correctional facilities have electronic medical records; however, it is the responsibility of the person with diabetes to release their information or ask for a printed copy to take to their next provider.

Transition to Rehabilitation Facilities

Individuals with diabetes who are transitioning to rehabilitation facilities should receive previously discussed discharge education with an added focus on checking blood glucose during planned or unplanned exercise. Rehabilitation facilities will have a formal exercise program, and a person with diabetes will have to learn how to check his or her blood glucose and eat according to the rehabilitation exercise schedule. The person with diabetes will have to document and learn his or her body's relationship between exercise and blood glucose. It is also important for the diabetes care and education specialist to provide goal ranges for blood glucose relative to exercise and advice for meal planning around rehabilitation activities. Individuals with diabetes should be educated to check their blood glucose before exercise and should have a modified plan for a value of 100 mg/dL (5.6 mmol/L) or less. They should also be educated to look for blood glucose patterns in response to different exercise regimens. If the individual has a higher rate of hypoglycemia unawareness during exercise, a higher pre-exercise blood glucose level may be targeted to prevent hypoglycemia.[83]

Individuals with diabetes should also be instructed to check their blood glucose 15 minutes after the exercise session. Hypoglycemia can occur up to 24 to 48 hours after an exercise session, so individuals should be educated to keep carbohydrate snacks available to prevent its occurrence. To prevent hypoglycemia, a snack of 15 to 30 g of carbohydrates should be consumed every 30 to 60 minutes during continuous physical activity. Meal planning, nutritional intake during exercise, and treatment of hypoglycemia are important components to avoid unnecessary caloric intake and weight gain during rehabilitation.[83]

The transition from rehabilitation facilities to home is as equally important as the transition to the center. Individuals with diabetes may have required a significant reduction in medication use from the hospital setting as exercise and activity hours were increased. The patient may have also experienced dramatic changes in weight. Frequent follow-up should be recommended upon discharge, especially in those patients whose rehabilitation plan included multiple hours of intense activity daily. Most patients will not perform the same amount and/or level of intensity exercise at home and will need more frequent medication adjustments as they resume their typical lifestyle.

Summary

Transitional care is an important component of the diabetes disease state management process. It starts at diagnosis and continues throughout the life span of the patient. It is crucial to take a proactive role in educating the patient and his or her family about the various transitions that may occur throughout his or her lifetime. Successful management of diabetes mellitus is dependent on collaboration between the patient and the healthcare team and their communication strategies to create an individualized plan. The diabetes care and education specialist's role should include a combination of care coordination and education focusing on the following:[70]

- Using an interdisciplinary team approach incorporating a patient- and family-centered model across the continuum of care
- Collaborating closely with other disciplines as needed, including social workers, care managers, and home care coordinators
- Establishing means of communicating the status of the diabetes self-management education plan of care and medication reconciliation to the next provider
- Empowering the patient and caregivers to actively participate in the patient's care regardless of the setting
- Promoting self-care

Focus on Education

Teaching Strategies

Create a timeline of teaching points for children, adolescents, and young adults in order to increase independence and improve diabetes self-management skills. The earlier you begin the checklist of skills, the easier the transition to an adult provider.

Education about disease management is one of the most important tools in reducing complications and readmissions. When transitioning adults from an inpatient to an outpatient setting, the best chance for success is to focus on survival skills first. Once in the outpatient setting, more detailed education can be initiated, based on individual need. The teach back method can help identify patient knowledge deficits and opportunities to provide further education.

Focus on Practice

Utilize checklists for education topics that are needed for adolescents and young adults to successfully transition to adult care.

For inpatient education, work with inpatient nursing staff to encourage teachable moments regarding the survival skills that are needed upon discharge.

References

1. Buschur EO, Glick B, Kamboj MK. Transition of care for patients with type 1 diabetes mellitus from pediatric to adult health care systems. Transl Pediatr. 2017;6(4):373-82.
2. Mixon AS, Myers AP, Leak CL, et al. Characteristics associated with postdischarge medication errors. Mayo Clin Proc. 2014;89(8):1042-51.

3. Forster A, Murff H, Peterson J, et al. The incidence and severity of adverse events affecting patients after discharge from the hospital. Ann Intern Med. 2003;138:161-7.
4. American Academy of Pediatrics. *Caring for Your Baby and Young Child: Birth to Age 5.* 6th ed. Elk Grove Village, Ill: American Academy of Pediatrics; 2014.
5. Winkelman TNA, Caldwell MT, Bertram B, et al. Promoting health literacy for children and adolescents. Pediatrics. 2016;138(6):e20161937.
6. Dovc K, Carnetutti K, Sturm A, et al. Continuous glucose monitoring use and glucose variability in pre-school children with type 1 diabetes. Diabetes Research and Clinical Practice. 2019;147:76-80.
7. Chiang JL, Kirkman MS, Laffel LMB, et al. Type 1 diabetes through the life span: a position statement of the American Diabetes Association. Diabetes Care. 2014:37:2034-54.
8. Abualula NA, Jacobsen KH, Milligan RA et al. Evaluating diabetes educational interventions with a skill development component in adolescents with type 1 diabetes: a systematic review focusing on quality of life. The Diabetes Educator. 2016;42(5): 515-27.
9. American Diabetes Association. Standards of medical care in diabetes—2020. Diabetes Care. 2019 Jan;43 Suppl 1:S1-212.
10. Scott LK. Developmental Mastery of Diabetes-Related Tasks in Children. Nurs Clin N Am. 2013;48:329-42.
11. Blum RW, Garrell D, Hodgman CH, et al. Transition from child-centered to adult health care systems for adolescents with chronic conditions: a position paper of the Society of Adolescent Medicine. J Adolesc Health. 1993;14:570-6.
12. Lyons SK, Becker DJ, Helgeson VS. Transfer from pediatric to adult health care: effects on diabetes outcomes. Pediatric Diabetes. 2014;15:10-17.
13. White PH, Cooley WC, TRANSITIONS CLINICAL REPORT AUTHORING GROUP, American Academy of Pediatrics, American Academy of Family Physicians, and American College of Physicians. Supporting the health care transition from adolescence to adulthood in the medical home. Pediatrics. 2018;142(5) e20182587.
14. Cooley, WC, Sagerman PJ. American Academy of Pediatrics; American Academy of Family Physicians; American College of Physicians; Transitions Clinical Report Authoring Group. Supporting the health care transition from adolescence to adulthood in the medical home. Pediatrics. 2011;128(1):182-200.
15. Peters A, Laffel L; American Diabetes Association Transitions Working Group. Diabetes care for emerging adults: recommendations for transition from pediatric to adult diabetes care systems. Diabetes Care. 2011;34(11):2477-85.
16. Cameron FJ, Garvey K, Hood KK, et al. ISPAD Clinical Practice Consensus Guidelines 2018: Diabetes in Adolescence. Pediatr Diabetes. 2018;19 (Suppl 27):250-61.
17. Spaic T, Robinson T, Goldbloom E, et al. Closing the gap: results of the multicenter Canadian randomized controlled trial of structured transition in young adults with type 1 diabetes. Diabetes Care. 2019;42(6):1018-26.
18. Shulman R, Chafe R and Guttmann A. Transition to adult diabetes care: a description of practice in the Ontario Pediatric Diabetes Network. Can J Diabetes. 2019;43:283-9.
19. O'Hara MC, Hynes L, O'Donnell M, et al. A systematic review of interventions to improve outcomes for young adults with type 1 diabetes. Diabet Med. 2017;34:753-69.
20. Iylengar J, Thomas IH, Soleimanpour SA. Transition from pediatric to adult care in emerging adults with type 1 diabetes: a blueprint from effective receivership. Clinical Diabetes and Endocrinology. 2019;(5)3. https://doi.org/10.1186/s40842-019-0078-7.
21. Lotstein DS, Seid M, Klingensmith G, et al; SEARCH for Diabetes in Youth Study. Transition from pediatric to adult care for youth diagnosed with type 1 diabetes in adolescence. Pediatrics. 2013;131(4):e1062-70.
22. Garvey KC, Foster NC, Agarwal S, et al. Health care transition preparation and experiences in the US National sample of young adults with type 1 diabetes. Diabetes Care. 2017;40: 317-24.
23. Simms MJ, Baumann K, Monaghan M. Health communication experiences of emerging adults with type 1 diabetes. Clin Pract Pediatr Psychol. 2017;5(4):415-25.
24. Garvey KC, Beste MG, Luff D, et al. Experiences of health care transition voiced by young adults with type 1 diabetes: a qualitative study. Adolesc Health Med Ther. 2014;5:191-8.
25. Garvey KC, Markowitz JT, Laffel LMB. Transition to adult care for youth with type 1 diabetes. Curr Diab Rep. 2012;12(5): 533-41.
26. Datye K, Bonnet K, Schlundt D, et al. Experiences of adolescents and emerging adults living with type 1 diabetes. The Diabetes Educator. 2019;45(2): 194-202.
27. National Health Service England. Diabetes transition service specification. January 2016. Found at https://www.england.nhs.uk/wp-content/uploads/2016/01/diabetes-transition-service-specification.pdf.
28. Allen D, Cohen D, Robling M, et al. The transition from paediatric to adult diabetes services: what works, for whom and in what circumstances? Final report. London: NIHR Service Delivery and Organisation programme; 2010.
29. Kaye J, Rapley P, Babel G, Brown S. Healthcare transition risk assessment for emerging adults with diabetes type 1. J Diabetes Mellitus. 2013;3(2):62-70.
30. Egan EA, Corrigan J, Shurpin K. Building the bridge from pediatric to adult diabetes care: making a connection. Diabetes Educ. 2015;41(4):432-43.
31. Agarwal S, Raymond JK, Schutta MH, et al. An adult health-care based pediatric to adult transition program for emerging adults with type 1 diabetes. The Diabetes Educator. 2017;43(1): 87-96.
32. Lugasi T, Achille M, Stevenson M. Patients' perspective on factors that facilitate transition from child-centered to adult-centered health care: a theory integrated metasummary of quantitative and qualitative studies. J Adolesc Health. 2011;48:429-40.

33. Findley MK, Cha ES, Wong E, Faulkner MS. A systematic review of transitional emerging adults with diabetes. J Pediatr Nurs. 2015;30:e47-62.

34. Garvey KC, Telo GH, Needleman JS, et al. Health care transition in young adults with type 1 diabetes: perspectives of adult endocrinologists in the United States. Diabetes Care. 2016;39(2):190-7.

35. Agarwal S, Garvey KC, Raymond JK, et al. Perspectives in care for young adults with type 1 diabetes transitioning from pediatric to adult health systems: a national survey of pediatric endocrinologists. Pediatr Diabetes. 2017;18(7):524-31.

36. Lewis K, Hermayer K. All grown up: moving from pediatric to adult diabetes care. Am J Med Sci. 2013;345(4):278-83.

37. Pew Research Center, May 2018, "Teens, Social Media & Technology 2018"–located at www.pewresearch.org.

38. Vaala SE, Hood KK, Laffel L, et al. Use of commonly available technologies for diabetes information and self-management among adolescents with type 1 diabetes and their parents: a web-based survey study. Interact J Med Res. 2015;4(4):e24. doi:10.2196/ijmr.4504.

39. Ramchandani N. Telemedicine services for emerging adults with type 1 diabetes. US Endocrinology. 2018;14(2):73-6.

40. Kaushal T, Montgomery KA, Simon R, et al. MyDiaText: Feasibility and functionality of a text messaging system for youth with type 1 diabetes. The Diabetes Educator. 2019;45(3): 253-9.

41. Ng AH, Crowe TC, Ball K, et al. Transitional Needs of Australian young adults with tytpe 1 diabetes: mixed methods study. JMIR Diabetes. 2017;2(2):e29. Doi:10.2196/diabetes.8315.

42. Prahalad P, Tanenbaum M, Hood K, et al. Diabetes technology: improving care, improving patient-reported outcomes and preventing complications in young people with type 1 diabetes. Diabet Med. 2018;35:419-29.

43. Tanenbaum ML, Hanes SJ, Miller KM, et al. Diabetes device use in adults with type 1 diabetes: barriers to uptake and potential intervention targets. Diabetes Care. 2016. doi:10/2337/dc16-1536.

44. Deans KJ, Minneci PC, Nacion KM, et al. A framework for developing healthcare quality measures for children and youth in foster care. Child Youth Serv Rev. 2015;58:146-52.

45. MacRae S, Brown M, Karatzias T, et al. Diabetes in people with intellectual disabilities: a systematic review of the literature. Res Dev Disabil. 2015;47:352-74.

46. Gangat M, Klein GW, Heptulla RA. Foster care and type 1 diabetes in the Bronx: a case series. J Pediatr Endocrinol Metab. 2012;25(7-8):775-9.

47. Williams EP, Seltzer RR, Boss RD. Language matters: identifying medically complex children in foster care. Pediatrics. 2017;140(4):e20163692.

48. Seltzer RR, Henderson CM, Boss RD. Medical foster care: what happens when children with medical complexity cannot be cared for by their families? Pediatr Res. 2016;79(1):191-6.

49. DiGiuseppe DL, Christakis DA. Continuity of care for children in foster care. Pediatrics. 2003;111(3):e208–13.

50. Donihi AC, Moorman JM, Abla A, Hanania R, Carneal D, MacMaster HW. Pharmacists' role in glycemic management in the inpatient setting: an opinion of the endocrine and metabolism practice and research network of the American College of Clinical Pharmacy. J Am Coll Clin Pharm. 2019; 2:167-76.

51. Kripalani S, Jackson A, Schnipper J, Coleman E. Promoting effective transitions of care at hospital discharge: a review of key issues for hospitalists. J Hosp Med. 2007 Sep;2(5):314-23.

52. Umpierrez GE, Hellman R, Korytkowski MT, et al. Management of hyperglycemia in hospitalized patients in non-critical care setting: an endocrine society practice guideline. J Clin Endocrinol Metab. 2012 Jan;97(1):16-38.

53. Moghissi E, Korytkowski M, DiNardo M, et al. American Association of Clinical Endocrinologists and American Diabetes Association consensus statement on inpatient glycemic control. Diabetes Care. 2009 Jun;32(6):1119-31.

54. Lupsa BC, Inzucchi SE. Use of SGLT2 inhibitors in type 2 diabetes: weighing the risks and benefits. Diabetologia. 2018;61:2118-25.

55. Burke K, Schumacher C, Harpe, S. SGLT2 Inhibitors: A systematic review of diabetic ketoacidosis and related risk factors in the primary literature. Pharmacotherapy. 2017;37:187-94.

56. Umpierrez GE, Gianchandani R, Smiley D, et al. Safety and efficacy of sitagliptin therapy for the inpatient management of general medicine and surgery patients with type 2 diabetes. Diabetes Care. 2013;36(11):3430-5.

57. Garg R, Schuman B, Hurwitz S, Metzger C, Bhandari S. Safety and efficacy of saxagliptin for glycemic control in non-critically ill hospitalized patients. BMJ Open Diabetes Res Care. 2017; 5(1):e000394.

58. Kilpatrick CR, Elliott MB, Pratt E, et al. Prevention of inpatient hypoglycemia with a real-time informatics alert. J Hosp Med. 2014;9(10):621-6.

59. Wesorick D, O'Malley C, Rushakoff R, et al. Management of diabetes and hyperglycemia in the hospital: a practical guide to subcutaneous insulin use in the non-critically ill, adult patient. J Hosp Med. 2008 Sep;3 Suppl 5:17-28.

60. Lansang C, Umpierrez G. Management of inpatient hyperglycemia in noncritically ill patients. Diabetes Spectr. 2008;21(4):248-55.

61. Bellido V, Suarez L, Rodriguez MG, et al. Comparison of basal-bolus and premixed insulin regimens in hospitalized patients with type 2 diabetes. Diabetes Care. 2015;38:2211-16.

62. Institute for Safe Medication Practices. Managing hospitalized patients with ambulatory pumps—Part 2: Guidelines for the use of insulin pumps during hospitalization (cited 2019 May 27). Available from: https://www.ismp.org/resources/managing-hospitalized-patients-ambulatory-pumps-part-2-guidelines-use-insulin-pumps.

63. Wallia A, Umpierrez GE, Rushakoff RJ, et al. DTS Continuous Glucose Monitoring in the Hospital Panel. Consensus statement on inpatient use of continuous glucose monitoring. J Diabetes Sci Technol. 2017;11:1036-44.

64. Umpierrez GE, Klonoff DC. Diabetes technology update: use of insulin pumps and continuous glucose monitoring in the hospital. Diabetes Care. 2018;41:1579-89.

65. Gomez AM, Umpierrez GE. Continuous glucose monitoring in insulin-treated patients in non-ICU settings. J Diabetes Sci Technol. 2014;8:930-6.

66. O'Malley C, Emanuele M, Halasyamani L, Amin A. Bridge over troubled waters: safe and effective transitions of the inpatient with hyperglycemia. J Hosp Med. 2008 Sep; 3 Suppl 5:55-65.

67. Bode B, Braithwaite S, Steed R, Davidson P. Intravenous insulin therapy: indications, methods, and transition to subcutaneous insulin therapy. Endocr Pract. 2004;10 Suppl 2:71-80.

68. Peterson G. Transitioning from inpatient to outpatient therapy in patients with in-hospital hyperglycemia. Hosp Pract. 2011 Oct;39(4):87-95.

69. Rogers S. Inpatient care coordination for patients with diabetes. Diabetes Spectr. 2008;21(4):272-5.

70. American Association of Diabetes Educators. AADE Position Statement. Diabetes inpatient management. Diabetes Educ. 2012;38:142-6.

71. Nettles A. Patient education in the hospital. Diabetes Spectr. 2005;18(1):44-8.

72. Laverna F. Treating hyperglycemia and diabetes with insulin therapy: transition from inpatient to outpatient care. Medscape J Med. 2008;10(9):216.

73. AHRQ Patient Safety Network. Electronic Health Records. (cited 2019 May 27) Available from: https://psnet.ahrq.gov/primers/primer/43/Electronic-Health-Records.

74. Magaji V, Johnston J. Inpatient management of hyperglycemia and diabetes. Clin Diabetes. 2011;29(1):3-9.

75. Donihi AC. Practical recommendations for transitioning patients with type 2 diabetes from hospital to home. Curr Diab Rep. 2017;17(7):52.

76. Umpierrez GE, Reyes D, Smiley D, et al. Hospital discharge algorithm based on admission HbA1c for the management of patients with type 2 diabetes. Diabetes Care. 2014; 37:2934-9.

77. Munshi MN, Florez H, Huang ES, et al. Management of diabetes in long-term care and skilled nursing facilities: a position statement from the American Diabetes Association. Diabetes Care. 2016;39:308-18.

78. Feldman SM, Rosen R, DeStasio J. Status of diabetes management in the nursing home setting in 2008: a retrospective chart review and epidemiology study of diabetic nursing home residents and nursing home initiatives in diabetes management. J Am Med Dir Assoc. 2009;10:354-60.

79. Migdal A, Yarandi SS, Smiley D, Umpierrez GE. Update on diabetes in the elderly and nursing home residents. J Am Med Dir Assoc. 2011;12:627-32.

80. Hass LB. Special considerations for older adults with diabetes residing in skilled nursing facilities. Diabetes Spectr. 2014; 27(1):37-43.

81. Federal Bureau of Prisons, Management of Diabetes, Federal Bureau of Prisons, Clinical Practice Guidelines (Washington, DC: Federal Bureau of Prisons, 2017; cited 2019 May 27). Available from: https://www.bop.gov/resources/pdfs/diabetes_guidance_march_2017.pdf.

82. American Diabetes Association. Diabetes management in correctional institutions. Diabetes Spectr. 2005;18(3):151-8.

83. Lopez-Jimenez F, Kramer V, Masters B, et al. Recommendations for managing patients with diabetes mellitus in cardiopulmonary rehabilitation. J Cardiopulm Rehabil Prev. 2012;32:101-12.

CHAPTER 13

Pathophysiology of the Metabolic Disorder

Jane K. Dickinson, RN, PhD, CDCES

Key Concepts

- Diabetes is a disease characterized by abnormal metabolism of carbohydrate, protein, and fat. An understanding of normal fuel metabolism and its hormonal control is necessary if one is to fully grasp the abnormalities that occur in diabetes.
- A progressive increase in our understanding of the hormones and systems that regulate the normal physiology of energy balance is enhancing our knowledge of the pathophysiology of diabetes. This is leading to improved pharmacologic treatment options for diabetes as well as more sensitive and accurate approaches to diabetes education.
- An estimated 9.4% of the US population (30.3 million people of all ages: 23 million diagnosed and 7.2 million undiagnosed) has diabetes, and, based on fasting glucose or hemoglobin A1C levels, 84.1 million (33.9%) US adults aged 20 years and older are predisposed to diabetes (have prediabetes). These disorders are increasingly prevalent in both children and adults, with even higher prevalence in certain racial and ethnic groups (Hispanics, Native Americans, African Americans, and Pacific Islanders).
- Reflecting the underlying pathophysiologic processes that result in diabetes, glycemic criteria are used to diagnose diabetes and prediabetes. The diagnosis for diabetes and prediabetes can be determined by any of the following: a fasting blood glucose of >126 mg/dl (7 mmol/L), a 2-hour 75-g oral glucose tolerance test of >200 mg/dL (11.1 mmol/L), and HbA1c value of >6.5% (48 mmol/mol). Confirmatory testing on a subsequent day is advised.
- Diabetes includes 4 clinical classes, which result from a variety of underlying pathophysiologic processes. These are type 1 diabetes, type 2 diabetes, gestational diabetes, and other specific types of diabetes (eg, caused by genetic defects in beta cell function or insulin action, diseases of the exocrine pancreas, or medications).
- Type 1 diabetes results from autoimmune beta cell destruction, leading to absolute insulin deficiency. Both genetic and environmental factors are implicated in type 1 diabetes. Type 1 diabetes is characterized by the abrupt onset of clinical signs and symptoms associated with marked hyperglycemia and a strong propensity for ketoacidosis.
- Type 2 diabetes results from multiple pathophysiologic abnormalities, the hallmark features of which are a progressive insulin secretory defect and insulin resistance. This disease progresses from an early asymptomatic state with insulin resistance, to mild postprandial hyperglycemia, to clinical diabetes requiring pharmacologic intervention, typically over many years. Obesity, weight gain in adulthood, and physical inactivity are environmental factors affecting this pathologic progression. There is substantial evidence for the role of genetics in both type 2 diabetes and obesity.
- Diabetes is characterized by elevated blood glucose levels, which can damage the large and small blood vessels of the body. The purpose of managing diabetes, therefore, is to maintain healthy blood vessels and lower the risk for micro- and macrovascular complications and comorbidities associated with diabetes.

State of the Problem

Diabetes is a chronic, progressive metabolic disorder characterized by abnormalities in the ability to metabolize carbohydrate, fat, and protein, leading to a hyperglycemic state. This chronic metabolic dysregulation is associated with long-term damage to blood vessels and various organ systems, including the eyes, kidneys, nerves, and heart.

Diabetes is an epidemic in the United States, with 30.3 million people (9.4% of the population) affected by the disorder. Approximately 23 million people are diagnosed, while 7.2 million people are unaware they have the disease.[1]

Epidemiology: Race and Ethnic Differences in the Prevalence of Diagnosed Diabetes

The national survey data for all Americans aged 20 years and older include the following prevalence of diagnosed diabetes by race/ethnicity:[1]

- 7.4% non-Hispanic white
- 8.0% Asian American
- 12.1% Hispanic
- 12.7% non-Hispanic black
- 15.1% American Indians/Alaska Natives

Among Hispanics, rates are as follows:

- 8.5% for Central and South Americans
- 9.0% for Cubans
- 12.0% for Puerto Ricans
- 13.8% for Mexican Americans

Table 13.1 provides a breakdown of diagnosed and undiagnosed diabetes among people aged 18 years and older in the United States in 2015.

An increase in body mass index (BMI) is generally associated with a significant increase in the prevalence of insulin resistance, hypertension, and dyslipidemia. Insulin resistance contributes to elevated blood glucose levels, the hallmark of diabetes. The prevalence of diabetes and hypertension, therefore, increases in an observable, linear fashion as BMI levels increase. Two national surveys, SHIELD and NHANES, showed the prevalence of diabetes mellitus was highest for those with morbid obesity (BMI ≥40 kg/m^2), with rates of 25% (SHIELD) and 27% (NHANES).[2]

The maps in Figure 13.1 show the trend in the age-adjusted prevalence of obesity and diagnosed diabetes among US adults aged 18 years and older from 1994 through 2015. During this period, the prevalence of obesity and diagnosed diabetes rose in all states. In 1994, all but 2 states had a prevalence of obesity less than 18%, and no state exceeded 22%. In 2015, no state had a prevalence of obesity less than 18%, and all but 1 state exceeded 22%. Similarly for diagnosed diabetes, in 1994, the majority of states had a prevalence less than 5.0%. In 2015, all states exceeded 6.0%; 29 of those exceeded 9.0%.[3]

Overweight and especially obesity, particularly at younger ages, substantially increase lifetime risk of diagnosed diabetes, while their impact on diabetes risk, life expectancy, and diabetes duration diminishes with age.

Characteristics used to identify people at risk for type 2 diabetes and prediabetes include the following:

- Obesity
- Sedentary lifestyle
- Hypertension
- Dyslipidemia
- Family history of diabetes
- Gestational history
- Race/ethnicity
- Age

TABLE 13.1 Diagnosed and Undiagnosed Diabetes Among People Aged 18 Years and Older, United States, 2015

Group	*Number or Percentage Who Have Diabetes*
Aged 18–44 years	3.0 million, or 2.6% of all people in this age group
Aged 45–64 years and older	10.7 million, or 12.7% of all people in this age group
Aged 65 years and older	9.9 million, or 20.8 % of all people in this age group
Men	11.3 million, or 9.2% of all men aged 18 years and older
Women	11.7 million, or 9.4% of all women aged 18 years and older

Note: Sufficient data are not available to estimate the total prevalence of diabetes—diagnosed and undiagnosed—for US racial/ethnic minority populations.

Source: National Center for Chronic Disease Prevention and Health Promotion/Centers for Disease Control and Prevention, Division of Diabetes Translation, *National Diabetes Statistics Report, 2017* (cited 2019 May 27), on the Internet at: http://www.cdc.gov/diabetes/pdfs/statistics/national-diabetes-statistis-report.pdf.

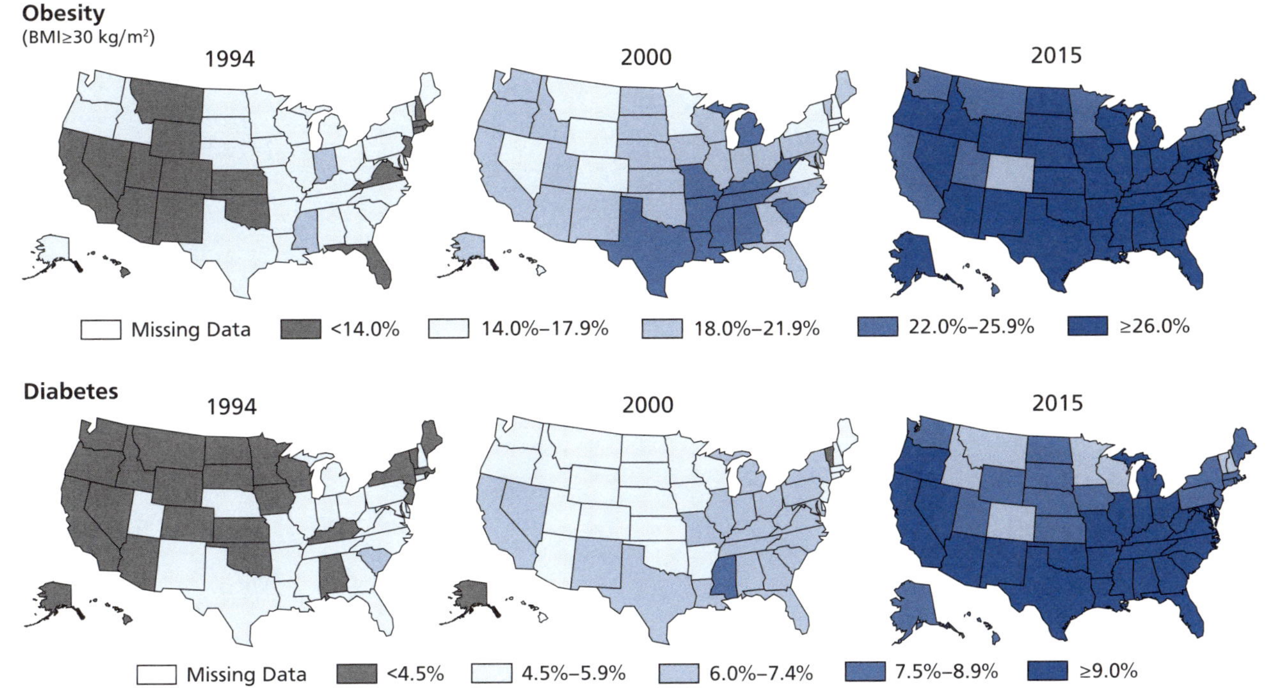

FIGURE 13.1 **Maps of Trends in Diagnosed Diabetes and Obesity, 1994–2015**

Source: Centers for Disease Control and Prevention, "Maps of trends in diagnosed diabetes and obesity," CDC's Division of Diabetes Translation, National Diabetes Surveillance System, 2017 Nov (cited 2019 May 27), on the Internet at: http://www.cdc.gov/diabetes/statistics/slides/maps_diabetesobesity_trends.pdf.

These risk factors may be assessed by various means, including community health screening, media campaigns, annual health maintenance exams, and risk assessment tools. Diabetes risk assessment tools have been validated for their ability to predict the likelihood of developing type 2 diabetes.[4,5] A variety of organizations, including the American Diabetes Association (ADA), the National Diabetes Education Program, and the Harvard School of Public Health, provide diabetes risk surveys on their Web sites.

Type 2 diabetes is more common among American Indian, African-American, Hispanic, and Latino children and adolescents.[1] Data from the 2015 Indian Health Service indicate that 15.1% of American Indians and Alaska Natives aged 18 years and older who received care from the Indian Health Service had diagnosed diabetes.[1] Type 1 diabetes may account for 5% to 10% of all diagnosed cases of diabetes in adults.[1] Risk factors for type 1 diabetes include genetic, autoimmune, and environmental factors.

Fuel Homeostasis: 5 Phases

An understanding of the phases of fuel homeostasis (Figure 13.2) will enable the diabetes care and education specialist to more fully understand how hormonal physiology is relevant to and must be considered in glucose management efforts undertaken with the person with diabetes. The following description is adapted from *Joslin Diabetes Mellitus*.[6]

Phase I is the fed state (0-3.9 hours after eating), in which circulating glucose predominantly comes from an exogenous source. Plasma insulin levels are high, glucagon levels are low, and triglycerides are synthesized in liver and adipose tissue. Insulin inhibits breakdown of glycogen (stored glucose) and triglyceride (stored fat) reservoirs. The brain and other organs use some of the glucose that has been absorbed from the gastrointestinal tract, with the remaining excess glucose stored in hepatic, muscle, adipose, and other tissue reservoirs.

Phase II is the fasting postabsorptive state (4 to 15.9 hours after food consumption), in which blood glucose originates mainly from glycogen breakdown and hepatic gluconeogenesis. Plasma insulin levels decrease and glucagon levels begin to increase. Energy storage (anabolism) ends in this phase and energy production (catabolism) begins. Carbohydrate and lipid stores are mobilized.

(continued)

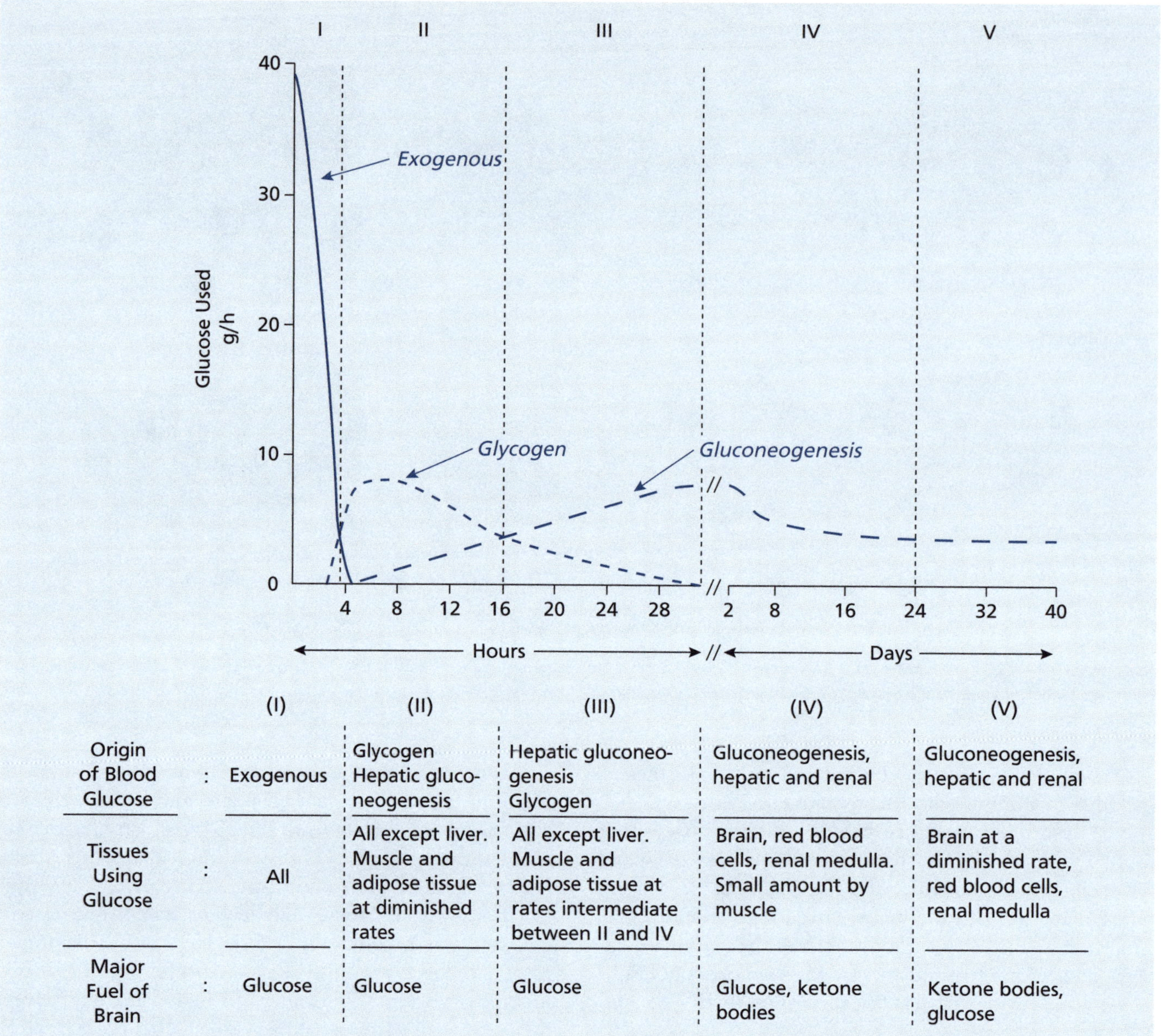

		(I)	(II)	(III)	(IV)	(V)
Origin of Blood Glucose	:	Exogenous	Glycogen Hepatic gluco-neogenesis	Hepatic gluconeo-genesis Glycogen	Gluconeogenesis, hepatic and renal	Gluconeogenesis, hepatic and renal
Tissues Using Glucose	:	All	All except liver. Muscle and adipose tissue at diminished rates	All except liver. Muscle and adipose tissue at rates intermediate between II and IV	Brain, red blood cells, renal medulla. Small amount by muscle	Brain at a diminished rate, red blood cells, renal medulla
Major Fuel of Brain	:	Glucose	Glucose	Glucose	Glucose, ketone bodies	Ketone bodies, glucose

FIGURE 13.2 Five Phases of Fuel Metabolism

Hepatic glycogen breakdown provides maintenance of plasma glucose and ensures an adequate supply of glucose to the brain and other tissues. Adipocyte triglyceride begins to break down, and free fatty acids (FFAs) are released into the circulation and used by the liver and skeletal muscle as a primary energy source and as a substrate for gluconeogenesis (making new glucose). The brain continues to use glucose, provided mainly by gluconeogenesis (35%-60%), because of its inability to use FFAs as fuel.

Phase III is the early starvation state (16-47.9 hours after food consumption), in which blood glucose originates from hepatic gluconeogenesis and glycogenolysis. Gluconeogenesis continues to produce most of the hepatic glucose. In this phase of starvation, lactate makes up half the gluconeogenic substrate. Amino acids, specifically alanine and glycerol, are other major substrates. Insulin secretion is markedly suppressed, and counterregulatory hormone (eg, glucagon, cortisol, growth hormone, and epinephrine) secretion is stimulated.

Phase IV is the preliminary prolonged starvation state (48 hours to 23.9 days after food consumption), in which blood glucose originates from hepatic and renal gluconeogenesis. By 60 hours of starvation, gluconeogenesis provides more than 97% of hepatic glucose output. Insulin secretion is markedly suppressed, and counterregulatory hormone (eg, glucagon, cortisol, growth hormone, and epinephrine) secretion is stimulated. In phases IV and V there is a progressive breakdown of proteins as the effective fat stores are depleted. This results in a severe catabolic state represented by muscle wasting.

Phase V is the secondary prolonged starvation state (24-40 days after food consumption), in which blood glucose originates from hepatic and renal gluconeogenesis, the same source as in phase IV. In phase V, the rate of glucose being used by the brain diminishes, as does the rate of hepatic gluconeogenesis.

Normal Fuel Metabolism

To understand the abnormalities in fuel metabolism characterized by diabetes, a basic understanding of normal fuel metabolism is needed.[6] Humans have a constant requirement for energy yet eat only intermittently. To offset this, food is ingested in excess of the immediate need of the vital organs and stored as extra calories in the form of hepatic and muscle glycogen, adipose tissue triglyceride, and to some extent tissue protein. In times of starvation and other stresses, these fuel stores are broken down to provide energy for organ metabolism and function.

The 2 main fuels—sources of energy—in humans are glucose and FFAs. Glucose is stored as glycogen in the skeletal muscle and the liver. Free fatty acids are stored as triglycerides primarily in adipose tissue.

The energy stores are utilized and replenished in response to hormones, depending on whether one is in a fasting or fed state. In the fed or anabolic state, where fuels are stored in the tissues, insulin levels increase, promoting glycogen synthesis in the liver and muscle, lipid storage in adipocytes, and amino acid uptake and protein synthesis in most cells. The net result is movement of glucose from the circulation into storage depots. Insulin thus acts as an anabolic, or storage, hormone. In the fasting state (8-12 hours without energy intake) or starvation (more than 12-24 hours), which occurs when the body no longer has any stored energy and begins breaking down fat and protein for an energy source, decreased insulin secretion enables glycogen breakdown, lipolysis, hepatic ketogenesis, and decreased synthesis and increased degradation of protein in order to meet the body's energy requirements.[6] Fasting and starvation represent a catabolic state where insulin secretion decreases, and glucagon, a catabolic hormone, enables glycogenolysis, lipolysis, and ketogenesis.

Counterregulatory hormones oppose insulin's actions. Glucagon and catecholamines (eg, epinephrine) stimulate glycogenolysis and gluconeogenesis in the liver, thereby raising blood glucose levels. Catecholamines are key regulators of lipolysis in adipose tissue and glycogenolysis in muscle and other tissues. Growth hormone and cortisol are also insulin counterregulatory hormones.

In normal glucose homeostasis, the balance between insulin and the counterregulatory hormones maintains normoglycemia. The serum glucose concentration depends on the rate at which the glucose enters and the rate at which it is utilized from the circulation. In adults without diabetes or impaired fasting glucose (IFG), the fasting plasma glucose (FPG) concentration remains within a narrow range of 70 to 100 mg/dL (3.88-5.55 mmol/L) despite varying rates of utilization. This maintenance occurs because glucose appearance and glucose disposal, which reflect the rate at which glucose is taken up by peripheral tissues, are well matched.

Insulin lowers plasma glucose levels both by stimulating glucose uptake in muscle and adipose tissue and by inhibiting hepatic glycogen breakdown and gluconeogenesis. The counterregulatory hormones balance these effects of insulin in order to maintain normogylcemia.[6]

The Role of Hormones

Multiple hormones play a key role in the regulation of fuel physiology. They may be broadly grouped as pancreatic (glucoregulatory), incretin (intestinal), and other hormones and factors affecting fuel metabolism. The knowledge and understanding of incretins and other hormones that diabetes care and education specialists need has grown tremendously. Therefore, the salient features relative to the role of each in the pathophysiology of diabetes will be reviewed below.

Pancreatic (Glucoregulatory) Hormones

Insulin Insulin is produced by the beta cells in the pancreas. It is highly regulated by glucose and the incretin system, including glucagon-like peptide-1 (GLP-1) and glucose-dependent insulin-releasing polypeptide (GIP).

Insulin regulates postprandial glucose via 2 mechanisms:

- Peripheral glucose utilization by insulin-sensitive tissues, mainly muscle and fat cells
- Direct inhibition of hepatic glucose production and glucagon secretion, thus further decreasing gluconeogenesis[7]

Amylin The discovery of amylin has contributed to the understanding of postprandial glucose homeostasis. This 37–amino acid polypeptide "neuroendocrine" hormone is co-secreted from the pancreatic beta cells with insulin in response to nutrient stimuli. It inhibits postprandial glucose exertions via 3 primary actions:[8]

- Regulation of food intake
- Slowing of gastric emptying
- Inhibition of digestive secretions (gastric acid, pancreatic enzymes, and bile)

Glucagon Glucagon is an alpha cell pancreatic hormone associated with maintaining glucose homeostasis. Glucagon increases glucose through glycogenolysis and gluconeogenesis during the fasting state and when blood glucose concentrations are low. Alpha cells are regulated by glucose, insulin, and the incretin system—mainly by GLP-1. Glucagon is secreted in response to low blood concentrations of glucose.[8] Glucagon-like peptide-1 suppresses glucagon secretion.[9]

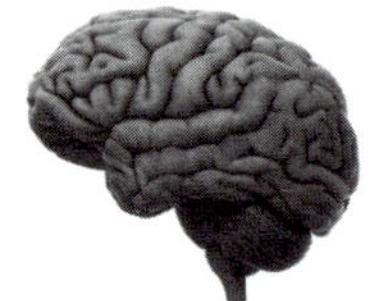

Brain:
Promotes satiety and reduces appetite

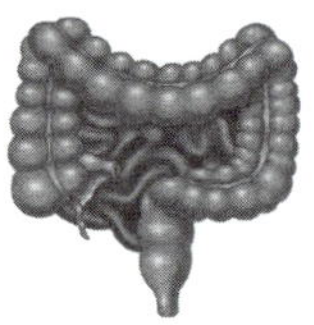

Intestines:
GLP-1 is secreted upon the ingestion of food

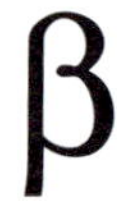

Beta cell:
Enhances glucose-dependent insulin secretion

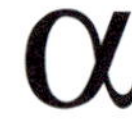

Alpha cell:
Lowers postprandial glucagon secretion

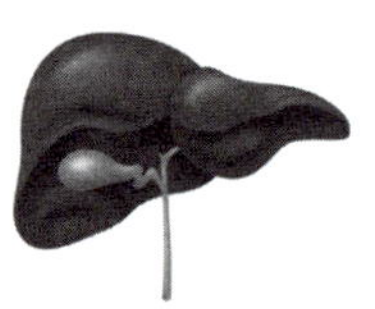

Liver:
Reduces hepatic glucose output

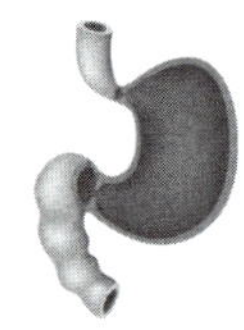

Stomach:
Helps regulate gastric emptying

FIGURE 13.3 **Functions of GLP-1**

Source: A Flint et al, *J Clin Invest.* 101 (1998): 515-20; H Larsson et al, *Acta Physiol Scand.* 160 (1997): 413-22; MA Nauck et al, *Diabetologia.* 39 (1996): 1546-53; DJ Drucker, *Diabetes.* 47 (1998): 159-69.

Incretin (Intestinal) Hormones

When meals are consumed, the gastrointestinal tract releases a number of hormones that aid in the absorption and disposition of nutrients. Among these hormones, GLP-1 and GIP are particularly important because of their regulation of hormone secretion. Glucagon-like peptide-1 and GIP augment glucose-stimulated insulin secretion, a process termed the *incretin effect*. The incretin effect accounts for approximately 50% of the insulin secreted after a meal and, therefore, has a prominent role in postprandial metabolism.[9] Figure 13.3 summarizes the effects of GLP-1 in humans.

In animal and in vitro studies, both GIP and GLP-1 also promoted beta cell proliferation and inhibited apoptosis, leading to expansion of beta cell mass. Glucagon-like peptide-1, but not GIP, controls glycemia via additional actions on glucose sensors, and inhibition of gastric emptying, food intake, and glucagon secretion.

Glucose-Dependent Insulin-Releasing Polypeptide Glucose-dependent insulin-releasing polypeptide is secreted by K cells from the upper small intestine. Along with GLP-1, GIP is released following a meal; together, these hormones act on the beta cells to increase their sensitivity to glucose. Glucose-dependent insulin-releasing polypeptide may help stimulate insulin secretion, but this is being studied and not yet conclusive.[9]

Glucagon-Like Peptide-1 Glucagon-like peptide-1 is predominantly produced in the enteroendocrine L cells located in the distal intestine.[9] As noted above, it is released after a meal and works with GIP to increase beta cell sensitivity to glucose. Glucagon-like peptide-1 appears to be the major mediator of the incretin effect in humans, and it potentiates the glucose-stimulated insulin secretion following a carbohydrate meal.

In addition to its effects on insulin secretion, GLP-1 exerts other significant actions to modulate intermediary metabolism, including stimulation of insulin biosynthesis, inhibition of glucagon secretion, delayed gastric emptying, reduced food intake, and trophic effects on the pancreatic islet cells.[10]

Dipeptidyl Peptidase-4 Both GIP and GLP-1 are rapidly metabolized in the circulation by the enzyme dipeptidyl peptidase-4 (DPP-4), which is produced by endothelial cells and circulates in the plasma. This protease cleaves the first 2 amino acids from GLP-1, leaving a metabolite that does not stimulate insulin secretion or glucose clearance. The short half-life of the incretins in the circulation (1-2 minutes for GLP-1 and 7 minutes for GIP) is due to the presence of DPP-4.[11]

Other Hormones and Factors Affecting Fuel Metabolism

Peptide-YY Peptide-YY (PYY) is secreted from the L cells of the gastrointestinal tract along with GLP-1. It is secreted postprandially in proportion to the calorie content of the meal. This gut hormone increases satiety through delayed gastric emptying.[9]

Leptin and Ghrelin Leptin and ghrelin are 2 hormones that have been recognized as having a major influence on energy balance. Leptin, the "satiety hormone," is a mediator of long-term regulation of energy balance, suppressing food intake and thereby inducing weight loss. Ghrelin, on the other hand, is a fast-acting hormone, often called the "hunger hormone." As a growing number of people experience obesity, understanding the mechanisms by which various hormones and neurotransmitters have influence on energy balance has been a subject of intensive research. In people with obesity, the circulating level of the anorexigenic hormone leptin is increased, whereas, surprisingly, the level of the orexigenic hormone ghrelin is decreased. It is now established that obese persons have leptin resistance. Low ghrelin also occurs in those with insulin resistance and after gastric sleeve procedures.[12] High ghrelin occurs during calorie restriction, weight loss, and Prader-Willi Syndrome. Low ghrelin levels are observed in women with gestational diabetes as well.[13] The manner in which both the leptin and ghrelin systems contribute to the development or maintenance of obesity continues to be studied.[14,15,16]

Endocannabinoid System The endocannabinoid system further contributes to the physiological regulation of energy balance, food intake, and lipid and glucose metabolism through both central and peripheral effects.[17]

Activation of the central endocannabinoid system increases food intake and promotes weight gain. The observation that endocannabinoid activation is not reversible with a 5% weight loss suggests that this activation may be a cause rather than a consequence of obesity. The endocannabinoid system is overactivated in response to exogenous stimuli, such as excessive food intake, leading experts to believe that overeating promotes more overeating.[17]

Exogenous cannabinoids and endocannabinoids increase food intake and promote weight gain by activating central endocannabinoid receptors. These normal endocrine processes provide the framework for research that may further our understanding of the pathophysiology leading to diabetes as well as insight into potential sites of pharmacologic intervention. Exploration of the potential for endocannabinoid blockers as diabetes and weight management agents is ongoing. To date, drugs investigated and/or under development have shown some promise; further investigation is under way.

Gut Microbiome There is new and ongoing research on the role of gut bacteria in obesity and diabetes. Studies have shown that gut microbes can increase or decrease the endocannabinoid system's activity in controlling glucose and energy metabolism. Gut bacteria are different in people who are lean versus obese and in those with and without type 2 diabetes.[18]

Bariatric surgery has led to improvements in glucose levels due to increased insulin sensitivity. While the exact mechanisms are still unclear, scientists believe bariatric surgery has a role in decreasing ghrelin, increasing secretion of gut hormones, and possibly changes in the gut microbiome.[19]

Diabetes Diagnostic Criteria

International diabetes organizations have determined categorical cutoff points in glucose and A1C to define diabetes.[20] These cutoff points correlate with the epidemiologic risk of developing microvascular complications, particularly diabetes-related retinopathy. However, vascular problems may pose a threat to individuals even at glycemic levels that do not approach the diagnostic definition of diabetes. These glycemic levels represent a high predisposition to diabetes and have been termed "prediabetes." Prediabetes can be defined in terms of impaired glucose tolerance (IGT) or IFG, depending on which test is used. Progression of prediabetes to type 2 diabetes may be delayed by lifestyle intervention and by some pharmacotherapeutic strategies. One study showed that 8.1% of subjects whose initial abnormal fasting glucose was 100 to 109 mg/dL (5.55-6.06 mmol/L) (added IFG subjects) and 24.3% of subjects whose initial abnormal fasting glucose was 110 to 125 mg/dL (6.11-6.94 mmol/L) (original IFG subjects) developed diabetes. Added IFG subjects who progressed to diabetes did so within a mean of 41.4 months, a rate of 1.34% per year. Original IFG subjects converted at a rate of 5.56% per year after an average of 29.0 months. A steeper rate of increasing fasting glucose; higher BMI, blood pressure, and triglycerides; and lower HDL cholesterol predicted diabetes development.[21]

A diagnosis of diabetes is made when presentation with a variety of clinical symptoms or results of a screening test lead to confirmation of its presence by formal diagnostic glycemic criteria.

The glycemic thresholds used to diagnose diabetes have been modified over the years largely on the basis of the current understanding of the epidemiologic relationship between glucose levels and diabetes-specific

TABLE 13.2 Diagnosing Diabetes—4 Testing Options	
A1C*	≥6.5% (48 mmol/mol)
Acute symptoms plus casual plasma glucose*	≥200 mg/dL (11.1 mmol/L)
Fasting plasma glucose*	≥126 mg/dL (7.0 mmol/L)
2-hour postprandial plasma glucose*	≥200 mg/dL (11.1 mmol/L) during OGTT (75-g glucose)

*Unless unequivocal symptoms of hyperglycemia are present, these criteria must be confirmed by repeat testing on a subsequent day.

Source: American Diabetes Association, *Standards of Medical Care in Diabetes—2019*, on the Internet at http//care.diabetesjournals.org/content/42/Supplement_1/S13.

microvascular complications (Table 13.2). As has been described earlier in this chapter, the processes by which diabetes occurs take place over a prolonged period of time, with a wide variety of compensating mechanisms. The disease is continuous, even though the glucose definitions are fixed.[20]

For decades, the diagnosis of diabetes has been based on glucose criteria, either an FPG or a 75-g oral glucose tolerance test (OGTT). In 1997, the first Expert Committee on the Diagnosis and Classification of Diabetes Mellitus revised the criteria using the association between FPG and the presence of retinopathy as the key factor with which to identify threshold glucose level. The additional analysis of FPG and 2-hour postprandial glucose set a new cutoff point of ≥126 mg/dL (7 mmol/L) for FPG and confirmed the long-standing 2-hour postprandial plasma glucose value of ≥200 mg/dL (11.11 mmol/L).[22]

In 2009 the International Expert Committee on the role of the A1C assay in the diagnosis of diabetes recommended the use of A1C ≥6.5% obtained using NGSP methodology for the diagnosis of diabetes.[23] It is important to be aware that A1C levels are not reliable in a variety of clinical circumstances. In people who have hemoglobin variants such as HbS (sickle cell trait) or thalassemia, some A1C tests give falsely high or low readings that can lead to the over- or undertreatment of diabetes. Individuals may be at risk for having a hemoglobin variant if they are of African, Mediterranean, or Southeast Asian heritage; members of their family have sickle cell trait or sickle cell anemia; laboratory or self-monitored blood glucose results don't match the results of their A1C; the A1C result is different from what was expected or is very high (above 15%); or the most recent A1C result is very different from the last A1C result.[24] A1C results may also be inaccurate in anemia due to other etiologies (eg, iron deficiency anemia) and in the setting of renal failure or liver disease. In addition, changes in A1C take place in pregnancy. A1C is significantly decreased early in pregnancy and further decreased in late pregnancy compared with age-matched nonpregnant women.[25] Recent blood donors can have a false low reading.[26]

The actual rate of diagnosis of type 2 diabetes remains poor, with 23.8% of those affected undiagnosed. Microvascular complications are often found in newly diagnosed individuals with type 2 diabetes. Type 2 diabetes may be present, on average, 6 to 12 years prior to identification and treatment. The prevalence of coronary artery disease in those with type 2 diabetes is twice that of the population without diabetes, and cardiovascular and total mortality are two- to threefold greater than that of individuals without diabetes.[27]

A diabetes diagnosis must be considered when encountering the classic acute symptoms associated with hyperglycemia, including blurred vision, excessive thirst and hunger, frequent urination, weight loss, fatigue, headache, and muscle cramps. A blood glucose ≥200 mg/dL (11.11 mmol/L) in the presence of these symptoms allows a formal diagnosis of diabetes. An acute presentation with diabetes-related ketoacidosis (DKA) or hyperosmolar hyperglycemic state (HHS) constitutes an endocrine emergency. The distinction between type 1 diabetes and type 2 diabetes generally can be made on the basis of laboratory testing at the time of such a presentation. However, increasing clinical evidence highlights significant overlap between type 1 diabetes and type 2 diabetes, and the classification into 2 main types has been challenged.

Diagnosis in Children

Distinguishing between type 1 diabetes and type 2 diabetes in children is important and can be difficult. The age of the person with diabetes at presentation is the main risk factor of delayed diagnosis, especially in children younger than age 2.[28] Ketosis may be present in those with otherwise straightforward type 2 diabetes (including obesity and acanthosis nigricans). Such a distinction at diagnosis is critical, because the natural history, treatment plans, educational approaches, and dietary counsel markedly differ between the 2 diagnoses.

Children should be screened for diabetes if they are overweight, have a family history of type 2 diabetes, are of a minority population, and have 2 of the following risk factors, which are signs of insulin resistance or conditions associated with insulin resistance: acanthosis nigricans, hypertension, dyslipidemia, polycystic ovary syndrome, or small-for-gestational-age birth weight. Children also should be screened if their mother had gestational diabetes during their gestation. Testing should begin at age 10, or younger if puberty has already occurred. Testing should be repeated every 3 years.[20]

Case—An African-American Woman at Risk for Diabetes

CS, a 29-year-old African-American woman, was noted to have a random glucose of 125 mg/dL (6.94 mmol/L) on a blood test obtained as part of a visit to the local health clinic. She has had no symptoms of diabetes and reports her blood glucose was "up a little" during her last pregnancy. She has been told to "watch her sugars" and to exercise. She has been healthy but recently complained of frequent yeast infections. Her family history includes a mother and 2 older sisters with type 2 diabetes. Her grandmother died from diabetes after she was started on "the shot." CS has been smoking one pack of cigarettes per day since age 18. She tried stopping because of the cost but has been unsuccessful. CS works evenings, her husband works days, and they have 2 children, ages 3 and 5 years old.

Physical Exam

- Height: 63 in
- Weight: 203 lb
- Blood pressure: 138/94 mm Hg
- Waist circumference: 40 in
- Skin: Acanthosis nigricans on neck, trace edema; otherwise normal
- A1C: 6.4%
- 1-hour postprandial glucose: 132 mg/dL (7.33 mmol/L)

Confirmation of Diagnosis

The test results that diagnose diabetes (see Table 13.2) should be repeated unless there is strong clinical evidence, such as classic signs of diabetes or a hyperglycemic crisis. Ideally, the same test should be used. However, if 2 tests are available for an individual and only 1 test's results are above the diagnosis point, the test that indicates results above the diagnostic point should be repeated. If the retest results are above the diagnostic point, then a diagnosis is made.

The emergency department may serve as a venue for the identification of previously unrecognized diabetes and/or prediabetes. Diagnostic criteria for use in people with diabetes and prediabetes presenting to the emergency department have not been well established. There are, however, some reports related to the potential for detection of these conditions in high-risk patients during emergency department visits.[29–31]

In the presence of signs and symptoms consistent with chronic hyperglycemia, including growth impairment; susceptibility to certain infections; and renal, retinal, macrovascular disease, connective tissue disorders, and neuropathic syndromes, it is contingent upon the provider to test for diabetes. Distinctions among the various conditions that encompass diabetes are described below.

Diabetes Classification

Prediabetes

The Expert Committee on the Diagnosis and Classification of Diabetes Mellitus[22] recognized an intermediate group of individuals whose glucose levels do not meet criteria for diabetes yet are higher than those considered normal (Table 13.3). These individuals, as well as those who have A1C levels above the laboratory normal (5.7%-6.4%) but below the diagnostic cutoff point[23] are referred to as being at high risk for developing diabetes. This condition has been described as prediabetes.

Impaired fasting glucose and IGT are not clinical entities but risk factors for diabetes as well as cardiovascular disease. They are associated with obesity (especially abdominal or visceral obesity), dyslipidemia with high triglycerides and/or low-density lipoprotein cholesterol (LDL-C), and hypertension.

Type 1 Diabetes

People with type 1 diabetes generally present with acute symptoms associated with markedly elevated blood glucose. Because of the acute onset of symptoms, type 1 diabetes usually is detected soon after symptoms develop, although the autoimmune process causing the disease may precede the clinical presentation by many years.[32] Approximately three-quarters of all cases of type 1 diabetes are diagnosed in individuals younger than age 18.[1] The following list describes characteristics of type 1 diabetes:

- Type 1 diabetes develops at any age, but in most cases is diagnosed before age 30.
- Type 1 diabetes is characterized by autoimmune destruction of the beta cells of the islets of Langerhans with resulting absolute insulin deficiency.
- Undiagnosed or untreated individuals experience significant weight loss, polyuria, and polydipsia

TABLE 13.3 Categories of Increased Risk for Diabetes (Prediabetes)

IFG	100–125 mg/dL (5.55–6.94 mmol/L)
IGT	2-hour OGTT values of 140–199 mg/dL (7.77–11.06 mmol/L)
A1C	5.7% to 6.4%

characterized by the abrupt signs and symptoms associated with marked hyperglycemia and the strong propensity for the development of ketoacidosis.

- People with type 1 diabetes are dependent on exogenous insulin to prevent ketoacidosis and sustain life.
- Coma and death can result from delayed diagnosis and/or treatment.
- Latent autoimmune diabetes in adults (LADA) is a slow onset form of type 1 diabetes that is diagnosed in adults and often mistaken for type 2 diabetes. Research has shown that as much as 50% of those who develop type 1 diabetes as adults are misclassified as having type 2 diabetes.[33]

Type 2 Diabetes

Type 2 diabetes frequently is not diagnosed until complications appear. This is because many of the symptoms are absent or attributed to other causes.[1] The following is a list of characteristics of type 2 diabetes:

- Approximately 90% of people in the United States with diabetes have type 2 diabetes, with disproportionate representation among the elderly and certain ethnic groups, including Native Americans, Alaskans and Hawaiians, South Asians, Hispanics, and African Americans.
- If present trends continue, as many as 1 in 3 adults in the United States will have diabetes in 2050.[3]
- Type 2 diabetes is usually diagnosed after age 30, but onset can occur at any age.
- Onset of type 2 diabetes in adolescence is becoming increasingly more common as obesity rates rise among youth. Type 2 diabetes now accounts for 30% to 50% of childhood-onset diabetes.[3]
- Type 2 diabetes is frequently asymptomatic at the time of diagnosis. Individuals may present with end-organ complications (eg, microvascular disease such as retinopathy, neuropathy, and nephropathy or macrovascular events such as stroke or myocardial infarction) due to delays in diagnosis of prediabetes and/or type 2 diabetes.
- Endogenous insulin levels may be normal, increased, or decreased, with a variable need for exogenous insulin.
- Insulin resistance occurs early and persists through prediabetes and subsequent clinical diabetes.
- Individuals with type 2 diabetes are not prone to ketosis except in rare cases of severe physiologic stress.

Test Selection

Which test to use is at the discretion of the healthcare professional. Factors to take into account include cost, practicality, and availability of the test.

Case—Part 2: Screening and Diagnostic Testing

With a random blood glucose of 125 mg/dL (6.94 mmol/L), CS did not meet the criteria for diabetes. However, she has several risk factors, physical evidence of insulin resistance, and an indication of hyperglycemia:

- High-risk racial group
- Family history of type 2 diabetes
- Likely history of gestational diabetes
- Obesity
- Acanthosis nigricans
- Recurrent yeast infections

Her family physician ordered a fasting blood glucose level:

- FPG: 112 mg/dL (6.22 mmol/L; when repeated, 108 mg/dL [6 mmol/L])

CS was identified as having prediabetes and counseled about healthy food choices, weight loss, and exercise.

Other Forms of Diabetes

Other forms of diabetes are diagnosed when diabetes occurs as a result of another disorder or treatment. Treatment of these underlying disorders or discontinuation of diabetogenic agents may result in amelioration of the diabetes. Frequently, however, reversing the underlying disorder or stopping the offending agent is not possible.[34] Therapy, then, is similar to diabetes therapy in general—using the modalities of nutrition, physical activity, and medications. The following disorders are classified as other kinds of diabetes:

- Known genetic defects associated with maturity-onset diabetes of the young (MODY), glycogen synthase deficiency, and mitochondrial DNA markers
- Pancreatic disorders, such as hemochromatosis, chronic pancreatitis, and pancreatectomy
- Hormonal disorders, such as Cushing's syndrome (excess amounts of corticosteroids), pheochromocytoma (excess catecholamines), and acromegaly (excess growth hormone)

- Other disorders, such as cystic fibrosis, congenital rubella syndrome, Down syndrome, and post-transplant diabetes mellitus
- Concomitant diabetogenic medications (eg, atypical antipsychotics, glucocorticoids, protease inhibitors, and pentamidine)[35]

Gestational Diabetes

Gestational diabetes (GDM) was traditionally defined as a diagnosis that applied to women in whom glucose intolerance developed or was first discovered during pregnancy.[36] Although most cases resolved with delivery, the definition applied whether or not the condition continued after pregnancy, and did not address the possibility that the pregnant women had preexisting undiagnosed diabetes. This definition facilitated a uniform strategy for detection and classification of GDM, but its limitations were recognized for many years. As the ongoing epidemic of obesity and diabetes has led to more cases of type 2 diabetes in women of childbearing age, the number of pregnant women with preexisting type 2 diabetes diagnosed during pregnancy has increased.[36]

After deliberations in 2008 and 2009, the International Association of Diabetes and Pregnancy Study Groups (IADPSG), an international consensus group with representatives from multiple obstetrical and diabetes organizations, recommended that high-risk women found to have diabetes at their initial prenatal visit (using standard criteria) receive a diagnosis of overt, not gestational, diabetes.[37]

Gestational diabetes, diagnosed between weeks 24 and 28 of pregnancy, is associated with insulin resistance due to pregnancy and perhaps obesity and genetic predisposition.[38] Failure to augment beta cell insulin response to the insulin resistance is the hallmark of the disorder. The condition is usually asymptomatic but is dangerous for the developing fetus. Maternal risks include hypertension, polyhydramnios, and cesarean delivery. There is mounting evidence that treating even mild GDM reduces morbidity for both mother and baby.[39] See chapter 24 for a complete discussion of GDM.

Pathophysiology

Type 1 Diabetes

Type 1 diabetes is an autoimmune disorder. It develops when the body's immune system generates antibodies that destroy the pancreatic beta cells, leading to the inability to produce the hormones insulin and amylin. Although type 1 diabetes is thought to be more commonly diagnosed in children and young adults, disease onset can occur at any age,[40] and up to 50% of adults with type 1 diabetes are initially misclassified with type 2 diabetes.[33] Type 1 diabetes is characterized by the abrupt onset of clinical signs and symptoms associated with hyperglycemia and a strong propensity for ketoacidosis. Decline in insulin secretion begins to develop long before the clinical signs become evident and may take place for as long as 9 years before the clinical presentation of type 1 diabetes. The 5 progressive stages of the natural history of the development of type 1 diabetes are shown in Table 13.4.

Genetic Propensity

Although most people with type 1 diabetes do not have a relative with the disease,[40] there is a genetic propensity for type 1 diabetes. That risk is substantially increased (from approximately 1 in 50 to 1 in 20) in the offspring of people with diabetes. Children with the human leukocyte

TABLE 13.4 Pathophysiologic Stages in the Development of Type 1 Diabetes

Stage	*Physiology and Events*	*Comments*
1	Genetic predisposition	Aggregates in families, but most do not have a relative with type 1 diabetes; strongly increased risk in monozygotic/identical twins
2	Precipitating event	Environmental trigger causes insulitis; congenital rubella, viruses implicated
3	Active autoimmunity	Antibodies to auto/self antigens lead to anti–islet cell antibodies that can be measured; insulin release remains normal
4	Progressive beta cell dysfunction	Progressive loss of beta cell function: loss of first phase of insulin release; glucose remains normal
5	Overt type 1 diabetes mellitus	C-peptide presents early, then lost; clinical onset of type 1 diabetes

Source: RA Insel, JL Dunne, MA Atkinson, et al., Staging: presymptomatic type 2 diabetes: a scientific statement of JDRF, the Endocrine Society, and the American Diabetes Association," *Diabetes Care*. 38(2015): 1964-74.

antigen (HLA)–risk genotypes HLA-DR3 and HLA-DR4 and DQ8 who have a family history of type 1 diabetes have more than a 1 in 5 risk for developing islet autoantibodies during childhood, and children with the same HLA-risk genotype but no family history have approximately a 1 in 20 risk. Children born with the high-risk genotype HLA-DR3 and HLA-DR4 and DQ8 compose almost 50% of children who develop anti-islet autoimmunity by 5 years of age.[41] Determining extreme genetic risk is a prerequisite for the implementation of primary prevention trials, which are now under way for relatives of individuals with type 1 diabetes.[42] The major susceptibility locus maps to the HLA class II genes at 6p21, although more than 40 non-HLA susceptibility genetic markers have been confirmed. The HLA class II alleles account for up to 30% to 50% of genetic type 1 diabetes risk. Multiple non–major histocompatibility complex loci contribute to disease risk with smaller effects; these include the insulin, PTPN22, CTLA4, IL2RA, IFIH1, and other loci.[41]

Not all individuals at genetic risk for type 1 diabetes develop the disease. Although 40% of Caucasian individuals express the DR3 or DR4 haplotype, less than 1% develops diabetes. Conversely, most people with type 1 diabetes do not even have the highest risk combination of HLA alleles.[40] A 50% discordance rate of type 1 diabetes exists between identical twins, suggesting that specific genes are necessary but not sufficient conditions for disease development.[43]

A trigger is necessary for expression of the genetic propensity for type 1 diabetes; environmental triggers have long been suspected. The pathogenesis of type 1 diabetes is believed to involve T-cell mediated autoimmune processes directed against the pancreatic beta cell. Increasing evidence suggests that environmental factors, including toxins, food antigens, and particularly viral infections, are implicated in the induction of type 1 diabetes.[34]

Viral triggers, such as enteroviruses, rubella, mumps, rotavirus, parvovirus, and cytomegalovirus, have been investigated in both laboratory and clinical studies to attempt to define their roles in the pathogenesis of type 1 diabetes. Enteroviruses are the most common cause of viral infection in humans worldwide. Enteroviruses have an affinity for islet cells and have been isolated from the islets of a person with type 1 diabetes and shown to be present in an individual concurrent with development of islet cell antibodies.[34] Enteroviral antigen-positive islet cells were shown to be present in 44 of 72 persons with recent-onset type 1 diabetes in an autopsy series.[44] All enterovirus serotypes (over 100) studied to date include strains with the ability to damage beta cells.[45] These findings reinforce the potential relevance of enteroviruses in the pathophysiology of this disease.

Bovine serum albumin (BSA), contained in cow's milk, has been reported as an environmental trigger. Antibodies specific to BSA have been found in the majority of children with newly diagnosed type 1 diabetes, leading to the hypothesis that early exposure to cow's milk may be a potential determinant of type 1 diabetes, with the potential to increase disease risk by as much as 1.5 times.[46] Structural similarities exist between BSA and an islet cell surface antigen referred to as ICA-69. The cross-reactivity of circulating anti-BSA antibodies with ICA-69 provides a link between the environmental trigger and subsequent development of autoimmunity. Longer duration of breastfeeding, exclusive breastfeeding in particular, and supplementation with vitamin D in infancy have been reported to confer partial protection against beta cell autoimmunity and type 1 diabetes.[47] Other researchers, however, have not been able to find data to support the hypothesis that infant diet is related to the occurrence of type 1 diabetes,[40] while still others have found a relationship between late introduction of rice/oats and type 1 diabetes.[48] Research on this topic is ongoing.

Oxidative Stress

Some researchers suggest that type 1 diabetes may be the result of oxidative stress, due to high local levels of nitric oxide (NO) and oxygen radicals (O_2) in the beta cells, which plays a role in their destruction.[49,50]

Furthermore, there is evidence suggesting that the incidence of type 1 diabetes is increased in both spring and fall and is coincidental with various viral disorders.[51]

One dilemma in identifying specific triggers for type 1 diabetes involves the apparent long latency period between the triggering of active autoimmunity and the subsequent clinical development of diabetes. Thus, identifying which specific insult over the past 7 to 10 years may have been the actual trigger of the disease process is challenging. It is also possible that a variety of viral or environmental agents play a role in triggering expression of the genetic predisposition to the disease.[34]

Autoimmunity

Regardless of the trigger, early type 1 diabetes is first identified by the appearance of active autoimmunity directed against pancreatic beta cells and their products. Fifty percent of relatives with high-titer islet cell antibodies (ICAs) have diabetes within 5 years of follow-up. Islet cell antibody negativity has a 99.9% probability of freedom from the development of type 1 diabetes. Additional ICAs that may play a permissive or pathologic role in causing type 1 diabetes include those related to insulin, glycolipids, ganglioside GT3, carboxypeptidase H, PM-1 polar antigen, additional islet cell proteins of varying sizes (37 kd or 40 kd, 38 kd, 52 kd, and 69 kd) and as yet undetermined function, peripherin, heat shock protein 65, insulin receptors, other endocrine cell antigens, cytoskeletal proteins (tubulin, actin, reticulin, nuclear antigens [single-stranded DNA and RNA]), and agonist islet tyrosine phosphatase (islet antigen A2 and A2 beta).[52]

Although the clinical onset of type 1 diabetes may be abrupt, the pathophysiologic insult occurs slowly and progressively. In the early stages of the disease, markers of immune destruction of the beta cells are found, including ICAs, insulin autoantibodies (IAAs), and autoantibodies to glutamic acid decarboxylase (GAD). Beta cell destruction occurs at varying rates and is usually faster among younger patients, accounting for the classic abrupt clinical manifestation. Beta cell destruction is slower in adults, which sometimes leads to an incorrect diagnosis of type 2 diabetes.[52] Evidence suggests autoantibodies are predictive of type 1 diabetes and help distinguish autoimmune type 1 diabetes and LADA from non-autoimmune diabetes.[54] Positivity to increasing numbers of autoantibodies indicates that the individual's autoimmune response is spreading and that the disease is progressing. The predictive ability of autoantibody tests therefore increases with the number of autoantibodies detected in an individual and may be influenced by the autoantibody titer, as well. There also appears to be a hierarchy of diabetes relevance in the autoantibody response against different antigenic targets within and between islet autoantigens. Circulating islet autoantibodies are present in sera from approximately 5% of children with new-onset diabetes and provide evidence of an active and disease-specific B lymphocyte response. The best-validated and most widely used predictive markers are autoantibodies directed against the biochemically defined target antigens insulin (IAA), GAD65 (GADA), IA-2 (IA-2A), and the zinc transporter ZnT8 (ZnT8A). Hyperglycemia and symptoms consistent with diabetes develop only after more than 90% of the secretory capacity of the beta cells has been destroyed.[52]

At any time during the progressive decline in beta cell function, overt diabetes may be precipitated by either acute illness or stress, which increases insulin demand beyond the reserve of the damaged islet cells. Hyperglycemia will ensue until such time as the acute illness or stress is resolved; then, the individual may revert to a compensated state for a variable time period in which the beta cells are able to maintain normal glycemia. This honeymoon period is a variable period of noninsulin dependency following acute decompensation. Ongoing progression of beta cell destruction continues, leading to absolute insulin deficiency and the need for insulin treatment, typically over 3 to 12 months.[55]

Case—Part 3: Inattention to Modifiable Risk Factors

For 2 years CS felt fine. Despite being encouraged to exercise and lose weight, she had been unable to incorporate this into her busy life. That summer she experienced progressive fatigue and found that she was often very thirsty. She assumed this was from the heat of summer. She noticed a shiny red patch of skin under her breasts and went to her local health clinic. A random blood glucose at that time was 203 mg/dL (11.27 mmol/L).

Type 2 Diabetes

The pathophysiology of type 2 diabetes is characterized as progressive and multifactorial. Both insulin resistance—the inability of insulin receptors to recognize insulin—in the liver and muscle and impaired insulin secretion play a major role in its pathogenesis. Increased and inappropriate hepatic glucose production is a hallmark feature. Initially, in the basal state, the liver overproduces glucose despite high fasting insulin levels, which leads to fasting hyperglycemia. At the same time, insulin promotes the production of lipids from the liver.[56] In addition, in the insulin-stimulated state after glucose ingestion, insulin resistance leads to reduction in muscle glucose uptake by more than 50%, which results in postprandial hyperglycemia.[57] The eight factors contributing to type 2 diabetes have been referred to as the "ominous octet" (see Figure 13.4).[58]

In the pancreas, in response to the hyperglycemia that results from increased hepatic glucose production and peripheral insulin resistance, beta cells increase their secretion of insulin. However, with persistent fasting hyperglycemia, the compensatory insulin response cannot be maintained, insulin secretion declines progressively, and diabetes emerges. About 70% of beta cell function has been lost when the 2-hour glucose value during the OGTT reaches 120 to 140 mg/dL (6.66-7.77 mmol/L). In addition, acquired defects in beta cell activity have been noted in response to hyperglycemia and are referred to as glucose toxicity. Beta cells chronically exposed to hyperglycemia and to increased FFAs become progressively less efficient in responding to subsequent glucose challenges. Thus, beta cell dysfunction may be either primary or acquired in the pathogenesis of type 2 diabetes. Further progression of the disease is marked in its later stages by an absolute insulin deficiency (see Figure 13.5).[59]

The islet in type 2 diabetes is characterized by a deficit in beta cell mass, increased beta cell apoptosis, and impaired insulin secretion. Some but not all studies suggest that a decrease in beta cell mass contributes to the

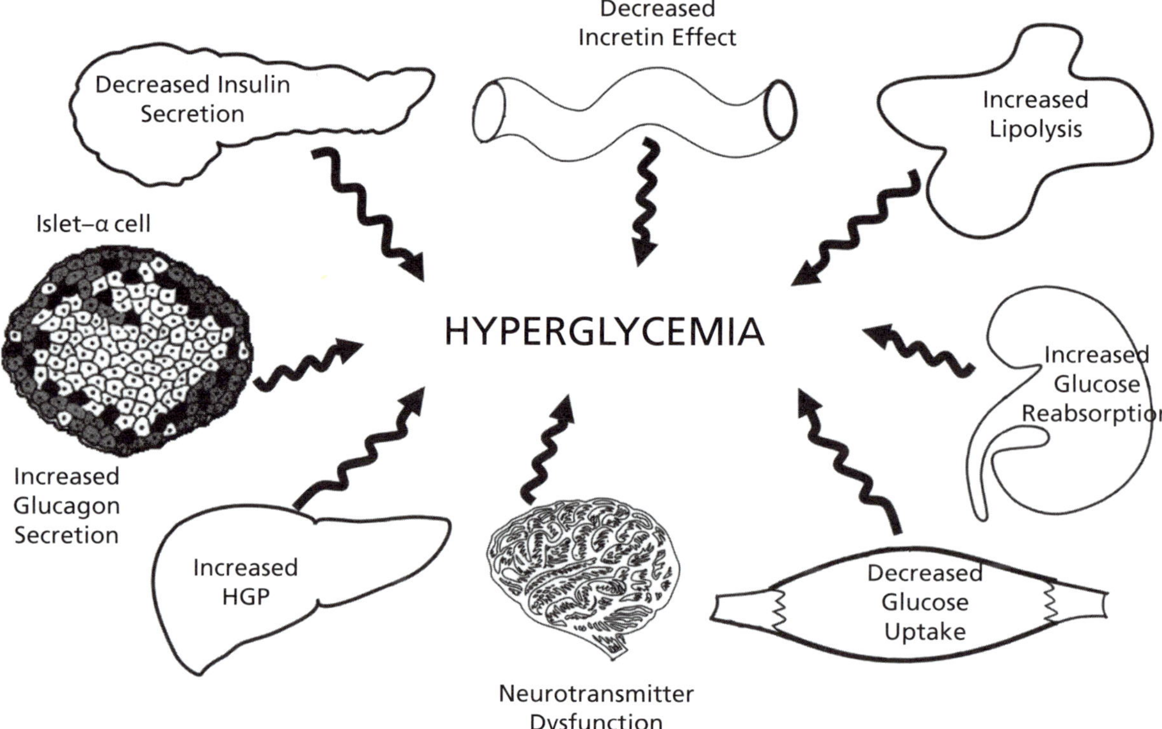

FIGURE 13.4 Ominous Octet

Source: RA Defronzo, "From the triumvirate to the ominous octet: a new paradigm for the treatment of type 2 diabetes mellitus," *Diabetes*. 58(2009): 773-95.

impaired insulin secretion of type 2 diabetes.[60] In sum, the beta cell mass is decreased in both obese and lean individuals with type 2 diabetes compared with their age- and weight-matched counterparts without diabetes. The net change in beta cell mass leads to a decrease in beta cell function. People with prediabetes have decreased beta cell mass, suggesting that this is an early process and mechanistically important in the development of type 2 diabetes. Finally, the decrease in beta cell mass may be caused by an increase in the frequency of beta cell apoptosis with the rate of new islet formation being unaffected. Thus, in striving to prevent type 2 diabetes, strategies to avoid beta cell apoptosis may be useful. Also, in people with established type 2 diabetes, inhibition of this three- to tenfold increased rate of apoptosis may lead to restoration of beta cell mass, because islet neogenesis appears intact.[60]

The major role genetics plays in the expression of type 2 diabetes is often overlooked. The function of genes may also be impacted through epigenetic changes that take place in the course of life. Epigenetic changes are described as external changes resulting from environmental influences that turn genes on or off. Epigenetic changes come about as a result of factors such as aging, chemicals, medication, diet, and exercise.[61,62]

Chemicals released by chemical-based agriculture, food production, and electronic waste are referred to as endocrine-disrupting chemicals (EDCs). There is evidence that these substances play a role in diabetes pathology including hyperglycemia, glucose intolerance, insulin resistance, gut microbiome changes, and more. Included in the list of EDCs are heavy metals, persistant organic pollutants, organophosphates, non-caloric artificial sweeteners, emulsifiers, and disinfection products.[62]

Researchers have now demonstrated that half of the known genetic risk variants for type 2 diabetes can be influenced by epigenetic changes that in turn influence the function of the insulin-producing cells. Most cases of type 2 diabetes involve many genes contributing small amounts to the overall condition. As of 2011, more than 36 genes have been found to contribute to the risk of type 2 diabetes. All of these genes together account for only 10% of the total genetic component of the disease.[63] Genetic research in type 2 diabetes is still ongoing.[64]

Offspring of individuals with type 2 diabetes have a ~40% chance of developing type 2 diabetes if one parent has the disease.[65] A greater than 90% concordance rate exists between monozygotic twins if one has type 2

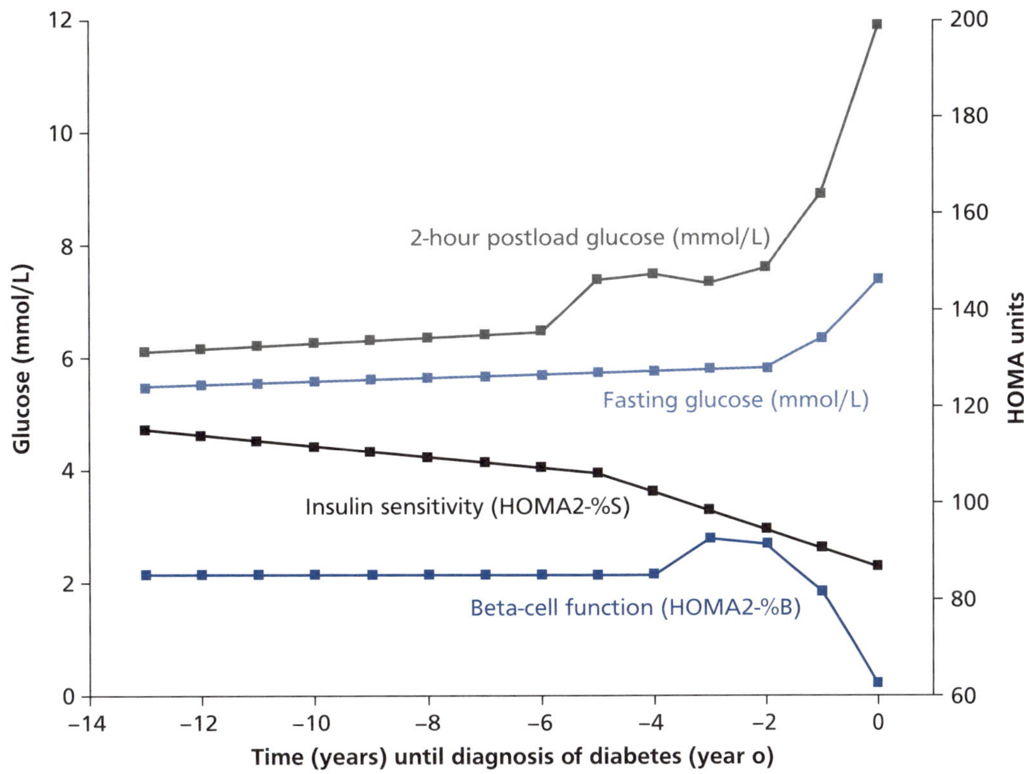

FIGURE 13.5 **The Homeostasis of Fasting and Postload Glucose During the Development of Type 2 Diabetes**

Source: AG Tabak, C Herder, W Rathmann, EJ Brunner, M Kivimaki, "Prediabetes: a high-risk state for diabetes development," *Lancet.* 2012;379(9833):2279–90. doi:10.1016/S0140-6736(12)60283-9.

diabetes, suggesting the primacy of the genetic defect in this form of the disease.[66]

In addition, in type 2 diabetes, adipocytes (fat cells) are resistant to the antilipolytic effect of insulin and pour fat into the bloodstream, resulting in elevated plasma FFA levels. These processes are referred to as lipotoxicity. In this component of the pathophysiology of type 2 diabetes, the elevated FFA levels exacerbate liver and muscle insulin resistance, drive gluconeogenesis in the liver, and impair beta cell insulin secretion, further exacerbating the tendency toward hyperglycemia. The dysfunctional adipocytes produce multiple cytokines that contribute to inflammation and atherosclerosis as well as insulin resistance.[67]

Gastrointestinal incretin hormones have been implicated as a factor in the pathogenesis of type 2 diabetes. Glucagon-like peptide-1 is deficient in people with type 2 diabetes and prediabetes, contributing to excessive hepatic glucose production, failure to suppress postprandial glucagon, and unrestrained eating. Dipeptidyl peptidase-4 activity is increased in the fasting state in people with type 2 diabetes. This is one reason type 2 diabetes may be associated with impaired postprandial GLP-1 secretion.[10]

Contributing to our understanding of the specific timing of changes in glucose metabolism before the occurrence of type 2 diabetes, a report characterized the trajectories of fasting and postload glucose, insulin sensitivity, and insulin secretion in the Whitehall II cohort of British civil servants. This study compared those who developed type 2 diabetes and those who did not over a 13-year follow-up. The study shows changes in glucose concentrations, insulin sensitivity, and insulin secretion as much as 3 to 6 years before the diagnosis of diabetes. Such information may contribute to more accurate risk prediction models that use repeated measures taken at serial checkups.[68]

Obesity, aging, weight gain in adulthood, and physical inactivity are environmental factors affecting the progression of diabetes at all points along the continuum. Type 2 diabetes progresses from an early asymptomatic state with insulin resistance, to mild postprandial hyperglycemia, to clinical diabetes requiring pharmacologic intervention. Additional factors contributing to a diagnosis of type 2 diabetes, which continue to be studied, include medications, smoking, and the role of kidney glucose reabsorption.

Risk Reduction and Intervention

Identifying people at risk for diabetes is the first step in preventing the disease. The landmark Diabetes Prevention Program (DPP) screened over 14,000 high-risk individuals for the presence of prediabetes. Interventions with intensive lifestyle modifications (eating habits, exercise, and subsequent weight loss) versus a pharmacologic intervention using metformin to improve endogenous insulin action were aimed at ameliorating the specific defects prior to progression to diabetes. The DPP showed that lifestyle intervention reduced incidence by 58% and metformin by 31% (95% confidence interval, 17%, 43%), as compared with placebo; the lifestyle intervention was significantly more effective than metformin. To prevent 1 case of diabetes during a 3-year period, 6.9 persons would have to participate in the lifestyle intervention program, and 13.9 would have to receive metformin.[17] A 10-year follow-up to the DPP showed that diabetes incidence was reduced by 34% in the lifestyle group and by 18% in the metformin group.[69]

The DPP Research Group continues to publish on the persistence of the effects and benefits of the study's intervention. During the 10-year follow-up since randomization to the DPP, the original lifestyle group lost and then partially regained weight. The modest weight loss with metformin was maintained. During the DPP follow-up, incidence rates in the former placebo and metformin groups fell to equal those in the former lifestyle group, and the cumulative incidence of diabetes remained lowest in the lifestyle group. These data demonstrate that delay of diabetes with lifestyle intervention or metformin can persist for at least 10 years.[69]

The Look AHEAD (Action for Health in Diabetes) study was a multicenter randomized clinical trial to examine the effects of a lifestyle intervention designed to achieve and maintain weight loss in people with diagnosed diabetes through decreased caloric intake and increased exercise. The Look AHEAD study tested whether a lifestyle intervention resulting in weight loss would reduce rates of heart disease, stroke, and cardiovascular-related deaths in overweight and obese people with type 2 diabetes.[70] Researchers at 16 centers across the United States studied 5,145 people, with half randomly assigned to an intensive lifestyle intervention and the other half to a general program of diabetes support and education. Both groups received routine medical care from their own healthcare providers. The intervention arm was stopped in 2012 because of the finding that the intervention did not reduce cardiovascular events. One positive finding was that both groups had a lower number of cardiovascular events compared with previous studies of people with diabetes.

Further analyses of the Look AHEAD data have shown lower risk of microvascular complications.[71] Look AHEAD showed other important health benefits of the lifestyle intervention, including decreasing sleep apnea, reducing the need for diabetes medications, helping to maintain physical mobility, and improving quality of life. Few, if any, studies of this size and duration have had comparable success in achieving and maintaining weight loss. Participants in the intervention group lost an average of more than 8% of their initial body weight after 1 year of intervention. They maintained an average weight loss of nearly 5% at 4 years, an amount that experts recommend to improve health. Participants in the diabetes support and education group lost about 1% of their initial weight after 1 and 4 years.[70] Genomic exploration may be the next step in determining effective therapies for risk reduction.[72]

Latent Autoimmune Diabetes in Adults

The clinical distinction between type 1 diabetes and type 2 diabetes is not always clear. There is increasing evidence that suggests significant overlap between type 1 diabetes and type 2 diabetes. It is important to note that both type 1 and type 2 diabetes are heterogeneous disorders and that LADA may account for as much as 10% of cases of insulin-requiring diabetes in older individuals and represents a slow, progressive form of type 1 diabetes that is frequently confused with type 2 diabetes.[33] Persons with LADA may remain insulin-independent for many years even though they experience the autoimmune beta cell deterioration associated with classic type 1 diabetes.[54] Independent risk factors for progression of beta cell failure in LADA are sulfonylurea treatment, ICA positive periods, and initial body weight. Whether agents that preserve islet cell function, stimulate beta cell proliferation and survival, and/or improve insulin sensitivity can delay progression of LADA (i.e., incretins and DPP-4 inhibitors) is being studied. Exenatide also may act as a regulator of the immune response in addition to its potential effects on beta cell proliferation.[65] When insulin therapy is required, the person with diabetes generally benefits from a basal-bolus insulin regimen, as it is part of the treatment spectrum for type 1 diabetes. The presence of autoantibodies suggests that LADA is, like type 1 diabetes, an autoimmune disease. There are, however, differences in autoantibody clustering, T-cell reactivity, and genetic susceptibility and protection between type 1 diabetes and LADA, suggesting important differences in the underlying disease processes. In LADA, diabetes occurs earlier in the process of beta cell destruction because a significant degree of insulin resistance is present.[74]

Persons with LADA are typically older than 35 years and non-obese. Their diabetes is managed initially with diet. Within a relatively short period of time, months to years, a need for oral agents and progression to insulin treatment occur. The eventual clinical features include weight loss, propensity for ketosis, unstable blood glucose, and low C-peptide reserves. As immune system modulating therapies that slow or halt the progression of type 1 diabetes are developed, consideration of their potential role in the treatment of LADA will be necessary.[75]

Maturity-Onset Diabetes of the Young

Some rare forms of diabetes result from mutations in a single gene and are called monogenic. Monogenic forms of diabetes account for about 1% to 5% of all cases of diabetes in young people. Maturity-onset diabetes of the young (MODY) is a monogenic form of diabetes that usually first occurs during adolescence or early adulthood. People with MODY may have mild or no symptoms of diabetes and their hyperglycemia may be discovered only through routine blood tests. This form of diabetes may be confused with type 1 diabetes or type 2 diabetes. People with MODY generally are not overweight and do not have other risk factors for type 2 diabetes, such as high blood pressure or abnormal blood fat levels. While both type 2 diabetes and MODY can run in families, people with MODY typically have a family history of diabetes in multiple successive generations, meaning that MODY is present in a grandparent, a parent, and a child. Treatment of MODY varies with the genetic mutation, therefore identification of the particular variant of MODY is important in determining not only the appropriate treatment plan but also in preventing suboptimal treatment. There are several cost-effective commercially available genetic tests to confirm the diagnosis. The presence of autoantibodies can help preclude additional testing for MODY.[20]

Identification of specific gene defects in certain groups with exceptionally high prevalence of type 2 diabetes has resulted in their designation as "other specific types of diabetes." These gene defects occur in a small percentage (<5%) of people with type 2 diabetes. Maturity-onset diabetes of the young is one monogenetic disorder that results from such defects. It is characterized by early onset and mild hyperglycemia. It is associated with distinct genetic defects of beta cell function and minimal or no defects in insulin action. Six genes on different chromosomes have been identified that cause MODY. Each abnormality leads to impaired insulin secretion. Numerous other specific mutations also have been identified in insulin, insulin receptor, and mitochondrial DNA that result in diabetes. Maturity-onset diabetes of the young can be suspected and recognized if a type 2 diabetes–like condition occurs in 2 or 3 or more generations and the pattern of inheritance is consistent with autosomal-dominant inheritance. The latter is the hallmark of MODY and distinguishes it from type 2 diabetes.[76]

Pathogenesis of Diabetes-Related Complications

Although hyperglycemia plays a key modifiable role in the complications associated with diabetes (which are caused by abnormalities in the structure and function of blood vessels and nerves and the impact of hyperglycemia on various factors, including platelet aggregation, inflammatory processes, and coagulation factors), other major, and sometimes independent, factors contribute to these complications. In a comprehensive approach to reducing risks for diabetes-related complications, the care team, including the person with diabetes, proactively manages not only hyperglycemia but also the complete spectrum of risk factors for complications. Other chapters in this book focus on management of nonglycemic risk factors.

Pathogenesis of Cardiovascular Disease in Diabetes

One cannot complete a discussion of the pathophysiology of the spectrum of diabetes as a metabolic disorder without mention of its links with cardiovascular disease (CVD). Diabetes clearly confers a strong increase in risk for CVD morbidity and mortality. While it is beyond the scope of this chapter to fully discuss this topic, further information may be found in chapter 25. Besides the coexistence of diabetes with other known risk factors for CVD, including family history, hypertension, dyslipidemia, and renal disease, hyperglycemia itself affects numerous processes that may be implicated in the pathogenesis of CVD. Hyperglycemia is pro-inflammatory and pro-thrombotic, causes platelet aggregation, impairs endothelial function and left ventricular function, and causes metabolic derangements, including an increase in FFAs. All these pathophysiologic mechanisms are closely interrelated and can lead to premature CVD morbidity and mortality.[77]

The strength of the association between diabetes and CVD has led to a search for data demonstrating the definitive impact of lifestyle and therapeutic interventions on CVD outcomes in people with diabetes. Since the UKPDS first suggested a trend toward reduction in CVD events when targeted glycemic levels are undertaken, definitive evidence that glycemic stability can improve CVD outcomes has proven to be elusive. The ACCORD trial for type 1 diabetes[78] and the ADVANCE[79] and VADT[80] studies (see chapter 25) of type 2 diabetes each sought to demonstrate that maintaining intensive A1C levels would reduce cardiovascular events and death. In none of these studies was it clear that lowering A1C alone resulted in definitive improvement in cardiovascular endpoints.

These studies do, however, provide some insights that may prove useful in aiding our understanding of the relationship between blood glucose and CVD. The VADT showed that intensified diabetes management reduced the risk of CVD events provided that therapy was started early, suggesting that it is necessary to intervene early in the underlying pathophysiologic processes if one is to have an impact on the course of CVD.[80] In ACCORD, while an increased risk of CVD death was observed in the intensively treated group, this increase was seen in those subjects with an A1C >7%, rather than in those reaching the intensive goal.[78] It would appear that those who responded more readily, as measured by lower A1C, did better than those whose blood glucose levels were more refractory to therapy. This finding raises the possibility that the responsiveness of the individual's blood glucose levels to treatment, which would reflect the underlying pathophysiologic status of his or her diabetes, might be pivotal in determining CVD outcomes.[80]

Stress and Diabetes

In the human body, the hypothalamic-pituitary-adrenal axis increases the secretion of glucocorticoids during times of stress.[81] These hormones naturally raise the blood glucose level, which is helpful for those without diabetes, but can contribute to the pathophysiology of diabetes. The stress response, which can be triggered by emotional or physical stress, is associated with elevated blood glucose levels.[82]

Diabetes and Cancer Risk

Epidemiologic evidence suggests that people with diabetes are at significantly higher risk for many forms of cancer. Furthermore, evidence from observational studies suggests that some medications used to treat hyperglycemia in diabetes may have an impact on cancer risk.[83] This evidence is discussed in the chapters on each antihyperglycemic medication, including metformin, GLP-1 agonists, and insulins. In addition, type 2 diabetes and certain cancers share a variety of risk factors, including advancing age, male gender (cancers and diabetes occur more often in men overall), racial/ethnic propensity, having excess weight, physical inactivity, smoking, and drinking more than 1 alcoholic drink per day for women or 2 for men. Biologic links between diabetes and cancer, however, are not well understood. A systematic review with meta analysis found that diabetes is a risk factor for cancer in all sites with women having a slightly higher risk than men.[84]

The summary and recommendations from the 2010 joint consensus report of the American Diabetes Association and the American Cancer Society on diabetes and cancer are shown in Table 13.5.

Case Wrap-Up

There were numerous clues that, if dealt with earlier, may have reduced the risk for or delayed the onset of type 2 diabetes for CS. Diabetes education could have played a vital role in risk reduction in this case. Care could have included recognizing the clues and intervening early to counsel CS about her risk factors (and her children's risk), treating her high risk for diabetes, and emphasizing the need for follow-up. The fact that this did not occur caused continued and progressive metabolic abnormalities that may have resulted in decreased beta cell function. Early intervention protects blood vessels, supporting the importance of early diagnosis and treatment.

Reducing Risks for Diabetes-Related Complications and the Role of the Diabetes Care and Education Specialist

The diabetes care and education specialist recognizes that the pathophysiology of diabetes is a problem not only of carbohydrate metabolism but also of abnormalities in fat metabolism, feeding behavior, and vascular biology.

Although advances in medications, technology, and scientific knowledge are providing more tools to enable people with diabetes to attain an optimal physiologic state to reduce risks of complications, the diabetes care and education specialist needs to be aware that responsibility for the lifestyle and self-management practices needed to maintain optimal physiology lies primarily with the person with diabetes. The person with diabetes owns the daily decisions that play a large role in the course of the disease. Healthcare professionals are challenged to understand the impact self-management has on the outcome of disease management. The Association of Diabetes Care and Education Specialists (ADCES), fomerly the American Association of Diabetes Educators (AADE), has defined 7 self-care behaviors—the AADE7 Self-Care Behaviors® as a framework for person-centered diabetes education and care. Diabetes education focuses on these

TABLE 13.5 Summary and Recommendations of the Diabetes and Cancer Risk Consensus Report
Diabetes (primarily type 2) is associated with increased risk for some cancers (liver, pancreas, endometrium, colon and rectum, breast, bladder). Diabetes is associated with reduced risk of prostate cancer. For some other cancer sites, there appears to be no association or the evidence is inconclusive.
The association between diabetes and some cancers may be partly due to shared risk factors between the 2 diseases, such as aging, obesity, diet, and physical inactivity.
Possible mechanisms for a direct link between diabetes and cancer include hyperinsulinemia, hyperglycemia, and inflammation.
Healthful diets, physical activity, and weight management reduce risk and improve outcomes of type 2 diabetes and some forms of cancer and should be promoted for all.
People with diabetes should be strongly encouraged by their healthcare professionals to undergo appropriate cancer screenings as recommended for all people of their age and sex.
The evidence for specific drugs affecting cancer risk is limited, and observed associations may have been confounded by indications for specific drugs, effects on other cancer risk factors such as body weight and hyperinsulinemia, and the complex progressive nature of hyperglycemia and pharmacotherapy in type 2 diabetes.
Although limited, early evidence suggests that metformin is associated with a lower risk of cancer and that exogenous insulin is associated with an increased risk of cancer. Further research is needed to clarify these issues and evaluate whether insulin glargine is more strongly associated with cancer risk compared with other insulins.*
Cancer risk should not be a major factor in choosing between available diabetes therapies for the average patient. For selected patients with very high risk for cancer occurrence (or for recurrence of specific cancer types), these issues may require more careful consideration.
Many questions remain regarding the association between diabetes and cancer risk.

*Additional studies have concluded that there is not sufficient evidence to say that insulin glargine is linked with cancer. GB Bolli, AD Hahn, R Schmidt, et al, "Plasma exposure to insulin glargine and its metabolites M1 and M2 after sub-cutaneous injection of therapeutic and supratherapeutic doses of glargine in subjects with type 1 diabetes," *Diabetes Care.* 35 (2012): 2626-30; P Lucidi, F Porcellati, P Rossetti, et al, "Metabolism of insulin glargine after repeated daily subcutaneous injections in subjects with type 2 diabetes," *Diabetes Care* 35 (2012): 2647-9; DR Owen, "Glargine and cancer: can we now suggest closure?," *Diabetes Care.* 35 (2012): 2426-8.

Source: E Giovannucci, DM Harlan, MC Archer, "Diabetes and cancer: a consensus report," *Diabetes Care* 33, no. 7 (2010; cited 2019 May 27): 1674-85. doi: 10.2337/dc10-0666. On the Internet at: http://care.diabetesjournals.org/content/33/7/1674/T1.expansion.html.

behaviors that are essential for health status and quality of life.[1] As understanding of the disease increases, health professionals can use this information to support clients in making their self-care behavior decisions.

In summary, knowledge of the pathophysiology of diabetes continues to grow. Diabetes care and education specialists can use this new knowledge to guide their clients in managing their diabetes to ameliorate complications.

Focus on Education

Teaching Strategies

As the diabetes epidemic broadens, the classic model of care has proven to be ineffective in slowing its spread. Recognize how other models and approaches can be implemented in order to effectively deal with all aspects of the continuum of care for those with or at risk for diabetes. Stay abreast of evolving concepts and new criteria.

Know all specific signs, symptoms, and classifications of the different types of diabetes. Recognize that the boundaries for traditional classifications are moving. More children are being diagnosed at a younger age. Adults with type 1 diabetes or LADA are still being misclassified as having type 2 diabetes. Teaching needs to be part of a widespread effort to focus on health in all parts of our community and society.

Stay informed about pathophysiology and implications for treatment. Attend local and national meetings and retain membership in organizations that provide frequent updates and the latest research. Bring this information back to the practice setting and inform peers and persons with diabetes when teaching. Use the information for educating persons with diabetes.

Heed diagnosing information. The diagnosis of diabetes may have major life-altering implications. Thus, the following steps are essential: follow diagnostic criteria, complete testing, and discuss test results and future implications (such as the need for follow-up or annual retesting).

Messages for Persons With Diabetes

Early diagnosis and treatment are important. Recognizing the risk of diabetes may be an opportunity to act. Lifestyle changes can reduce the risk for or delay diabetes. Healthy lifestyles can be integrated throughout the entire family. Recognize also that having diabetes or even having risk factors for diabetes increases the chances that relatives may also have the same problem. Healthy lifestyles can improve the future health of the entire family.

You are at the center of the care team. The more you know, the better prepared you are to be an active participant on the healthcare team. Being involved from the beginning is the first step toward implementing preventive health care and can revolutionize health management through lifestyle modification.

Staying up-to-date can help your health. Keep current with new ideas on diabetes management, treatment options, and other pertinent information. Attend education sessions annually. Use reputable Web sites, the diabetes care and education specialist on the team, and diabetes publications to learn the latest about diabetes management.

Health Literacy

Information on the pathophysiology of the metabolic disorder is complex even for healthcare professionals. Persons with diabetes need to understand what is happening in their bodies, how it relates to diabetes symptoms, and what can be done about it. It is hard for people with diabetes to follow recommendations and do all that needs to be done without understanding why and what will change as a result. Use analogies and a simple explanation of pathophysiology and how it affects glucose levels. For example, "Your body cannot operate without glucose just as your car cannot drive without gasoline." People need to visualize the connections between the functionality of glucose regulation and its impact on the body and treatment.

Use simple language to communicate the relevant information about pathophysiology and how it affects diabetes management. Think about being on an elevator and having only 1 minute to convey important information about the pathophysiology of diabetes to a person with diabetes. What would you say? What would be the most important information to convey? How would you explain it?

It is better to have 3 important messages and repeat them 3 times than it is to have 9 messages but repeat them only once. Choose the most important concepts to understand and relate them to persons with diabetes frequently to indicate the importance and increase recollection.

When communicating a lot of complex information, choose 3 or 4 messages that you think are most important for your listener to hear and remember. For each message, focus your audience by first stating the main point or "headline" (1 engaging statement), back up the message with facts or data, provide an anecdote to help your audience visualize what you are saying, use a personal example to humanize your story, and end by restating your main point or headline.

Focus on Practice

Utilize evidence-based interventions. Stay current on the pathophysiology of diabetes and how it relates to diagnosis and care. Create systems for addressing advances in care and the expectations of persons with diabetes. Examine whether your healthcare system can efficiently support the advancements, their cost-effectiveness, and the expected outcomes.

As clinical leaders, communicate with administrative departments and operational leaders to provide system integration of metabolic care. Monitoring and improving metabolic care outcomes is an ongoing and necessary process for every shift and corresponding department. Developing a continuous quality improvement plan with specific performance and markers of success indicators will provide a road map and destination points for all involved.

Existing healthcare systems are becoming competitive because of a focus on high quality, cost-effectiveness, and continuous improvement. Diabetes care clinicians self-reflect on their practices and how they relate to the hospital, clinical, public health, and other applicable deliverables.

References

1. Centers for Disease Control and Prvention, National Diabetes Statistics Repot, 2017. Atlanta, GA: Centerse for Disease Control and Prevention, U.S. Dept of Health and Human Services; 2017 https://www.cdc.gov/diabetes/pdfs/data/statistics/national-diabetes-statistics-report.pdf (cited May 27, 2019).
2. Bays HE, Chapman RH, Grundy S, et al. The relationship of body mass index to diabetes mellitus, hypertension and dyslipidaemia: comparison of data from two national surveys. Int J Clin Pract. 2007 May 1;61(5):737-47. doi: 10.1111/j.1742-1241.2007.01336.x. PMCID: PMC1890993.
3. Centers for Disease Control and Prevention. Maps of trends in diagnosed diabetes and obesity. CDC's Division of Diabetes Translation. National Diabetes Surveillance System. 2017 Apr (cited 2019 May 27). On the Internet at: http://www.cdc.gov/diabetes/statistics/slides/maps_diabetesobesity_trends.pdf.
4. Wijdenes M, Henneman L, Dondorp WJ, Cornel MC, Timmermans DRM. Users evaluate a detailed familial risk questionnaire as valuable and no more time consuming than a simple enquiry in a web-based diabetes risk assessment tool. Public Health. 2016;130:87-90.
5. Buijsse B, Simmons RK, Griffin SJ, Schulze MB. Risk assessment tools for identifying individuals at risk of developing type 2 diabetes. Epidemiol Rev. 2011;33(1):46-62.
6. Ruderman NB, Myers M, Chipkin SR, et al. Hormone–fuel interrelationships: fed state, starvation, and diabetes mellitus. In: Joslin EP, Kahn CR, eds. *Joslin Diabetes Mellitus*. 14th ed. Baltimore: Lippincott Williams & Wilkins; 2005:128-44.
7. Ferrannini E, DeFronzo R. Insulin actions in vivo: glucose metabolism. In: DeFronzo R, Ferrannini E, Zimmet P, Alberti KGMM, eds. *International Textbook of Diabetes Mellitus*. 4th ed. Chichester, West Sussex, UK: Wiley; 2015:211-31.
8. Hieronymus L, Griffin S. Role of amylin in type 1 and type 2 diabetes. Diabetes Educ. 2015 Dec;41 Suppl 1:S47-56. doi 10.1177/0145721715607642.
9. Lean MEJ, Malkova D. Altered gut and adipose tissue hormones in overweight and obese individuals: cause or consequence? Int J Obes. 2016;40:622-32.
10. Gautier JF, Fetita S, Sobngwi E, et al. Biological actions of the incretins GIP and GLP-1 and therapeutic perspectives in patients with type 2 diabetes. Diabetes Metab. 2005;31(3 pt 1): 233-42.
11. Richter B, Bandeira-Echtler E, Bergerhoff K, et al. Dipeptidyl peptidase-4 (DPP-4) inhibitors for type 2 diabetes mellitus. Cochrane Database Syst Rev. 2008;2:CD006739.
12. Heppner KM, Tong J. Mechanisms in Endocrinology: regulation of glucose metabolism by the ghrelin system: multiple players and multiple actions. European Journal of Endocrinology. 2014;171:R21-32. doi: 10.1530/EJE-14-0183.
13. Gomez Diaz RA, Gomez Medina MP, Ramirez Soriano E, et al. Journal of Clinical Research in Pediatric Endocrinology. 2016;8(4): 425-31. doi: 10.4274/jcrpe.2504.
14. Otto-Buczkowska E, Chobot A. Role of ghrelin and leptin in the regulation of carbohydrate metabolism. Part I. Ghrelin. Postepy Hig Med Dosw. (online). 2012;66:795-8.
15. Otto-Buczkowska E, Chobot A. Role of ghrelin and leptin in the regulation of carbohydrate metabolism. Part II. Leptin. Postepy Hig Med Dosw. (online). 2012;66:799-803.
16. Insert/add Rehman, K., Akash, M.S.H., & Alina, Z. (2017). Leptin: a new therapeutic target for treatment of diabetes mellitus. Journal of Cellular Biochemistry, 119, 5016-27.
17. Gruden G, Barutta F, Kunos G, Pacher P. Role of the endocannabinoid system in diabetes complications. Br J Pharmacol. 2016;173(7):1116-27.
18. Cani PD, Geurts L, Matamoros S, Plovier H, Duparc T. Glucose metabolism: focus on gut microbiota, the endocannabinoid system and beyond. Diabetes Metab. 2014;40:246-57.
19. Azim S, Kashyap SR. Bariatric surgery: Pathophysiology and outcomes. Endocrinol Metab Clin N Am. 45 (2016) 905-92120. American Diabetes Association. Standards of medical care in diabetes—2019. Diabetes Care. 2019;42 Suppl 1:S1-112. doi: 10.2337/dc16-S001.
21. The Diabetes Prevention Program Research Group. The Diabetes Prevention Program: baseline characteristics of the randomized cohort. Diabetes Care. 2000;23:1619-29.
22. Expert Committee on the Diagnosis and Classification of Diabetes Mellitus. Report of the Expert Committee on the Diagnosis and Classification of Diabetes Mellitus. Diabetes Care. 1997;20:1183-97.
23. International Expert Committee. International Expert Committee report on the role of the A1C assay in the diagnosis of diabetes. Diabetes Care. 2009;32:1327-34.
24. National Diabetes Clearinghouse, National Institute of Diabetes and Digestive and Kidney Disease, National Institutes of Health. For people of African, Mediterranean, or Southeast Asian heritage: important information about diabetes blood tests (cited 2016 May 9). On the Internet at: http://diabetes.niddk.nih.gov/dm/pubs/traitA1C.
25. Nielsen LR, Ekbom P, Damm P, et al. HbA1c levels are significantly lower in early and late pregnancy. Diabetes Care. 2004 May;27:1200-1.
26. https://www.ncbi.nlm.nih.gov/pmc/articles/PMC5261611/ (cited Aug 18, 2019).
27. https://www.heart.org/en/health-topics/diabetes/why-diabetes-matters/cardiovascular-disease–diabetes accessed 5/28/2019 Section title Cardiovascular Disease and Diabetes.
28. Pawłowicz M, Birkholz D, Niedźwiecki M, et al. Difficulties or mistakes in diagnosing type 1 diabetes in children?—demographic factors influencing delayed diagnosis. Pediatr Diabetes. 2009;10:542-9.
29. Charfen MA, Ipp E, Kaji AH, et al. Detection of undiagnosed diabetes and prediabetic states in high-risk emergency department patients. Acad Emerg Med. 2009;16:394-402.

30. Magee MF, Nassar C. Hemoglobin A1C testing in an emergency department. J Diabetes Sci Technol. 2011;5:1437-43.

31. Magee MF, Nassar CM, Copeland J, et al. Synergy to reduce emergency department visits for uncontrolled hyperglycemia. Diabetes Educ. 2013;39:354-64. doi: 10.1177/0145721713484593.

32. Atkinson MA, Eisenbarth GS. Type 1 diabetes: new perspectives on disease pathogenesis and treatment. Lancet. 2010;358:221-9.

33. Thomas NJ, et al. Type 1 diabetes defined by severe insulin deficiency occurs after 30 years of age and is commonly treated as type 2 diabetes. Diabetologia. 2019; DOI: 10.1007/s00125-019-4863-8.

34. Vaarala O, Hyoty H, Akerblom HK. Environmental factors in the etiology of childhood diabetes. Diabetes Nutr Metab. 1999;12:75-85.

35. National Institute of Diabetes and Digestive and Kidney Diseases (NIDDK). What else causes diabetes? (cited 2019 May 28) On the Internet at: http://www.niddk.nih.gov/health-information/health-topics/diabetes/overview/symptoms-causes.

36. Feig DS, Hwee J, Shah BR, et al. Trends in incidence of diabetes in pregnancy and serious perinatal outcomes: a large, population-based study in Ontario, Canada, 1996-2010. Diabetes Care. 2014;37:1590-6.

37. International Association of Diabetes and Pregnancy Study Groups Consensus Panel. International Association of Diabetes and Pregnancy Study Groups recommendations on the diagnosis and classification of hyperglycemia in pregnancy. Diabetes Care. 2010;33:676-82.

38. Lawrence JM, Contreras R, Chen W, et al. Trends in the prevalence of preexisting diabetes and gestational diabetes mellitus among a racially/ethnically diverse population of pregnant women, 1999-2005. Diabetes Care. 2008;31:899-904.

39. Sipetic S, Vlajinac H, Kocev N, Bjekic M, Sajic S. Early infant diet and risk of type 1 diabetes mellitus in Belgrade children. Nutrition. 2005;21:474-9.

40. DiMeglio LA, Evans Molina C, Oram RA. Type 1 diabetes. The Lancet. 2018; 391, 2449-62.

41. Achenbach P, Warncke K, Reiter J, et al. Stratification of type 1 diabetes risk on the basis of islet autoantibody characteristics. Diabetes. 2004;53:384-92.

42. Steck AK, Rewer MJ. Genetics of type 1 diabetes. Clin Chem. 2011;57:176-85.

43. Redondo MJ, Jeffrey J, Fain PR, Eisenbarth GS, Orban T. Concordance for islet autoimmunity among monozygotic twins. N Engl J Med. 2008; 359: 2849-50.

44. Dotta F, Censini S, van Halteren AG, et al. Coxsackie B4 virus infection of beta cells and natural killer cell insulitis in recent-onset type I diabetic patients. Proc Natl Acad Sci USA. 2007;104:5115-20.

45. van der Werf N, Kroese FG, Rozing J, Hillebrands JL. Viral infections as potential triggers of type 1 diabetes. Diabetes Metab Res Rev. 2007;23:169-83.

46. Wasnuth HE, Kolb H. Cow's milk and immune-mediated diabetes. Proc Nutr Soc. 2000;59:573-9.

47. Knip M, Akerblom HK. Early nutrition and later diabetes risk. Adv Exp Med Biol. 2005;569:142-50.

48. Frederiksen B, Kroehl M, Lamb MM, et al. Infant exposures and development of type 1 diabetes: the Diabetes Autoimmunity Study in the Young (DAISY). JAMA Pediatr. 2013;167:808-15.

49. Franco R, Panayiotidis MI. Environmental toxicity, oxidative stress, human disease and the "black box" of their synergism: how much have we revealed? Mutat Res. 2009;674:1-2. doi: 10.1016/j.mrgentox.2009.01.005.

50. Lenzen S. Oxidative stress: the vulnerable beta-cell. Biochem Soc Trans. 2008;36(Pt 3):343-7. doi: 10.1042/BST0360343.

51. Moltchanova EV, Schreier N, Lammi N, Karvonen M. Seasonal variation of diagnosis of type 1 diabetes mellitus in children worldwide. Diabet Med. 2009;26:673-8.

52. Knip M, Siljander H. Autoimmune mechanisms in type 1 diabetes. Autoimmun Rev. 2008;7:550-7.

53. Insel RA, Dunne JL, Atkinson MA, et al. Staging: presymptomatic type 2 diabetes: a scientific statement of JDRF, the Endocrine Society, and the American Diabetes Association. Diabetes Care. 2015; 38, 1964-74.

54. Laugesen E, Ostergaard JA, Leslie RDG. Latent autoimmune diabetes of the adult: current knowledge and uncertainty. Diabet Med. 2015; published online doi: 10.1111/dme.1270.

55. Abdul-Rasoul M, Habib H, Al-Khouly M. "The honeymoon phase" in children with type 1 diabetes mellitus: frequency, duration, and influential factors. Pediatr Diabetes. 2006;7:101-7.

56. Cook JR, Langlet F, Kido Y, Accili D. Pathogenesis of selected insulin resistance in isolated hepatocytes. J Biol Chem. 2015;290:13972-80.

57. Nichols GA, Hillier TA, Brown JB. Progression from newly acquired impaired fasting glucose to type 2. Diabetes Care. 2007;30:228-33.

58. Defronzo, R.A. (2009). From the triumvirate to the ominous octet: A new paradigm for the treatment of type 2 diabetes mellitus. Diabetes 58, 773-95.

59. Bays H, Mandarino L, DeFronzo RA. Role of the adipocyte, free fatty acids, and ectopic fat in pathogenesis of type 2 diabetes mellitus: peroxisomal proliferator-activated receptor agonists provide a rational therapeutic approach. J Clin Endocrinol Metab. 2004;28:463-78.

60. Triangle Butler AE, Janson J, Bonner-Weir S, et al. Beta-cell deficit and increased beta-cell apoptosis in humans with type 2 diabetes. Diabetes. 2003;52:102-10.

61. Lund University. New clues in hunt for heredity in type 2 diabetes. ScienceDaily. 2013 Mar 19 (cited 2016 May 11). On the Internet at: http://www.sciencedaily.com/releases/2013/03/130319091144.htm.

62. Velmurugan G, Ramprasath T, Gilles M, Swaminathan K, Ramasamy S. Gut microbiota, endocrine-disrupting chemicals,

and the diabetes epidemic, Trends in Endocrinology and Metabolism, 28, 612-25.

63. Drong AW, Lindgren CM, McCarthy MI. The genetic and epigenetic basis of type 2 diabetes and obesity. Clin Pharmacol Ther. 2012 Dec;92(6):707-15. doi: 10.1038/clpt.2012.149. Epub 2012 Oct 10.

64. Fuchsberger C, Flannick J, Teslovich TM, Mahajan A, Agarwala V, et al. (2019) The gentic artchitecture of type 2 diabetes. Nature. 2019;536(7614), 41-47V doi:10.1038 /nature18642.

65. Skyler J, Bakris GL, Bonifacio E, et al. Differentiation of diabetes by pathophysiology, natural history, and prognosis. Diabetes. 2017; 66, 241-55.

66. Meigs J, Cupples LA, Wilson PW. Parental transmission of type 2 diabetes: the Framingham Offspring Study. Diabetes. 2000;49(12):2201-7.

67. Bauters C, Ennezat PV, Tricot O, et al. Stress hyperglycaemia is an independent predictor of left ventricular remodelling after first anterior myocardial infarction in non-diabetic patients. Eur Heart J. 2007;28:546-52.

68. Tabak AG, Jokela M, Akbaraly TN, et al. Trajectories of glycaemia, insulin sensitivity, and insulin secretion before diagnosis of type 2 diabetes: an analysis from the Whitehall II study. Lancet. 2009;373:2215-21.

69. Diabetes Prevention Program Research Group. 10-year follow-up of diabetes incidence and weight loss in the Diabetes Prevention Program Outcomes Study. Lancet. 2009;374:1677-86.

70. The Look AHEAD Research Group. Cardiovascular effects of intensive lifestyle intervention. N Engl J Med. 2013;369:145-54.

71. Wing RR; for the Look AHEAD Research Group. Implications of Look AHEAD for clinical trials and clinical practice. Diabetes Obes Metab. 2014;16:1183-91.

72. Srinivasan S, Florez JC. Therapeutic challenges in diabetes prevention: we have not found the "exercise pill." Clin Pharmacol Ther. 2015;98:162-9.

73. Protective effects of sitagliptin on β cell function in patients with adult-onset latent autoimmune diabetes (LADA) (cited 2016 May 11). On the Internet at: http://www.bioportfolio.com/resources/trial/63001/Protective-Effects-Of-Sitagliptin-On-Cell -Function-In-Patients-With-Adult-onset.html.

74. Groop L, Tuomi T, Rowley M, et al. Latent autoimmune diabetes in adults (LADA)—more than a name. Diabetologia. 2006;49:1996-8.

75. Pozzilli P, Di Mario U. Autoimmune diabetes not requiring insulin at diagnosis (latent autoimmune diabetes of the adult): definition, characterization, and potential prevention. Diabetes Care. 2001;24:1460-7.

76. Fajans SS, Bell GI. MODY: history, genetics, pathophysiology, and clinical decision making. Diabetes Care. 2011;34:1878-84.

77. Laakso M, Kuusisto J. Insulin resistance and hyperglycaemia in cardiovascular disease development. Nat Rev Endocrinol. 2014;10:293-302.

78. The Action to Control Cardiovascular Risk in Diabetes Study Group. Effects of intensive glucose lowering in type 2 diabetes. N Engl J Med. 2008;358:2545-59.

79. Patel A, MacMahon S, Chalmers J, et al; for the ADVANCE Collaborative Group. Intensive blood glucose control and vascular outcomes in patients with type 2 diabetes. N Engl J Med. 2008;358:2560-72.

80. Duckworth W, Abraira C, Moritz T, et al; for the VADT Investigators. Glucose control and vascular complications in veterans with type 2 diabetes. N Engl J Med. 2009;360:129-39.

81. Chrousos GP. The hypothalamic-pituitary-adrenal axis and immune-mediated inflammation. N Engl J Med. 1995;332:1351-62.

82. Siddiqui A, Madhu SV, Sharma SB, Desai NG. Endocrine stress responses and risk of type 2 diabetes mellitus. Stress. 2015 Aug 13:1-9.

83. Giovannucci E, Harlan DM, Archer MC, et al. Diabetes and cancer: a consensus report. Diabetes Care. 2010;33:1674-85.

84. Ohkuma T, Peters SAE, Woodward M. Sex differences in the association between diabetes and cancer: a systematic review and meta-analysis of 121 cohorts including 20 million individuals and one million events. Diabetologia, 2018;61(10):2140–54.

CHAPTER 14

Type 1 Diabetes Throughout the Life Span

Carolyn Banion, RN, MN, CPNP, CDCES
Virginia Valentine, APRN, BC-ADM, CDCES, FADCES

Key Concepts

- Clinical management of diabetes relies on the person with diabetes and family self-management.
- Diabetes education is an essential and crucial component of the care and management of individuals with type 1 diabetes. Education must be ongoing throughout the course of the disease.
- There are important differences between children/adolescents and adults in diabetes education and management. Learning materials, content, demonstration of skills, and expectations must be appropriate for the age, abilities, and attention span of each child, adult, and family member.
- The primary goals of treatment are achievement of optimal glycemic goals, avoidance of acute and chronic complications, positive psychosocial adjustment to diabetes, and normal growth and development in children.
- To achieve the desired goals of diabetes management, the person with diabetes and the person's family must integrate a comprehensive and rigorous diabetes regimen into their daily lives. In caring for children and adolescents with diabetes, healthcare providers need to understand the importance of involving adults in diabetes management for these youths.

Introduction

Type 1 diabetes affects all ages, and management and education are ongoing processes throughout an individual's life span. There are a variety of issues, situations, and physical and emotional differences that present at distinct ages and life stages. The diabetes care education specialist must appreciate that diabetes self-management education (DSME) in children, adolescents, and adults presents challenges. The goals for treatment are twofold: (1) to promote normal physical and psychological growth and development, and (2) to avoid both acute and chronic complications of diabetes. This chapter focuses on DSME in type 1 diabetes throughout the life span. Issues in providing care to children and teens are given primary attention. As appropriate, though, information pertinent to adults with type 1 diabetes is provided throughout the chapter. Transition to adult care and development of type 1 diabetes in adults are addressed at the end of the chapter.

State of the Disease

Type 1 diabetes is an autoimmune disease in which hyperglycemia is secondary to insulin deficiency, which is caused by destruction of pancreatic beta cells. Type 1 diabetes accounts for 5% to 10% of all diagnosed cases of diabetes.[1] Age at diagnosis was the initial classification criterion used to describe what was clearly a distinct form of diabetes. Recent classification systems abandoned both age and treatment as criteria and now attempt to identify etiology of disease in order to classify different types of diabetes.[1]

Seventy percent of type 1 diabetes cases are diagnosed before the person reaches 30 years of age, but onset can occur at any age. Type 1 diabetes is one of the most common childhood illnesses, and in the United States approximately 1 in every 400 to 500 children and adolescents under 20 years of age has type 1 diabetes.[1] The worldwide prevalence and incidence of type 1 diabetes vary from one geographic location to another, with the highest incidence occurring in the Scandinavian countries of Sweden, Finland, and Norway, and the lowest incidence occurring in Japan. Evidence suggests that the incidence of type 1 diabetes is increasing globally at a rate of about 3% per year. In some regions, this increase is reported to be greater in children under the age of 5 years.[2] This trend has been speculated to be more likely related to environmental changes, such as exposure to viral infections, than to differences in genetic susceptibility.[3]

The current standards for diabetes management reflect the need to maintain glucose levels as near to normal as safely possible in both children and adults. The Diabetes Control and Complications Trial (DCCT) and the follow-up Epidemiology of Diabetes Interventions and Complications study have shown that intensive treatment and maintenance of glucose concentrations close to the normal range clearly decrease the frequency and severity of the macrovascular and microvascular complications of diabetes.[4,5] These trials have involved adults and only a small cohort of adolescent patients.

Evidence indicates that near normalization of blood glucose levels is not often attained in children and adolescents after the honeymoon (remission) period.[6] Special consideration must be given to the unique aspects of care and management of children and adolescents, such as changes in insulin sensitivity related to sexual maturity and physical growth, ability to provide self-care, supervision in child care and school, and unique neurological vulnerability to hypoglycemia. Glycemic goals may need to be modified, because most children less than 6 to 7 years of age have a form of "hypoglycemic unawareness." Their counter regulatory mechanisms are immature, and they may lack the cognitive capacity to recognize and respond to hypoglycemic symptoms, placing them at greater risk for severe hypoglycemia and its sequelae. Children under the age of 5 years are at risk for permanent cognitive impairment following episodes of severe hypoglycemia.[7] Table 14.1 shows the glycemic targets–plasma blood glucose, A1C, and time in range–across the lifespan for persons with type 1 diabetes.

Diagnosis

The onset of type 1 diabetes is usually acute, with symptoms ranging from incidental glycosuria to life-threatening diabetic ketoacidosis (DKA). The diagnosis of diabetes in infants is rare, and children less than 4 years of age more often present in DKA than do older children or adults. About 25% of children with new-onset type 1 diabetes present in DKA, requiring intravenous rehydration and insulin.[8] Many require treatment in an intensive care unit. At the time of diagnosis, 80% to 90% of the beta cells have been destroyed. Most children present with complaints of nocturia and enuresis and a several-week history of polyuria, polydipsia, and weight loss. Adults with type 1 diabetes often present with polyphagia, but this is rarely seen in children. Other common symptoms include blurred vision, drowsiness, poor stamina, nausea and vomiting, frequent skin and bladder infections, and vaginitis in females. Laboratory values indicate hyperglycemia, glycosuria, and often but not always ketonemia and ketonuria.

Diagnosis of type 1 diabetes in children is usually clear-cut and requires little or no specialized testing. An elevated blood glucose concentration or A1C ≥6.5%

TABLE 14.1 Glycemic Targets for Type 1 Diabetes Across the Lifespan

Preprandial Plasma Blood Glucose		*A1C*	*Time in Range (70-180)**
Ages 0-17	80-130 mg/dl (4.4-7.2 mmol/L)	**7-7.5%** 154 mg/dL – 169 mg/dL (8.6 mmol/L) – (9.4 mmol/L)	**>60-70%**
Ages 18+	80-130 mg/dl (4.4-7.2 mmol/L)	**<7.0%** 154 mg/dL (8.6 mmol/L)	**>70%**

GOALS MUST BE INDIVIDUALIZED. When working with individuals to set targets, factors to consider include, but are but not limited to:

- Age
- History of severe hypoglycemia and/or hypoglycemia unawareness
- Other comorbidities
- Activity level
- Social support
- Access to technology and care
- History of regimen engagement

Glucose Ranges	*Targets (% of Readings)*
>250 mg/dL (13.9 mmol/L)	<5%
>180 mg/dL (10 mmol/L)	<25%
70-180 mg/dL (3.9-10 mmol/L)	>70%
<70 mg/dL (3.9 mmol/L)	<4%
<54 mg/dL (3.0 mmol/L)	<1%

Source: American Diabetes Association, "Clinical practice recommendations 2020" *Diabetes Care* 43 Suppl 1 (2020); Clinical Targets for Continuous Glucose Monitoring Data Interpretation: Recommendations from the International Consensus On Time in Range. Diabetes Care 2019; 42: 1593-1603;

See Chapter 24 for Pregnancy Goals

*Calculated from CGM or fingerstick blood glucoses (if 4 or more/day).

Case: Type 1 Diabetes—Infancy to Young Adulthood

JJ is a 22-year-old college student who was diagnosed with type 1 diabetes at 9 months of age.

- His diabetes was diagnosed when his parents took him to his primary care physician because he was waking frequently and soaking through many diapers during the night, and would drink anything given to him.
- He was in moderate diabetic ketoacidosis (DKA) and was hospitalized at a children's hospital for metabolic stabilization, initiation of insulin therapy, and education of his family.
- Family history includes a maternal aunt with type 1 diabetes, who incidentally had been a subject in the DCCT before JJ's diagnosis.

The case study in this chapter follows a young male from diagnosis at infancy through young adulthood. Issues that the boy and his family faced at different stages are highlighted.

must be documented to diagnose diabetes. The American Association of Clinical Endocrinologists does not recommend the A1C as a diagnostic test for type 1 diabetes. The incidental discovery of hyperglycemia in the absence of classic symptoms does not necessarily indicate new-onset diabetes, especially in young children with acute illness.[6]

The criteria for the staging and diagnosis of diabetes are presented in Table 14.2. In the absence of unequivocal hyperglycemia, these criteria should be confirmed by repeat testing. The oral glucose tolerance test is not recommended for routine clinical use but may be required in the evaluation of patients when diabetes is still suspected despite a normal fasting plasma glucose.[7] Glucose tolerance testing is rarely required to diagnose type 1 diabetes, except in atypical cases or at the beginning of the disease. Because of the risk of rapid clinical deterioration, especially in untreated children with type 1 diabetes, unnecessary delays in the diagnosis must be avoided, and a definitive diagnosis should be made promptly.[6]

As the incidence of type 2 diabetes in children and adolescents increases, differentiating newly diagnosed type 1 diabetes from type 2 diabetes has become more important. In the slender prepubertal child, type 2 diabetes would be very unlikely. In the overweight adolescent, measurement of islet autoantibodies and C-Peptide levels may be necessary to differentiate the diagnosis. Between 85% and 95% of individuals with type 1 diabetes have circulating antibodies directed against 1 or more islet cell components. Regardless of the type of diabetes, insulin will be required for the child who presents with significant fasting hyperglycemia, metabolic derangement, and ketonemia.[6]

The diagnosis of diabetes, as in other chronic illnesses, often causes individuals to grieve the loss of their health, or parents to grieve the loss of their healthy child. Frequently, parents feel guilty about the diagnosis of diabetes in their child because of the genetic component of the disease. Parents may have numerous unexpressed questions, and they may fear they did something to cause the diabetes.

The diabetes care and education specialist can be instrumental in initiating discussion of and normalizing

TABLE 14.2 Diagnosing Type 1 Diabetes

4 Options			
A1C*	**Fasting Plasma Glucose†**	**2-Hour Plasma Glucose**	**Acute Symptoms§ Plus Casual¶ Plasma Glucose**
≥6.5%	≥126 mg/dL (7.0 mmol/L)	≥200 mg/dL (11.1 mmol/L) during oral glucose tolerance test (75 g glucose)‡	≥200 mg/dL (11.1 mmol/L)

Note: Unless unequivocal symptoms of hyperglycemia are present, these criteria must be confirmed by repeat testing on a subsequent day.

*Performed in a laboratory using a method that is National Glycohemoglobin Standardization Program certified and standardized to the Diabetes Control and Complications Trial assay. The American Association of Clinical Endocrinologists does not recommend the A1C as a diagnostic test for type 1 diabetes mellitus.

†Fasting is defined as no caloric intake for at least 8 hours.

‡See text for discussion of when the oral glucose tolerance test is appropriate.

§Classic symptoms of diabetes include polyuria, polydipsia, and unexplained weight loss.

¶Casual is defined as any time of day without regard to time since last meal.

Source: American Diabetes Association, "Clinical practice recommendations 2016," *Diabetes Care* 39 Suppl 1 (2016): S13.

these feelings. Parents and family must be reassured that there is nothing they could have done to prevent the disease. The combination of genes from both parents increases the risk for type 1 diabetes in their offspring. New technology, medications, and treatment strategies have changed diabetes management dramatically in recent years; explaining this to families is usually reassuring. The parents and family need to understand the difference in pathophysiology and treatment of type 1 diabetes and that of type 2 diabetes. Diabetes self-management education is essential for all individuals with newly diagnosed diabetes. Planning and provision of diabetes education should recognize the following:

Infants and preschoolers. Education is directed toward the parents and primary caregivers (babysitters, day care personnel, grandparents, older siblings). The tremendous responsibility of care and the fear of hypoglycemia are extremely stressful for these families.[9]

School-aged children. Parents need to assume most of the responsibility, but the child will be able to perform some of the skills of self-management with adult supervision. School/day care personnel must also be educated since the child spends a great deal of the day in the school setting.[6]

Adolescents. When diabetes is diagnosed during adolescence, both the parent and child must be educated. Part of the education should be guiding parents and teens to work together as a team, and when appropriate, transitioning more responsibility to the teen. Independence is not age specific and is a gradual process.

Adults. Spouses or significant others should be included in self-management education.

Survival Skills: The Focus of the First Week

Because of the strong emotions (shock, anger, grief, fear) felt at this time, most persons with diabetes and their families do not comprehend much more than survival skills in the first week. Others may seem to adapt more quickly and move forward at a quicker pace, but may experience

Case—Part 2: Provision of Family Education and Support

Once JJ's DKA was treated, the educational process with his family was initiated by a team of healthcare professionals, including a pediatric endocrinologist, diabetes nurse educator, dietitian, and medical social worker. JJ's parents experienced the usual shock, grief, anger, sadness, and denial that most parents do when their child is diagnosed. JJ's mother grew up with a sibling with type 1 diabetes, so she had some preconceived ideas about diabetes management. Other family members and friends who had experience with type 2 diabetes offered conflicting advice about the management of JJ's diabetes. This heightened JJ's parents' fears. Both parents had a real fear of hypoglycemia because of the increase in frequency of hypoglycemia the mother's sister had experienced with intensive insulin therapy during her participation in the DCCT. The diagnosis can be particularly devastating for families who have experienced the complications of diabetes. It is important for the healthcare team to know a family's past experience with diabetes.

Education needed to be individualized and communicated in a way that addressed JJ's age and developmental stage, family dynamics, past experiences with diabetes, and issues facing the entire family. In JJ's case, his family needed to understand that there are different types of diabetes and that everyone's experience with diabetes is different. The family needed to be reassured that they could not have prevented the diagnosis of diabetes. Diabetes education regarding survival skills was foremost, and this education included JJ's siblings and other caretakers, such as his grandparents. The pace of teaching followed the progress the family was making in learning the necessary skills.

The art of diabetes education and care is in the delivery and effectiveness. Although the biomedical aspects of type 1 diabetes are similar across people, the experience of having diabetes can be very different in different cultural and ethnic groups. The majority of people with type 1 diabetes are non-Hispanic whites, 10% are Hispanic, and 7% are other ethnic backgrounds.[3] Assessments should include cultural values and language skills, including health literacy. Healthcare providers need to be familiar with the normative cultural values that may affect the health care of ethnic and cultural groups and be understanding about these values. For example, in some cultures, diabetes is seen as a death sentence, so why take care of it? Sometimes diabetes is thought to be the result of some traumatic event, and there is tremendous guilt. In some cultures, insulin is thought to be a drug that can cause blindness, kidney problems, amputations, or death.

To provide appropriate education for the family, the diabetes care and education specialist must carefully evaluate the meaning of the diagnosis, assess family members' comfort with using insulin, ensure that they understand that insulin is necessary, encourage the person with diabetes/family to share whether they are using any alternative therapies, and assess family routines and schedules. It is also important to have educational materials available to meet the language, cultural, and literacy needs of persons with diabetes and families. Frequent contact in the weeks after the diagnosis and the initial education will be necessary.

the grief and anger at a later time. The initial teaching focuses on the following survival skills:

- Testing blood glucose and urine or blood ketones
- Measurement and administration of insulin
- Understanding insulin actions and peaks
- Meal planning
- Preventing, recognizing, and treating hypoglycemia

The education provided must be culturally appropriate, personalized to the needs of its recipients (child, individual, family), sensitive to family resources, paced to accommodate individual needs, and provided for all caregivers. Siblings should not be overlooked, as they sometimes feel left out because of the attention being given to the child with diabetes.

The educational process needs to be an open-ended, ongoing experience between the individual with diabetes and the individual's family, friends, and diabetes team. Developing effective stress management/coping skills and problem-solving skills is considered as important to successful therapy as insulin administration, nutrition therapy, monitoring, and exercise.[10]

The content provided will be the same whether the individual with new-onset diabetes is in the inpatient or outpatient setting. About 75% of children and adults with new-onset diabetes are not acutely ill and do not require hospitalization for medical management.[8] However, hospitalization may be necessary if there is not an outpatient facility equipped to provide this care. To do initial management successfully, a multidisciplinary team must teach the patient and family how to monitor blood glucose and how to safely use insulin at home, and must be available to troubleshoot by phone if problems arise. Initial outpatient care and education costs are substantially lower than those associated with inpatient care. Families may be directed to additional educational support through the Association of Diabetes Care and Education Specialists (ADCES) the American Diabetes Association (ADA), and Juvenile Diabetes Research Foundation (JDRF), which can refer them to a diabetes care education specialist or diabetes education team.

To achieve the desired goals for glycemic levels, persons with diabetes and families must integrate a comprehensive and rigorous diabetes management plan into their daily lives.

Management of type 1 diabetes includes the following key components:

- *Monitoring:* Measurement of blood glucose 6 to 8 times per day or use of continuous glucose monitor
- *Taking medication:* Insulin infusion therapy or 4 to 6 injections of insulin per day
- *Healthy eating:* Attention to food intake
- *Being active:* Regular exercise

Monitoring

Blood Glucose Monitoring

Regular self-monitoring of blood glucose is essential for optimal glycemic stability for all individuals with Type 1 Diabetes. This can be achieved by accurate fingerstick blood glucose measurements, continuous glucose monitoring (CGM), or intermittently scanned glucose monitoring.

When fingerstick blood glucose monitoring is used, frequent monitoring (6-10 measurements/day) is essential in determining patterns of hypoglycemia and hyperglycemia and in enabling individuals to make adjustments in food, exercise, scheduling, and/or insulin.

The ADA recommends blood glucose checks prior to meals and snacks, occasionally postprandially, at bedtime, prior to exercise, when the individual suspects low blood glucose, after treating low blood glucose, and prior to critical tasks (such as driving) for persons with diabetes using multiple daily injections (MDIs) or insulin pump therapy.[1]

- *Preprandial blood glucose:* To determine premeal insulin dose; pre-breakfast fasting glucose also assists in determining appropriateness of basal insulin dosing
- *Postprandial blood glucose:* Important in determining whether premeal insulin dose was correct
- *Overnight blood glucose:* Valuable in determining doses and detecting nocturnal hypoglycemia, especially after exercise that is greater than usual intensity, duration, or frequency; illness; poor food intake or if nocturnal hypoglycemia is a problem
- *Frequent testing:* Essential in young children or anyone who has hypoglycemic unawareness

Meters

Many good blood glucose meters are available. Often, third-party payers dictate which meter the individual uses. The diabetes care and education specialist can play an important role in assisting individuals with choosing the best blood glucose meter to fit their needs and optimize accuracy and safety.[11]

The sides of the fingertips are the most frequently used site for blood samples. Some individuals may find alternate sites (forearm or palm of the hand) more acceptable. The results from fingertips and forearms are usually similar in the fasting state. Alternate-site testing may not reflect arterial glucose values as quickly as finger-stick capillary blood glucose measurements, so it is advised that fingertips be used when symptoms of hypoglycemia are present.

Data Log

It is important for blood glucose test results to be documented using a monitoring logbook, smart meter, app, or cloud-based program. Interpretation of results and use of this information for calculating insulin doses are essential in achieving good metabolic stability. Individuals and families should be taught to review these data frequently to look for blood glucose patterns and make appropriate dose adjustments or call their healthcare provider for assistance. These tools should be reviewed during visits with healthcare providers to discuss causes of variability and strategies for improving metabolic stability, being careful not to use them judgmentally.

Continuous Glucose Monitoring

Continuous glucose sensors track glucose levels every few minutes, 24 hours a day, and CGM is a more sophisticated monitoring method than fingerstick blood glucose. CGM can identify times of consistent hyperglycemia and times of increased risk for hypoglycemia. These devices have proven to improve metabolic management and assist in the avoidance of hypoglycemia, which is often the most significant barrier to optimal stability. The use of CGM allows for the achievement of lower blood glucose targets, thus improving HbA1c levels without increasing hypoglycemia.[12] Continuous glucose monitoring devices may dramatically alter the management of type 1 diabetes in individuals who are motivated to use this technology and capable of incorporating it into their own daily diabetes management. Continuous glucose monitoring may be particularly useful in those with hypoglycemia unawareness, frequent episodes of hypoglycemia, nocturnal hypoglycemia, unexplained glucose excursions, or gastroparesis.[13]

The range of diabetes technology and connected health devices is growing rapidly. Staying current on the data, assessing all of the options, and finding reliable training is often a challenge. Diabetes Advanced Network Access has been designed and built specifically to support the technology-based needs of the diabetes healthcare professional. Members of ADCES can access danatech.org for the latest information and training on devices, review of apps, continuing education and much more.

Ketone Testing

The general recommendation for ketone testing is to test when blood glucose levels exceed 250 mg/dL (13.9 mmol/L) and during illness.

Some centers advise routine ketone testing before breakfast as an indicator of overnight or antecedent insulin deficiency. Overnight (antecedent) insulin deficiency—referred to as the "dawn phenomenon"—is fasting hyperglycemia related to the normal rise in growth hormone, cortisol, and other hormones that can raise blood glucose levels in the absence of insulin.[14]

Ketones can be tested in either urine or blood. Blood ketone testing gives more current results, but the blood testing strips are more expensive than the urine testing strips. Testing the urine for ketones is a commonly taught skill; however, meters are now available that test both blood glucose and blood ketones.[1] Some families may find this meter more convenient for those times when obtaining a urine sample is difficult.

The presence of persistent moderate or large amounts of ketones in the urine or concentrations of greater than 0.6 mmol/L in the blood suggests the possibility of impending DKA and should prompt individuals to adjust their insulin or seek assistance from their healthcare provider. Additional fluids and/or insulin are often required to clear ketosis. See chapter 23 for more information on management of hyperglycemia.

Considerations for Insulin Injections in Children and Teens[15,16]

- Usual injection sites for children are the abdomen, legs, arms, and buttocks. Because children usually have less subcutaneous tissue than adults, appropriate sites must be used to ensure subcutaneous injection and avoid administration into underlying muscle. Abdominal injections may not be advisable in young children with little subcutaneous fat.
- Rotating sites in a consistent manner (eg, legs in the morning, arms in the evening, buttocks at bedtime) may provide a more consistent rate of absorption. It may also prevent lipohypertrophy of sites.
- Avoid giving injections into hypertrophied areas, to achieve the best absorption possible.

- Use 31-gauge, 6-mm syringe needles and 4 mm pen needles for more comfortable injections and to avoid intramuscular injection. The use of a two-finger lift up and/or a 45-degree needle insertion can also prevent inadvertent intramuscular injection.
- Use the smallest barrel possible (eg, 30-unit syringe for doses less than 30 units, 50-unit syringe for doses between 30 and 50 units) for the most accurate dosing.
- Half-unit increment insulin syringes are available
- Both reusable insulin pens and disposable half-unit insulin pens are available for pediatric patients.
- An automatic injector (eg, Inject-Ease® or similar device) may be useful for some individuals. Subcutaneous indwelling catheters (eg, Insuflon®, iport®) may also be helpful.
- Needle phobias are common in children and adults (parents or persons with diabetes). *Always* assess.
- By giving each other practice saline injections, parents can reassure themselves that giving insulin injections to their child is not the trauma they envision.
- For older children, seeing family members give themselves a practice saline injection may be supportive, making it less frightening for the child.

Taking Medication

Insulin Injection Therapy

Insulin is the mainstay of treatment of type 1 diabetes. Subcutaneous insulin injections are begun at the time of diagnosis, or once ketoacidosis is resolved in those in whom it was present. There are many different insulin preparations available. The various preparations are genetically engineered to have different onsets, peaks, and duration of activity (see chapter 17). These insulins are used in combination or individually and can be delivered by syringe, pen, or pump.

Regimen and Dose Determinations

For all persons with newly diagnosed diabetes, a basal-bolus regimen, consisting of a long-acting insulin plus rapid-acting insulin before meals, is recommended. Some persons with diabetes are started on insulin pump therapy very soon after diagnosis.

Infants and Toddlers

Because of their need for frequent food intake, infants and toddlers may require frequent small injections. The small insulin needs of infants and toddlers may require diluted insulin to allow for more precise dosing and measurement of insulin in less than 1-unit increments. Diluents are available for specific types of insulin from the insulin manufacturers. Insulin can be diluted either at a pharmacy or at home, once parents are trained. Insulin pump therapy is another option since most pumps can infuse insulin in very small increments.

Children/Adolescents

Children's insulin requirements are based on body weight, age, and pubertal status. Children with newly diagnosed type 1 diabetes usually require an initial total daily dose of 0.5 to 1.0 units per kilogram. Younger and prepubertal children usually require lower doses, while the presence of ketoacidosis, use of steroids, and onset of puberty all dictate the need for higher doses.

Adults

Adults, on average, require 0.5 to 1 unit per kilogram per day.[1]

Decreased Insulin Needs During Honeymoon Period

Once blood glucose levels are normalized and endogenous insulin production increases during the first few weeks after diagnosis, most individuals with type 1 diabetes enter a honeymoon, or remission, period. During the honeymoon phase, insulin requirements will be less (0.2-0.6 units per kilogram of body weight per day) compared with the requirements at the initial diagnosis of diabetes.[1] The duration of the honeymoon period varies, but it typically lasts between 3 and 12 months. Parents and persons with diabetes need to be prepared for this period of decreasing insulin needs and minimal fluctuation in blood glucose values so that they do not question the diagnosis of diabetes. Beta cell destruction continues during the honeymoon period. The end of this remission period is characterized by the following:

- Increased variability of blood glucose levels
- Increased insulin requirements
- Greater need to attend to diabetes management

Case—Part 3: Tools of Therapy

During baby JJ's hospitalization, his parents were taught survival skills for diabetes management.

Monitoring

- Blood glucose
- Blood or urine ketones

JJ's parents were instructed on the use of a blood glucose meter that uses a small sample of blood. They were also instructed on record keeping and the importance of using these data for pattern management. (Current practice would be to initiate continuous glucose monitoring as soon after diagnosis as possible.)

Insulin Therapy

JJ was started on MDIs, using a long-acting insulin analog for basal insulin and a rapid-acting insulin analog with all food intake. JJ's parents were instructed on the measurement of insulin and the administration and rotation of insulin injection sites. When JJ's mother expressed reluctance because she did not want to hurt her baby, the diabetes care and education specialist had the parents practice giving each other saline injections.

Meal Planning

Ensuring adequate nutrition and calories was a primary consideration, as it is essential in the growing child. At the time JJ was diagnosed, his parents met with a pediatric registered dietitian. Food was one of their biggest concerns, as is often the case for parents of infants and toddlers. The diabetes care and education specialist explained that because infants require a frequent feeding schedule, getting glucose values with even a 2-hour fast is often difficult, and feedings often do not match the peaks of insulin.

Physical Activity

The activity level of a 9-month-old, such as JJ at the time of his diagnosis, is unpredictable and in general cannot be planned for or controlled—this is just one of the many challenges of managing diabetes in an infant. It was important for JJ's parents to understand how his activity level, sleep, and nap patterns affected his blood glucose levels so they could make appropriate adjustments in food and insulin.

Hypoglycemia

The fear of hypoglycemia is both one of the major barriers to achieving optimal glycemic stability for all individuals with diabetes and one of the biggest fears of parents of children with diabetes. Severe hypoglycemia can affect the growing brain of the child, and recognizing the early warning signs of hypoglycemia in a very young child may be difficult. However, due to the seriousness of hypoglycemia, the importance of prevention and early adequate treatment must be stressed. JJ's parents were instructed on the signs, symptoms, and treatment of hypoglycemia, including the use of glucose gel and glucagon. They were encouraged to do frequent monitoring of blood glucose to validate hypoglycemic episodes.

When baby JJ was discharged from the hospital, his parents had learned an entire new set of skills and had the challenge of raising a child with diabetes.

Some persons with diabtes who have had a prolonged and significant honeymoon period have described the end of this period as "getting diabetes all over again."

Increased Insulin Needs With Growth and Puberty

Insulin requirements increase with growth, and particularly during puberty. Insulin requirements during puberty may increase to as much as 1.5 units per kilogram per day due to the hormonal influences of increased growth hormone and sex hormone secretion. Insulin therapy regimens must be based on the individual needs of the child, adolescent, adult, and family and must also consider meal, school, and work schedules, supervisory issues, and glycemic patterns.

Metabolic Management

The DCCT demonstrated that individuals on basal-bolus insulin therapy with MDI or a continuous subcutaneous insulin infusion (pump therapy) achieved better metabolic stability compared with those on twice-daily insulin dosing.[4]

Regimen Flexibility

A basal-bolus insulin regimen uses a long-acting insulin analog (most often given at bedtime, although it can be given at other times) combined with a rapid-acting insulin analog given before meals and snacks. Using an insulin-to-carbohydrate ratio, along with correction factor to determine the rapid-acting insulin dose before meals and snacks allows for flexibility in the timing and amount of food consumed. Other factors involved in determining the dose are the current blood glucose level and the anticipated level of physical activity in the coming hours.

To prevent postprandial hyperglycemia, the premeal rapid-acting insulin analog should be given 10 to 20 minutes before the meal, when the premeal blood glucose is at or above the target range. The higher the blood glucose, the earlier the insulin should be given so that it begins to lower the blood glucose before the meal is ingested. If the blood glucose is greater than 300 mg/dL (16.6 mmol/L), it may be necessary to give the insulin even earlier than 20 minutes before the meal. If the premeal blood glucose is below target range, food may need to be consumed before insulin is administered. This regimen must be individualized and may also need to be specific for meals. One of the most difficult times to manage postprandial glucose is after the morning meal, perhaps because of some insulin resistance early morning and because of the high carbohydrate content of most breakfast meals.

For children, whose intake is unpredictable, giving the insulin immediately after the meal, so that actual food intake and insulin are matched more closely, may be efficacious in minimizing the potential for hypoglycemia. However, when insulin is given after the meal, postprandial glucose level will not be as good.

Case—Part 4: Insulin Infusion Therapy to Improve Glycemic Stability

When JJ was 14 years old, he was using MDIs, and his A1C was in the 8% to 9% range. He had one severe nocturnal hypoglycemic episode and was experiencing fairly frequent mild to moderate hypoglycemic episodes, often related to his competitive ski racing. JJ and his parents decided to pursue pump therapy (continuous subcutaneous insulin infusion).

Insulin pump therapy should be a joint decision by the person with diabetes, family, and diabetes management team. It requires more in-depth self-management education and performance of self-care behaviors. JJ and his family received extensive DSME, including adequate nutrition for his activity, the need for more frequent blood glucose monitoring, problem solving, calculating insulin dosages, and mechanics of the insulin pump. JJ had to demonstrate his ability to operate the pump and manage his diabetes safely and appropriately. With help from the diabetes management team, JJ learned to adjust his pump for his skiing and reduced the number of hypoglycemic episodes. JJ and his parents also discussed the use of pump therapy with JJ's ski coach.

The multiple snacks consumed by some children and adolescents may translate into multiple injections (5 or more) if the basal-bolus plan is strictly followed. The number of insulin injections may be a barrier to good management using an MDI regimen with carbohydrate counting, even though it allows for flexibility of eating times and amounts. This practice can also lead to stacking of insulin doses, resulting in hypoglycemia. Omission of injections may increase when the regimen becomes too difficult. Some persons with diabetes and families may consider insulin infusion therapy when injections are required too frequently.

Premixed Insulins

Commercially prepared, premixed insulins do not allow for flexibility of daily dosage adjustment based on blood glucose values and exercise levels, which are especially variable in children, and therefore may not be appropriate for people with type 1 diabetes. However, these insulins may be useful for those who are unable or unwilling to regularly adjust insulin doses.

Continuous Subcutaneous Insulin Infusion

Continuous subcutaneous insulin infusion (CSII) has been demonstrated to improve stability, decrease fluctuations in blood glucose, decrease the risk of severe hypoglycemia, allow for more flexibility in food intake, and improve quality of life. These advantages make CSII a safe, effective, and appealing option for infants, children and adults with type 1 diabetes.[7,17]

Glucose Target Levels

CSII does not always result in improved glucose targets. The primary reasons for suboptimal glucose levels in children and adults using CSII are missed meal boluses and lack of attention to blood glucose levels, resulting in blood glucose levels not being corrected.

Some pump issues are unique to children, including use at school or camp and adjustments for sports.

Use at School, Day Care, or Camp

One issue with CSII is management of the pump in the school setting, at day care, or at camp. The child may need help counting carbohydrates, correctly bolusing, and troubleshooting the pump (eg, what to do for air bubbles, alarms, dislodgement of insulin infusion sets). Either the school nurse or other school or camp staff will require training to perform these tasks for or with the child. Camp counselors, camp nurses, and day care staff should be familiar with the mechanics of the insulin pump and know how to problem solve and who to contact if there is a problem with the pump.

Adjusting for Sports

Managing insulin infusion therapy during sports requires some special adjustments, whether the pump is worn or disconnected during the sport. Pumps without tubing and waterproof pumps can be worn during most sports. However, individuals often prefer to be "untethered" to avoid pump damage, or discomfort if the site is hit and it is often difficult to secure the pump adequately. Diabetes care and education specialists can provide guidance, but the individual often learns by trial and error how to adjust for the missed basal. If history proves that the blood glucose is above target after an activity, a starting place is to give one half of the missed basal prior to disconnecting. It is best if the pump is disconnected for no longer than 2 hours. If the pump must be disconnected for longer periods (eg, a day of water sports), it is possible to simultaneously use an insulin pump and a long-acting insulin analog by injection.[18] Frequent blood glucose monitoring is essential so that the individual can learn what adjustments work. For sports that do not require the pump to be disconnected, temporary basal rates and decreasing boluses usually work well.

Healthy Eating

Eating is usually one of the biggest concerns for all individuals with new-onset diabetes. Common misbeliefs have instilled a fear in some people with diabetes that they will never again eat sweets or other foods they like. An important role of the diabetes care education specialist is to help the person with diabetes and the family of the person with diabetes understand how to incorporate foods the person with diabetes likes into a healthful food plan. The clinical goals of medical nutrition therapy (MNT) are the same for all individuals with type 1 diabetes, with the addition of maintenance of normal growth and development for children and adolescents.[19]

Medical Nutrition Therapy

All individuals with type 1 diabetes should receive individualized MNT as needed to achieve treatment goals. Nutrition recommendations are based on a nutritional assessment that involves evaluating parameters such as age, weight, height, growth percentiles on a growth chart for children and adolescents, body mass index (BMI), gender, recommended daily allowances (RDAs) for caloric range, schedules, treatment modalities, and blood glucose patterns for each individual.[20]

Calorie Consumption and Normal Growth in Children

Children need sufficient calories for growth and pubertal development without excessive hypoglycemic episodes. Meal-time routines with some limitations on snacking help improve dietary quality and optimize glycemic outcomes. The child's height and weight should be plotted on a growth chart at each visit to determine trends. If the child's growth patterns are appropriate for his or her age, then the child's meal plan includes calories adequate for growth and development. Children and teens who are of normal weight do not need to focus on weight-management issues, other than to follow prudent recommendations important for the general population. For children and adults who are above an ideal weight range, encouraging alterations in food selection and physical activity levels can help decrease possible insulin resistance and improve metabolic status.[19]

Meal Plan and Insulin Regimen

The meal plan must be individualized to match food preferences, cultural influences, family eating patterns and schedules, age, weight, activity level, and insulin action peaks. Insulin therapy can be integrated into usual eating and exercise habits. Therefore, it is important to determine the meal plan before determining an insulin regimen. The individual's appetite should be considered when determining the total caloric level provided in the meal plan. Young children require smaller portions of food and need to eat more frequently than adults. Infants and toddlers have changing and unpredictable eating patterns.

Most children and adults newly diagnosed with type 1 diabetes experience some weight loss that will be restored with insulin initiation, hydration, and adequate energy intake. Once their weight is restored to normalcy, their appetite and caloric intake will decrease significantly.

When the person with diabetes recovers from the acute onset of diabetes and his or her appetite decreases, the insulin dose must be decreased to avoid hypoglycemia. The person with diabetes and/or family should be forewarned that this may occur and must be alerted to watch for this.

Adolescents, especially girls, are often pleased with the weight loss they incur as diabetes develops and do not want to regain the weight. As appropriate, these teens should be given guidance to help them minimize their weight gain.

Using an insulin-to-carbohydrate ratio to determine the premeal insulin dose allows for more flexibility in food intake, whereas food intake will need to be more consistent for individuals on fixed insulin regimens. In children, withholding food can feel punitive to the child and eventually promote reluctance to honestly report extra food or high glucose values. This can also result in inadequate caloric intake for growth. Forcing children to eat when they are not hungry or when they are no longer hungry should also be avoided.

Carbohydrate-counting principles are the same for children and adults. Carbohydrate counting can allow for greater flexibility and alternatives in meal planning in MDI and CSII (see chapter 16, on nutrition therapy, for more detail). Children under the age of 6 typically want 3 meals per day plus 3 snacks. Most children over the age of 6 want 3 meals per day plus midafternoon and bedtime snacks. Additional carbohydrate intake is often needed before physical activity to decrease the risk of a hypoglycemic episode during or after exercise.

Chapters 5 and 16, on self-management behavior related to healthy eating and nutrition therapy, respectively, provide more information.

Being Active

Physical activity has many benefits, but in type 1 diabetes increased attention must be given to age, consistency, insulin dosing, and changes in blood glucose levels. Increased frequency in checking blood glucose is a requirement, as is education on how to respond before, during, and after the period of physical activity.

Adjusting for Activity Levels

The activity level of the very young child is unpredictable and in general cannot be planned for or controlled—this is just one of the many challenges of managing diabetes in infants and children. Individuals of all ages with diabetes need to make adjustments in their diabetes regimen for changes in activity levels.

Benefits of Physical Activity

Intervention strategies that promote lifelong physical activity should be encouraged for all individuals with diabetes because of the health-promoting benefits of a regular exercise program. The benefits of exercise in type 1 diabetes are detailed in an ADA Position Statement[21] and include the following:

- Lower plasma glucose levels
- Greater sense of well-being
- Weight management
- Improved physical fitness
- Improved cardiovascular fitness with lower pulse and blood pressure
- Improved lipid profile

These benefits apply to children as well as adults. All individuals with type 1 diabetes should strive to meet the physical activity recommendations of the American Diabetes Association.[1]

- Children: At least 60 minutes of physical activity daily
- Adults: 150 minutes a week over at least 3 days a week, with no more than 2 consecutive days with no exercise
- All persons, including those with diabetes, should avoid being sedentary and avoid prolonged sitting (more than 90 minutes)

Hypoglycemia Prevention

More frequent blood glucose monitoring (before, during, and after exercise) may be necessary to avoid hypoglycemia during or after exercise. The decision of whether to adjust food or insulin is determined by the individual's diabetes management goals and is further affected by whether the exercise was planned. When exercise is planned sufficiently in advance, the preference is to adjust the insulin acting during the period of physical activity to minimize hypoglycemia risk. If exercise is not planned far enough ahead to modify the relevant insulin dose, a carbohydrate snack should be consumed. Planning or predicting physical activity in very young children is especially difficult. For school-aged children and adolescents, the intensity and duration of a sports practice, physical education period, or sports game may vary greatly from day to day, so adjusting insulin may be difficult for them as well. With the increasing prevalence of obesity in all age groups, exercise is often important for weight management, and if additional food is consumed to cover increases in activity, the benefits of exercise for weight management are lost.

Depending on the glucose value at the start of exercise and the intensity and duration of the activity, carbohydrate intake may be necessary before, during, and/or after exercise. Recommendations must be individualized, but a general guideline is to consume 10 to 20 g of carbohydrate for every 30 minutes of moderate activity.

In the pediatric population, 10% to 20% of hypoglycemic episodes are associated with exercise that is of greater-than-usual intensity, duration, or frequency. Increased hepatic glucose output in association with vigorous exercise secondary to both beta- and alpha-adrenergic stimulation may cause hyperglycemia during and immediately after exercise. Hypoglycemia may follow within

1 to 16 hours of completion of exercise due to glucose transport into skeletal muscle tissue and hepatic glycogen depletion.[22,23] School-aged children and adolescents are frequently involved in different sports at various times of the year, all requiring different adjustments in their diabetes regimen. Their activities are often during the late afternoon and evening, and the delayed hypoglycemia that can occur is likely to occur during the night if appropriate adjustments are not made in insulin or carbohydrate intake. Blood glucose monitoring or attention to CGM at bedtime is crucial.

In a study examining the effect of exercise on overnight hypoglycemia in children with diabetes, 36% of the 50 study participants experienced nocturnal hypoglycemia even when their blood glucose was greater than 130 mg/dL (7.2 mmol/L) at bedtime.[24]

Consuming an electrolyte-containing sports drink or other source of a readily absorbable carbohydrate may be helpful in preventing hypoglycemia both during and after exercise. Chapter 6 offers more information on encouraging fluid intake.

See chapter 6 for more information on physical activity and self-management behaviors related to being active.

Healthy Coping

When a child or adult is diagnosed with type 1 diabetes, developing effective stress management/coping skills and problem-solving skills is as important as insulin administration, nutrition therapy, monitoring, and exercise. Many parents equate having a newly diagnosed child with diabetes with leaving the hospital with their firstborn child. The adult or child/parent can be overwhelmed with fears and the stress of learning new skills and having new responsibilities associated with having to deal with a chronic illness. The stressful, changed situation may create tension among family members. The parents/significant others may argue, and family members may feel frightened and can become resentful as all the attention is directed toward the family member with diabetes. The potential for family dysfunction is great. Psychosocial issues for the person with diabetes and the entire family change throughout the lifetime. The diabetes care and education specialist needs to understand normal developmental stages in order to identify and circumvent potential problems. Major developmental issues and their effect on diabetes in children and adolescents are summarized in Table 14.3.

The diabetes care and education specialist or can be instrumental in assisting individuals and families dealing with these issues by initiating discussion about these feelings and suggesting referral for family counseling. Many diabetes teams include a social worker or psychologist to help deal with these issues. Including the entire family in the diabetes education process helps support all family members and provides everyone the opportunity to participate in the care of the person with diabetes.

Peer group activities such as diabetes camp, support groups, and group clinic visits may be helpful in improving acceptance of diabetes, management skills, quality of life, and glycemic stability. Stress management, problem-solving, and coping skills training delivered in small groups has been shown to reduce diabetes-related stress, improve social interaction, increase glucose monitoring, and improve glycemic stability.[15]

Increased access to the internet and social media has allowed individuals across the globe to connect in ways not possible decades ago. There are many social media platforms and online communities that individuals with diabetes or parents of children with diabetes may find helpful for diabetes-related support and information. The ADA and ADCES have endorsed the importance of peer support through Diabetes online communities.[25]

Peer connections and support are especially important during adolescence and the young adult period. The college diabetes network is a non-profit organization whose mission is focused on providing young adults an avenue of peer support and the expert resources they need to successfully manage the challenging transitions to independence. The positive and realistic advice from others can be helpful but they must understand the pros and cons of such sources and be encouraged to discuss the information with their healthcare providers.

Primary Treatment Goals for All Individuals With Type 1 Diabetes

- To achieve optimal glycemic goals with a flexible, individualized diabetes management plan
- To avoid severe hypoglycemia, symptomatic hyperglycemia, and ketoacidosis
- To promote and maintain day-to-day clinical and psychological well-being[1]

Adults newly diagnosed with diabetes often employ a basal-bolus regimen, using a long-acting insulin plus a rapid-acting insulin before meals. Adults, on average, require between 0.4 and 1.0 units per kilogram per day.[1]

TABLE 14.3 Major Developmental Issues and Their Effect on Diabetes in Children and Adolescents

Developmental Stage (Approximate Ages)	*Normal Developmental Tasks*	*Type 1 Diabetes Management Priorities*	*Family Issues in Type 1 Diabetes Management*
Infancy 0–12 months	Developing a trusting relationship/"bonding" with primary caregiver(s)	Preventing and treating hypoglycemia Avoiding extreme fluctuations in blood glucose levels	Coping with stress Sharing the "burden of care" to avoid parent burnout
Toddler 13–36 months	Developing a sense of mastery and autonomy	Preventing and treating hypoglycemia Avoiding extreme fluctuations in blood glucose levels due to irregular food intake	Establishing a schedule Managing the "picky eater" Setting limits and coping with toddler's lack of cooperation with regimen Sharing the burden of care
Preschooler and Early Elementary School Age 3–7 years	Developing initiative in activities and confidence in self	Preventing and treating hypoglycemia Managing unpredictable appetite and activity Positive reinforcement for cooperation with regimen Trusting other caregivers with diabetes management	Reassuring child that diabetes is no one's fault Educating other caregivers about diabetes management
Older Elementary School Age 8–11 years	Developing skills in athletic, cognitive, artistic, and social areas Consolidating self-esteem with respect to the peer group	Making diabetes regimen flexible to allow for participation in school/ peer activities Child learning short- and long-term benefits of optimal control	Maintaining parental involvement in insulin and blood glucose monitoring tasks while allowing for independent self-care for "special occasions" Continuing to educate school and other caregivers
Early Adolescence 12–15 years	Managing body changes Developing a strong sense of self-identity	Managing increased insulin requirements during puberty Diabetes management and blood glucose control become more difficult Weight and body image concerns	Renegotiating parents' and teen's roles in diabetes management to be acceptable to both Learning coping skills to enhance ability to self-manage Preventing and intervening with diabetes-related family conflict Monitoring for signs of depression, eating disorders, risky behaviors
Later Adolescence 16–19 years	Establishing a sense of identity after high school (decisions about location, social issues, work, education)	Begin discussion of transition to a new diabetes team Integrating diabetes into new lifestyle	Supporting the transition to independence Learning coping skills to enhance ability to self-manage Preventing and intervening with diabetes-related family conflict Monitoring for signs of depression, eating disorders, risky behaviors

Source: JL Chiang, MS Kirkman, LMB Laffel, AL Peters; on behalf of the *Type 1 Diabetes Sourcebook* authors, "Type 1 diabetes through the life span: a position statement of the American Diabetes Association," *Diabetes Care 37*, no. 7 (2014): 2034-54. http://dx.doi.org/10.2337/dc14-1140.

Psychosocial: Infants and Toddlers

Normal characteristics in the development of young children must be taken into account when diabetes management regimens are determined. Normal growth and development for infants and toddlers (from birth to age 3) progress rapidly and predictably. An understanding of normal developmental tasks of children is essential when developing the diabetes management plan.

One of the developmental tasks of infancy is to build a trusting relationship with caregivers. Parents often worry that "hurting" their child (finger pokes and injections) will hamper this bonding process. Parents should be encouraged to develop a matter-of-fact attitude for the management tasks with the provision of incentives, like hugs, positive verbal reinforcement, or reading a book immediately after the poke or injection. Infants become much more mobile when they begin crawling at around 9 months of age and walking at about 10 to 15 months of age. Their energy expenditure increases greatly once they become mobile; insulin dose adjustments or extra snacks may thus be necessary to prevent hypoglycemia. In infancy, feedings not only provide nutrition to maintain life and physiologic well-being but also build a relationship. A positive feeding interaction between the infant and the caregiver fosters the ingestion of an appropriate amount of food. Infants usually nurse or eat predictably, but for breastfed infants it is difficult to know how much breast milk they are getting. A feeding pattern that imitates family mealtimes should evolve by the end of the first year of life, to incorporate the infant into the family's normal meal schedule.[26]

Toddlers develop a sense of mastery and autonomy, and they begin to separate and individuate, testing their separateness by saying "no" and behaving in an oppositional manner. Most parents know this as the "terrible twos." Providing choices can give the toddler with diabetes some control, but the choices need to be framed in such a way that the child is not allowed to make important decisions. For example, asking "Which finger shall we use?" works better than asking "Do you want to do your blood test now?" Some families have "cute" names for finger pokes and injections. Naming the meter and decorating it with stickers can take some of the fear out of the testing procedure. Injections should not be called "shots," because children may confuse this with the shot of a gun.

Appetite may become erratic in toddlers when rapid growth begins to subside. Food can become problematic for parents and caretakers. If a toddler will not eat, favorite foods or alternatives can be offered, but parents should avoid becoming short-order cooks for a demanding toddler. A basal-bolus regimen, adjusting insulin for food intake, and giving insulin immediately after consumption of food may work best. Insulin infusion therapy is also an option in this age group. Normal activity in toddlers is sporadic and spontaneous, interspersed with sudden bursts of whole body movement. To prevent hypoglycemia, activity needs to be balanced with extra food or beverages such as milk or juice.

Hypoglycemia is a constant fear for parents of infants and toddlers with diabetes. Parents must rely on frequent blood glucose monitoring to distinguish normal infant and toddler behaviors from symptoms of hypoglycemia. Infants and toddlers are often defiant, demanding, sleepy, or cranky as part of their normal development. Temper tantrums cannot be ignored until hypoglycemia has been ruled out with a blood test.

Psychosocial Issues: Preschool Years

The preschool years are from ages 3 to 5. Physical growth slows after the toddler stage but is still relatively rapid. Development of fine motor skills continues, and cognitive language is rapid. Children engage in magical thinking: they believe that if they think or wish something, they can cause it to happen. Separation-individuation continues as children learn to distinguish themselves as separate from their parents. Body integrity and confidence in their ability to accomplish tasks are important. Fear of intrusive procedures is characteristic of this age, and children may act out their anxieties when insulin injections and blood testing are done. The use of adhesive bandages is helpful to the preschool child and helps address concerns about body integrity. Even though they often lack the fine motor skills, cognitive development, and impulse control to do diabetes management tasks independently, allowing preschoolers to do "bits and pieces" of procedures is important; examples include placing the meter and lancing device on the table or getting the syringe out of the box.

Preschoolers have difficulty understanding the need for insulin injections and blood tests, particularly if they are feeling well. Describing the need in terms of "keeping you healthy" fosters a positive outlook. Allowing the child to have some control by providing limited choices can be helpful; for example, asking "Do you want mashed potatoes or macaroni for dinner?" Preschoolers need positive reinforcement for cooperating with the regimen; this may include verbal praise and/or sticker charts. Diabetes management tasks should not be used as rewards or punishment.

Children establish a balance between their inner life and reality by continually exploring and testing through their play. Guided play, or play therapy, provides a forum and vehicle for children to express their concerns. Play therapy provides a mechanism for emotional release by helping the child learn to deal with these issues through creative expression. Giving a child a "safe" syringe, family and health professional dolls, a meter, and other diabetes supplies provides an opportunity for the child to play out personal life issues and concerns about having diabetes. A stuffed bear with colored patches for injections and finger pokes is useful for this and is available from the JDRF. Forms of artwork also help young children express themselves.

A preschool child's appetite may be erratic and is often unpredictable. Variability in eating is not considered harmful but, rather, normal from a developmental point of view. Children may eat only a few foods or may want the same item meal after meal; for example, children may want to eat only bananas and peanut butter for days at a time, and then they will switch to grilled cheese sandwiches and apples. These eating patterns typically last a few days or weeks. When treated casually, the behaviors are forgotten after a brief period. Increased appetites tend to precede growth spurts, and food intake is usually balanced over a period of weeks.[26] This erratic eating makes glucose stability difficult for this age group, and parents worry about hypoglycemia when their child will not eat. Parents can allow the child some control over eating by providing reasonable choices without allowing the child to control eating situations. By giving young children limited choices, parents may avoid a battle of wills.

Many preschool-aged children are able to identify symptoms of hypoglycemia and can at least alert adults that they do not feel well. This is especially important since many children are in preschool or day care settings at this age. Undetected hypoglycemia is still a risk in the preschool years and is especially worrisome to parents when their child is in the care of others.

The responsibility of caring for a young child with diabetes and the fear of hypoglycemia are extremely stressful for families. In 2-parent families, both parents should be involved in the day-to-day management of the child's diabetes. In single-parent families, the parent needs to identify others who can provide support and respite care. Healthcare providers can often assist parents in identifying support systems that can be helpful in easing the burden of care and avoiding parental burnout. Professional organizations such as the ADA and the JDRF and local organizations may be a source of support for families, not only those with young children but those with children of all ages.

Psychosocial Issues: School-Aged Children

A school-aged child (6-11 years old) is physically well coordinated, has a vivid fantasy life, speaks fluently, has a conscience, and is able to share and cooperate. The child has concrete reasoning and likes repetition, which is played out in sports, games, and skills. Although the school-aged child has an increasing need for independence, the power and protection of the parent are very important to the child's well-being. One of the greatest drives of school-aged children is to avoid failure. They acquire strategies to keep from feeling different from peers.

Young people with diabetes have a greater incidence of depression, anxiety and psychological distress compared to their peers without diabetes. This commonly occurs in the initial adjustment period after diagnosis or with the end of the honeymoon period, when children come to realize that the disease will not go away and that it is more difficult to manage. When depression persists it can have a negative impact on diabetes self management. Intervention should be initiated early and be a part of follow-up care.[27] Support groups, individual counseling, or diabetes camps can also be useful in assisting the child in resolving these feelings. Chapter 4 provides more information on depression and anxiety in the child with diabetes.

Parent and Child Roles in Diabetes Management

The parent's role in diabetes management is to perform diabetes care tasks while moving the child toward independence through supervision, encouragement, and support. At times, the child may be willing and able to perform blood glucose monitoring, prepare his or her own snacks, and administer insulin (and may do so with supervision). At other times, a parent will need to perform the test or administer insulin. Parent-child sharing of these responsibilities is essential during the school-age years and beyond. When a child is given more responsibility for their diabetes management than they are ready to assume, metabolic stability may suffer. Parents of the school-aged child with diabetes may be more protective than other parents. Although this is understandable, this attitude can make it difficult for the child with diabetes to attain the same level of independence as a child of the same age without diabetes. Diabetes management planning for special events and activities is important to promote independence and minimize differences. By planning ahead, most children with diabetes can safely participate in all childhood activities.

Monitoring, assessing sensor values, eating special snacks, taking injections, and fearing that peers will witness symptoms of hypoglycemia can alter diabetes self-care routines and ultimately affect self-esteem. Helping the child fit diabetes management into normal routines both at home and at school can minimize feelings of being different. For example, a snack break can be implemented for all children in the classroom. Children who need to check their glucose in the classroom should be able to do so. However, school policies vary, and not all schools allow blood glucose testing in the classroom. Some are concerned about other children coming into contact with another student's blood and the school's liability if the blood test result is not reported correctly. Children should carry a source of fast-acting carbohydrate with them at all times and need to be able to treat hypoglycemia in the classroom. An adult or other student should accompany the student with diabetes to the clinic if the student is not feeling well.

Blood glucose values are often seen as "good" or "bad," and a child's level of stability can also affect self-esteem. Because of their desire to please adults and their fear of failure, school-aged children sometimes falsify blood glucose results or report results when tests were omitted. When a child's A1C result is incompatible with the day-to-day glucose testing results, there is a high level of suspicion that this is occurring.

Care in School Settings

Because school-aged children spend a large portion of their day in school, expecting school personnel to become informed about diabetes care is reasonable. The school can either present significant challenges or be a source of support to the child with diabetes.[6] This topic is well covered in the ADA's position statement on diabetes care in the school and day care settings[7] and in another publication, Helping the Student With Diabetes Succeed: A Guide for School Personnel, by the National Diabetes Education Program, which is available on the Internet (https://niddk.nih.gov/health-information/communication-programs/ndep/health-professionals/helping-student-diabetes-succeed-guide-school-personnel). School districts and personnel are obligated to provide an individualized plan to accommodate a child's special healthcare needs. Certain federal laws address these issues. The Education for All Handicapped Act of 1975, commonly referred to as Public Law No. 94-142, is a federal mandate that entitles all physically, developmentally, emotionally, and other health-impaired children to free, appropriate public education.[48] Any school that receives federal funding or a facility that is considered open to the public must reasonably accommodate the special needs of children with diabetes.[48] The other law, Section 504, is a more general civil rights law that makes it illegal for any agency or organization that receives federal funds to discriminate in any way against qualified people with disabilities.[48] See the sidebar summarizing key points on facilitating appropriate diabetes care in school settings.

The current standards for diabetes management reflect the need to maintain glucose stability as near to normal as safely possible. To achieve this level of stability, many children will be on intensified management. Intensified therapy requires the following:

1. 1 to 3 blood glucose checks during the school day, or the use of a CGM
2. insulin administration by injection or infusion pump
3. attention to food intake and carbohydrate content of foods, and
4. knowledgeable school staff to observe for and treat hypoglycemia. This requires flexibility and close communication among the child, parents, school personnel, and the healthcare team.

Each school year should begin with a conference involving the child with diabetes, his or her parents, and school personnel to establish a plan of care, communication, and a means of addressing important issues and concerns.

Key Points on Arranging Diabetes Care in School Settings

Information from parent. Parents need to provide the school with basic information about diabetes, the causes of hypoglycemia, the specific requirements of their child's daily management plan, and their child's usual signs and symptoms of hypoglycemia and hyperglycemia.

Plan of care. The information provided by the parents is used to develop a plan of care that satisfies the needs of the child, the child's parents, and school policies.[26] This written plan includes who will administer the care, the location of the supplies, and where the treatment will take place in the school setting.

Glucagon administration. The administration of glucagon must be provided if recommended by the student's healthcare provider.[7] When an order is issued by the healthcare provider, the school must designate a person to administer glucagon in the written plan of care.

Scheduling changes. When scheduling changes occur in the daily school routine (eg, field trips or parties), the school needs to notify parents prior to the event so appropriate care can be administered or arranged. However, parents cannot be required to attend all field trips.

Meal plan. A review of the food/meal plan basics provides school personnel with a general awareness of what the child eats. Providing a plan to enable the child to manage parties and snacks in school is also beneficial.[45] Some instruction on carbohydrate counting will be necessary if the student is using an insulin-to-carbohydrate ratio for calculating the insulin dose for lunch and snacks.

Psychosocial Issues: Adolescence

There are many differences in behavior and development between early, middle, and late adolescence, the time between 12 and 21 years of age. Characteristics of each of these 3 stages are outlined in Table 14.4.

Adolescence is a period of rapid biological change and increasing physical, cognitive, and emotional maturity. These changes may occur slowly or rapidly and are determined by genetic factors, the economy, nutrition, health, and habitat.

Identity and self-image concerns can revolve around diabetes concerns such as the appearance of the injection site or self-identification as "a diabetic." Normal independence issues may be thwarted as a result of parental protectiveness or the teen's failure to assume responsibility for self-care. Adolescents with diabetes can become particularly concerned about their physical growth and sexual maturation even though they usually display normal growth patterns and normal onset and progression of pubertal development.

TABLE 14.4 Developmental Characteristics at Each Stage of Adolescence

Early adolescence, 11–13 years old:
The child becomes acutely aware of body image
Dependent versus independent struggles begin between parent and child
There may be great vacillation between childlike and adult behaviors
There is less social involvement with family and more with peers
Parental criticism becomes difficult to accept
Turmoil and conflict within the parent-child relationship may begin
Middle adolescence, 14–18 years old:
Peer group allegiance develops
Greater experimentation and risk taking occur
Physical and social activity increases
Opposite-sex relationships emerge and are important
Formal operational thinking begins along with abstract reasoning
Late adolescence, 19–21 years old:
Teens and parents experience conflict in their relationship
Cognitive abilities and abstract morals develop
The peer group loses its primary importance
There is increasing separation from the family unit
Teens become future oriented
Conscience can stand without support or validity from others

Source: M Grey, ME Cameron, TH Lipman, et al, "Psychosocial status of children with diabetes in the first 2 years after diagnosis," *Diabetes Care* 18 (1995): 1330-6.

Metabolic stability tends to deteriorate in adolescence. Attitudes of experimentation and rebellion and risk-taking behaviors normally associated with adolescence can affect diabetes issues such as taking insulin regularly, monitoring, and the quality and quantity of food consumption.

Risky Behaviors

Healthcare providers must be aware of and address issues of substance abuse (tobacco, alcohol, and drug use), use of steroids or other supplements to enhance muscle growth, and sexual practices and attitudes in their assessment of adolescent diabetes management. Risk taking and lack of health-promoting behaviors are widespread. Alcohol use can result in severe hypoglycemia several hours after drinking if adequate food is not ingested. Some individuals may need to lower their basal insulin through the night. Alcohol can also affect judgment and impair an individual's ability to recognize and adequately treat the symptoms of hypoglycemia.

Eating Habits

Food intake becomes less consistent due to issues such as participation in athletics, busier schedules, preoccupation with body weight and/or appearance, and the search for self-identity. Proper eating habits are still important to ensure continued growth and development and to develop good practices over the lifetime. Adolescents give low priority to their nutritional needs regarding recommended amounts and types of food. Typical food-related behaviors include skipping meals, eating away from home, experimenting with fad diets, and attempting to change their weight.[45] Educating adolescents, especially boys, about the effect of poor metabolic stability on growth can sometimes be a motivating factor for improving management.

Issues Involving Reproductive Health

Issues of sexuality, sexual functioning, and reproductive health should be addressed with teens and young adults, as well as adults, in a relaxed, comfortable manner. Reproductive health must be discussed with those of childbearing age. Comfort in discussing sexual topics comes with practice and a sense of control over the subject matter. The comfort level of the healthcare provider is communicated to the person with diabetes and sets the tone for discussions. Sex education should begin in the preteen years so that it becomes a routine part of diabetes assessment and education. Use of unbiased, gender-neutral language is important when assessing sexual orientation, practice, frequency, use of contraceptives, and consistency of contraceptive practices.

Females with diabetes must be taught the importance of planning pregnancy and meticulously using contraception to avoid an unwanted pregnancy. Their instruction should include a frank dialogue about the potential fetal/maternal health risks of an unplanned pregnancy in a woman with diabetes.(See chapter 24, on pregnancy.)

Females may experience vaginal candidiasis, especially if glucose levels are less than optimal. Males may have concerns about sexual dysfunction, since this is a fairly common complication in adults with diabetes. Discussing this with them can sometimes be a motivating factor to strive for good management. Teens should be reminded that abstinence is the only 100% effective contraceptive method for preventing pregnancy, sexually transmitted diseases (STDs), and acquired immune deficiency syndrome (AIDS). They need to be taught that use of a condom during sexual activity will help prevent STDs and AIDS, but it is not the most effective method of preventing pregnancy. Table 25.7, in chapter 24, summarizes the efficacy and safety of female contraceptive methods for those with diabetes.

Case—Part 5: Acute Complications: Hypoglycemia and DKA

JJ was never hospitalized again in DKA. He did, however, experience one nocturnal hypoglycemic seizure, at the age of 13, after a very active day of skiing.

Conditions Associated With Glucose Levels Above Target and/or Poor Health Outcomes[26]

- Biologically, the adolescent's heightened insulin resistance combined with earlier and greater epinephrine responses to drops in blood glucose concentrations may contribute to some of the lability in metabolic stability.
- Adolescent rebellion/experimentation, a chaotic home environment, chronic family stress, parent-child conflicts, and degree of parental involvement can contribute to poor metabolic stability for children and adolescents. While adolescents can perform the tasks necessary for diabetes management, they may not always follow the treatment regimen and may still need help making decisions about insulin dose adjustments. Adolescents whose parents maintain some guidance and supervision in the management of diabetes have better metabolic stability.[43,47]
- Developmental delays or learning disabilities in either the adolescent child or a parent may hamper understanding of diabetes care and thus self-management.
- Emotional disturbance can cause disequilibrium and precipitate frequent episodes of DKA. Insulin insufficiency may occur by insulin omission, pump malfunction, intentional disconnection from pump, or in response to physical or emotional stress, resulting in overproduction of counterregulatory hormones.[43] Repeated episodes of DKA warrant investigation, as DKA can be deliberately induced to displace family tensions. Family patterns of interaction may reveal family enmeshment, rigidity, poor communication, and overprotectiveness.[48] Treatment may include family counseling and aggressive insulin therapy when illness, stress, or ketones appear. Adolescents sometimes develop DKA because they fail to take their insulin. Insulin doses can be missed when parents are not involved in an adolescent's diabetes management.[48,49]
- Adolescents and adults may decide to skip injections for the purpose of weight management, which is a variant of an eating disorder. This most often occurs in females but can also occur in males. Diabetes and the treatment regimen may provide the right conditions for those who are at risk of developing an eating disorder because of the focus on food and discipline required. Healthcare providers need to be aware of the possibility of pathologic eating behaviors, particularly among adolescent and young adult females.
- Needle anxiety occurs in almost everyone to some degree. If this anxiety is severe or persistent and left unresolved, diabetes stability may suffer because of missed injections, inadequate testing, and avoidance of healthcare follow-up visits. When a parent has needle fears, the child will most likely have the same fears. Any person with diabetes who has a persistently high A1C should be evaluated for needle phobias. Desensitization therapy, biofeedback, assistance with relaxation, distraction, and use of an automatic injector (Inject-Ease® or similar device) have proven helpful.[50]

TABLE 14.5 Safe Driving for Persons With Diabetes

Issues to Discuss:
Practicing responsible diabetes self-care
Considering the safety of self and others
Monitoring blood glucose levels before driving
Stopping to check blood glucose at 2-hour intervals while driving
Carrying appropriate supplies, including fast-acting carbohydrates
Wearing a medical ID
Never driving with signs or symptoms of hypoglycemia

Source: JB Roemer, T McGee, "Type 1 diabetes in youth," in MJ Franz, ed., *A Core Curriculum for Diabetes Education: Diabetes Management Therapies*, 5th ed (Chicago: American Association of Diabetes Educators, 2003), 36-7.

Driver Safety

Driving is a serious adult responsibility that can be given as a privilege to teens. The use of appropriate self-care skills and safety precautions must be taught and reinforced in teens and adults who drive themselves to school or work or otherwise operate a motorized vehicle. Healthcare professionals and parents of teens who are approaching legal driving age should begin discussions with the teen about the responsibility of safety when driving. Students heading off to college with a car should be frequently reminded to drive responsibly and take the self-care steps necessary to ensure safety of the driver, passengers, and those on the road. Guidelines for safety while driving are summarized in Table 14.5.

Hypoglycemia

The fear of hypoglycemia is one of the major barriers to achieving optimal glycemic levels for all individuals with diabetes, and it is one of the biggest fears for parents of children with diabetes. The definition of hypoglycemia is typically recognized as a blood glucose level less than 70 mg/dL (3.86 mmol/L), but studies have shown cognitive impairment at blood glucose concentrations of less than 60 mg/dL (3.3 mmol/L).[28] Mental function is reduced somewhat during the acute phase of hypoglycemia, and sometimes this persists beyond the acute phase. Hypoglycemia that interferes with normal thinking can make schoolwork difficult. It also makes riding a bicycle, driving a car, or operating machinery dangerous. While diabetes itself is not associated with cognitive deficits, some investigations have found an increase in cognitive dysfunction in individuals who have experienced repeated or prolonged episodes or severe hypoglycemia before the age of 5 years.[29]

Glycemic goals are higher for children under 5 years of age because of the deleterious effects of hypoglycemia in this age group.

Hypoglycemia is more frequent in individuals with lower A1C levels, a prior history of severe hypoglycemia, or higher insulin doses and in younger children.[29]

Frequent hypoglycemia, even if it is mild, can cause hunger and overeating, thus contributing to excessive weight gain and subsequent hyperglycemia. Repeated episodes of hypoglycemia or long diabetes duration may result in abnormality of the counterregulatory system and loss of adrenergic symptoms, leading to hypoglycemia unawareness. Frequent blood glucose monitoring is necessary to avoid recurrent episodes.

Hypoglycemia can be categorized according to severity. The precise blood glucose level at which persons with diabetes develop symptoms or the level at which they experience a mild, moderate, or severe hypoglycemic episode is difficult to define. Symptoms generally occur when the blood glucose is less than 60 mg/dL (3.3 mmol/L).

Mild Hypoglycemia

Mild hypoglycemia is associated with mild adrenergic symptoms (sweating, pallor, palpitations, and tremors) and occasionally mild neuroglycopenic symptoms (headache and behavior change). Except in infants and toddlers, these can usually be self-treated with 10 to 15 g of easily absorbed carbohydrate, such as 3 to 4 glucose tablets or 4 oz of juice or regular soda. Additional intake of a more complex carbohydrate may be necessary, depending on timing for the next meal or snack. Treatment is individualized, and most individuals learn what and how much works best for them. Excessive intake should be avoided.

Moderate Hypoglycemia

Moderate hypoglycemia requires that someone else help with treatment, but the treatment can be administered orally. Typical symptoms are aggressiveness, drowsiness, and confusion. Usually, at least 15 to 30 g of an easily absorbed glucose in a gel form is required, with an additional snack to follow.

Severe Hypoglycemia

Severe hypoglycemia is associated with altered states of consciousness, including coma or seizure, and requires treatment with glucagon or intravenous glucose.[56] Glucagon may be required when the person with diabetes cannot safely swallow, is combatant to efforts to intervene, or is

TABLE 14.6 Recommended Doses for Glucagon

Adults and children >20 kg	*Children <20 kg*
1 mg subcutaneously (SQ) or intramuscularly (IM)*	0.5 mg SQ or IM or 20–30 mcg per kilogram (9.1–13.6 mcg per pound) of body weight*

*If necessary, the dose may be repeated after 15 minutes.

Source: HP Chase, D Maahs, "Hypoglycemia," in *Understanding Diabetes*, 13th ed (Denver, Colo: Paros Press, 2015).

unable to cooperate with treatment. Doses for infants and children are significantly different from those for adults. Table 14.6 lists recommended doses. Glucagon can be given intramuscularly or subcutaneously in the deltoid or anterior thigh region. Parents, roommates, spouses, and significant others should be taught how to mix, draw up, and administer glucagon. Stabilized glucagon solutions are now available with improved delivery systems such as nasal delivery or autoinjector. These should be considered and discussed with healthcare providers.

Following a hypoglycemic episode, the plasma glucose threshold for autonomic activation is lowered, thus increasing the potential for further hypoglycemic events. Any severe episode of hypoglycemia should be reported to the healthcare provider so that changes in therapy can be made when indicated.

A reasonable individualized glycemic goal is the lowest A1C that does not cause severe hypoglycemia and preserves awareness of hypoglycemia, preferably with little or no symptomatic or even asymptomatic hypoglycemia. The selection of a glycemic goal should be linked to the risk of hypoglycemia.[57]

Also see the section on hypoglycemia in chapter 17, Pharmacotherapy for Glucose Management.

Case—Part 6: Associated Autoimmune Disorders

When he was 11 years old, JJ was diagnosed with hypothyroidism on a routine screening test. He denied symptoms (fatigue, dry skin, constipation), his physical exam did not reveal thyromegaly, and his linear growth was normal. He was started on thyroid replacement therapy. At age 13, he was diagnosed with celiac disease after 2 positive TG antibodies, which was confirmed by a gastroenterologist via a small-bowel biopsy. JJ also had no symptoms of celiac disease.

The dietitian instructed JJ and his parents on a gluten-free diet. The diagnosis of another chronic illness can be difficult for persons with diabetes and their families. The affected individual often feels that his or her entire body is failing. This may be especially difficult for adolescents, who are working to develop a strong sense of identity.

Diabetic Ketoacidosis

Diabetic ketoacidosis is a result of insulin deficiency leading to hyperglycemia, an accumulation of ketone bodies in the blood, dehydration, and subsequent metabolic acidosis. Diabetic ketoacidosis is potentially a life-threatening emergency and occurs in a variety of circumstances. Approximately 25% of children with new-onset diabetes present in ketoacidosis.[8] In the person with known diabetes, the most common cause is omitted insulin injections or mismanagement of insulin infusion therapy. Diabetic ketoacidosis also results when inadequate dose adjustments are made for intercurrent illnesses, trauma, surgery, or other physiological stress. Recurrent episodes of DKA in the child or adolescent/adult are frequently due to insulin omission. These persons with diabetes have a higher incidence of psychiatric illness, especially depression, and are more likely to omit insulin, come from single-parent homes, and be underinsured than their peers.[30]

Because of the significant morbidity and mortality associated with DKA, prevention is of paramount importance. Prevention can be achieved by the following:

- Public awareness of the signs and symptoms of untreated diabetes
- Education of friends, roommates, and other caregivers about the signs and symptoms of early DKA
- Increased recognition that insulin omission due to psychological problems and lack of financial resources is the most common cause of DKA in persons with established diabetes
- Improved detection of families at risk
- Education about ketone monitoring
- 24-hour telephone availability and encouragement to contact the healthcare team when blood glucose levels are high, when there is ketonuria or ketonemia, and especially during intercurrent illnesses[6]

Chapter 23 provides detailed information on hyperglycemia.

Associated Autoimmune Disorders

There are several autoimmune disorders associated with type 1 diabetes.

Thyroid Disorders

Thyroid disorders are the most common autoimmune disorder associated with type 1 diabetes, with an incidence of about 17%. Persons with thyroid autoimmunity may be euthyroid, hypothyroid (most common), or hyperthyroid.[31]

Individuals with type 1 diabetes should be screened for autoimmune thyroid disease shortly after diabetes diagnosis, when metabolic stability has been established. Thyroid antibodies are measured to identify thyroid autoimmunity and persons at risk for developing thyroid disease. Measurement of thyroid-stimulating hormone (TSH) may be the most sensitive way to identify persons with thyroid dysfunction. Subclinical hypothyroidism has been associated with an increased risk of symptomatic hypoglycemia and with reduced linear growth. Persons with elevated TSH levels should be treated with thyroid replacement therapy. Persons with a normal TSH who have no thyromegaly or growth abnormality should be screened every 1 to 2 years.[6]

Celiac Disease

Celiac disease is an immune-mediated disorder that is also more common in individuals with type 1 diabetes, with a prevalence of 1% to 16%.[32]

Individuals with type 1 diabetes should be screened for celiac disease by measuring tissue transglutaminase or antiendomysial antibodies, with documentation of normal serum IgA levels, soon after the diagnosis of diabetes. Testing should be repeated if growth failure, failure to gain weight, weight loss, or gastroenterolic symptoms occur. Consideration should be given to periodic rescreening of asymptomatic individuals.[7] In individuals with gluten intolerance, immune-mediated damage to the mucosa of the small intestine occurs after exposure to gluten, leading to destruction of the villi of the small intestine. Symptoms of celiac disease include diarrhea, constipation, weight loss or poor weight gain, growth failure, abdominal pain, chronic fatigue, irritability, an inability to concentrate, malnutrition due to malabsorption, and other gastrointestinal problems. In individuals with diabetes, the maldigestion and malabsorption of nutrients, vitamins, and minerals in the gastrointestinal tract may lead to unpredictable blood glucose levels, unexplained hypoglycemia, and deterioration in glycemic stability. Although positive antibody test results can be supportive of a diagnosis, a small intestinal biopsy is the gold standard for the diagnosis of celiac disease.[32] Individuals with confirmed celiac disease should be provided guidance so that they are able to follow a gluten-free diet to prevent unexpected hypoglycemia due to absorptive abnormalities and to prevent the other nutritional, metabolic, and oncologic consequences of celiac disease.[6]

There are no controlled trials to guide recommendations for asymptomatic individuals with elevated autoantibody levels and normal small-bowel biopsies.

Case—Part 7: Ongoing Care

JJ's most recent A1C was 6.9%. Over the years, he has had regular quarterly visits, and his parents have always been involved in his care. His most recent eye exam was normal, as were his urine microalbumin excretion tests. He is successfully using continuous insulin infusion therapy and has experienced infrequent hypoglycemia. He has been following a gluten-free diet. Since starting college, he has experienced some depression and has been taking an antidepressant.

Ongoing Care

Individuals with type 1 diabetes should see their diabetes healthcare provider every 3 months for evaluation of therapy and ongoing education. Studies suggest that delivery of intensive diabetes care management, telephone availability of the healthcare team, and regular in-person care improve A1C and decrease hospitalizations.[7]

Knowledge and skills of the person with diabetes should be evaluated regularly by a diabetes care and education specialist. Frequency of hypoglycemia and the presence of hypoglycemia unawareness should be assessed at every visit. If hypoglycemia unawareness is present, blood glucose targets should be reassessed and continuous glucose monitoring may be an appropriate recommendation. For children, height and weight measurements are essential and should be plotted on growth charts at each visit. Poor diabetes management can lead to poor linear growth and poor weight gain, as well as a delay in pubertal and skeletal maturation. Poor growth with adequate metabolic stability should raise suspicion of hypothyroidism or celiac disease.

Quarterly Follow-Up With Healthcare Provider

- Each quarterly follow-up visit with the healthcare provider should include the following:[7] Height, weight, and BMI calculation (and comparison with age- and sex-specific norms)
- Blood pressure determination (and comparison with age-, sex-, and height-related norms)[33]
- A1C determination
- Evaluation of results of blood glucose monitoring, ketone testing, and person with diabetes' use of data
- Physical examination with specific emphasis on injection or pump sites (lipoatrophy or lipohypertrophy) and finger or alternative sites for blood glucose testing; physical examination should also

include funduscopic, oral, cardiac, abdominal (hepatosplenomegaly), hand/finger, foot, skin (acanthosis nigricans, necrobiosis lipoidica diabeticorum), and neurological examinations

- Interval history should include recent or current infections or illnesses; current or recent use of medications; frequency and treatment of hypoglycemia; presence of hypoglycemia unawareness; physical activity and exercise habits; meal plan; psychosocial factors that may influence diabetes management; use of tobacco, alcohol, and/or recreational drugs; and contraception and sexual activity (if applicable)
- Review of symptoms should include gastrointestinal function (including symptoms of gluten intolerance) and symptoms of other endocrine disorders, especially thyroid and Addison disease
- Assessment of knowledge, skills, and coping level with referral to appropriate diabetes healthcare provider (diabetes nurse educator, dietitian, behavioral specialist) for intervention
- Assessment of emergency preparedness, including availability of glucagon to parents, roommates, and significant others knowledgeable about administering it; wearing of diabetes identification (wallet cards are not adequate); testing before driving, and the availability of a source of glucose in the car; for those living alone, identification of someone to check in if the individual fails to show for work or school

A plan for continuity of care is critical for successful transition. Adolescents leaving their pediatric team and starting afresh with a new physician and new team were more likely to be hospitalized for DKA than those whose adult team included some of the members of their pediatric team.[66]

Care management and coordination could help with the transition process so that the adolescent young adult does not get lost to follow-up and care during this process.

Yearly Assessments and Screenings

- Ophthalmologic evaluation: Starting at 10 years of age with diabetes duration of 3 to 5 years[6]
- Microalbuminuria: Starting at 10 years of age with diabetes duration of 5 years[6]
- Lipid profile: Starting at 2 years of age if positive or unknown family history for cardiovascular disease; starting at puberty if family history is negative
- Celiac and adrenal antibodies, TSH: Every 1 to 2 years (more frequently if symptomatic or poor growth)
- Depression screening: Starting at 10 years of age
- Diabetes nurse educator and dietitian: Yearly visit is the minimum; many individuals may benefit from this quarterly or even more frequently, especially during the first year of diagnosis
- Behavioral specialist: To enhance support and empowerment, to identify and discuss ways to overcome barriers in successful diabetes management, and, in pediatrics, to maintain family involvement in diabetes care tasks[6]

Vaccinations

Children and adults with type 1 diabetes should receive all immunizations in accordance with the recommendations of the Centers for Disease Control and Prevention. This includes the annual influenza vaccine and a one-time pneumococcal polysaccharide vaccine to all individuals with diabetes over 2 years of age. A one-time revaccination is recommended for individuals over 64 years of age who were previously immunized when they were less than 65 years of age if the vaccine was administered more than 5 years ago.[7] Large studies have shown no causal relationship between childhood vaccination and type 1 diabetes.

Transition to Adult Care

Adolescents growing into young adulthood need to transfer from pediatric to adult diabetes providers at a time determined by the individual with diabetes, the family, the pediatric diabetes team, and the adult care providers. The developmental stage from the late teens through the 20s has been defined as "emerging adulthood," a period of significant competing educational, social, work, and financial priorities. As young adults with Type 1 diabetes experience competing life priorities and decreased parental support, engagement with regimens and glycemic management sometimes declines.[34] The transition from a pediatric to an adult-orientated service should not involve a sudden unanticipated transfer but an organized process of preparation and adaptation. The appropriate age for transfer from a pediatric or adolescent service to adult care varies depending on the maturity of the adolescent, preferences of the person with diabetes and family preferences, and the availability of appropriate services for the young person in an adult clinic.[35]

Primary Treatment Goals for All Individuals With Type 1 Diabetes

- To achieve optimal glycemic goals with a flexible, individualized diabetes management plan
- To avoid severe hypoglycemia, symptomatic hyperglycemia, and ketoacidosis
- To promote and maintain day-to-day clinical and psychological well-being[1]

Adults newly diagnosed with diabetes often employ a basal-bolus regimen, using a long-acting insulin plus a rapid-acting insulin before meals. Adults, on average, require between 0.4 and 1.0 units per kilogram per day.[1]

Type 1 Diabetes in Adults

Although type 1 diabetes is most frequently diagnosed in children, 30% to 50% of people are diagnosed over the age of 30, and the diagnosis can occur at any age. When diabetes is diagnosed in adults, differentiating type 1 diabetes from type 2 diabetes is sometimes more difficult. One way to identify the person with the autoimmune type of diabetes (type 1) versus the insulin-resistant form (type 2) is to look for the presence or absence of islet autoantibodies. Laboratory markers of immune destruction of the beta cell include islet cell autoantibodies, autoantibodies to glutamic acid decarboxylase (GAD), tyrosine phosphatase–related islet antigen 2, and insulin autoantibodies. One and usually more of these autoantibodies are present in 85% to 90% of individuals when fasting hyperglycemia is initially detected.[36]

See chapter 13, on pathophysiology, for a more in-depth discussion on latent autoimmune diabetes in adults (LADA).

The rate of beta cell destruction can be rapid in some adults (as it almost always is in infants and children) and slow in others. While some authors differentiate rapid-onset type 1 diabetes in adults from LADA, most clinicians now recognize the term *LADA* to describe the adult form of type 1 diabetes. Adults with LADA have similar human leukocyte antigen genetic susceptibility as well as autoantibodies to islet antigens. However, they may retain sufficient residual beta cell function so that treatment of their diabetes does not require insulin initially, and they appear to be clinically affected by type 2 diabetes. Adults with LADA usually require insulin for survival after about 6 years, and they are at risk for ketoacidosis at that time. At this latter stage of the disease, there is little or no insulin secretion, as manifested by low or undetectable levels of plasma C-peptide.[7]

Associated Autoimmune Disorders

Adults with type 1 diabetes are also prone to other autoimmune disorders, such as Graves disease, Hashimoto thyroiditis, Addison disease, vitiligo, celiac sprue, autoimmune hepatitis, myasthenia gravis, and pernicious anemia.[37] In one study, the proportion of persons with diabetes testing negative for all autoantibodies was lower among the children than among the adults. The adults were characterized by a higher proportion of males, a longer duration of symptoms, and a lower frequency of infections during the preceding 3 months.

Clinical Presentation

The clinical presentation of adults with rapid-onset type 1 diabetes and the initial management of their diabetes and treatment with insulin are similar to the presentation and management of children with new-onset diabetes, as discussed earlier in this chapter. The clinical presentation of the adult with LADA may include the following:

- Lean body mass
- Family history of type 1 diabetes or autoimmune disease
- Age over 35 years

Diagnosis

In addition to the usual glucose diagnostic tests, the clinician may want to measure anti-GAD antibodies; if positive, this confirms the diagnosis of LADA. Subsequent measurement of C-peptide can delineate progression to insulin dependency. Attention should be paid to diagnose such individuals because therapy may influence the speed of progression toward insulin dependency, and in this respect, efforts should be made to protect residual C-peptide secretion.

Treatment[38]

No specific guidelines for management of LADA currently exist, but treatment to achieve normoglycemia to prevent complications is warranted. Most individuals with LADA become insulin dependent within 6 to 8 years, and many clinicians progress to insulin sooner rather than later, although in the initial stages, LADA can be managed with therapies used for type 2 diabetes.

Summary

Type 1 diabetes is not just a disease of the very young. It affects people throughout the life span and presents many challenges to both the person with diabetes and the family and friends of that person. The self-management behaviors and skill sets required to be successful and effective are very demanding, and this is in addition to the issues and stages that an individual goes through as he or she ages. It is important to not only make normal physical growth and development a goal for this population, but also address emotional growth and development. In addition, self-management depends on socioeconomic support as well as emotional and physical support. Wishing to participate in intensive management but not being able to afford the supplies needed may be one of many barriers the individual with type 1 or type 2 diabetes and the family will face. More and more people with type 1 diabetes are reaching senior age and qualifying for Medicare and must learn to navigate the requirements for Medicare reimbursement. Seniors with type 1 diabetes face all the challenges of advancing age with the added complications of type 1 diabetes, such as labile glucose levels. Focusing only on blood glucose values and judging blood glucose numbers as "good" or "bad" will only lead to resentment and can affect self-esteem. The diabetes care and education specialist is a very important part of the diabetes care team and plays a crucial role in helping families cope with the many anticipated and unanticipated events and changes that occur.

Focus on Education

Teaching Strategies

Individualize self-management teaching plans and approaches. There is no *one* right way to provide DSME in type 1 diabetes, whether working with children or adults. Focus on the "need to know" and "need to do" first. Build on practical and essential daily function needs to keep glucose levels within desirable ranges.

Focus on the person with diabetes' needs and expectations. Assess what is the most difficult daily diabetes management task. Explore reasonable solutions to the most challenging tasks so that they come as routine. Evaluate the accomplishments in successful problem solving.

Provide age-appropriate clinical therapies and care. Healthy growth, nutritional needs, and lifestyle trends need to be evaluated on an ongoing basis. Allow for a healthy relationship with food and diabetes self-care to develop.

Collaborate with family members to build needed assistance or support in care. Whether it's a child, an adolescent, or an adult, each age group has a different support network. An infant, toddler, preschooler, older elementary child, early adolescent, or later adolescent is able to do different tasks at different stages. Parental involvement varies at different stages, and normal characteristics in the development of young children must be considered when determining needs and self-management strategies.

Respect that all persons have different desires, needs, and expectations. Flexibility, creativity, and options for different learning styles and ages are needed—for example, use of games and puppets for small children; demonstrations and media-based materials (videos, handheld and electronic games) for teens and young adults; and models, problem-solving discussions, and demonstrations for adults.

Teach the person to become the "expert." Coach children or adults to be the "expert" in their diabetes management. Assist them in planning a topic-specific presentation in their school or support group (in a safe environment). Include family and friends. This teaching activity reinforces information and may help self-esteem.

Messages for Persons With Diabetes

Knowledge is power. Learn as much as possible about taking care of diabetes. Attend classes offered through a local clinic or diabetes-affiliated organizations at every reasonable opportunity.

Change is inevitable. Expect that at different stages of life and in different situations glucose stability will change and require adjustments in how it is managed. The diabetes care and education specialist and care team will help with these unexpected or unanticipated events. Include your child with diabetes in care issues and teaching school personnel.

Diabetes is often unpredictable. Everything can be done "right," and still perfection is not achieved. Generally speaking, life is not perfect and often not predictable. The focus should not be on making life perfect and being in total stability; rather, it needs to be more about how to cope with change and how to prioritize effectively. The same thing may be handled differently, under a different circumstance. Keep on strategizing and reevaluating the ability to handle things on an ongoing basis.

Everyone needs support. Use friends, family, and your medical team for support. Ask for help; ask for necessities to achieve short- and long-term goals. Use the diabetes care and education specialist and the health team as consultants. Diabetes care needs to be flexible, dynamic, and individualized. There are many different ways to achieve optimal stability. If one method or plan does not work, try a different approach.

Utilize peer-to-peer social support networks. Sharing experiences with others can help both the person with diabetes and others. Other benefits may include learning effective and practical diabetes management strategies, validating assumptions, sharing successes, and getting others' perspectives on things. Everyone needs to be around peers and people who share similar interests.

Embrace yourself and your diabetes. Allow the challenges with diabetes to become opportunities. You can do what you desire in your life when managing diabetes. Remember that diabetes is manageable, and every day is a new day!

Health Literacy

Health literacy in pediatrics, young adults, and adults with type 1 diabetes varies greatly per multiple contributing factors. It means that different age groups understand information about health, know how to perform daily self-care, and make good decisions differently based on their age.

Everyone is at risk for low health literacy. Be careful not to make assumptions about health literacy levels on the basis of an individual's age, race, ethnicity, education, or income. Regardless of health literacy level, each individual should know where to get health information, understand the health information he or she finds, and apply the information to make good decisions about health.

Assess the attitude and belief system of the person with diabetes toward diabetes care. The following questions will help persons with diabetes explore their attitudes and focus on effective care:

- What is important to you about your diabetes?
- What would you like to be different about your diabetes?
- What is the most difficult thing for you about managing your diabetes on a daily basis?
- What can I do to help you accomplish your diabetes care goals?
- What are you going to do differently until I see you next time?
- How are you going to monitor your daily self-management?

Effective communication with persons with diabetes can minimize the challenge of health literacy:

- Avoid miscommunication by finding the right words to say, as well as the right questions to ask
- Take the time to assess recall and comprehension in all persons with diabetes
- Achieve true agreement with person with diabetes on goals and strategies to care for their diabetes
- Problem + Solution = Strategy
- Put a meaning to the numbers
- Use phrases to remember: simple, concrete, emotional
- Use real stories with real examples and demonstration/hands-on experience

Focus on Practice

Type 1 diabetes affects all ages; consequently, management and education are ongoing processes throughout an individual's life span. Healthcare professionals involved in care need to be specialized in clinical and age-appropriate behavioral therapies.

Clinical management of type 1 diabetes relies on person with diabetes and family self-management. Continuous reassessment of needs and the support network is part of ongoing DSME.

The primary goals for type 1 diabetes management in children include glycemic management, avoidance of acute and chronic complications, positive psychosocial adjustment to diabetes, and normal growth and development. The functionality of healthcare systems needs to provide access to the qualified healthcare team.

Situational problem solving needs to be incorporated into all interactions with persons with diabetes. Persons with diabetes need to know how to handle daily glucose management emergencies and learn from each experience. Proactive behaviors and attitudes need to be assessed on an ongoing basis.

Type 1 diabetes self-management requires ongoing care with careful consideration of multiple factors such as the following: state of the disease, age of person with diabetes, survival skills, glucose management, insulin taking, healthy eating, carbohydrate counting, activity, sports, hypoglycemia, appetite changes, bedtime, school, parties, friends, peer pressure, glucagon, driving, anxiety, depression, DKA, short-term versus long-term metabolic stability, thyroid disorders, celiac disease, ongoing care, screening, and vaccinations. Diabetes care and education specialists are instrumental in helping persons with diabetes maximize their potential in living a healthy and self-fulfilling life.

Make a paradigm shift to the empowerment model of care by learning to ask questions instead of offering advice. Time spent offering recommendations that are not relevant for persons with diabetes or will never be implemented is time wasted.

References

1. American Diabetes Association. Clinical practice recommendations 2016. Diabetes Care. 2016;39 Suppl 1:S13-22.
2. Dabelea D, Mayer-Davis EJ, Saydah S, et al. Prevalence of type 1 and type 2 diabetes among children and adolescents from 2001 to 2009. JAMA. 2014;311:1778-86.
3. Cho NH, Shaw JE, Karuranga S, et al. IDF diabetes atlas: global estimates of diabetes prevalence for 2017 and projections for 2045. Diabetes Res Clin Pract. 2018;138: 271-81.
4. Diabetes Control and Complications Trial Research Group. The effect of intensive treatment of diabetes on the development and progression of long-term complications in insulin-dependent diabetes mellitus: the Diabetes Control and Complications Trial Research Group. N Engl J Med. 1993;329:977-86.
5. The Epidemiology of Diabetes Interventions and Complications (EDIC) Study. Sustained effect of intensive treatment of type 1 diabetes mellitus on development and progression of diabetic nephropathy. JAMA. 2003;290:2159-67.
6. Chiang JL, Kirkman MS, Laffel LMB, Peters AL; on behalf of the Type 1 Diabetes Sourcebook authors. Type 1 diabetes through the life span: a position statement of the American Diabetes Association. Diabetes Care. 2014;37(7): 2034-54. On the Internet at: http://dx.doi.org/10.2337/dc14-1140.
7. Children and Adolescents: Standards of Medical Care in Diabetes—2019. American Diabetes Association. Diabetes Care 2019 Jan; 42 (Supplement 1): S148-S164. https://doi.org/10.2337/dc19-S013.
8. Dabelea D, Rewers A, Stafford JM, et al. Trends in the prevalence of ketoacidosis at diabetes diagnosis: the SEARCH for diabetes in youth study. Pediatris. 2014;133(4):e938-45.
9. Driscoll KA, Raymond J, Naranjo D, et al. Fear of hypoglycemia in children and adolescents and their parents with type 1 diabetes. Curr Diab Rep. 2016;16:77.
10. Kemmis K. Turning a vision into action in 2019 and beyond. AADE in Practice. Jan 2019;(7)1: 8-9.
11. American Association of Diabetes Educators. Diabetes Educator Guide to Blood Glucose Meter Selection and Monitoring for Accuracy and Safety. Chicago: American Association of Diabetes Educators; 2017:1-6.
12. Danne T, Nimri R, Battelino T, et al. International consensus on use of continuous glucose monitoring. Diabetes Care. 2017;40:1631-1640.
13. DiMeglio LA, Acerini CL, Codner E, et al. 2018 ISPAD Practice Consensus Guidelines: glycemic control targets and glucose monitoring for children, adolescents, and young adults with diabetes. Pediatr Diabetes. 2018:19(Suppl 27):105-14.
14. Deeb A, Yousef H, Abdelrahman L, et al. Implementation of a diabetes educator care model to reduce paediatric admission for diabetic ketoacidosis. J Diabetes Res. 2016;2:1-5.
15. American Association of Diabetes Educators. Subcutaneous Injection Guidelines for the Educations of Persons with Diabetes. Chicago: American Association of Diabetes Educators; 2019:1-6.
16. Frid AH, Kreugel G, Grassi G, et al. New insulin delivery recommendations. Mayo Clin Proc. 91(9):1231-55.
17. Danne T, Moshe P, Buckingham B. ISPAD Clinical Practice Consensus Guidelines 2018: Insulin treatment in children and adolescents with diabetes. Pediatr Diabetes. 2018;19(Suppl 27):115-35.
18. Edelman S. The un-tethered regimen. Children With Diabetes. Last reviewed 2010 Jan 6 (cited 2012 May). On the Internet at: http://www.childrenwithdiabetes.com/clinic/untethered.htm.
19. Smart, C Annan, F Higgins, L et al. ISPAD Clinical Practice Consensus Guidelines 2018: Nutritional management in children and adolescents with diabetes. Pediatr Diabetes 2018: 19(Suppl 27): 136-154.

20. American Association of Diabetes Educators. Healthy Eating. Chicago: American Association of Diabetes Educators; 2015:1-10.

21. Colberg SR, Sigal RJ, Yardley JE, et al. Physical activity/exercise and diabetes: a position statement of the America Diabetes Association. Diabetes Care. 2016 Nov;39(11):2065-79.

22. Galassetti P, Riddell MC. Exercise and Type 1 diabetes. Compr Physiol. 2013;3(3):1309-36.

23. Shetty V, Fournier P, Davey R, et al. Effect of exercise intensity on glucose requirements to maintain euglycemia during exercise in type 1 diabetes. J Clin Endocrinol Metab. 2016;101(3):972-80.

24. Taplin CE, Cobrye E, Messer L, et al. Preventing Post-exercise nocturnal hypoglycemia in children with type 1 diabetes. J Pediatr. 2010:157(5): 784-8.

25. Litchman ML, Walker HR, Ng AH, et al. State of the science: a scoping review and gap analysis of diabetes online communities. J Diabetes Sci Tech. 2019;13(3):466-92.

26. Satter E. Child of Mine: Feeding with Love and Good Sense, Boulder, CO: Bull Publishing Co; 2018:2-4.

27. Delamater A, deWit M, McDarby V. ISPAD Clinical Practice Consensus Guidelines 2018: psychological care of children and adolescents with type 1 diabetes. Pediatr Diabetes 2018;19(Suppl. 27):237-49.

28. Cameron F. Pediatr Clin N Am. 2015;62:911-27. http://dx.doi.org/10.1016/j.pcl.2015.04.003

29. Jones TW, ISPAD Hypoglycemia Guidelines Writing Group. Defining relevant hypoglycemia measures in children and adolescents with type 1 diabetes. Pediatr Diabetes. 2018; 19:354.

30. ISPAD Clinical Practice Consensus Guidelines 2018: Diabetic ketoacidosis and the hyperglycemic hyperosmolar state. Pediatric Diabetes. 2018 Oct;19(Suppl. 27):155-77.

31. Shun CB, Donaghue KC, Phelan H, Twigg SM, Craig ME. Thyroid autoimmunity in type 1 diabetes: systematic review and meta-analysis. Diabet Med. 2014;31:126-35.

32. Cohn A, Sofia A, Kupfer S. Type 1 Diabetes and Celiac Disease: Clinical Overlap and New Insights into Disease Pathogenesis. Curr Diab Rep. 2014 Aug;14(8):517. doi: 10.1007/s11892-014-0517-x.

33. Clinical Practice Guidelines for Screening and Management of High Blood Pressure in Children and Adolescents at https://pediatrics.aappublications.org/content/140/3/e20171904.

34. Peters A, Laffel L. Diabetes care for emerging adults: recommendations for transition from pediatric to adult diabetes care systems. Diabetes Care. 2011;34:2477-85.

35. Pihoker C, Forsander G, Fantahun B, et al. ISPAD Clinical Practice Consensus Guidelines 2018: the delivery of ambulatory diabetes care to children and adolescents with diabetes. Pediatr Diabetes. 2018 Oct;(Suppl 27):84-104.

36. O'Neal KS, Johnson JL, Panak RL. Recognizing and appropriately treating latent autoimmune diabetes in adults. Diabetes Spectrum. Nov 2016;29(4):249-52. DOI: 10.2337/ds15-0047.

37. Bao YK, Weide LG, Ganesan VC, et al. High prevalence of comorbid autoimmune diseases in adults with type 1 diabetes from the HealthFacts Database [published online September 18, 2018]. J Diabetes. doi:10.1111/1753-0407.12856.

38. Chiang JL, Maahs DM, Garvey KC, Hood KK, Laffel LM, Weinzimer SA, Wolfsdorf JI, Schatz D. Type 1 diabetes in children and adolescents: a position statement by the American Diabetes Association. Diabetes Care. Sep 2018;41(9):2026-44. DOI: 10.2337/dci18-0023.

CHAPTER 15

Type 2 Diabetes Throughout the Life Span

Eva M. Vivian, PharmD, MS, CDCES, BC-ADM, FADCES

Key Concepts

- Type 2 diabetes, while historically a disease affecting older individuals, is affecting children, teenagers, young adults, and older adults at alarming rates. Each age group has specific problems requiring unique and customized strategies.
- Risk factors for developing type 2 diabetes include ethnic background, family history, obesity, and a sedentary lifestyle.
- Type 2 diabetes is also associated with hypertension, hyperlipidemia, and cardiovascular disease. Other complications associated with this disease include diabetic retinopathy, painful neuropathy, and nephropathy.
- Treatment primarily consists of physical activity, healthy eating, and multiple medications, which present challenges to the diabetes care and education specialist, the individual with diabetes, and family.

Introduction

The discussion of type 2 diabetes across the life span begins with the concept of diabetes as a progressive disease. A case study is used to provide a brief overview of the pathophysiologic deficits and diagnostic criteria for type 2 diabetes. Next, treatment is discussed, using the clinical practice recommendations of the American Diabetes Association (ADA). The basic principles of care are then outlined for 2 age groups with numerous special considerations: (1) elderly adults and (2) children and adolescents. Similarities and differences in approaches to care for each of these age-specific populations are explored.

State of the Problem

Clinical Presentation

Type 2 diabetes is a disease characterized by hyperglycemia. The dual defects of insulin resistance, primarily at the cell receptor sites of muscle tissue, and a progressive decrease in insulin secretory capacity result in hyperglycemia.[1]

The deficiency of pancreatic beta cell function, which progresses over time, limits insulin production. Without adequate amounts of insulin to compensate for insulin resistance, the transportation of glucose from the bloodstream into the cell cannot occur. Insulin resistance and a reduction in insulin production and secretion are present in varying degrees, depending on the duration of the disease.

- *Phase 1:* The natural progression of type 2 diabetes appears to start with insulin resistance and impaired insulin sensitivity, followed by compensatory insulin hypersecretion.
- *Phase 2:* Impairment of pancreatic beta cell secretion of insulin produces an abnormal rise in post-meal and fasting glucose levels (now referred to as prediabetes).
- *Phase 3:* Overt diabetes appears due to progressive impairment of beta cell insulin secretion and lack of insulin sensitivity accompanied by increased hepatic glucose production.[2]

In the third phase, fasting glucose levels are greater than or equal to 126 mg/dL (7.0 mmol/L); however, many people with type 2 diabetes are unaware they have the disease since the mild elevations in glucose levels do not produce physical signs and symptoms prompting medical evaluation. Because of the number of persons who have long-term complications at initial presentation, scientists have estimated that diabetes may have been present for 4 to 7 years prior to the clinical diagnosis.[2,3]

Unlike the abrupt onset of type 1 diabetes, which presents with the classic symptoms of polyuria, polydipsia, and polyphagia, type 2 diabetes is usually insidious and progresses gradually. The first symptoms may be fatigue, poor wound healing, recurrent yeast or skin infections, dry mouth, blurred vision (persons with diabetes are often diagnosed during or after a visit with their eye doctor and often have just gotten new glasses), or other poorly differentiated symptoms. Alternately, type 2 diabetes that has gone undetected for a period of time can present with many of the overt symptoms usually attributed to type 1 diabetes. This wide range of presenting symptoms reflects the level of insulin resistance and the degree of beta cell dysfunction at diagnosis.[2,3]

Incidence and Prevalence

Diabetes is reaching epidemic proportions throughout the world. It is estimated that by the year 2045, 693 million people will have diabetes, predominately type 2 diabetes. The greatest areas of growth are in Asia and Africa, where the shift to more industrialized economies, sedentary lifestyles, and Westernized diets has increased the incidence of type 2 diabetes dramatically.[4]

The 2017 National Diabetes Statistics Report announced that 30.3 million people, or 10% of the US population, have diabetes. Approximately 7.2 million of these Americans are undiagnosed. Of those diagnosed, 85% to 90% have type 2 diabetes. The number of adults aged 20 years and older at risk for diabetes with prediabetes is 84.1 million. There were 1.5 million new cases of diabetes diagnosed in people aged 18 years and older during 2015.[5]

Generally Increases With Age

In looking at how type 2 diabetes affects the demographic groups, the fastest-growing segment of the population diagnosed with this disease is individuals aged 65 years and older. The prevalence of diabetes increases with age. In 2015 it was estimated that 12.0 million people aged 65 years and older (25.2% of all people in this age group) have diabetes.[4] The incidence may vary between the sexes from one population to another, but in general, men and women are afflicted equally.[5]

Children and Adolescents Now Also a Concern

The National Diabetes Statistics Report indicates that type 2 diabetes in children is still rare but of growing concern.[5,6] Although type 2 diabetes typically presents in adults over 30 years old, diagnosis of children with type 2 diabetes, particularly among the high-risk ethnic groups (ie, Hispanic, African American, and Native American), continues to increase. The SEARCH study, which estimated diabetes mellitus (DM) incidence in youth under 20 years old according to race/ethnicity and DM type, found that while type 2 DM is still relatively infrequent among children under 10 years of age, the highest rates (17.0 to 49.4 per 100,000 person-years) were observed among adolescent minority populations.[7] Two million adolescents (or 1 in 6 overweight adolescents) aged 12 to 19 years have prediabetes.[5] As this explosion in the number of persons with diabetes reaches epidemic proportions, healthcare economics will be seriously affected. The healthcare system will be straining its capacity to effectively and efficiently diagnose, treat, and educate those affected. Prevention and early detection of diabetes play a significant role in controlling this epidemic.

Risk Factors for Type 2 Diabetes

The most important risk factors for type 2 diabetes are the following:

- Heredity, which is non-modifiable
- Obesity, which is modifiable
- Physical inactivity, which is also modifiable

Family studies have revealed that first-degree relatives of individuals with type 2 diabetes are about 3 times more likely to develop the disease than individuals without a positive family history of the disease. It has also been shown that concordance rates for monozygotic twins, which have ranged from 60% to 90%, are significantly higher than those for dizygotic twins. Thus, it is clear that type 2 diabetes has a strong genetic component.[8,9]

Unlike type 1 diabetes, type 2 diabetes can generally be prevented by maintaining an age-appropriate body weight and engaging in physical activity.[8,9]

Obesity is also a heritable trait that arises from the interaction of multiple genes and lifestyle factors. Obesity is the most powerful predictor for the development of type 2 diabetes. In high-risk populations, such as the Pima Indians, members of the at-risk group who are not obese have a lower incidence of diabetes. The interplay of other risk factors, however, such as family history with obesity, can increase incidence.[9,10]

Habitual physical inactivity is a contributor to obesity and the rising rates of diabetes. Physical activity has been found to decrease insulin resistance, lower blood glucose levels, and decrease the risk of disease. Cohort studies have documented the lower risk of incident diabetes even for everyday activities such as walking.[11,12] Physical activity is now recognized as a major component of type 2 diabetes prevention.

The following list summarizes commonly accepted risk factors.[1]

Testing should be considered in all adults who have the following factors:

- Overweight (body mass index [BMI] ≥25 kg/m^2*)
- Age of at least 45 years: The elderly especially have increased risk
- First-degree relative with diabetes
- Habitual physical inactivity
- Member of a high-risk ethnic population: African American, Hispanic, Native American, Asian American, Pacific Islander
- Previously identified prediabetes: impaired glucose tolerance (IGT) or impaired fasting glucose (IFG)
- History of gestational diabetes mellitus or delivery of a baby weighing more than 4.1 kg (9 lb)
- Hypertension ≥140/90 mm Hg or on therapy for hypertension
- High-density lipoprotein level less than 35 mg/dL (1.94 mmol/L) or a triglyceride level of at least 250 mg/dL or greater (13.87 mmol/L)
- Polycystic ovarian syndrome
- A1C greater than or equal to 5.7%, IGT or IFG on previous testing
- Conditions associated with insulin resistance, such as acanthosis nigricans, a thickening of the stratum corneum that becomes pigmented (obesity), or spontaneous or eruptive xanthomas often from unmanaged high triglyceride levels that arise more when the glucose levels are elevated
- History of cardiovascular disease

In addition, some public health experts and planners have noted that the economically disadvantaged have increased risk, and some groups are targeting public health programs to this group. Low-income persons with diabetes are at higher risk of type 2 diabetes compared to middle- or high-income persons with diabetes.[13] In addition once low-income persons with diabetes are diagnosed with diabetes they are much more likely to suffer complications. Most low-income persons with diabetes live in high-poverty neighborhoods that contributes to the risk of developing diabetes. These under-resourced neighborhoods are characterized by an overall lack of grocery stores, parks, recreation facilities, quality schools, and accessible and integrated health care. Residents of lower-income neighborhoods often find it difficult to access fresh, healthy foods and programs that promote physical activity, both of which are key to managing stress, managing weight, and preventing disease.[13,14] While obesity, physical inactivity and other health problems are key risk factors, the diabetes care and education specialist should pay closer attention to the socioeconomic conditions that can lead to them.

Diagnosis of Type 2 Diabetes

The ADA has outlined 4 options for diagnosing type 2 diabetes. See Table 15.1 for a summary. Findings should be confirmed by repeat testing on a different day.

Another option, especially used for those people with diabetes who also have anemia, anemia of chronic disease, or a blood dyscrasia, is the fructosamine lab result. This test does not involve the hemoglobin molecule, which can often skew the HgbA1c results.

Treatment of Type 2 Diabetes

At diagnosis of type 2 diabetes, the person with diabetes and the healthcare professional work together to create an individually tailored management plan that focuses

TABLE 15.1 Diagnosing Type 2 Diabetes in Nonpregnant Adults

4 Options			
A1C ≥6.5%*	**Acute Symptoms† Plus Casual‡ Plasma Glucose** ≥200 mg/dL (11.1 mmol/L)	**Fasting Plasma Glucose§** ≥126 mg/dL (7.0 mmol/L)	**2-Hour Postload Glucose** ≥200 mg/dL (11.1 mmol/L) during oral glucose tolerance test (75-g glucose)¶

*Test is performed in a laboratory using a method that is NGSP (National Glycohemoglobin Standardization Program) certified and standardized to the DCCT (Diabetes Control and Complications Trial) assay.

†Classic symptoms of diabetes include polyuria, polydipsia, and unexplained weight loss.

‡Casual is defined as any time of day without regard to time since last meal.

§Fasting is defined as no caloric intake for at least 8 hours.

¶The oral glucose tolerance test is not recommended for routine clinical use.

Source: Data from the American Diabetes Association. 2. Classification and diagnosis of diabetes: Standards of Medical Care in Diabetes 2020. Diabetes Care 2020;43(Suppl. 1):S14–S31.

on the treatment of hyperglycemia present as well as the underlying physiologic deficits, self-management, and behavior change. The plan addresses the following:

- Healthy eating
- Being active
- Taking medication
- Monitoring
- Problem solving
- Healthy coping
- Reducing risks

This multifaceted approach requires that the person with diabetes and the provider consider a significant range of options. Much of the initial treatment aims to reduce troublesome symptoms such as polyuria and dry mouth and restore physiologic balance. Treatment should also include the psychosocial aspects of the diagnosis, which affect the person with diabetes as well as every member of the person's family.

Lifestyle Interventions

For persons newly diagnosed with diabetes, medical nutrition therapy (MNT) is an essential first step in managing glucose levels. Increasing physical activity is also important to reduce insulin resistance and manage weight. The case in this chapter exemplifies this; more information on these topics can be found in chapters 5 and 16 (on nutrition) and 6 (on physical activity).[1]

Reducing Complications

Diabetes can affect major organs in the body including heart, blood vessels, nerves, eyes, and kidneys. Maintaining a normal blood sugar level can dramatically reduce the risk of many complications. Cardiovascular disease (CVD) is the major cause of mortality and morbidity in persons with type 2 diabetes.[15,16] Adults with diabetes have heart disease death rates about 2 to 4 times higher than adults without diabetes. In 2004, heart disease was noted on 68% of diabetes-related death certificates among people aged 65 years and older.[5] Heart disease risk rises for everyone with diabetes as they age, but for women symptoms can become more evident after the onset of menopause.

Both nutrition plans and exercise plans for individuals with type 2 diabetes must incorporate prevention of CVD. Reducing saturated fat, limiting sodium use, and encouraging physical fitness and weight reduction when appropriate are all components of a healthy-heart strategy. After the diagnosis of diabetes, screening for hypertension and hypercholesterolemia is appropriate; if these comorbidities are present, aggressive treatment is initiated.

The ADA recommendations for glycemic, blood pressure, and lipid target levels for adults with diabetes follow:[1]

- A1C: <7.0%[†]
- Blood pressure: <140/80 mm Hg
- Lipids: LDL cholesterol: <100 mg/dL (5.56 mmol/L)[‡]

Blood Glucose Management

The ADA established the following target goals to minimize the effects of the disease and its chronic complications:[1]

- Preprandial capillary plasma glucose: 80 to 130 mg/dL (7.2 mmol/L)
- Peak postprandial capillary plasma glucose: <180 mg/dL (9.99 mmol/L)[§]
- A1C: below 7%

The Diabetes Control and Complications Trial (DCCT)[17] and the UK Prospective Diabetes Study (UKPDS)[18] demonstrated that maintaining glycemic levels with an A1C of <7% significantly reduced the microvascular complications associated with diabetes. Most of the microvascular complications of diabetes are related to the degree and length of exposure to hyperglycemia. New data from the follow-up study of the DCCT, the Epidemiology of Diabetes Intervention and Complications (DCCT/EDIC) study,[19] and the UKPDS stressed the importance of glycemic stability early in the course of the disease and its value in prevention of later complications. The ongoing beneficial effects on diabetic complications after a period of improved glycemic stability, even if followed by a return to usual (often poorer) metabolic stability, have been described as representing "metabolic memory" by the DCCT/EDIC investigators and as a "legacy effect" by the UKPDS investigators.

Self-Monitoring Self-monitoring of blood glucose (SMBG) and continuous glucose monitoring (CGM) are essential components of self-care. It empowers those with diabetes to make needed adjustments in their daily care and gives them the necessary data to evaluate those changes. Continuous glucose monitoring is recommended for all persons with diabetes who have hypoglycemia unawareness and/or frequent hypoglycemia.

See Table 18.7 in chapter 18 for a comparison of the ADA and the American Association of Clinical Endocrinologists (AACE) target blood glucose goals.

Pharmacologic Interventions

The pathways to managing optimal blood glucose levels and achieving target goals vary for each person with diabetes. Initially, lifestyle modifications may be sufficient, but as the disease progresses, the pathophysiologic changes diminish insulin sensitivity and beta cell production, requiring medications to reach target goals.

Individualized Plan

The healthcare professional must tailor the medication regimen to the individual and adjust it as necessary to maintain glycemic stability. Metformin should be started at the time type 2 diabetes is diagnosed unless there are contraindications. Metformin in combination with lifestyle modification may reduce the risk of cardiovascular events and death. If the A1C target is not obtained after approximately 3 months and the person with diabetes does not have atherosclerotic cardiovascular disease (ASCVD) or chronic kidney disease (CKD), then any of the 6 preferred treatment options—sulfonylurea, thiazolidinedione, dipeptidyl peptidase 4 (DPP-4) inhibitor, SGLT2 Inhibitor, GLP-1 receptor agonist, or basal insulin—can be selected based on specific person with diabetes and drug-specific factors. Persons with diabetes with established ASCVD, CKD, or heart failure may benefit from a GLP-1 receptor agonist or SGLT2 inhibitor with demonstrated cardiovascular risk reduction.

Medications (discussed in depth in chapter 17) used for the treatment of diabetes address the various pathophysiologic deficits:

Biguanides (metformin):	Reduce hepatic glucose output
Sulfonylureas (glyburide, glipizide):	Improve insulin secretion
Thiazolidinediones (rosiglitazone, pioglitazone):	Increase insulin sensitivity
Meglitinides (repaglinide, nateglinide):	Increase circulating insulin levels but have a shorter duration than the sulfonylureas
Alpha-glucosidase inhibitors (miglitol, acarbose):	Act within the intestinal wall to prevent/delay the breakdown of certain carbohydrates
Dipeptidyl peptidase-4 (DPP-4) inhibitors (sitagliptin, saxagliptin, alogliptin, linagliptin):	Act within the gut to inhibit the breakdown of GLP-1, an incretin hormone that improves insulin secretion, reduces hepatic glucose production, and slows gastric emptying
SGLT2 inhibitors (canagliflozin, dapagliflozin, empagliflozin):	Lower blood sugar by blocking reabsorption of glucose and increasing its excretion in urine
GLP-1 agonists (exenatide, liraglutide, dulaglutide, albiglutide):	Enhance glucose-dependent insulin secretion by the pancreatic beta cell, suppress inappropriately elevated glucagon secretion, and slow gastric emptying
Bile acid sequestrants (colesevelam):	Bind bile acids in the intestine, impeding their reabsorption. However, the exact mechanism by which Welchol improves glycemic stability is unknown.
Dopamine agonists (bromocriptine):	Inhibit excessive sympathetic tone within the central nervous system, resulting in a reduction in postmeal plasma glucose levels due to enhanced suppression of hepatic glucose production

With increasing duration of the disease, many people with type 2 diabetes require insulin therapy to remain in a healthy glycemic range. Both the person with diabetes and the healthcare professional need to determine when to add or convert to insulin therapy.

Case—Part 1: An Adult Develops Type 2 Diabetes

AA, a 52-year-old widowed African American woman, noted that in the past year she gained 15 lb, had recurrent vaginitis, and tended to become fatigued after her main meal. She attributed these problems to her stressful life, which includes caring for both her ill mother and a new grandchild in her home. Her past medical history was significant for hypertension and dyslipidemia, notably an elevated LDL-cholesterol level. Her social history revealed that she has never smoked and that she drinks red wine approximately 1 to 2 times per month. She has not been sexually active since the death of her husband 3 years prior. During the medical evaluation for urinary tract infection (UTI) and the

(continued)

Case—Part 1: An Adult Develops Type 2 Diabetes (continued)

subsequent follow-up laboratory testing, the following data were gathered:

- Urine analysis: glycosuria
- BMI: 35 kg/m^2
- Blood pressure: 120/80 mm Hg
- Skin: marked acanthosis nigricans in folds of neck and axillae
- Fasting glucose: 199 mg/dL (11 mmol/L) and 233 mg/dL (12.93 mmol/L)
- A1C: 8.2%
- LDL cholesterol: 140 mg/dL (7.78 mmol/L)

The lab data confirmed the diagnosis of diabetes. AA was upset but not surprised by the diagnosis. Her mother, 2 sisters, and a brother all have type 2 diabetes; in the past, she had wondered if she, too, had diabetes. During the course of the visit, AA stated she knows very little about managing diabetes and cannot see herself incorporating changes in diet or exercise into her already busy life. She expressed fear at the possible development of blindness and kidney disease and is worried that her children will be burdened with her care.

Discussion

The diagnosis of type 2 diabetes in AA signifies the increased incidence of the disease among certain ethnic groups, in this case among African Americans. With a significant family history, AA had a genetic predisposition: 4 first-degree relatives already diagnosed with diabetes. A history of obesity with further weight gain, diminished exercise, and significant life stressors may have been the environmental and behavioral triggers that led to the manifestation of type 2 diabetes. The presence of acanthosis nigricans, a thickening of the stratum corneum that becomes pigmented, was a marker for the presence of insulin resistance. This hyperinsulinemia promotes keratinocyte proliferation, resulting in acanthosis nigricans and/or skin tags.[1]

AA had a significant number of risk factors for diabetes. She was obese with a BMI of 35 kg/m^2 and, although active, rarely exercised. Her family history was strongly positive for diabetes, and her ethnicity further increased her risk. AA also had a past medical history of hypertension and elevated lipid values.

In those with underlying pathophysiologic changes indicative of prediabetes, the overt presentation of type 2 diabetes often occurs after an illness or other stressor. In AA's case, she had the physical stress and exhaustion of being a multigenerational caregiver. Determining whether the underlying and as-yet untreated diabetes exacerbated the urinary tract symptoms, which brought her to the clinic, or whether the UTI was an initial symptom of the diabetes is difficult. Often, UTI or vaginitis is the presenting symptom in a woman with abnormal glucose levels.

The presence of glucose in the urine indicated that the level of serum glucose had exceeded approximately 180 mg/dL (9.99 mmol/L), the level considered the usual adult renal threshold where the kidneys begin to excrete glucose into the urine. Urine results are not diagnostic but heighten the suspicion for the diagnosis of diabetes. Renal threshold is reduced in children and pregnant women and elevated in the aged. Applying the diagnostic criteria (Table 15.1) to AA's lab results shows that her glucose values are indicative of diabetes.

In the future, it will be important for AA to track her blood glucose values at home. (See the Self-Monitoring section.)

The decision to start an injectable therapy, particularly insulin, can be a difficult one. Fear of needles or injections, myths and fallacies about insulin therapy, concerns about hypoglycemia when using insulin, and alterations in lifestyle due to the use of injectable therapies all can present barriers to initiation of this therapy. (See chapters 4 and 10 for more information on anxieties and diabetes-specific fears.) Those who did not engage with their diabetes regimen may have been threatened with the prospect of insulin therapy, further compounding their reluctance to switch to this therapy when the time was appropriate. Coercion of this type increases fear and resistance to using this safe and effective drug.

There are many different types of insulin and various delivery devices. Education for the person with diabetes is a critical component of management of type 2 diabetes with insulin therapy. Not only must the individual with diabetes and the ancillary caregivers understand how to administer the insulin; they must also learn about the type, timing, and action of insulin. Chapters 7 and 17 provide detailed information.

Case—Part 2: Implementing a Treatment Plan for an Adult

Although AA had stated her reservations about attempting lifestyle changes, the individualized approach to nutrition, presented in a stepwise manner, addressed these concerns so that the necessary adjustment could be made.

Culturally Sensitive Plan

AA's interaction with a culturally sensitive diabetes care and education specialist provides comfort and helps her to trust her providers. Given that stress is commonly experienced by patients in the process of experiencing health care as evidenced by the "white coat hypertension" phenomenon, and given that African Americans are at risk for perceived or experienced racism related stress from likely unintentional racial bias in the healthcare process it is important to consider physical stress in AA's case. It is understandable how patients who experience mistrust of their healthcare providers, racial bias in health care received, unsatisfactory patient-provider interactions (e.g., interactions in which providers are rushing in order to see many patients), and/or who lack the perceived interpersonal control needed to discuss healthcare dissatisfaction with their providers may experience healthcare-associated stress. Such stress as well as other healthcare circumstances (eg, receiving negative test results) can impede patients' understanding of treatment recommendations and/or willingness to follow these recommendations, resulting in lack of engagement with the treatment. Conversely, AA's satisfaction with her health care and perceived interpersonal control in interactions with her healthcare providers can contribute to her experiencing lower stress, and these experiences can promote the mental health needed to understand and follow recommended treatment regimens, including health-promoting lifestyle behaviors and medication and nutrition plans.

Nutrition Plan

Medical nutrition therapy (MNT) involves a thorough assessment of the person's current lifestyle, eating patterns, and ethnic, cultural, or traditional food preferences, as well as nutritional requirements for stages of growth and development. MNT also incorporates nutritional changes necessary to prevent or treat other health conditions, such as dyslipidemia or osteoporosis. AA's nutrition plan incorporates the following key elements:

- She can eat the traditional foods she loves but is encouraged to limit portion sizes where appropriate to enhance weight loss.
- During early phases of treatment, carbohydrates such as juices and concentrated sweets will be reduced in order to lower the glycemic load, which will help reduce insulin resistance from glucose toxicity, a condition where pancreatic beta cells are inactive as a result of chronic exposure to high concentrations of glucose.

Physical Activity Plan

AA's life was very active, but she was doing little to improve her cardiovascular system or increase her metabolism to burn calories and contribute to weight loss. An increase in aerobic exercise would address both of these concerns. In addition, weight loss and exercise might improve her lipid values—raising HDL and lowering triglycerides. Exercise would also provide a healthy outlet for the stress AA experiences in her role as caregiver. Although beginning an exercise program can be daunting, helping AA identify an activity she enjoys will increase the likelihood that she will engage with her exercise program. Most persons with diabetes find a walking program an easy and effective way to increase aerobic activity. Brief, 10- to 15-minute periods of walking throughout the day will help improve insulin sensitivity, reduce weight, and improve cardiovascular fitness. For some persons with diabetes, the use of a pedometer that records the number of steps taken in a day promotes an increase in physical activity.

Blood Glucose Management

A significant part of AA's treatment plan focused on obtaining and maintaining blood glucose ranges in accordance with target goals established by the ADA.[1] The role of maintaining glycemic stability in reducing microvascular complications was an important and empowering message for AA, who feared blindness and renal disease.

Monitoring

To monitor changes in blood glucose levels and the response to treatment, AA needed to learn to check her blood glucose (often referred to as blood sugar by older African Americans) at home. AA had been checking her mother's blood glucose level at home sporadically. She had never self-tested. She told the diabetes care and education specialist she felt confident using the brand of meter she used for her mother and did not feel the need for further instructions. AA demonstrated proper technique in the use of her glucose meter and agreed to test before breakfast and again before supper. Training her daughter in use of the meter and the medications will be critical in AA's success, as the daughter can help reinforce the training and provide support to her mother when she is on her own at home.

AA was given an instruction sheet written in Spanish that delineated the steps needed to periodically check the accuracy

(continued)

Case—Part 2: Implementing a Treatment Plan for an Adult (continued)

of the meter. The instructions include the toll-free help-line number for the meter manufacturer, which is available 24/7 with interpreters if needed. AA may need help filling out the warranty card that came with her meter and sending it in. Registering her meter will make it easier for the manufacturer to pull up her information should she need to call the help line.

Medication

Because of her elevated blood glucose levels, AA needed not only MNT but also medication. She was started on metformin (Glucophage®, Bristol-Myers Squibb Co.). She received all written instructions and materials in both Spanish and English.

After receiving a prescription to treat the UTI, a sample of metformin, and instructions to increase her fluid intake while on the antibiotics, AA was scheduled for a follow-up appointment the next week. She was asked to bring her glucose test results diary for discussion and to participate in further dietary instruction. AA may be a candidate for high-intensity statin therapy since she is between 40 and 75 years of age with additional CVD risk factors (LDL cholesterol greater than 100 mg/dL [5.55 mmol/L]).[14] EB's blood pressure and cholesterol should be regularly monitored to decrease her risk of macrovascular complications.

Health Literacy and Numeracy

In chronic disease management, the person with diabetes becomes a partner in care and is responsible for day-to-day management of the disease. Education for the person with diabetes, the cornerstone of self-management, requires the dissemination of information, most of which occurs by the written word.

Health literacy, the ability to perform basic reading and numerical tasks required to function in a health environment, significantly impacts diabetes self-management: the ability to read medication labels, appointment cards, and medical nutrition plans. Problems with health literacy are more common among immigrants, older persons with diabetes, those with disrupted schooling, and those for whom English is not their primary language. However, low literacy can affect anyone. It is not limited to the inability to read but includes comprehension and synthesis of new information. Low health literacy is common among those with diabetes and has been associated with having less knowledge about diabetes and worse glycemic levelsl.[20]

Low numeracy skills, or the inability to use numbers, is a significant part of health literacy. Understanding measurements, time, and multistep operations is important in assessing portion sizes, understanding insulin action curves, and performing capillary glucose testing and other basic diabetes self-care management.

To ascertain understanding of the information, the provider must present the person with diabetes with simple tasks that involve the use of information taught, such as selecting the correct insulin dosage from a blood glucose–based algorithm or demonstrating the use of an insulin pen. The educational literature given to AA should have large colorful pictures with simple explanations that provide clear instructions. For example, the use of the plate method for MNT gives an excellent visual representation of the distribution of food type and portion for a meal that is readily understood with limited explanation.

At the follow-up visit, the provider will need to assess blood glucose logs and food and activity diaries not only for issues of blood glucose stability but for signs that suggest low health literacy or numeracy problems.

Type 2 Diabetes in Older Adults

The prevalence of diabetes among US adults aged 65 years and older varies from 22% to 33%, depending on the diagnostic criteria used.[21] Postprandial hyperglycemia is a prominent characteristic of type 2 diabetes in older adults,[22–24] contributing to observed differences in prevalence depending on which diagnostic test is used.[23] Using the hemoglobin A1C (A1C) or fasting plasma glucose (FPG) diagnostic criteria, as is currently done for national surveillance, one third of older adults with diabetes are undiagnosed.[5] The epidemic of type 2 diabetes is clearly linked to increasing rates of overweight and obesity in the US population, but projections by the CDC suggest that even if diabetes incidence rates level off, the prevalence of diabetes will double in the next 20 years, in part due to the aging of the population.[25] Other projections suggest that the number of cases of diagnosed diabetes in those aged 65 years and older will increase by more than fourfold (compared to threefold in the total population) between 2005 and 2050.[26]

Physiologic changes in fuel regulation combined with genetic, behavioral, and environmental interactions place this population at risk for diabetes. The elderly metabolism has alterations in glucose counterregulation affecting glucagon, epinephrine, and growth hormone. Declines in adiponectin, leptin, and GLP-1 also affect glucose regulation.[22,23]

Screening and Diagnosis of Older Adults

Diagnostic criteria for diabetes are not altered or made less stringent for older adults. The same set of criteria is applied to the non-pregnant adult regardless of age. Only in the case of pregnancy do guidelines for screening and diagnosing gestational diabetes change, relying on an oral glucose tolerance test (OGTT) to determine the diabetes state.

In the physiology of aging, glucose tolerance declines, with fasting plasma glucose levels increasing by 1 to 2 mg/dL (0.6-0.11 mmol/L) per decade after age 30. Postprandial glucose levels increase by approximately 15 mg/dL (.83 mmol/L) per decade. While there is a loss of first-phase insulin response, second-phase insulin release that is glucose induced may be normal. A reduced frequency and amplitude of pulsatile insulin release results in disruption in hepatic glucose inhibition.[24]

Clinical Presentation

As in the younger adult population, type 2 diabetes is more common than type 1 diabetes in older adults. Older adults with diabetes rarely present with the typical symptoms of hyperglycemia.[21] Physiologic changes associated with aging may diminish thirst and increase dehydration. Glycosuria at the usual levels may not be seen, because of the advance in renal threshold associated with aging.

Lean, Older Persons With Diabetes Obese and lean older adults may have impairment of beta-cell secretory capabilities associated with aging. Lean, older adults may also exhibit signs of autoimmune changes like those usually seen in type 1 diabetes. Latent autoimmune diabetes of adults (LADA) does occur, presenting in older adults who are not obese. Often, this presentation creates a confusing clinical picture of acute hyperglycemia because this population normally is diagnosed with type 2 diabetes. To be well managed, LADA requires insulin treatment to preserve beta cell function and promote euglycemia. Although the rates of occurrence are small, the healthcare professional must be aware of the possibility of this diagnosis in lean, older persons with diabetes. A laboratory blood test to measure antiglutamic acid decarboxylase (anti-GAD) or islet cell antibodies (ICAs) can confirm the autoimmune state and improve treatment of the person with LADA.[21]

Other Presentations Others may present with glucose elevations due to an acute illness, a transient medical condition, or the introduction of a certain medication (steroids, antihypertensives, cardiac medications). This increase in plasma glucose levels may reveal previously undiagnosed diabetes, IGT, or IFG and present an opportunity for further assessment and treatment.[21,26,27]

> **Caring for Older Adults**
>
> Interventions must carefully consider nutrition and exercise limitations and medication side effects that are pertinent to the older adult's situation.

Considerations Regarding Older Adults

Older adults are a heterogeneous group; some may be active and functional, providing their own self-care, while others may suffer from multiple comorbidities and require assistance or total care. The following factors must be carefully considered in planning education and care for the unique needs of individuals in this age group:

- Medical complications
- Physical limitations
- Other prescribed medications
- Effects of aging
- Greater risk of hypoglycemia

Complications

Older persons with type 2 diabetes may have a long duration of diabetes with an increase in complications, both macrovascular and microvascular. The UKPDS showed that macrovascular complications of diabetes are 1.5 to 2 times more prevalent in the older diabetic populations than in the nondiabetic population.[28,29] From the diabetes mortality and morbidity rates collected from Medicare claims data on the elderly population in the United States, the following conclusions have been drawn[29]:

- Leading causes of morbidity are ischemic heart disease and stroke.
- Gangrene, amputation, and lower extremity infection make up the next cohort of diseases associated with morbidity.
- Acute complications (hypoglycemia, ketoacidosis, hyperosmolar syndrome) make up the last group.

Physical Limitations

Older adults with diabetes are about 1.5 times more likely to have physical limitations and alterations in daily living activities than those without diabetes.[30,31] Disabilities may be directly linked to eye disease, stroke, CVD, neuropathies, and peripheral vascular disease. Older persons with diabetes may also respond more symptomatically to both hyperglycemia and hypoglycemia. Coupled with additional comorbidities, the long tenure of diabetes may contribute to frailty. Physical limitations necessitate adjustments in management goals and interventions.

Polypharmacy

Older adults with diabetes may also be on multiple medications for a variety of ailments. This can lead to not only dosing and timing errors but also the heightened possibility of drug interactions. The healthcare professional must use caution when prescribing certain diabetes medications for older adults.

Aging

Physiologic changes in aging affect signs and symptoms associated with diabetes and its complications. Below are facets of normal aging that can significantly impact diabetes care:

- Diminished taste and olfactory sense
- Reduced metabolic rate that alters digestion
- Decreased renal clearance
- Altered pain perception

Cautions With Diabetes Medication in Older Adults[19]

- *Metformin.* In persons with diabetes >80 years of age, evaluate renal function with creatinine clearance; if <60 mg/dL (3.33 mmol/L), do not administer drug. Serum creatinine is a poor correlate of renal health because of the low muscle mass characteristic of the elderly person.
- *Thiazolidinediones.* Contraindicated in Class 3 and Class 4 congestive heart failure (CHF); avoid if CHF is present, determine benefit versus risk.
- *Sulfonylureas.* Beware of long half-life and propensity for hypoglycemia; caution in liver and renal dysfunction. Glyburide also decreases preischemic conditioning and, therefore, should not be used in the elderly.
- *Insulin.* Risk of severe hypoglycemia increases with age.

Higher Risk for Hypoglycemia

Slowed counterregulation of hormones, erratic food intake, certain medications (beta-blockers), and slowed intestinal absorption place the older adult at higher risk for hypoglycemia. The adrenergic response to low blood glucose levels may be diminished or absent. Instead, the initial symptoms, such as lack of motor skills or confusion, represent a neuroglycopenia that may be misdiagnosed or pose a safety risk to the individual.

In light of all the changes in the older adult's health, close attention must be paid to nutrition and exercise interventions and medication side effects. The healthcare professional must keep in mind the individual's preferences and physiologic alterations. The ADA goal for glycemic levels in many adults is an A1C <7%, but less stringent goals are recommended for elderly persons with limited life expectancy, advanced diabetes complications, or extensive comorbid conditions.[1]

Factors Influencing Education Strategies

For those with diabetes who are still hardy, diabetes self-care and management goals must reflect their capabilities. Despite the fact that age can affect the processing of information, the capacity to learn and integrate new information remains intact throughout the life cycle. In the educational process, accommodations should be made for the following:

- Hearing changes
- Visual changes
- Cognitive status

Paced Learning and Feedback Like all adult learners, older persons with diabetes benefit from a stepwise approach to education that recognizes their past experience and builds on it. In addition, several studies have demonstrated that some older adults with type 2 diabetes may experience some mental slowing that affects the ability to perform diabetes self-care behaviors.[30,31] The diabetes care and education specialist must assess older persons with diabetes for comprehension and memory through both verbal and skills feedback.

Equipment Difficulties Self-care devices that require technical skill and manipulation, such as those for self-monitoring of glucose and insulin administration, have become much easier for the older adult with diabetes to use.

- *Self-monitoring of glucose.* Glucose meters have larger display screens, audible beeping prompts, reduced sample size, and ergonomically designed easy-to-grip bodies to facilitate ease of use. Some meters have test strips in drums or cartridges that are easier for arthritic hands to maneuver.
- *Insulin administration.* Insulin pens have made self-administration of insulin safer for the older person with diabetes. Since it is easier to read dosage marks on insulin pens than on syringes, dosing is more accurate. These devices reduce dosage errors and do not require the manual dexterity of the vial and syringe method. However, the diabetes care and education specialist must assess the person with diabetes' ability to push hard enough on the end of the pen to adequately deliver the

entire dose. The person with diabetes also needs enough hand strength to be able to screw the pen needle on and off.

Since some third-party payers do not routinely reimburse for some of these devices, the diabetes care and education specialist must endeavor to educate third-party payers regarding the need for these devices and to advocate in behalf of the person with diabetes.

Other Barriers In an older, retired population, financial concerns, insurance issues, and transportation difficulties can become staggering problems, confounding the delivery of health care and health maintenance. For the person with type 2 diabetes, expenses can be a concern—both the expense of medication for diabetes and its comorbidities and the cost of coverage for multiple medical visits plus podiatric, dental, and eye care. The healthcare provider must be aware of these issues and seek to ameliorate them whenever possible. For example, prescribing medications that are preferred and offer maximal reimbursement or coverage whenever possible reduces the financial burden of the person with diabetes.

Institutional Settings Many older adults live in long-term care facilities, and a large proportion of these individuals have diabetes. In addition to all the usual therapeutic considerations for type 2 diabetes, skin care takes on heightened importance in this population so that infections, ulcerations, and amputations can be avoided. Reduced circulation, neurological impairment, diminished range of motion, and compromised nutritional status contribute to the fragility of the skin. People with diabetes who are no longer capable of self-care depend on healthcare providers to develop effective care strategies to maintain glycemic target levels and prevent or reduce health-altering consequences. The diabetes care and education specialist can help establish strategies to ensure the following:

- Glucose levels are appropriately monitored and acted upon.
- Acute complications of hypoglycemia and hyperglycemia are avoided when possible and treated if present.
- Insulin and other diabetes medications are given accurately and in a timely manner; other medications are checked for potential negative interactions.
- Nutrition intervention supplies sufficient calories and is delivered in a manner that best suits the person with diabetes' needs and preferences.
- Skin and foot care become an integral part of the daily care regimen to promote circulation and avoid breakdown.

Type 2 Diabetes in Children and Adolescents

In 2010, 22,820 youth under the age of 20 were diagnosed with type 2 diabetes. This number is estimated to quadruple to 84,131 in 2050 with Hispanics representing 50% of all youth with type 2 diabetes and African Americans representing 27%.[32]

Diagnosis of Type 2 Diabetes in Children and Teens

Risk Factors

Type 2 diabetes in children and adolescents has increased as the frequency of obesity has risen in the United States. At diagnosis, 85% of children with type 2 diabetes are overweight or obese.[33] Nearly all children diagnosed have a positive family history of type 2 diabetes, with 74% to 100% having a first- or second-degree relative with type 2 diabetes and 45% to 80% having a parent with diabetes. Many of these children are of non-European descent (eg, African American, Hispanic, or Native American).

Clinical Presentation

In general, children and adolescents diagnosed with type 2 diabetes have glycosuria without ketonuria, mild thirst, some increase in urination, and little-to-no weight loss; however, up to 33% will have ketonuria at diagnosis, with 5% to 25% having ketoacidosis unrelated to stress, illness, or infection.[34] Polycystic ovarian syndrome (PCOS) and acanthosis nigricans, disorders associated with insulin resistance, are commonly seen,[34,35] as well as lipid disorders and hypertension. At onset 10% to 32% have hypertension, 14% to 22% have microalbuminuria, 10% have retinopathy, and 18% to 83% have dyslipidemia.[32,33] There are ethnic differences in lipids, lipoproteins, and blood pressure with further indications of the metabolic syndrome in this high-risk population. Other clinical problems that arise in this population are sleep apnea associated with obesity, hepatic steatosis, orthopedic complications, and psychosocial concerns.[34–38]

As obesity in this age group rises, the clinical picture of the child with diabetes can be confusing, making it difficult to differentiate type 1 diabetes from type 2 diabetes without laboratory studies. A variation on the presentation of type 2 diabetes occurs in children with a positive family history of early-onset diabetes. Although the child presents in diabetic ketoacidosis, which is usually seen in type 1 diabetes, the antibody tests are negative (both anti-GAD and ICA), and insulin is not required once the acute episode is resolved. These children have elevated C-peptide levels, which indicates a hyperinsulinemia as opposed to reduced insulin levels found in type 1 diabetes. Many of these children are of African-American descent.[36–38]

Due to the difficulty of establishing the type of diabetes in children by presentation alone, in an ideal situation, type 1 diabetes would be confirmed by a test for auto-antibodies, while type 2 diabetes would use a test for insulin resistance such as the fasting C-peptide.[39]

Insulin Resistance The pattern for development of type 2 diabetes in children appears to follow the insidious pathway seen in type 2 diabetes in adults. Insulin levels may be normal or elevated, but first-phase insulin release is not sufficient to compensate for insulin resistance, which leads to hyperglycemia. Just as in adults with type 2 diabetes, obesity and a lack of physical activity promote overt diabetes. Both of these lifestyle factors promote insulin resistance. The onset of type 2 diabetes frequently occurs around the time of puberty, a time when insulin sensitivity declines. This evidence further supports the importance of insulin resistance in the pathogenesis of the disease.[34,36–38]

Intrauterine Environment The intrauterine environment, specifically birth weight and maternal hyperglycemia, may have links to type 2 diabetes in children. Low birth weight predicts type 2 diabetes in middle age[37] and has also been associated with the development of diabetes in teens and adolescents. Higher levels of amniotic fluid insulin at 33 to 38 weeks' gestation were a strong predictor of later IGT.[38] Children born to mothers with gestational diabetes also appear to have a higher risk of developing type 2 diabetes.[40,41]

Diagnostic Criteria

With the current explosion in the number of new cases of diabetes and the importance of screening, controversies concerning the criteria and the most effective method for screening for diabetes, particularly type 2 diabetes in children, abound. At present, the same diagnostic criteria that are applied to adults are applied to children; however, whether these established cut points are valid in a younger population is not known.

Public Health Interventions The advent of type 2 diabetes in children and adolescents carries with it a significant public health problem. The onset of the disease in younger populations leads to earlier onset of complications, both macrovascular and microvascular. The estimated financial costs and loss of productivity resulting from these health problems represent a significant economic burden. Earlier diagnosis and aggressive treatment may help in preventing or delaying these costly complications, making a strong case for screening. The ADA outlined recommendations for testing children at substantial risk for type 2 diabetes. See Table 15.2.

TABLE 15.2 Diagnosing Type 2 Diabetes in Children

Criteria for Considering Screening for Diabetes:*
Overweight (BMI 85th percentile) for age and sex; or obese > 95th percentile for age and sex;
Plus any 2 of the following risk factors:
• Family history of type 2 diabetes in first- or second-degree relative
• Maternal history of diabetes or gestational diabetes mellitus during the child's gestation
• Race/ethnicity (American Indian, African American, Hispanic, Asian/Pacific Islander)
• Signs of insulin resistance or conditions associated with insulin resistance (acanthosis nigricans, hypertension, dyslipidemia, PCOS)
Age of Initiation: Age 10, or at onset of puberty if puberty occurs at a younger age
Testing Frequency: Every 3 years
Test: Fasting plasma glucose, oral glucose tolerance test, A1C

*Clinical judgment should be used to test for diabetes in high-risk subjects who do not meet these criteria.

Source: Data from the American Diabetes Association. 2. Classification and diagnosis of diabetes: Standards of Medical Care in Diabetes 2020. Diabetes Care 2020;43(Suppl. 1):S14–S31.

Considerations Regarding Children and Teens

Once a child or adolescent learns he or she has type 2 diabetes, the approach to care must incorporate the youth's developmental needs and psychosocial concerns. Since many of the children and teens diagnosed with type 2 diabetes are overweight or obese, they may have already faced issues that separate them from their peers. Personal appearance (issues of both style and size), participating in competitive athletics, and congregating at fast-food restaurants or malls are often integral aspects of growing up in the United States. Lifestyle adjustments that help reduce weight and manage diabetes can seem to run counter to the norm and become problematic. Striving for independence and developing a sense of self are important developmental tasks that are made more difficult in the presence of diabetes. While parental support and guidance are a necessary part of dealing with a medical condition such as diabetes, at this time of life, the adolescent desires less parental involvement.

For adolescents and children with type 2 diabetes, the goals of therapy are the same as for any person with diabetes:

- To achieve physical and psychological well-being while maintaining long-term glycemic stability, and to avoid microvascular and macrovascular complications[31,37]

Lifestyle Interventions[41,42]

Medical nutrition therapy and increased physical activity are the cornerstone of therapy for all age groups; however, weight management in children and adolescents must consider healthy growth and development needs. Thus, aggressive weight-loss programs are not recommended for these age groups. The approach must be one of substitution and reduction, rather than elimination. The following important dietary adjustments still leave room for the adolescent lifestyle:

- Learning to make healthy choices at fast-food restaurants
- Eating fewer fatty, calorie-dense foods
- Drinking less sugary beverages
- Choosing healthy snacks

Obese youth may lack the stamina and athletic prowess to compete in sports. Therefore, physical activities can be a source of self-degradation and ridicule by peers and can contribute to low self-esteem. In the treatment of type 2 diabetes, physical activity lowers insulin resistance and helps maintain weight loss. The challenge is to make this important therapy agreeable to an audience that usually eschews it.

The child should be encouraged to improve fitness through individual activities such as roller-blading, biking, or dancing rather than through competitive activities.[41,42] Also, replacing television and computer time with any type of physical movement has benefits.

Pharmacologic Interventions

Many children with type 2 diabetes will require medication in addition to lifestyle modification to achieve glucose goals. Some will need medication at diagnosis. However, the compendium of medications available for use is limited due to lack of pharmacologic clinical trials in this age group. The US Food and Drug Administration has approved 2 pharmacologic agents for use in children and adolescents:

- Metformin (an oral agent)
- Insulin (injectable formulations)

Metformin The oral agent metformin (Glucophage®, Bristol-Myers Squibb Co.), a biguanide, has been approved for use in children 10 to 16 years of age with type 2 diabetes. In controlled trials in subjects aged 8 to 16 years with type 2 diabetes, metformin significantly decreased fasting plasma glucose and A1C levels when compared with placebo.[43,44] The drug has 3 common adverse effects:

- Diarrhea, or abruptly loose stool
- Nausea
- Upper abdominal pain from gas

To minimize adverse effects, metformin should be taken with food and the dosage titrated slowly, starting with one 500-mg tablet per day until the effective dosage is achieved. The extended-release preparation of metformin may lessen or minimize the adverse effects. For children, the maximum dosage is 2,000 mg (in adults it is 2,550 mg).

In girls with type 2 diabetes and PCOS, use of metformin may normalize ovulatory abnormalities and increase the risk of unplanned pregnancy; therefore, girls of childbearing age using this therapy should be counseled regarding this risk.[42,44] See also the section on teens in chapter 24, on pregnancy with diabetes.

Insulin Insulin therapy has a long history of usage in the pediatric population. Healthcare professionals prescribe insulin for children with type 1 diabetes or type 2 diabetes who present with diabetic ketoacidosis, hyperosmolar hyperglycemic state, moderate ketosis, or symptomatic glycemic levels. The need for insulin in the hyperglycemic state complicated by insulin resistance may persist for weeks after diagnosis. However, once glycemic levels decrease and lifestyle measures are in place, some children are able to maintain euglycemic levels with metformin.

Insulin therapy should be used if oral agents are not effective or when the disease worsens and clinical goals are no longer met with oral agents alone. Insulin can be used as monotherapy or in combination with metformin.

Some children have been able to meet target goals with 1 injection of a long-acting insulin per day, such as insulin glargine (Lantus®, Sanofi-Aventis US, LLC) or detemir (Levemir®, Novo Nordisk), while others have needed multiple daily injections (MDIs) using a basal-bolus regimen. Insulin therapy must be tailored to the physical as well as psychosocial needs of the person with diabetes. Despite the flexibility of an MDI regimen, adolescents may at times feel encumbered by it and switch to prefilled mixed insulin pens to maximize convenience and have a respite from the demands of self-care.[39] In the presence of insulin resistance in type 2 diabetes, larger amounts of insulin are necessary to adequately manage glycemic levels. This is also true in children and particularly in adolescents who have type 2 diabetes. During puberty and growth spurts, insulin resistance increases, necessitating compensatory dosing of insulin. Irrespective of ethnicity, insulin sensitivity is reduced while fasting levels are increased in both obese and nonobese children during Tanner stages II through IV of pubertal development.[36,37]

Other Medications Sulfonylureas, glucosidase inhibitors, and meglitinides may be effective in treating type 2 diabetes in children, but more research must be conducted to determine the risks of using these drugs in this population. In particular, researchers must explore whether insulin secretagogues such as sulfonylureas accelerate beta cell demise in this group, especially in the presence of autoimmunity.[36,37]

Social Support

No matter the therapy selected, education and family support are vital components of diabetes management in children and teens. For children and adolescents at risk, healthcare professionals can encourage, support, and educate the entire family to make lifestyle changes that may delay or lower the risk for the onset of type 2 diabetes. Studies show that parents are particularly important as role models, encouragers, and facilitators of physical activity and healthy nutrition in children and adolescents.[45,46] Their roles include everything from buying sports equipment, to taking kids to practice, to doling out praise. Other important factors in raising active children include paternal activity levels and positive reinforcement, maternal participation, sibling involvement, time spent outdoors, and family income. Helping families find ways to utilize the resources that are available in their community is vital to sustaining healthy lifestyle behaviors.[47]

Ideally, a diabetes care team will be able to assess, treat, evaluate, and support the youth and family during the initial stages of the disease. Not all communities have access to such services. In many cases, school counselors and nurses, coaches, teachers, family friends, and peers can assist in providing information, supporting dietary changes, encouraging physical activity, and becoming a sounding board for the frustrations and concerns of the young person with diabetes.

Self-Care Behaviors

The AADE7 Self-Care Behaviors® are applicable throughout the life span for those with type 2 diabetes. Each behavior is critical in attaining self-sufficiency in the management of diabetes. However, each behavior must be modified to incorporate the particular developmental needs of the person with diabetes to reflect the individual's physical capabilities and self-care responsibilities. Strategies pertinent to each behavior are covered more fully in chapters 4 through 10 of this book.

Being Active

All persons with type 2 diabetes need to maintain a program of physical fitness, the definition of which will vary according to age and ability. Creating a program that is sustainable and integrating it into a daily routine may be quite different for a child compared with a nursing home resident; yet for both, exercise is an integral factor in reducing insulin resistance and improving cardiovascular health.

Healthy Eating

Nutritional management skills such as knowing what, when, and how much to eat are the basis of self-care in diabetes. Modifications for age, caloric requirements, and activity level individualize this therapy.

Adults and Older Adults

Adults with diabetes must learn to replace harmful dietary habits with healthy ones. Selecting nutritious foods that are easy to chew and digest and that are also appetizing may pose a problem for some older adults. The elderly adult may also experience social isolation and have a reduced appetite. Financial limitations can also affect healthy eating behaviors.

Teens

Learning how to cope with the typical diet of their peers while maintaining glycemic stability is a daunting task for teens. Alcohol consumption and eating disorders, particularly overeating, may also pose a threat (see chapters 4 and 5).

Taking Medication

Polypharmacy in adults and older persons with diabetes can create problems in accuracy and engagement with medication taking. Issues of vision and manual dexterity complicate this task. For children, medications can be dispensed by a responsible adult or taken under supervision. Despite this, the child needs an age-appropriate understanding of the importance of the medication regimen and the ability to recognize and treat possible side effects such as hypoglycemia.

Monitoring

Learning to accurately monitor glucose levels is a basic skill that is integral to self-managing diabetes, regardless of age. Both the young and the old experience lifestyle changes that can radically alter glucose levels. In such cases, SMBG is an important safety tool for avoiding critically low or high levels.

Problem Solving

Understanding glucose data or interpreting signs and symptoms of acute complications and being able to make appropriate therapeutic adjustments are complex skills that require education and mentoring. Caregivers for those who are homebound or in nursing facilities may assume this task when the person with diabetes is unable to make these decisions alone. In these situations, diabetes healthcare professionals need to educate and support ancillary care providers to ensure that standards of diabetes care are upheld.

Reducing Risks

For the young, much of self-care education focuses on improving glycemic stability to prevent future complications. Risk reduction for CVD is of paramount importance in obese children with type 2 diabetes. Smoking abstinence or cessation and management of lipids and blood pressure are also important in reducing risk. Diabetes care and education specialists have the task of informing communities of the lifestyle modifications necessary to prevent and treat diabetes in youth. For older persons with diabetes, vigilance in screening is important to delay or prevent complications. Eye exams, prophylactic foot care, flu and pneumonia vaccines, and dental care all help maintain functional status among elderly adults.

Healthy Coping

Psychosocial adaptations are required. Living with a chronic disease requires support, creative coping skills, and a certain hardiness. Remaining motivated in the face of a somewhat capricious disease such as diabetes can be very difficult.

The life stressors present for young and old add considerable burden, and it is not uncommon for persons with diabetes to become depressed. Healthcare providers must help persons with diabetes learn a variety of coping skills to meet the challenges of life with diabetes, and be ready to appropriately screen for and treat depression. Chapter 4 provides more information on depression.

Summary

Type 2 diabetes is a major problem affecting all ages. With the incidence and prevalence of this disease rising to epidemic proportions, the healthcare professional must address the factors that contribute to the development of diabetes as well as those that contribute to the development of diabetic complications. Obesity, genes, and family history are the prime risk factors; however, attention to interpersonal, intrapersonal, community, and societal issues can help promote healthy lifestyles for those with diabetes.

- To prevent type 2 diabetes, interventions at the individual, family, and community levels are crucial to reduce the levels of obesity in Western society.
- Important steps to improve diabetes care include community awareness of lifestyle modifications necessary to reduce risk, appropriate screening for diabetes among those at highest risk, and promotion of and engagement with diabetes standards of care.
- To be effective, education and medical management must be tailored to the individual, taking into consideration age, socioeconomic status, and cultural and religious affiliations.

By recognizing the needs of individuals with type 2 diabetes throughout the life span, the health professional is better prepared to offer appropriate treatment and guidance.

Focus on Education

Teaching Strategies

Be sensitive to issues of age and culture. Type 2 diabetes affects a wide range of age groups. Give simple, clear information and messages in a stepwise approach. Tailor content to the specific concerns of that age group. Seek out questions that need to be answered first. Become familiar with various cultural norms and incorporate them into teaching as appropriate. Ask about food staples in the diet and forms of preparation. What is the hierarchy of the family? A child may be cared for by a relative other than the parents.

Establish a relationship in order to determine a person with diabetes' knowledge, find out the person with diabetes' agenda, find out what he or she already knows, and then offer information and handouts. Being a guide and partner in diabetes care is an important component in individualizing care. Persons with diabetes must be able to openly discuss their concerns to create a successful plan of care. Asking open-ended questions (eg, What challenges do you face when trying to manage your diabetes?) you demonstrate an interest in the person with diabetes and allow the person with diabetes to express concerns about the management of their disease.

Provide culturally sensitive person with diabetes care. Providing culturally sensitive health care that is relevant to a person with diabetes' needs and expectations can influence their engagement with their treatment plans and improve health outcomes. Culturally sensitive health care has been described as "the ability to be responsive to the attitudes, feelings, or circumstances of groups of people that share a common and distinctive racial, national, religious, linguistic, or cultural heritage."[48] Studies have found that person with diabetes' satisfaction their health care provider is positively associated with various provider behaviors that show sensitivity and caring such as empathy, warmth, genuineness, support, and acknowledgment of cultural values and beliefs. Cultural sensitivity has evolved from making assumptions about persons with diabetes on the basis of their background to the implementation of the principles of person-centered care. Communication skills such as exploration, empathy, and other techniques are the gateway to understanding needs, values, and preferences of the person with diabetes. The following questions are examples of effective cross cultural communication:

- Belief about health (What do you think has caused your problem? Why do you think it started when it did? What do you fear most about diabetes? What kind of treatment do you think you should receive?)
- Explanation (Why did diabetes happen at this time in your life?)
- Learn (Help me to understand your belief/opinion about diabetes?)
- Impact (How is diabetes impacting your life? What are the chief problems your sickness has caused for you?)

Create a milieu. Think about a wide range of ages, previous experience with diabetes in the family or with friends, and how to deliver content with more than a single approach. For example, teens and adults who drink soft drinks benefit from measuring teaspoons of sugar that equal the amount of sugar found in a "real" soft drink. This gives a visual of the calorie and glycemic value of a commonly consumed beverage. Adults and teens also respond to seeing test tubes filled with fat that equal the amount of fat in food products such as hamburger, steak, and chicken.

Identify polypharmacy problems. Polypharmacy may be a problem for persons with diabetes, particularly in older adults. Routinely review all medications the person is taking, including over-the-counter products and dietary supplements. Discuss use and misuse (for example, use in combination with other medicines and street drugs).

Recognize psychological concerns. Changes in self-esteem, for example, are a concern for all age groups. Accepting diabetes as a chronic disease may be especially difficult for younger individuals, but belief in the chronicity and care needed is of concern to all age groups. As an elderly person's medical and mental status changes, the person may be placed at risk for adverse events. Family involvement is advised for support.

Person-centered pedagogy versus andragogy. When working with persons with diabetes throughout their life span, the diabetes care and education specialist should consider his or her teaching style and people's learning style. The pedagogical approach happens when a learner is dependent on the instructor for all learning; the experience of the instructor is most influential; students are told what they have to learn in order to advance; learning is a process of acquiring prescribed content; and motivation is based on external pressures, competition for grades, and the consequences of failure.

The andragogical approach happens when the learner is self-directed, experience becomes the source of self-identity, and change is likely to trigger a readiness to learn. Learning must have relevance to real-life tasks, and students are internally motivated via self-esteem, recognition, better quality of life, self-confidence, and self-actualization.

In summary, pedagogy is when diabetes care and education specialists believe that they know what the person with diabetes needs to know and what to do about it. It is a very conservative strategy of education by providing lecture with the information persons with diabetes need to know. On the other hand, andragogy is a more liberal approach to education. In an andragogical approach, diabetes care and education specialists provide learning opportunities that are organized around life/work situations rather than content.

What can persons with diabetes teach diabetes care and education specialists? Each education visit should be an opportunity for diabetes care and education specialists to learn from persons with diabetes. Only when they learn from a person with diabetes can they effectively provide accurate teaching. By carefully listening to persons with diabetes, diabetes care and education specialists can assess gaps between where they are now and where they need to be.

Person-centered education. The theory of multiple intelligences was developed in 1983 by Dr. Howard Gardner and suggests that the traditional interpretation of being smart, based on IQ testing, is not indicative of one's capacity to learn and utilize the knowledge. Diabetes care and education specialists can utilize multiple theories of learning and approaches to deliver effective education. There is no one formula for empowering, influencing, and moving one from wanting to learn to actually learning and doing something with the information. Diabetes care and education specialists can use words, logic, pictures, music, self-reflection, physical activities, and social interactions to convey information effectively to people with diabetes. The common denominator is to focus on the learner and his or her needs and desires and consequently deliver a person-centered education.

Messages for Persons With Diabetes

Screening visits protect health longer. Schedule health visits for screening and then schedule any needed follow-up appointments without delay. Doing so will help you know what you are most at risk for, avoid or delay complications related to having diabetes, and improve the chances for effective treatment.

Physical activity helps at every age. All age groups should engage in fitness. Although competitive sports may be culturally encouraged, fitness and endurance are the true primary focus. Walking and workout programs are examples.

Involve family. Involving family and/or significant others at all levels of self-care diabetes management is encouraged.

Focus on Practice

Multidimensional strategies for a multidimensional problem. Multiple factors within type 2 diabetes management require special attention: ethnic background, family history, obesity, and a sedentary lifestyle. Population-specific education strategies, clinical interventions, public health policies, and media influences are among many factors that impact how an individual internalizes and approaches diabetes care. Diabetes care specialists need to be involved in all aspects of diabetes care, spectrums of delivery, and dimensions of information dissemination.

Quality improvement needs to be an easy and welcoming process. It takes a long time to change systems and the way that diabetes care is practiced. Later, it takes a while to realize that things do not work anymore. Once it is realized that things do not work, it takes a long time to change them. As a result, diabetes care and education specialists are often stuck implementing unnecessary processes and practices that do not produce optimal outcomes. Diabetes care and education specialists need to question what they do and ask those involved in diabetes self-management education (DSME), "What does not work?" and "What needs to be done to fix it?"

Evidence-based DSME does not always need to be based on randomized clinical trials. Consider exploratory investigations to identify problems and corresponding solutions, constructive research to develop solutions to a problem, and empirical research to test the feasibility of a solution. Each DSME practice needs to look at the program deliverables: Are you achieving the desired metabolic markers? Are you cost-effective? Are persons with diabetes choosing your center as a preferred method of care? Share your successes and challenges with others, allow others to learn from your experience, and model and adapt strategies that work.

References

1. American Diabetes Association. 2. Classification and diagnosis of diabetes: Standards of Medical Care in Diabetes 2020. Diabetes Care 2020;43(Suppl. 1):S14–S31.
2. Skyler JS, Bakris GL, Bonifacio E, et al. Differentiation of diabetes by pathophysiology, natural history, and prognosis. Diabetes. 2017;66:241-55.
3. Phillips LS, Ratner RE, Buse JB, Kahn SE. We can change the natural history of type 2 diabetes. Diabetes Care. 2014; 37(10): 2668-76.
4. Cho NH, Shaw JE, Karuranga S, Huang Y, da Rocha Fernandes JD et al. IDF Diabetes Atlas: Global estimates of diabetes prevalence for 2017 and projections for 2045. Diabetes Res Clin Pract. 2018 Apr;138:271-81. doi: 10.1016/j.diabres.2018.02.023. Epub 2018 Feb 26.
5. Centers for Disease Control and Prevention. *National Diabetes Statistics Report, 2017*. Atlanta, GA: Centers for Disease Control and Prevention, US Department of Health and Human Services; 2017.
6. National Diabetes Education Program. Overview of diabetes in children and adolescents. 2011 Jun (cited 2013 Jun 10). On the Internet at: http://ndep.nih.gov/media/youth _factsheet.pdf.
7. The SEARCH for Diabetes in Youth Study Group. The many faces of diabetes in American youth: type 1 and type 2 diabetes in five race and ethnic populations. Diabetes Care. 2009;32 Suppl 2:S99-147.
8. Pociot F, Akolkar B, Concannon P, et al. Genetics of type 1 diabetes: what's next? Diabetes. 2010;59:1561-71.
9. Lyssenko V, Jonsson A, Almgren P, et al. Clinical risk factors, DNA variants, and the development of type 2 diabetes. N Engl J Med. 2008;359:2220-32.
10. Mora-Rodriguez R, Ortega JF, Ramirez-Jimenez M, Moreno-Cabañas A, Morales-Palomo F. Insulin sensitivity improvement with exercise training is mediated by body weight loss in subjects with metabolic syndrome. Diabetes Metab. 2019 May 31. pii: S1262-3636(19)30086-2. doi: 10.1016/j.diabet .2019.05.004.
11. American Diabetes Association. Lifestyle Management: Standards of Medical Care in Diabetes—2019. Diabetes Care 2019;42(Suppl.1): S46-60.
12. Haskell WL, Lee IM, Pate RR, et al. Physical activity and public health: updated recommendation for adults from the American College of Sports Medicine and the American Heart Association. Med Sci Sports Exerc. 2007;39:1423-34.
13. Gaskin DJ, Thorpe RJ, McGinty EE, Bower K, Rohde C, LaVeist TA, et al. Disparities in Diabetes: The Nexus of Race, Poverty, and Place Am J Public Health. 2014; 104(11): 2147–55.
14. Ludwig J, Sanbonmatsu L, Gennetian L et al. Neighborhoods, obesity, and diabetes—a randomized social experiment. N Engl J Med. 2011;365(16):1509–19.
15. American Diabetes Association. Prevention or delay of type 2 diabetes: standards of medical care in diabetes—2019. Diabetes Care. 2019;42(Suppl.1):S29-33.
16. American Diabetes Association. Cardiovascular disease and risk management: Standards of Medical Care in Diabetes—2019 Diabetes Care. 2019;42; Suppl 1:S103-23.
17. The DCCT Research Group. The effect of intensive treatment of diabetes on the development and progression of long-term complications in insulin-dependent diabetes mellitus. N Engl J Med. 1993;329:977-86.
18. UK Prospective Diabetes Study Group. Intensive blood glucose control with sulphonylureas or insulin compared with conventional treatment and risk complications in patients with type 2 diabetes (UKPD 33). Lancet. 1998;352:837-53.
19. Ranjit Unnikrishnan I, Anjana RM, Mohan V. Importance of controlling diabetes early—the concept of metabolic memory, legacy effect and the case for early insulinisation. J Assoc Physicians India. 2011 Apr;59 Suppl:8-12.
20. Kim SH, Lee A Health-Literacy-Sensitive Diabetes Self-Management Interventions: A Systematic Review and Meta-Analysis. Worldviews Evid Based Nurs. 2016 Aug;13(4):324-33. doi: 10.1111/wvn.12157. Epub 2016 Apr 22.
21. Kirkman SM, Briscoe VJ, Clark N, Florez H, Haas LB, Halter JB. Diabetes in older adults: a consensus report. J Am Geriatr Soc. 2012 Dec;60(12):2342-56.
22. Bandeen-Roche K, Seplaki CL, Huang J, et al. Frailty in older adults: a nationally representative profile in the United States. J Gerontol A Biol Sci Med Sci. 2015;70:1427–34.
23. Westacott MJ, Farnsworth NL, St. Clair JR, Poffenberger G, Heintz A, Ludin NW, et al. Age-dependent decline in the coordinated [Ca^{2+}] and insulin secretory dynamics in human pancreatic islets. Diabetes. 2017; 66(9): 2436–45.
24. Centers for Disease Control and Prevention. National Diabetes Statistics Report [Internet], 2017. Available from https://www.cdc.gov/diabetes/data/statistics/statistics-report.html. Accessed 20 May 2019.
25. Narayan KM, Boyle JP, Geiss LS, et al. Impact of recent increase in incidence on future diabetes burden: US, 2005-2050. Diabetes Care. 2006;29:2114-6.
26. Bertoni AG, Krop JS, Anderson GF, Brancati FL. Diabetes-related morbidity and mortality in a national sample of US elders. Diabetes Care. 2002;25(3):471-5.
27. Stratton IM, Adler AI, Neil HA, et al. Association of glycaemia with macrovascular and microvascular complications of type 2 diabetes (UKPDS 35): prospective observational study. BMJ. 2000;321(7258):405-12.
28. Huang ES. Appropriate application of evidence to the care of elderly patients with diabetes. Curr Diabetes Rev. 2007;3(4): 260-3.

29. Feinkohl I, Aung PP, Keller M, et al.; Edinburgh Type 2 Diabetes Study (ET2DS) Investigators. Severe hypoglycemia and cognitive decline in older people with type 2 diabetes: the Edinburgh Type 2 Diabetes Study. Diabetes Care. 2014;37: 507–15.

30. McCrimmon RJ, Ryan CM, Frier BM. Diabetes and cognitive dysfunction. Lancet. 2012;379(9833):2291-9.

31. Imperatore G, Boyle JP, Thompson TJ, et al; SEARCH for Diabetes in Youth Study Group. Projections of type 1 and type 2 diabetes burden in the US population aged <20 years through 2050: dynamic modeling of incidence, mortality, and population growth. Diabetes Care. 2012;35(12):2515-20.

33. American Diabetes Association. Children and adolescents. Standards of medical care in diabetes—2019. Diabetes Care. 2019;42(Suppl. 1):S148-64.

34. Arslanian S, Bacha F, Grey M, Marcus MD, White NH, Zeitler P. Evaluation and management of youth-onset type 2 diabetes: a position statement by the American Diabetes Association. Diabetes Care. 2018;41:2648-68.

35. Nadeau KJ, Anderson BJ, Berg EG, et al. Youth-onset type 2 diabetes consensus report: current status, challenges, and priorities. Diabetes Care. 2016;39:1635-42.

36. Styne DM, Arslanian SA, Connor EL, et al. Pediatric obesitydassessment, treatment, and prevention: an Endocrine Society clinical practice guideline. J Clin Endocrinol Metab. 2017;102: 709–57.

37. Michalsky MP, Inge TH, Simmons M, et al.; Teen-LABS Consortium. Cardiovascular risk factors in severely obese adolescents: the Teen Longitudinal Assessment of Bariatric Surgery (Teen-LABS) study. JAMA Pediatr. 2015;169: 438–44.

38. Hannon TS, Arslanian SA. The changing face of diabetes in youth: lessons learned from studies of type 2 diabetes. Ann N Y Acad Sci. 2015;1353: 113–37.

39. Phillips DI. Birthweight and the future development of diabetes: a review of the evidence. Diabetes Care. 1998;21 Suppl 2:B150-5.

40. Silverman BL, Metzger BE, Cho NH, Loeb CA. Impaired glucose tolerance in adolescent offspring of diabetic mothers: relationship of fetal hyperinsulinism. Diabetes Care. 1995; 18:611-7.

41. Van Name MA, Guandalini C, Steffen A, Patel A, Tamborlane W The present and future treatment of pediatric type 2 diabetes. Expert Rev Endocrinol Metab. 2018 Jul;13(4):207-12. doi: 10.1080/17446651.2018.1499467.

42. Atkin AJ, Sharp SJ, Harrison F, Brage S, Van Sluijs EM. Seasonal variation in children's physical activity and sedentary time. Med Sci Sports Exerc. 2016;48:449–56.

43. Jones KL, Arslanian S, Peterokova VA, et al. Effect of metformin in pediatric patients with type 2 diabetes: a randomized controlled trial. Diabetes Care. 2002;25:89-94.

44. Kendall D, Vail A, Amin R, et al. Metformin in obese children and adolescents: the MOCA trial. J Clin Endocrinol Metab. 2013;98(1):322-9.

45. Poulsen MN, Knapp EA, Hirsch AG, Bailey-Davis L, Pollak J, Schwartz BS. Comparing objective measures of the built environment in their associations with youth physical activity and sedentary behavior across heterogeneous geographies. Health Place. 2018; 49:30-8.

46. Hingle M.D., Turner T., Kutob R., Merchant N., Roe D.J., Stump C., Going S.B. The EPIC kids study: a randomized family-focused YMCA-based intervention to prevent type 2 diabetes in at-risk youth. BMC Public Health. 2015;15:1253.

47. Colberg SR, Sigal RJ, Yardley JE, et al. Physical activity/exercise and diabetes: a position statement of the American Diabetes Association. Diabetes Care. 2016;392065-79.

48. Tucker CM, Marsiske M, Rice KG, Nielson JJ, Herman K. Patient-centered culturally sensitive health care: model testing and refinement. Health Psychology. 2011:30(3), 342-50. http://dx.doi.org/10.1037/a0022967

CHAPTER 16

Nutrition Therapy

Alison B. Evert, MS, RDN, CDCES

Key Concepts

- There is not an ideal percentage of calories from carbohydrate, protein, and fat for all people with or at risk of diabetes. Therefore, nutrition therapy for persons with diabetes and prediabetes should be individualized on the basis of the person's metabolic needs (i.e., glucose, lipid, blood pressure), preferences, and willingness and ability to make lifestyle changes.
- A variety of eating patterns (combinations of different foods or food groups) are acceptable for the management of diabetes and prediabetes. Key factor that are common among the patterns:
  - —Emphasize non-starchy vegetables
  - —Minimize added sugars and refined grains
  - —Choose whole foods over highly processed foods to the extent possible
  - —Replace sugar-sweetened beverages with water as often as possible
  - —There is no "one-size-fits-all" answer to diet and diabetes
- Strong evidence supports that medical nutrition therapy (MNT) provided by a registered dietitian nutritionist (RDN) can improve A1C, with absolute reductions of up to 1.9% (in type 1 diabetes) and up to 2% (in type 2 diabetes) at 3 to 6 months. Ongoing MNT support can assist with maintenance of glycemic improvements.
- Reducing overall carbohydrate intake and consistency in food intake are key strategies in achieving glucose goals in persons with type 2 diabetes or type 1 diabetes and can be applied in a variety of eating patterns. Adults with overweight/obesity and prediabetes or diabetes should have MNT and diabetes self-management and support (DSMES) or diabetes prevention services to support weight loss and improve A1C, cardiovascular (CVD) risk factors, and quality of life. The eating plan should be individualized in a format that results in an energy deficit. In the absence of contraindications, physical activity should be encouraged in all persons with diabetes to decrease insulin resistance and assist in achieving individualized glucose, lipid, and blood pressure goals. While physical activity alone does not result in significant weight loss, it plays an important role in prevention of weight regain and reduces the risk of CVD.
  - —For people with prediabetes, the goal is to lose 7% to 10% of body weight for preventing progression to type 2 diabetes.
  - —For people with type 2 diabetes with overweight and obesity, losing at least 5% body weight to see a meaningful benefit, and the benefits are progressive. The goal for optimal benefit is weight loss of 15% or more, assuming it can be feasibly and safely accomplished.
  - —Because weight loss through lifestyle changes is difficult to maintain long-term, ongoing support and additional therapeutic options may be needed.
  - —When counseling all individuals with diabetes or prediabetes about weight management, special attention also must be given to prevent, diagnose, and treat disordered eating.
- Replacing intake of saturated fat, *trans* fat with unsaturated fats reduces both cholesterol and LDL-cholesterol and also benefits CVD risk.
- The recommendation for the general public to consume less than 2,300 mg/day of sodium is also appropriate for people with diabetes and prediabetes.

Introduction

Nutrition therapy has been essential in the treatment of diabetes since diabetes was first discovered to be the "sweet urine" disease centuries ago. Nutrition recommendations have changed over the years based on theories of the era. Today, nutrition guidelines are based on available scientific evidence, which has dispelled many of the nutrition myths and misinformation of earlier times. Diabetes nutrition therapy, like medicine, remains an ever-changing field as researchers and clinicians learn more about the human body and how various components and combinations of foods and nutrients affect disease risk and management. The Diabetes Mellitus Types 1 and 2 Systematic Review and Guideline 2015 from the Academy of Nutrition and Dietetics (Academy)[1] and the Nutrition Therapy for Adults With Diabetes or Prediabetes: A Consensus Report published by American Diabetes Association (ADA)[2] as well as the ADA's Standards of Medical Care in Diabetes—2019[3] provide healthcare providers and persons with diabetes with the latest information on beneficial nutrition therapies and outcomes. In addition, an Association of Diabetes Care and Educations Specialist (ADCES) practice synopsis is available to summarize key message about healthy eating practices as a cornerstone of self-management care that leads to improved quality of life in persons with diabetes.[4]

MNT is defined as an evidence-based application of the Nutrition Care Process provided by the RDN and is the legal definition of nutrition counseling by an RDN in the United States.[5] Medical nutrition therapy involves a nutrition assessment, nutrition diagnosis, nutrition intervention, and nutrition monitoring and evaluation.[1–3] According to the Institute of Medicine (IOM), nutrition therapy is the treatment of a disease or condition through the modification of nutrient or whole-food intake and does not specify that nutrition therapy must be provided by an RDN.[6] For persons with type 1 diabetes or type 2 diabetes, the recommended number of RDN encounters during the first 6 months is 3 to 6, with the RDN to determine whether additional encounters are needed. A minimum of 1 annual MNT follow-up encounter is also recommended.[1,7] During this time it can be determined whether target goals can be achieved by implementation of MNT in combination with physical activity or whether medication(s) will need to be combined with MNT.

The ADCES recommends that diabetes care and education specialists be knowledgeable about diabetes nutrition therapy, as they may participate in the delivery of nutrition education in group classes or one-on-one sessions as part of DSMES or collaborate in the development of an individualized eating plan and support its implementation.[4] A joint position statement was co-published by the ADCES, ADA, and the Academy of Nutrition and Dietetics (Academy) to assist all members of the health care team to know when to refer people with type 2 diabetes to accredited DSMES programs.[8] The four essential times for assessing the need for DSMES referral: 1) at time of diagnosis, 2) on an annual basis, 3) when new complicating factors influence self-management, and 4) at times of transitions in care. The joint statement includes a DSMES *Algorithm of Care* for healthcare professionals (HCPs) and integrates with MNT delivered by a RDN as well as emotional health provider by a mental health professional, if needed. Another section of the algorithm identifies areas of focus and action steps that should be considered by both the HCP and diabetes care and education specialist, as well as the RDN or mental health professional, if indicated at these critical times.

Historically, eating plans for people with diabetes were calorie-controlled diets with specified macronutrient percentages prescribed by the healthcare provider. Nutrition therapy now focuses on the needs and preferences of the individual with diabetes to collaboratively develop an eating plan that can be followed long-term.[3,9] This focus sets the stage for the adoption of small, incremental lifestyle changes that include food/nutrition and physical activity to improve overall health, reduce the risk of diabetes complications, and manage complications if necessary. Evidence from clinical trials and observational studies supports the effectiveness of nutrition therapy in the primary, secondary, and tertiary prevention of diabetes (ie, preventing or delaying the development of diabetes, and preventing or controlling the complications of diabetes).[1–4] Unfortunately, national data in the United States indicate that only about half of persons with diabetes receive diabetes education, and even fewer see an RDN.[10] One study of over 18,000 people with diabetes revealed that only 9.1% had at least 1 nutrition visit within a 9-year time period.[11]

This chapter discusses the role of nutrition therapy in the following areas: glucose management; energy balance and weight management; prevention and treatment of CVD (including hypertension and dyslipidemia) and diabetic kidney disease; and intervention strategies to achieve nutrition therapy goals for youth and adults with diabetes. Evidence-based systematic reviews of diabetes nutrition therapy are the basis for the majority of the recommendations cited in this chapter.[1,2,3]

Goals of Diabetes Nutrition Therapy

Persons with type 1 or 2 diabetes and those at risk for diabetes should receive individualized or group nutrition therapy at diagnosis and as needed throughout the lifespan and during times of changing health status to achieve treatment goals.[1,2,8] Diabetes-focused MNT is provided by an RDN, preferably one who has comprehensive knowledge and experience with diabetes care.[2] The person with diabetes should be involved in the decision-making process.

Goal of Nutrition Therapy for Persons at Risk for Diabetes:[2]

- Refer people with prediabetes and overweight/obesity to an intensive lifestyle intervention program that includes individualized goal-setting components, such as the Diabetes Prevention Program (DPP) and/or individualized MNT.

Goals of Nutrition Therapy for All Persons With Diabetes:[2]

- Promote and support healthful eating patterns, emphasizing a variety of nutrient-dense foods in appropriate portion sizes, in order to improve overall health and specifically to:
  - —Decrease A1C, blood pressure, and cholesterol levels (goals differ for individuals based on age, duration of diabetes, health history, and other present health conditions.
  - —Achieve and maintain body weight goals
  - —Delay or prevent complications of diabetes
- Address individual nutritional needs, based on personal and cultural preferences, health literacy and numeracy, access to healthful food choices, willingness and ability to make behavioral changes, as well as barriers to change
- Maintain the pleasure of eating by providing positive messages about food choices, while limiting food choices only when indicated by scientific evidence
- Provide the individual with diabetes with practical tools for day-to-day meal planning

A Healthy Eating Pattern

Optimal nutrition through healthy food choices remains the underlying principle of diabetes nutrition recommendations.[1,2,4] In general, a healthful eating pattern recommended by the USDA Dietary Guidelines for Americans emphasizes a variety of vegetables from all the subgroups, fruits, especially whole fruits; grains, at least half of which are whole intact grains, lower-fat dairy; a variety of protein foods; and oils. This eating pattern limits intake of saturated fats and *trans* fats, added sugars, and sodium.[12]

The recently published ADA Nutrition Therapy for Adults With Diabetes and Prediabetes: A Consensus Report reviewed research studies on persons with diabetes following

Case: Type 2 Diabetes Treated With Glucose-Lowering Medications

LW, a 51-year-old woman with type 2 diabetes of 5 years' duration, was referred for diabetes medical nutrition therapy.

Nutrition Assessment

- Height: 64 in
- Weight: 175 lb
- Body mass index (BMI): 31 kg/m^2

Medical Diagnosis

- Type 2 diabetes, obesity, hypertension, dyslipidemia

Lab Data

- A1C: 8.1%
- Low-density lipoprotein cholesterol (LDL-C): 160 mg/dL (8.879 mmol/L)
- High-density lipoprotein cholesterol (HDL-C): 43 mg/dL (2.39 mmol/L)
- Triglycerides (TG): 234 mg/dL (12.99 mmol/L)
- Blood pressure: 148/88 mm Hg

Medications

- Glimepiride (Amaryl®, Sanofi Aventis) 4 mg daily, for diabetes; metformin (Glucophage®, Bristol-Myers Squibb) 1000 mg bid, for diabetes
- Simvastatin (Zocor®, Merck) 20 mg daily, for dyslipidemia
- Quinapril (Accupril®, Pfizer) 20 mg daily, for hypertension

Nutrition History

LW stated that she either skips breakfast or eats a light breakfast in her car, eats lunch primarily at fast-food restaurants, and eats out for dinner about half of the time. She occasionally snacks on chips or other salty snacks in the afternoon and usually eats a bowl of sugar-free ice cream in the evening after dinner. She does not drink alcoholic beverages. A brief evaluation of LW's usual food/nutrition history reveals that her diet

(continued)

Case: Type 2 Diabetes Treated With Glucose-Lowering Medications (continued)

is high in total and saturated fat, is high in sodium, contains few fruits and vegetables, and appears low in fiber and calcium. LW asked if a low-carbohydrate, high-protein eating plan would help her lose weight and achieve glucose management goals. LW's job is sedentary. She said she does not have the time or energy to go to the gym after work.

Assessment of LW's metabolic status reveals that she exhibits characteristics common in type 2 diabetes. Markers of LW's increased cardiovascular risk are a pattern of dyslipidemia that includes elevated LDL-C, low HDL-C, and hypertriglyceridemia along with hypertension and obesity (BMI ≥30 kg/m^2).

Nutrition Diagnosis

Excessive intake of calories, sodium, and saturated fat related to eating frequently in restaurants and lack of portion control; low energy expenditure due to sedentary job and lack of regular physical activity.

As the chapter progresses, readers will gain insight into the following regarding LW's case: What initial lifestyle changes can be suggested to improve her glycemic management? What aspects of nutrition therapy can reduce her cardiovascular risk? What are the risks and benefits of using a low-carbohydrate diet to achieve her goals?

different types of eating patterns, including Mediterranean-style, vegetarian and vegan, low-fat, low-carbohydrate and very low carbohydrate, DASH (dietary approaches to stop hypertension) and Paleo. It concluded that a variety of eating patterns are acceptable for the management of diabetes.[2] Personal preferences (eg, tradition, culture, religion, health beliefs and goals, economics) and metabolic goals should be considered when implementing one eating pattern over another. Based on their review of evidence, the ADA Nutrition Therapy in Adults with Diabetes and Prediabetes: A Consensus Report suggests, "reducing overall carbohydrate intake for individuals with diabetes that have demonstrated the most evidence for improving glycemia and may be applied in a variety of eating patterns that meet individual needs and preferences. For select adults with type 2 diabetes not meeting glycemic targets or where reducing antihyperglycemic medications is a priority, reducing overall carbohydrate intake with a low- or very low-carbohydrate eating plans is a viable approach.[2]" Further research is needed to determine the most effective strategies to help persons with diabetes adopt new eating patterns.

> With nutrition therapy and increased physical activity, the effect on blood glucose level is evident almost immediately.

Nutrition Therapy and Glycemic Management

A primary goal in the management of diabetes is the regulation of blood glucose to achieve individualized blood glucose goals. With changes in lifestyle, the effect on blood glucose levels is evident almost immediately. Clinical trials and outcome studies of diabetes MNT provided by an RDN can improve A1C, with absolute reductions of up to 1.9% (in type 1 diabetes) and up to 2% (in type 2 diabetes) at 3 to 6 months, depending on the type and duration of diabetes and level of glycemia.[1,7] Studies have demonstrated that ongoing RDN provided follow-up encounters ranging from 3 to 6 sessions, with a minimum of 1 follow-up session annually can be helpful in maintaining glycemic improvements.[1,7]

> Clinical trials and outcome studies of diabetes MNT provided by an RDN can improve A1C, with absolute reductions of up to 1.9% (in type 1 diabetes) and up to 2% (in type 2 diabetes) at 3 to 6 months, depending on the duration of diabetes and level of glycemia.

Attempts are often made to identify one approach to diabetes nutrition therapy; however, a single approach does not exist, just as there is no one medication or insulin plan that applies to all persons with diabetes. A variety of nutrition therapy interventions—such as carbohydrate counting utilizing carbohydrate or "carb" choices or insulin-to-carbohydrate ratios (ICRs), simplified meal plans such as the plate method, individualized meal-planning strategies with prescribed amounts of energy/fat, vegetarian or Mediterranean-style eating patterns, or *Choose Your Foods* or *Exchange Lists for Meal Planning*—are all reported to be effective when implemented appropriately.[1,7] In order for the nutrition therapy intervention to be effective it must be implemented in collaboration with the person with diabetes. In reviewing consistent themes for nutrition interventions, it appears that, for individuals with type 2 diabetes, reducing the energy content of usual food intake is central to successful outcomes.[1,2,7] For individuals with type 1 diabetes, adjusting insulin doses for planned carbohydrate intake is of primary importance.[1,2] Appropriate implementation of nutrition therapy is similar to other therapies which require regular follow-up and evaluation of effect, ease of implementation, engagement, and need for adjustment in therapy. Due to the need for daily engagement, continuous intervention to increase support and maintenance is also an essential component of nutrition care. The number and duration of nutrition encounters may need to be greater if the patient has language, ethnic, or cultural concerns or if the person's medications have changed (such as the addition of anti-hyperglycemic agents or insulin therapy in type 2 diabetes, or changes in insulin plans in type 1 diabetes or type 2 diabetes).[1,7] To make DPPs more accessible, digital health tools are an area of increasing interest.[2] Evolving research reveals that delivery of DPP interventions through technology-enabled platforms and digital health tools can result in reduced risk of diabetes and CVD, weight loss, and improved glycemia.[2]

RDNs providing diabetes MNT should assess and monitor medication use and changes in relation to the eating plan.[2] Research studies and practice papers report the role of the RDN in organization-approved medication adjustment protocols.[13–15] The experienced RDN that has demonstrated competency in medication adjustment and practicing within their scopes of practice can help to reduce clinical inertia and/or reduce risk of hypoglycemia and hyperglycemia.[2]

Macronutrients

Because all 3 macronutrients (carbohydrate, protein, and fat) require insulin for metabolism and influence the attainment of nutrition therapy goals, including healthy eating, they must be addressed. In the United States, the majority of persons with type 1 diabetes or type 2 diabetes report eating moderate amounts of carbohydrate (~45% of total energy intake) and getting ~35% to 40% of energy intake from fat, with the remainder (~16%-18%) from protein.[16] Generally, as carbohydrate intake decreases, total fat (usually saturated fats) increases. A number of studies have reported on differing percentages of carbohydrate intake in adults with diabetes. The Strong Health Study reported that a lower intake of carbohydrate and higher consumption of total and saturated fats was associated with poorer glycemic outcomes.[17] Similarly, in subjects receiving intensive treatment in the Diabetes Control and Complications Trial (DCCT), diets lower in carbohydrate and higher in total and saturated fats were associated with worse glycemic management, independent of exercise and BMI.[18] However, in clinical trials, both high- and low-carbohydrate diets led to similar changes in body weight and A1C.[1,2] It appears likely that the total energy intake outweighs the amount of carbohydrate in the eating pattern. Higher carbohydrate eating plans, which are generally low in fat, tend to have beneficial effects on LDL-C and total cholesterol, whereas lower carbohydrate diets tend to have beneficial effects on triglycerides and HDL-C.[19] Evidence suggests that there is not an ideal percentage of calories from carbohydrate, protein, and fat for all persons with diabetes.[1,2] Therefore, because of the benefits and/or similarities in outcomes, it would seem prudent to recommend an eating pattern that should include an assessment of current dietary intake followed by individualized guidance on self-monitoring of carbohydrate intake to optimize meal timing and food choices to guide medication and physical activity recommendations.[2] When recommending carbohydrate-containing foods for people with diabetes and those at risk of diabetes, higher fiber foods, instead of processed foods with added sodium, fat, and sugars, should be encouraged whenever possible.

The dietary reference intakes (DRIs) from the Food and Nutrition Board of the IOM provide guidance for macronutrient distribution in healthy adults and recommend 45% to 65% of calories from carbohydrate, 10% to 35% from protein, and 20% to 35% from fat.[20] The Recommended Daily Allowance (RDA) for carbohydrate for adults without diabetes (19 years and older) is 130 grams per day and is determined in part by the brain's requirement for glucose, although this energy requirement can be fulfilled via glycogenolysis, gluconeogenesis, and/or ketogenesis in the setting of very low carbohydrate intake. The actual amount of carbohydrate intake required for optimal health in humans is unknown. In situations of reduced carbohydrate intake that are unintentional (eg, illness or food insecurity) or planned (eg, low carbohydrate eating plan), glucose can be derived from endogenous sources through metabolism of the glycerol component of fat and from gluconeogenic amino acids in protein.

Carbohydrate and Glycemia

Historically, it was a commonly held belief that sugars, such as sucrose, must be restricted on the assumption that they are more rapidly digested and absorbed than starches and thus aggravate hyperglycemia. However, scientific evidence does not support restricting sucrose based on this belief. In people with diabetes, research consistently reports that the total amount of carbohydrate consumed and available insulin response after eating, regardless of the type or source (sucrose or starch), is the primary determinant of postprandial glucose levels.[1,2] In approximately 20 studies in which sucrose was substituted for equal amounts of other carbohydrate (starches), the glucose response was nearly identical.[21] Monitoring total grams of carbohydrate, whether by carbohydrate counting or experience-based estimation, is a key strategy in achieving glycemic targets.[1,2]

The acute impact on eating non-starchy vegetables and/or protein 5 to 15 minutes before carbohydrate foods was shown to reduce postprandial glucose and insulin excursion in 3 randomized crossover studies in people with type 2 diabetes.[22–24] When compared to eating carbohydrates first or eating carbohydrates together with non-starchy vegetables and protein such as a sandwich over a 30-minute period, eating carbohydrates last led to significantly lower postprandial glucose and insulin excursions.[24] Checking glucose levels after eating by use of self-monitoring of blood glucose (SMBG) or continuous glucose monitoring (CGM) may help to help to guide treatment decisions or adjustments in carbohydrate intake.[3] Day-to-day consistency in the amount of carbohydrate consumed at breakfast, lunch, and dinner and in snacks can also improve glucose levels, particularly in persons on nutrition therapy alone, anti-hyperglycemic agents, or fixed insulin doses.[1,2]

For persons using multiple daily insulin doses or insulin pumps, adjusting the prandial insulin dose to match planned carbohydrate intake results in achievement of glucose targets.[2] Insulin-to-carbohydrate ratios indicate how many grams of carbohydrate are "covered" or "matched" with 1 unit of rapid- or short-acting insulin.[25] A typical ICR for a normal-weight adult is 1:10 (1 unit of rapid-acting insulin is expected to cover 10 g of carbohydrate).[25] A glucose correction factor (insulin sensitivity factor [ISF]) is the estimated drop in blood glucose (mg/dL) expected from the administration of 1 unit of rapid- or short-acting insulin. The ISF is also related to the individual's insulin sensitivity and body size. A typical ISF for a normal-weight adult with type 1 diabetes is 1:40 mg/dL (1 unit of rapid-acting insulin is expected to drop the blood glucose level 40 mg/dL [2.2 mmol/L]). An overweight insulin-resistant individual may have an ICR of 1:5 and ISF of 1:20 (1 unit of rapid-acting insulin is expected to "cover" 5 g carbohydrate and drop the blood glucose level 20 mg/dL [1.11 mmol/L]).[25]

After reviewing the evidence, the Academy's Diabetes Mellitus Types 1 and 2 Systematic Review and Guideline and the ADA Nutrition Therapy Consensus Report in adults made the following nutrition therapy recommendations regarding carbohydrate intake:[1,2]

- In persons with diabetes on nutrition therapy alone or non-insulin secretagogues, educate on carbohydrate management strategies such as reducing overall carbohydrate intake or portion sizes; a simplified eating such as plate method; or food lists (such as *Choose Your Foods* or *Exchange Lists for Meal Planning*) or carbohydrate counting using carbohydrate choices.
- In persons with diabetes on fixed insulin doses or insulin secretagogues, educate on carbohydrate consistency (timing and amount) using carbohydrate counting alone; plate method, portion control, simplified meal plan; or food lists (such as *Choose Your Foods* or *Exchange Lists for Meal Planning*) or carbohydrate choices or grams of carbohydrate.
- In persons with diabetes on multiple daily injections of insulin or insulin pump therapy, educate on carbohydrate counting using ICRs.

These interventions can be accomplished by comprehensive nutrition education and counseling with the person with diabetes based on his or her individual abilities, preferences, and management skills in collaboration with the RDN or provided by a diabetes care and education specialist as part of a DSMES program.

Achieving Glycemic Targets

Monitoring carbohydrate intake is a key strategy in achieving glycemic targets in people with type 1 diabetes or type 2 diabetes.

Sugars

Sugars include glucose, fructose, sucrose (table sugar), and lactose (milk sugar). When consumed separately, glucose causes the highest glycemic peak response compared with other sugars. This is because sugars such as sucrose and lactose are metabolized into only 50% glucose and the other 50% into fructose or galactose. Fructose and galactose are metabolized by the liver into glucose, glycogen, and/or triglycerides (in the case of fructose), but very little, if any, of the glucose enters into the general circulation.[26]

Two reviews of studies conducted in persons with diabetes showed that naturally occurring "free fructose," found in fruit, may result in more optimal glycemic control compared with isocaloric intake of sucrose or starch and is not likely to have detrimental effects on triglycerides (ie, if it is not consumed in excess amounts: >12% of total energy).[27,28] Excessive consumption of products marketed to individuals with diabetes that contain large amounts of fructose, such as agave nectar, is not recommended.[7]

For the use of carbohydrate in treating low blood glucose levels under 70 mg/dL (3.9 mmol/L), the ADA recommends 15 to 20 g of sucrose or glucose in the form of tablets, liquid, or gel over fruit snacks or fruit juice, although cost, availability, and convenience should be considered.[3] The blood glucose level should be rechecked in 15 minutes; if hypoglycemia persists, then retreat until blood glucose level is above 70 mg/dL.

Starches

The digestive tract is very efficient in breaking down starches into glucose. It is the ability of digestive enzymes to break down the starch, rather than the size of the starch molecule, that determines the glycemic effect of a particular starch. It also depends on the structure of the starch, the source of the starch, and the types of processing and cooking used. Starches composed of higher proportions of amylopectin, such as potatoes, have a greater effect on blood glucose levels than starchy foods that contain more resistant starch or high-amylose foods, such as beans, legumes, and certain types of specially formulated cornstarch. Another form of indigestible fiber is fructan (inulin or chicory root), which has been reported to have glucose-lowering effects. Limited research has been conducted in people with diabetes on resistant starches and fructans.[1]

Glycemic Index

The glycemic index (GI) is a system of ranking carbohydrate foods according to their effect on postprandial glycemia.[29] The glycemic effect (measured as the area under the curve) of 50 g of digestible carbohydrate from a single food is measured over a 2-hour period in people without diabetes. The food is then assigned a percentage value compared with the response of a reference food (glucose or bread). For example, if the area under the curve for a food is three fourths of that of the reference food, it has a GI of 75, or 75%. Diet books and health professionals often claim that the GI measures how rapidly blood glucose levels increase after eating carbohydrate foods, implying that high-GI foods peak rapidly and low-GI foods have a more gradual peak response. However, although the area under the curve for various foods may differ, the general curve shape, including the peak response, is similar within each food category.[29] Therefore, it is incorrect to state that a high-GI food peaks very rapidly and a low-GI food peaks more gradually.

Glycemic load (GL) is another method of predicting the postprandial glucose response.[30] The GL of foods takes into account both the quantity of carbohydrate food consumed and the GI value of the food. The GL is determined by multiplying the GI of the food by the grams of carbohydrate in a serving of food (or for meals by totaling the values for all foods in the meal). There has been no assessment of efficacy of GL in children or adults with type 1 diabetes.[31]

GI and GL research studies are complicated by differing definitions of "high GI" and "low GI" diets or quartiles. Although GI results are commonly interpreted as low GI <55, moderate GI 56 to 69, and high GI >70, these categories have not been used consistently in research studies. GIs in the low-GI diets range from 38% to 77% and in the high-GI diets from 63% to 98%. There is a need to standardize definitions of low, moderate, and high GIs. It should also be noted, that the GI is not always an indicator of healthy food or meal choices. Very early, Wolever et al noted that one of the strongest correlates of overall diet GI is the intake of simple sugars—low-GI diets are associated with significantly higher sugar intakes than high-GI diets.[32] Many high-sugar foods fall into the moderate- or low-GI categories. For example, Coke (GI = 58), a Snickers bar (GI = 56), whereas premium ice cream (GI = 37) has a low GI value.[33] Sugars have moderate to low GI values because they are only 50% glucose (the other 50% being fructose or lactose, depending on the sugar), while starches have higher GIs because they are polymers of glucose and have the potential to be metabolized to 100% glucose. Wolever further reports that whole wheat, brown rice, and brown spaghetti have the same GI values as their refined white versions, and whereas fruits generally have a low GI, whole fruits and juice have the same GI.[34]

The Diabetes Mellitus Types 1 and 2 Systematic Review and Guideline 2015 from the Academy reviewed GI and GL research in adults with type 1 and type 2 diabetes.[1] In studies in participants with type 2 diabetes, the authors reported no significant impact on A1C, mixed results on fasting glucose, no significant effect on LDL-C or blood pressure, whereas the effect of GI on total cholesterol, HDL-C, and triglycerides were mixed. No studies were identified that met search criteria in adults with type 1 diabetes. In a recent systematic review, the authors reported it is unlikely that the GI of a food or diet is linked to disease risk or health outcomes.[35] Other measures of dietary quality, such as fiber or whole grains, may be more likely to predict health outcomes.

Despite the confounding variables and mixed results from GI research studies as described in the preceding paragraphs, use of the GI continues to be very popular worldwide by many people with diabetes and at risk of diabetes. The use of the GI may provide some additional benefit to glucose management over that observed when total carbohydrate is considered alone.[36–38] Based on evidence-review in youth with type 1 diabetes, the International Society of Pediatric and Adolescent Elliott Diabetes (ISPAD) Clinical Practice Consensus Guidelines 2018: Nutritional Management in Children and Adolescents With Diabetes recommends that GI should not be used in isolation, but with a method of carbohydrate quantification.[31] A controlled study in children substituting low-GI for high-GI foods found the lower GI diet improved glucose management after 12 months compared to prescriptive dietary advice.[39]

Fiber

The average amount of fiber a person without diabetes in the United States consumes is 17 g per day, with only 5% of the population meeting the adequate intake (14 g total fiber per 1,000 kcal, or 25 g for adult women and 38 g for adult men).[40] Fiber studies that have shown improved glycemia included diets containing ~44 to 50 g of fiber per day,[1,2] an amount that may be difficult for many Americans to consume due to the palatability and gastrointestinal side effects. It is recommended that persons with diabetes include foods containing 21 to 25 g (women) or 30 to 38 g (men) of fiber per day, which is the amount recommended for the general public (14 g/1,000 calories).[2,20] An emphasis on soluble fiber sources (7-13 g) is recommended.[1] Fiber-containing foods such as fruits, vegetables, whole grains, and legumes are encouraged because they provide vitamins, minerals, and other nutrients important for good health.[12]

Of interest is how to account for the fiber in carbohydrate for carbohydrate counting, as it is incompletely digested, absorbed, and metabolized. In deriving energy values for food labeling, the dietary fiber portion of carbohydrate is calculated as having about half the energy (2 kcal/g) of most other carbohydrates (4 kcal/g).[41] Adjustment in total carbohydrate is practical only if the amount per serving of dietary fiber is >5 g. In that case, subtract half of the fiber grams from the total carbohydrate. This calculation is only practical for individuals who are using ICRs for managing their insulin-requiring diabetes and should not be recommended for all people with diabetes as it can add an additional degree of complexity to diabetes meal planning.[41]

Sugar-Sweetened Beverages

The 2019 ADA Nutrition Consensus Report and the 2018 American Heart Association (AHA) science advisory both recommend avoiding sugar-sweetened beverages (SSBs) such as soft drinks, fruit drinks, and energy and vitamin water drinks containing sucrose, high-fructose corn syrup, and/or fruit juice concentrates; replacing with water as often as possible should be encouraged.[2,42] Large quantities of SSBs should be avoided to reduce the risk of type 2 diabetes, heart disease, weight gain, non-alcoholic liver disease, and tooth decay.[43] In a meta-analysis of cohort studies, individuals in the highest versus lowest quartile of SSB intake had a 26% greater risk of developing diabetes.[44] Energy intake in those with diabetes can be reduced in some individuals by replacing SSBs with sugar-free beverages.

Nonnutritive and Hypocaloric Sweeteners

The safety and role of nonnutritive sweeteners in a diabetes eating plans continue to be frequently asked questions by people with diabetes, and it is important for diabetes healthcare professionals to provide evidence-based answers rather than personal opinion. It should be noted that terms for non-nutritive sweeteners also include the following artificial sweeteners, sugar substitutes, high-intensity sweeteners, and low-calorie sweeteners. The Food and Drug Administration (FDA) has approved the use of acesulfame potassium, advantame aspartame, neotame, saccharin, and sucralose as food additives; stevia is approved as "generally recognized as safe" (GRAS).[45] The FDA also determined an acceptable daily intake (ADI) for each nonnutritive sweetener. The ADI is the amount that can be safely consumed on a daily basis over a person's lifetime without adverse effects and generally includes a hundredfold safety factor.

The 2018 scientific advisory from the AHA that was supported by the ADA concluded that there was not enough evidence to determine whether non-nutritive sweetener use definitively leads to long-term reduction in cardiometabolic risk factors or body weight, including glycemia.[42] An earlier AHA scientific statement advised when used judiciously, non-nutritive sweeteners could facilitate reductions in added sugars intake, thereby resulting in decreased total energy and weight loss/weight control, and promoting beneficial effects on related metabolic parameters. They noted, however, that potential benefits will not be achieved if there is a compensatory increase in energy intake from other sources.[46] The review of literature for the Academy's Diabetes Mellitus Types 1 and 2 Systematic Review and Guideline in adults found that beverages sweetened with non-nutritive sweeteners have no significant impact on A1C, insulin, or fasting glucose levels in adults with diabetes.[1] Sugar-Sweetened Beverages and Risk of Metabolic Syndrome and Type 2 Diabetes: A Meta-Analysis revealed that replacing intake of SSBs with products containing hypocaloric or non-nutritive sweeteners can help with weight loss,[44] as long as individuals do not replace those calories through other sources.

Food products that contain sugar alcohols do impact glycemia. Studies have shown that most sugar alcohols—including erythritol, hydrogenated starch hydrolysates, isomalt, lactitol, maltitol, mannitol, sorbitol, and xylitol—produce a small rise in blood glucose. However, there is no evidence that sugar alcohols in amounts likely to be consumed improve long-term glycemia, energy intake, or weight, and although safe to use, they may cause gastrointestinal side effects such as bloating, flatulence, and diarrhea, especially in children.[1]

Protein and Fat and Glycemia

Ingestion of protein results in an acute stimulation of insulin secretion similar to that of carbohydrate and has historically been thought to have no long-term effect on insulin requirements. Although 50% to 60% of ingested protein undergoes gluconeogenesis in the liver, studies have also historically demonstrated that glucose produced by the liver does not increase blood glucose concentrations.[19] However, it is a widely held belief that high-protein meals can alter the predicted postprandial response to a carbohydrate-containing meal. Dietary fats are also said to slow glucose absorption and delay the peak glycemic response to the ingestion of carbohydrate foods. These observations are supported by evidence from clinical practice in people with type 1 and type 2 diabetes, particularly from the increasing use of personal CGM, that meals with larger amounts of protein and fat prolong the postprandial glucose excursions up to several hours. Evolving research is providing strategies on how to adjust prandial insulin doses for high-fat and high-protein meals.

A systematic review in adults and youth with type 1 diabetes examined the evidence for the impact of fat and protein on postprandial blood glucose levels.[47] The review concluded that meals high in protein and/or fat increase delayed hyperglycemia (up to 3–6 hours) after eating the meal as well as reduce early (1–2 hours) postprandial rise.[47,48] The authors of the systematic review suggested incremental dose increases up to 30% to 35% for meals high in fat and/or protein, accompanied by a combination bolus if using an insulin pump or split dose injection, if utilizing mealtime injections. Another study has suggested up to 65% more insulin for a meal high in fat or protein.[49] However, it has been shown that due to the substantial interindividual differences that exist in insulin dose requirements for protein and fat, individualized advice based on postprandial glucose monitoring up to 6 hours is required.[49,50] Novel algorithms have been proposed to reduce the postprandial excursions resulting from high-fat and/or high-protein meals; however, a higher rate of clinically significant hypoglycemia was a limitation of this method.[51] A conservative starting point for incremental bolus dose increases is an additional 15% to 20% for high-fat, high-protein meals.[31] The ADA now recommends that people with type 1 diabetes who have mastered carbohydrate counting be educated on prandial (bolus) insulin adjustment strategies to manage the glycemic excursions caused by fat and protein.[3] However, it is important that other aspects of diabetes management be addressed first, such as the optimization of basal insulin doses and ICRs, before insulin adjustment is considered for protein and fat.

Because protein stimulates the release of insulin, protein should not be used to treat or prevent hypoglycemia.[1,2] For persons with diabetes, there is insufficient evidence to suggest that the usual protein intake (15%-20% of energy), the same amount recommended for people without diabetes, be changed.[12] For individuals with diabetic kidney disease with either micro- or macroalbuminuria, reducing the amount of protein does not alter the course of glomerular filtration rate, glycemic measures, or CVD risk measures[2,52] and therefore is not recommended.

Epidemiological data and clinical trials implicate chronic intake of higher levels of total dietary fat, especially saturated fats, in the development of insulin resistance.[53,54] Studies suggest that reduced intake of fat, particularly saturated fat, may improve insulin sensitivity independent of energy restriction.[54,55] In addition, unsaturated fats may have a beneficial effect on insulin action.

Vitamin and Mineral Supplementation and Glycemia

Nutrition therapy should include education on how to acquire adequate amounts of vitamins and minerals from food sources. There is no clear evidence of benefits from vitamin and mineral supplementation in individuals with diabetes who do not have underlying deficiencies.[2] For select groups of individuals, such as the elderly, pregnant or lactating women, vegetarians, and those on energy-restricted diets, a multivitamin supplement may be necessary. Supplementation above the tolerable upper intake level (UL) established by the IOM increases the risk of adverse effects and should be considered only after review of safety and efficacy determined by controlled clinical trials.[20] Routine supplementation of antioxidants such as vitamins C and E and beta-carotene is not advised due to possible adverse effects and the lack of efficacy shown in large placebo-controlled clinical trials.[2]

Recent attention on the prevalence of vitamin D deficiency has raised questions about intake recommendations and supplemental needs for people with diabetes and at risk of diabetes. A meta-analysis of observational studies assessing the association between blood levels of 25(OH)D and risk of type 2 diabetes reported an inverse and significant association.[56] However, a randomized controlled trial (RCT) in persons with prediabetes and hypovitaminosis D using high doses of vitamin D for 1 year reported no effect of the supplement on insulin secretion, insulin sensitivity, or the development of diabetes compared with the placebo.[57] Most recently, the Vitamin D and Type 2 Diabetes (D2d) Study enrolled 2,423 adults and was conducted at 22 sites across the United States. The study was funded by National Institute of Diabetes and Digestive and Kidney Diseases (NIDDK), part of the National Institutes of Health. The study included adults aged 30 or older and assigned participants randomly to either take 4,000 International Units of the D3 (cholecalciferol) form of vitamin D or a placebo pill daily. All study participants had their vitamin D levels measured at the start of the study. At that time, about 80% of participants had vitamin D levels considered sufficient by US nutritional standards. Results of the study reported that taking a daily vitamin D supplement does not prevent type 2 diabetes in adults at high risk.[58]

Chromium supplementation has been studied for its potential influence on glycemia, insulin resistance, and body weight. Current studies have not conclusively demonstrated efficacy.[59] Evidence from clinical studies that evaluated magnesium supplementation to improve glycemia in people with diabetes is also conflicting. Evolving evidence is suggesting that magnesium status may be related to diabetes risk in people with prediabetes.[60] Many micronutrients are involved in carbohydrate and/or glucose metabolism as well as with insulin release and sensitivity. This information, however, is frequently extrapolated beyond what is supported by research findings.[2] Evidence is lacking to support the routine use of micronutrients and other herbs/supplements for the treatment of diabetes.

For information on the use of herbal preparations, see chapter 21, on biological complementary therapies in diabetes.

Physical Activity and Glycemia

Physical activity and nutrition therapy should be considered complementary therapies that together promote optimal glycemic control and reduced risk for chronic diseases. In persons with type 2 diabetes, studies have reported improvements in glucose control and insulin sensitivity, reduced cardiovascular risk, assistance with weight management, and improved well-being from regular physical activity.[3] In persons with type 1 diabetes, physical activity confers significant health benefits such as improving insulin sensitivity, increasing cardiovascular fitness, and improving muscle strength.[3] However, it also has potential negative effects related to hypo- and hyperglycemic excursions unless variations in activity are carefully monitored and planned for. In individuals at risk for diabetes, a combination of regular physical activity and weight loss significantly reduces the risk of developing diabetes.[61] In overweight and sedentary persons and in persons with type 2 diabetes, both exercise and energy restriction independently and additively reduce glucose and insulin levels.[62]

In most persons with type 1 and type 2 diabetes, in the absence of contraindications, 150 minutes of accumulated moderate-to-vigorous intensity aerobic physical activity spread over at least 3 days with no more than 2 consecutive days without activity is recommended.[3,61] If not contraindicated, people with type 2 diabetes should also be encouraged to perform resistance training with free weights or weight machines at least 2 to 3 times per week on nonconsecutive days.[3,63] Both improve glycemic control, independent of weight loss. To accommodate physical activity, safety guidelines to prevent hypoglycemia are important. These include frequent glucose monitoring, possible adjustments in insulin dose or carbohydrate intake, and carrying carbohydrate while exercising. For all adults with diabetes, reducing sedentary time should be encouraged, and prolonged sitting should be interrupted every 30 minutes for glucose benefits, in particular in adults with type 2 diabetes.[3,64]

See chapter 6, on the self-care behaviors related to being active and exercise prescription, for more information.

When to Expect Results

Evaluation of the effectiveness of nutrition therapy on glucose should be done between 6 weeks and 3 months. During this time it can be determined whether target goals have been achieved by implementation of nutrition therapy or whether medication(s) will need to be combined with nutrition therapy.

Alcohol and Glycemia

Moderate amounts of alcohol (1 drink or less per day for adult women and 2 drinks or less per day for adult men) ingested with food have minimal, if any, effect on glucose and insulin concentrations.[2,65] The type of alcohol-containing beverage consumed does not appear to make a difference. One alcohol-containing beverage is defined as 12 oz beer, 5 oz wine, or 1.5 oz distilled spirits. Each contains approximately 15 g of alcohol. Excessive amounts of alcohol (3 or more drinks per day) on a consistent basis can contribute to hyperglycemia.[5] Individuals using insulin or insulin secretagogues should consume food with alcohol to reduce risk of hypoglycemia. Blood glucose testing should be used to determine whether extra carbohydrate and/or a reduction in diabetes medication (such as insulin or insulin secretagogues) will be needed to reduce the risk of hypoglycemia during the night or the next morning following consumption of alcohol the previous evening.[66]

There is a U-shaped relationship between alcohol consumption and risk for diabetes.[67] Compared with nondrinkers, moderate drinkers have a lower risk for diabetes, while those who consume more than 3 drinks daily have a greater risk for diabetes. A systematic review and a dose-response meta-analysis of over 38 observational studies reported reduced risk of type 2 diabetes at all levels of alcohol intake <63 g per day with peak reduction at a daily alcohol intake of 10 to 14 g (approximately 1 drink) in non-Asian populations and woman.[66–68] People with a history of alcohol abuse or dependence, women who are pregnant, and people with medical problems such as liver disease, pancreatitis, advanced neuropathy, or severe hypertriglyceridemia should abstain from alcohol.

Personalized Nutrition and Glycemia

The use of nutrition counseling approaches aimed at personalizing guidance based on microbiome, genetic, or metabolomics information is an area of interest to many people with diabetes and at risk of diabetes. Direct to consumer advertising has become readily available, making access to this information and request for interpretation by diabetes care team more common. Evolving research has revealed that there is wide interpersonal variability in glucose response to standardized meals. However at this point in time, no clear conclusions can be made regarding their utility owing to wide variation in markers used for predicting outcomes, in the populations and nutrients studied, and in the associations found.[2]

Case—Part 2: Improving Glycemic Control

Nutrition Intervention

One of LW's initial short-term goals is to reduce her A1C from 8.1% to less than 7%. In evaluating her usual meals and food choices, she can make a few small changes that may make a significant difference in her glucose levels. LW appears to be consuming the bulk of her calories and carbohydrate later in the day, often skipping breakfast, eating a light lunch, and eating a larger dinner.

LW can begin with a basic carbohydrate-counting meal-planning approach with carbohydrate spaced throughout the day. With LW's regular consumption of "sugar-free" ice cream, education on how to interpret food label information to determine the total carbohydrate, sugar content, and serving size would help her evaluate nutrition claims on packaged foods. Information obtained during LW's nutrition history regarding frequent intake of fast-food lunches shows that she would benefit from healthy, quick-to-fix lunches that she could prepare at home. Also encourage increased consumption of non-starchy vegetables at lunch and dinner. Spend a few minutes searching a variety of online recipe Web sites for quick-to-fix meals and non-starchy vegetable recipes.

Monitoring her glucose levels utilizing a "paired" approach, checking pre-meal and then 2 hours after eating will reinforce the effect of varying amounts of carbohydrates on her blood glucose levels. (Chapter 5, on healthy eating, provides a basic explanation of carbohydrate counting.)

LW is also encouraged to begin some type of physical activity, such as brisk walking, to assist in achievement of her personal glucose management goals. She is instructed to begin slowly and work toward a goal of accumulating 150 minutes of physical activity per week. An activity tracker such as a step counter or an app on her smartphone is recommended as a motivational tool to encourage LW to increase her activity as well as reduce sedentary time each day. She is also encouraged to add muscle-strengthening activities. Her glucose response will be evaluated initially with blood glucose records, but after she has implemented her lifestyle changes, an A1C test will be done (in ~8-12 weeks) to determine whether she needs to make any changes in her glucose-lowering medication(s).

Nutrition and Physical Activity Goals

Follow carbohydrate-counting plan to include a carbohydrate budget of approximately 45 g to 60 g per meal and 15 g for evening snack if hungry; record food/carbohydrate intake and exercise performed for 7 days prior to return visit; walk briskly for at least 30 minutes 4 days per week; and monitor blood glucose twice a day, alternating before and 2 hours after breakfast, lunch, and dinner.

Monitoring and Evaluation

Follow up in 3 weeks to evaluate and assess food and blood glucose records, review food and activity records, and monitor weight status.

Nutrition Therapy and Weight Management

A major challenge in diabetes care is the high incidence of overweight and obesity in persons with or at risk for type 2 diabetes. Weight loss is an important goal for overweight or obese persons at risk for diabetes, as it prevents or delays the onset of diabetes. In persons with diabetes, the role of weight loss is controversial. Obesity prevalence is also increasing in people with type 1 diabetes.[69] Providers need to be alert to any weight increases and intervene early to assist their patients in weight management.

Weight Loss Effectiveness

A moderate weight loss of 7% to 10% can reduce the risk of developing type 2 diabetes and improve glycemia, primarily in individuals who are insulin resistant, including those with prediabetes and early-onset type 2 diabetes.[3,70] The 2019 ADA Nutrition Therapy for Adults with Diabetes and Prediabetes: A Consensus Report, review of the literature reported that there is not a threshold of weight loss for maximal clinical outcomes.[2] In type 2 diabetes, the goal for optimal outcome is ≥15% when it can be feasibly and safely accomplished. However, as the disease progresses and individuals become more insulin deficient, weight loss may or may not significantly improve glycemia.[2,71] With insulin deficiency, additional glucose-lowering medications combined with nutrition therapy are necessary, and prevention of weight gain rather than weight loss becomes the priority.

A systematic review and meta-analysis of randomized clinical trials of lifestyle interventions for weight loss in persons with diabetes conducted by Franz et al found that lifestyle interventions <5% weight loss had less effect on A1C or CVD risk factors compared with studies that achieved ≥5%.[71] Weight losses from interventions ranged from 1.9 to 8.4 kg at 12 months; however, 9 of the studies reported weight losses ranging from 2.4 to 4.8 kg. Two study groups achieved weight loss of >5% and reported significant A1C decrease (range 0.6%-1.2%) and significant beneficial effects on lipids and blood pressure; one was a Mediterranean-style diet (MED) implemented in subjects with newly diagnosed diabetes, and the other was the Look AHEAD (Action for Health in Diabetes) intensive lifestyle intervention (ILI). These 2 studies reported the largest weight loss at 1 year, 6.2 kg and 8.4 kg, respectively,[72,73] and a low-carbohydrate intervention reported the smallest, 1.9 kg.[74] It appears likely that many persons with type 2 diabetes, unless they are newly diagnosed or receive an intensive intervention as provided in the Look AHEAD trial, find it difficult to lose sufficient weight at 1 year to experience improvements in A1C values, lipids, and blood pressure.

Because of its size and duration, the Look AHEAD trial is of importance. It was conducted in 16 centers across the United States in an attempt to determine the effectiveness of intentional weight loss interventions in reducing rates of heart disease, stroke, and CVD deaths in overweight and obese persons with type 2 diabetes.[73] Half of the 5,145 participants randomized to the ILI received meal replacements or structured food plans, were encouraged to achieve 175 minutes of physical activity a week, and attended 3 to 4 education/counseling sessions per month. The other half, the control group, received a general program of diabetes support and education. The trial was stopped early on the basis of a futility analysis with a median follow-up of 9.6 years.[75] The ILI resulted in greater weight loss at study end (6.0% vs. 3.5%) as well as greater improvements in fitness and all CVD risk factors, except for LDL-C. However, the ILI intervention did not reduce the rate of CVD events in the participants.

Although much smaller in scale, a recent study found similar results at 1 year for a lifestyle intervention with frequent in-person visits and use of pre-packed foods.[76] The intervention group lost 8.2% of their baseline weight, compared with 2.5% in a usual care group. Intervention subjects had significant improvements in A1C, HDL-C, and triglycerides while also decreasing use of oral diabetes medicine, insulin, and blood pressure and cholesterol-lowering medications. Structured weight loss programs with regular visits and use of meal replacements have also been shown to enhance weight loss in persons with type 2 diabetes.[77]

In general, weight loss intervention studies in people without diabetes report that individuals lose, on average, 5% to 10% of their starting weight by 6 months, at which time weight loss reaches a plateau.[78] Adaptive mechanisms occur with a reduced energy intake (eg, hormonal regulation, adaptive thermogenesis leading to a decrease in energy expenditure, and decline in basal energy requirement), and, at this point, maintenance of the weight loss should become the focus of the ongoing care and intervention. In studies extending to 48 months, a 3% to 6% weight loss from starting weight was maintained.[78] A systematic review and meta-analysis of RCT in people with type 2 diabetes show a pattern of weight loss that is similar for persons without diabetes, but in the majority of the studies, weight loss was less than 5% between 6 and 12 months in persons with diabetes.[63] Therefore, energy restriction, with or without weight loss, and healthy eating should be the focus of nutrition therapy interventions for persons with type 2 diabetes.

Diabetes remission, defined as euglycemia (complete remission) or prediabetes level glycemia (partial remission) with no diabetes medication for at least 1 year in people undergoing weight loss treatment is an area of heightened interest.[79] The Look AHEAD trial[75] and the Diabetes Remission Clinical Trial (DiRECT)[80] both provided varying degrees of diabetes remission. In the Look AHEAD trial, the intensive treatment arm when compared to the control group resulted in at least partial remission in 11.5% of the participants versus 2% in the control group.[75] The DiRECT trial research hypothesis is that type 2 diabetes is caused by excess fat in the liver and pancreas and that drastic loss of weight reduces fat in the pancreas and helps to remit type 2 diabetes. The results of DiRECT suggest that type 2 diabetes of up to 6 years' duration can be reversed by weight loss with help of an evidence-based structured weight management program delivered in a community setting, by routine primary care staff.[80] Almost a quarter of participants who followed the intervention achieved at least 15 kg of weight loss at 12 months, and half maintained at least 10 kg reduction. Almost half (46%) of participants in the intervention group showed remission of diabetes and were off antidiabetic medication. Remission rates were closely related to the degree of weight loss, from 7% to 86%, as weight loss at 12 months increased from <5% to ≥15%.

Metabolic surgery has also been identified as an approach for weight loss and remission of type 2 diabetes compared to lifestyle intervention or conventional therapy at ≥12 months.[81] A multisite study of long-term remission and relapse in persons with type 2 diabetes following gastric bypass reported that the gastric bypass surgery was associated with durable remission of type 2 diabetes in many but not all persons; about one third experienced a relapse within 5 years of initial remission.[82] Predictors of relapse were poor glycemic control prior to surgery, insulin use, and longer diabetes duration, suggesting aggressive and early obesity treatment is warranted for people with type 2 diabetes.

Nutrition Therapy for Weight Management

Nutrition therapy interventions that use a behavioral approach, combine a reduction in energy intake with an increase in physical activity, and provide ongoing counseling and support are needed for beneficial outcomes. Evidence supports the fact that weight loss is primarily associated with engagement with an energy-reduced eating plan rather than macronutrient composition or type of eating pattern.[3,83,84] Advice for reducing energy intake should be individualized to account for the individual's food preferences and preferred approach for reducing energy intake. Weight loss interventions for people with diabetes and those at risk of diabetes can also be provided in traditional settings such as one-on-one or group visits, and evolving research reveals alternately in telehealth programs.[85,86] When counseling individuals with diabetes and at risk of diabetes about weight management, special attention needs to be given to prevent, diagnose, and treat disordered eating.[2] The prevalence of disordered eating varies, estimated to affect 18% to 40% of individuals with diabetes. When identified by screening, referral to a mental healthcare professional and an RDN with expertise in disordered eating is recommended.[87] Other strategies such as intuitive eating and non-diet approaches may also be options for overweight and obese persons with diabetes and prediabetes in achievement of glucose and weight goals.[88]

In people with diabetes, nutrition interventions shown to be effective in weight management programs include the following: (1) an individualized reduced-energy diet, (2) total energy intake distributed throughout the day, (3) consumption of breakfast, (4) portion control emphasized, and (5) meal replacements (eg, liquid meals, meal bars, calorie-controlled packaged meals) for persons who have difficulty with self-selection and/or portion control.[89] In addition, a variety of behavioral strategies that have shown to be helpful can be employed (eg, self-monitoring, stress management, stimulus control, problem solving, contingency management, cognitive restructuring, and social support).[89]

Energy Restriction

Energy restriction, with or without weight loss, and healthy eating should be the focus of nutrition therapy interventions for persons with type 2 diabetes.

Physical Activity and Weight Management

Physical activity is a key component of a comprehensive weight management program. Physical activity and exercise, by themselves, have only a modest weight loss effect. They are to be encouraged because they improve insulin sensitivity independent of weight loss, acutely lower blood glucose, and greatly improve the prospects for long-term weight maintenance.[90] Guidelines for physical activity should take into account a person's ability, safety, willingness, age, previous physical activity level, and conditions that might contraindicate certain types of exercise or predispose the person to injury.[3,61] Individuals should gradually increase duration and frequency of moderate-intensity aerobic physical activity to 150 minutes per week and resistance training to 3 times per week, when possible. Longer activity levels of at least 1 to 1½ hours per day of moderate activity may be needed to achieve successful long-term weight loss and maintenance.

Chapter 6 on the self-management behaviors related to being active and exercise prescription provides more information.

Challenges With Anti-hyperglycemic Therapy

Diabetes pharmacotherapy often presents an additional challenge to the diabetes care team—in that weight gain often accompanies glucose-lowering pharmacologic therapy, hampering the individual's efforts at weight loss. Diabetes medications that can increase weight include sulfonylureas, thiazolidinediones, meglitinides, and insulin. GLP-1 agonists, sodium-glucose co-transporter 2 (SGLT-2) inhibitors, and pramlintide can result in weight loss, and metformin, alpha-glucosidase inhibitors, and dipeptidyl peptidase-4 (DPP-4) inhibitors are weight neutral.[9] Decisions are often made to accept some weight gain in exchange for improved glycemic control.

Some clinicians assume that weight gain with the addition of insulin therapy is inevitable. For this reason, clinicians and people with diabetes are often reluctant to initiate insulin or intensify treatment despite the need shown by elevated A1C levels. This delay in starting insulin can cause a greater increase in weight gain once insulin is initiated than if insulin was initiated in a timely manner.[91] Weight gain may also occur as a return to previous body weight prior to weight loss due to inadequate insulin. In addition, the introduction of anti-hyperglycemic agents may be responsible for resolution of hyperglycemia, thereby reducing glucosuria and retaining calories otherwise lost. Engaging patients in nutrition therapy can help them avoid or minimize weight gain so that glycemic control is optimized, long-term complications are minimized, and quality of life is maintained.[92] After anti-hyperglycemic agents are initiated, nutrition therapy continues to be an important part of the diabetes treatment plan.[9]

Weight Loss Medications and Bariatric Surgery

Five weight loss medications have been approved by the FDA for long-term treatment of overweight and obesity: orlistat, phentermine/topiramate extended release (ER), lorcaserin, naltrexone/bupropion ER, and liraglutide/saxenda. All 5 weight loss medications are approved for nonpregnant adults with a BMI ≥30 kg/m^2, or ≥27 kg/m^2 in the presence of other risk factors (eg, diabetes, hypertension, dyslipidemia). Only orlistat has been well studied in persons with diabetes. Medication side effects, cost, and insurance coverage vary, and these factors impact initiation and continuation of any weight loss medication. After weight loss medications are started, side effects and early outcomes need to be monitored. Individuals who lose <5% of their baseline weight in 3 months should have therapy discontinued and an alternate weight loss medication should be considered, since they have different mechanisms of action. Use of weight loss medications was found to result in a reduction of antidiabetic medications, fewer dose increases, and fewer additional antidiabetes agents.[80–82] Research reveals that there were CVD risk factor benefits with some of the medications,[93–95] and no worsening of CVD risk factors with any of the medications.

Metabolic surgery—either gastric banding or procedures that bypass, transpose, or resect sections of the small intestine—when part of a comprehensive team approach, has been shown to be an effective treatment for severe obesity.[3] A recent joint statement by several international diabetes organizations on metabolic surgery in the treatment of type 2 diabetes was published by the ADA.[96] Metabolic surgery was recommended as an option to treat type 2 diabetes with the following conditions: Class III obesity (BMI ≥40 kg/m^2) regardless of the level of glycemic control or complexity of glucose-lowering regimens; or Class II obesity (BMI 35.0-39.9 kg/m^2) with inadequately controlled hyperglycemia despite optimized lifestyle and medical therapy. The BMI thresholds should be reduced by 2.5 kg/m^2 for Asian patients. These patients will need lifelong lifestyle support and medical monitoring. Surgical weight loss also appears to have a positive impact on CVD risk factors such as blood pressure and lipid profile,[97] even with reduced medication use.[98]

Case—Part 3: CVD Risk Reduction

LW's weight puts her at risk for CVD and other comorbidities. Weight loss and maintenance are difficult to achieve. Nutrition therapy interventions might not significantly improve LW's blood glucose levels, due to the duration of her diabetes and any significant beta cell dysfunction she may have. The diabetes care team might consider the use of antidiabetic medications that can result in weight loss and the use of GLP-1 agonists in place of the sulfonylurea (glimepiride) that LW is currently taking that can increase weight.

Nutrition Therapy and the Prevention and Treatment of CVD

Persons with diabetes are at a three- to fourfold increased risk of CVD, which is particularly evident in younger age groups and in women. They have the equivalent CVD risk of persons with preexisting CVD and no diabetes.[99] Closely linked to prediabetes and type 2 diabetes is the metabolic syndrome, the clustering of risk factors including abdominal obesity, physical inactivity, hypertension, atherogenic dyslipidemia, a prothrombotic state, and glucose intolerance. Nutrition therapy and aerobic physical activity are integral to the prevention and treatment of CVD in diabetes. Both glycemic control and cardioprotective nutrition interventions improve the lipid profile and blood pressure and should be addressed in counseling all individuals with prediabetes or type 2 diabetes.[1,2] The Academy's Diabetes Mellitus Types 1 and 2 Systematic Review and Guideline in adults reported that subjects in the systematic review did not have or were not described as having any disorders of lipid metabolism.[1] Evidence for the effectiveness of MNT on CVD risk factors was found to be mixed, likely due to many of the subjects being on lipid-lowering medications. Additional long-term studies of the effectiveness of MNT on lipid profiles in adults with diabetes and disorders of lipid metabolism are needed.[1] Pharmacotherapy for dyslipidemia and hypertension is the topic of chapter 20.

Nutrition Therapy and Dyslipidemia

In persons with prediabetes or diabetes, triglycerides are often elevated, HDL-C is generally decreased, and LDL-C may be elevated, borderline, or normal. LDL particles are small and dense, resulting in more LDL particles for any cholesterol concentration. In addition, these small, dense particles are more atherogenic, as they may be more readily oxidized and glycated. The primary goal in persons with diabetes or prediabetes is to achieve LDL-C goals to reduce cardiovascular risk.[3]

The 2019 ADA Standards of Care recommend lifestyle modification and application of a Mediterranean-style eating pattern or Dietary Approaches to Stop Hypertension (DASH) dietary pattern, focusing on weight loss (if indicated); reducing saturated and *trans* fatty acids, and dietary cholesterol; increasing viscous fiber (such as oats, legumes, and citrus) and plant stanols/sterols, and n-3 fatty acids; and increased physical activity.[3,100] Lifestyle therapy and glycemic management should be intensified in individuals with elevated triglycerides (≥150 mg/dL) and/or low HDL cholesterol (<40 mg/dL for men, <50 mg/dL for women).[3] Intensive lifestyle intervention focused on weight loss through increased physical activity and decreased caloric intake as performed in the Look AHEAD trial may also be considered for improvement in some CVD risk factors, glucose control, and fitness.[73] The nutrition intervention should be individualized according to the person's diabetes type, age, lipid levels, pharmacologic treatment, and medical conditions. Glycemic control is also important, especially for persons with diabetes with very high triglycerides and poor glycemic control. The 2019 ADA Standards of Care also recommend for individuals of all ages with diabetes and ASCVD or 10 year ASCVD risk of >20%, high intensity statin therapy should be added to lifestyle therapy.[3] Individuals with diabetes <40 years and additional ASCVD risk factors, the individual and healthcare provider should consider using moderate-intensity statin in addition to lifestyle therapy.[3] The evidence is lower for individuals aged >75 years of age. If LDL-cholesterol is ≥70 mg/dL on maximally tolerated statin dose, an additional LDL-lowering agent (such as ezetimibe or PCSK9 inhibitor) should be considered. Although fewer studies examining these benefits have been conducted in persons with diabetes, since the 2 groups have equivalent CVD risks, the nutrition therapy recommendations for persons with diabetes are the same as for individuals with preexisting CVD and the general public.

Dietary Fat and Cholesterol

There is insufficient evidence to support the recommendation of a specific amount of total fat intake for people with diabetes; therefore, the goals should be individualized.[1–3] Data suggest that quality of fat is more important than quantity in attaining metabolic goals and reducing the risk of CVD.[2,101]

Saturated and *trans* fats are the major components in the diet that increase LDL-C levels. Due to limited research regarding optimal dietary saturated fat, cholesterol, and *trans* fat in persons with diabetes, recommendations are the same as for the general population. Saturated fat should be reduced to <10% of total energy intake and *trans* fat limited as much as possible.[2,3,12] Previously, the Dietary Guidelines for Americans (DGAC) recommended that cholesterol intake be limited to no more than 300 mg per day. However, the 2015 DGAC report did not bring forward this recommendation because available evidence shows no appreciable relationship between consumption of dietary cholesterol and serum cholesterol, consistent with the conclusions of a report by the American Heart Association and the American College of Cardiologists.[12,100,102]

Unsaturated fats, including both monounsaturated fatty acids (MUFA) and polyunsaturated fatty acids, have been shown to improve blood lipid levels.[1,2] Evidence from large prospective cohort studies, clinical trials, and two systematic reviews of RCTs reports that high-MUFA diets are associated with improved glycemic control and CVD risk.[52,101,103] Replacing calories from saturated fats with unsaturated fats has been shown to lower LDL-C.[104]

Dietary intake of omega-3 fatty acids from both plant sources (alpha-linolenic acid) and marine sources (eicosapentaenoic [EPA] and docasahexanoic [DHA] acids) as is recommended for the general public; however, evidence does not support recommending omega-3 supplements.[2,105] Also recommended is 2 or more servings of fish per week (with the exception of commercially fried fish filets), particularly fatty fish (ie, salmon, herring, and mackerel), along with food sources of alpha-linolenic acid (ie, canola and soybean oil, flaxseed, and English walnuts [the type most commonly sold in the United States]).[106]

Fiber

The addition of fiber, especially soluble fiber, can further reduce LDL-C levels. A fat-modified eating plan that provides 25 to 30 g of total dietary fiber, including at least 7 to 13 g of soluble fiber (such as oatmeal or oat bran, apples, pears, psyllium, barley, and legumes), is recommended.[106]

Plant Stanols/Plant Sterols

Plant stanols and sterols and their esters come from different plant sources but are all cholesterol-reducing food ingredients that lower LDL-C in a similar way. Because of their similarity to cholesterol, they interfere with dietary and biliary cholesterol absorption in the intestinal tract and thus lower LDL-C levels.[2,106] The amounts naturally present in foods are small, and therefore stanol- or sterol-fortified foods or supplements are necessary. Use of fortified food products that provide ~2 g per day of plant stanols or sterols has been shown to reduce LDL-C and total cholesterol levels.[107] Individuals with hypercholesterolemia can consume 2 to 3 g of plant sterols or stanols to improve LDL-C and total cholesterol levels. Two to four servings of various foods fortified with plant stanols/sterols, such as spreads, orange juice, cheese, and yogurt, are needed to provide 2 g per day. Calories from these foods need to be considered in the overall food plan.

Mediterranean-Style Eating Pattern/CVD Risk

A systematic review concluded that a Mediterranean-style eating pattern may improve CVD risk and glycemic control in persons with diabetes.[108] Improvements in CVD risk factors included HDL-C ratio of total cholesterol to HDL-C, triglycerides, and systolic blood pressure. The PREDIMED trial, compared a Mediterrean-style eating pattern with a low-fat eating plan. After 4 years, the PREDIMED trial showed that a Mediterranean-style eating pattern intervention including olive oil or nuts significantly reduced CVD risk incidence in both people with diabetes and those at risk of diabetes.[109] Characteristics of a Mediterranean-style eating pattern are a high ratio of monounsaturated fats (mainly olive oil) to saturated fats; moderate alcohol consumption; high consumption of legumes, fruits, vegetables, and nonrefined cereals, including bread; low consumption of meat and meat products; and moderate consumption of milk and dairy products.[110]

Alcohol and Dyslipidemia/CVD Risk

In persons with type 2 diabetes, studies show that mild to moderate alcohol consumption (≤1 to 2 drinks per day) is associated with a decreased risk of coronary heart disease,[111,112] and reduced total mortality rates from coronary heart disease and total mortality rates,[100] likely related to improved insulin sensitivity.[113] A limited number of studies have examined the effect of alcohol consumption on triglycerides in persons with diabetes. Moderate amounts of alcohol have not been shown to have a detrimental effect on triglyceride levels and may even have a beneficial effect.[114,115] However, it is recommended that individuals with severe hypertriglyceridemia (>500 mg/dL) abstain from alcohol along with a reduced saturated fat intake to reduce risk of pancreatitis.[116] The available evidence does not support recommending alcohol consumption in persons who do not currently drink. However, for the majority of people who choose to drink alcohol in moderation, alcohol consumption does not need to be discouraged.

Physical Activity and Dyslipidemia/CVD Risk

Strong evidence supports the role of exercise and physical activity in reducing the risk factors for CVD in adults without diabetes. In persons with diabetes, physical activity improves insulin sensitivity and decreases risk for CVD and all-cause mortality.[117,118] Fitness attenuates, but does not completely eliminate, risk, underscoring the importance of promoting regular physical activity, following a cardioprotective eating pattern, and maintaining a healthy weight. A review of the effects of aerobic exercise in participants without diabetes reported increases in HDL-C and reductions in triglycerides, LDL-C, and total cholesterol.[119] However, in a meta-analysis examining the effects of aerobic exercise on lipids and lipoproteins in adults with type 2 diabetes, the authors concluded that exercise lowers LDL-C by about 5%, but no significant improvements were found on other lipid values.[120]

Nutrition Therapy and the Prevention and Treatment of Hypertension

Randomized controlled trials have demonstrated unequivocally that treatment of hypertension to blood pressure <140 mm Hg systolic and <90 mm Hg diastolic reduces cardiovascular events as well as microvascular complications in persons with diabetes.[3,121] Management of hypertension has been demonstrated to reduce the rate and progression of diabetic nephropathy and to reduce complications of hypertensive nephropathy, CVD, and cerebrovascular disease.[99] Adoption of healthy lifestyle strategies is critical for the prevention of high blood pressure and is an indispensable part of the management of high blood pressure for those with hypertension.[121] Lifestyle modifications effective in preventing and managing hypertension include weight loss, the DASH eating plan, high potassium intake, reduced sodium intake, moderate alcohol intake, and physical activity.[3,122–124] Several studies have demonstrated the additive effects of combining lifestyle interventions.[125–128]

Weight Loss and Hypertension

Obesity and overweight, particularly abdominal obesity, have consistently correlated closely with increased blood pressure independent of other risk factors for hypertension.[116] In almost all weight-reduction studies in the general population, systemic blood pressure was reduced, even if the degree of weight loss was small.[129,130] A 2015 systematic review and meta-analysis of RCTs found that in overweight/obese individuals with type 2 diabetes, a weight loss of >5% at 1 year was associated with improved blood pressure.[71] However, in persons with diabetes, there is variability in the blood pressure response to weight loss.[71]

DASH Eating Plan

The DASH Trial showed that restricting sodium intake (<2,300 mg per day), increasing consumption of fruits and vegetables (8-10 servings per day) and low-fat dairy foods (2 or 3 servings per day), and reducing the amounts of total fat, saturated fat, and cholesterol significantly reduced blood pressure in the absence of weight change.[131] The beneficial effect on blood pressure from the DASH eating plan is likely due to a combination of factors, none of which can be specifically identified from this study. In a small study in people with type 2 diabetes, the DASH eating plan, which included a sodium restriction of 2,300 mg per day, improved A1C, blood pressure, and other CVD risk factors.[124]

Sodium and Hypertension

Moderate sodium restriction (~2,300 mg per day) has been shown to be an effective strategy in the prevention and treatment of hypertension among the general population.[12] The ADA and the Academy agree that the recommendation for the general public to reduce sodium to less than 2,300 mg per day is appropriate for adults with diabetes.[1,2] The DASH-Sodium Trial showed that lower sodium intakes resulted in greater reductions in blood pressure. Combining sodium restriction and the DASH eating plan had the greatest effect on blood pressure.[131] Sodium reduction appears to have linear dose-response to blood pressure in adults; lowering sodium may have a similar blood pressure-lowering effect as some medications.[122] However, in both persons with type 2 diabetes and persons with type 1 diabetes, a lower 24-hour urinary sodium excretion (suggesting a lower sodium intake) was associated with increased all-cause and cardiovascular mortality or end-stage renal disease.[125,126] In the absence of clear scientific evidence for the benefit of individuals with both hypertension and diabetes, a further reduction in sodium intake goals that are significantly lower than 2,300 mg/day should be considered only on an individualized basis.[2] Although associations do not demonstrate causality, these findings suggest that recommendations for a lower sodium intake in people with diabetes should be individualized and made with caution.[2] If blood pressure is consistently above 140/90 mmHg, antihypertensive medications should be initiated promptly in conjunction with lifestyle modifications.[122]

Physical Activity and Hypertension

Physical activity is an important strategy for the prevention and treatment of high blood pressure. Persons who are less active and less fit have a greater risk for high blood pressure. Clinical trials have demonstrated that regular aerobic activity reduces blood pressure in hypertensive and normotensive persons, independent of weight loss.[132] The underlying mechanisms responsible for an exercise-induced reduction in blood pressure are unclear. Insulin resistance and hyperinsulinemia may contribute to the pathogenesis of hypertension, and physical activity reduces insulin resistance and insulin levels in individuals with hypertension.

Alcohol and Hypertension

There has been limited research conducted on hypertension and moderate alcohol intake in people with diabetes. A J-shaped relationship was observed between alcohol intake and blood pressure in people with diabetes.[134]

Another study comparing moderate alcohol consumption with no alcoholic beverage intake found no effect on blood pressure.[134] A large cross-sectional study conducted in men with and without diabetes revealed light alcohol intake was not associated with increases in blood pressure, whereas blood pressure was significantly higher in participants with moderate and heavy alcohol intake.[135] In a 2-year RCT, alcohol abstainers at baseline reported no differences in blood pressure when they consumed either mineral water or red wine or white wine with dinner across the 3 groups.[112]

Hypertension is also discussed in chapter 25, on macrovascular disease, and pharmacotherapy for hypertension is the focus of chapter 20.

Case—Part 4: CVD

LW's hyperglycemia, dyslipidemia, and uncontrolled hypertension put her at considerable risk for CVD. Her food history and 24-hour recall revealed that her usual diet is high in total fat and saturated fat (2 factors that increase LDL-C) and high in sodium.

The next goal is to help LW reduce her risk of CVD by improving her blood lipids and blood pressure. A major focus is on reducing her LDL-C to <100 mg/dL. In addition to her walking program and moderate caloric restriction, she may be able to lower her blood pressure by reducing her sodium intake and adopting an eating plan similar to the DASH eating plan that incorporates more fruits, vegetables, and low-fat dairy foods and reduces the total fat, saturated fat, and *trans* fats. This, along with adding at least 2 servings of fish each week to provide omega-3 fatty acids, can also help improve her lipid profile. Adding a margarine-type spread containing a plant sterol/stanol might further reduce her LDL-C.

Since LW does not currently drink alcoholic beverages, she is not encouraged to start, despite the reported benefits of light to moderate alcohol consumption on blood pressure and CVD risk. Alcoholic beverages add calories, and excess intake could potentially result in less attention to diabetes self-care management.

An initial strategy to help LW achieve her goals is for her to choose what she is willing and able to try: eat out less frequently, eat less when eating out, or make more healthful food choices. The RDN can discuss organizational techniques to help LW with the time constraints involved in preparation of lunches that she could take to work. Web sites with healthful, quick, and easy recipes for lunches could be shared with LW.

Regular physical activity is encouraged at each of LW's visits to improve lipids, blood pressure, and glycemia. LW is encouraged to perform resistance exercises 3 times a week (she has no contraindications). She was also taught to keep a record of her physical activity along with her blood glucose values to observe the effect on glycemia.

LW was instructed to self-monitor her blood pressure, in addition to blood pressure checks on follow-up visits, to assess the effect of her lifestyle changes and any need for medication additions or changes. The RDN told her that the impact of lifestyle changes on blood lipids could be observed in a lipid profile in just 6 to 12 weeks.

Nutrition Therapy and the Prevention and Treatment of Diabetic Kidney Disease

Optimizing glucose levels and effective treatment of hypertension have been shown to delay the onset and progression of diabetic kidney disease (DKD).[3,136] In general, every 1% drop in A1C can reduce the risk of microvascular complications such as kidney disease by 40%, and lowering blood pressure can reduce the decline in kidney function by 30% to 70%.[137] Therefore, management of blood glucose levels and blood pressure is strongly recommended.[3,136]

Although low-protein diets have traditionally been recommended for persons with diabetes and DKD, engagement with them is poor and malnutrition is a reported concern.[136] Based on the review of evidence conducted for the 2019 ADA Nutrition Consensus Report and previous systematic reviews, in people with diabetes and non-dialysis-dependent DKD, reducing the amount of dietary protein below the recommended daily allowance (0.8 g/kg body weight per day) does not meaningfully alter glycemic measures, cardiovascular risk measures, or the course of glomerular filtration rate decline.[2,52,138] Low-protein diets were not significantly associated with a change in glomerular filtration rates (GFRs) or the creatinine clearance rate, but they did result in a decline in urinary protein excretion.Therefore, reducing the amount of protein for people with diabetes and DKD (either micro- or macroalbuminuria) is not recommended.[2] For people with DKD and macroalbuminuria, changing to a more soy-based source of protein may improve CVD risk measures but does not appear to alter proteinuria.[139]

For further information on DKD, see chapter 28.

Nutrition Therapy in Youth

Nutrition goals for youth with diabetes focus on optimal glycemic goals, lipid and blood pressure goals, and normal growth and development.[140,141] Children and adolescents with diabetes have nutritional needs similar to those without diabetes. Energy needs can be estimated based on DRIs[20] and a history of the child's or adolescent's usual food intake. Growth and weight gain should be evaluated on a regular basis by recording height and weight on a pediatric growth chart. As energy requirements change with age, physical activity, and growth rate, an evaluation of height, weight, BMI, and the nutrition therapy plan is recommended at least every year.[140,141] The meal plan must be individualized based on food preferences, cultural practices, family schedules and eating patterns, age, weight, activity level, and insulin action. Macronutrient composition of the meal plan should be based on blood glucose, lipids, and requirements for growth and development. Education in problem solving based on blood glucose monitoring results is important for all youth with diabetes.

Youth With Type 1 Diabetes

Blood glucose goals for children and adolescents with type 1 diabetes are accomplished by balancing food intake, insulin, and physical activity and should emphasize achieving glycemic goals without excessive hypoglycemia.[3] Initial nutrition therapy by a pediatric diabetes dietitian should be provided as soon as possible after diagnosis to promote a secure, trusting, and supportive relationship.[31] Providing adequate caloric intake for normal development and growth is an important goal for youth with type 1 diabetes. Height and weight should be recorded on growth charts and evaluated regularly. Withholding food to prevent hyperglycemia or having a child eat without an appetite to avoid hypoglycemia should be discouraged. A flexible insulin regimen with long-acting basal and rapid-acting boluses or insulin pump therapy precludes the need for a rigid meal plan, allowing the child or adolescent more flexibility in food choices and timing of meals and snacks. Carbohydrate counting using ICRs is a meal-planning approach often used with youths with type 1 diabetes on physiological insulin regimens because it offers more flexibility than matching carbohydrate to a set insulin dose.[142] Recent practice guidelines for youth with diabetes recommend administration of the prandial dose before meals to diminish the post-prandial blood glucose excursion and to reduce the likelihood of the dose being forgotten.[31] Physical activity is recommended for all youth with type 1 diabetes with the goal of 60 minutes of moderate-to vigorous-intensity activity daily, with vigorous muscle-strengthening activities at least 3 times per week.[3]

Youth With Type 2 Diabetes

Treatment of youth onset type 2 diabetes should include lifestyle management, diabetes self-management education, and pharmacologic treatment.[3] Youth with type 2 diabetes and their caregivers need to prioritize lifestyle modifications such as achieving and maintaining a healthy weight by following an individualized eating plan that is culturally appropriate and sensitive to the available resources. Nutrition for youth with type 2 diabetes, like all children, should be encouraged to decrease consumption of calorie-dense, nutrition-poor foods, particularly sugar-added beverages. A multidisciplinary team that includes an RDN with expertise in pediatric populations is recommended.[141] Since these behaviors are generally family behaviors, family involvement in the behavior-change process is encouraged.[3] All youth, including those with diabetes, should be encouraged to perform at least 30 to 60 minutes of moderate to vigorous physical activity at least 5 times per week (and strength training on at least 3 days/week) and to decrease sedentary behavior.[3] Comorbidities such as hypertension and hyperlipidemia must also be addressed. A number of meal-planning approaches can be used to facilitate the selection of a variety of healthy foods in appropriate portions. Emphasis on carbohydrate consistency can improve blood glucose levels. Successful nutrition therapy must include regular follow-up and is defined as the cessation of excessive weight gain with normal linear growth and near-normal fasting blood glucose and A1C values.[141]

Nutrition Therapy in Pregnancy

See chapter 24, on pregnancy with preexisting diabetes and gestational diabetes.

Nutrition Therapy in Older Adults

Nutrition therapy in older adults with diabetes presents unique challenges. Barriers to the adoption of a healthy eating pattern can be attributed to changes in taste and smell, changes in appetite, difficulty chewing and swallowing, physical disabilities, food availability, difficulty preparing food, changes in mental ability, and side effects from medications.[143,144] In addition, changes in body composition or function in older adults can directly influence nutrient requirements. Reductions in muscle mass, bone density, nutrient absorption, and metabolism make it difficult for older adults to meet nutrition requirements, especially when energy needs are reduced.[145] The Mini-Nutritional Assessment is a widely used, validated screening tool specifically designed for assessing the nutritional status of older adults.[145,146] A thorough nutrition history and an assessment of psychosocial needs are necessary to determine the appropriate nutrition interventions.[143] Nutrition therapy must address adequacy of nutritional needs, glycemic stability, and nutrition-related cardiovascular risk factors that are common in this age group. Weight change is the most reliable indicator of poor nutritional status in older adults.[144] Weight loss, both intentional and unintentional, has been associated with an increase in mortality.[147] Overweight and obesity are prevalent in older adults. Older persons can be overweight or obese due to increased fat mass, yet still be malnourished.[144] Body mass index may not be an accurate predictor of the degree of adiposity in some older adults due to changes in body composition with aging.[147] Most studies have reported a U-shaped relationship with increased mortality at lower and higher BMI levels.[148] Aggressive caloric restriction in older adults can potentially worsen sarcopenia, bone mineral density, and nutrition deficits.[146,147,149,150] A modest caloric reduction with an emphasis on nutrient-dense foods may be beneficial along with physical activity to reduce the loss of muscle mass while improving physical function and reducing cardiometabolic risk.[146,149]

Although energy needs decrease for older adults due to loss of lean body mass and less physical activity, requirements for other nutrients remain the same or increase with age.[150] Data suggest that dietary protein intake declines with age and, due to the contribution of protein undernutrition to sarcopenia and morbidity, older adults may need to be encouraged to consume more foods containing high-quality protein.[148] Meeting micronutrient needs with lower calorie intake is challenging as vitamin and mineral needs often remain constant or may increase, resulting in an increased risk for deficiencies in older adults with diabetes.[146] Evidence on dietary trends indicates that older adults are at risk for not meeting the recommended dietary allowance or adequate intake values for calcium; vitamins D, E, and K; potassium; and fiber.[150,151] Nutrient deficiencies can occur with lower than recommended intakes or as a result of malabsorption, such as in vitamin B_{12} malabsorption that occurs in an estimated 6% to 15% of older adults.[150]

When nutrition needs are not met through usual intake, additional interventions may include encouraging smaller, more frequent meals, fortifying usual foods, changing food texture, or adding liquid nutrition supplements (either regular or diabetes-specific formulas) between meals.[146] Adequate intake of calcium and vitamin D are difficult for older adults to achieve from food alone; therefore, supplements may be necessary to meet recommended amounts.[150] An evidence-based analysis of the literature found that supplementation of vitamin D-3 with calcium resulted in small increases in bone mineral density and reduced fall risk in older adults.[152,153] Either supplementation or food fortification of vitamin B_{12} is recommended for adults older than 50 years due to decreased absorption.[150,154] Nutrition recommendations for older adults include restricting sodium to <2,300 mg per day, although this can result in decreased food intake if the taste is undesirable.[2,12]

Elderly individuals with severely insulin deficient type 2 diabetes and individuals with long-term type 1 diabetes are particularly vulnerable to severe hypoglycemia due to their reduced ability to recognize symptoms of low blood glucose and effectively communicate their needs.[3] A study found that 16% of elderly individuals with long-standing type 1 diabetes experienced at least 1 seizure or episode of unconsciousness in the past year due to severe hypoglycemia.[155] Other studies have found the elderly's high risk of hypoglycemia increases the risk of falls, fractures, and related complications.[156]

Physical activity should be encouraged for older adults to minimize the loss of muscle mass, decrease bone loss, decrease central adiposity, improve insulin sensitivity, and improve cardiovascular risk factors.[157] Physical activity improves functional status in older adults with diabetes and is associated with higher self-rated physical health and psychosocial well-being.[146] The care and education of older adults is complicated by their clinical and functional heterogeneity. Some individuals are limited cognitively or physically with multiple comorbidities, yet others are relatively healthy, physically active, and active learners. A thorough assessment followed by an individualized plan for supporting personal, social, and cultural needs, along with respecting the individual's vision of quality of life, is key to successful outcomes in older adults.

Focus on Education

Teaching Strategies

Modest weight loss. Overweight and obese persons benefit from weight loss and increases in physical activity for the prevention or delay of type 2 diabetes. Weight loss also assists with decreasing cardiovascular risk factors and is likely to improve glycemia in individuals with newly diagnosed type 2 diabetes who are primarily insulin resistant. Help patients set realistic weight loss goals.

Glycemia is less likely to be reduced through weight loss in individuals with long-standing diabetes who are insulin deficient. It appears that weight loss is more difficult to achieve in persons with diabetes compared with persons without diabetes. Studies report less weight loss from similar weight loss interventions in persons with diabetes compared with persons without diabetes.

Weight maintenance. Teach strategies that will assist the person with diabetes in weight loss maintenance such as (1) an individualized reduced-energy diet, (2) total energy intake distributed throughout the day, (3) consumption of breakfast, (4) portion control emphasized, and (5) meal replacements (eg, liquid meals, meal bars, calorie-controlled packaged meals) for persons who have difficulty with self-selection and/or portion control. Other key elements of weight maintenance include ongoing behavioral support and regular physical activity. When counseling individuals with diabetes and at risk of diabetes about weight management, special attention needs to be given to prevent, diagnose, and treat disordered eating. When identified by screening, referral to a mental health care professional and an RDN with expertise in disordered eating is recommended. Other strategies such as intuitive eating and non-diet approaches may also be options for overweight and obese persons with diabetes and prediabetes in achievement of glucose and weight goals.

Glucose monitoring. Encourage the use of premeal and postmeal (paired) blood glucose results or personal CGM data to reinforce understanding of the glycemic effect of food and beverage choices. This can be especially helpful for persons with type 1 diabetes, but it can also help persons with type 2 diabetes if they have questions about certain foods. Additionally, it can help reinforce positive behavior related to portion control and physical activity. Monitoring blood pressure and lipid levels is as important as monitoring blood glucose.

Involvement. Set and prioritize nutrition therapy goals involving each person, and family member if appropriate, to individualize meal plans. Encourage use of food records to evaluate actual food and beverage intake and eating patterns, and determine the individual's understanding of meal-planning principles and food and beverages choices. Understanding the impact of portion sizes is critical for both glucose and weight management. Measure progress in behavior changes related to more healthful choices, amount of food/beverage intake, and timing of meals/snacks. Have participants use food models to demonstrate portion sizes at meals, and provide feedback about their choices. Teach selecting foods from a variety of food groups. Demonstrating meal planning, preparing menus, and selecting meals from restaurant menus during a teaching event are useful in role-playing the selection of healthy food choices and identifying potential barriers and facilitators to implementing the individual's meal plan. Ask persons with diabetes what their questions, concerns, priorities, and goals are and focus on these to capture their interest and promote continued involvement and success.

Type 2 diabetes is progressive. Since diabetes is a progressive disease, over time the use of medications will likely be necessary to achieve glycemic goals, in addition to lifestyle interventions. However, nutrition therapy still continues to be an integral component of the diabetes treatment plan as the pharmacotherapy regimen intensifies to include oral and/or injectable diabetes medications.

Messages for Patients

Healthy food choices. Instead of focusing on weight loss, collaborate with an RDN or other healthcare professional to set short-term goals that include more healthful food choices in place of highly processed foods with added fat, sugar, and/or sodium. Involve a friend or family member to assist in creating an individualized eating plan and how to evaluate food labels and food products.

Carbohydrate. Learn to identify sources of carbohydrate in the diabetes eating plan. Use some type of carbohydrate management strategy such as the plate method or carbohydrate counting to plan meals and snacks. Learning "how much" carbohydrate is found in the portions or servings that are consumed may help to achieve individual glucose and metabolic goals. Whenever possible, choose whole, unprocessed carbohydrate foods rather than highly processed foods with added sodium, fat, and sugars. Planning which meals and snacks to eat is an effective strategy for improving blood glucose, lipids (cholesterol), and blood pressure.

Glucose monitoring. Glucose levels can be checked before and after meals using SMBG or CGM to observe the glucose response to the type and amount of carbohydrate in a meal. However, discourage choosing foods solely on the basis of their effect on blood glucose; food selection to optimize glycemia should not compromise healthy eating. Diabetes medications frequently need to be combined with a food plan to achieve glucose goals. This is not "diet failure" but failure of the beta cells of the pancreas to produce adequate insulin to maintain normal blood glucose levels.

Physical activity. Take energy expenditure as seriously as food (nutritional) intake. Use an activity tracker such as a step counter or an app on a smartphone or smartwatch to keep track of the number of steps taken in a day. The baseline and progressive steps provide a goal and motivation. If it has been a long time since you have been physically active, ask your healthcare provider for a referral to a physical therapist or exercise physiologist to develop a personal plan.

Goal setting and support. Setting goals and taking ownership for meeting them are important strategies. Let your healthcare team know your questions, concerns, priorities, and goals. Seek the support you need to make and maintain lifestyle choices that are best for you.

Health Literacy

Health literacy is not just about persons with diabetes skills. Consider the following when examining your skills and your practice approach to health literacy: general health literacy practice strategies, how to recognize people with low literacy, how to improve communication, and factors to consider when creating documents.

Use plain language in order for your patient to understand the information (written and verbal). Some of the techniques include logical organization of the content (ie, a long-term goal and how you will accomplish it). Use "you" and other pronouns, use the active voice, use short sentences, use everyday words, and use easy-to-read design materials. *No one technique defines plain language. Rather, plain language is defined by results—it is easy to read, understand, and use.* The following is an example of plain-language conversion:

- Before: "The Dietary Guidelines for Americans recommends a half hour or more of moderate physical activity on most days, preferably every day. The activity can include brisk walking, calisthenics, home care, gardening, moderate sports exercise, and dancing."
- After: "Do at least 30 minutes of physical activity, like brisk walking, most days of the week."[158]

Use specific rather than vague suggestions:

- Instead of "exercise regularly," use "exercise 3 to 5 days per week for 40 minutes."
- Instead of "don't lift anything heavy," use "don't lift anything over 10 pounds."
- Instead of "get adequate rest," use "get at least 7 hours of sleep each night."

Use written materials that are easy to understand. Use short sentences (10-15 words) and simple language (monosyllable words), be consistent with words and terminology, define technical or difficult words, put important concepts first, use bulleted lists instead of blocks of text, use headings and subheadings, use a readable type style, use 12- to 14-point type for text and 16- to 18-point bold type for headings, use uppercase and lowercase for the text (do not use all capitals, as they are harder to read), have a 50/50 blend of white space and type, use dark text against a light background for sharp contrast, use summary techniques, do not justify the right margin, use columns that are 50 to 60 characters wide, and use pictures.

Use verbal communication that the patient understands. State concepts in logical order, one step at a time; define healthcare terms and explain acronyms; verify understanding: rephrase message and have the patient explain instructions back to you (teach-back method: "How would you explain this to your friends with diabetes?"); adjust to patient needs; allow your patient to talk; pay attention to nonverbal communication; and be positive.

Take time to assess health literacy and health numeracy skills. Multiple health literacy assessment tools are available.[159]

Focus on Practice

Monitor the quality and outcomes of your nutrition therapy. Examine how your clients' care outcomes compare with nutrition therapy expectations. Demonstrate the effectiveness of your nutrition therapy to providers to increase referrals.

Integrate nutrition therapy into the Chronic Care Model. Allow for ongoing access, assessment, and reassessment of needs. Recognize a possible nutrition therapy relapse and provide services to identify and treat accordingly.

References

1. Academy of Nutrition and Dietetics. Diabetes mellitus types 1 and 2 systematic review and guideline 2015. Academy of Nutrition and Dietetics Evidence Analysis Library Web site. (cited on 2019 May 31). On the Internet at: http://www.andeal.org/topic.cfm?menu=5305.

2. Evert AB, Dennison M, Gardner C, et al. Nutrition therapy for adults with diabetes and prediabetes. A consensus report. Diabetes Care. 2019;42:731-54.

3. American Diabetes Association. Standards of medical care in diabetes—2019. Diabetes Care. 2019;42 Suppl 1:S1-193.

4. American Association of Diabetes Educators. Practice Synopsis: Healthy Eating. 2015. (cited on 2019 May 31). On the internet at: https://www.diabeteseducator.org/docs/default-source/default-document-library/practice-synopsis-final_healthy-eating.pdf?sfvrsn=0

5. Lacey K, Pritchett E. Nutrition care process and model: ADA adopts road map to quality care and outcomes management. J Am Diet Assoc. 2003;103:1061-72.

6. Institute of Medicine. The Role of Nutrition in Maintaining Health in the Nation's Elderly: Evaluating Coverage of Nutrition Services for the Medicare Population. Washington, DC: National Academies Press; 2000.

7. Franz MJ, MacLeod J, Evert A, et al. (2017) Academy of Nutrition and Dietetics Nutrition Practice Guideline for Type 1 and Type 2 Diabetes in Adults: systematic review of evidence for medical nutrition therapy effectiveness and recommendations for integration into the nutrition care process. J Acad Nutr Diet. 2017; 117:1659-79.

8. Powers MA, Bardsley J, Cypress M, et al. Diabetes self-management education and support in type 2 diabetes: a joint position statement of the American Diabetes Association, American Association of Diabetes Educators, and the Academy of Nutrition and Dietetics. Diabetes Care. 2015;38:1372-82.

9. Davies MJ, D'Alessio DA, Franklin J, et al; Management of hyperglycemia in type 2 diabetes, 2018: a consensus report by the American Diabetes Association (ADA) and the European Association for the Study of Diabetes (EASD). Diabetes Care. 2018;41:2669-2701.

10. Ali MK, Bullard KM, Saaddine JB, Cowie CC, Imperatore G, Gregg EW. Achievement of goals in US diabetes care. N Engl J Med. 2013;368:1613-24.

11. Robbins JM, Thatcher GE, Webb DA, Valdmanis VG. Nutritionist visits, diabetes classes, and hospitalization rates and charges: the Urban Diabetes Study. Diabetes Care. 2008;31:655-60.

12. Department of Health and Human Services and US Department of Agriculture. 2015-2020 Dietary Guidelines for Americans. 8th ed. June 2015. On the Internet at: http://health.gov/dietaryguidelines/2015/guidelines/.

13. Benson GA, Sidebottom, A, Hayes J, et al. Impact of ENHANCED (diEtitiaNs Helping pAtieNts CarE for Diabetes) telemedicine randomized controlled trial on diabetes optimal care outcomes in patients with type 2 diabetes. J Acad Nutr Diet. 2019; 119:585-98.

14. Marincic PZ, Salazar MV, Hardin A, et al. Diabetes self-management education and medical nutrition therapy: a multisite study documenting the efficacy of registered dietitian nutritionist interventions in the management of glycemic control and diabetic dyslipidemia through retrospective chart review. J Acad Nutr Diet. 2019: 119:449-63.

15. Davidson P, Ross T, Casor, C. Academy of Nutrition and Dietetics: Revised 2017 Standards of Practice and Standards of Professional Performance for the Registered Dietitian Nutritionist (Competent, Proficient, and Expert) in Diabetes Care. J Acad Nutr Diet. 2018:118;932-46.

16. Oza-Frank R, Cheng YJ, Narayan KM, Gregg EW. Trends in nutrient intake among adults with diabetes in the United States: 1988-2004. J Am Diet Assoc. 2009;109:1173-8.

17. Xu J, Eilat-Adar S, Loria CM, et al. Macronutrient intake and glycemic control in a population-based sample of American Indians with diabetes: the Strong Health Study. Am J Clin Nutr. 2007;86:480-7.

18. Delahanty LM, Nathan DM, Lachin JM, et al; for the Diabetes Control and Complications Trial/Epidemiology of Diabetes. Association of diet with glycated hemoglobin during intensive treatment of type 1 diabetes in the Diabetes Control and Complications Trial. Am J Clin Nutr. 2009;89:518-24.

19. MacLeod JS, Franz MJ. Macronutrients and nutrition therapy for diabetes. In: Evert AB, Franz MJ eds. American Diabetes Association Guide to Nutrition Therapy for Diabetes. 3rd ed. Alexandria, Va: American Diabetes Association; 2017:17-43.

20. Institute of Medicine. Dietary Reference Intakes: Energy, Carbohydrate, Fiber, Fat, Fatty Acids, Cholesterol, Protein, and Amino Acids. Washington, DC: National Academies Press; 2002.

21. Franz MJ, Bantle JP, Beebe CA, et al. Evidence-based nutrition principles and recommendations for the treatment and prevention of diabetes and related complications (technical review). Diabetes Care. 2002;25:148-98.

22. Kuwata H, Iwasaki M, Shimizu S, et al. Meal sequence and glucose excursion, gastric emptying and incretin secretion in type 2 diabetes: a randomised, controlled crossover, exploratory trial. Diabetologia. 2016; 59:453-61.

23. Imai S, Fukui M, Kajiyama S. Effect of eating vegetables before carbohydrates on glucose excursions in patients with type 2 diabetes. J Clin Biochem Nutr. 2014;54(1):7-11. doi:10.3164/jcbn.13-67.

24. Shukla AP, Andono J, Touhamy SH, et al. Carbohydrate-last meal pattern lowers postprandial glucose and insulin excursions in type 2 diabetes. BMJ Open Diabetes Research and Care 2017;5:e000440. doi: 10.1136/bmjdrc-2017-000440.

25. Evert AB. Nutrition therapy for adults with type 1 and insulin-requiring type 2 diabetes. In: Evert AB, Franz MJ eds. American Diabetes Association Guide to Nutrition Therapy for Diabetes. 3rd ed. Alexandria, Va: American Diabetes Association; 2017:107-32.

26. Feinman RD, Fine EJ. Fructose in perspective. Nutr Metab. 2013;10:45-56.

27. Sievenpiper JL, Carleton AJ, Chatha S, et al. Heterogeneous effects of fructose on blood lipids in individuals with type 2 diabetes: systematic review and meta-analysis of experimental trials in humans. Diabetes Care. 2009;32:1930-7.

28. Livesey G, Taylor R. Fructose consumption and consequences for glycation, plasma triacylglycerol, and body weight: meta-analyses and meta-regression models of intervention studies. Am J Clin Nutr. 2008;88:1419-37.

29. Brand-Miller JC, Stockmann K, Atkinson F, et al. Glycemic index, postprandial glycemia, and the shape of the curve in healthy subjects: analysis of a database of more than 1000 foods. Am J Clin Nutr. 2009;89:97-105.

30. Barclay AW, Petocz P, McMillan-Price J, et al. Glycemic index, glycemic load, and chronic disease risk—a meta-analysis of observational studies. Am J Clin Nutr. 2008;87:627-37.

31. Smart CE, Annan F, Higgins LA, et al. ISPAD clinical practice consensus guidelines 2018: Nutritional management in children and adolescents with diabetes. Pediatr Diab. 2018; Suppl 27: 136-54.

32. Wolever TMS, Nguyen PM, Chiasson J-L, et al. Determinants of diet glycemic index calculated retrospectively from diet records of 342 individuals with non-insulin-dependent diabetes mellitus. Am J Clin Nutr. 1994;59:1265-9.

33. Atkinson FS, Foster-Powell K, Brand-Miller JC. International tables of glycemic index and glycemic load values: 2008. Diabetes Care. 2008;31:2281-3.

34. Wolever TMS. Physiological mechanisms and observed health impacts related to the glycaemic index: some observations. Int J Obes. 2006;30 Suppl 3:S72-8.

35. Vega-Lopez S, Venn BJ, Slavin JL. Relevance of the glycemic index and glycemic load for the body weight, diabetes, and cardiovascular disease. Nutrients. 2018; 10:E1361.

36. Thomas D, Elliott E. Low glycaemic index, or low glycaemic loads, diets for diabetes mellitus. Cochrane Database Syst Rev. 2009. https://doi.org/10.1002/14651858.CD006296.pub2.

37. Brand-Miller J, Hayne S, Petocz P, Colagiuri S. Low-glycemic index diets in the management of diabetes: a meta-analysis of randomized controlled trials. Diabetes Care. 2003;26:2261-7.

38. Craig ME, Twigg SM, Donaghue KC, et al. National Evidence-Based Clinical Care Guidelines for Type 1 Diabetes in Children, Adolescents and Adults. Canberra: Australian Government Department of Health and Ageing; 2011.

39. Gilbertson HR, Brand-Miller JC, Thorburn AW, Evans S, Chondros P, Werther GA. The effect of flexible low glycemic index dietary advice versus measured carbohydrate exchange diets on glycemic control in children with type 1 diabetes. Diabetes Care. 2001;24:1137-43.

40. Academy of Nutrition and Dietetics. Position statement: health implications of dietary fiber. J Acad Nutr Diet. 2015;115:1861-70.

41. Wheeler ML, Daly A, Evert A, et al. Choose your foods: exchange lists for diabetes, sixth edition, 2008: description and guidelines for use. J Am Diet Assoc. 2008;108:883-8.

42. Johnson RK, Lichtenstein AH, Anderson CAM, et al. American Heart Association Nutrition Committee on the Council on Lifestyle and Cardiometabolic Health; Council on Cardiovascular and Stroke Nursing; Council on Clinical Cardiology; Council on Quality of Care and Outcomes Research; Stroke Council. Low-calorie sweetened beverages and cardiometabolic health: a science advisory form the American Heart Association. Circulation. 2018; 138:e126-40.

43. Malik vs. Sugar sweetened beverages and cardiometabolic health. Curr Opin Cardiol. 2017; 32:572-9.

44. Malik VS, Popkin BM, Bray GA, Despres JP, Willett WC, Hu FB. Sugar-sweetened beverages and risk of metabolic syndrome and type 2 diabetes: a meta-analysis. Diabetes Care. 2010;33:2477-83.

45. Food & Nutrition Information Center, National Agricultural Library, U.S. Department of Agriculture. Nutritive and non-nutritive sweetener resources. (cited on 2019 May 26). On the Internet: https://www.nal.usda.gov/fnic/nutritive-and-nonnutritive-sweetener-resources.

46. Gardner C, Wylie-Rosett J, Gidding SS, et al; on behalf of the American Heart Association Nutrition Committee of the Council on Nutrition, Physical Activity and Metabolism, Council on Arteriosclerosis, Thrombosis and Vascular Biology, Council on Cardiovascular Disease in the Young, and the American Diabetes Association. Nonnutritive sweeteners: current use and health perspectives. A scientific statement from the American Heart Association and the American Diabetes Association. Diabetes Care. 2012;35:1798-808.

47. Bell KJ, Smart CE, Steil GM, Brand-Miller JC, King B, Wolpert HA. Impact of fat, protein, and glycemic index on postprandial glucose control in type 1 diabetes: implications for intensive diabetes management in the continuous glucose monitoring era. Diabetes Care. 2015;38(6):1008-15.

48. Smart CE, Evans M, O'Connell SM, et al. Both dietary protein and fat increase postprandial glucose excursions in children with type 1 diabetes and the effect is additive. Diabetes Care. 2013;36:3897-902.

49. Bell KJ, Toschi E, Steil GM, et al. Optimized mealtime insulin dosing for fat and protein in type 1 diabetes: application of a model-based approach to derive insulin doses for open-loop diabetes management. Diabetes Care. 2016;39:1631-4.

50. Wolpert HA, Atakov-Castillo A, Smith SA, Steil GM. Dietary fat acutely increases glucose concentrations and insulin requirement in patients with type 1 diabetes. Diabetes Care. 2013;36:810-6.

51. Piechowiak K, Dżygało K, Szypowska A. The additional dose of insulin for high-protein mixed meal provides better glycemic control in children with type 1 diabetes on insulin pumps: randomized cross-over study. Pediatr Diabetes. 2017;18(8):861-8.

52. Wheeler ML, Dunbar SA, Jaacks LM, et al. Macronutrients, food groups, and eating patterns in the management of diabetes. A systematic review of the literature, 2010. Diabetes Care. 2012;35:434-45.

53. Galgani JE, Uauy RD, Aguirre CA, Diaz EO. Effect of the dietary fat quality on insulin sensitivity. Br J Nutr. 2008;100:471-9.

54. Vessby B, Unsitupa M, Hermanses K, et al. Substituting dietary saturated for monounsaturated fat impairs insulin sensitivity in healthy men and women: the KANWU Study. Diabetologia. 2001;44:312-9.

55. Rosenfalck AM, Almdal T, Viggers L, et al. A low-fat diet improves peripheral insulin sensitivity in patients with type 1 diabetes. Diabet Med. 2006;23:384-92.

56. Song Y, Wang L, Pittas AG, et al. Blood 25-hydroxy vitamin D levels and incident type 2 diabetes. A meta-analysis of prospective studies. Diabetes Care. 2013;36:1422-8.

57. Davidson MB, Duran P, Lee ML, Friedman TC. High-dose vitamin D supplementation in people with prediabetes and hypovitaminosis D. Diabetes Care. 2013;36:260-6.

58. Pittas AG, Dawson-Hughes B, Sheehan P, et al. Vitamin D supplementation and the prevention of type 2 diabetes. N Engl J Med. 2019 Jun 7. doi: 10.1056/NEJMoa1900906. [Epub ahead of print]

59. Balk EM, Tatsioni A, Lichtenstein AH, Lau J, Pittas AG. Effect of chromium supplementation on glucose metabolism and lipids: a systematic review of randomized controlled trials. Diabetes Care. 2007;30:2154-63.

60. Veronese N, Watutantrige-Fernando S, Luchini C, et al. Effect of magnesium supplementation on glucose metabolism in people with or at risk of diabetes: a systematic review and meta-analysis of double-blind randomized controlled trials. Eur J Clin. 2016; 70:1354-9.

61. American College of Sports Medicine. Exercise and type 2 diabetes: a joint position statement of the American Diabetes Association and the American College of Sports Medicine. Med Sci Sports Exerc. 2010;42:2282-303.

62. Duncan GE, Perri MG, Teriaque DW, et al. Exercise training without weight loss increases insulin sensitivity and postheparin plasma lipase activity in previously sedentary adults. Diabetes Care. 2003;26:557-62.

63. Church TS, Blair SN, Cocreham S, et al. Effects of aerobic and resistance training on hemoglobin A1c levels in patients with type 2 diabetes: a randomized controlled trial. JAMA. 2010; 304:2253-62.

64. Dempesy PC, Larsen RN, Sethi P, et al. Benefits for type 2 diabetes of interrupting prolonged sitting with brief bouts of light walking or simple resistance training activities. Diabetes Care. 2016; 39:964-72.

65. Franz MJ. Alcohol and diabetes. In: Evert AB, Franz MJ, eds. American Diabetes Association Guide to Nutrition Therapy for Diabetes. 2nd ed. Alexandria, Va: American Diabetes Association; 2017:87-106.

66. Turner BC, Jenkins E, Kerr D, et al. The effect of evening alcohol consumption on next-morning glucose control in type 1 diabetes. Diabetes Care. 2001;24:1888-93.

67. Howard AA, Amsten JH, Gourevitch MN. Effect of alcohol consumption on diabetes mellitus. A systematic review. Ann Intern Med. 2004;140:211-9.

68. Knott C, Bell S, Britton A. Alcohol consumption and the risk of type 2 diabetes: a systematic review and a dose-response meta-analysis of more than 1.9 million individuals from 38 observational studies. Diabetes Care. 2015;38;1804-12.

69. Powers MA, Gal RL, Connor CG, et al. Eating patterns and food intake of persons with type 1 diabetes with the T1D Exchange. Diabetes Res Clin Pract. 2018;141;217-28.

70. The Diabetes Prevention Program Research Group. Reduction in the incidence of type 2 diabetes with lifestyle intervention or metformin. N Engl J Med. 2002;346:393-403.

71. Franz MJ, Boucher JL, Rutten-Ramos S, VanWormer JJ. Lifestyle weight-loss intervention outcomes in overweight and obese adults with type 2 diabetes: a systematic review and meta-analysis of randomized clinical trials. J Acad Nutr Diet. 2015;115:1447-63.

72. Esposito K, Maiorino MI, Ciotola M, et al. Effects of a Mediterranean-style diet on the need for antihyperglycemic drug therapy in patients with newly diagnosed type 2 diabetes: a randomized trial. Ann Intern Med. 2009;151:306-14.

73. The Look AHEAD Research Group. Reduction in weight and cardiovascular disease risk factors in individuals with type 2 diabetes. One-year results of the Look AHEAD trial. Diabetes Care. 2007;30:1374-83.

74. Guldbrand H, Dizdar B, Bunjaku B, et al. In type 2 diabetes, randomization to follow a low-carbohydrate diet transiently improves glycaemic control compared with advice to follow a low-fat diet producing similar weight loss. Diabetologia. 2012;55:2118-27.

75. The Look AHEAD Research Group. Cardiovascular effects of intensive lifestyle intervention in type 2 diabetes. N Engl J Med. 2013;369:145-54.

76. Rock CL, Flatt SW, Pakiz B, et al. Weight loss, glycemic control, and cardiovascular disease risk factors in response to differential diet composition in a weight loss program in type 2 diabetes: a randomized controlled trial. Diabetes Care. 2014;37:1573-80.

77. Hamdy O, Mattalib A, Morsi A, et al. Long-term effect of intensive lifestyle intervention on CVD risk factors in patients with diabetes in real-world clinical practice: a 5-year longitudinal study. BMJ Open Diabetes Res Care. 2017;5:e000259.

78. Franz MJ, VanWormer JJ, Crain LA, et al. Weight loss outcomes: a systematic review and meta-analysis of weight loss clinical trials with a minimum 1-year follow-up. J Am Diet Assoc. 2007;107:1755-67.

79. Buse JB, Caprio S, Cefalu WT, et al. How do we define cure of diabetes? Diabetes Care. 2009;32;2133-5.

80. Lean ME, Leslie WS, Barnes AC, et al. Primary care-led weight management for remission of type 2 diabetes (DiRECT): an open-label, cluster-randomized trial. Lancet. 2018;391:541-51.

81. Sjostrom I, Peltonen M, Jacobson P et al. Association of bariatric surgery with long-term remission of type 2 diabetes and with microvascular disease and macrovascular complications. JAMA. 2014; 311:2297-2304.

82. Arterburn DE, Bogart A, Sherwood NE, et al. A multisite study of long-term remission and relapse of type 2 diabetes mellitus following gastric bypass. Obes Surg. 2013;23:93-102.

83. Dansinger ML, Gleason JA, Griffith JL, et al. Comparison of the Atkins, Ornish, Weight Watchers, and Zone diets for weight loss and heart disease risk reduction: a randomized trial. JAMA. 2005;293:43-53.

84. Sacks FM, Gray GA, Carey VJ, et al. Comparison of weight-loss diets with different compositions of fat, protein, and carbohydrates. N Engl J Med. 2009;360:859-73.

85. Goode AD, Winkler EAH, Reeves MM et al. Relationship between intervention dose and outcomes in living well with diabetes—a randomized control trial of a telephone-delivered lifestyle-based weight loss intervention. Am J Health Promot. 2015; 30:120-9.

86. Vanheim LM, Patch K, Brokaw SM et al. TeleHealth delivery of the Diabetes Prevention Program to rural communities. Transl Behav Med. 2017; 7:286-91.

87. Young-Hyman D, de Groot M, Hill-Briggs F, et al. Psychological care of people with diabetes: a position statement of the American Diabetes Association. Diabetes Care. 2016; 39:2126-40.

88. Willig AL, Richardson BS, Agne A, et al. Intuitive eating practices among African-American women living with type 2 diabetes: a qualitative study. J Acad Nutr Diet. 2014;114(6):889-96.

89. American Dietetic Association. Position of the American Dietetic Association: weight management. J Am Diet Assoc. 2009;109:330-46.

90. Klein S, Burke LE, Bray GA, et al. Clinical implications of obesity with specific focus on cardiovascular disease: a statement for professionals from the American Heart Association Council on Nutrition, Physical Activity, and Metabolism. Circulation. 2004;110:2952-67.

91. Larger E, Rufat P, Dubois-Laforgue D, Ledoux S. Insulin therapy does not itself induce weight gain in patients with type 2 diabetes. Diabetes Care. 2001;24:1849-50.

92. Daly A. Use of insulin and weight gain: optimizing diabetes nutrition therapy. J Am Diet Assoc. 2007;107:1386-93.

93. Hollander P, Gupta AK, Plodkowski R, et al; COR-Diabetes Study Group. Effects of naltrexone sustained-release/bupropion sustained-release combination therapy on body weight and glycemic parameters in overweight and obese patients with type 2 diabetes. Diabetes Care. 2013;36:4022-9.

94. Garvey WT, Ryan DH, Bohannon NJV, et al. Weight-loss therapy in type 2 diabetes: effects of phentermine and topiramate extended release. Diabetes Care. 2014;37:3309-16.

95. Kelley DE, Bray GA, Pi-Sunyer FX, et al. Clinical efficacy of orlistat therapy in overweight and obese patients with insulin-treated type 2 diabetes: a 1-year randomized controlled trial. Diabetes Care. 2002;25:1033-41.

96. Rubino F, Nathan DM, Eckel RH, et al. Metabolic surgery in the treatment algorithm for type 2 diabetes: a joint statement by international diabetes organizations. Diabetes Care. 2016;39:861-77.

97. Mor A, Omotosho P, Torquat A. Cardiovascular risk in obese diabetic patients is significantly reduced one year after gastric bypass compared to one year of diabetes support and education. Surg Endosc. 2014;28:2815-20.

98. Mingrone G, Panunzi S, De Gaetano A, et al. Bariatric–metabolic surgery versus conventional medical treatment in obese patients with type 2 diabetes: 5 year follow-up of an open-label, single-centre, randomised controlled trial. Lancet. 2015;386:964-73.

99. Buse JB, Ginsberg HN, Bakris GL, et al. Primary prevention of cardiovascular diseases in people with diabetes mellitus. Diabetes Care. 2007;30:162-72.

100. Schwingshackl L, Strasser B, Joffmann G. Effects of monounsaturated fatty acids on glycaemic control in patients with abnormal glucose metabolism: a systematic review and meta-analysis. Ann Nutr Metab. 2011;58:290-6.

101. Eckel RH, Jakicic JM, Ard JD, et al. 2013 AHA/ACC guideline on lifestyle management to reduce cardiovascular risk: a report of the American College of Cardiology/American Heart Association Task Force on Practice Guidelines. Circulation. 2014;129(25 Suppl 2):S76-99.

102. Shin JY, Xun P, Nakamura Y, He K. Egg consumption in relation to risk of cardiovascular disease and diabetes: a systematic review and meta-analysis. Am J Clin Nutr. 2013;98(1):146-59.

103. Huo R, Du T, Xu Y, et al. Effects of Mediterranean-style diet on glycemic control, weight loass and cardiovascular risk factors among type 2 diabetes individuals: a meta-analysis. Eur J Clin Nutr. 2015; 69:1200-8.

104. Summers LK, Fielding BA, Bradshaw HA, et al. Substituting dietary saturated fat with polyunsaturated fat changes abdominal fat distribution and improves insulin sensitivity. Diabetologia. 2002;45:369-77.

105. O'Mahoney LL, Matu J, Price OJ, et al. Omega-3 polyunsaturated fatty acids favourably modulate cardiometabolic biomarkers in type 2 diabetes: a meta-analysis and meta-regression of randomized controlled trials. Cardiovasc Diabetol. 2018;17:98.

106. Academy of Nutrition and Dietetics. Disorders of lipid metabolism evidence-based nutrition practice guidelines. 2011 (cited 2019 June 26). On the Internet at: http://adaevidencelibrary.com/topic.cfm?cat=4528.

107. Lee YM, Haastert B, Scherbaum W, Hauner H. A phytosterol-enriched spread improves the lipid profile of subjects with type 2 diabetes mellitus—a randomized controlled trial under free-living conditions. Eur J Nutr. 2003;42:111-7.

108. Esposito K, Maiorino MI, Ceriello A, Giugliano D. Prevention and control of type 2 diabetes by Mediterranean diet: a systematic review. Diabetes Res Clin Pract. 2010;89:97-102.

109. Estruch R, Ros E, Salas-Salvado J, et al. PREDIMED Study Investigators. Primary prevention of cardiovascular disease with a Mediterranean-diet supplemented with extra-virgin olive oil or nuts. N Engl J Med. 2018;378:e34.

110. Brill JB. The Mediterranean diet and your health. Am J Lifestyle Med. 2009;3:44-56.

111. Blomster JI, Zoungas S, Chalmers J, et al. The relationship between alcohol consumption and vascular complications and mortality in individuals with type 2 diabetes. Diabetes Care. 2014;37:1353-59.

112. Gepner Y, Golan R, Harman-Boehm I, et al. Effects of initiating moderate alcohol intake on cardiometabolic risk in adults with type 2 diabetes. Ann Intern Med. 2015;163:569-79.

113. Bantle AE, Thomas W, Bantle JP. Metabolic effects of alcohol in the form of wine in persons with type 2 diabetes mellitus. Metabolism. 2008;57:241-5.

114. Pownall HJ, Ballantyne CM, Kimball KT, et al. Effect of moderate alcohol consumption on hypertriglyceridemia. Arch Intern Med. 1999;159:981-7.

115. Nanchahal K, Ashton WD, Wood DA. Alcohol consumption, metabolic cardiovascular risk factors and hypertension in women. Int J Epidemiol. 2000;29:57-64.

116. Miller M, Stone NJ, Ballantyne C, et al. Triglycerides and cardiovascular disease. A scientific statement from the American Heart Association. Circulation. 2011;123:2292-333.

117. Wei M, Gibbons LW, Kampert JB, et al. Low cardiorespiratory fitness and physical inactivity in men with type 2 diabetes. Ann Intern Med. 2000;132:605-11.

118. Church TS, Cheng YJ, Earnest CP, et al. Exercise capacity and body composition as predictors of mortality among men with diabetes. Diabetes Care. 2004;27:83-8.

119. Leon AS, Sanchez OA. Response of blood lipids to exercise training alone or combined with dietary intervention. Med Sci Sports Exerc. 2001;33:S502-15.

120. Kelley GA, Kelley KS. Effects of aerobic exercise on lipids and lipoproteins in adults with type 2 diabetes: a meta-analysis of randomized-controlled trials. Public Health. 2007;9:643-55.

121. Xie X, Atkins E, Lv J, et al. Effects of intensive blood pressure lowering on cardiovascular disease and renal outcomes: updated systematic review and meta-analysis. Lancet. 2016;387-435-43.

122. Benson G, Hayes J. Nutrition therapy for diabetes and hypertension. In: Evert AB, Franz MJ eds. American Diabetes Association Guide to Nutrition Therapy for Diabetes. 3rd ed. Alexandria, Va: American Diabetes Association; 2017:361-76.

123. Harsha DW, Lin PH, Obarzanek E, Karanja NM, Moore TJ, Caballero B; DASH Collaborative Research Group. Dietary Approaches to Stop Hypertension: a summary of study results. J Am Diet Assoc. 1999;99 Suppl:S35-9.

124. Azadbakht L, Fard NR, Karimi M, et al. Effects of the Dietary Approaches to Stop Hypertension (DASH) eating plan on cardiovascular risks among type 2 diabetic patients: a randomized crossover clinical trial. Diabetes Care. 2011;34:55-7.

125. Thomas MC, Moran J, Forsblom C, et a. FinnDiane Study Group. The association between dietary sodium intake, ESRD, and all-cause mortality in patients with type 1 diabetes. Diabetes Care. 2011; 34:861-6.

126. Ekinci El, Clarke S, Thomas MC, et al. Dietary salt intake and mortality in patients with type 2 diabetes. Diabetes Care. 2011; 34:703-9.

127. Appel LJ, Champagne CM, Harsha DW, et al; Writing Group of the PREMIER Collaborative Research Group. Effects of comprehensive lifestyle modification on blood pressure control: main results of the PREMIER clinical trial. JAMA. 2003;289:2083-93.

128. Miller ER III, Erlinger TP, Young DR, et al. Results of diet, exercise, and weight loss intervention trial (DEW-IT). Hypertension. 2002;40:612-8.

129. Kaplan NM. Lifestyle modification for prevention and treatment of hypertension. J Clin Hypertens. 2004;6:716-9.

130. Blumenthal JA, Babyak MA, Hinderliter A, et al. Effects of the DASH diet alone and in combination with exercise and weight loss on blood pressure and cardiovascular biomarkers in men and women with high blood pressure: the ENCORE study. Arch Intern Med. 2010;170:126-35.

131. Appel LJ, Moore TJ, Obarzanek E, et al; for the DASH Collaborative Research Group. A clinical trial of the effects of dietary patterns on blood pressure. N Engl J Med. 1997;336:1117-24.

132. Delahanty LM, Nathan DM. Implications of the Diabetes Prevention Program and Look AHEAD clinical trials for lifestyle interventions. J Am Diet Assoc. 2008; 108(Suppl 1):S66-72. doi:10.1016/j.jada.2008.01.026.

133. Pitsavos C, Makrilakis K, Panagiotakos DB, et al. The J-shape effect of alcohol intake on the risk of developing acute coronary syndromes in diabetic subjects: the CARDIO2000 II Study. Diabet Med. 2005;22:243-8.

134. Marfella R, Cacciapuoti F, Siniscalchi M, et al. Effect of moderate red wine intake on cardiac prognosis after recent myocardial infarction of subjects with type 2 diabetes mellitus. Diabet Med. 2006;23:974-81.

135. Wakabayashi I. Comparison of the relationships of alcohol intake with atherosclerotic risk factors in men with and without diabetes mellitus. Alcohol Alcohol. 2011;46:301-7.

136. Munson L. Nutrition therapy for diabetic kidney disease. In: Evert AB, Franz MJ. eds. American Diabetes Association Guide to Nutrition Therapy for Diabetes. 3rd ed. Alexandria, Va: American Diabetes Association; 2017:377-90.

137. Centers for Disease Control and Prevention. National diabetes fact sheet: national estimates and general information on diabetes and prediabetes in the United States, 2017. Atlanta, Ga: US Department of Health and Human Services, Centers for Disease Control and Prevention; 2017. (cited on 2019 June 26). On the internet: https://www.cdc.gov/diabetes/pdfs/data/statistics/national-diabetes-statistics-report.pdf.

138. Pan Y, Guo LL, Jin HM. Low-protein diets for diabetic nephropathy: a meta-analysis of randomized controlled trials. Am J Clin Nutr. 2008;88:660-6.

139. Teixeira SR, Tappenden KA, Carson L, et al. Isolated soy protein consumption reduces urinary albumin excretion and improves the serum lipid profile in men with type 2 diabetes mellitus and nephropathy. J Nutr. 2004;134:1874-80.

140. Chiang JL, Maahs DM, Garvey KC, et al. Type 1 diabetes in children and adolescents: a position statement by the American Diabetes Association. Diabetes Care. 2018;41:2026-44.

141. Arslanian S, Bacha F, Grey M, et al. Evaluation and management of youth-onset type 2 diabetes: a position statement by the American Diabetes Association. Diabetes Care. 2018;41:2648-68.

142. Spiegel G. Nutrition therapy for youth with diabetes. In: Evert AB, Franz MJ. eds. American Diabetes Association Guide to Nutrition Therapy for Diabetes. 3rd ed. Alexandria, Va: American Diabetes Association; 2017:159-82.

143. Stanley K. Nutrition therapy for older adults with diabetes. In: Evert AB, Franz MJ eds. American Diabetes Association Guide to Nutrition Therapy for Diabetes. 3rd ed. Alexandria, Va: American Diabetes Association; 2017:183-201.

144. Academy of Nutrition and Dietetics. Position of the Academy of Nutrition and Dietetics: Food and nutrition for older adults: promoting health and wellness. J Acad Nutr Diet. 2012;112:1255-77.

145. Well JL, Dumbrell AC. Nutrition and aging: assessment and treatment of compromised nutritional status in frail elderly patients. Clin Interv Aging. 2006;1:67-79.

146. Kirkman MS, Briscoe VJ, Clark N, et al. Diabetes in older adults (consensus report). Diabetes Care. 2012;35:2650-64.

147. Miller SL, Wolfe RR. The danger of weight loss in the elderly. J Nutr Health Aging. 2008;12:487-91.

148. Villareal DT, Banks M, Siener C, Sinacore DR, Klein S. Physical frailty and body composition in obese elderly men and women. Obes Res. 2004;12:913-20.

149. Shapses SA, Riedt CS. Bone, body weight, and weight reduction; what are the concerns? J Nutr. 2006;136:1453-6.

150. Academy of Nutrition and Dietetics. Food and nutrition for older adults promoting health and wellness evidence analysis project. 2012 (cited 2019 June 26). On the Internet at: http://www.andevidencelibrary.com/topic.cfm?cat=3987.

151. Lichtenstein AH, Rasmussen H, Winifred Y, Epstein S, Russell R. Modified MyPyramid for older adults. J Nutr. 2008;138:5-11.

152. Academy of Nutrition and Dietetics. Position of the American Dietetic Association: Nutrient supplementation. J Acad Nutr Diet. 2009;109:2073-84.

153. Cranney A, Horsley T, O'Donnell S, et al. Effectiveness and safety of vitamin D in relation to bone health. Evidence Report/Technology Assessment No. 158. Rockville, Md: Agency for Healthcare Research and Quality; 2007. AHRQ Publication No. 07-E013.

154. Institute of Medicine, Food and Nutrition Board. Dietary Reference Intakes: Thiamin, Riboflavin, Niacin, Vitamin B6, Folate, Vitamin B12, Pantothenic Acid, Biotin, and Choline. Washington, DC: National Academy Press; 1998.

155. Chaliwal R, Weinstock RS. Management of type 1 diabetes in older adults. Diabetes Spectr. 2014;27:9-20.

156. Chu E, Meinel N. Severe hypoglycemia and complications in elderly people with diabetes, hypoglycemia in hospitalized patients, and hypoglycemia and falls related to fractures. Diabetic Hypoglycemia. 2012;5:24-8.

157. McLaughlin S. Diabetes in older adults. In: Ross TA, Boucher JL, O'Connell BS, eds. Diabetes Medical Nutrition Therapy and Education. Chicago: American Dietetic Association; 2005:179-88.

158. Public Health Service, Department of Health and Human Services. Losing weight safely (cited 2019 June 26). On the Internet at: http://www.plainlanguage.gov/examples/before_after/pub_hhs_losewgt.cfm.

159. Diabetes Related Literacy/Numeracy Scales. (cited 2019 June 26). On the internet at: https://labnodes.vanderbilt.edu/resource/view/id/10654/community_id/1136.

CHAPTER 17

Pharmacotherapy for Glucose Management

Lauren G. Pamulapati, PharmD, BCACP
Evan M. Sisson, PharmD, MSHA, BCACP, CDCES, FADCES

Key Concepts

- The pathophysiology of hyperglycemia helps determine the appropriate therapy for persons with different types of diabetes.
- In the management of hyperglycemia associated with type 2 diabetes, combination therapies that target different aspects of the metabolic abnormality are often employed.
- Preference for specific drug therapies relies on their proven benefit to improve cardiovascular and renal outcomes in addition to glycemic control.
- The goal of insulin therapy, regardless of diabetes type, is to replace lost capacity and mimic normal physiology.
- The various insulin preparations differ in onset, action, and duration after subcutaneous injection.
- The role of the diabetes care and education specialist is to help those with diabetes understand the medications they take and to provide guidance for monitoring and effective use of the drug therapies.

Introduction

This chapter primarily reviews pharmacologic therapies for glucose management in type 2 diabetes. Although local preferences determine specific practice patterns, the generally accepted approach to therapy is described in complementary documents from the American Diabetes Association (ADA) and the American Association of Clinical Endocrinologists (AACE).[1,2,3] Both documents emphasize the need to individualize therapy based on person with diabetes-specific characteristics, such as age and affordability, and presence of comorbid conditions, such as atherosclerotic cardiovascular disease (ASCVD), chronic kidney disease (CKD), or heart failure with reduced ejection fraction (HFrEF). Further information is available from the Endocrine Society and the American Geriatric Society regarding treatment goals and therapy in older adults.[4,5]

In the past decade, several new drug therapy choices received approved labeling from the US Food and Drug Administration (FDA) for use in people with diabetes. In addition to oral agents, there are several peptide substances that mimic endogenous hormones.[1] Insulin administration technology continues to be refined, with the ultimate goal of closely approximating the physiologic action of endogenous insulin. New approaches to improve glycemic control involve gastrointestinal enzyme alteration and use of products that enhance insulin action.[1,2] Because diabetes drug regimens can be very complex, the diabetes care and education specialist who remains knowledgeable about current standards of care can be extremely valuable to the person with diabetes.

Obesity Management

Approach to Obesity Management

Because obesity and type 2 diabetes are linked, the 2019 AACE and 2019 ADA guidelines offer nearly identical recommendations for care of the overweight and obese person with diabetes.[2,6] The first step of the AACE algorithm includes evaluation of complications (presence of cardiometabolic disease such as diabetes, hypertension, or dyslipidemia and biomechanical problems) and staging of obesity and pre-obesity (BMI ≥30 kg/m^2 and 25–29.9 kg/m^2). Step 2 includes selection of therapeutic targets, treatment modality, and treatment intensity based on weight loss staging. All persons with diabetes are enrolled in lifestyle modification, while those with more severe obesity-related complications are considered for medication therapy and surgical interventions. Addition of drug therapy in combination with lifestyle therapy may be considered for all persons with diabetes with a BMI greater than or equal to 27 kg/m^2, and bariatric surgery should be considered for persons with diabetes with a BMI greater than or equal to 35 kg/m^2.[2,7] Step 3 of the algorithm includes intensification of interventions for those persons with diabetes who fail to meet therapeutic targets or whose complications do not improve.

Pharmacologic Treatment Options for Obesity

There are currently 5 classes of orally administered agents used for obesity management (see Table 17.1). Of the 8 medications approved for weight loss adjunct to lifestyle, 3 are approved for short-term use over several weeks (diethylpropion, phendimetrazine, and phentermine), and the remaining 5 are approved for long-term use. Of the agents approved for long-term use, lorcaserin, orlistat, and naltrexone/bupropion are associated with modest weight loss rates (approximately 30%-50% of persons with diabetes achieve a 5% weight loss and 15%-35% of persons with diabetes achieve a 10% weight loss).[9–11] Phentermine/topiramate and liraglutide are associated with a greater degree of weight loss (approximately 45%-70% of persons with diabetes achieve a 5% weight loss and 20%-50% of persons with diabetes achieve a 10% weight loss).[12,13]

TABLE 17.1 Medications for Obesity Management

Sympathomimetic Agents: Short-Term Therapy	
Action: Central nervous system (CNS) effects similar to amphetamines. Reduce appetite by stimulation of the hypothalamus to release norepinephrine. *Expected weight loss:* Agents approved for short-term treatment as adjunct to low-calorie diet and increased physical activity. Weight loss amount varies. Person with diabetes weight may return to baseline after discontinuation. *Contraindications:* History of cardiovascular disease (arrhythmias, heart failure, coronary artery disease, stroke, uncontrolled hypertension), hyperthyroidism, glaucoma, agitated states, history of drug abuse, monoamine oxidase inhibitor (MAOI) therapy.	
Phentermine • Adipex-P® (Teva Pharmaceuticals USA) • Lomaira (KVK Tech, Inc.)	*Contraindications.* Pregnant women (excreted in breast milk). *Interactions.* Numerous drug-drug interactions related to the stimulatory effects of amphetamines (especially increased blood pressure and heart rate). Alcohol may enhance CNS adverse effects. Use of MAO inhibitors within 14 days may result in hypertensive crisis. *Precautions.* Amphetamines may impair the ability to engage in potentially hazardous activities. Discontinue in persons with diabetes experiencing new-onset chest pain, shortness of breath, or lower extremity edema. May be associated with development of valvular heart disease. Significant abuse potential (C-IV controlled substance).
Diethylpropion • Tenuate® (Aventis Pharmaceuticals, Inc.)	*Interactions.* Use of MAO inhibitors within 14 days may result in hypertensive crisis. *Precautions.* Symptomatic cardiovascular disease, including arrhythmia and severe hypertension, may occur. Risk for seizure in persons with epilepsy. Significant abuse potential (C-IV controlled substance). Excreted in human milk: caution should be used in nursing mothers.
Phendimetrazine • Bontril (Sandoz Inc.)	*Contraindications.* Pregnant women (excreted in breast milk). *Interactions.* Use of MAO inhibitors within 14 days may result in hypertensive crisis. Avoid use with alcohol. *Precautions.* Caution should be exercised even in mild hypertension. Significant abuse potential (C-III controlled substance).
Sympathomimetic Agents: Long-Term Therapy	
Phentermine with Topiramate • Qsymia™ (Vivus Inc.)	*Action.* Phentermine as above. Topiramate may suppress appetite, but exact mechanism is unknown. *Expected weight loss.* Approved for chronic weight management as adjunct to low-calorie diet and increased physical activity. Persons with diabetes may lose 5% to 10% of baseline weight. Person with diabetes weight typically returns to baseline after discontinuation.

TABLE 17.1 Medications for Obesity Management (continued)	
Phentermine with Topiramate • Qsymia™ (Vivus Inc.) (*continued*)	*Contraindications.* Phentermine as above. Topiramate—Pregnancy associated with cleft palate. Phentermine/Topiramate—avoid use in pregnancy (excreted in breast milk). *Interactions.* Phentermine as above. Topiramate—Hypokalemia if used with non-potassium-sparing diuretics. Phentermine/Topiramate—May decrease estrogen component of oral contraceptives by 16% and increase the progestin component by 22%. *Precautions.* Cognitive dysfunction and psychiatric disturbances may result from rapid titration and higher doses. In addition to concerns with phentermine above, the following precautions are related to topiramate use: Associated with acute myopia and glaucoma (typically within 1 month of initiation). Severe hyperthermia may result during strenuous exercise or during exposure to high environmental temperatures. May raise serum creatinine and increase risk of kidney stone formation. Increased seizure risk with abrupt withdrawal; taper doses over at least 1 week. Significant abuse potential (C-IV controlled substance).
Selective-Serotonergic Agents	
Lorcaserin • Belviq® (Arena Pharmaceuticals GmbH)	*Action.* Agonist of selective serotonin (5-HT2c) receptors in the hypothalamus, resulting in decreased appetite. *Expected weight loss.* Approved for chronic weight management as adjunct to low-calorie diet and increased physical activity. Persons with diabetes may lose 5% of baseline weight, or 3 kg. *Contraindications.* Pregnant women (unknown if excreted in breast milk). *Interactions.* Use with other serotonergic drugs (selective serotonin reuptake inhibitors [SSRIs], serotonin-norepinephrine reuptake inhibitors [SNRIs], MAOIs) may increase risk of serotonin syndrome. May increase serum concentrations of cytochrome P450 2D6 substrates. *Precautions.* May be associated with development of valvular heart disease. May cause cognitive disturbances (attention or memory, euphoria, dissociation, depression, or suicidal thoughts). May cause priapism. Significant abuse potential (C-IV controlled substance).
Lipase Inhibitors	
Orlistat • Xenical® (Genentech USA Inc.) • Alli® (GlaxosmithKline Consumer Healthcare)	*Action.* Inhibits gastrointestinal lipases, resulting in decreased hydrolysis of dietary fat necessary for fat absorption. *Expected weight loss.* Approved for chronic weight management as adjunct to low-calorie diet and increased physical activity. Persons with diabetes may lose 2.8% of baseline weight. Persons with diabetes may regain weight after discontinuation. *Contraindications.* Chronic malabsorption syndrome, cholestasis. Pregnant women (unknown if excreted in breast milk). *Interactions.* Decreased vitamin K absorption may prolong bleeding for persons with diabetes taking warfarin. Decreased absorption of cyclosporine and levothyroxine (administration of orlistat should be separated by at least 3 to 4 hours from interacting target drugs). *Precautions.* Gastrointestinal events (spotting, flatus with discharge, fecal urgency, oily stool, fecal incontinence) may increase with high-fat diets (>30% of calories from fat).
Opioid Agonist/Aminoketone Antidepressant	
Naltrexone/bupropion HCl • Contrave® (Takeda Pharmaceuticals America, Inc.)	*Action.* Unknown for weight loss; suggested to impact the hypothalamus (appetite regulatory center) and dopamine system (reward system) *Expected weight loss.* Approved as an adjunct agent for chronic weight management with a BMI ≥30 kg/m^2 or ≥27 kg/m^2 and at least 1 weight-related comorbidity. Weight loss is variable; most persons with diabetes can expect a 5% reduction in body weight.

(continued)

TABLE 17.1 Medications for Obesity Management (continued)	
Naltrexone/bupropion HCl • Contrave® (Takeda Pharmaceuticals America, Inc.) (*continued*)	*Contraindications.* Uncontrolled hypertension, seizure disorder, anorexia nervosa or bulimia, abrupt discontinuation of substance misuse, chronic opioid use, MAO inhibitor use. Pregnant women (excreted in breast milk). *Interactions.* Extensive interactions including with antipsychotics, beta-blockers, antiarrhythmics, platelet-inhibitors, and dopamine agonists. *Precautions.* Combination product—may cause heart rate and blood pressure increases, and pupillary dilation may precipitate angle-closure glaucoma. Bupropion—persons with diabetes with depression may experience worsening of symptoms and/or suicidal thoughts or behaviors. May lower seizure threshold and increase seizure risk.
GLP-1 Receptor Agonist	
Liraglutide • Saxenda® (Novo Nordisk Inc.)	*Action.* GLP-1 agonist acts as a physiological regulator of appetite and calorie intake. *Expected weight loss.* Approved as an adjunct agent for chronic weight management with a BMI ≥30 kg/m^2 or ≥27 kg/m^2 and at least 1 weight-related comorbidity. Variable results; most persons with diabetes can expect a 5% to 10% reduction in body weight. *Contraindications.* Personal or family history of medullary thyroid carcinoma or multiple endocrine neoplasia syndrome type 2. Pregnant women (unknown if excreted in breast milk). *Interactions.* Slowing of GI emptying may alter absorption of oral medications; serious hypoglycemia with secretagogues. *Precautions.* May increase risk of thyroid tumors, acute pancreatitis, gallbladder disease.

Sympathomimetic Agents

Agents in the sympathomimetic class include phentermine, diethylpropion, phendimetrazine, benzphetamine, and phentermine with topiramate (PHEN/TPM). Dosing for phentermine, diethylpropion, and phendimetrazine is noted in the table.[14–16] The combination product is unique in that both components provide weight reduction benefits; however, both are associated with significant side effects, especially at higher doses. The value of the combination product is achievement of maximum weight loss while using the lowest dose to minimize risk of side effects. The maximum weight loss benefit with PHEN/TPM in clinical trials was 5% to 10% from baseline.[7] The percentage of persons with diabetes able to achieve 5% weight loss was 44.9% to 75.2% with low-dose PHEN/TPM, compared with 66.7% to 79.3% with high-dose PHEN/TPM. Unfortunately, weight loss benefits typically reverse upon discontinuation.

Mechanism of Action The sympathomimetic agents have activity similar to amphetamines and reduce appetite by stimulation of the hypothalamus to release norepinephrine.[7] Topiramate originally received FDA-approved labeling in 1996 as an anticonvulsant. The exact mechanism by which it produces weight loss is unknown. Topiramate is thought to suppress appetite and enhance satiety by a combined effect in the hypothalamus that includes inhibition of carbonic anhydrase.

Dosing Phentermine, diethylpropion, and PHEN/TPM are classified as C-IV controlled substances, and phendimetrazine is classified as a C-III controlled substance. Because of the long list of serious adverse effects associated with PHEN/TPM (especially fetal harm with topiramate), this combination is available only from certified pharmacies according to an FDA risk evaluation and mitigation strategy (REMS). Therapy with PHEN/TPM is usually started at the lowest dose (PHEN/TPM 3.75 mg/23 mg) to avoid cognitive impairment issues associated with the topiramate component. The once-daily dose is taken once daily in the morning without regards to meals; it is preferred to avoid evening dosing to prevent insomnia. The dose is gradually increased as noted in the table. If weight loss of at least 5% is not achieved by 12 weeks on the maximum dose, PHEN/TPM should be tapered down and discontinued. A slow taper (taking PHEN/TPM every other day for 1 week) is recommended due to the risk of seizures with rapid discontinuation.

Precautions These agents can increase resting heart rate, which may exacerbate symptoms in persons with diabetes with coronary artery disease or hypertension. Concomitant use with alcohol may exacerbate central nervous system effects.

Topiramate is associated with cognitive dysfunction, psychiatric disturbances (mood disorders), and sedation

Sympathomimetic Agents: Dosage Information

Drug	*Trade Name*	*Common Dose/Frequency and Available Strengths*
Benzphetamine	–	25 mg–50 mg once daily; may increase to 25 mg to 50 mg 1 to 3 times daily based on response *Tabs*: 25 mg, 50 mg
Phentermine	Adipex-P®; Lomaira®	Adipex®: 15–37.5 mg once daily before breakfast or 1–2 hours post-breakfast Lomaira®: 8 mg 3 times daily *Tabs/Capsules:* 15 mg, 30 mg, 37.5 mg Caps (Lomaira®): 8 mh
Diethylpropion	Tenuate®	Immediate release (IR): 25 mg 3 or 4 times daily before meals (may administer one mid-evening to control overnight hunger) Controlled release (CR): 75 mg daily, administered mid-morning *Tabs/Capsules:* IR 25 mg, CR 75 mg
Phendimetrazine	Bontril	IR: 35 mg two or three times daily, 1 hour before meals ER: 105 mg daily, 30–60 minutes before food (morning meal)
Phentermine with topiramate	Qsymia™	Initiate at 3.75 mg/23 mg once daily for 14 days Increase to 7.5 mg/46 mg once daily If 3% weight loss has not been achieved at 12 weeks, either discontinue therapy or escalate the dose Increase to 11.25 mg/69 mg for 14 days Increase dose to maximum dose of 15 mg/92 mg If 5% weight loss has not been achieved at 12 weeks on the maximum dose, then taper drug to discontinuation *Capsule:* Phentermine 3.75 and topiramate 23 mg PHEN/TPM 7.5/46 mg PHEN/TPM 11.25/69 mg PHEN/TPM 15/92 mg

(somnolence or fatigue). Topiramate is also associated with acute myopia and glaucoma that typically occur within 1 month of initiation. Severe hyperthermia due to oligohydrosis may result during strenuous exercise or during exposure to high environmental temperatures. Because topiramate is a weak carbonic anhydrase inhibitor, it may increase the risk of kidney stones by approximately 2 to 4 times that of the untreated population.

Contraindications Phentermine, diethylpropion, and PHEN/TPM are contraindicated in pregnancy women due to known fetal risks. These agents should also be avoided in breastfeeding women or in children. Topiramate is also known to cause cleft palate in children of mothers who took the drug during pregnancy. The combination drug may decrease the estrogen component of oral contraceptives by 16% and increase the progestin component by 22%.

Because of their sympathomimetic activity, these agents should be avoided in persons with diabetes with a history of cardiovascular disease, including arrhythmias, heart failure, coronary artery disease, stroke, or uncontrolled hypertension. Phentermine is also contraindicated in persons with diabetes with hyperthyroidism, glaucoma, agitated states, and a history of drug abuse. Concomitant use with monoamine oxidase inhibitors (MAOIs) may exacerbate the hypertensive effect of phentermine. No specific contraindications are listed for topiramate; however, persons with diabetes should be carefully selected due to the many potential adverse effects.

Monitoring Monitoring parameters for persons with diabetes on sympathomimetic agents include resting heart rate, blood pressure, visual acuity and symptoms of glaucoma, and renal function. For persons with diabetes taking phentermine with topiramate, additional monitoring parameters include serum bicarbonate, potassium, and creatinine; suicidal thoughts and mood disorders; symptoms of acute acidosis; and weight. Sympathomimetic agents should be discontinued if weight loss is not observed within the first 4 weeks of therapy. As noted above, the combination drug should be discontinued if weight loss of at least 5% is not achieved by 12 weeks on the maximum dose. Overall, sympathomimetics, with the exception of Qsymia (phentermine/topiramate) are only approved for short-term duration (≤12 weeks).

Instructions for Persons With Diabetes Persons with diabetes should be advised of the side effects related to therapy and encouraged to communicate any changes to their healthcare provider, especially those related to the heart or mood. Because glycemic control may be affected by weight loss, persons with diabetes should be educated on symptoms of hypoglycemia and its treatment. Persons with diabetes should be counseled about the risks for birth defects and to use effective contraception while on these agents.

Selective-Serotonergic Agents

The neurotransmitter serotonin helps regulate many body functions, including mood, appetite, and sleep.[7] Lorcaserin is a selective agonist of 5-HT_{2C}, which promotes satiety and weight loss.[7] In clinical studies, 37.5% to 47.2% of persons with diabetes taking 10 mg twice daily of lorcaserin lost 5% of weight from baseline; however, persons with diabetes regained most of their weight upon discontinuation.[7] Lorcaserin's affinity for other serotonin receptor subtypes contributes to side effects such as changes in mood, hallucinations, valvulopathy, and hypertension.

Selective-Serotonergic Agents: Dosage Information

Drug	*Trade Name*	*Common Dose/Frequency and Available Strengths*
Lorcaserin	Belviq®	IR: 10 mg twice daily
	Belviq XR®	XR: 20 mg once daily
		Tabs: 10 mg (IR), 20 mg (XR)

Mechanism of Action Lorcaserin is a selective-serotonin agonist of receptors in the hypothalamus.[9] Activation of these receptors increases satiety and promotes weight loss. Although the drug may activate off-target receptor subtypes, selectivity for the 5-HT_{2C} subtype is high, corresponding to the low rates of toxicity in clinical trials. However, with higher than recommended doses, a greater risk for psychiatric effects resulting from this off-target activation may be seen.

Dosing Lorcaserin is classified as a C-IV controlled substance. The dose of 10 mg twice daily may be taken with or without food. If weight loss of at least 5% is not achieved after 12 weeks, therapy should be discontinued.

Precautions Concomitant administration of lorcaserin with serotonergic agents (eg, selective serotonin reuptake inhibitors [SSRIs], serotonin-norepinephrine reuptake inhibitors [SNRIs], tricyclic antidepressants [TCAs], bupropion, St John's wort, tryptophan), agents that impair metabolism of serotonin (eg, MAOIs, dextromethorphan, tramadol, lithium), or antidopaminergic agents (eg, antipsychotics) may increase the risk of serotonin syndrome.[9] Symptoms of serotonin syndrome may include agitation, hallucinations, tachycardia, hyperthermia, nausea, and vomiting.

In clinical trials, valvular regurgitation was observed in 2.4% of persons with diabetes taking lorcaserin, compared with 2% of persons with diabetes taking placebo.[9] Lorcaserin has not been studied in persons with diabetes with heart failure; thus, it should be avoided due to possible cardiac risks. Routine echocardiogram evaluations are not recommended in the absence of symptoms.

The following rare adverse effects were observed in persons with diabetes taking lorcaserin: hematologic changes (decreased white blood cell or red blood cell count), increased prolactin, pulmonary hypertension, and priapism. Periodic evaluation of complete blood count (CBC) is likely helpful, but other follow-up laboratory tests and examinations are determined by risk and symptom presentation.

Lorcaserin may cause cognitive impairment (attention and memory), confusion, somnolence, and fatigue. Persons with diabetes may also experience euphoria, hallucinations, and dissociation; however, these effects typically occur at doses greater than the recommended 10 mg twice daily.

Contraindications Lorcaserin is contraindicated in pregnant women and is not indicated for use during pregnancy, for breastfeeding women, or for children.

Monitoring Monitoring parameters for persons with diabetes on lorcaserin include CBC (periodically during use), blood glucose (in individuals with diabetes), and prolactin levels (if galactorrhea, gynecomastia, or other signs and symptoms of hyperprolactinemia arise). Persons with diabetes should be monitored for signs and symptoms of depression, suicidal thoughts, serotonin syndrome, and valvular heart disease (dyspnea, dependent edema). As noted above, lorcaserin should be discontinued if weight loss of at least 5% is not achieved by 12 weeks on therapy.

Instructions for Persons With Diabetes Persons with diabetes should be advised of the side effects related to therapy and encouraged to communicate any changes to their healthcare provider, especially those related to the heart or mood. Because glycemic control may be affected by weight loss, persons with diabetes should be educated on symptoms of hypoglycemia and its treatment. Women of reproductive age should be counseled about the risks of fetal harm while taking this agent and to use adequate contraception to prevent pregnancy while taking this agent.

Lipase Inhibitors

Originally approved as a prescription-only product, orlistat is available in a lower dose over the counter.[7] Weight loss associated with orlistat is only 2.8% compared with placebo, which is significantly less than other agents. Almost 10% of persons with diabetes discontinue orlistat due to gastrointestinal complaints related to the inability to absorb dietary fat. Because most of the side effects associated with orlistat are related to dietary indiscretions, the value of orlistat lies in its ability to reinforce positive behavior modification.

Lipase Inhibitors: Dosage Information

Drug	*Trade Name*	*Common Dose/Frequency and Available Strengths*
Orlistat	Xenical®	60–120 mg 3 times daily
	Alli®	*Xenical Tabs:* 120 mg
		Alli Tabs: 60 mg

Mechanism of Action Orlistat is a reversible inhibitor of gastrointestinal lipases, resulting in decreased fat absorption from the small intestine.[10] The resulting decrease in caloric intake promotes weight loss.

Dosing Prescription orlistat (the 120-mg dose) and over-the-counter orlistat (Alli® 60 mg) should be given 3 times daily with each main meal containing fat. Doses should be omitted if a meal is missed or if the meal does not contain fat.

Precautions Concomitant administration of orlistat with lipophilic drugs may reduce serum concentrations by as much as 30%.[10] Persons with diabetes taking cyclosporine should administer the dose 3 hours after orlistat, while persons with diabetes taking levothyroxine should separate the dose by at least 4 hours from orlistat administration. Persons with diabetes taking fat-soluble vitamins (A, D, E, and K) should separate the administration time by at least 2 hours before or after the orlistat dose.

The most common complaints with orlistat are associated with its mechanism of action, especially in persons with diabetes consuming >30% of total daily calories from fat. Gastrointestinal complaints during the first year of treatment include oily spotting (27%), flatus with discharge (24%), fecal urgency (22%), and oily stool (20%). These complaints decreased significantly in persons with diabetes who continued orlistat into the second year, possibly due to better avoidance of dietary fat.[10]

Rare cases of severe liver injury and increased urinary oxalate have been reported with orlistat.

Contraindications Orlistat is contraindicated in pregnant women and is not indicated for use during pregnancy, for breastfeeding women, or for children. It should also be avoided in persons with diabetes with chronic malabsorption or those with cholestasis.

Monitoring In addition to weight loss, persons with diabetes should be monitored for thyroid function if receiving supplementation. Evaluation of liver function should be performed in persons with diabetes exhibiting symptoms of hepatic dysfunction. If weight loss of at least 5% is not achieved by 12 weeks on the maximum dose, orlistat should be discontinued.

Instructions for Persons With Diabetes Persons with diabetes should be advised of the relationship between the mechanism of orlistat, dietary fat, and the side effects. Because orlistat may decrease the absorption of dietary fat-soluble vitamins (A, D, E, and K), persons with diabetes should take a multivitamin containing fat-soluble vitamins at least 2 hours before or after the orlistat dose. Persons with diabetes should monitor blood glucose levels while taking orlistat because of its ability to directly inhibit calorie absorption. Persons with diabetes should be encouraged to communicate any changes to their healthcare provider, especially those related to thyroid therapy or liver injury (severe nausea, inability to eat, discolored urine, or jaundice).

GLP-1 Receptor Agonists

This details of this class of drugs will be discussed in the diabetes treatment section. However, there is one agent in this class that is FDA-approved for weight loss only, Saxenda® (liraglutide). Weight loss should be monitored. If there is not a reduction of 4% to 5% of baseline body weight achieved after 12 weeks at the maximum tolerated dose (or 16 weeks after initiation), liraglutide should be discontinued.

GLP-1 Receptor Agonists

Drug	*Trade Name*	*Common Dose/Frequency and Available Strengths*
Liraglutide	Saxenda®	0.6 mg once daily, may titrate weekly up to maximum dose of 3 mg
		Pen auto-injector: 18 mg/3 mL

Diabetes Treatment Goals

The goals of treatment of both type 1 diabetes and type 2 diabetes are to achieve near-normal glucose levels in order to avoid short- and long-term complications. The AACE guidelines recommend an A1C goal of <6.5%, whereas the ADA standards of care recommend an A1C goal of <7.0%.[2,3] The more aggressive AACE recommendation attempts to overcome clinical inertia among providers, while the ADA recommendation is based on clinical trial evidence of reduced microvascular and macrovascular outcomes. The ADA position statement acknowledges the benefit of more aggressive goals in selected persons with diabetes, and both guidelines suggest less stringent goals in persons with diabetes who will not benefit from or may be harmed by lower A1C goals (eg, persons with diabetes with a history of severe hypoglycemia, limited life expectancy, or advanced microvascular or macrovascular complications).[3] The 2019 Treatment of Diabetes in Older Adults: An Endocrine Society Clinical Practice Guidelines emphasizes the importance of setting a glycemic goal that minimizes the risk of hypoglycemia.[4] Similar to the 2012 Diabetes in Older Adults: A Consensus Report by the ADA/American Geriatric Society, A1C goals in older adults are based on illness burden, cognitive impairment, functional impairment, and placement in long-term care.[4,5] Mounting evidence suggests that prolonged hyperglycemia and delayed time to goal increases the risk of both microvascular and macrovascular disease. Diabetes care and education specialists are in a unique role to counsel persons with diabetes on their goals of therapy and the importance of overcoming clinical inertia (ie, lack of treatment intensification in a person with diabetes not at evidence-based goals for care) to achieve these goals and prevent further complications.

Approach to Antihyperglycemic Management

Many different pharmacologic treatment options are currently available to treat type 2 diabetes. The 2020 AACE algorithm recommends pharmacotherapy interventions based on the presenting A1C level (see Figure 17.1).[2] The foundation of therapy rests on therapeutic lifestyle change, and metformin is presented as the preferred first agent among the hierarchy of options. For persons with diabetes with an A1C level less than 7.5%, reasonable alternatives to metformin (depicted with a check mark in the algorithm in order of preference) include glucagon-like peptide-1 (GLP-1) receptor agonists, sodium-glucose co-transporter 2 (SGLT2) inhibitors, dipeptidyl peptidase-4 (DPP-4) inhibitors, and alpha-glucosidase inhibitors. Caution is advised for the use of thiazolidinediones, sulfonylureas, and meglitinides (depicted with a "use with caution" triangle in the algorithm). New in the 2020 algorithm is the recommendation to add a GLP-1 receptor agonist or SGLT2 inhibitor for people with established ASCVD or at high risk, CKD, or HFrEF, regardless of glycemic control. Because many diabetes providers are accustomed to selecting agents based on the degree of A1C lowering, addition of therapeutic agents independent of glycemic control may take time to integrate into practice. Persons with diabetes with A1C levels greater than or equal to 7.5% are recommended to start dual or triple drug therapy with metformin as the base. Persons with diabetes with an entry-level A1C greater than 9% plus symptoms are recommended to start insulin in addition to other agents.

The 2020 ADA algorithm continues its person with diabetes–centered approach to drug therapy selection.[1] Determination of a treatment plan begins with establishing glycemic targets of care. The domains of consideration when choosing between a more stringent treatment plan and a less stringent one include the following: person with diabetes attitude and expected treatment effort, risks potentially associated with hypoglycemia and other adverse events, disease duration, life expectancy, important comorbidities, established vascular complications, and person with diabetes resources or support system. As with the AACE algorithm, the foundation of therapy according to ADA remains healthy eating, weight control, and increased activity; however, metformin is suggested as the single monotherapy option (see Figure 17.2). This recommendation is based on its low cost, low risk of hypoglycemia, potential cardiovascular benefit and ability to achieve glycemic goals in most persons with diabetes. Furthermore, data suggest that initiation of metformin within 3 months of diagnosis may preserve pancreatic beta cell function and delay the progression of diabetes.[8] The 2020 ADA guideline recommendations for two- and three-drug combinations in addition to metformin shifted away from glycemic control to prioritize agents with proven efficacy to help persons with diabetes and evidence or ASCVD or at high risk, CKD or HFrEF. The ADA algorithm establishes a tiered approach that starts by recommending either a GLP-1 for persons with diabetes in whom ASCVD predominates. The second step of the five tiers recommends SGLT2 inhibitors with proven evidence of reducing heart failure or CKD progression. In persons with diabetes without established disease, subsequent drug selection is based on compelling need to: 1) minimize hypoglycemia; 2) minimize weight gain or promote weight loss; and, 3) decrease person with diabetes costs. Regardless of the drug combinations chosen, it should be noted that all persons with type 2 diabetes eventually arrive at a regimen that includes intensive insulin.

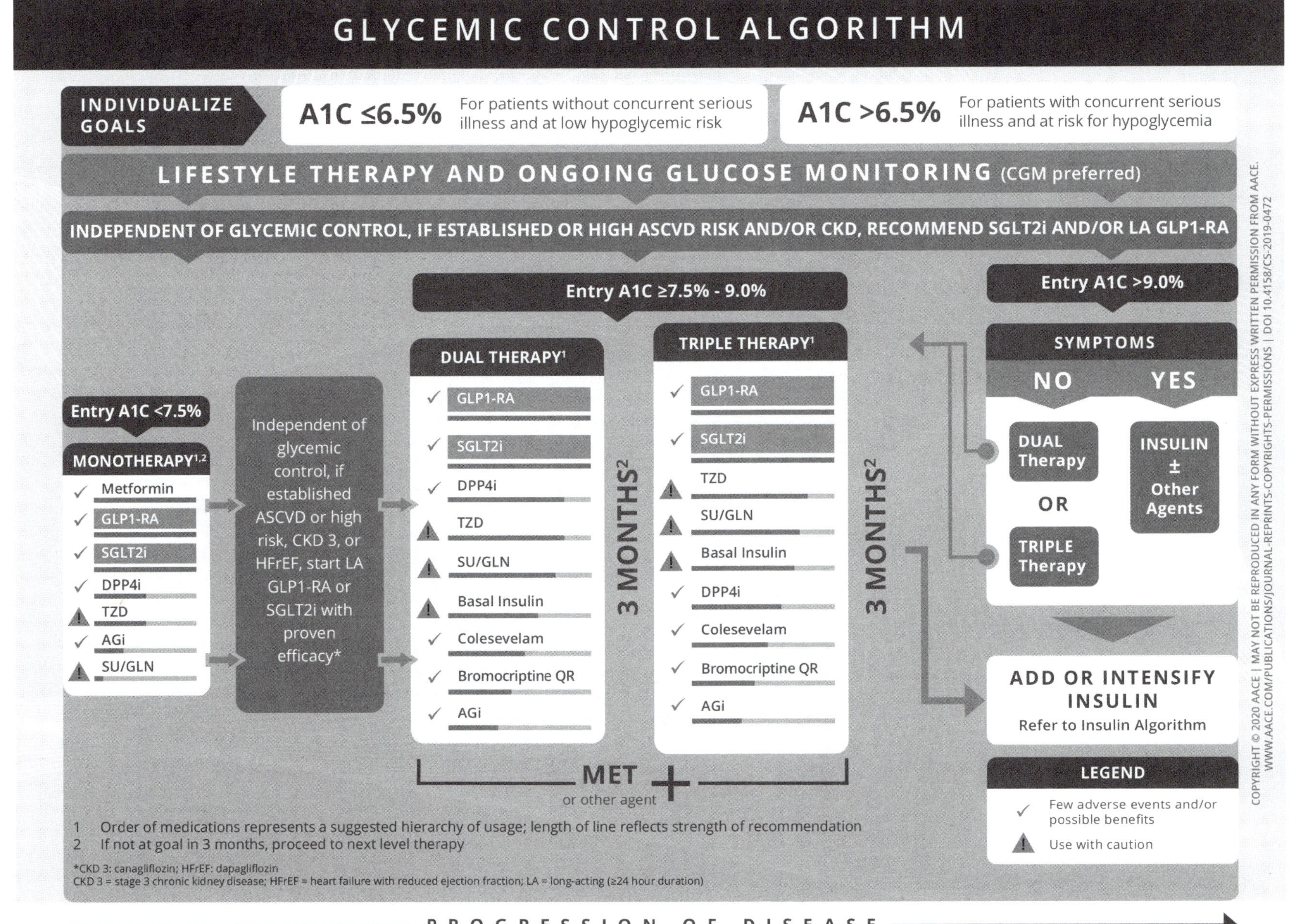

FIGURE 17.1 **AACE Algorithm for the Medical Management of Type 2 Diabetes**

Source: Reprinted with permission from American Association of Clinical Endocrinologists. Garber AJ, Handelsman Y, Grunberger G, et al. Consensus statement by the American Association of Clinical Endocrinologists and American College of Endocrinology on the comprehensive type 2 diabetes management algorithm—2020 executive summary. Endocr Pract. 2020 Jan;26(1):107-139. doi:10.4158/CS-2019-0472.

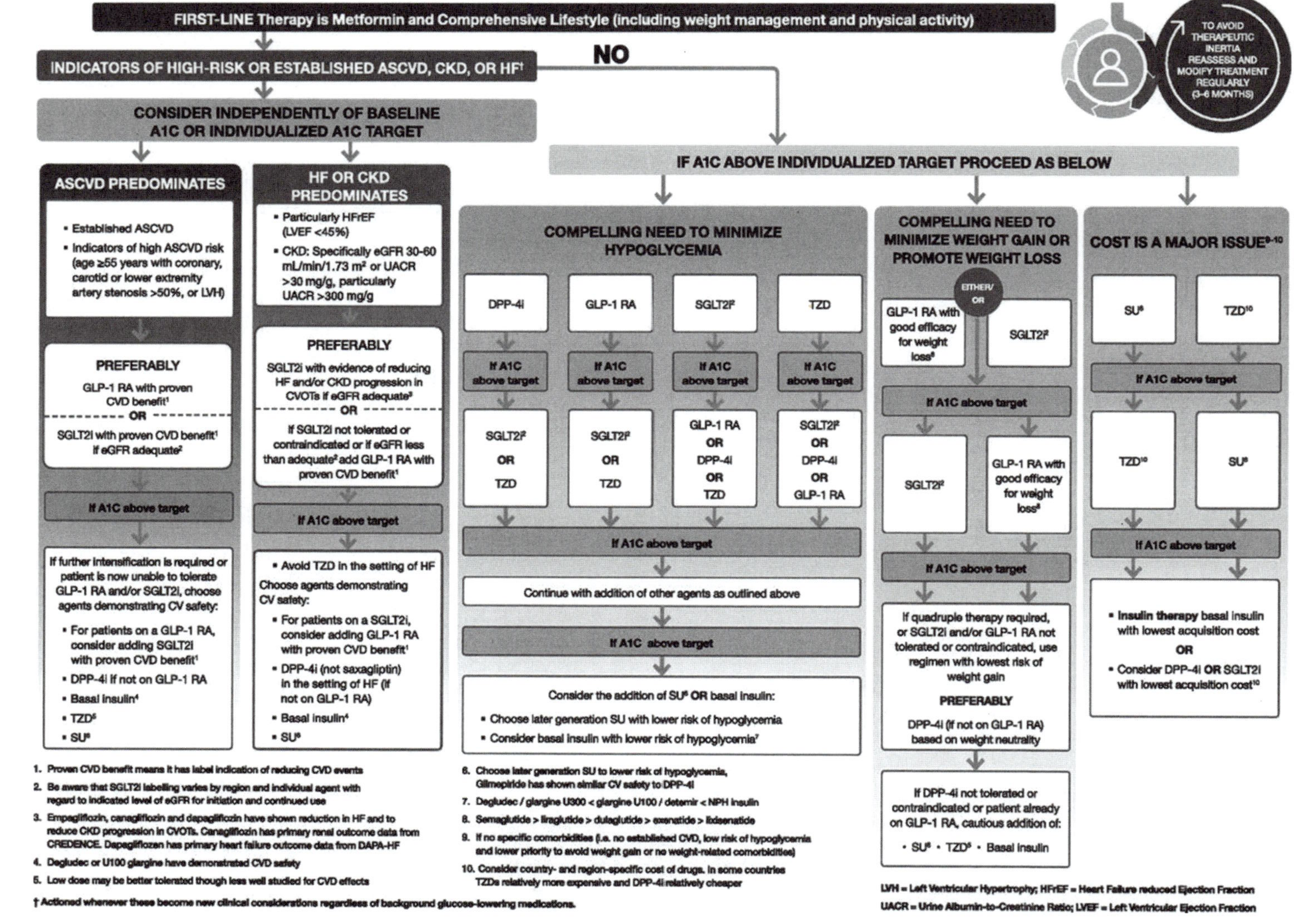
FIRST-LINE Therapy is Metformin and Comprehensive Lifestyle (including weight management and physical activity)
TO AVOID THERAPEUTIC INERTIA REASSESS AND MODIFY TREATMENT REGULARLY (3-6 MONTHS)
INDICATORS OF HIGH-RISK OR ESTABLISHED ASCVD, CKD, OR HF†
NO
CONSIDER INDEPENDENTLY OF BASELINE A1C OR INDIVIDUALIZED A1C TARGET
IF A1C ABOVE INDIVIDUALIZED TARGET PROCEED AS BELOW
ASCVD PREDOMINATES
• Established ASCVD
• Indicators of high ASCVD risk (age ≥55 years with coronary, carotid or lower extremity artery stenosis >50%, or LVH)
PREFERABLY
GLP-1 RA with proven CVD benefit¹
OR
SGLT2i with proven CVD benefit¹ if eGFR adequate²
If A1C above target
If further intensification is required or patient is now unable to tolerate GLP-1 RA and/or SGLT2i, choose agents demonstrating CV safety:
• For patients on a GLP-1 RA, consider adding SGLT2i with proven CVD benefit¹
• DPP-4i if not on GLP-1 RA
• Basal insulin⁴
• TZD⁵
• SU⁶
HF OR CKD PREDOMINATES
• Particularly HFrEF (LVEF <45%)
• CKD: Specifically eGFR 30-60 mL/min/1.73 m² or UACR >30 mg/g, particularly UACR >300 mg/g
PREFERABLY
SGLT2i with evidence of reducing HF and/or CKD progression in CVOTs if eGFR adequate³
OR
If SGLT2i not tolerated or contraindicated or if eGFR less than adequate² add GLP-1 RA with proven CVD benefit¹
If A1C above target
• Avoid TZD in the setting of HF
Choose agents demonstrating CV safety:
• For patients on a SGLT2i, consider adding GLP-1 RA with proven CVD benefit¹
• DPP-4i (not saxagliptin) in the setting of HF (if not on GLP-1 RA)
• Basal insulin⁴
• SU⁶
COMPELLING NEED TO MINIMIZE HYPOGLYCEMIA
DPP-4i
GLP-1 RA
SGLT2i²
TZD
If A1C above target
SGLT2i² OR TZD
SGLT2i² OR TZD
GLP-1 RA OR DPP-4i OR TZD
SGLT2i² OR DPP-4i OR GLP-1 RA
If A1C above target
Continue with addition of other agents as outlined above
If A1C above target
Consider the addition of SU⁶ OR basal insulin:
• Choose later generation SU with lower risk of hypoglycemia
• Consider basal insulin with lower risk of hypoglycemia⁷
COMPELLING NEED TO MINIMIZE WEIGHT GAIN OR PROMOTE WEIGHT LOSS
GLP-1 RA with good efficacy for weight loss⁸
EITHER/OR
SGLT2i²
If A1C above target
SGLT2i²
GLP-1 RA with good efficacy for weight loss⁸
If A1C above target
If quadruple therapy required, or SGLT2i and/or GLP-1 RA not tolerated or contraindicated, use regimen with lowest risk of weight gain
PREFERABLY
DPP-4i (if not on GLP-1 RA) based on weight neutrality
If DPP-4i not tolerated or contraindicated or patient already on GLP-1 RA, cautious addition of:
• SU⁶ • TZD⁵ • Basal insulin
COST IS A MAJOR ISSUE⁹⁻¹⁰
SU⁶
TZD¹⁰
If A1C above target
TZD¹⁰
SU⁶
If A1C above target
• Insulin therapy basal insulin with lowest acquisition cost
OR
• Consider DPP-4i OR SGLT2i with lowest acquisition cost¹⁰
1. Proven CVD benefit means it has label indication of reducing CVD events
2. Be aware that SGLT2i labelling varies by region and individual agent with regard to indicated level of eGFR for initiation and continued use
3. Empagliflozin, canagliflozin and dapagliflozin have shown reduction in HF and to reduce CKD progression in CVOTs. Canagliflozin has primary renal outcome data from CREDENCE. Dapagliflozen has primary heart failure outcome data from DAPA-HF
4. Degludec or U100 glargine have demonstrated CVD safety
5. Low dose may be better tolerated though less well studied for CVD effects
6. Choose later generation SU to lower risk of hypoglycemia. Glimepiride has shown similar CV safety to DPP-4i
7. Degludec / glargine U300 < glargine U100 / detemir < NPH insulin
8. Semaglutide > liraglutide > dulaglutide > exenatide > lixisenatide
9. If no specific comorbidities (i.e. no established CVD, low risk of hypoglycemia and lower priority to avoid weight gain or no weight-related comorbidities)
10. Consider country- and region-specific cost of drugs. In some countries TZDs relatively more expensive and DPP-4i relatively cheaper
† Actioned whenever these become new clinical considerations regardless of background glucose-lowering medications.
LVH = Left Ventricular Hypertrophy; HFrEF = Heart Failure reduced Ejection Fraction
UACR = Urine Albumin-to-Creatinine Ratio; LVEF = Left Ventricular Ejection Fraction

FIGURE 17.2 **ADA Algorithm for the Medical Management of Type 2 Diabetes**

*Consider beginning at this stage in patients with very high HbA1c (eg, ≥9%).

†Consider rapid-acting nonsulfonylurea secretagogues (meglitinides) in patients with irregular meal schedules or who develop late postprandial hypoglycemia on sulfonylureas.

‡Usually a basal insulin (NPH, glargine, detemir) in combination with noninsulin agents.

§Certain noninsulin agents may be continued with insulin. Consider beginning at this stage if patient presents with severe hyperglycemia (≥300-350 mg/dL [≥16.7-19.4 mmol/L]; HbA1c ≥10.0-12.0%) with or without catabolic features (weight loss, ketosis, etc).

Source: American Diabetes Association. 9. "Pharmacologic approaches to glycemic treatment: standards of medical care in diabetes–2019," *Diabetes Care.* (2019) Jan;42(Suppl 1):S90-102. doi: 10.2337/dc19-S009.

Case: Type 2 Diabetes

CR is a 52-year-old African-American male with type 2 diabetes. When diagnosed, he had a casual glucose of 226 mg/dL (12.4 mmol/L) and an A1C of 9.3%. He was started on 500 mg of metformin twice daily. Two weeks later, he presented to the clinic with continued, though decreased, polyuria and nocturia. He denied stomach upset or other gastrointestinal disturbance. His blood pressure was 128/82 mm Hg. His fasting glucose was 184 mg/dL (10.2 mmol/L).

Past Medical History

- Hypertension for 3 years
- Hyperlipidemia for 4 months
- Obesity

Family History

- Father: history of cardiovascular disease (CVD)/hypertension; deceased
- Mother: history of type 2 diabetes, hypertension; still living

Social History

- Tobacco: 24 pack-years, currently smokes
- Illicit drug use: none
- Alcohol: occasional/socially

Current Medications

- Metformin (Glucophage®, Bristol-Myers Squibb) 500 mg twice daily
- Atorvastatin (Lipitor, Pfizer) 40 mg daily
- Metoprolol succinate (Toprol® XL, AstraZeneca) 50 mg twice daily
- Lisinopril (Zestril, AstraZeneca) 40 mg daily
- Hydrochlorothiazide (HCTZ) 25 mg daily

Engagement in Taking Drug Therapy

CR picked up his prescription for metformin the day after his appointment 2 weeks ago. He stated taking all of his medications as prescribed.

Physical Exam

- Height: 69 in
- Weight: 241 lb
- Body mass index (BMI): 35 kg/m^2
- Waist circumference: 42 in

Vitals

- Blood pressure: 128/82 mm Hg
- Heart rate: 72 beats per minute

Lab Data

- Alanine aminotransferase (ALT): 24 international units per liter
- Serum creatinine: 1.4 mg/dL (0.124 mmol/L)
- Fasting blood glucose: 184 mg/dL (10.2 mmol/L)
- A1C: 9.3%
- Total cholesterol: 218 mg/dL (5.6 mmol/L)
- Low-density lipoprotein cholesterol (LDL-C): 131 mg/dL (3.4 mmol/L)
- Triglycerides: 162 mg/dL (1.8 mmol/L)
- High-density lipoprotein cholesterol (HDL-C): 37 mg/dL (1 mmol/L)

As this case continues throughout the chapter, the focus will be on pharmacologic interventions to optimize glycemic control.

Management of Type 2 Diabetes

As suggested by the chapter case, type 2 diabetes is a chronic disorder with multiple metabolic abnormalities. Poor glycemic control in type 2 diabetes is associated with two defects: insulin resistance (decreased response to insulin action) and diminished insulin secretion (also known as pancreatic beta cell failure). Individuals with type 1 diabetes have only one defect resulting in hyperglycemia: lack of insulin production due to pancreatic beta cell destruction. Behavioral interventions (medical nutrition therapy, physical activity, lifestyle changes) are the basis of initial and ongoing treatment of both types of diabetes; however, all individuals with type 1 diabetes also require supplemental insulin beginning at diagnosis. Because worsening hyperglycemia progresses more slowly in type 2 diabetes than in type 1 diabetes, many clinicians may choose to begin intensive lifestyle change prior to starting drug therapy to improve glycemic control, particularly in those near their A1C goal. However, most individuals with type 2 diabetes require medication by the end of the first year due to progression of the disease.[1] Dual therapy should be considered for those with an A1C ≥9%, and combination injectable therapy should be considered when blood glucose is ≥300 to 350 mg/dL and/or A1C is ≥10% to 12%, especially in symptomatic persons with diabetes.[2]

Medications for Antihyperglycemic Management

Pharmacologic Treatment

There are currently 9 classes of orally administered agents used for type 2 diabetes (see Table 17.2):

- Sulfonylureas
- Meglitinides
- Biguanides
- Thiazolidinediones
- Alpha-glucosidase inhibitors
- Dopamine receptor agonists
- Sodium-glucose co-transporter 2 inhibitors
- Dipeptidyl peptidase-4 inhibitors
- Bile acid sequestrants

Generally, monotherapy with any of these agents is associated with a reduction in A1C level of approximately 0.5% to 2.0%.[1] When combination therapy is used (2 or more oral agents or an oral agent combined with insulin), an additive effect is observed, as demonstrated by a further decrease in the A1C level. Several fixed-dose combination products are available, which may improve person with diabetes engagement in taking their medications.

Insulin is considered first-line therapy for pregnant women; however, metformin or glyburide may also be considered in those women who are unable or unwilling to use insulin.[1,17,18] Of all the oral medications for type 2 diabetes, only metformin and Victoza® (liraglutide) has FDA-approved labeling for use in children ≥10 years of age.[19] The lack of alternate oral drug therapy options

TABLE 17.2 Oral and Non-Insulin Injectable Medications for Management of Type 2 Diabetes

Sulfonylureas	
Glimepiride • Amaryl® (sanofi-aventis U.S.) Glipizide • Glucotrol® (Roerig, division of Pfizer) • Glucotrol XL® (Roerig, division of Pfizer) Glyburide • Micronase® (Pharmacia and Upjohn Co., division of Pfizer) • Glynase® (Pharmacia and Upjohn Co., division of Pfizer)	*Action.* Reduce glucose by increasing insulin secretion from pancreatic beta cells in persons with diabetes with residual beta cell function. *Expected decrease in A1C with monotherapy.* 1%–2% *Contraindications.* Documented hypersensitivity; diabetic ketoacidosis (DKA); type 1 diabetes; caution in pregnancy (positive retrospective data exist with glyburide). *Interactions.* Numerous possible drug interactions, few clinically significant. Sulfonamides may enhance hypoglycemic effect. *Precautions.* Hypoglycemia. Risk factors are older age, malnutrition, and irregular eating. Caution in hepatic or renal impairment. May cause rash, sun sensitivity, nausea, vomiting, leukopenia, agranulocytosis, aplastic anemia (rare), intrahepatic cholestasis (rare), disulfiram-like reaction, flushing, headache, and SIADH (syndrome of inappropriate antidiuretic hormone) causing hyponatremia.
Meglitinides	
Nateglinide • Starlix® (Novartis Pharmaceuticals Corp.) Repaglinide • Prandin® (Novo Nordisk)	*Action.* Short-acting insulin secretagogues; stimulate insulin release from pancreatic beta cells. *Expected decrease in A1C with monotherapy.* 0.5%–1.5% *Contraindications.* Documented hypersensitivity; DKA; type 1 diabetes. *Interactions.* CYP3A4 inhibitors (eg, clarithromycin, ketoconazole, miconazole, erythromycin) decrease metabolism, increasing serum levels and effects. Thiazide diuretics, corticosteroids, estrogens, oral contraceptives, nicotinic acid, calcium channel blockers, phenothiazines, and thyroid products may lower glycemic control. Toxicity increased with highly protein-bound drugs (eg, nonsteroidal anti-inflammatory drugs [NSAIDs], sulfonamides, anticoagulants, hydantoins, salicylates, phenylbutazone). *Precautions.* Hypoglycemia, especially if carbohydrate not eaten after drug. Caution in hepatic impairment.

TABLE 17.2 Oral and Non-Insulin Injectable Medications for Management of Type 2 Diabetes (continued)

Biguanides	
Metformin • Glucophage® (Bristol-Myers Squibb) • Glucophage XR® (Bristol-Myers Squibb)	*Action.* Decrease hepatic gluconeogenesis (primary effect) and increase peripheral insulin sensitivity (secondary effect). Do not increase insulin levels or weight. Monotherapy does not cause hypoglycemia. *Expected decrease in A1C with monotherapy.* 1%–2% *Contraindications.* eGFR below 30 mL/min/1.73 m^2; starting metformin in eGFR between 30 and 45 mL/min/1.73 m^2 not recommended; hepatic dysfunction; acute or chronic acidosis; local or systemic tissue hypoxia; excessive alcohol intake; drug therapy for congestive heart failure. *Interactions.* Numerous possible drug interactions, few (if any) clinically significant. Can cause gastrointestinal (GI) upset, nausea, and diarrhea; take with food or milk to minimize GI effects. Metformin may cross the placenta (positive retrospective data exist with metformin). *Precautions.* Fatal lactic acidosis if given with contraindication (rare without contraindication). Discontinue before IV contrast enhancement; do not restart until renal function stable. Withhold in acute hypoxia. Check renal function regularly and discontinue if abnormal. Adverse effects, including GI, especially diarrhea (30%), may cause discontinuation (5%).
Thiazolidinediones	
Pioglitazone • Actos® (Takeda Pharmaceuticals America) Rosiglitazone • Avandia® (GlaxoSmithKline)	*Action.* Increase peripheral insulin sensitivity by increasing transcription of nuclear proteins that help increase uptake of glucose, probably with effects on free fatty acid levels. About 12 to 16 weeks to achieve maximal effect. May restore ovulation in anovulation due to insulin resistance. Improve target cell response to insulin without increasing insulin secretion from pancreas. Decrease hepatic glucose output and increase insulin-dependent glucose use in skeletal muscle and possibly liver and adipose tissue. *Expected decrease in A1C with monotherapy.* 0.5%–1.4%. *Contraindications.* Documented hypersensitivity; active liver disease; DKA; type 1 diabetes; class III or IV congestive heart failure. *Interactions.* With insulin or oral hypoglycemics (eg, sulfonylureas), may increase risk of hypoglycemia. *Precautions.* Monitor transaminases at baseline and as clinically indicated; discontinue if alanine aminotransferase is above 3X upper limit of normal. Caution in edema and congestive heart failure. May decrease hemoglobin, hematocrit, and white blood cell (WBC) counts (dilution). Effects on lipids neutral or beneficial (decreased triglyceride, increased HDL levels). May increase fracture risk. Increased risk of cardiovascular events with rosiglitazone.
Alpha-Glucosidase Inhibitors	
Acarbose • Precose® (Bayer HealthCare Pharmaceuticals) Miglitol • Glyset® (Pharmacia and Upjohn Co., a division of Pfizer)	*Action.* Inhibit action of alpha-glucosidase (carbohydrate digestion), delaying and attenuating postprandial blood glucose peaks. Undigested sugars are delivered to the colon, where they are converted into short-chain fatty acids, methane, carbon dioxide, and hydrogen. Do not increase insulin levels or inhibit lactase; major effect is to lower postprandial glucose levels (lesser effect on fasting levels). Do not cause weight gain. May restore ovulation in anovulation due to insulin resistance. *Expected decrease in A1C with monotherapy.* 0.5%–0.8%

(continued)

TABLE 17.2 Oral and Non-Insulin Injectable Medications for Management of Type 2 Diabetes (continued)	
Acarbose • Precose® (Bayer HealthCare Pharmaceuticals) Miglitol • Glyset® (Pharmacia and Upjohn Co., a division of Pfizer) *(continued)*	*Contraindications.* Documented hypersensitivity, DKA, or cirrhosis; inflammatory bowel disease; colonic ulceration; serum creatinine level >2 mg/dL; elevated liver enzyme levels; partial or predisposition to intestinal obstruction. *Interactions.* Hypoglycemia with insulin or sulfonylurea agents (give glucose as dextrose, as absorption of long-chain carbohydrates is delayed). May decrease absorption and bioavailability of digoxin, propranolol, and ranitidine. Digestive enzymes (eg, amylase, pancreatin) may reduce effects. *Precautions.* May cause GI symptoms; not recommended in significant renal dysfunction.
Dopamine Receptor Agonists	
Bromocriptine mesylate • Cycloset® (Salix Pharmaceuticals)	*Action.* Ergot derivative that is a dopamine receptor agonist improves glycemic control by an unknown mechanism. *Expected decrease in A1C with monotherapy.* 0.1%–0.4% *Contraindications.* Documented hypersensitivity to ergot-related drugs; history of syncopal migraines; nursing women; DKA or type 1 diabetes. *Interactions.* Orthostatic hypotension with antihypertensive medications. May exacerbate psychotic disorders or reduce effectiveness of antipsychotic medications. Interaction with dopamine antagonists such as neuroleptic agents. May increase ergot-related side effects or reduce ergot effectiveness for migraines. Dopamine antagonists (such as metoclopramide) may decrease the effectiveness of bromocriptine. May increase unbound fraction of highly protein-bound therapies, altering their safety and efficacy. Extensively metabolized by CYP3A4. Use caution when coadministered with strong inhibitors, inducers, or substrates for CYP3A4. *Precautions.* May cause somnolence.
Sodium-Glucose Co-transporter 2 (SGLT2) Inhibitors	
Canagliflozin • Invokana® (Janssen) Dapagliflozin • Farxiga® (AstraZeneca) Empagliflozin • Jardiance® (Boehringer) Ertugliflozin • Steglatro® (Pfizer)	*Action.* Inhibit reabsorption of filtered glucose in the kidney. *Expected decrease in A1C with monotherapy.* 0.8%–1% *Contraindications.* Documented hypersensitivity; severe renal impairment (GFR <30 mL/min/1.73 m^2), end-stage renal disease, or on dialysis; nursing women. *Interactions.* Use caution when canagliflozin is coadministered with UGT inducers (rifampin)—rifampin may decrease dapagliflozin concentrations, but impact of UGT induction has not been established with empagliflozin. Digoxin concentrations may increase with canagliflozin use. *Precautions.* Hypotension related to hypovolemia especially in persons with diabetes >65 years old. Hyperkalemia in persons with diabetes with renal impairment. Increased risk of genital mycotic infections and urinary tract infections; increased urination. Increased risk of ketoacidosis. May cause increase in LDL-C. Dapagliflozin and empagliflozin may increase hematocrit. Association of bladder cancer with dapagliflozin. Potential increased risk of lower extremity amputation with canagliflozin and ertugliflozin.
Dipeptidyl Peptidase-4 Inhibitors (DPP-4i)	
Alogliptin • Nesina® (Takeda Pharmaceuticals America) Linagliptin • Tradjenta® (Boehringer Ingelheim Pharmaceuticals)	*Action.* Slow inactivation of incretin hormones (GLP-1) by the enzyme DPP-4. Prolonged action of endogenous GLP-1 increases insulin release and decreases glucagon secretion from pancreatic cells, resulting in lower circulating glucose levels. *Expected decrease in A1C with monotherapy.* 0.5%–0.8% *Contraindications.* Documented hypersensitivity; history of pancreatitis; DKA or type 1 diabetes.

TABLE 17.2 Oral and Non-Insulin Injectable Medications for Management of Type 2 Diabetes (continued)

Sitagliptin • Januvia® (Merck Sharp & Dohme Corp, a subsidiary of Merck & Co.) Saxagliptin • Onglyza® (Bristol-Myers Squibb)	*Interactions.* With insulin secretagogues (eg, sulfonylurea) may increase risk of hypoglycemia; not studied in combination with insulin. Coadministration of saxagliptin with strong CYP3A4/5 inhibitors (eg, ketoconazole) significantly increases saxagliptin concentrations. *Precautions.* Reduced dose recommended with decreased renal function (creatinine clearance <50 mL/min) for all except linagliptin. Postmarketing reports of increased risk of acute pancreatitis (including fatal and nonfatal hemorrhagic or necrotizing pancreatitis) and severe joint pain associated with incretin mimetics. Saxagliptin and alogliptin may increase heart failure risk, particularly in those with existing heart or kidney disease.
Bile Acid Sequestrants	
Colesevelam • Welchol® (Daiichi Sankyo)	*Action.* Not well understood; believed to be from alterations in hepatic glucose production. *Expected decrease in A1C with monotherapy.* 0.3%–0.5% *Contraindications.* Persons with diabetes with triglyceride levels >500 mg/dL, past medical history of acute pancreatitis due to elevated triglyceride levels, or bile obstruction. *Interactions.* Decrease absorption of fat soluble vitamins (ie, A, D, E, K); separate by 4 hours. Drugs with narrow-therapeutic indices may have altered concentrations (ie, warfarin, levothyroxine, phenytoin), as well as decrease absorption of oral contraceptives. *Precautions.* Increase in triglyceride levels; due to increased constipation, caution in persons with diabetes with gastroparesis, other gastrointestinal motility disorders, and in those who have had major gastrointestinal tract surgery and who may be at risk for bowel obstruction.
Glucagon-Like Peptide-1 Receptor Agonists (GLP-1 RA)	
Exenatide • Byetta® (Lilly) Liraglutide • Victoza® (Novo Nordisk) Lixisenatide • Adlyxin® (Sanofi) Exenatide LAR • Bydureon® (Lilly) Semaglutide • Ozempic® (Novo Nordisk) Dulaglutide • Trulicity® (Lilly)	*Action.* Increased insulin synthesis and secretion in the presence of elevated glucose concentrations, improvement of first-phase insulin response, reduced glucagon concentrations during hyperglycemic swings, slowed gastric emptying, and reduced food intake. *Expected decrease in A1C with monotherapy.* 0.5%–1.5% *Contraindications.* Not recommended for use in pregnancy or breastfeeding; Severe renal impairment (CrCl <30 mL per minute) or end-stage renal disease; personal or family history of medullary thyroid cancer (MTC) and in persons with diabetes with multiple endocrine neoplasia syndrome type 2 (MEN 2); type 1 diabetes; ketoacidosis. *Interactions.* Drugs with narrow therapeutic indices should be carefully monitored (eg, warfarin, digoxin, oral contraceptives, statins). *Precautions.* Increased risk for acute pancreatitis (avoid in persons with diabetes with past history of pancreatitis); increased hypoglycemia risk when used with secretagogues or insulin; potential for acute or worsening renal failure.
Amylin Analog	
Pramlintide • Symlin® (AstraZeneca)	*Action.* Slows gastric emptying and suppresses glucagon secretion. *Expected decrease in A1C with monotherapy.* 0.1%–0.7% *Contraindications.* Gastroparesis; concomitant use with drugs that alter gastrointestinal motility or slow absorption of nutrients. *Interactions.* May enhance hypoglycemic effects of hypoglycemia agents or insulin. *Precautions.* Hypoglycemia (especially when given in persons with diabetes prescribed concomitant insulin).

Note: Under each class of orally administered agents, the generic drug is listed, followed by the brand name(s) of that drug.

presents a concern with the increased incidence of type 2 diabetes among young people.

Persons with diabetes should be reminded that any pharmacologic treatment of type 2 diabetes is only a supplement to lifestyle changes. These changes include adequate person with diabetes engagement to a medical nutrition therapy plan, regular appropriate physical activity, and alteration of other specific health habits (eg, smoking cessation). Prior to initiating therapy, the healthcare provider should review the drug mechanism of action, proper dose, daily schedule of when to take each dose, and expected effects. The provider should also review and emphasize the importance of routine self-monitoring of blood glucose. Finally, every person with diabetes should be able to identify the signs and symptoms of major side effects and the appropriate action to take when these reactions occur.[1,20]

Sulfonylureas

Sulfonylureas are classified as first- and second-generation oral hypoglycemic agents. The first-generation agents are described as rapid-acting, intermediate-acting, or long-acting products based on their onset and duration.[21] Sulfonylureas are known as hypoglycemic agents because their major pharmacologic action has the potential to reduce blood glucose levels below normal (ie, cause hypoglycemia). As a result of their high renal dependency and risk for hypoglycemia, use of the first-generation agents (tolbutamide) has fallen out of favor. Sulfonylurea agents are useful only in persons with diabetes who still produce endogenous insulin; hence, they are used exclusively in type 2 diabetes.

According to the 2019 ADA and 2019 AACE treatment algorithms, sulfonylureas may be considered as second-line agents behind metformin in treating type 2 diabetes and for those for whom cost is a major issue. A typical candidate for sulfonylurea monotherapy is an individual with type 2 diabetes without dyslipidemia who is not overweight and when hypoglycemia is not of concern.[1,2] Some individuals will not respond at all to sulfonylureas, and most over time will experience treatment failure with sulfonylureas as the disease progresses, primarily due to the mechanism of action that puts increased workload on the beta-cells.

Mechanism of Action/Effects Sulfonylureas increase the release of insulin from the pancreas, especially at the onset of therapy. These agents close the energy-sensitive potassium channel in the cell membrane of the beta cells. This effect causes an increase in the available insulin for action throughout the body, although these agents may be less effective in those with impaired first-phase insulin release.[1,2] Absorption of sulfonylureas is generally rapid, fairly complete, and unaffected by food, except for short-acting glipizide, which may be delayed. Significant variance in metabolism and excretion of these agents helps determine product choice. Second-generation sulfonylureas are metabolized in the liver to active or inactive metabolites. Caution must be exercised in individuals with liver disease or renal insufficiency.

Dosing Sulfonylureas should be started at the lowest dose and titrated as needed to reach target blood glucose levels. Outlined in the sulfonylurea chart are the most commonly used dosages.

Precautions Sulfonylureas are known to cross the placenta. Prospective studies with glyburide in rats and rabbits revealed no harm to the fetus, and older retrospective human data suggested that glyburide may be a suitable option for pregnant women unable or unwilling to use insulin.[1,17] However, more recent data demonstrate glyburide concentrations in the umbilical cord plasma may be up to 70% higher than maternal levels. Furthermore,

Sulfonylureas: Dosage Information

Drug	*Trade Name*	*Common Dose and Available Strengths*	*Common Frequency*
Second Generation			
Glimepiride	Amaryl®	1–2 mg to 8 mg daily *Tabs:* 1 mg, 2 mg, 4 mg	Daily or twice daily
Glipizide	Glucotrol® Glucotrol XL®	2.5–5 mg to 40 mg daily/max 20 mg with XL daily *Tabs:* 5 mg, 10 mg; XL 2.5 mg, 5 mg, 10 mg	Daily or twice daily
Glyburide	Diabeta® Micronase®	2.5–5 mg to 20 mg daily *Tabs:* 1.25 mg, 2.5 mg, 5 mg	Daily or twice daily
Glyburide, micronized	Glynase®	1.5–3 mg to 12 mg daily *Tabs:* 1.5 mg, 3 mg, 4.5 mg, 6 mg	Daily or twice daily

a systematic review and meta-analysis showed higher rates of neonatal hypoglycemia or macrosomia compared to insulin or metformin.[18] Based on these findings, the utility of sulfonylureas in pregnancy is uncertain compared to other alternatives, such as metformin and insulin. Additionally, because many drugs are excreted in human milk creating a potentially dangerous mixture, sulfonylureas should not be administered to nursing women. Safety and efficacy of sulfonylureas have not been established for children.

People with diabetes can experience a sulfonylurea hypersensitivity reaction. This reaction does not indicate a cross-sensitivity with sulfonamide agents. Rarely, diabetic ketoacidosis (DKA), altered glucose control from a severe infection, surgery, trauma, or other severe metabolic stressors may induce toxicity in persons with diabetes receiving sulfonylureas. Elderly, debilitated, or malnourished persons with diabetes and those with adrenal, pituitary, or hepatic insufficiency who are particularly susceptible to the hypoglycemic effects of glucose-lowering agents should be monitored closely when using a sulfonylurea.[19]

Contraindications Contraindications to sulfonylureas include type 1 diabetes, ketoacidosis, allergy, or documented hypersensitivity to these agents.

Side Effects Perhaps the most common and most serious adverse reaction is hypoglycemia.[19] An additional complicating factor is a progressive age-related decline in renal function that alters drug clearance of highly renally dependent agents, such as the first-generation agents and second-generation glyburide, and predisposes the person to hypoglycemia. The updated Beers criteria strongly recommends that elderly persons with diabetes avoid long-acting sulfonylureas to mitigate this concern in elderly persons with diabetes.[19] Weight gain likely secondary to increased insulin secretion will occur, and skin rashes can be seen in about 2% of persons with diabetes using the medication. The skin rashes usually resolve and the sulfonylurea can be continued. Usually mild gastrointestinal disturbances are reported in approximately 5% of users.[22]

Drug Interactions Sulfonylureas may interact with a variety of medications. These interactions may alter the effect of the sulfonylurea or the other medication or both. It is commonly accepted that more drug-drug interactions occur with the first-generation agents than with the second-generation agents. One of the principal mechanisms of these interactions is a competition for protein-binding sites, allowing more sulfonylurea to circulate freely in the bloodstream, capable of causing hypoglycemia. Altered hepatic enzyme activity may also alter clearance of sulfonylureas.

Monitoring Baseline renal and hepatic function levels should be documented prior to starting sulfonylurea therapy. People with diabetes who use sulfonylureas should self-monitor their blood glucose daily. They should be able to detect and treat hypoglycemic episodes. The number of tests and timing each day, usually preprandial and/or at bedtime, should be determined by the goals of therapy, concomitant medications, and information needs to assess control.

Continued monitoring and follow-up visits should occur to assess the ongoing effectiveness of the agent. Up to 20% of people with diabetes will not respond to sulfonylureas. This is termed a *primary failure* of therapy. *Secondary failure* is defined as a significantly diminished or missing response to the sulfonylurea following an initial therapeutic response. People with diabetes who experience this treatment failure should be changed to another class of medication.[1]

Instructions for Persons With Diabetes Sulfonylureas may enhance sensitivity to sunlight, so persons with diabetes should be advised to use appropriate sun protection. Prevention, recognition, and treatment of hypoglycemia should be included in person with diabetes education for people taking these medications (see the section on hypoglycemia in this chapter).

Meglitinides

Meglitinides, which include repaglinide and nateglinide, are similar to sulfonylureas in that they also increase insulin secretion from the pancreas. Although meglitinides share many of the pharmacologic actions and side effects of sulfonylureas, their duration of action is very short.

Meglitinides are often used in combination with other oral agents, especially in persons with diabetes who experience hypoglycemia on sulfonylureas.[1] Adding meglitinides to concurrent sulfonylurea therapy offers no benefit, and meglitinides should not be used in persons with diabetes who previously experienced primary or secondary failure on a sulfonylurea. Transition to insulin may be considered when treatment using these medications approaches the maximum dose without achieving target blood glucose levels.

Meglitinides are used as monotherapy in people with type 2 diabetes or in individuals with secondary diabetes with substantial capacity for insulin production. A typical candidate for initial repaglinide monotherapy has type 2 diabetes, without dyslipidemia, with or without renal failure, without being overweight, and with a fasting plasma glucose level >20 mg/dL (1.1 mmol/L) above the target concentration.

Nateglinide can be effectively used as monotherapy in people with type 2 diabetes who have a capacity for insulin production, whose hyperglycemia is not adequately controlled by nutrition therapy and physical activity, and who have not been treated long-term with other oral glucose-lowering agents.

Meglitinides: Dosage Information

Drug	*Trade Name*	*Common Dose/Frequency and Available Strengths*
Repaglinide	Prandin®	0.5–1.0 mg 3 times per day before meals to 16 mg daily *Tabs:* 0.5 mg, 1 mg, 2 mg
Nateglinide	Starlix®	60–120 mg 3 times per day before meals to 360 mg daily *Tabs:* 60 mg, 120 mg

Mechanism of Action Meglitinides increase the release of insulin from the pancreas in a glucose-dependent manner and are therefore effective in helping restore first-phase insulin release. Treatment with repaglinide and nateglinide is effective in individuals with type 2 diabetes close to target A1C and in those with type 2 diabetes whose control is suboptimal.[1,2] These agents act as very rapid-acting oral insulin secretagogues that stimulate insulin secretion when needed (postprandial) and then allow insulin concentrations to return to normal basal concentrations.[1,2]

Persons with diabetes treated with repaglinide or nateglinide who miss or delay a meal have less risk of hypoglycemia compared with persons with diabetes treated with longer acting sulfonylurea drugs. Absorption of repaglinide from the gastrointestinal tract is rapid and complete, and food slightly decreases absorption.[23]

Dosing The number of daily doses taken is determined by the number of meals eaten. This type of meal-based dosing frequency may offer advantages for persons with diabetes who vary the frequency of daily meals.

The usual initial and maintenance dose of nateglinide is 120 mg taken just before meals (1-30 minutes before). Titration of dose is usually not necessary. The 60-mg dose may be used in those who are near their A1C goal.[24] Dose adjustment is not needed in the elderly, in persons with diabetes with mild to severe renal insufficiency, or in those with mild hepatic insufficiency.[24]

Repaglinide is initiated at a low, single daily dose, with gradual increases to reach glucose goals, and taken 15 minutes (but no longer than 30 minutes) before each meal. The initial dosage does not need to be adjusted for persons with diabetes with renal dysfunction, but upward titration should proceed cautiously. The initial dose for those previously treated with glucose-lowering drugs and with an A1C level >8% is usually 1 or 2 mg with each meal. The dose may be adjusted weekly, perhaps doubling each preprandial dose until the desired effect is attained. The maximum dose is 16 mg daily.

Precautions Information regarding the safety of repaglinide and nateglinide in certain populations is limited, thus these agents are not indicated for use during pregnancy, for breastfeeding women, or for children. Repaglinide should be used with caution in persons with diabetes with impaired hepatic function, with careful monitoring and adjustment of dosing.[23] Elderly, debilitated, or malnourished persons with diabetes and those with adrenal, pituitary, or hepatic insufficiency are particularly susceptible to the hypoglycemic effects of repaglinide and nateglinide.

Contraindications Contraindications to meglitinides include type 1 diabetes, DKA, severe infection, surgery, trauma, or other severe stressors.

Side Effects Side effects associated with repaglinide include gastrointestinal disturbances in approximately 4% of persons with diabetes receiving the drug. Upper respiratory infection or congestion problems have been noted along with back pain. Hypoglycemia is the most common serious adverse effect. Different studies document the incidence to be between 16% and 31%.[23] Also, similar to sulfonylurea use, primary or secondary treatment failure occurs when an individual is insensitive to the effects of repaglinide. No clinically significant interactions are noted with nateglinide.

Side effects associated with nateglinide include hypoglycemia, usually mild, in approximately 2.4% of persons with diabetes in clinical trials. There were no reports of hypoglycemia requiring third-party assistance or nocturnal hypoglycemia in the phase III trials (2,400 persons with diabetes). Dizziness was reported in approximately 3.6% of users with a weight gain of <1 kg from baseline. This weight gain is lowered with concomitant use of metformin.[24]

Monitoring Blood glucose monitoring should include some premeal and postmeal readings to assess the effectiveness of the medications. Maximum concentrations are reached within 1 hour, but administration with food reduces maximum concentrations for both agents and delays time to reach maximum concentration of nateglinide.

Instructions for Persons With Diabetes Meglitinides should be taken right before eating. Due to the potential for hypoglycemia, those taking this medication should be advised to monitor blood glucose levels for confirmation and subsequent treatment with fast-acting carbohydrate.

Biguanides

Biguanides are not considered hypoglycemic agents, because their major pharmacologic action does not increase insulin secretion and thus does not increase the risk of hypoglycemia. Currently, metformin is the only biguanide marketed in the United States. Metformin is indicated for use in type 2 diabetes as a Step 1 drug or adjunct to other therapy.[1,2] With the introduction of new agents for the treatment of diabetes, metformin has remained the first-line agent, in the absence of contraindications to therapy, due to its high efficacy, cardiovascular benefit, and relatively low cost. However, metformin requires endogenous insulin production for its effectiveness.[25] An ideal candidate for initial metformin monotherapy has type 2 diabetes with preserved kidney function, dyslipidemia, obesity or genetic factors favoring insulin resistance, and an elevated fasting plasma glucose level.[1,2]

Mechanism of Action Metformin improves glycemic control primarily by decreasing hepatic glucose production through reduced gluconeogenesis. Metformin may also decrease intestinal absorption of glucose and improve insulin sensitivity in skeletal muscle.

The oral bioavailability is 50% to 60%, and food decreases the bioavailability with a slight delay in the absorption of metformin. Metformin does not bind to liver or plasma proteins and is primarily excreted by the kidneys, largely unchanged, through an active tubular process.

Dosing Metformin therapy is initiated at a low dose, with gradual increases to obtain desired control. The usual initial dose for the standard formulation is 500 mg or 850 mg daily or twice daily, with doses taken just prior to a meal. The extended-release (ER) formulation dose is usually adjusted every week until the goal is met, while the standard formulation is usually adjusted every 1 or 2 weeks. The maximum daily dose is 2,550 mg (850 mg three times daily), but the maximal effective dose is achieved with 2,000 mg daily. Metformin has FDA-approved labeling for use in children 10 years of age and older.[25] Children's therapy should be started with 250 mg twice daily and titrated slowly until treatment goals are attained.

Biguanides: Dosage Information

Drug	*Trade Name*	*Common Dose/ Frequency and Available Strengths*
Metformin Metformin extended release	Glucophage® Fortamet® Glucophage XR®	500 mg twice daily to 2,550 mg daily (max. effective: 2,000 mg daily); dose split daily to twice daily *Tabs:* 500 mg, 850 mg, 1 g *XR:* 500 mg, 750 mg, 1 g
Metformin liquid	Riomet®	500 mg twice daily *Solution:* 100 mg/mL

Precautions Metformin may restore ovulation in women who were previously anovulatory due to insulin resistance in conditions such as polycystic ovary syndrome. Metformin has the potential to cross the placenta with umbilical cord levels higher than maternal levels. However, prospective studies with metformin in rats and rabbits revealed no harm to the fetus, and retrospective human data suggest that metformin may be a suitable option for pregnant women unable or unwilling to use insulin. Compared to insulin, metformin has less risk of neonatal hypoglycemia or maternal weight gain, but may be associated with higher risk of prematurity. It is not known whether metformin is excreted in human milk; however, it is excreted unchanged in the milk of lactating rats. Nursing women should either discontinue the drug or discontinue nursing to avoid hypoglycemia in breastfeeding infants.

In acute illness or in any situation that would predispose the individual to acute renal dysfunction or tissue hypoperfusion, metformin should be temporarily withheld. Included in this set of conditions are acute myocardial infarction, acute exacerbation of congestive heart failure, use of iodinated contrast media, and major surgical procedures.[25] People with diabetes using this medication should be instructed to stop the metformin the day of the use of the iodinated contrast media and restart the metformin in 2 days when renal function has returned.[25]

Contraindications Metformin is contraindicated in persons with diabetes with an estimated glomerular filtration rate (eGFR) below 30 mL/min/1.73 m^2, and its initiation is not recommended in those with an eGFR of 30 to 45 mL/min/1.73 m^2.[26] Consideration for a 24-hour creatinine clearance for a more precise assessment of renal function may be appropriate for persons with diabetes

80 years of age and older.[19] Because metformin is excreted by the kidneys, it can accumulate in persons with diabetes with renal dysfunction.

The presence of hepatic dysfunction can predispose persons with diabetes receiving metformin to lactic acidosis because lactate metabolism is carried out in the liver. Persons with diabetes with a history of severe or decompensated hypoxic conditions (chronic obstructive pulmonary disease or a history of cardiac function decline) are not good candidates due to the potential for lactate accumulation. Persons with diabetes with a history of alcoholism or binges of alcohol intake are not good candidates for the therapy.

Side Effects Metformin produces some side effects that can be beneficial for those with diabetes. Frequently, a slight weight loss of 2 to 5 kg is seen with metformin therapy, though the mechanistic cause of weight loss is not known. Metformin reduces triglyceride concentrations by approximately 16%, low-density lipoprotein cholesterol (LDL-C) by approximately 8%, and total cholesterol by approximately 5%. Metformin is associated with an increase in high-density lipoprotein cholesterol (HDL-C) of approximately 2%.[27]

Metformin does not directly induce hypoglycemia, though a few persons with diabetes reported mild symptoms necessitating dose reductions as their nutrition and physical activity programs became more effective in lowering glucose levels.[25] Persons with diabetes using metformin in combination with sulfonylureas, meglitinides, or insulin may experience hypoglycemia secondary to the hypoglycemic agent.[25] Gastrointestinal effects such as abdominal bloating, nausea, cramping, feeling of fullness, and diarrhea are experienced in up to 30% of users.[28] A metallic taste in the mouth is also a common complaint. Up to 4% of persons with diabetes using metformin stop taking the drug due to gastrointestinal effects; however, these effects are usually self-limiting and transient (7–14 days).[25] To minimize gastrointestinal side effects, persons with diabetes should start with a low dose and slowly titrate the dose upward. Persons with diabetes may also consider taking metformin with food or switching from the IR to ER formulation for less gastrointestinal disturbances.

Metformin therapy is associated with a reduction in vitamin B_{12} levels, contributing to anemia or neuropathic symptoms. Lactic acidosis can occur with the administration of metformin but is rare (0.03 cases per 1000 person with diabetes years).[21]

Monitoring Due to the deterioration of renal function in the elderly, assessment of glomerular filtration rate (GFR) testing should be done prior to initiation and periodically during therapy, particularly in those with renal dysfunction or in those over age 80. Metformin therapy should be monitored with self-monitoring of blood glucose and follow-up visits to achieve target glycemic control. Continual review with the person with diabetes who has the potential for the aforementioned renal or hepatic effects should be undertaken, with encouragement concerning the possible time-limited gastrointestinal side effects. As with the other oral agents, combination therapy or transition to insulin monotherapy is considered when metformin therapy approaches the maximum effective dose.[1,2] Due to the risk of vitamin B_{12} deficiency, monitoring of B_{12} should occur in persons with diabetes on long-term metformin therapy. The frequency of monitoring has been debated and should be a clinician-based decision accounting for the other person with diabetes-specific factors.

Drug interactions with metformin may include the effect that intravenous contrast media have on renal function, enzyme induction in the liver by cimetidine, and alcohol potentiation of lactate production.

Instructions for Persons With Diabetes Persons with diabetes should be instructed to take metformin with meals to reduce gastrointestinal side effects. They should also be told that a metallic taste may occur but will subside in time. While metformin itself does not cause hypoglycemia, combination therapy with sulfonylureas, meglitinides, or insulin can be associated with hypoglycemia. Women of reproductive age should be advised of the risk of pregnancy, as metformin can restore ovulation in anovulation due to insulin resistance.

Thiazolidinediones

Thiazolidinediones (TZDs) are not hypoglycemic agents; the major pharmacologic action does not increase insulin secretion and thus does not intrinsically increase the risk of hypoglycemia. However, use with secretagogues or insulin may increase hypoglycemia risk. Currently, the 2 compounds with FDA-approved labeling are pioglitazone and rosiglitazone. These agents may best be described as insulin sensitizers.

Thiazolidinediones: Dosage Information

Drug	*Trade Name*	*Common Dose/Frequency and Available Strengths*
Pioglitazone	Actos®	15–45 mg once daily *Tabs:* 15 mg, 30 mg, 45 mg
Rosiglitazone	Avandia®	2–8 mg daily or twice daily *Tabs:* 2 mg, 4 mg, 8 mg

Mechanism of Action Thiazolidinediones are synthetic ligands for peroxisome proliferator-activated receptor gamma (PPAR-g).[29] Activation of PPAR-g by TZDs alters transcription of genes responsible for carbohydrate and lipid metabolism, resulting in improved insulin sensitivity of peripheral muscle cells and adipose and hepatic cells. Both rosiglitazone and pioglitazone retain FDA-approved labeling for use as monotherapy or in combination with other agents to treat type 2 diabetes. An earlier agent, troglitazone, was removed from the market in 2000 due to reports of hepatotoxicity. As a result of early meta-analyses suggesting increased risk of cardiovascular disease with rosiglitazone, a comprehensive review of these data by the FDA in 2010 led it to restrict the use of rosiglitazone to persons with type 2 diabetes who were unable to achieve glycemic control on other medications. This restriction has since been removed. The same risks have not been identified for pioglitazone.

Dosing Therapy is usually started at the lowest dose, with gradual increases to reach plasma glucose goals. Thiazolidinediones can be taken with or without food. Several weeks (8–12) are necessary to assess the full benefit from a dose level for the medication secondary to its mechanism. The doses may be titrated upward until the desired therapeutic effect is reached. Dose increases are not recommended more frequently than every 4 weeks.

Both of these medications are well absorbed without regard to meals. Both medications are extensively bound (>99%) to serum albumin and are extensively metabolized in the liver. Metabolites and parent compounds are eliminated primarily in the feces with minor amounts in the urine.

Precautions Thiazolidinediones may cross the placenta and are not indicated for use during pregnancy, for breastfeeding women, or for children. Thiazolidinediones may restore ovulation in women who are anovulatory due to insulin resistance; thus women of reproductive age should be cautioned to use adequate contraception

Thiazolidinediones cause fluid retention and edema, especially when used in combination with insulin, predisposing persons with diabetes to a twofold increase in the risk of heart failure in those with and without previous history. Due to plasma volume expansion, small reductions in hemoglobin, hematocrit, and neutrophil counts may occur with TZD use. Dose-related weight gain occurs with TZDs alone and in combination with other hypoglycemic agents. The mechanism of weight gain may be related to a combination of fluid retention and subcutaneous fat accumulation.

Small increases in HDL-C and LDL-C may occur with rosiglitazone, while reductions in triglycerides and elevations of HDL-C have been reported with pioglitazone. The clinical significance of the lipid effects of this class of drugs is unclear.[30]

Several meta-analyses suggest that rosiglitazone may increase the relative risk of myocardial infarction by 30% to 40%. These data differ from studies with pioglitazone, which suggest a beneficial effect on cardiovascular disease risk.[1] In 2011, the FDA announced a REMS that severely restricted access and distribution of drugs containing rosiglitazone. However, the FDA eliminated the REMS program for rosiglitazone-containing products in 2015 upon review of data suggesting no increased cardiovascular risk of rosiglitazone compared with metformin or sulfonylureas.

A concern specific to pioglitazone is the possible increased risk of bladder cancer. A meta-analysis of six studies found that use of pioglitazone resulted in higher incidence of bladder cancer, concluding that the number needed to harm was five additional cases of bladder cancer per 100,000 people.[31]

Increased risk for fracture in women and risk for macular edema have also been observed with TZD therapy. Both adipocytes and osteoblasts arise from mesenchymal stem cells. Activation of PPAR-g by TZDs may shift cell differentiation away from osteoblast formation in favor of new adipocytes.

Thiazolidinediones should be used with caution in persons with diabetes with hepatic dysfunction. Thiazolidinedione therapy can cause elevated hepatic enzymes. Rare cases of severe idiosyncratic hepatocellular injury occurred with troglitazone, prompting its removal from the market; however, pioglitazone and rosiglitazone do not appear to carry the same risk of hepatotoxicity.[29]

Contraindications Thiazolidinediones are contraindicated in persons with diabetes with NYHA (New York Heart Association) class III and class IV heart failure and active liver disease. Rosiglitazone is metabolized by CYP2C9 and CYP2C8.[30] In vitro studies have suggested that inhibition of these isoenzymes by rosiglitazone does not occur at concentrations usually encountered clinically.[30] The isoenzyme CYP3A4—which is responsible for the metabolism of several drugs, including erythromycin, calcium channel blockers, corticosteroids, and HMG-CoA reductase inhibitors—is also partially responsible for the metabolism of pioglitazone. Therefore, the possibility of altered safety or efficacy should be considered when using these agents with pioglitazone.

Monitoring Persons with diabetes who receive either of these medications may perform routine self-monitoring of blood glucose multiple times daily as their condition and glucose control dictate. Serum transaminase levels should be monitored prior to initiating therapy and periodically thereafter per the clinical judgment of the healthcare provider.[19] Liver function studies should also be obtained in the presence of hepatic dysfunction symptoms such as abdominal pain, fatigue, nausea, vomiting, and dark urine. Thiazolidinedione therapy should be discontinued in the presence of jaundice. Edema, shortness of breath, rapid weight gain, and other signs and symptoms of heart failure should be included in assessing TZD therapy.

Instructions for Persons With Diabetes Thiazolidinediones require several weeks to achieve the maximum benefit from a dosage level, and those taking it should be encouraged to continue the therapy. Persons with diabetes experiencing edema/swelling, shortness of breath, or muscle aches should contact their healthcare provider for assessment of the side effect. Women should be cautioned regarding the risk of pregnancy, as ovulation may be restored in women who have been anovulatory due to insulin resistance.

Alpha-Glucosidase Inhibitors

Alpha-glucosidase inhibitors are used as adjunctive therapy in type 2 diabetes or secondary diabetes with substantial capacity for insulin production.[32] Good candidates for initial alpha-glucosidase inhibitor therapy have type 2 diabetes, dyslipidemia or obesity, and symptoms or blood glucose levels demonstrating significant postprandial hyperglycemia. Due to their limited ability to lower A1C and their side effect profile, these drugs are not commonly used as monotherapy but rather as adjuncts to existing therapy. Individuals demonstrating significant premeal hyperglycemia without a significant premeal-to-postmeal glucose rise would not be expected to respond optimally to alpha-glucosidase inhibitor monotherapy.

Alpha-Glucosidase Inhibitors: Dosage Information

Drug	*Trade Name*	*Common Dose/Frequency and Available Strengths*
Acarbose	Precose®	Start: 25 mg (25 mg to 100 mg) three times daily *Tabs:* 25 mg, 50 mg, 100 mg
Miglitol	Glyset®	Start: 25 mg once to 3 times daily *Tabs:* 25 mg, 50 mg, 100 mg

Mechanism of Action Alpha-glucosidase inhibitors are not hypoglycemic agents, as their major pharmacologic action does not increase insulin secretion and thus does not increase the risk of hypoglycemia. These agents may best be described as antihyperglycemic agents. They inhibit alpha-glucosidase enzymes in the brush border of the small intestine and pancreatic alpha-amylase, leading to a reduction in carbohydrate-mediated postprandial blood glucose elevation. Alpha-glucosidase enzymes (maltase, isomaltase, glucoamylase, and sucrase) hydrolyze oligosaccharides, trisaccharides, and disaccharides to glucose and other monosaccharides in the brush border of the small intestine. Alpha-amylase enzymes hydrolyze complex starches to oligosaccharides in the lumen of the small intestine. This enzyme inhibition reduces the rate of digestion of starches and the subsequent absorption of glucose.

Dosing Alpha-glucosidase inhibitor therapy is initiated at low doses to minimize gastrointestinal side effects, with gradual increases to reach glucose goals. The usual initial dose is 25 mg with meals, and each dose should be taken with the first bite of the meal for the drug to be most effective. The dose is increased upward as person with diabetes tolerance to the gastrointestinal effects allows, until the desired therapeutic effect is reached. Combination therapy should be considered when the maximum dose is reached.

Precautions Alpha-glucosidase inhibitors are not absorbed systemically; thus there is presumed minimal fetal exposure. Because animal reproduction studies are not always predictive of the human response, this drug should be used during pregnancy only if clearly needed. Because many drugs are excreted in human milk, neither acarbose or miglitol should be administered to nursing women. Safety and efficacy of acarbose have not been established for children.

Alpha-glucosidase inhibitor monotherapy is not associated with hypoglycemia.[1,2] Persons with diabetes using combination therapy with insulin or sulfonylureas may experience hypoglycemia secondary to the insulin or sulfonylurea. Hypoglycemia in this situation is best managed with oral glucose (if the person is conscious) or intravenous glucose or glucagon (if the person is unconscious). Alpha-glucosidase inhibitors blunt the digestion and conversion of complex sugars to glucose; oral sugar sources other than glucose or lactose (eg, cane sugar, sucrose, milk) are unsuitable for rapid correction of hypoglycemia.[33]

Elevation of serum transaminases (AST or ALT) has been observed in clinical trials in persons with diabetes taking acarbose at a dose of 200 to 300 mg daily.[33] Liver function should be periodically monitored. The effect of alpha-glucosidase inhibitors may be altered by charcoal, and these agents may in turn also decrease the bioavailability of ranitidine, propranolol, and digoxin.

Contraindications Persons with diabetes with inflammatory bowel disease, colonic ulceration, obstructive bowel disorders, or chronic intestinal disorders of digestion or absorption should not use these agents.[33] Acarbose is contraindicated in persons with diabetes with cirrhosis of the liver and not recommended in persons with diabetes with serum creatinine levels >2.0 mg/dL or a creatinine clearance of <25 mL/min/1.73 m^2.

Side Effects Gastrointestinal effects, occurring primarily at initiation of therapy or when dosage is increased, are abdominal pain, diarrhea, and flatulence secondary to the drugs' mechanism. These effects are usually self-limiting and transient and can be minimized by starting with a low dose and titrating upward slowly. Redistribution of the inhibited enzymes usually occurs after several weeks of therapy, resulting in a mitigation of side effects.[33]

Monitoring Alpha-glucosidase is often monitored by using 2-hour postprandial glucose measurements. This allows an assessment of the rapid effects and timing of the action of the medication. Serum transaminase levels should be checked every 3 months during the first year and periodically thereafter to monitor for liver toxicity with acarbose.

Instructions for Persons With Diabetes Persons with diabetes using alpha-glucosidase inhibitors should be encouraged to maintain physical movement, especially after a meal, to limit the buildup of gastrointestinal tract gas from the fermenting carbohydrate, as the drug limits carbohydrate absorption. The medication should be taken with the first bite of food at mealtime or with a large snack. While this medication will not induce hypoglycemia, those taking it should be instructed on the products of choice for hypoglycemic episodes if this agent is used in combination with an agent that can induce hypoglycemia (see the section on hypoglycemia near the end of this chapter).

Dopamine Receptor Agonists

Dopamine receptor agonists are used as adjunctive therapy in people with type 2 diabetes or secondary diabetes with substantial capacity for insulin production.[34] Good candidates for dopamine receptor agonist therapy have type 2 diabetes with only mildly elevated blood glucose levels. Due to their limited ability to lower A1C and their side effect profile, these drugs are not commonly used as monotherapy but rather as adjuncts to existing therapy.

Dopamine Receptor Agonists: Dosage Information

Drug	*Trade Name*	*Common Dose/Frequency and Available Strengths*
Bromocriptine mesylate	Cycloset®	1.6–4.8 mg once daily within 2 hours of waking *Tabs:* 0.8 mg

Mechanism of Action The mechanism by which dopamine receptor agonists improve glycemic control is unknown. Following morning administration of bromocriptine mesylate, postprandial glucose levels improve without increasing plasma insulin concentrations.

Dosing The usual initial dose of bromocriptine mesylate is 0.8 mg taken 2 hours after waking with the first meal of the day. The dose may be increased by 0.8 mg each week until the maximal tolerated daily dose of 1.6 to 4.8 mg is achieved. Dose adjustment is not needed in the elderly, in persons with diabetes with mild to severe renal insufficiency, or in those with mild hepatic insufficiency.[34]

Precautions Bromocriptine mesylate crosses the placenta. Because animal reproduction studies are not always predictive of the human response, this drug should be used during pregnancy only if clearly needed. Bromocriptine inhibits lactation and should not be administered to nursing women. Safety and efficacy of bromocriptine have not been established for children. Risk of hypotension and syncope may be increased with bromocriptine upon initiation or dose escalation, especially in those persons with diabetes with a history of orthostasis or those taking antihypertensive medications. Bromocriptine may exacerbate psychotic disorders or reduce the effectiveness of drugs used to treat psychosis. Dopamine receptor antagonists (eg, clozapine, olanzapine, ziprasidone) may reduce the effectiveness of bromocriptine.

Concomitant use of bromocriptine with other dopamine receptor agonists indicated for the treatment of Parkinson's disease, hyperprolactinemia, restless leg syndrome, acromegaly, and other disorders is not recommended. Combining bromocriptine with ergot-related drugs may increase the risk of ergot-related side effects such as nausea, vomiting, and fatigue; bromocriptine may also decrease the effectiveness of these agents to treat migraine headaches.

Contraindications Bromocriptine should not be used to treat type 1 diabetes or DKA. Persons with diabetes with syncopal migraines should avoid bromocriptine mesylate due to the potential increased risk of hypotension. Nursing women should also avoid this agent due to its ability to inhibit lactation and potential for increased stroke risk in this population while taking bromocriptine. Dopamine receptor agonists are not recommended for persons with diabetes with severe psychotic disorders.

Side Effects Side effects associated with bromocriptine include somnolence, nausea, fatigue, dizziness, vomiting, and headache.

Drug Interactions Bromocriptine is highly bound to serum proteins and may increase the unbound fraction of other highly protein-bound drugs (eg, salicylates, sulfonamides, chloramphenicol, and probenecid), resulting in altered effectiveness and risk of side effects.

Bromocriptine is extensively metabolized by the liver isoenzyme CYP3A4. Coadministration of bromocriptine with strong inhibitors of CYP3A4, erythromycin, or ketoconazole increases bromocriptine exposure, as measured by area under the curve (AUC), by 2.8-fold.

Monitoring Blood glucose monitoring should include some premeal and postmeal readings to assess the effectiveness of the medication. Persons with diabetes should also be assessed for signs and symptoms of orthostatic hypotension.[34]

Instructions for Persons With Diabetes Bromocriptine should be taken 2 hours after waking with the first meal of the day. Persons with diabetes should notify their healthcare provider regarding symptoms of orthostatic hypotension such as dizziness, nausea, or diaphoresis.[34]

Sodium-Glucose Co-Transporter 2 Inhibitors

Sodium-glucose co-transporter 2 inhibitors are used as glycemic lowering agents in people with type 2 diabetes, as well as used for cardiovascular and renal protection based on recent evidence. Good candidates for sodium-glucose co-transporter 2 inhibitors are persons with diabetes with moderately elevated glucose levels, cardiovascular risk or history, chronic kidney disease, and weight loss desired.

Sodium-Glucose Co-Transporter 2 Inhibitors: Dosage Information

Drug	*Trade Name*	*Common Dose/Frequency and Available Strengths*
Canagliflozin	Invokana®	100 mg–300 mg once daily in the morning *Tabs:* 100 mg, 300 mg
Dapagliflozin	Farxiga®	5 mg–10 mg once daily in the morning *Tabs:* 5 mg, 10 mg
Empagliflozin	Jardiance®	10 mg–25 mg once daily in the morning *Tabs:* 10 mg, 25 mg
Ertugliflozin	Steglatro®	5 mg–15 mg once daily in the morning *Tabs:* 5 mg, 15 mg

Mechanism of Action Approximately 90% of filtered glucose is reabsorbed through the sodium-glucose co-transporter 2 (SGLT2) transport system in the proximal tubule of the kidney.[35] Normal glucose load in the tubules is approximately 120 mg per minute with almost no glucose excreted in the urine. Glucosuria occurs when the plasma glucose concentration rises above 180 mg/dL (10 mmol/L). Sodium-glucose co-transporter 2 inhibitors block the action of SGLT2, resulting in increased excretion of glucose in the urine. The reduced ability to reabsorb tubular glucose results in lower plasma glucose and potentially excess calories for fat accumulation. These agents reduce A1C levels by 0.5% to 1%, cause modest weight loss (approximately 2 kg), and contribute to blood pressure reduction (up to 4 mm Hg systolic/2 mm Hg diastolic). Use of SGLT2- inhibitors has primarily risen due to the proven cardiovascular benefits, especially reductions in hospitalizations for heart failure, observed in randomized controlled trials with empagliflozin, canagliflozin, and dapagliflozin.[36] Based on emerging evidence from cardiovascular outcomes trials and renal outcomes trials, many of the drugs in the SGTL-2 inhibitor class are seeking or have current approval for reducing cardiac events or slowing the progression of chronic kidney disease in persons with diabetes with T2D. Based on the cardiovascular and renal benefits, the ADA 2020 Standards of Care recommends these agents for persons with diabetes especially if heart failure or chronic kidney disease predominates.[1]

Dosing Currently, use of these agents is limited by renal function; however, more recent trials have demonstrated improvement in renal outcomes, even when the agent is used below the recommended eGFR cut-offs.[36] Canagliflozin, dapagliflozin, and empagliflozin should not be started in persons with diabetes with an eGFR ≤45 ml/min/1.73 m^2. In those with an eGFR ≤60 ml/min/1.73 m^2, use of ertugliflozin should be avoided, and doses of canagliflozin should be limited to 100 mg.[37–40] The initial doses of canagliflozin, dapagliflozin, empagliflozin, and ertugliflozin are 100 mg, 5 mg, 10 mg, and 5 mg, respectively; these doses may be increased to 300 mg, 10 mg, 25 mg, and 15 mg daily in persons with diabetes with normal kidney function.[37–40] Dapagliflozin, empagliflozin, and ertugliflozin can be administered once daily without regard to meals.[37–39] Dapagliflozin and ertugliflozin, however, are recommended to be dosed in the morning, and canagliflozin should be dosed once daily with the first meal of the day.[38–40]

Precautions These agents are classified as not recommended in the second or third trimester due to the potential for fetal effects on renal development. In the absence of adequate trials in humans, this drug should be avoided during pregnancy unless clearly needed. The agents should not be administered to nursing women or children.

Risk of hypotension may be increased in persons with diabetes with low volume status, especially those persons with diabetes with a history of orthostasis or renal dysfunction or the elderly. Persons with diabetes taking diuretics, angiotensin-converting enzyme inhibitors, or angiotensin receptor blockers should be carefully monitored and have their fluid status corrected before starting an SGLT2 inhibitor. Additionally, these medications may increase the risk for acute kidney injury—caution and monitoring should be used in situations where predisposing factors may be present.[38,40]

All agents may increase the risk of euglycemic ketoacidosis (diabetic ketoacidosis with blood glucose levels <300 mg/dL). Canagliflozin may cause hyperkalemia, especially in persons with diabetes with decreased kidney function.[40] Increases in LDL-C levels have also been observed. Increases in hematocrit have been observed with the use of dapagliflozin and empagliflozin.[37,38] The increased glucose excretion is associated with increased urinary frequency. The high urinary glucose concentration also predisposes persons with diabetes to genital mycotic infections and urinary tract infections. Dapagliflozin use has been associated with an increase in bladder cancer.[38] An increased risk of bone fracture and/or lower limb amputation (black box warning) has been observed in persons with diabetes using canagliflozin.[40] The amputation risk, although unclear in both cases due to varying degrees of reporting in clinical trials,[41] is also mentioned for ertugliflozin.[39]

Contraindications These agents should not be used to treat type 1 diabetes or DKA. Persons with diabetes with severe kidney disease (eGFR <30 mL/min/1.73 m^2) or on hemodialysis should not use these agents.

Side Effects Side effects commonly associated with these agents include hypotension, mycotic infections, urinary tract infections, and renal insufficiency. Canagliflozin may also contribute to hyperkalemia.[40]

Drug Interactions Coadministration of these agents with inducers of UDP-glucuronosyl transferase (UGT), such as rifampin, phenobarbital, phenytoin, and ritonavir, may decrease exposure. While no recommendations are made for dapagliflozin or empagliflozin, canagliflozin use may require a dose increase to 300 mg in persons with diabetes with normal renal function if continuation of the UGT inducer is required. Canagliflozin itself increases the exposure and peak of digoxin by 20% and 36%, respectively.[40]

Monitoring Routine A1C monitoring should be accompanied by potassium and LDL-C monitoring. Blood pressure and symptoms of mycotic infection should also be checked.

Instructions for Persons With Diabetes Increased urination is expected in about 5% of persons with diabetes. Persons with diabetes should notify their healthcare provider regarding symptoms of orthostatic hypotension; dysuria or urinary retention; ketoacidosis symptoms including difficulty breathing, nausea, vomiting, abdominal pain, confusion, and unusual fatigue or sleepiness; and signs of acute kidney injury such as decreased urine, edema, and dehydration. Persons with diabetes may decrease risk of acute kidney injury or genital infections by staying well-hydrated.

Bile Acid Sequestrants

Bile acid sequestrants are often used as add-on therapy for persons with diabetes with type 2 diabetes who have not responded to other therapy.[42] Good candidates for bile acid sequestrant therapy have type 2 diabetes with elevated LDL-C. Due to their limited ability to lower A1C and their side effect profile, these drugs are not commonly used as monotherapy but rather as adjuncts to existing therapy.

Bile Acid Sequestrants: Dosage Information

Drug	*Trade Name*	*Common Dose and Available Strengths*	*Common Frequency*
Colesevelam	Welchol	3.75 g/day Packet: 3.75 g Tabs: 625 mg	Once daily (or can divide total daily dose into 2 doses)

Mechanism of Action The mechanism of action in regards to glucose control is not well understood. It is proposed that bile acids may act as signaling molecules in the liver and GI tract, thus affecting glucose metabolism.[42] When ingested, bile acid sequestrants bind to bile acids in the intestine, thus impeding their reabsorption. With the removal of bile acids from the intestines, the liver produces more by taking cholesterol from the bloodstream, which ultimately lowers LDL, thus making these agents good for persons with diabetes with need for additional cholesterol lowering. These agents are not absorbed systemically.[42]

Dosing Colesevelam can be taken once or twice daily. It comes supplied as 3.75mg powder packets and tablets. The powder packets are emptied into a 4 ounce or 8-ounce glass of liquid (eg, water, juice) and stirred until the contents are well distributed (they will not completely dissolve). Persons with diabetes should drink this glass completely with a well-balanced meal. The dry powder should not be ingested in its dry form to avoid esophageal distress. The powder is available as a sugar-free option for persons with diabetes with diabetes. If persons with diabetes prefer tablets, they may take three 625 mg tablets twice a day with a meal and liquid or six 625 mg tablets once a day with a meal and liquid.[42]

Precautions Because bile acid sequestrants are not absorbed systemically, fetal exposure should be minimal. However, bile acid sequestrants may interact with vitamins that pregnant women take for supplementation, thus resulting in inadequate vitamin supplementation. Due to the availability of other agents for glycemic control during pregnancy, bile acid sequestrants should be reserved when the benefits clearly outweigh the risks and when other agents are unable to be utilized. Due to the lack of systemic absorption, these agents may be considered when breastfeeding, since the drug is not expected to be present in breast milk.[42]

Bile acid sequestrants may increase triglyceride levels; therefore, the agents should be avoided in persons with diabetes who have elevated triglyceride levels >500 mg/dL. In persons with diabetes with type 2 diabetes, greater increases in triglyceride levels were seen when colesevelam was combined with pioglitazone, sulfonylureas, or insulin. Triglyceride levels should be monitored throughout therapy.[42]

Colesevelam may cause constipation; therefore, it should be used with caution in persons with diabetes with gastroparesis, other gastrointestinal motility disorders, and in those who have had major gastrointestinal tract surgery and who may be at risk for bowel obstruction.[42]

Contraindications Bile acid sequestrants should be avoided in persons with diabetes with triglyceride levels >500 mg/dL, past medical history of acute pancreatitis due to elevated triglyceride levels, or bile obstruction.[42]

Side Effects The most common side effects observed with colesevelam in persons with diabetes with type 2 diabetes are constipation, dyspepsia, nausea, hypoglycemia, and high blood pressure. In clinical trials, colesevelam resulted in a median placebo-corrected increase serum triglycerides of 5%, 22%, and 18% when added to metformin, insulin and sulfonylureas, respectively.[42]

Drug Interactions Bile sequestrants can decrease absorption of fat soluble vitamins (ie, A, D, E, K). Persons with diabetes should be counseled to take colesevelam and fat-soluble vitamins at least 4 hours apart. Additionally, persons with diabetes who are taking vitamin K antagonists, such as warfarin, should be monitored clearly, as there may be decreased absorption of warfarin, leading to potentially sub-therapeutic INR levels. Colesevelam may also reduce absorption of phenytoin, leading to decreased phenytoin levels and increased seizure activity when this agent. Increased TSH levels have also been observed for persons with diabetes taking concomitant levothyroxine and colesevelam. Any medications that have narrow therapeutic indices should be monitored closely. Women on oral contraceptives should be counseled on the potential for decreased effectiveness, thus back-up contraception may be needed.[42]

Monitoring Routine monitoring of blood glucose, A1c, LDL-C, and triglycerides and non-HDL should occur. Drug levels for potential interacting medications should be closely monitored to ensure adequate efficacy.[42]

Instructions for Persons With Diabetes Persons with diabetes should expect to see some glycemic lowering in 4 to 6 weeks, with maximum effect seen in 12 to 18 weeks. Due to potential for drug interactions, persons with diabetes should take medications 4 hours apart from colesevelam. If persons with diabetes experience difficulty swallowing colesevelam tablets, they may switch to powder packets. Persons with diabetes should be counseled on the risk of increased triglyceride levels and the importance of monitoring cholesterol levels.[42]

Incretin-Based Therapies

Over the past several years, a great deal of research and attention have been focused on the impact of incretin hormones on glycemic control. Following ingestion of a meal, gut hormones including glucose-dependent insulinotropic peptide (GIP) and glucagon-like peptide-1 (GLP-1) are released into the circulation. Increased GLP-1 levels exert multiple actions that affect plasma glucose. These actions include (1) promotion of satiety in the brain, (2) decreased or slowed gastric emptying rate, (3) increased glucose-dependent insulin release from beta cells, and (4) decreased glucagon release from pancreatic alpha cells. Although naturally occurring GLP-1 is essential in glucose regulation, its utility as a therapeutic target is limited by its rapid inactivation (half-life of 1 to 2 minutes) by the ubiquitous enzyme dipeptidyl peptidase-4 (DPP-4). Recently, two therapeutic approaches have emerged which successfully address this barrier. These new agents to treat type 2 diabetes include glucagon-like peptide-1 receptor agonists (GLP-1 RA) and dipeptidyl peptidase-4 inhibitors (DPP-4i), which block activity of the DPP-4 enzyme.

Of note, these agents are not typically used together due to similar mechanism of action.

GLP-1 Receptor Agonists

Glucagon-like peptide-1 receptor agonists are used as glycemic lowering agents in people with type 2 diabetes, as well as used for cardiovascular benefits based on recent evidence. Good candidates for GLP-1 RAs are persons with diabetes who are overweight with moderately elevated glucose levels and cardiovascular risk or history, without a history of pancreatitis or gastroparesis

Mechanism of Action/Effects In 2005, the first GLP-1 RA, exenatide, received FDA-approved labeling for use in people with type 2 diabetes.[43] Exenatide is a synthetic form of a protein found in the saliva of the Gila monster, a lizard that is native to Mexico and the southwestern United States. Since the introduction of exenatide, its long-acting formulation and five new GLP-1 RAs have been approved for type 2 diabetes management. As noted above, one of these agents, once-weekly liraglutide (Saxenda®), is not approved for management of type 2 diabetes; this agent is only approved for weight reduction. Another GLP-1 RA, albiglutide (Tanzeum®) was voluntarily discontinued by the manufacturer in the United States due to limited prescribing, leaving six available options for persons with diabetes, three of which are dosed daily (liraglutide, lixisenatide, exenatide) and three of which are dosed once weekly (exenatide ER, dulaglutide, and semaglutide). These agents bind to and activate GLP-1 receptors, resulting in a drop in fasting and postprandial glucose concentrations. They improve glycemic control in type 2 diabetes through several mechanisms, including increased insulin synthesis and secretion in the presence of elevated glucose concentrations, improvement of first-phase insulin response, reduced glucagon concentrations during hyperglycemic swings, slowed gastric emptying, and reduced food intake.

Concurrent use of insulin, metformin, sulfonylureas, or a combination of these drugs with GLP-1 RA is recommended. However, all agents have not been studied with all types of diabetes. Use of these agents should not be a substitute or replacement for insulin therapy in type 1 diabetes. Significantly reduced A1C levels have been observed in persons with diabetes using these agents, with a reduction in both fasting and postprandial plasma glucose concentrations. A reduction in body weight may also be noted.[1] Cardiovascular risk reduction has been demonstrated in randomized controlled trials with liraglutide, semaglutide, and dulaglutide.[44] Like with the SGLT-2 inhibitors, many of these agents have approval for risk reduction or major cardiovascular events (ie, cardiovascular death, nonfatal MI, or nonfatal stroke) or are seeking approval for these cardiovascular benefits. Neutral (no harm or benefit) cardiovascular effects have been shown with exenatide and lixisenatide.[1,45]

Dosing All GLP-1 RAs are administered by subcutaneous injection in the thigh, upper arm, or abdomen. With the exception of exenatide IR and lixisenatide, all agents can be administered at any time of day, without regard to meals. Exenatide IR should be administered anytime within the 60 minutes before morning and evening meals and should not be given after a meal. The extended-release formulation of exenatide (Bydureon®) is dosed once weekly without regard to meals.[46] Lixisenatide should be administered within 1 hour before the first meal of the day, preferably the same meal each day. Weekly agents are dosed without regard for meals, and missed doses can be given within 3 days of scheduled dose for dulaglutide and exenatide LAR and 5 days of scheduled dose for semaglutide.

GLP-1 Receptor Agonists: Dosage Information

Drug	*Trade Name*	*Common Dose and Available Forms*	*Storage/administration notes*
Exenatide	Byetta® (Lilly)	5–10 mcg twice daily within 60 minutes of meals *Pen injectors:* multi-dose 5 or 10 mcg pens (1.2 mL, 2.4 mL)	Refrigerate until opened Once opened, may remain unrefrigerated for 30 days
Exenatide LAR	Bydureon® (Lilly) Bydureon BCise® (Lilly)	Bydureon LAR Pen: 2 mg once weekly without regard to meals Bydureon BCise (auto-injector): 2 mg once weekly without regard to meals	Refrigerate until opened Administer immediately after dose prepared (must mix contents in pen to ensure even suspension)

(continued)

GLP-1 Receptor Agonists: Dosage Information (continued)

Drug	*Trade Name*	*Common Dose and Available Forms*	*Storage/administration notes*
Liraglutide	Victoza® (Novo Nordisk)	0.6–1.8 mg daily *Pen injectors:* multi-dose pens (6 mg/mL; 3 mL)	Refrigerate until opened Once opened, may remain unrefrigerated for 30 days
Lixisenatide	Adlyxin® (Sanofi)	20 mcg daily (titrated up from 10 mcg × 14 days then increased to 20 mcg on day 15) *Pen-injector kit:* 10 mcg/0.2 mL; 20 mcg/0.2 mL *Solution pen-injector:* 20 mcg/0.2 mL	Refrigerate until opened Once opened, may remain unrefrigerated for 14 days
Semaglutide	Ozempic® (Novo Nordisk)	0.5–1 mg once weekly (must start with 0.25 mg × 4 weeks for adjustment to gastrointestinal side effects, then increase to 0.5 mg once weekly) *Pen injectors:* 2 mg/1.5 mL multi-dose pens (starter pen with dose markers for 0.25 mg and 0.5 mg, and second pen with 1mg dose marker); (32G, 4-mm needles)	Refrigerate until opened Once opened, may remain unrefrigerated for 56 days
Dulaglutide	Trulicity® (Lilly)	0.75–1.5 mg once weekly *Pen injectors:* 0.75 mg, 1.5 mg single-dose pens	Refrigerate until opened Once opened, may remain unrefrigerated for 14 days

Precautions All agents are have potential to cause harm to the fetus and should be used during pregnancy only if the potential benefit justifies the risk.[46–50] Labeling for Ozempic® states that the medication should be discontinued ≥2 months prior to planned pregnancy.[48] It is not known whether these drugs are excreted in human milk; however, they are excreted unchanged in the milk of lactating rats. Nursing women should either discontinue the drug or discontinue nursing. Pediatric effectiveness and safety have also not been demonstrated with any agent.

The GLP-1 RAs have been shown to increase risk for acute pancreatitis, including fatal and nonfatal hemorrhagic or necrotizing pancreatitis. Alternate agents should be considered in persons with diabetes with a history of pancreatitis, and if new onset symptoms are suspected or confirmed, these agents should be discontinued. The GLP-1 RAs may also increase the risk of hypoglycemia when used with secretagogues or insulins. If combination therapy is utilized, doses of secretagogues or insulin should be reduced to decrease the risk. There have been postmarketing reports of acute and worsening of chronic renal failure with the GLP-1 RAs. Reported events often occurred in persons with diabetes who had experienced adverse gastrointestinal symptoms. Approved labeling for both exenatide formulations include recommendations to avoid use in persons with diabetes with severe renal impairment (IR: creatinine clearance [CrCl] <30 mL per minute, LAR: eGFR <45 mL/min/1.73 m^2) or end-stage renal disease. Lixisenatide also recommends avoiding use in severe renal impairment (eGFR <15 mL/min/1.73 m^2). No renal dose adjustment is recommended for any of the other GLP-1 RAs. The GLP-1 RAs have also been found to cause thyroid C-cell tumors in both male and female mice and rats.[47] It is unknown whether these agents cause thyroid C-cell tumors in humans; however, all agents except Byetta® carry a boxed warning for this risk. As a result of the ability to slow gastric emptying, both exenatide formulations should be avoided in persons with diabetes with severe gastrointestinal disease and caution used with the other agents.

Drug Interactions Due to the ability of GLP-1 RAs to slow gastric emptying, the extent and absorption rate of orally administered drugs should be considered. In general, drugs with narrow therapeutic indices should be carefully monitored in persons with diabetes taking GLP-1 RAs. Medications such as warfarin, digoxin, oral contraceptives, and the statins may be impacted. Agents have not been consistent in their reductions to pharmacokinetic parameters. For example, exenatide has been shown to increase the international normalized ratio in persons with diabetes taking warfarin. To avoid acute effects of GLP-1 RAs on gastric emptying, persons with diabetes may consider taking oral medications that depend on achieving threshold concentrations at least 1 hour before the injection, especially with exenatide IR and lixisenatide.

Contraindications Contraindications to GLP-1 RAs are similar across the class and include type 1 diabetes, ketoacidosis, allergy, or documented hypersensitivity to these agents. Persons with diabetes with a personal or family history of medullary thyroid carcinoma (MTC) or multiple endocrine neoplasia syndrome type 2 (MEN 2) should not take these agents.[46–50]

Side Effects Gastrointestinal side effects such as nausea, vomiting, diarrhea, and dyspepsia are common, occurring in up to 40% of persons with diabetes taking these agents. Head-to-head studies suggest that nausea is more common with shorter acting agents (25%-35% with exenatide twice daily,[48] and 20%-25% with liraglutide once daily) and decreases with extended-acting agents (9%-26% with exenatide once weekly,[46] 15%-20% with semaglutide once weekly,[49] and 16%-28% with dulaglutide once weekly).[50] Mild to moderate nausea is reported most often when therapy is started, with frequency and severity decreasing as treatment is continued. Other common side effects occurring in ≥5% of persons with diabetes include headache and injection site reactions.

Monitoring The potential for GLP-1 RAs to promote antibody formation must be considered in persons with diabetes whose glycemic control is unresponsive to therapy, especially those receiving exenatide or exenatide LAR. Persons with diabetes who developed these antibodies in clinical trials of exenatide and liraglutide did not experience a difference in glucose control compared with persons with diabetes who did not develop measurable antibody levels. Among the long-acting GLP-1 RAs, antibodies to varying degrees were observed with all agents except dulaglutide.

The effectiveness of orally administered medications taken concomitantly with GLP-1 RAs should be carefully monitored, especially medications such as antibiotics, oral contraceptives, and agents with a narrow therapeutic index.[51]

After initiation of therapy or dose increases with GLP-1 RAs, persons with diabetes should be monitored for signs and symptoms of pancreatitis. Symptoms include persistent severe abdominal pain, sometimes radiating to the back, which may or may not be accompanied by vomiting. If pancreatitis is suspected, GLP-1 RAs and other potentially suspect medications should be promptly discontinued.

For persons with diabetes taking these agents, it is unknown whether routine monitoring of serum calcitonin, a marker for MTC, or thyroid ultrasound decreases the risk of thyroid C-cell tumors. Persons with diabetes should be counseled regarding the risk of MTC and symptoms of thyroid tumors, such as a mass in the neck, dysphagia, dyspnea, or persistent hoarseness.

Instructions for Persons With Diabetes Gastrointestinal side effects, primarily nausea, vomiting, diarrhea, and dyspepsia, are the most common side effects; persons with diabetes should be counseled about this side effect. If the symptoms do not improve, persons with diabetes should let their healthcare provider know, as this may be a sign of pancreatitis. Persons with diabetes should be advised on the potential signs of pancreatitis and instructed to call their healthcare provider if these occur.

DPP-4 Inhibitors

Dipeptidyl peptidase-4 inhibitors (DPP-4i) are used as glycemic lowering agents in people with type 2 diabetes. Good candidates for DPP-4is are persons with diabetes who are with mildly elevated glucose levels that are in need of additional post-prandial blood glucose lowering.

Mechanism of Action/Effects In 2006, the first DPP-4i, sitagliptin, received FDA-approved labeling for use in people with type 2 diabetes.[52] Sitagliptin improves glycemic control by competitive inhibition of the enzyme responsible for GLP-1 inactivation, thus prolonging the effects of endogenous GLP-1. Since approval of sitagliptin, three more DPP-4i have come to market. These drugs improve glycemic control in type 2 diabetes through prolonged half-life of GLP-1, which increases insulin synthesis and secretion, reduces glucagon concentration, slows gastric emptying, and reduces food intake.[52] The main advantage of DPP-4i drugs over GLP-1R agonists is their oral formulation. However, because DPP-4i drugs depend on endogenous GLP-1 to exert their effect, they produce less weight loss and less glycemic lowering than GLP-1 RAs, which achieve supraphysiologic levels of GLP-1.

Dosing These agents are administered once daily with or without food. With the exception of linagliptin, doses of these agents should be reduced in the presence of renal dysfunction.

Precautions Because animal reproduction studies are not always predictive of the human response, DPP-4i drugs should be used during pregnancy only if clearly needed. All agents have been found excreted into milk in available animal data. As a result, DPP-4i drugs should not be administered to nursing women. Safety and efficacy of DPP-4i drugs have not been established for children.

The DPP-4i agents share similar warnings and precautions. When DPP-4i drugs are used in combination with secretagogues or insulin, doses of the medication may need to be reduced to avoid hypoglycemia.[52,53] These agents have been associated with acute pancreatitis, including fatal and nonfatal hemorrhagic or necrotizing pancreatitis based on postmarketing data. Hypersensitivity reactions (eg, urticaria, facial edema) are reported more commonly with DPP-4i drugs than with placebo. Postmarketing data with sitagliptin include serious allergic reactions such as anaphylaxis, angioedema, and exfoliative skin conditions including Stevens-Johnson syndrome. As a result of increased risk for congestive heart failure in at-risk persons with diabetes taking alogliptin or saxagliptin, assessment for heart failure history or risk factors should be completed prior to initiation. As there have been postmarketing reports of fatal and nonfatal hepatic failure in persons with diabetes taking alogliptin, symptoms should be investigated immediately. In 2015, the FDA warned "sitagliptin, saxagliptin, linagliptin, and alogliptin may cause joint pain that can be severe and disabling." Although the exact mechanism of this adverse effect is unknown, symptoms resolved with discontinuation and reappeared upon rechallenge.[54]

Drug Interactions Saxagliptin is primarily metabolized by the isoenzyme CYP3A4/5. Coadministration of saxagliptin with the inhibitors of CYP3A4/5, diltiazem, and ketoconazole increases saxagliptin peak concentration by 63% and 62%, respectively. Saxagliptin exposure, as measured by AUC, increases by more than twofold with the CYP3A4/5 inhibitors. Therefore, the dose of saxagliptin should be limited to 2.5 mg when given with strong CYP3A4/5 inhibitors. Saxagliptin does not appear to affect exposure of other concomitantly administered drugs. Sitagliptin may increase the peak concentration and AUC of digoxin.[52] Strong inducers of CYP3A4 or PCP such as rifampin may significantly decrease linagliptin exposure, and other DPP-4i should be considered. Alogliptin does not appear to carry clinically meaningful drug interactions.

DPP-4 Inhibitors (DPP-4i): Dosage Information

Drug	*Trade Name*	*Common Dose and Available Forms*	*Common Frequency*
Alogliptin	Nesina®	6.25 mg to 25 mg daily CrCl ≥60 mL/minute: No dosage adjustment necessary. CrCl ≥30 to <60 mL/minute: 12.5 mg once daily CrCl ≥15 to <30 mL/minute: 6.25 mg once daily ESRD (CrCl <15 ml/min or requiring hemodialysis): 6.25 mg once daily; administered without regard to timing of hemodialysis *Tabs:* 25 mg, 12.5 mg, and 6.25 mg	Once daily
Linagliptin	Tradjenta®	2.5 mg to 5 mg daily *Tabs:* 5 mg	Once daily
Saxagliptin	Onglyza™	2.5 mg to 5 mg daily eGFR >45 mL/min/1.73 m²: No dosage adjustment necessary. eGFR ≤45 mL/min/1.73 m²: 2.5 mg once daily *Tabs:* 2.5 mg, 5 mg	Once daily
Sitagliptin	Januvia®	100 mg daily eGFR ≥45 mL/min/1.73 m²: No dosage adjustment necessary. eGFR ≥30 to <45 mL/min/1.73 m²: 50 mg once daily eGFR <30 mL/min/1.73 m²: 25 mg once daily *Tabs:* 25 mg, 50 mg, and 100 mg	Once daily

Contraindications Contraindications to DPP-4i include type 1 diabetes, ketoacidosis, allergy, and documented hypersensitivity to these agents.

Side Effects Common side effects in DPP-4i drugs include upper respiratory tract infection and headache; urinary tract infections were also more commonly reported with saxagliptin than with placebo. Occurrence of peripheral edema was more common with saxagliptin than with placebo when used with a thiazolidinedione.

Monitoring In addition to routine measurements of blood glucose and A1C for efficacy, kidney function (serum creatinine) should be monitored to evaluate the need for dose adjustment. After initiation of therapy or dose increases with DPP-4i, persons with diabetes should be monitored for signs and symptoms of pancreatitis. Symptoms include persistent severe abdominal pain, sometimes radiating to the back, which may or may not be accompanied by vomiting. If pancreatitis is suspected, the DPP-4i and other potentially suspect medications should be promptly discontinued. Baseline liver function tests (serum transaminases) are recommended when initiating alogliptin.

Instructions for Persons With Diabetes When used with a hypoglycemic agent (eg, sulfonylurea), DPP-4i drugs may cause hypoglycemia; therefore, persons with diabetes should be cautioned to monitor blood glucose levels carefully. Persons with diabetes should be advised of the risks and symptoms of pancreatitis. Persons with diabetes should also be advised how to respond in the event of a severe hypersensitivity reaction with any DPP-4i drug.

Amylin Analog

In 1987 amylin was discovered to be produced and co-secreted with insulin from pancreatic beta cells in response to food intake.[55] In people with type 1 diabetes and those with type 2 diabetes who require insulin, secretion of both insulin and amylin is diminished due to pancreatic cell dysfunction or damage. A recombinant form of amylin, pramlintide (Symlin®), is now available for clinical use.[9]

Case—Part 2: Pharmacologic Intervention

The choice of drug products is generally made by considering individual characteristics and agent specific effects. Cardiovascular and renal benefits take precedence; however, the effect on weight, hypoglycemia, drug interaction potential, required number of daily doses, age-related issues, and cost are also important considerations. Metformin is a good choice for CR because he has good kidney function; as monotherapy, metformin has a low incidence of hypoglycemia and may have favorable effects on his lipids and blood pressure. Although oral agents are easier for persons with diabetes to start and require much less person with diabetes education at diagnosis, insulin and GLP-1 RAs are also rational choices for therapy. Initiation of insulin should be strongly considered if blood glucose levels are above 300 mg/dL (16.7 mmol/L), A1C is ≥10%, or symptoms of catabolism exist suggesting insulin deficiency.[1]

Metformin was initiated concurrently with a nutrition and physical activity plan at diagnosis due to the high blood glucose level and presence of clinical symptoms. Despite CR's engagement with taking metformin and lifestyle modifications, his glycemic control was not in the recommended target range 2 weeks later. Each of the oral agents, except TZDs, which take up to 3 months, reach their maximum benefit within 2 weeks of initiation. For persons with diabetes who regularly monitor their blood glucose, changes to therapy can reliably be made between weeks 2 and 4. Once an optimal dose is identified by self-monitored blood glucose, then an A1C can be scheduled 3 months later to verify glycemic control in between SMBG testing. For persons with diabetes who do not self-monitor, the guidelines recommend therapy changes with each subsequent A1C level. Because CR is tolerating metformin without gastrointestinal disturbance but produces self-monitored blood glucose values above goal, increasing the dose to 1000 mg twice daily is appropriate.

Although CR does not have established ASCVD, his estimated 10-year ASCVD risk is 31.3%, which is very high. If his A1C remains uncontrolled after 3 months, dual therapy with either a GLP-1 RA or an SGLT2 inhibitor would be preferred. When choosing an agent, providers must consider the whole person with diabetes, including their ability to afford the medications. Currently, DPP-4 inhibitors, SGLT2 inhibitors, and GLP-1 receptor agonists are fairly expensive; thus if the person with diabetes does not have insurance, a sulfonylurea or TZD might be preferred due to lower cost.

Amylin Analog: Dosage Information		
Drug	*Trade Name*	*Common Dose/Frequency and Available Strengths*
Pramlintide	Symlin®	Type 1 DM: 15 mcg to 60 mcg before meals Type 2 DM: 60 mcg to 120 mcg before meals *Pen-injector:* 2700 mcg/2.7 mL; 1500 mcg/1.5 mL

Mechanism of Action Pramlintide affects the rise of postprandial glucose by slowing gastric emptying, suppressing glucagon secretion, and reducing total caloric intake. Some research and discussion of this satiety sensation have led to the possible conclusion of a central effect.[19] Pramlintide is administered subcutaneously just before major meals, defined as having at least 250 calories or 30 grams of carbohydrates, and is indicated for both type 1 diabetes and type 2 diabetes therapy in people who use mealtime insulin therapy. People with type 2 diabetes who take pramlintide may also take metformin or a sulfonylurea.[56–59]

Dosing People with type 1 diabetes should receive a starting dose of 15 mcg before major meals; the dose can be titrated in 15-mcg increments up to 60 mcg as tolerated with nausea. People with type 2 diabetes using insulin usually receive an initial dose of 60 mcg before major meals. Pending glycemic control and the tolerance to nausea, the dose can be titrated to 120 mcg. The bioavailability of a single subcutaneous dose is approximately 40%, and its half-life is 48 minutes with a 3-hour duration after injection. Pramlintide is primarily metabolized in the kidneys to an active metabolite with a short half-life. Clearance of the drug was not altered in persons with diabetes with moderate or severe renal impairment.[57,58]

Precautions Despite low risk for crossing the placenta, there have been observed adverse events in animal reproduction studies; therefore, pramlintide should be used in pregnancy only if the potential benefit justifies the risk. The major concern with pramlintide use is the risk of hypoglycemia; careful monitoring and person with diabetes instruction for monitoring this action are mandatory. This effect is not actually due to the pramlintide but rather secondary to the pramlintide, making the insulin more effective, which can induce the blood glucose swing.[57,58]

Contraindications Gastroparesis is a contraindication to the use of pramlintide due to its effect in slowing gastric emptying. Further, pramlintide should not be considered for persons with diabetes taking drugs that alter gastrointestinal motility (eg, anticholinergic agents) or slow absorption of nutrients (eg, alpha-glucosidase inhibitors). Pramlintide can slow the rate of absorption of orally administered medications. Mixing pramlintide with insulin products can alter the pharmacokinetics of both agents and result in hypoglycemia. As a result, pramlintide and insulin should be administered separately. It is also recommended to reduce current mealtime insulin by approximately 50% (depending on person with diabetes's current overall glucose control) to avoid hypoglycemia. Because pramlintide slows gastric emptying, medications that depend on rapid concentrations or specific thresholds, such as antibiotics, analgesics, and oral contraceptives, should be administered 1 hour before or 2 hours after pramlintide injection.

Side Effects Nausea is the most common side effect noted with use of pramlintide, ranging up to 48% of persons with diabetes, though the incidence is higher at the start of therapy and decreases with time. Gradual titration to the recommended dose reduces this reaction. Other side effects include anorexia, vomiting, fatigue, and headache.[57,58]

Instructions for Persons With Diabetes Medications that demand a prompt or rapid onset of action should be taken at least 1 hour before or 2 hours after a pramlintide dose. The dose is adjusted to reach the desired glycemic control and tolerance to nausea.[58] Pramlintide vials require refrigeration, though the vial in use can be stored at room temperature at a temperature of less than 77°F. Opened vials must be used within 28 days and then discarded. Pramlintide should be administered subcutaneously into the abdomen or thigh at sites distinctly different from concomitant insulin injections. Pramlintide should not be administered into the upper arm due to variable absorption.

Insulin

Physiology of Insulin in Diabetes

Insulin is a hormone produced in the beta cells of the islets of Langerhans in the pancreas; it is formed from a substance called proinsulin. When the pancreas is stimulated, primarily by an elevated blood glucose level, the proinsulin is cleaved at 2 sections of the molecule. When the proinsulin molecule is broken apart, insulin and the connecting peptide (C-peptide) are both secreted and enter the bloodstream in equimolar amounts.[60] Normal daily insulin secretion in a healthy, nonpregnant adult without obesity is approximately 0.5 to 0.7 units of insulin per kilogram of body weight. Exogenous insulin is manufactured to be chemically identical to human insulin through recombinant DNA technology.[60] Another polypeptide, amylin, is also produced in the pancreas and released with insulin to assist in regulating the effects of insulin and to attenuate the actions of insulin.[61]

Mechanism of Action

The physiologic actions of insulin on body tissues include the following:[62]

- Stimulates entry of amino acids into cells and enhances protein synthesis
- Enhances fat storage (lipogenesis) and prevents mobilization of fat for energy (lipolysis and ketogenesis)
- Stimulates entry of glucose into cells for use as an energy source and promotes the resultant storage of glucose as glycogen (glycogenesis) in muscle and liver cells
- Inhibits production of glucose from liver or muscle glycogen (glycogenolysis)
- Inhibits formation of glucose from noncarbohydrates, such as amino acids (gluconeogenesis)

Several hormones in the body exert antagonistic effects to the hypoglycemic actions of insulin. These hormones are collectively referred to as counterregulatory hormones. The primary counterregulatory hormones include glucagon (produced in the alpha cells of the pancreas), epinephrine, norepinephrine, growth hormone, and cortisol. Blood glucose management in diabetes needs to take into account, and compensate for, the release of one or more of these hormones throughout the day in response to a variety of stimuli.

Indications for Use

Insulin is indicated in all people with type 1 diabetes and in many people with type 2 diabetes when other forms of therapy do not effectively achieve glycemic goals. Insulin may also be indicated in those with type 2 diabetes who may be well controlled on oral agents but experience periods of physiological stress, such as surgery or infection, which cause severe hyperglycemia that is not responsive to oral agents. Women with gestational diabetes may need insulin if medical nutrition therapy alone does not adequately control blood glucose levels. Persons with diabetes receiving parenteral nutrition or high-caloric supplements to meet an increased energy need may require exogenous insulin to maintain normal glucose levels during periods of insulin resistance or increased insulin demand. Insulin is necessary in treating DKA and often needed in treating hyperosmolar hyperglycemic state.[63]

Types of Insulin

Insulin harvested from animal sources is no longer manufactured in the United States. A key factor stimulating this decision is that human insulin is less antigenic than beef insulin and pork insulin. Insulin analogs and concentrated insulin products (U-200, U-300, and U-500 insulin) all require a prescription, although other insulin preparations are available without a prescription.[19]

The concentrations of insulin currently available in the United States are U-100, U-200, U-300, and U-500, indicating 100 units/mL, 200 units/mL, 300 units/mL, and 500 units/mL, respectively. Most persons with diabetes use U-100 insulin; however, persons with diabetes requiring large doses of insulin may benefit from the more concentrated insulin products. Concentrated insulin preparations allow higher doses to be administered in a smaller volume, resulting in less injection site discomfort and potentially more consistent absorption.

Insulin products are classified according to onset, peak effect, and duration of action (see Table 17.3). Once absorbed into the bloodstream, all insulin products exert the same effect on insulin receptors. The difference between insulin products depends on the ability of each molecule to dissociate and be absorbed into the bloodstream following subcutaneous administration. When regular insulin is injected under the skin, it forms hexamers that break into dimers, then into monomers. Because insulin is a large protein, only the monomeric insulin molecules are small enough to be absorbed into the systemic circulation. Rapid-acting insulin preparations possess changes in their amino acid sequences that decrease the likelihood of forming hexamers. By reducing the number of dissociation steps leading to the monomeric form, the rapid-acting insulin products are absorbed into the bloodstream very quickly. Conversely, long-acting insulin preparations possess properties that promote the formation of hexamers and delay absorption, allowing them to mimic endogenous basal insulin.

Short- or Rapid-Acting Insulin

The currently available rapid-acting insulin products are insulin lispro, insulin aspart, and insulin glulisine.[59] The short-acting agent is regular insulin. Generally, these insulin products are administered into the subcutaneous tissue, although they may also be given intravenously or inhaled.[19] Injectable regular insulin and the insulin analogs

TABLE 17.3 Time Action for Insulin Preparations

Insulin Type	*Preparations (generic)**	*Onset*	*Peak*	*Effective Duration*
Rapid-acting	Humalog®; Admelog® (lispro) Novolog®; Fiasp® (aspart) Apidra® (glulisine) Afrezza® (insulin human)	5–15 min	30–90 min	<5 h
Short-acting	Humulin-R®; Novolin R® (Regular, human)	30–60 min	2–3 h	5–8 h
Intermediate-acting	Humulin-N®; Novolin-N® (NPH, human)	2–4 h	4–10 h	10–16 h
Long-acting	Lantus®; Basaglar®; Toujeo® (glargine)	2–4 h	No peak	20–24 h
	Levemir® (detemir)	3–8 h	Nearly peakless	5.7–23.2 h
	Tresiba® (degludec)	1 h	No peak	25–42 h
Fixed combination	70/30 (NPH/regular ratio)	30–60 min	Dual	10–16 h
	50/50 (NPL/lispro ratio)	5–15 min	Dual	10–16 h
	75/25 (NPL/lispro ratio)	5–15 min	Dual	10–16 h
	70/30 (NPA/aspart ratio)	5–15 min	Dual	10–16 h

*Most branded products are available via pen delivery systems.

Source: Adapted from *Facts and Comparisons* eAnswers. Accessed 6/3/2019.

are clear solutions; insulin preparations that include protamine are cloudy suspensions. Insulin lispro, aspart, and glulisine are generally preferred over regular insulin for postprandial coverage because of their very rapid onset and short duration of action. Several studies show reduced risk of late-onset hypoglycemia in people with type 1 diabetes treated with insulin lispro compared with those treated with regular human insulin due to its longer 4- to 6-hour duration of action.[21] Rapid-acting insulin can be injected immediately prior to eating (generally less than 15 minutes preprandially); however, injecting rapid-acting insulin too early (30-60 minutes prior to meals) may result in profound hypoglycemia. All three rapid-acting insulin analogs and regular insulin may be used in insulin pumps. When compared with regular insulin, lispro reduced A1C levels in pump users; however, both products reduced the incidence of hypoglycemia compared with injected insulin.[63]

Intermediate-Acting Insulin

Neutral protamine Hagedorn (NPH) insulin is an intermediate-acting insulin named for the researcher who derived the formulation. This insulin suspension contains the protein protamine (as well as zinc) and is at a neutral pH. Addition of the zinc/protamine complex to regular insulin adds an extra step in the dissociation of insulin molecules, causing increased duration of effect. Both protamine and zinc have occasionally been implicated as the causative agents of immunologic reactions such as urticaria or other allergic-type reactions at the injection site. Since protamine is the antidote for heparin toxicity, some have expressed concerns about sensitizing persons with diabetes to protamine with NPH insulin, but these concerns have not proven to be warranted.

Long-Acting Insulin

Long-acting insulin analogs are glargine (Lantus®, Basaglar®, Toujeo®), detemir (Levemir®), and degludec (Tresiba®). The long-acting analogs provide a peakless (glargine and degludec) or near-peakless (detemir) pharmacokinetic or drug effect pattern. Interestingly, the three agents differ in terms of the biochemical explanation for their extended basal insulin action curve.

Insulin glargine is a clear solution with a pH of 4.0. Following injection, glargine forms microcrystalline precipitates that act as a depot in the subcutaneous fat. These microprecipitates must first dissolve before the subsequent progression through hexamers, dimers, and monomers can take place. This extended dissociation process is responsible for the long duration of action with glargine. Insulin glargine can be given at bedtime or at any time of the day, but it should be given consistently at the same time each day.[1] Glargine must not be mixed in the same syringe with other insulin products, and the syringe must not contain any other medicine or residue.[1] Converting from a once-daily long-acting insulin may be done at the same dose; however, a dose reduction is recommended for euglycemic persons with diabetes needing to convert from NPH to glargine.

Because of the high peak and subsequent valley associated with NPH insulin, there is a potential for hypoglycemia when converting to glargine, which is nearly peakless. The recommendation is to reduce the glargine, dose to 80% of the previous NPH dose, to avoid filling the previous glycemic valley with insulin and inducing hypoglycemia.

Insulin detemir is a clear solution whose protracted duration of action is due to increased self-aggregation and albumin binding both in the subcutaneous compartment and in the plasma.[1] Although considered relatively peak-less, detemir reaches a peak effect in 6 to 8 hours and has a duration of 24 hours at doses greater than 0.4 units per kilogram following subcutaneous administration.[1] Like all insulin preparations, the duration of action of insulin detemir extends with higher doses due to greater self-aggregation in the subcutaneous tissue. Insulin detemir must not be diluted or mixed with any other insulin preparations.

Insulin degludec is the newest addition to the family of long-acting insulin products. Insulin degludec has a long fatty acid side chain attached to a human insulin molecule. Similar to detemir, the fatty acid side chain promotes formation of hexamers and binds to albumin, resulting in a degludec half-life of over 25 hours and a 42-hour duration of action.

Premixed Insulin Products

Commercially available premixed insulin products (70/30, 50/50, 75/25) are manufactured and stabilized by altered buffering.[1,19] These products may be appropriate for persons with diabetes who have difficulty mixing their own insulin, for those who do not want to commit to a strict basal/bolus regimen, or for those in whom these ratios are effective. For example, persons with diabetes with type 2 diabetes and modest residual beta cell function may benefit from a fixed-dose combination of insulin before meals. By slightly underdosing the fixed-dose insulin in persons with type 2 diabetes, the endogenous insulin can respond to variations in carbohydrate intake and avoid hypoglycemia from the short-acting or rapid-acting portion of the premixed insulin. The intermediate portion of the premixed insulin provides basal insulin support, allowing the pancreas to store endogenous insulin between meals. However, for intensive insulin regimens requiring full replacement of insulin requirements, such as for persons with type 1 diabetes, premixed insulin products are usually not recommended due to lack of dosing flexibility.

Fixed-Dose Combination of Basal Insulin with GLP-1 RA

There are two commercially available fixed-dose combinations of basal insulin with a GLP-1 RA; Soliqua® (insulin glargine/lixisenatide) and Xultophy® (insulin degludec/liraglutide).[64,65] Like other fixed-dose combinations, these products offer simplified administration at the cost of decreased flexibility. The 2019 ADA treatment algorithm recommends that these agents be considered for persons with diabetes on dual or triple therapy if the A1C is greater than 10% or 2% above target.[1] Compared with traditional basal/bolus regimens, inclusion of a GLP-1 RA with basal insulin offers similar glycemic control but is less likely to cause weight gain.

Approach to Insulin Dosing

The starting dose and schedule of insulin administration are based on several factors, including the type of diabetes, the clinical assessment of insulin deficiency and suspected insulin resistance, and individual person with diabetes preferences for eating times, meal composition, physical activity, and waking/sleeping patterns.[1,21] Target blood glucose levels for before meals, after meals, bedtime, and during sleep should be established with the person with diabetes. Setting targets enhances acceptance, understanding, and decision making as the person with diabetes observes changes in blood glucose levels in relation to changes in food, exercise, stress, or illness. Subsequent adjustments in dose or timing of the insulin are based on self-monitoring of blood glucose results and clinical signs and symptoms of hypoglycemia or hyperglycemia. Other parameters used to refine the insulin dose and schedule include A1C levels, achievement of weight or lipid goals, and variability of lifestyle or activities from day to day.

Insulin Regimens

Insulin regimens vary and should be designed with regard to a person's meals, exercise program, medications, work or activity schedule, and emotional factors. Appropriate alterations can be made in the insulin regimen to accommodate a midnight shift or rotating work schedule or other lifestyle preferences. Figure 17.3 shows some different types of insulin regimens using 2 to 4 or more injections a day. Although the typical split and mixed 2-injection daily regimen is often used (1 basal insulin injection and 1 bolus insulin injection timed with the largest meal), it may not be adequate to reach glycemic targets. Multiple injections of insulin (3 or more) are components of the system called flexible or intensive insulin therapy. With 3-injection regimens, insulin is administered in the morning before breakfast, before the evening meal, and at bedtime or administered before each meal. Before breakfast, rapid-acting or short-acting insulin is often mixed in the same syringe with intermediate-acting insulin. Before the evening meal, rapid-acting or short-acting insulin is often used alone. At bedtime, intermediate-acting insulin

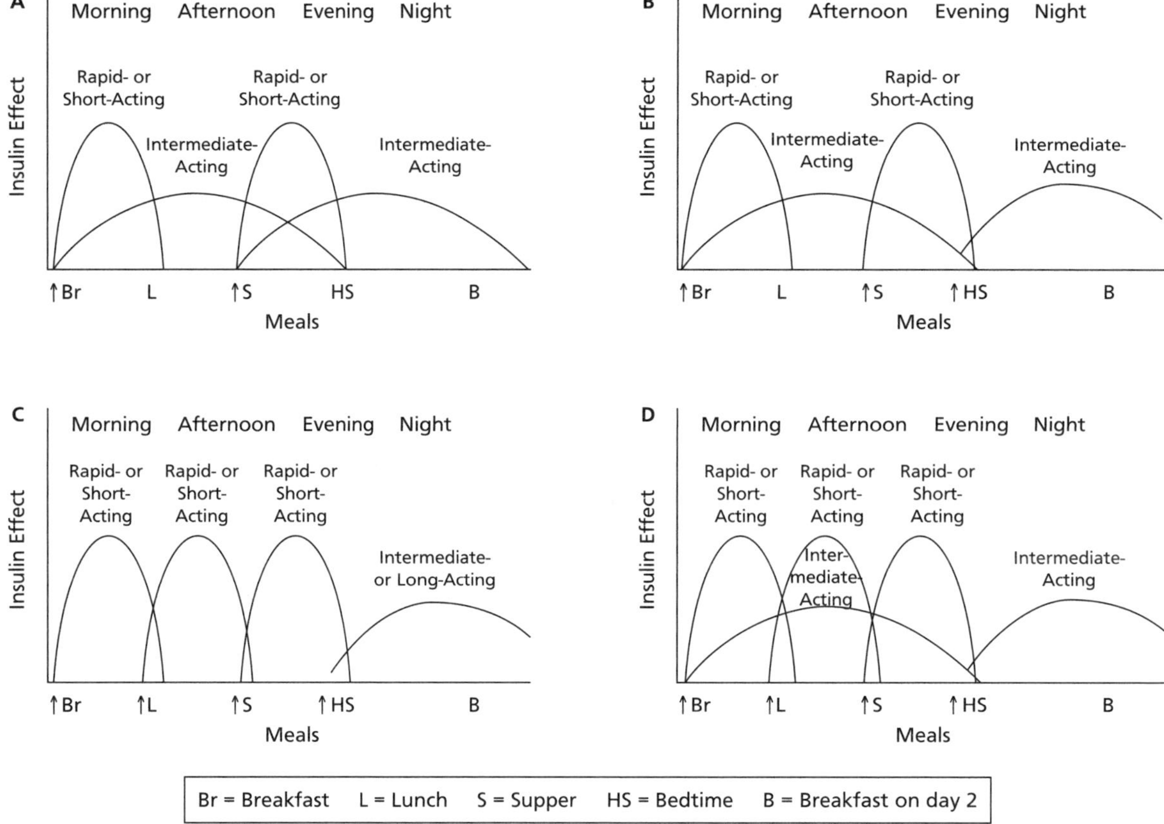

FIGURE 17.3 **Potential Multiple-Injection Insulin Regimens**

Source: Reprinted with permission from HE Lebovitz, *Therapy for Diabetes Mellitus and Related Disorders*, 5th ed. (Alexandria, Va: American Diabetes Association, 2009), 283.

is often used. This type of therapy can reduce the risk of nocturnal (2-4 AM) hypoglycemia, allow for better insulin coverage for early-morning (5-10 AM) hyperglycemia from the release of cortisol and growth hormone (the dawn phenomenon), and, in some cases, may accommodate sleeping in.[1]

With four-injection regimens, a long-acting insulin such as insulin glargine, insulin detemir, or insulin degludec is administered once a day and a rapid-acting or short-acting insulin is administered at mealtimes, but these must be administered as separate injections due to lack of compatibility in the same syringe. If a snack contains more than 15 g of carbohydrate, an injection of rapid-acting insulin may be needed before the snack. This regimen is illustrated in Figure 17.3. The rapid-acting or short-acting insulin provides postmeal glycemic control, while the long-acting insulin dose ensures a low, steady rate of insulin throughout the day. This type of regimen or use of an insulin pump can best duplicate normal physiologic insulin action.[1] In people with type 1 diabetes, physiologic replacement using basal insulin and a mealtime rapid-acting insulin improves A1C levels and results in fewer episodes of hypoglycemia than previous regimens.[59] This regimen can provide individuals with diabetes the flexibility in insulin doses necessary for busy and active lifestyles.

Insulin Therapy in Type 2 Diabetes

For persons with type 2 diabetes, insulin therapy may be employed in 2 ways. First, insulin may supplement or be added to 1 or more oral agents, usually including metformin. Typically, a single daily injection of long-acting insulin, commonly starting at 10 units or 0.2 units per kilogram, is administered in the morning or at bedtime.[1,2] The 2019 AACE algorithm also considers A1C level when determining dose (0.1-0.2 units per kilogram for A1C <8%, and 0.2-0.3 units per kilogram for A1C >8%).[2] Regardless of the starting dose, increases can be made every two to three days in fixed increments (2-4 units) or as a percentage of the current dose (10%-20%).[1,2] Due to the presence of insulin resistance in type 2 diabetes, the ultimate total daily dose of long-acting (basal) insulin is often very high (usually 0.5 units per kilogram per day, but may range from 0.7 to 2.5 units per kilogram per day).

Second, type 2 diabetes can also be treated with insulin as the sole pharmacologic agent. With insulin as the sole source of glycemic control, persons with diabetes often require at least 2 or more injections per day. The wide range of insulin products allows various permutations of 2-injection regimens depending on the pattern of person with diabetes glycemic excursions. The 3 most commonly used approaches are (1) twice-daily intermediate insulin, (2) split-mixed insulin, and (3) a semi-intensive insulin regimen. Many persons with diabetes eat only 2 meals per day (breakfast and dinner), making them good candidates for 2 doses of intermediate insulin, or mixed doses of regular or rapid-acting insulin and long-acting or intermediate-acting insulin (mixed by the person with diabetes or premixed) at 1 or both injection times. Usually two thirds of the total daily dose of insulin is given before breakfast (using a ratio of 1 part rapid-acting or short-acting insulin to 2 parts intermediate-acting insulin), and one third is given before the evening meal (using a ratio of 1:1 or 1:2, rapid-acting or short-acting to intermediate insulin). A semi-intensive regimen combines 1 dose of long-acting (basal) insulin with 1 dose of rapid-acting insulin with the largest meal.

Because type 2 diabetes is a progressive disease, the drug therapy regimen of most persons with diabetes evolves from oral therapy, to 2 or 3 oral agents plus GLP-1 RA, to combination therapy plus basal insulin, to basal insulin plus prandial insulin with or without oral agents. For persons with diabetes who progress to semi-intensive insulin and require the addition of prandial insulin (identified by FPG values at goal with elevated A1C or PPG levels), both the 2019 ADA and 2019 AACE algorithms suggest stopping insulin secretagogues (sulfonylureas and meglitinides). When adding rapid-acting insulin for prandial coverage of the largest meal, the recommended dose is 0.1 unit per kilogram, or 10% of the basal insulin dose, or 4 to 5 units.[1,2] Subsequent dose adjustments of the rapid-acting insulin can be made based on the 2-hour postprandial blood glucose level (goal <140 mg/dL) by either 1 to 2 units, or 10% to 15% of the dose.[1,2] If the person with diabetes becomes hypoglycemic (2-hour postprandial blood glucose <70 mg/dL), then determine the cause and if consistent, consider reducing the rapid-acting insulin by 2 to 4 units or 10% to 20%.[1,2]

Insulin Therapy in Type 1 Diabetes

A goal of contemporary insulin therapy is to mimic, as nearly as possible, the physiologic profile of insulin secretion (basal/bolus).[1,2] To optimize glycemic control, the pharmacology and pharmacokinetics of insulin require that a person with type 1 diabetes receive insulin continuously (basal, also referred to as *background insulin*), with boluses of insulin before meals and snacks (often called *mealtime insulin*).[1,2] Physiologic insulin secretion typically occurs at a rate of 0.5 to 1.0 units per hour. The metabolic balance among basal insulin, the counterregulatory hormones, hepatic glucose production, and circulating glucose normally provides the body with sufficient glucose to function between meals. Bolus insulin is rapidly released in response to nutrient intake from a meal, and under normal circumstances it reduces postprandial glycemic excursions back to baseline in 60 to 90 minutes.[1]

Insulin requirements for individuals with type 1 diabetes or who are within 20% of ideal body weight are usually 0.5 to 1.0 units per kilogram of body weight per day. Insulin requirements may be higher (even double) in the presence of intercurrent illness or other metabolic instability. Insulin requirements will be less (0.2-0.6 units per kilogram of body weight per day) during the honeymoon phase, the period of relative remission early in the course of the disease.

Although persons with type 1 diabetes may choose to inject insulin subcutaneously, continuous insulin infusion via an insulin pump is considered the standard of care. For further discussion of evaluation and management of persons with diabetes receiving insulin via an insulin pump, see chapter 18.

Insulin Therapy in Pregnancy

Preexisting Diabetes

Insulin requirements for women with preexisting diabetes increase early in the pregnancy followed by a decrease during weeks 9 to 16. During the second and third trimesters of pregnancy, insulin resistance gradually increases by about 5% per week and may result in insulin demands of 0.9 to 1.2 units per kilogram of body weight per day (as much as twice the total daily dosage of insulin needed before pregnancy).[17,18] These increases in plasma insulin demand result from placental production of counterregulatory hormones, which diminish responsiveness to insulin action. Women with preexisting diabetes should be treated with an intensive insulin regimen, 3 to 4 injections or an insulin pump, to provide the basal/bolus regimen.

Gestational Diabetes Mellitus

Insulin is the drug treatment of choice for glycemic control during pregnancy; however, approaches to insulin therapy for gestational diabetes differ greatly. A total dose of 20 to 30 units given before breakfast is commonly used to initiate therapy.[17,18] The total dose is usually divided into two-thirds intermediate-acting insulin and one-third rapid-acting or short-acting insulin. For obese women, a higher starting dose of insulin is usually needed due to insulin resistance. The total initial dosage may be as high as 0.8 to 1.0 units per kilogram of body weight per day.[17,18] Pregnant women should be counseled to inject the insulin in their thigh or back of the arm.

Insulin Delivery Devices

Syringe

Disposable insulin syringes for use with U-100 insulin are available in different sizes, chosen according to the dose of insulin to be injected: 0.25 mL (for doses <25 units), 0.3 mL (for doses <30 units), 0.5 mL (for doses <50 units), or 1 mL (for doses 50-100 units). The attached needle length may be 6 mm (15/64-in), 8 mm (5/16-in), or 12.7 mm (1/2-in). The "short needle" (either the 6-mm or the 8-mm length) is appropriate for all persons with diabetes regardless of BMI. A study of 388 individuals with diabetes divided participants into BMI categories (<25, 25-29.9, and ≥30 kg/m^2) and measured skin thickness at 4 different injection sites.[66] The authors concluded that needle lengths greater than 8 mm were likely to penetrate underlying muscle if inserted perpendicularly. A separate study in 173 persons with diabetes concluded that a 4-mm (32 gauge) insulin pen needle provided equivalent glycemic control compared with 5-mm and 8-mm (31 gauge) needles.[67] In most situations, persons with diabetes may safely reuse syringes and needles during a single day; however, reuse may carry an increased risk of infection for some individuals.[68] Advise those persons with diabetes who choose to reuse syringes that the markings on the syringe may rub off and that the needle becomes dull with repeated use. Instruct persons with diabetes to safely recap the needle and store at room temperature.

Used insulin syringes should not be discarded in regular trash cans or recycling bins or flushed down the toilet, due to the risk of harming others. The safest way to dispose of used syringes is with a sharps disposal container immediately after use. Sharps disposal containers that are three-quarters full should be closed and discarded according to community guidelines. Persons with diabetes who do not have access to sharps disposal containers may use household containers with similar characteristics, such as a thick-walled plastic liquid detergent bottle. The container should be clearly marked "sharps" and have the cap sealed closed with duct tape once it is three fourths full. Persons with diabetes may also elect to recap the syringe using a one-handed technique (see "Safely Using Sharps [Needles and Syringes] at Home, at Work and on Travel" on the FDA Web site for details: www.fda.gov/MedicalDevices/ProductsandMedicalProcedures/HomeHealthandConsumer/ConsumerProducts/Sharps/). Alternatively, persons with diabetes may use needle clippers to make syringes unusable. Note that scissors should not be used to cut insulin syringe needles due to the risk of flying debris.

Pump

Continuous subcutaneous insulin infusion (CSII) pumps became available in 1974. An insulin pump consists of a reservoir filled with insulin, a small battery-operated pump, and a computer chip that allows the user to control the insulin delivery (see chapter 19, on intensifying insulin therapy, for more on insulin pump therapy). Pump therapy is a continuous basal amount of insulin (0.5-1.0 units per hour) that is usually administered in addition to bolus doses given prior to meals.[1]

Jet Injector

Jet injectors are a novel, needle-free system that delivers insulin transcutaneously. Jet injectors release a fine stream of insulin at high speed and under high pressure to penetrate the skin. These may represent an option for persons with diabetes with needle phobia; however, the device expense, injection site pain, and required weekly maintenance limit widespread adoption.

Pen Device

Pen devices have been a popular insulin delivery option in Europe for many years and were introduced in the United States in 1987. They combine the insulin container and the syringe into a single modular unit that allows for convenient insulin delivery. Insulin pens are available for almost all branded insulin products in a variety of types and styles (see Table 17.4). Pens are either reusable or prefilled, and both types hold cartridges of insulin. With the reusable pen, the person with diabetes must first load an insulin cartridge; however, this step is eliminated with prefilled pen devices. Compared with traditional 10 mL insulin vials, insulin pen cartridges (1.5-3 mL) have a relatively large surface area relative to the volume of insulin. Consequently, insulin pens may be more sensitive to heat and light than insulin vials. Regardless of the container, unopened insulin should be stored in the refrigerator and not frozen. In general, "in use" insulin pens and vials may be stored at room temperature, protected from extreme heat and light, for up to 28 days; however, providers should check specific product labeling. Some agents may be able to be stored out of the refrigerator for longer, such as insulin degludec that can be kept out of the refrigerator for 56 days.

Inhalation Device

An inhalable powdered form of recombinant human insulin (Exubera®) received FDA-approved labeling in January 2006, but the manufacturer halted its production in October 2007 due to poor sales. At the time, many attributed poor adoption by person with diabetes adoption to the

TABLE 17.4 Summary of Insulin Formulations

	*Brand Name (generic)**	*Manufacturer*	*Strength*
Rapid-acting	***Human Insulin Analog***		
	Humalog® (lispro)*	Lilly	U-100, U-200
	Admelog® (lispro)*	Sanofi-Aventis	U-100
	Novolog®; Fiasp® (aspart)*	Novo-Nordisk	U-100
	Apidra® (glulisine)*	Sanofi-Aventis	U-100
	Afrezza® (human)	Sanofi	4- and 8-unit cartridges w/inhaler
Short-acting	***Human***		
	Humulin® R (regular)*	Lilly	U-100, U-500
	Novolog® R (regular)*	Novo Nordisk	U-100
	Novolin® R (regular)*, ReliOn R+	Lilly	U-100
Intermediate-acting	***Human***		
	Humulin® (NPH)*	Lilly	U-100
	Novolin® (NPH)*, ReliOn N+	Novo Nordisk	U-100
Long-acting	***Human Insulin Analog***		
	Lantus® (glargine)	Sanofi-Aventis	U-100
	Basaglar® (glargine)	Lilly	U-100
	Levemir® (detemir)	Norvo Nordisk	U-100
	Tresiba® (degludec)	Novo Nordisk	U-100, U-200
	Toujeo® (glargine)*	Sanofi-Aventis	U-300
Fixed combination	***Human***		
	Humulin® 70/30*	Lilly	70/30 (NPH/regular ratio)
	Novolin® 70/30	Novo Nordisk	70/30 (NPH/regular ratio)
	ReliOn 70/30†	Lilly	70/30 (NPH/regular ratio)
	Human Insulin Analog		
	Humalog® Mix 75/25*	Lilly	75/25 (NPL/lispro ratio)
	Novolog® Mix 70/30*	Novo Nordisk	70/30 (NPA/aspart ratio) 70/30 (NPH/regular ratio)
	Humalog® Mix 50/50*	Lilly	50/50 (NPL/lispro ratio)
	Soliqua® (100/33)*	Sanofi	Glargine/Lixisenatide
	Xultophy® (100/3.6)*	Novo Nordisk	Degludec/Liraglutide

*Available in a pen-style delivery system.

†Available only at Walmart.

large delivery system, which approximated a paper towel roll. A second, smaller inhaled insulin delivery system (Afrezza®) received FDA-approved labeling in June 2014. This device, which is the size of a whistle, delivers regular insulin in 4-unit, 8-unit, and 12-unit increments. Conversion to Afrezza® from insulin injections requires providers to round the dose according to recommendations in the product labeling. Like Exubera®, Afrezza® adversely affects lung function. In clinical trials with Afrezza®, pulmonary function declined within the first 3 months and persisted over 2 years in persons with diabetes without a history of chronic lung disease. Consequently, Afrezza® requires monitoring of forced expiratory volume in the first second (FEV1) at baseline, at 6 months, and then annually thereafter even in the absence of symptoms. In clinical trials, cough was reported in 27% of persons with diabetes using Afrezza®, and the product labeling contains a black box warning of acute bronchospasm in persons with diabetes with asthma and chronic obstructive pulmonary disease (COPD). The need for ongoing spirometry (FEV1) and concerns about adverse lung function also limit the acceptance of inhaled insulin.[69]

Future Possibilities

In the future, insulin may be delivered by implantable insulin pumps, transdermal systems, or oral tablets. Technical barriers to the market development of implantable insulin pumps include the requirement for surgical placement, relatively short battery life, and occlusion of the insulin delivery catheter. Transdermal and oral insulin delivery systems represent novel attempts to bypass gastric degradation of insulin and provide systemic insulin absorption without injections. All 3 modalities continue to be investigated.

Insulin Use

Monitoring

Self-monitoring of blood glucose and periodic A1C levels (every 3 months until goal level is attained, then every 6 months) should be the primary monitors for insulin therapy. Inquiries about hypoglycemic episode severity and frequency should also be included in the assessment. Because insulin and C-peptide are jointly secreted, measurement of C-peptide levels is useful to determine endogenous insulin production and type of diabetes. Direct measurement of insulin secretion is difficult, except under controlled or research conditions, because insulin is rapidly removed from the blood after it exerts its pharmacologic action.[70] Initial measurement of C-peptide is useful to confirm the diagnosis of diabetes type in persons with diabetes without a clear presentation and when the absolute need for exogenous insulin is uncertain.

Precautions

The major adverse effect of insulin therapy is hypoglycemia. Virtually all persons with diabetes who inject insulin will experience hypoglycemia at some time. Common causes of hypoglycemia include excessive doses of insulin; delayed, missed, or insufficient food intake; or too much (unplanned) physical activity.[61]

Side Effects

Various problems or complications may arise from insulin characteristics. Insulin impurity can cause lipodystrophies (atrophy and/or hypertrophy). Atrophy, which is a concavity or pitting of the fatty tissue, is an immune phenomenon that occurs in a small number of persons with diabetes and is related to species/source or purity. Use of highly purified insulin preparations such as human insulin or purified pork insulin reduces the occurrence of atrophy. Persons with diabetes who develop this problem may benefit from injecting human or highly purified insulin around the periphery of the atrophied areas.[71] Many clinicians recommend reviewing the insulin dose and injection technique with persons with diabetes when lipodystrophy occurs. Hypertrophy, which is a fatty thickening of the lipid tissue, is best prevented by rotating injection sites.

Allergies to insulin are possible but rare. Insulin allergy may occur as local reactions (rash, urticarial cutaneous reaction) or systemic reactions (serum sickness, anaphylaxis). Prior to insulin purification, local cutaneous reactions were more common. Zinc or protamine in the insulin, preservatives, and rubber or latex stoppers have all been implicated in inducing allergic reactions. Both local and systemic reactions appear to be immunologically mediated through induction of high titers of IgG and IgE antibodies. If a systemic reaction occurs, desensitization to the insulin will be necessary. If desensitization is needed, the attending physician should be encouraged to contact the insulin manufacturer for the desensitization kit and the procedure to follow.[72]

Instructions for Persons With Diabetes

Insulin mixing standards are based on published data.[68] Varying the time delay for injecting after mixing may result in a different insulin action. As a general rule, both insulin products to be mixed should be of the same brand. Rapid-acting or regular insulin is usually drawn up first, followed by the intermediate-acting insulin. This practice limits the potential for contamination, which may result in dose variance.

All insulin mixtures must be thoroughly resuspended immediately prior to an injection or after storage for any time period. Individuals using these products should be instructed to gently roll the vial or prefilled syringe or pen device between the palms of the hands several times to thoroughly mix the insulin component.

Strategies to reduce the risk of hypoglycemia include performing routine self-monitoring of blood glucose levels and watching for and responding quickly to early symptoms of hypoglycemia. Insulin users are instructed to ingest appropriate quantities and choices of a pre-exercise carbohydrate supplement and apply a consistent food/meal plan and pattern.[73]

Those using insulin should be instructed to take extra supplies when traveling to foreign countries, as some countries may still use U-40 insulin preparations.

Insulin users should be taught to store insulin according to the manufacturer's recommendations. Generally, insulin should be refrigerated at 36°F to 46°F (2°C-8°C). Unopened insulin products may be stored under refrigeration until the expiration date noted on the product label. Injecting a cold insulin preparation can produce local irritation and increased pain at the injection site; therefore, persons with diabetes should be counseled that to bring the insulin to room temperature, the prepared syringe should be rolled between the palms of the hands. Other options include returning the vial of insulin to room temperature before withdrawing the dose or storing the insulin at room temperature. Opened or unopened vials of insulin may be stored at a controlled room temperature of 59°F to 86°F (15°C-30°C) for 28 days (longer duration may be appropriate depending on the product); unused insulin should be discarded after that time.[68] Storage guidelines differ for used (punctured) or unused cartridge insulin and disposable prefilled insulin pens:

- Used or unused insulin cartridges or regular prefilled insulin pens may be kept unrefrigerated for 28 days (1.5-mL or 3.0-mL cartridges); longer depending on manufacturer guidelines
- Humalog Mix 75/25 may be used for 10 days capped at room temperature (72°F) and out of direct sunlight; the unused portion can be stored without refrigeration for 28 days but should be stored in the refrigerator to preserve its effectiveness until the labeled expiration.
- 70/30 insulin cartridges or prefilled insulin pens may be kept and used unrefrigerated for 10 days; unused units should be refrigerated, but if not refrigerated, they should be discarded in 10 days.
- NPH insulin cartridges or prefilled insulin pens may be kept and used unrefrigerated for 14 days; unused units should be refrigerated, but if not refrigerated, they should be discarded in 14 days.

Manually prefilled syringes of either single formulations or mixtures of insulins are to be refrigerated and used within 21 to 30 days.[68] Availability of insulin and supplies may vary; teach persons with diabetes to carry insulin and supplies when traveling. Due to the variance of temperature, insulin should not be left in a car or checked through in airline baggage. Instruct those using insulin to examine vials for sediment or other visible changes before withdrawing the insulin into the syringe. Cloudiness or discoloration of clear insulin, clumping of insulin suspensions, or flocculation (frosting) of insulin suspensions indicates that the insulin has lost potency and should not be used; it should be returned to the pharmacy for exchange. The incidence of frosting may be minimized if temperature is stabilized through refrigeration and if agitation or shaking of the vial is minimized.

Teach persons with diabetes using insulin to follow a specific routine for insulin injections, including consistent technique, priming the needle, accurate dosage, and site rotation. The insulin is injected into the subcutaneous tissue. Most individuals are able to lightly grasp a fold of skin and inject at a 90-degree angle. Thin individuals

Case—Part 3: Combining Agents

CR returned to the diabetes clinic 3 months after metformin was increased to 1000 mg twice daily. At that visit his A1C was still above goal, so empagliflozin was added to his metformin. To simplify his regimen and decrease his pill burden, a fixed-dose combination of empagliflozin 5 mg plus metformin 1000 mg twice daily was selected. Today, his A1C is elevated at 8.8%, and he continues to have fasting glucose levels over 200 mg/dL (11.1 mmol/L). He lost about 10 lb since his diagnosis by increasing his physical activity and paying more attention to his eating habits. He reports some tingling in his hands and feet and wants better control of his diabetes.

Because of his high ASCVD risk, a GLP-1 RA is recommended in addition to his fixed-dose oral therapy. The advantage of this regimen is low risk of hypoglycemia and convenience of once weekly dosing for the GLP-1 RA. For persons with diabetes on dual or triple oral drug therapy, with an A1C greater than 10%, or 2% above their target, the ADA algorithm recommends consideration of combination injectable therapy preferably with a GLP-1 RA plus basal insulin. For these persons with diabetes, fixed-dose combinations of liraglutide/degludec or lixisenatide/glargine might be options.

After discussion with the diabetes team, CR decided to add 20 units (0.2 units per kg) of glargine insulin at bedtime to help lower his fasting blood glucose due to the significant proximity from his glucose goals. Insulin degludec and detemir were also viable therapeutic options; also, NPH insulin could be chosen to minimize out-of-pocket expenses for CR depending on his insurance coverage. Weight-based insulin dosing was chosen due to the presence of symptoms and continued significantly elevated blood glucose levels. CR received diabetes education regarding prevention, recognition, and treatment of hypoglycemia; proper injection technique; and proper storage. A plan for the frequency of self-monitoring of blood glucose was agreed upon, and monthly follow-up was scheduled with the diabetes care and education specialist. CR's target is to achieve an A1C of <7%.

or children may need to pinch the skin and inject at a 45-degree angle to avoid intramuscular injection.[68] Insulin may be injected into the subcutaneous tissue of the upper arm, the anterior and lateral aspects of the thigh, the buttocks, and the abdomen (with the exception of a 2-in radius around the navel).[68] These sites are chosen because of general person with diabetes acceptability and accessibility. Once the thumb button is depressed completely, persons with diabetes should be instructed to count to 5 for low doses and at least 10 for higher doses to ensure adequate insulin absorption and distribution under the skin.

Areas for injection must be determined individually, with consideration for scar tissue and areas with less subcutaneous fat, as well as individual preference. Both the person with diabetes and the health professional need to examine injection areas at regular intervals to detect bruising, redness, infection, lipoatrophy, or lipohypertrophy. Due to the acidic pH, insulin glargine may cause a mild burning when injected, whereas other insulin products retain normal pH in solution. Teach persons with diabetes to rotate injection sites to prevent local irritation. Rotating within a single area is recommended (eg, rotating injections systematically within the abdomen) rather than rotating to a different area with each injection. This practice may decrease variability in absorption from day to day.[68] Insulin absorption may vary depending on several parameters. Abdominal injection provides the most rapid absorption, followed by the arms, thighs, and buttocks.[68] However, note that insulin glargine does not display this difference of absorption rates at different sites.[58] Deeper intramuscular injections induce faster absorption and shorter duration of action. High levels of insulin antibodies can also inhibit insulin action following injection. Exercise or massage of the injection site may induce more rapid absorption.

Medication Side Effects: Self-Management Considerations

Certain drug side effects have an impact on diabetes self-management. People with diabetes who are taking medication must be taught to be attentive to particular signs and symptoms that may indicate impending hypoglycemia or hyperglycemia.

In addition, certain procedures and aspects of diabetes care require the person with diabetes to be alert, coordinated, and capable of making self-management decisions. A drug that mimics an individual's usual warning signs of hypoglycemia or hyperglycemia, or one that impairs a person's ability to perform necessary self-care tasks, may adversely affect glycemic control.

Hypoglycemia

Defining hypoglycemia on the basis of a specific plasma glucose level is difficult. Absolute blood glucose levels cannot be used to describe the severity of hypoglycemic episodes, because glycemic thresholds for the onset of symptoms, as well as symptom magnitude, differ greatly among individuals and from episode to episode, depending on various mediating variables. Some individuals remain alert with only a few symptoms at a plasma glucose level less than 70 mg/dL (3.9 mmol/L), while others become stuporous at the same glucose concentration. Even the same person may tolerate low glucose levels differently on different occasions. The American Diabetes Association Workgroup on Hypoglycemia concluded that hypoglycemic events should be reported on the basis of the following definitions:

- *Severe hypoglycemia* is characterized by an inability to self-treat due to mental confusion, lethargy, or unconsciousness. Because the individual is unable to self-treat, others must provide treatment to raise the blood glucose level out of a dangerously low range.
- *Documented symptomatic hypoglycemia* is characterized by a documented blood glucose level less than or equal to 70 mg/dL with symptoms such as sweating, trembling, difficulty concentrating, lightheadedness, and a lack of coordination. These symptoms are usually alleviated quickly by drinking beverages or eating foods containing carbohydrates.
- *Documented asymptomatic hypoglycemia* is characterized by a documented blood glucose less than or equal to 70 mg/dL without symptoms.[74]

Causes of Hypoglycemia

The first step in determining the cause of frequent hypoglycemia is to carefully examine the treatment regimen, including insulin and non-insulin agents. Hypoglycemia resulting from insulin excess is more likely to occur at those times of the day when insulin action is peaking. Some of the newer insulin analogs, including rapid-acting insulins (eg, insulin lispro, aspart, and glulisine) and long-acting insulins (glargine, detemir, and degludec), appear to reduce some of the problems with hypoglycemia but still carry risk.

Hypoglycemia is more of a risk when an individual has taken insulin or a medication that promotes insulin secretion and has not eaten for several hours, or when an individual has significantly increased physical activity. Alcohol consumption, without food intake, may also result in hypoglycemia, as gluconeogenesis by the liver is impaired.

Prevention of Hypoglycemia

Prevention is the best intervention. Treatment regimens may be developed that include intake of carbohydrate coinciding with insulin or medication peak if necessary and snacks prior to increased physical activity. In addition, the individual should understand that foods high in fat or protein and very low in carbohydrate will not prevent hypoglycemia. Similarly, foods high in fat or protein in conjunction with carbohydrate may delay the absorption of carbohydrates and have implications for the timing of medication and carbohydrate peaks and treatment of hypoglycemia.

Treatment of Hypoglycemia

To treat hypoglycemia, individuals should eat or drink 15 to 20 g of glucose or any form of carbohydrate that contains glucose, such as the following:

- 3 or 4 glucose tablets (follow package instructions)
- glucose gel (follow package instructions)
- 8 to 10 hard candies
- 2 tablespoons raisins
- 1 tablespoon sugar, honey, or corn syrup
- 4 to 6 oz non-diet soft drink
- 4 to 6 oz fruit juice
- 1 piece of fruit
- 1 cup low-fat or nonfat milk

In the management of hypoglycemia, the challenge is to treat but not overtreat. Overtreating hypoglycemia is relatively common and causes post-treatment hyperglycemia. Some persons with diabetes may continue eating until all symptoms disappear. Others may overeat because they are fearful of the symptoms (often feeling as though they are losing control). Using commercially available portion-controlled glucose products may help individuals avoid overtreatment.

The choice of glucose or carbohydrate-containing product should be based on its ability to raise blood glucose levels quickly. Drinks or foods that are high in fat content slow gastric emptying and absorption of carbohydrate and, therefore, take longer to raise blood glucose levels. Adding protein to the treatment of hypoglycemia does not raise blood glucose levels and does not prevent subsequent hypoglycemia.

If possible, blood glucose levels should be tested before treatment and again 15 to 20 minutes after initiating treatment. If blood glucose levels remain low (less than 70 mg/dL), treatment should be repeated regardless of symptom presence. If a meal or snack is not scheduled within the next hour, individuals should be cautioned that their blood glucose level may fall again.

General guidelines for treating hypoglycemia are the following:

- Do not keep eating after the initial treatment; wait 15 to 20 minutes and then test blood glucose level to determine whether further treatment is needed.
- Do not keep eating until symptoms disappear.
- Avoid using high-fat foods for treatment.
- Always carry some type of carbohydrate.
- Keep something at your bedside to treat nocturnal hypoglycemia.
- Keep something in the car at all times to treat episodes of hypoglycemia that might occur while driving.
- Always wear diabetes identification.

Treatment of hypoglycemia may need to be given by others. A person with type 1 diabetes who is experiencing hypoglycemia often has to be treated by others because hypoglycemia may affect the individual's judgment and behavior. Family members and significant others should be taught how to cope with episodes of severe hypoglycemia and what to expect in terms of the person's behavior (eg, stupor or possible resistance). Coworkers, friends, and teachers also need to know how to respond to symptoms of hypoglycemia, which can be a problem if individuals do not want to reveal their diabetes to others. In cases where others are too anxious or frightened to treat the hypoglycemia, they should be instructed to call 911.

Severe hypoglycemia occurs when the individual is unable to self-treat. The following basic guidelines are recommended for treating severe hypoglycemia:

- *Able to swallow.* Persons with diabetes who are able to swallow without risk of aspiration may be coaxed into drinking juice or a non-diet soft drink. If this is not possible, place some glucose gel, honey, syrup, or jelly inside the individual's cheek.
- *Unable to swallow.* Persons with diabetes who are unable to swallow without risk of aspiration can be given glucagon by subcutaneous or intramuscular injection (see Table 17.5). Glucagon is a hormone that stimulates hepatic glucose production. Glucagon will produce substantial hyperglycemia, but its effects are very short lived. As soon as the individual is able to swallow, liquid carbohydrates should be given to maintain normoglycemia.

TABLE 17.5 Recommended Doses for Glucagon
Adults and children >20 kg:
1 mg SQ (subcutaneously) or IM (intramuscularly)*
Children <20 kg:
0.5 mg SQ or IM, or 20–30 mcg per kilogram (9.1–13.6 mcg per pound) of body weight*

*If necessary, the dose may be repeated after 15 minutes.

Source: Glucagon [package insert], Indianapolis, Ind: Eli Lilly and Company, 2012.

The person with diabetes and those likely to be involved in treatment need to know that glucagon may cause nausea and vomiting. Therefore, it is important to place the individual on their side to prevent choking or aspiration of vomit.

Frequent blood glucose monitoring is needed over the next several hours to detect whether blood glucose levels fall again or to detect hyperglycemia due to overtreatment.

Family and significant others should be taught how and when to administer glucagon. Persons with diabetes should keep glucagon in their homes at all times. Individuals who may be required to administer the injection need to know how to use the glucagon kit; this may include a teacher, coworker, roommate, friend, or neighbor. Glucagon kits are obtained by prescription. Persons with diabetes also need to be aware of the expiration date on their glucagon.

Treating Hypoglycemia in Type 2 Diabetes

Individuals with type 2 diabetes who are taking oral glucose-lowering medication also need to be taught about hypoglycemia, even though they appear to be at less risk for severe hypoglycemia.

Persons with diabetes who are changing from oral medications to insulin may have considerable fears and concerns about hypoglycemia and need to be taught to monitor themselves for warning symptoms, especially at those times of the day when they are most at risk (eg, just before lunch). These persons with diabetes may also need to increase the frequency of self-monitoring of blood glucose.

Many people with type 2 diabetes are not adequately educated about hypoglycemia and are not aware of the risks that hypoglycemia can impose. Knowledge about hypoglycemia, including warning symptoms, needs to be assessed even in persons with diabetes who have been taking medication for a long period of time. Hypoglycemia is treated by carbohydrate consumption, following the guidelines prescribed for people with type 1 diabetes.

People with diabetes also need to be educated about the risk of hypoglycemia in other potentially dangerous situations, such as when caring for young children or when using heavy tools (eg, electric saws, lawn mowers).

Medication Taking: Combination Oral Medications for Type 2 Diabetes

Adequate medication taking to oral agents for type 2 diabetes may be as low as 65% to 85%.[75] The medication burden associated with advancing disease may contribute to the low rates of person with diabetes engagement in taking their medications. Several fixed-dose combination products of two different drug classes are available to treat type 2 diabetes, which may reduce medication burden and improve person with diabetes engagement in taking their medications. Fixed-dose combinations are generally started after a person with diabetes has failed to reach his or her glycemic goals on one drug alone. This stepwise titration is often necessary because the combination products are only available in specific doses (see Table 17.6). In addition, starting combination therapy in drug-naïve persons with diabetes can create problems determining the specific cause of drug-induced side effects or allergic reactions. In some cases, these combination drug products cost more than each drug separately; therefore, the provider must weigh the risks and benefits of using combination medications.

Drug Interactions

Other drugs can interact with medications used for diabetes control. Certain drugs or foods can have an effect on blood glucose levels by altering the action, the effect, or the outcome from a particular drug regimen. These actions are generally categorized as follows:

- Drug-drug (or pharmacokinetic) interaction
- Drug-disease (or pharmacodynamic) interaction
- Drug-food interaction

A drug-drug interaction is said to occur when a medication is added to an individual's regimen that alters the effect of another medication the person is taking. Some of these interactions are listed in Table 17.7. This type of interaction can occur with changes anywhere along

TABLE 17.6 Selected Combination Oral Medications for Type 2 Diabetes

Medication (generic)	*Available Dosages*	*Initial Dose*
ACTOplus met® (pioglitazone/metformin)	15 mg/500 mg 15 mg/850 mg	*Already on Metformin:* 15 mg/500 mg or 15 mg/850 mg once or twice a day *Already on Pioglitazone:* 15 mg/500 mg twice a day, or 15 mg/850 mg daily *Maximum Dose:* pioglitazone 45 mg/metformin 2,550 mg
Avandaryl® (rosiglitazone/glimepiride)	4 mg/1 mg 4 mg/2 mg 4 mg/4 mg	*Already on Rosiglitazone or Glimepiride:* 4 mg/1mg or 4 mg/2 mg daily *Maximum Dose:* rosiglitazone 8 mg/glimepiride 4 mg
Avandamet® (rosiglitazone/metformin)	1 mg/500 mg 2 mg/500 mg 4 mg/500 mg 2 mg/1,000 mg 4 mg/1,000 mg	*Already on Rosiglitazone:* usual rosiglitazone dose/metformin 1,000 mg divided dose twice daily *Already on Metformin:* rosiglitazone 4 mg/usual metformin dose divided dose twice daily *Maximum Dose:* rosiglitazone 8 mg/metformin 2,000 mg
Duetact® (pioglitazone/glimepiride)	30 mg/2 mg 30 mg/4 mg	*Already on Glimepiride:* 30 mg/2 mg or 30 mg/4 mg daily *Already on Pioglitazone:* 30 mg/2 mg once daily *Maximum Dose:* pioglitazone 30 mg/glimepiride 4 mg
Glucovance® (glyburide/metformin) generic available	1.25 mg/250 mg 2.5 mg/500 mg 5 mg/500 mg	*As Initial Therapy:* 1.25 mg/250 mg daily or twice daily *As Second-Line Therapy:* 2.5 mg/500 mg or 5 mg/500 mg twice daily *Maximum Dose:* glyburide 20 mg/metformin 2,000 mg
Metaglip™ (glipizide/metformin)	2.5 mg/250 mg 2.5 mg/500 mg 5 mg/500 mg	*As Initial Therapy:* 2.5 mg/250 mg daily or twice daily *Maximum for Initial Therapy:* glipizide 10 mg/metformin 2,000 mg *As Second-Line Therapy:* 2.5 mg/500 mg or 5 mg/500 mg twice daily *Maximum for Second-Line Therapy:* glipizide 20 mg/metformin 2,000 mg
Prandimet (repaglinide/metformin)	1 mg/500 mg 2 mg/500 mg	*As Initial Therapy:* 1 mg/500 mg twice daily *Already on Repaglnide:* usual repaglinide dose/500 mg metformin twice daily *Maximum Dose:* 10 mg/2,500 mg daily or 4 mg/1,000 mg per meal

(continued)

TABLE 17.6 Selected Combination Oral Medications for Type 2 Diabetes (continued)		
Medication (generic)	*Available Dosages*	*Initial Dose*
Janumet™ (sitagliptin/metformin)	50 mg/500 mg 50 mg/1,000 mg	*As Initial Therapy:* 50 mg/500 mg twice daily *Already on Metformin 850 mg or 1,000 mg twice daily:* 50 mg/1,000 mg twice daily *Already on Sitagliptin:* 50 mg/500 mg twice daily *Maximum Dose:* sitagliptin 100 mg/metformin 2,000 mg
Kombiglyze XR (saxagliptin/metformin)	5 mg/500 mg 5 mg/1,000 mg 2.5 mg/1,000 mg	*Already on Saxagliptin:* 5 mg/500 mg once daily with gradual titration *Maximum for Initial Therapy:* 5 mg/2,000 mg once daily with evening meal
Invokamet (canagliflozin/metformin)	50 mg/500 mg 10 mg/1,000 mg 150 mg/500 mg 150 mg/1,000 mg	*Already on Canagliflozin:* usual canagliflozin dose/metformin 500 mg *Already on Metformin:* canagliflozin 50 mg/usual metformin dose *Maximum Dose:* 300 mg/2,000 mg per day
Xigduo XR (dapagliflozin/metformin)	5 mg/500 mg 5 mg/1,000 mg 10 mg/500 mg 10 mg/1,000 mg	*Already on Dapagliflozin:* usual dose of dapagliflozin/metformin 500 mg *Already on Metformin:* dapagliflozin 5 mg/usual dose of metformin *Maximum Dose:* 10 mg/2,000 mg per day
Glyxambi (empagliflozin/linagliptin)	10 mg/5 mg 25 mg/5 mg	*As Initial Therapy:* 10 mg/5 mg once daily in the morning

Note: An FDA REMS severely restricts the access and distribution of drugs containing rosiglitazone.

Source: Adapted from "Drugs for type 2 diabetes," *Pharmacist's Letter/Prescriber's Letter* (2015): 310601.

TABLE 17.7 Drug-Disease and Drug-Drug Interactions				
Interacting Drug	*Drug-Disease (Intrinsic Effect)*	*Drug-Drug Interaction**	*Net Effect on Blood Glucose*	*Notes*
Allopurinol	No	Sulfonylureas and Meglitinide	↓	Decreased renal tubular secretion of chlorpropamide
Androgens/ anabolic steroids	Yes	—	↓	Mechanism unknown
Anticoagulants, vitamin K antagonists	No	Sulfonylureas and Meglitinide	↓	Unknown, may display medication from binding site

TABLE 17.7 Drug-Disease and Drug-Drug Interactions (continued)

Interacting Drug	*Drug-Disease (Intrinsic Effect)*	*Drug-Drug Interaction**	*Net Effect on Blood Glucose*	*Notes*
Aspirin	Yes[3]	Sulfonylureas and Meglitinide	↓	Large daily doses (~4 g/d): Increase basal and stimulated release of insulin Displace sulfonylurea from protein binding; decrease urinary excretion of sulfonylurea
Atypical antipsychotics	Yes		↑	Increase insulin resistance, decrease insulin secretion, weight gain Greatest risk with olanzapine and clozapine; lowest risk with aripiprazole and ziprasidone
β-Adrenergic antagonists	Yes	—	↑↓	Both hypoglycemic and hyperglycemic responses have been reported; may alter physiologic response to, and subjective symptoms of, hypoglycemia; may reduce hyperglycemia-induced insulin release or decrease tissue sensitivity to insulin
Calcium channel blockers	Yes	—	↑↓	Hypoglycemia reported with verapamil Hyperglycemia reported with diltiazem, nifedipine
Cholestyramine	No	TZD and Acarbose	↑↓	Cholestyramine reduces absorption of coadministered TZD Cholestyramine may enhance effects of acarbose; interactions may be avoided by administering cholestyramine 2 hours apart from other medications
Cimetidine/ possible other H2 antagonists	No	Sulfonylureas, Meglitinide, and Metformin	↓	Increased absorption and/or decreased clearance of glipizide and glyburide Decreased renal tubular secretion of metformin; other drugs excreted via renal tubular transport may similarly interfere with metformin clearance
Corticosteroid	Yes	—	↑	Increased gluconeogenesis; transient insulin resistance
Cyclosporine	Yes	—	↑	—
Disopyramide	Yes	—	↑	Most susceptible: elderly or persons with diabetes with renal or liver impairment
Diuretics	Yes	—	↑	—
Estrogen products	Yes	—	↑	Mechanism unknown
Ethanol	Yes	Sulfonylureas and Meglitinide	↑↓	Disulfiram-like reaction may occur, especially with chlorpropamide; not noted with second-generation sulfonylureas Chronic alcohol ingestion may increase metabolism of sulfonylurea; alcohol ingestion, especially with carbohydrate-based drink (beer, mixed drink), has caloric effect Intrinsic hypoglycemic effect; impairs gluconeogenesis and increases insulin secretion; effect is potentiated if alcohol consumed without food or in fasting state
Fluconazole	No	Sulfonylureas and Meglitinide	↓	

(continued)

TABLE 17.7 Drug-Disease and Drug-Drug Interactions (continued)

Interacting Drug	*Drug-Disease (Intrinsic Effect)*	*Drug-Drug Interaction**	*Net Effect on Blood Glucose*	*Notes*
Fluoxetine	Yes	—	↑↓	Hypoglycemia and hyperglycemia have been reported
Fibrates	Yes	—	↑	Possible pharmacokinetic OATP inhibition and displacement from protein binding sites; possible pharmacodynamics modulation of insulin secretion and resistance
Glyburide	Yes	Acarbose and Miglitol	↑	Miglitol reduces the area under the curve (AUC) and peak concentration of glyburide
Isoniazid	Yes	—	↑	Increases glycogenolysis
Ketoconazole	Yes	Pioglitazone	↑	In vitro studies suggest that ketoconazole inhibits the metabolism of pioglitazone and saxagliptin
Metformin	No	Alpha-glucosidase inhibitors	↑	Acarbose reduces metformin bioavailability by ~35% when coadministered; separate doses to avoid interaction
Monoamine oxidase inhibitors	Yes[19]	Sulfonylureas and Meglitinide	↓	May stimulate insulin secretion (beta-adrenergic stimulation) or may be secondary to hepatotoxicity May interfere with metabolism of sulfonylurea
Nicotinic acid (niacin)	Yes	—	↑	Dose dependent, when lipid-lowering doses are used Insignificant effect at vitamin supplement dose
NSAIDs (nonsteroidal anti-inflammatory drugs)	Yes	Sulfonylureas and Meglitinide	↑	Possible intrinsic hypoglycemic effect Protein-binding displacement
Oral contraceptives	Yes	Pioglitazone and Rosiglitazone	↑	Pioglitazone has not been evaluated; however, caution should be used No clinically significant effect on oral contraceptives with rosiglitazone
Pancrelipase/ pancreatic enzymes	Yes	—	↑	Do not administer these agents concurrently with acarbose
Phenothiazines	Yes	—	↑↓	Hypoglycemia observed with some phenothiazines, hyperglycemia with others
Phenytoin	Yes	—		Decreased insulin secretion
Probenecid	Yes	Sulfonylureas and Meglitinide	↓	Intrinsic glycemic effect Decrease urinary excretion of chlorpropamide
Protease inhibitors	Yes	—	↑	—
Rifampin	Yes[25]	Sulfonylureas[26], Meglitinides and SGLT2-inhibitors	↑↓	Possible intrinsic hypoglycemic effect Increased metabolism of sulfonylureas Induction SGLT-2 inhibitor metabolism by UGT induction

TABLE 17.7 Drug-Disease and Drug-Drug Interactions (continued)

Interacting Drug	*Drug-Disease (Intrinsic Effect)*	*Drug-Drug Interaction**	*Net Effect on Blood Glucose*	*Notes*
Salicylates	Yes[27]	Sulfonylureas and Meglitinide	↓	Large daily doses (~4 g/d): Increase basal and stimulated release of insulin Displace sulfonylurea from protein binding; decrease urinary excretion of sulfonylurea
Sulfonamides, highly protein-bound	No	Sulfonylureas and Meglitinide	↓	Various effects upon chlorpropamide, tolbutamide kinetics: displacement from protein binding, decreased urinary excretion, and/or altered metabolism
Tacrolimus	Yes	—	↑	—
Thyroid products	Yes	—	↑	Once euthyroid status is achieved, diabetes medications may need to be adjusted to compensate for glycemic effect of thyroid product

*Interactions with sulfonylureas, meglitinide, metformin, pioglitazone and rosiglitazone (both thiazolidinediones), alpha-glucosidase inhibitors, DPP-4 inhibitors, and insulin are listed.

Note: This listing is not intended to be all inclusive. Before any new medication is initiated, consult the package labeling (insert) or other reference. In general, these interactions are based on moderate to severe clinical significance and/or possible or established documentation.

Sources: Adapted from "Drug-Disease and Drug-Drug Interactions," in E Sisson, ed, *Quick Guide to Medications*, 6th ed. (Chicago: American Association of Diabetes Educators, 2016), 51-56; C Triplett, "Drug Interactions of Medications Commonly Used in Diabetes," *Diabetes Spectr* 19, no. 4 (2006): 202-11.

the map of drug transport through the body. Specifically, a drug can have its absorption into the body, distribution through the body, metabolism by the body—usually the liver or kidneys—and elimination from the body changed by another agent. The effect may be an increase or decrease in the rate of a particular step or an altered level of protein binding in the bloodstream, resulting in either a decreased or increased net action by the medication. This type of interaction is also termed a *pharmacokinetic interaction*, since the alteration is on the flow of the drug through its normal kinetic movement through the body.

A drug-disease interaction has an intrinsic physiologic effect, as a particular medication may alter the level of control of a particular disorder. The interaction can either improve or worsen the level of control of a particular problem and is termed a *pharmacodynamic interaction.*

Drug actions can also be altered by concurrent ingestion of certain foods. A common mechanism of this interaction is to alter the absorption of a medication from the gastrointestinal tract, although other mechanisms of interactions (eg, effect on hepatic enzymes) may also occur.

Summary

Treatment Plan for Diabetes

Diabetes management requires prompt attention to achieve glycemic control in a timely manner. Quick return to optimal blood glucose levels appears to predict more positive long-term outcomes for the person with diabetes.[76] The foundation of an effective treatment plan relies on sound person with diabetes education and support for good nutrition and physical activity habits. Each person with diabetes's treatment regimen must be individualized based on the history of drug allergies, renal and/or hepatic function, and the cost of medications. Consideration should also be given to the ability and willingness of the individual to actively participate in his or her care. With a good understanding of each person with diabetes's needs, plans can be developed that maximize glycemic control while limiting any lifestyle intrusions.

Rather than waiting for extended periods of time to evaluate drug regimen effectiveness, clinicians should aggressively advance drug therapy to achieve the desired glycemic goals. The effectiveness of any drug therapy regimen and nutrition/physical activity plan should be assessed at least every 3 months to reduce chronic complications.[1,2]

Focus on Education

Teaching Strategies

Multiple medications. Emphasize the unique function of each drug—oral agents, injection therapies, and insulin—and the options available for best control. Encourage monitoring of premeal and postmeal blood glucose levels only as necessary to observe changes and determine medication effectiveness.

New medicines. Many new products are available. Know the dosing, side effects, and population-specific issues of each agent in order to individualize drug therapy. To stay abreast of the changing landscape of agents to treat diabetes, you may find it beneficial to utilize the resources at your institution for staying up to date on new medications that come to market.

Involvement in decision making. Empowering persons with diabetes to make good decisions requires person with diabetes-appropriate presentation of factual information and honest discussion of the pros and cons for each medication. Shared documentation of results as a team also helps determine the need for medication changes. In addition, prompt attention to achievement of glycemic goals is important to long-term diabetes success.

Messages for Persons With Diabetes

Consider lifestyle changes. Aim for good nutritional intake, portion control, and a wide variety of foods when planning meals. Make scheduled physical activity and modest lifestyle adjustments part of the plan, as these will assist in weight control and blood glucose management.

Consider all the options. Seek information about each medication, including its function in your diabetes care and side effects. Ask for specific instructions as to the timing of medications; the effect of the medications on blood glucose, kidneys, and bodily functions; how to manage missed doses; and the timing of blood glucose testing. Knowing this information enables you to judge the effects of taking the medication.

Follow the prescribed medication plan. All medicines have a timed action. Many of them rely on consistency and take time to build up in the system in order to work. Some require laboratory monitoring to make certain they are tolerated by the body. The importance of following "the plan" cannot be stressed enough.

Health Literacy

Low health literacy impacts medication safety and contributes to medication errors. One study indicated that approximately half of the persons with diabetes were unable to read and correctly state 1 or more of the label instructions on 5 common prescriptions. Rates of misunderstanding were higher among persons with diabetes with marginal and low literacy. Nevertheless, more than one third of persons with diabetes with adequate literacy skills misunderstood at least 1 of the label instructions.[77]

Even when the instructions were written at a first-grade level—eg, "Take with food"—not all persons with diabetes (84%) understood them. Only 56% of persons with diabetes understood the simple instruction, "This medication should be taken with plenty of water."[77]

Health literacy is not just about reading level, plain language, and numeracy. It also relates to the problem-solving and decision-making capacity. A person with adequate health literacy can read, understand, and act appropriately on health information.

You can help your persons with diabetes understand the medications they take and provide strategies for monitoring and effective use of the drug therapies. Consider the following communication strategies:

1. Ask your person with diabetes to explain what he or she understands about the medication, why it needs to be taken, how it is being taken, and when does it not have to be taken. This way you can discover misunderstandings, gaps in knowledge, and misinterpretations.
2. Ask your person with diabetes how he or she would like to receive information or learn about a topic: by reading about it, watching a video, attending a class, or getting reminders.
3. Suggest that a support person accompany the person with diabetes on appointments. Another person's perspective may provide insight into possible barriers to effective self-care and provide ongoing support as needed.
4. Advise the person with diabetes to review medication-taking instructions with a family member or friend.
5. Ask the person with diabetes to carry his or her medication list at all times.
6. Troubleshoot existing medication-taking behaviors. Any challenges can become an opportunity to change therapy to increase engagement.

7. Reevaluate the medication-taking strategy on an ongoing basis. As the circumstances of the daily schedule change, so will the medication-taking behaviors. For example: "Now that you have to get up earlier, how will you remember/have time to take your medication?"

Successful diabetes care requires two-way communication between healthcare providers and persons with diabetes. Diabetes care and education specialists need to examine their communication skills and how they impact health literacy. Low-literacy-level literature will not provide adequate education without the diabetes care and education specialist's verbal support. When communicating with the person with diabetes, consider the following:

1. Involve the person with diabetes in treatment decisions—explore options for and what is important important to the person with diabetes.
2. Get true agreement on short- and long-term goal setting; examine whether the person with diabetes is stating a goal just to please you or whether the goal really is important to him or her.
3. Assess not just the knowledge but the skills necessary to implement the tasks needed; people with inadequate literacy may lack the skills to accomplish specific tasks and find it difficult to access and understand healthcare information.
4. Identify possible barriers of language, culture, and a healthcare system that is difficult to navigate. State some of the challenges that are common to other persons with diabetes to minimize a sense of embarrassment by the person with diabetes. Nobody wants to admit that this information is impossible to implement; by normalizing the barriers and challenges you can open a trust between you and a person with diabetes and work as a team to strategize accordingly.
5. Celebrate the successes of treatment accomplishments and build a foundation for advancement in therapy. Persons with diabetes are more likely to add additional behaviors and self-care if they have successfully accomplished something in the past. They need to feel that they can do it and that the change is a good thing in diabetes care.

Focus on Practice

Interprofessional teams. Interprofessional teamwork involves different health and/or social care professions that work closely together in an integrated and interdependent manner to solve complex care problems and deliver services. Because of the breadth and depth of issues related to diabetes, effective care management requires a highly functioning interprofessional team.

The complexity of drug therapy options demands inclusion of an interprofessional team member who is focused on medication management. Collaborative drug therapy management (CDTM) is a collaboration among the pharmacist, the person with diabetes, and other healthcare professionals that permits the clinical pharmacist to assume responsibility for performing person with diabetes assessments; ordering drug therapy-related laboratory tests; administering drugs; and selecting, initiating, monitoring, continuing, and adjusting drug regimens. The value of CDTM is to leverage the drug-therapy knowledge of pharmacists to achieve optimal medication-related outcomes, while allowing other interprofessional team members to contribute at the top of their professional skill and training.

Rate of engagement in taking medications for persons with type 2 diabetes range from 65% to 85% for oral agents and 60% to 80% for insulin.[76] The barriers to medication engagement include understanding of the treatment regimen, complexity of the treatment regimen, perception of the benefits of treatment, adverse effects, costs of medications, and emotional well-being. Engagement with taking medications should be assessed at every person with diabetes care visit. When persons with diabetes are started on new medications, it is important to address how this medication will help them control their diabetes, what are potential side effects, and how to manage missed doses. Providing this information will enable the person with diabetes to feel empowered with the appropriate information that is needed for self-management and ensure they are involved in their medical decision making as a member of the team.

References

1. American Diabetes Association. 9. Pharmacologic approaches to glycemic treatment: standards of medical care in diabetes—2020. Diabetes Care. 2020 Jan; 43(Suppl 1): S98-110. https://doi .org/10.2337/dc20-S009.
2. Garber AJ, Handelsman Y, Grunberger G, et al. Consensus statement by the American Association of Clinical Endocrinologists and American College of Endocrinology on the comprehensive type 2 diabetes management algorithm—2020 executive summary. Endocr Pract. 2020 Jan;26(1):107-139. doi:10.4158 /CS-2019-0472.
3. American Diabetes Association. 6. Glycemic targets: standards of medical care in diabetes—2019. Diabetes Care 2019 Jan; 42 (Supplement 1): S61-S70. doi.org/10.2337/dc19-S006.
4. LeRoith D, Biessels GJ, Braithwaite SS, et al. Treatment of diabetes in older adults: an endocrine society* clinical practice guideline. J Clin Endocrinol Metab. 2019;104(5): 1520-74. doi:10.1210/jc.2019-00198.
5. Kirkman MS, Jones Briscoe V, Clark N, et al. Diabetes in older adults: a consensus report. J Am Geriatr Soc. 2012;60(12):2342-56.
6. American Diabetes Association. 8. Obesity management for the treatment of type 2 diabetes: standards of medical care in diabetes—2019. Diabetes Care 2019 Jan; 42(Supplement 1): S81-S89. doi.org/10.2337/dc19-S008.
7. Fleming JW, McClendon KS, Riche DM. New obesity agents: lorcaserin and phentermine/topiramate. Ann Pharmacother. 2013;47:1007-16.
8. Brown JB, Conner C, Nichols GA. Secondary failure of metformin monotherapy in clinical practice. Diabetes Care. 2010;33:501-6.
9. Belviq [package insert]. Zofingen, Switzerland: Arena Pharmaceuticals GmbH; 2012.
10. Xenical [package insert]. San Francisco: Genentech, Inc.; 2012.
11. Contrave [package insert]. La Jolla, Calif: Orexigen Therapeutics, Inc.; 2014.
12. Qysmia [package insert]. Mountain View, Calif: Vivus, Inc.; 2014.
13. Saxenda [package insert]. Plainsboro, NJ: Novo Nordisk; 2014.
14. Adipex [package insert]. Sellersville, Pa: Teva Pharmaceuticals USA; 2012.
15. Tenuate [package insert]. Bridgewater, NJ: Aventis Pharmaceuticals Inc.; 2003.
16. Phendimetrazine [package insert]. Princeton, NJ: Sandoz Inc.; 2011.
17. Committee on Practice Bulletins Obstetrics. ACOG Practice Bulletin No. 190: Gestational Diabetes Mellitus. Obstet Gynecol 2018;131:e49–64.
18. Balsells M, Garcia-Patterson A, Sola I, Roque M, Gich I, Corcoy R. Glibenclamide, metformin, and insulin for the treatment of gestational diabetes: a systematic review and meta-analysis. BMJ 2015;350:h102.
19. American Geriatrics Society 2019 Updated AGS Beers criteria for potentially inappropriate medication use in older adults. J Am Geriatr Soc. 2019 Apr;67(4):674-94.
20. Burden M. Culturally sensitive care: managing diabetes during Ramadan. Br J Community Nurs. 2001;6:581-5.
21. Nathan DM, Buse JB, Davidson MB, et al. Medical management of hyperglycemia in type 2 diabetes: a consensus algorithm for the initiation and adjustment of therapy. Diabetes Care. 2009;32:193-203.
22. Stenman S, Melander A, Groop PH, Groop LC. What is the benefit of increasing the sulfonylurea dose? Ann Intern Med. 1993;118:169.
23. Prandin [package insert]. Princeton, NJ: Novo Nordisk; 2008.
24. Starlix [package insert]. East Hanover, NJ: Novartis Pharmaceuticals Corporation; 2013.
25. Glucophage [package insert]. Princeton, NJ: Bristol-Myers Squibb Company; 2009.
26. US Food and Drug Administration. FDA drug safety communication: FDA revises warnings regarding use of the diabetes medicine metformin in certain persons with diabetes with reduced kidney function. Last updated 2016 Apr 20 (cited 2016 May 26). On the Internet at: http://www.fda.gov/Drugs/DrugSafety/ ucm493244.htm.
27. UK Prospective Diabetes Study Group. Effect of intensive blood-glucose control with metformin on complications in overweight persons with diabetes with type 2 diabetes (UKPDS 34). Lancet. 1998;352:854-65.
28. Aviles-Santa L, Sinding J, Raskin P. Effects of metformin in persons with diabetes with poorly controlled, insulin-treated type 2 diabetes. Ann Intern Med. 1999;131:182-8.
29. Yale JF, Valiquett TR, Ghazzi MN, et al. The effect of a thiazolidinedione drug, troglitazone, on glycemia in persons with diabetes with type 2 diabetes mellitus poorly controlled with sulfonylurea and metformin: a multimember, randomized, double-blind, placebo-controlled trial. Ann Intern Med. 2001;134:737-45.
30. Avandia [package insert]. Research Triangle Park, NC: GlaxoSmithKline; 2019.
31. Ferwana M, Firwana B, Hasan R, et al. Pioglitazone and risk of bladder cancer: a meta-analysis of controlled studies. Diabet Med. 2013;30:1026-32.
32. Campbell LK, Baker DE, Campbell RK. Miglitol: assessment of its role in the treatment of persons with diabetes with diabetes mellitus. Ann Pharmacother. 2000;34:1291-301.

33. Precose [package insert]. Wayne, NJ: Bayer Pharmaceuticals Inc; 2011.
34. Cycloset [package insert]. Tiverton, RI: Veroscience; 2009.
35. Nisly SA, Kolanczyk DM, Walton AM. Canagliflozin, a new sodium-glucose cotransporter 2 inhibitor, in the treatment of diabetes. Am J Health Syst Pharm. 2013;70:311-9.
36. Zelniker, Wiviott SD, Raz I, et al. SGLT2 inhibitors for primary and secondary prevention of cardiovascular and renal outcomes in type 2 diabetes: a systematic review and meta-analysis of cardiovascular outcome trials. *Lancet.* 2019; 393:31-9.
37. Jardiance [package insert]. Ridgefield, Conn: Boehringer Ingelheim Pharmaceuticals Inc.; 2016.
38. Farxiga [Package insert]. Wilmington, Del.: AstraZeneca Pharmaceuticals LP; 2016.
39. Steglatro [package insert]. Whitehouse Station, NJ: Merck & Co. Inc.; 2017.
40. Invokana [package insert]. Titusville, NJ: Janssen Pharmaceuticals Inc.; 2013.
41. Fadini GP, Avogaro A. SGTL2 inhibitors and amputations in the US FDA Adverse Event Reporting System. Lancet Diabetes Endocrinol. 2017; 5:680–681. doi: 10.1016/S2213-8587(17)30257-7.
42. Welchol [package insert]. Parsippany, NJ. Daiichi Sankyo, Inc.; 2011.
43. Vilsboll T, Krarup T, Deacon CF, Madsbad S, Holst JJ. Reduced postprandial concentrations of intact biologically active glucagon-like peptide in type 2 diabetic persons with diabetes. Diabetes. 2001;50:609-13.
44. Pfeffer MA, Claggett B, Diaz R, Dickstein K, et al. Lixisenatide in persons with diabetes with type 2 diabetes and acute coronary syndrome. N Engl J Med. 2015;373(23):2247-57.
45. Lytvyn Y, Bjornstad P, Udell JA, Lovshin JA, Cheney DZI. Sodium glucose transporter-2 inhibition of heart failure: potential mechanisms, cllinical applications, and summary of clinical trials. *Circulation.* 2017;136:1643-58.
46. Bydureon [package insert]. Princeton, NJ: Bristol-Myers Squibb Company; 2013.
47. Victoza [package insert]. Princeton, NJ: Novo Nordisk; 2010.
48. Byetta [package insert]. Wilmington, Del: AstraZeneca Pharmaceuticals Inc.; 2015.
49. Ozempic [package insert]. Plainsboro, JN: Novo Nordisk; 2019.
50. Trulicity [package insert]. Indianapolis, Ind: Eli Lilly and Company; 2015.
51. Barnett AH. Exenatide. Drugs Today. 2005;41:563-78.
52. Januvia [package insert]. Whitehouse Station, NJ: Merck & Co Inc; 2009.
53. Onglyza [package insert]. Princeton, NJ: Bristol-Myers Squibb Company; 2009.
54. US Food and Drug Administration. FDA drug safety communication: FDA warns that DPP-4 inhibitors for type 2 diabetes may cause severe joint pain. Last updated 2016 Apr 20 (cited 2016 Aug 29). On the Internet at: http://www.fda.gov/Drugs/DrugSafety/ucm459579.htm.
55. Nolte MS, Karam JH. Pancreatic hormones and antidiabetic drugs. In: Katzung B, ed. Basic and Clinical Pharmacology. 8th ed. New York: Lange Medical Books/McGraw Hill; 2001:711.
56. Weyer C, Fineman MS, Strobel S, et al. Properties of pramlintide and insulin upon mixing. Am J Health Syst Pharm. 2005;62:816-20.
57. Schmitz O, Brock B, Rungby J. Amylin agonists: a novel approach in treatment of diabetes. Diabetes. 2004;53 Suppl:S233-8.
58. Symlin [package insert]. Wilmington, DE: AstraZeneca Pharmaceuticals LP; 2014.
59. Comparison of insulins. Pharmacist's Letter/Prescriber's Letter. 2006;22(3):220309.
60. Ratner RE, Hirsch IB, Neifing JL, Garg SK, Mecca TE, Wilson CA. Less hypoglycemia with insulin glargine in intensive insulin therapy for type 1 diabetes: US study group of insulin glargine in type 1 diabetes. Diabetes Care. 2000;23:639-43.
61. McQueen J. Pramlintide acetate. Am J Health Syst Pharm. 2005;62:2363-72.
62. Guyton AC, Hall JE, eds. Textbook of Medical Physiology. 10th ed. Philadelphia: WB Saunders; 2000:884.
63. American Diabetes Association. Hyperglycemic crises in diabetes. Diabetes Care. 2004 Jan;27 Suppl 1: S94-102.
64. Xultophy [package insert]. Plainsboro, NJ: Novo Nordisk, Inc.; 2019.
65. Soliqua [package insert]. Bridgewater, NJ: Sanofi-aventis U.S. LLC; 2019.
66. Gibney MA, Arce CH, Byron KJ, Hirsch LJ. Skin and subcutaneous adipose layer thickness in adults with diabetes at sites used for insulin injections: implications for needle length recommendations. Curr Med Res Opin. 2010;26:1519-30.
67. Hirsch LJ, Gibney MA, Albanese J, Qu S, Kassler-Taub K. Comparative glycemic control, safety and person with diabetes ratings for a new 4 mm × 32G insulin pen needle in adults with diabetes. Curr Med Res Opin. 2010;26:1531-41.
68. American Diabetes Association. Insulin administration (position statement). Diabetes Care. 2004;27 Suppl 1:S106-7.
69. Afrezza [package insert]. Danbury, Conn: MannKind Corporation; 2016.
70. Powers AC, D'Alessio D. Endocrine pancreas and pharmacotherapy of diabetes mellitus and hypoglycemia. In Brunton LL, Chabner BA, Knollmann BC, eds. Goodman & Gilman's: The Pharmacological Basis of Therapeutics, 12 ed. 2011 (cited 2016 Sep 1). On the Internet at: http://accesspharmacy.mhmedical.com.proxy.library.vcu.edu/content.aspx?bookid=1613&Sectionid=102162253.

71. Griffin ME, Feder A, Tamborlane WV. Lipoatrophy associated with lispro insulin in insulin pump therapy: an old complication, a new cause? Diabetes Care. 2001;24:174.

72. Bodtger U, Wittrup M. A rational clinical approach to suspected insulin allergy: status after five years and 22 cases. Diabet Med. 2005;22:102-6.

73. American Diabetes Association. Nutrition recommendations and interventions for diabetes. Diabetes Care. 2008;31 Suppl 1:S61-78.

74. Agiostratidou G, Anhalt H, Ball D, et al. Standardizing clinically meaningful outcome measures beyond HbA1c for type 1 diabetes: a consensus report of the American Association of Clinical Endocrinologists, the American Association of Diabetes Educators, the American Diabetes Association, the Endocrine Society, JDRF International, The Leona M. and Harry B. Helmsley Charitable Trust, the Pediatric Endocrine Society, and the T1D Exchange. Diabetes Care 2017;40:1622-30.

75. Rubin RR. Adherence to pharmacologic therapy in persons with diabetes with type 2 diabetes mellitus. Am J Med. 2005;118:27 S-34 S.

76. Krentz AJ, Bailey CJ. Oral hypoglycemic agents: current role in type 2 diabetes mellitus. Drugs. 2005;65:385-411.

77. Davis TC, Wolf MS, Bass PF III, et al. Literacy and misunderstanding prescription drug labels. Ann Intern Med. 2006;145(12):887-94.

CHAPTER 18

Glucose Monitoring

Mary M. Austin, MA, RDN, CDCES, FADCES
Beth A. Olson, MHA, RN, CDCES

Key Concepts

- Glucose monitoring includes self-monitoring of blood glucose (SMBG) and continuous glucose monitoring (CGM) which measures interstitial glucose. Both methods provide data that is beneficial for glucose pattern management. In addition, CGM is a useful tool for filling glucose data gaps.
- Glucose monitoring plays a key role in supporting self-care behaviors and decision-making. Structured, accurate monitoring plays a role in achieving target glucose levels and reducing complications.
- Structured glucose monitoring schedules are essential in order to interpret the effects of food, physical activity, and medications on glycemic goals.
- Diabetes care and education specialists need to recognize the value of glucose monitoring as a tool for prevention and early diagnosis and to delay progression of the related complications and comorbidities that result in disabilities that may compromise effective self-management and reduce quality of life.
- Diabetes care and education specialists need to be aware of the operational and interpretive aspects of SMBG and CGM as well as the key teaching components and skill set requirements of each.

Introduction

Monitoring is one of the AADE7 Self-Care Behaviors® and thereby is recognized as an important component of the treatment plan for persons with diabetes. Although diabetes is mostly a self-managed disease, the individual still relies on healthcare professionals for monitoring, advice, and support as life changes and health needs change.[1] Healthcare professionals need to understand the parameters that require monitoring, as well as recognize those that must be monitored by them and those that are or can be self-monitored by the individual.[2,3] The 2019 Standards of Medical Care in Diabetes by the American Diabetes Association (ADA) and the 2016 Consensus Statement on Glucose Monitoring by the American Association of Clinical Endocrinologists (AACE) and the Academy of Clinical Endocrinologists (ACE) provide guidance and direction regarding best practices for monitoring in diabetes.[4,5] This chapter primarily focuses on SMBG and CGM; other aspects of diabetes management that require monitoring are discussed in appropriate chapters throughout this book.

Self-Monitoring of Blood Glucose

Self-monitoring of blood glucose provides people with diabetes the information they need to assess how food, physical activity, and medications affect their blood glucose levels. The ADA 2019 Standards of Care states, "Glucose monitoring allows individuals to evaluate their individual response to therapy and assess whether glycemic targets are being safely achieved. Integrating results to diabetes management can be a useful tool for guiding medical nutrition therapy and physical activity, preventing hypoglycemia, and adjusting medications (particularly prandial insulin doses)."[4] Persons performing SMBG and utilizing SMBG results need to understand how to properly operate the meter and utilize supporting apps, if provided, interpret the results, and take appropriate action. Self-monitoring of blood glucose in itself is not a therapeutic intervention. The action taken as a result of utilizing the SMBG data becomes the therapeutic intervention.

Diabetes care and education specialists can play a pivotal role in helping individuals incorporate blood glucose monitoring into their self-management and care. In 2018 the American Association of Diabetes Educators (AADE)–as of January 2020, the Association for Diabetes Care & Education Specialists (ADCES)–released the Practice Paper, "Self-Monitoring of Blood Glucose Using Glucose Meters in the Management of Type 2 Diabetes," which identifies the following practices for the diabetes care and education specialist:[6]

- SMBG readings are to be used in clinical decision-making by every member of the individual's healthcare team.
- Diabetes self-management education and support must include instruction on recognizing blood glucose levels that are out of the target range and taking the appropriate action steps in response to such readings.
- In appropriate cases where barriers such as cognitive limitations impede effective use of SMBG, diabetes care and education specialists and people with type 2 diabetes need to individualize regular performance of SMBG, based on the person's needs and abilities.

SMBG provides immediate feedback and data. SMBG not only refers to the checking of blood glucose levels but also utilizing the results to make lifestyle and medication decisions. Specifically, obtaining and using this data help with the following:[4,5]

- Achieving and maintaining target goals for blood glucose
- Preventing and detecting hypoglycemia, including hypoglycemia unawareness
- Preventing and detecting hyperglycemia and avoiding diabetic ketoacidosis (DKA) or hyperosmolar hyperglycemic nonketotic syndrome (HHNS)
- Evaluating the glycemic response to types and amounts of food and physical activity
- Evaluating the glycemic response to stress, eg, illness, injury
- Determining appropriate insulin-to-carbohydrate ratios, correction factors, and basal insulin rates for intensive management (multiple daily injections and insulin pumps)
- Adjusting treatment in response to changes in lifestyle and the need to add, subtract, increase, or decrease dosages or types of pharmacologic therapies
- Determining the need for adjustment in insulin dosages during illness
- Determining the need for pharmacologic therapy in gestational diabetes

Two skill sets are required in order to successfully perform SMBG with the goal of improving diabetes outcomes. The person performing SMBG or the caregiver must be competent and confident in obtaining a blood sample and (1) operating the meter and (2) interpreting the SMBG data to make behavior changes. The latter is considered a "problem-solving" self-care behavior. Depending on how, when, and where the person initially receives a blood glucose meter, the diabetes care and education specialist may or may not be directly involved in teaching both of these skill sets. However, it is important for the diabetes care and education specialist to assess both of these skill sets at the time of diabetes education and to be aware of potential barriers to implementing SMBG.

Using the Meter—Operational Skills

As with other self-care behaviors, if individuals with diabetes or caregivers are to integrate and embrace SMBG as part of their diabetes management, they must first learn the operational (technical) skills, understand their value, and be able to replicate the skill sets, as applicable.[7] The checklist for SMBG education outlines the operational skills required for successful SMBG (see Table 18.1).

Select a Meter

Choice of meter will depend on factors such as insurance coverage, an assessment of manual dexterity and visual acuity, and the individual's unique needs or desires. The diabetes care and education specialist can assist individuals with meter selection by reviewing the following factors that affect choice:

- *Availability and cost:* specific meter(s) covered by insurance or governmental plans, coverage for cost of lancets, lancing device, test strips, meter, and out-of-pocket expense
- *Overall size and shape of the meter and strips*
- *Ease of use:* physical dexterity, number of steps to check blood glucose, size of the readout, and required blood sample size
- *Optional features:* screen font size and high-contrast backlighting, audio capability, memory capacity, required blood sample size, calibration (no coding), computer download features, average glucose data display, flagging of events, and incorporated bolus calculator, smartphone app compatibility, and ability to share data through Bluetooth or cellular technology
- *General preference of the individual*

More often than not, for those who have healthcare insurance, either private or governmental, meter selection

TABLE 18.1 Checklist for SMBG Education

Using the Meter—Operational Skills	*Using the Data—Interpretation Skills*
• Select a meter • Ensure meter accuracy • Obtain adequate blood sample • Perform the glucose check • Access the SMBG data (personally documented or electronically downloaded) • Address individual needs, eg, dexterity, visual or cognitive limitations	• Know blood glucose targets or goals • Understand frequency and timing of glucose checks • Use pattern management

is limited to certain meters covered by the health insurance plan or mail order service. Checking which meters are covered prior to the diabetes education visit saves time and prevents frustration. Some insurance plans provide coverage for a variety of meters and supplies.

This could be done at the pharmacy when the prescription for diabetes glucose monitoring supplies is presented. In the best-case scenario, several meters can be demonstrated and the person with diabetes can be given the opportunity to "practice" using them. More often than not, sampling meters is not possible; however, it is important for the diabetes care and education specialist to evaluate whether the choice of the meter provided is in itself a potential barrier to the individual using the meter. Sometimes individuals require a feature or meter that partners with another device that they use (eg, insulin pump) that is not preferred by the insurance company. It is important to know that the diabetes care and education specialist and the prescriber can appeal to the insurance company for coverage for the medical necessity.

Medicare Coverage If individuals have Medicare Part B coverage, the following supplies are covered for all people with diabetes: blood glucose meters, test strips, lancing devices and lancets, replacement batteries, and control solutions for checking the accuracy of glucose monitoring equipment, and test strips. Medicare will cover self blood glucose monitoring equipment and supplies only if individuals have a prescription from their prescriber that includes the following information: the individual's diagnosis of diabetes, the kind of meter needed and why (eg, a special meter because of low vision), whether the individual uses insulin, and how often the individual should check his or her blood glucose.

It is important for diabetes care and educations specialists to be aware of continual changes to Medicare regulations regarding coverage of meters, strips, and supplies. For example, for persons using insulin, Medicare currently covers 100 glucose monitoring test strips and lancets per month and 1 lancing device every 6 months. If not using insulin, individuals will receive 100 glucose monitoring test strips and 100 lancets every 3 months and 1 lancing device every 6 months.[8] Coverage for additional strips is possible if requested by the prescribing healthcare provider and medical necessity is documented, such as a change in medication class or frequent hypoglycemia. On July 1, 2013, the Centers for Medicare & Medicaid Services (CMS) implemented a National Mail Order Program for Diabetes Testing Supplies as part of a DMEPOS (Durable Medical Equipment, Prosthetics, Orthotics, and Supplies) Competitive Bidding Program. This is part of a larger effort to change the way Medicare pays for items considered as durable medical equipment (DME), ie, wheelchairs, oxygen, hospital beds, blood glucose meters, etc. The intent of the program is to lower the out-of-pocket expense for the user.[9] In February, 2018 Congress took action on the Protecting Access to Diabetes Supplies Act whereby language was added to the National Mail Order Program to provide individuals greater access and choice in diabetes glucose monitoring supplies. The DMEPOS Program expired on December 31, 2019 and a temporary gap program is in effect until December 31, 2020.[10] Detailed information on the National Mail-Order Program for Diabetes Testing Supplies as well as other blood glucose monitoring resources can be found on the ADCES Web site (www.diabeteseducator.org).[11]

Private Insurance Most private insurance plans follow Medicare guidelines for coverage of diabetes supplies. Some insurance plans consider the meter and glucose monitoring supplies as part of an individual's pharmacy benefit while others consider them a DME benefit. Individuals may be directed by their insurance carrier to obtain their meter and supplies from a local pharmacy or place an order with a DME supplier that will ship the supplies directly to the individual. Refills for subsequent mailed supplies need to be requested by the individual; auto shipment of supplies is not allowed.

Individuals should be encouraged to learn about the specifics of their insurance plan coverage for blood glucose meters and supplies. Obtaining the meter and supplies from the insurance plan's specified supplier will ensure that the glucose monitoring supplies are covered and at the least cost to the individual. This should be a cost savings for the individual, which will help reduce the financial barrier to blood glucose monitoring. There are times when the insurance co-pay is greater than the full price of some of the large store brand meters; options should be discussed with the individual.

Ensure Meter Accuracy

Meaningful utilization of SMBG data are dependent on the accuracy of the glucose measurement, which depends on multiple factors.[12,13] Some meters are more accurate than others. The International Organization for Standardization (ISO) sets minimum accuracy requirements for blood glucose meters. The US Food and Drug Administration (FDA) requires that glucose meters meet ISO performance standards. In 2013, ISO released ISO/FDIS 15197:2013: In Vitro Diagnostic Systems—Requirements for Blood-Glucose Monitoring Systems for Self-Testing in Managing Diabetes Mellitus. The updated standard requires that 95% of readings be (1) within +15% of reference for glucose levels >100 mg/dL (5.5 mmol/L) and (2) within +15 mg/dL (.8 mmol/L) of the reference for glucose levels <100 mg/dL (5.5 mmol/L). Additionally, 99% of readings must be within Zones A and B of the survey-derived consensus grid for type 1 diabetes.[14] This standard took effect in May 2016; this standard will apply to all FDA-cleared meters released into the marketplace going forward. Meters cleared by the FDA prior to 2013 which meet the 2003 ISO 15197:2003 Standard are grandfathered and do not need to meet the more stringent 2013 ISO Standard.[15] In 2017, the Diabetes Technology Society's Blood Glucose Monitoring System (BGMS) Surveillance Program tested 18 FDA-cleared popular meters and found that only 6 meters met the 2013 ISO standard for accuracy.[13,16] Since this study, one additional meter has met the accuracy standard (see Table 18.2).[17] The product specification section of a meter's user manual should indicate what percent of the time (5%, 10%, or 15%) the meter is with the reference lab value. If unavailable in the user manual, contact customer service for the specific meter to request this information.

Human errors can contribute to inaccurate data. To ensure meter accuracy, individuals should be encouraged to do the following:

- Use clean, dry fingers that have been washed with soap and water, *not* alcohol.
- Apply an adequate size blood droplet.
- Use a properly stored meter and strips (avoid temperature extremes, high humidity, or open vial).
- Use in-date, compatible, and defective-free strips.
- Code the meter (aligning strip lot and meter), if required.
- Perform control solution checks on a regular basis and when starting a new box of strips, if required.
- Keep meter clean and free of dried blood or debris.

TABLE 18.2 Blood Glucose Meters Meeting Current ISO Standards for Accuracy (16)

Manufacturer	*Blood Glucose Meter*	*Connectivity*
Ascensia (formerly Bayer)	Contour Next	Computer download through micro USB cable
Roche	Accu-Chek Aviva Plus	Bluetooth
Arkray	Walmart ReliOn Confirm (Micro)	Cable
AgaMatrix	CVS Advanced	Bluetooth
Abbott	Free-Style Lite	Computer download through USB cable
Roche	Accu-Chek Smart View	Bluetooth
Smart Meter	iGlucose (17)	Cellular, smartphone app

Other factors that may influence blood glucose results are listed in Table 18.3.

An individual's safety is always foremost when evaluating glucose results. If physical symptoms are not consistent with blood glucose results (eg, hypoglycemic symptoms with in-target SMBG values), a repeat SMBG check should be performed. However, if hypoglycemic symptoms persist regardless of SMBG values obtained, the individual should treat the hypoglycemia promptly.

Details on the use of strips, control solution, and meters as well as the correct technique for obtaining the blood sample are given in the paragraphs that follow.

Guidelines for teaching individuals how to operate their blood glucose meters are summarized in Table 18.4.

Identifying Barriers to SMBG

Potential user barriers to implementation of SMBG are important to identify up front so discussion of how to resolve these barriers may ensue. Table 18.5 provides examples of potential barriers and possible solutions.

Use of Strips

To yield accurate results, the strips must be compatible with the meter being used, be stored according to the manufacturer's guidelines, be coded correctly (if required), and be within the expiration date. Once opened, the strips will expire within 3 to 6 months (check manufacturer's guide for recommendation).

TABLE 18.3 Common Factors Affecting Accuracy of Blood Glucose Results

Problem	*Result*	*Recommendation*
Test strip not fully inserted into meter	False low	Always be sure strip is fully inserted into meter
Sample site (eg, the fingertip) is contaminated with a glucose source (eg, juice)	False high	Always clean site with soap and water, alcohol wipe, or non-fragrant, non-glucose hand cleaner before sampling
Not enough blood applied to strip	False low	Warm finger, rub finger to bring blood to the fingertip; have lancing device at appropriate depth setting; repeat check with a new sample
Batteries low on power	Error codes	Change batteries and repeat sample collection
Strips/control solution stored at temperature extremes	False high/low	Do not use; obtain new strips/solution and store according to directions
Person is dehydrated	False high	Stat venous sample on main lab analyzer
Person is in shock	False low	Stat venous sample on main lab analyzer
Squeezing fingertip too hard because blood is not flowing	False low	Repeat check with a new sample from a new site
Sites other than fingertips	High/low	Results from alternative sites may not match finger-stick results
Strip/solution vial cracked	False high/low	Do not use; obtain new strips/solution
Anemia/decreased hematocrit	False high	Venous sample on main lab analyzer
Polycythemia/increased hematocrit	False low	Venous sample on main lab analyzer
Defective strips (giving inaccurate and erratic results)	False low/high	Report to the manufacturer and your distributor for replacement

Source: Adapted from US Food and Drug Administration (FDA), "How to Safely Use Glucose Meters and Test Strips for Diabetes" (Current as of 04/10/2019), on the Internet at: https://www.fda.gov/consumers/consumer-updates/how-safely-use-glucose-meters-and-test-strips-diabetes.

TABLE 18.4 Guidelines for Teaching Individuals How to Operate a Blood Glucose Meter

- Use universal precautions: change lancets, end-caps, and gloves for each person seen. Additionally, follow your institution's policies regarding use of a multiuse/patient device with regard to device quality checks.
- Encourage the individual to lance the finger or alternative site at the beginning of the session to minimize anxiety about the discomfort involved.
- Demonstrate how to check blood glucose using control solution first and then using the individual's blood.
- After demonstrating this technique, ask the individual to provide a return demonstration before you begin teaching about control solution, calibration (if required), cleaning, and how to log blood glucose results.
- Explain how to dispose of lancets in an appropriate sharps container.
- Demonstrate how to document blood glucose in a logbook or download software to retrieve blood glucose data.
- Evaluate the individual's technique at every opportunity.
- Consider using a "demo only" meter using control solution only.

Sources: American Association of Diabetes Educators, "Position statement: educating providers and persons with diabetes to prevent the transmission of bloodborne infections and avoid injuries from sharps," *Diabetes Educ* 23 (1997): 401-3; American Association of Diabetes Educators, "Preventing infection and injury during blood glucose monitoring and injectable medication administration," AADE practice advisory, issued 2013 Dec 19.

All meters have companion strips made by the same manufacturer. Generic or "third-party" strips are made by a different manufacturer and are typically less expensive. It is important that the generic strips work with the meter for which they are used. The generic strip may *look* like the meter manufacturer's strip, but that does not mean it is compatible with the meter. If inconsistent results occur when using generic strips, it may be better to use the

TABLE 18.5 Identifying Barriers to SMBG

Type of Potential Barrier	*Description*	*Possible Solution (depends on the real cause of the barrier)**
Physical	Lack of manual dexterity or visual deficits	• Select meter and strips that are an easy size to handle and maneuver • Select meter with large numbers and high-contrast backlighting or a talking meter for the visually impaired
Financial	Inadequate or lack of insurance coverage for glucose monitoring supplies	• Focus monitoring times to maximize use of strips • Ensure monitoring technique does not waste strips • Explore programs offered by meter companies and social service agencies to provide supplies • Find a pharmacy or medical equipment supplier that is enrolled in Medicare (as applicable) and accepts assignment • Compare cash price of supplies from various pharmacies for the best price • Explore assistance programs sponsored by device and medication manufacturers
Cognitive	Cognitive deficits that make it impossible to carry out the monitoring procedure without assistance	• Engage caregivers or assistants in education and provide written directions at the level of the user and assistants • Adjust monitoring time and frequency to fit schedule of the assistants • Suggest reminder aids
Time constraints	Real or perceived lack of time to perform blood glucose checks	• Review operational skills to increase confidence in technique • Reinforce that the SMBG results are not a "test" but rather feedback to be used along with other information • Engage caregivers to help perform the blood glucose check
Health literacy/ numeracy[1]	Difficulty understanding steps, recording SMBG data, and interpreting results	• Ask the individual how to do SMBG and record the description using his/her own words and/or pictures • Practice completing a logbook that the individual designs with you • Consider the meter's download capabilities so that the individual doesn't have to record data that you can easily obtain • Assess numeracy skills[2]
Inconvenience	Choosing not to stop current activity to check blood glucose, limited access to hand-washing facilities, working in climate extremes that make access to blood glucose meter challenging	• Problem-solve what would help the individual to do the blood glucose check • Provide suggestions to keep the meter and strips within recommended temperature guidelines
Emotional	Fear of performing SMBG checks due to anticipated pain, fear of being noticed as being different, denial of diabetes, lack of support from family or caregivers	• Listen for fears and concerns and acknowledge that others have felt the same way • Discuss options to decrease fear, eg, less frequent glucose checking, assistance with checking • Suggest accessing support by joining a diabetes support group or by receiving counseling to address concerns

*Be sure to determine the root cause of the barrier to ensure the solution addresses the appropriate need. Additionally, ask the individual how he or she feels about doing the blood glucose check and whether he or she is confident in performing the check and using the results. Determine whether the individual has the basic operational and interpretive skills necessary for successful SMBG.

Sources:

1. CY Osborn, K Cavanaugh, KA Wallston, RO White, RL Rothman, "Diabetes numeracy: an overlooked factor in understanding racial disparities in glycemic control," *Diabetes Care*. 32(9)(2009):1614-9. Epub 2009 Apr 28.
2. K Cavanugh, MM Huizinga, KA Wallston, et al, "Association of numeracy and diabetes control," *Ann Intern Med*. 148(2008):737-46.

manufacturer's strips so it can be determined whether the strips are the problem or whether the inconsistent results are due to some other reason.

The expiration date of the strips should be checked prior to use, as expired strips may be inaccurate and the manufacturer will not guarantee or warrantee the accuracy of the results. Strips should be stored appropriately. Users should be instructed to store the strips in a dry place and to always make sure the strip bottle is properly sealed so strips are not exposed to light, moisture, and temperature variations. Additionally, to avoid introducing moisture into the strip vial, fingers should be completely dry when dispensing strips. Each meter and set of strips has its own storage requirements which are found in the user manual, and these should be reviewed with the individual.

Code the Meter

Coding is performed to align strip lot and meter. The majority of meters available today do this automatically, whereas some meters require setting a code or inserting a chip or strip. If this is required, coding should be performed with each new box of strips per manufacturer instructions. Using an incorrect code can give the user false low or high blood glucose values.

Control Solution

Control solution is a product provided by manufacturers to verify the integrity of the glucose monitoring strips. A control solution check should be performed every time a new box of strips is opened. This is an underused method of verifying strip accuracy. A drop of control solution is placed on a strip, or enters the strip, in the same manner as when a drop of blood is used. Every manufacturer provides at least 1 control solution vial, and some have low-, normal-, and high-level control solutions to the meter at extremes.

Follow-up discussions or initial visits with a person newly referred for education may reveal that the person has not been using control solution for a variety of reasons: its use or importance was not explained, the person did not want to "waste" a strip (because strips are costly) that could have been used to check his or her own blood, or the person's insurance plan does not cover the cost of the control solution. It is important that the individual's prescription for monitoring include not only the meter, strips, and lancets but also an order for control solution. An insurance plan that covers control solution will do so only with a prescription for it. The diabetes care and education specialist can discuss these needs with the person and problem solve regarding this aspect of ensuring meter accuracy.

Care of Meter

The manufacturer's instructions should be followed for cleaning the meter. When traveling, the individual should take extra care to keep the meter and all other monitoring supplies safe; usually this means carried with them and not packed in a suitcase. The cargo compartments of buses, airplanes, and trains, as well as automobile trunks, may be too hot or too cold to store a meter and supplies. Extreme temperatures may damage the meter, render the test strip enzyme inactive, or cause a delay in its readiness to function (eg, requiring several hours for the meter to warm up in very cold weather). Current Transportation Security Administration regulations allow meters, blood glucose test strips, lancets, alcohol swabs, control solution, and sharps disposal containers past the security checkpoint after screening.[18]

Obtain an Adequate Blood Sample

It is important that the individual provide an adequate blood sample. Some meters reject an inadequate sample, whereas other meters have a feature (usually an error message) that signals the user when the blood sample is not large enough to provide an accurate reading. Unfortunately, this feature creates a false sense of security because users assume that if they do not get an error message, they have given an adequate sample. The meter will only signal the user about a blood sample it cannot process; any other sample, even an inadequate one, registers a reading, but the reading can be inaccurate. Diabetes care and educations specialists have the opportunity at each visit to ask the individual to demonstrate his or her meter techniques. This demonstration gives the diabetes care and education specialist an opportunity to verify technique, provide guidance, or clean a soiled unit. Universal precautions should be followed by the diabetes care and education specialist when handling a used blood glucose meter.

Some individuals have difficulty securing a drop of blood and may require guidance in obtaining an adequate blood droplet, in choosing a lancing device, and/or in selecting a puncture depth. Most lancing devices are spring-loaded and release a lancet at the push of a button. The smaller the lancet needle's gauge and the shallower its penetration, the less pain occurs. Lancets are usually available in 28, 30, and 33 gauge with 28 gauge being the thicket lancet. Typically, in a lancing device, the higher the setting, the deeper the lancet with penetrate. Lancets are intended for onetime use and will dull with repeated use, resulting in more pain and possible inadequate blood sample. Careful and safe disposal of used lancets is critical. Used lancets should be disposed of in an appropriate sharps container (regulations vary from state to state).

When monitoring blood glucose away from home, used lancets can be place in an empty pill bottle for appropriate disposal later. Providing individualized guidance for each person's needs minimizes waste of glucose monitoring strips due to inadequate blood sample size and promotes a positive approach to blood glucose monitoring.

Securing an Adequate Blood Sample

It is important for the diabetes care and education specialist to provide specific directions to follow for securing an adequate blood sample.[19] For example, when using the fingertips as a puncture site, the person should be aware of the following procedures to help increase sample size:

- Vigorously wash hands with warm water to increase circulation to fingertips.
- Hang the hand at your side for 30 seconds so blood pools in that hand.
- Shake the hand to be pricked as though you were shaking down a thermometer.
- Use either a smaller gauge lancet or a lancing device or end-cap that will allow a deeper puncture.
- Puncture the sides of the fingertips rather than the pads in the center of the fingers, as this produces less pain.
- After your finger is punctured, gently milk the blood from the base of the finger to the tip of the finger until the blood sample is the correct size. Milking the finger with a press/release, press/release repetition assists blood flow, whereas just squeezing the fingertip may obstruct blood flow.

Use Alternative Sites Appropriately

Some meters and strips are designed to use alternative sites such as the forearm, palm of the hand, upper arm, or thigh for puncture. However, a few precautions are important for users to understand.

There is wide discordance between fingertip and alternative-site samples when blood glucose levels are changing rapidly due to circulatory physiology. Blood circulation in the skin of the fingers and palm of the hand is distinctly different from that in the arms and legs. The blood flow through the arteriovenous shunts in the fingertips proceeds at a higher velocity than the flow through other capillaries of the skin. Therefore, the transient difference between the alternative site and the fingertip during rapid blood glucose changes is a result of this decreased velocity of blood flow to sites such as the forearm. When blood glucose concentration is falling rapidly, this lag between the alternative site and the fingertip could cause a delay in detection of hypoglycemia if an alternative site is being used for measuring glucose levels. In preprandial monitoring, glucose levels are in a relatively steady state, so the difference between alternative-site and fingertip samples is small and often not clinically significant; but for up to 2 hours postprandial, the blood glucose is in flux.[20] The following are key points about when to use alternative sites:

- Alternative sites should not be used
  - —when the person is hypoglycemic
  - —if the person is prone to hypoglycemia (during peak activity of a short- or intermediate-acting injected insulin or up to 2 hours after injecting rapid-acting insulin)
  - —after exercise
  - —during illness
  - —during a time when blood glucose levels are rapidly increasing or decreasing (such as any time less than 2 hours after a meal)
  - —before driving
  - —during pregnancy
  - —if required for calibration of CGM
- Persons with a history of hypoglycemia unawareness should not use alternative sites

Because between-site differences of up to 100 mg/dL (5.6 mmol/L) have been reported, the person performing the blood glucose check must document not only the result, time, medication, and relevant comments but also the sampling site used.[21] Some pediatric endocrinologists prefer that children and adolescents use only the fingertips as puncture sites because of the rapid changes in blood glucose levels often seen in these age groups due to spontaneous activity and glucose uptake into the muscle.

Document Results

Individuals should be encouraged to use a documenting system they are comfortable with, which enables assessment of relationships of food, physical activity, medications, if taken, and stressors such as illness or injury. Note that this can occur on paper using a log book or form, or by using a smartphone app. This will be critical when the individual begins to interpret the blood glucose results, as the results need to be readily available and in a format that is easily reviewed. During meter training, the diabetes care and education specialist should observe the individual document blood glucose results to ensure that the data (ie, date, time, and actual result) are correctly entered. Many meters have a memory feature that the diabetes care and education specialist can use to verify the accuracy of the individual's documentation. The diabetes care and education specialist should also explore how to download the meter from home when this is an option for the individual, and how to look at the data produced by the download. Most meters have data download and analysis capabilities as well and this feature should be utilized.

Although a written record and graph of blood glucose readings yield important information, recording comments or explanations can be more helpful for teaching the impact of certain decisions related to food, activity, and medication, if taken, and stress. Additionally, the individual, healthcare provider, and diabetes care and education specialist may find that documenting food intake, physical activity, and stress/illness provide greater insight as to how these variables affect blood glucose. This is especially important for people who are new to monitoring. The person who finds value in performing SMBG will be more likely to continue to monitor. Keep in mind that these features can be documented in a smartphone app as well as some meters. It's important to find the platform that works best for the individual and that the diabetes care and education specialist is familiar with an app that is used.

It is important to remind individuals to bring their meter and logbook to every medical visit and present their logbook or smartphone app to their healthcare provider for review. The meter can be cleaned, the strips and control solution can be checked, if required, codes can be verified, and an actual blood glucose measurement can be performed. Ask if more than one blood glucose meter is being used. For example, some individuals prefer the convenience of having an additional meter at their workplace. Results of SMBG will be most consistent if the same meter model is used each time. If an individual chooses to use more than one type of meter, the readings obtained from each should be identified as such in their logbook, download, or smartphone app. Correctly and consistently performing SMBG and documenting blood glucose results lay the foundation for pattern management (described later in this chapter).

Meet Individual Needs for Operational or Interpretation Skills

Certain populations of people with diabetes have unique needs relating to meter selection and use. Issues specific to the elderly, children, the visually impaired, and those with special needs are discussed in the paragraphs that follow.

Elderly Elderly adults with diabetes remain an underserved population despite the prevalence of diabetes in this population. Age should not be the sole criterion for decisions concerning SMBG. Indeed, research has shown that many older individuals perform as well as, and in some cases better than, younger individuals in their follow-through with SMBG. The elderly are a heterogeneous population requiring personalized therapy and monitoring schedules. Diabetes care and education specialists need to consider the unique needs of some of the elderly that may influence the choice of products, such as potential limitations in manual dexterity, slowed reaction time, or low vision. For example, individually wrapped strips may be more difficult for some people to handle than strips dispensed from a vial. How an elderly person receives meter supplies may also influence the level of consistency to the scheduled SMBG plan. Many elderly individuals find that receiving meter supplies through mail order is both convenient and cost-effective. Reordering of blood glucose monitoring supplies must be requested and/or authorized by the individual, as auto shipment of blood glucose monitoring supplies no longer complies with current Medicare regulations. A relative or caregiver may need to help obtain the needed supplies.

Children Children also have unique needs that influence product choice. Children especially benefit from strips that require a small sample of blood and lancing devices that hide the lancet and minimize discomfort. Parents often prefer meters that yield results quickly, have a backlight (for checking blood glucose in the middle of the night), and store multiple values in memory. At a very young age, many children begin to take responsibility for doing their blood glucose *pokes* or *checks*. When speaking with children, these terms are preferred over *tests*, which often has a pass/fail or good/bad negative connotation. Emphasize the value of the information the numbers provide, "like clues of a puzzle." It is important that children be verbally praised for participating in this critical part of their diabetes management. However, even after children have mastered the technique, it is important for parents and other caregivers to supervise the checking procedure so that data are recorded for use in treatment and pattern management.

Visually Impaired Visually impaired individuals who have diabetes, including those with fluctuating vision and nonfunctional vision, need products that are fully accessible for them. Beneficial equipment features include tactile markings on the strip; clear speech output on a small, portable meter; and a method of consistent placement of the blood sample.[22] A limited number of products are currently available that meet these recommendations. The National Federation of the Blind continually evaluates and provides updates on products and services for people with diabetes who are blind. For the most current list of available products, contact the National Federation of the Blind (www.nfb.org).

Special Needs It is also important to recognize that due to age limitations, physical or cognitive disabilities, and other factors, some individuals may need to rely on family members or caregivers to help them with or to perform these tasks. Prior to the initial teaching session, the diabetes care and education specialist should ask who may be involved with facilitating diabetes management so that the appropriate individuals may be invited to attend the initial and subsequent sessions. These individuals must be part of the teaching and skills process. Also, as life's circumstances change, so does the level of involvement by others. For example, as the young child with type 1 diabetes grows and matures, the parents and other caregivers release increasingly greater amounts of the diabetes management skills to the child; conversely, as older adults age, physical limitations such as a decline in visual acuity or manual dexterity may result in the need for more assistance by others.

Using the Blood Glucose Data—Interpretation Skills

Many persons with diabetes are trained in the mechanics of operating a meter and in how to record or retrieve the blood glucose results, but not on how to use the data or why they are of value. Harris and associates found that the frequency of monitoring was related to having attended a diabetes education class.[23] Diabetes education was associated with an almost threefold increase in the probability that study participants would monitor their blood glucose at least once per day.

Once individuals are competent and confident in their ability to operate a blood glucose meter, diabetes education on utilizing or interpreting the blood glucose data to improve glycemic stability can begin. Performing blood glucose checks without either the individual or the healthcare provider using the data obtained is of no value and a waste of resources.

Diabetes education on SMBG should provide the individual with guidance on blood glucose targets, monitoring frequency, and interpretation of the results in order to see a link between blood glucose values and factors known to contribute to glucose variability (eg, food, physical activity, stress, and medication), as well as reinforce positive outcomes. Situations in which more frequent monitoring may be needed are shown in Table 18.6.

TABLE 18.6 Situations That May Require More Frequent Monitoring

SMBG may need to be performed more frequently in the following situations:

- Identifying and treating hypoglycemia
- Making decisions concerning food intake or medication adjustment when exercising
- Determining the effect of food choices or portions on blood glucose levels
- Managing intercurrent illness
- Managing hypoglycemia unawareness
- Prior to performing critical tasks, eg, driving
- Monitoring recommended glucose management during preconception and pregnancy

Blood Glucose Targets

Individuals need to be clear regarding their blood glucose goal targets. It is not uncommon to find individuals dutifully performing SMBG but not be aware of their target blood glucose goals. Target goals for fasting, premeal, and postmeal times should be determined based on recommended guidelines. Table 18.7 lists 2 organizations' therapeutic goals for glycemia for nonpregnant adults. (See chapter 24 for specifics on blood glucose targets for pregnancy.) However, more or less stringent glycemic goals may be appropriate; goals should be individualized based on multiple factors such as duration of diabetes, age/life expectancy, comorbid conditions, hypoglycemia unawareness, known cardiovascular disease (CVD) or microvascular complications, and individual's considerations.

Target blood glucose differs between the ADA and the AACE. The glycemic guidelines of the ADA can be applied to all persons given that more stringent individualized targets are possible within its recommendations. The ADA postprandial "peak" level can best be explained to individuals as aiming for a blood glucose value no higher than 180 mg/dL (10.0 mmol/L), 1 to 2 hours after the start of a meal. For individuals who find it difficult to check their blood glucose exactly 2 hours after the start of a meal, the "peak" provides a target limit within the 1- to 2-hour postmeal window.

All meters use a drop of whole blood on the glucose monitoring strip, and results are expressed as plasma glucose levels; this allows for easy comparison with a laboratory's plasma results.

Encourage individuals to write their target goals in their logbook or on their form; this helps remind them of their target goals while at the same time reinforcing them. Some glucose meters allow for setting individual target ranges, which are then used in personalized graphic printouts.

Frequency of Monitoring The timing (the "when") and frequency (how often) of glucose checks depend on multiple factors. There are no universally accepted

TABLE 18.7 ADA and AACE Target Blood Glucose Goals for Nonpregnant Adults

	American Diabetes Association (ADA)	*American Association of Clinical Endocrinologists (AACE)*
A1C	<7.0%. Individualized based on duration of disease, age/life expectancy, comorbid conditions, known CVD or advanced microvascular complications, hypoglycemia unawareness, individual considerations. • More (<6.5%) or less (8.0%) stringent glycemic goals may be appropriate for some individuals.	≤6.5% for most. Individualized based on age, comorbidities, duration of disease. • Closer to normal for healthy • Less stringent for "less healthy"
Fasting and preprandial blood glucose*	80–130 mg/dL (4.4–7.2 mmol/L)	<110 mg/dL (<6.1 mmol/L)
Postprandial blood glucose*	<180 mg/dL (<10.0 mmol/L) at "peak" levels, 1–2 hours after start of meal • Postprandial glucose may be targeted if A1C goal not met despite reaching preprandial glucose goals.	<140 mg/dL (<7.8 mmol/L) 2 hours after start of meal

*Capillary plasma glucose values.

Sources: Adapted from American Diabetes Association, "Standards of medical care in diabetes—2019," *Diabetes Care* 42, Suppl 1(2019):S61-70; American Association of Clinical Endocrinologists, "AACE medical guidelines for clinical practice for developing a diabetes comprehensive care plan," *Endocr Pract* 21, Suppl 1(2015):1-87.

standard guidelines; professional organizations such as the ADA and the AACE have made their own recommendations, which are regularly revised and updated.

The 2016 consensus statement from the AACE/ACE on glucose monitoring encourages "meaningful monitoring" whereby glucose monitoring should be done in the context of therapy and with specific goals.[4] In general, SMBG is viewed from 2 perspectives: (1) SMBG results utilized by the individual to make behavior and lifestyle changes related to diet and exercise and (2) results utilized by the individual and the healthcare provider to adjust medications, usually insulin.[24,25] These perspectives affect timing and frequency recommendations. The current consensus is that SMBG should be utilized by persons who are using an intensive insulin schedules such as multiple daily injections (MDI), or insulin pump therapy. However, there is less consensus for persons who are on less intensive insulin schedules or oral medications. Table 18.8 summarizes the recommendations for SMBG frequency for type 1 and type 2 diabetes from the ADA and the AACE/ACE. These recommendations are also recommended by ADCES.[26]

For persons with type 1 diabetes or type 2 diabetes on intensive insulin therapy, the 2016 ADA Standards of Care recommend that blood glucose checking be done prior to meals and snacks, occasionally postprandially, at bedtime, prior to exercise, when low blood glucose is suspected, after treating a hypoglycemic event until normalized, and prior to performing critical tasks such as driving. This recommendation may require checking 6 to 10 times per day or more. Additionally, the ADA recommends that persons who are prescribed SMBG receive instruction in and routine follow-up evaluation of SMBG technique and their ability to use the data to adjust therapy.

For persons with type 2 diabetes using less intensive insulin schedules such as basal insulin, the ADA does not give a specific frequency schedule but does state that a number of studies have indicated that fasting SMBG provides guidance for the titration of basal insulin. Additionally, the ADA states that when SMBG is prescribed as part of a broader educational context, SMBG results may be helpful to guide treatment decisions and/or self-management.

The AACE/ACE consensus statement recommends that persons with type 1 diabetes should monitor their glucose at least twice per day, up to 6 to 10 times per day, including before meals, occasionally postprandially, before exercise or driving, and at bedtime. For persons with type 2 diabetes using basal and bolus insulin, monitoring is recommended at fasting, premeal, bedtime, and periodically in the middle of the night. For less intensive insulin schedules, monitoring is recommended less often, but at a minimum fasting and bedtime. For persons with type 2 diabetes using insulin, sulfonylureas, or glinides, "structured" blood glucose monitoring is recommended depending on how the medication is used. For individuals with type 2 diabetes who are at low risk for hypoglycemia, the AACE/ACE consensus statement does not recommend glucose monitoring but acknowledges that monitoring may help individuals understand how food and exercise affect their blood glucose levels.

TABLE 18.8 SMBG Frequency Recommendations

Type of Diabetes Mellitus	*ADA*	*AACE/ACE*
Type 1 Adult: Risk of hypoglycemia	**6–10 times per day to include:** prior to meals and snacks, occasionally postprandially, at bedtime, prior to exercise, when hypoglycemia is suspected, after treating hypoglycemia until normoglycemic, prior to critical tasks such as driving	**At least twice a day to 6–10 times per day to include:** before meals, occasionally postmeal, before exercise or critical tasks such as driving, and at bedtime
Type 2: Risk of hypoglycemia	**On intensive insulin plan:** 6–10 times per day to include: prior to meals and snacks, occasionally postprandially, at bedtime, prior to exercise, when hypoglycemia is suspected, after treating hypoglycemia until normoglycemic, prior to critical tasks such as driving **On less intensive insulin therapy:** more frequent SMBG (eg, fasting, before/after meals) may be helpful, as increased frequency has been shown to be inversely correlated with glycemic management	**On intensive insulin plan:** fasting, premeal, bedtime, and periodically in the middle of the night **On basal insulin alone or with additional diabetes medications:** at minimum, fasting and at bedtime **On basal insulin plus 1 daily mealtime insulin injection or premixed insulin injection**: at minimum, fasting and before the preprandial or premixed insulin; periodically at other times such as premeal, bedtime, 3 AM Additional glucose monitoring before exercise or critical tasks, such as driving
Type 2: Low risk of hypoglycemia	**Insufficient evidence to recommend when or how often to monitor in individuals on orals or basal insulin***	**Daily blood glucose monitoring not recommended** Initial periodic structured monitoring (at meals and bedtime) may be useful. Once at A1C goal, less frequent monitoring is acceptable.

*A1C reduction seen in individuals who use monitoring results to adjust insulin dose to attain fasting target.

Sources: American Diabetes Association, "Standards of medical care in diabetes—2019," *Diabetes Care* 42, Suppl 1 (2019): S61-70.; "AACE/ACE glucose monitoring consensus statement," *Endocr Pract* 22, no. 2 (2016): 22.

For persons with type 2 diabetes who are not on oral medications or noninsulin injections, there is less clarity regarding the timing and frequency of SMBG. Neither the ADA nor the AACE gives any specific SMBG frequency or timing recommendations, but both agree that SMBG may be helpful and useful in guiding treatment decisions and/or self-management. Numerous studies on the use of SMBG in persons with noninsulin type 2 diabetes and the positive effect on clinical outcomes, particularly A1C, have been published.[27–31] Recent studies found that SMBG in noninsulin-using individuals correlated positively with weight loss and lower A1C when SMBG results were utilized to follow healthier dietary recommendations.[32–33]

Monitoring schedules are based on the person's needs, desires, and use of the data. It is important that the diabetes care and education specialist assess how SMBG results are going to be used by the person with diabetes. Is the intent of SMBG to use the results to guide behavior and lifestyle change, to guide medication efficacy, or both?

From a practical point of view, the number of blood glucose checks performed per day is often based on the number of strips covered by health insurance plans. The following factors should be considered when helping individuals determine their blood glucose monitoring frequency and time:

- Type of diabetes
- Individual's willingness to perform SMBG
- Level of glycemic stability
- Medication schedule
- Consistency of food intake
- Lifestyle and daily schedule with regard to activity, food, and work
- Physical ability to check blood glucose

- Ability to problem solve and take action
- Financial limitations
- Comorbid conditions

In type 1 diabetes and in individuals on MDI, checking blood glucose levels 4 or more times per day is an accepted standard. Typically, these individuals are encouraged to check their fasting and premeal blood glucoses prior to mealtime insulin dosing. Additionally, postprandial glucose checks may be performed to monitor the glucose-rising effects of meals. Any hypoglycemic symptom also warrants performing a blood glucose check. Some individuals check their glucose level prior to bedtime and before driving to ensure their safety. More frequent monitoring is beneficial during insulin dose adjustment, illness, pregnancy, heavy periods of exercise or physical activity, and when an oral medication and/or injectable medication or insulin is prescribed. There is little doubt of the value of SMBG for individuals who take multiple insulin injections per day, as the SMBG results are used to dose insulin or detect hypoglycemia. In fact, more frequent glucose checking is correlated with an improved A1C level.[34,35]

In type 2 diabetes, most diabetes care and education specialists find SMBG a valuable tool, even for those not taking insulin. There is evidence that SMBG data can be used in this population to reinforce therapy decisions and therapeutic lifestyle changes. A study by Schwedes et al showed that meal-related blood glucose monitoring within a structured counseling program significantly improved glycemic stability in the majority of non-insulin-using individuals with type 2 diabetes.[29] Utilizing SMBG also resulted in improvement in A1C in persons with type 2 diabetes on oral glucose-lowering medications in a study by Barnett et al.[36]

For all persons with diabetes, it is recommended that "SMBG should be used only when individuals with diabetes (and/or their caregivers) have the knowledge, skills, and willingness to incorporate SMBG monitoring and therapy adjustments into their diabetes care plan in order to attain agreed treatment goals."[35] In terms of frequency and timing of SMBG, a number of sources recommend starting with "focused" SMBG schedules based on what blood glucose information is desired.[1,4,5,37]

- An everyday 5- or 7-point blood glucose profile (ie, preprandial and postprandial plus bedtime blood glucose performed in 1 day) repeated for 5 to 7 days can provide insight as to when out-of-target blood glucoses are occurring on a given day.
- A staggered 2 or 3 blood glucose checks per day for 5 to 7 days—whereby 1 mealtime is selected and premeal and postmeal blood glucose checks are performed—can be useful. A different mealtime is selected on subsequent days. Over the course of a week, the individual has blood glucose values for 2 premeal and postmeal blood glucose pairings to evaluate in light of blood glucose goals. Both the 5- or 7-point schedule and the staggered frequency schedule are considered meal-based plans. Individuals can use the results from these schedules to gain insight into the effects of meals on blood glucose excursions.
- A 3-point SMBG schedule—whereby fasting, pre-largest-meal, and post-largest-meal blood glucoses are taken—can be very helpful to an individual newly diagnosed with type 2 diabetes. This schedule provides information regarding reaching glycemic targets at fasting and the glycemic response to the largest meal of the day.[38]

Ideally, individuals who find their postmeal blood glucose values out of target range will have the opportunity to work with a registered dietitian, who can evaluate the meal composition and corresponding blood glucose results to individualize a meal plan. A more detailed discussion on the significance of checking postprandial blood glucose can be found in the Utilizing Glucose Pattern Management section. See the examples in Figure 18.1. This approach is in stark contrast to what is often seen in noninsulin-using individuals with type 2 diabetes who are instructed to check their blood glucose once a day, fasting, first thing in the morning. For individuals with type 2 diabetes whose fasting values are typically in target range, checking only fasting blood glucose offers little insight into overall blood glucose stability and, therefore, offers a false sense of achieving glycemic targets.

A term that is becoming more commonly used when discussing SMBG is *structured monitoring*. This refers to a schedule for checking blood glucoses that is specifically prescribed to discover the effects of food, medication, and physical activity on daily glucose levels. The SMBG profiles provided in Figure 18.1 are examples of structured monitoring schedules that provide "meaningful monitoring." A number of studies have used structured monitoring in their research protocol to determine the effects of SMBG on clinical outcomes.[29–31,39,40] In a consensus report regarding the use of SMBG in noninsulin-using type 2 diabetes, the panel recommended that SMBG be performed in a structured format and used to guide treatment. Additionally, the panel noted that both persons with diabetes and healthcare providers require education on how to respond to SMBG data in order for SMBG to be an effective tool.[41]

Regardless of the ideal structured monitoring recommendation, it is key to keep in mind that persons with

3-point SMBG profile to check fasting and effect of largest meal							
	Pre-breakfast	Post-breakfast	Pre-lunch	Post-lunch	Pre-supper	Post-supper	Bedtime
Monday	X				X	X	
Tuesday	X				X	X	
Wednesday	X				X	X	
Thursday	X				X	X	
Friday	X				X	X	
Saturday	X				X	X	
Sunday	X				X	X	

5-point SMBG profile							
	Pre-breakfast	Post-breakfast	Pre-lunch	Post-lunch	Pre-supper	Post-supper	Bedtime
Monday	X	X		X	X	X	
Tuesday	X	X		X	X	X	
Wednesday							
Thursday							
Friday							
Saturday							
Sunday	X	X		X	X	X	

7-point SMBG profile							
	Pre-breakfast	Post-breakfast	Pre-lunch	Post-lunch	Pre-supper	Post-supper	Bedtime
Monday							
Tuesday							
Wednesday							
Thursday	X	X	X	X	X	X	X
Friday	X	X	X	X	X	X	X
Saturday	X	X	X	X	X	X	X
Sunday							

Meal-based SMBG profile (less intensive)							
	Pre-breakfast	Post-breakfast	Pre-lunch	Post-lunch	Pre-supper	Post-supper	Bedtime
Monday	X	X					
Tuesday							
Wednesday			X	X			
Thursday							
Friday							
Saturday					X	X	
Sunday							

FIGURE 18.1 **Examples of SMBG Plans**

(continued)

"Staggered" SMBG profile							
	Pre-breakfast	Post-breakfast	Pre-lunch	Post-lunch	Pre-supper	Post-supper	Bedtime
Monday	X	X					
Tuesday			X	X			
Wednesday					X	X	
Thursday	X	X					
Friday			X	X			
Saturday					X	X	
Sunday	X	X					

SMBG profile to assess or detect fasting hyperglycemia							
	Pre-breakfast	Post-breakfast	Pre-lunch	Post-lunch	Pre-supper	Post-supper	Bedtime
Monday							X
Tuesday	X						
Wednesday							X
Thursday	X						
Friday							X
Saturday	X						
Sunday							

Note: Ensure that the person's food and activity tracking are consistent in order to appropriately interpret the glucose data.

FIGURE 18.1 **Examples of SMBG Plans *(continued)***

Source: Type 2 Diabetes BASICS Curriculum Guide, 3rd ed (Minneapolis, Minn: International Diabetes Center, 2009).

noninsulin-using type 2 diabetes will most likely have only 100 strips over 3 months (100 strips for ~90 days) available as a covered benefit, unless the physician prescribes and justifies the need for a greater quantity. The diabetes care and education specialist should work with the individual to determine how the strips will be used to gain the most actionable information; there will be days where blood glucose checks are not performed.

Interpreting SMBG Results—Utilizing Glucose Pattern Management

Blood glucose monitoring data provide the individual and the healthcare team with information to make lifestyle or therapeutic decisions. Some decisions (eg, treating hypoglycemia, determining the need for a snack, or calculating insulin correction units) require instant feedback for taking action; however, pattern management requires 3 or 4 readings to establish a pattern (eg, adjusting medication dosages, changing the meal plan, or recognizing the impact of exercise). Glucose pattern management (GPM) is the process of recognizing, analyzing, and acting on repeated out-of-target readings to move them into target range.[42] The process requires the application of a systematic review and analysis of data by both persons with diabetes and their healthcare team in the daily, weekly, and long-term management of blood glucose levels. Integrating SMBG and GPM into a diabetes self-management education (DSME) program requires 3 essential components: (1) a guiding belief that SMBG and GPM are necessary for the understanding of the effects of food, physical activity, and medications on daily glucose levels (and ultimately on A1C); (2) a staff with expertise on how to teach individuals to interpret and use glucose data to problem-solve behaviors related to food, physical activity, and medication taking; and (3) tools that guide data collection and interpretation. A checklist for integrating SMBG and GPM into a DSME program has been developed by Powers et al.[43]

Steps in GPM As one begins to review and interpret SMBG data, a series of questions need to be asked: What medications are currently being taken and what are their intended effects on blood glucose?[44] (See Table 18.9.) Have enough blood glucose checks been recorded? Are

TABLE 18.9 Medication Effects on Blood Glucose

Medication	*Fasting*	*Postprandial*
Biguanides (metformin)	X	X (mild)
Insulin secretagogues:		
• Sulfonylureas (glyburide, glimepiride, glipizide, chlorpropamide, tolazamide, tolbutamide)	X	X
• Meglitinides (nateglinide, repaglinide)	X (mild)	X
Alpha-glucosidase inhibitors (acarbose, miglitol)		X
Thiazolidinediones (pioglitazone, rosiglitazone)	X	X (mild)
Sodium-glucose co-transporter 2 (SGLT2) inhibitors (canagliflozin, dapagliflozin, empagliflozin)	X	X (mild)
Incretin mimetics:		
• GLP-1 receptor agonists (exenatide, exenatide XR, liraglutide, dulaglutide, albiglutide)	X (mild)	X
• Amylin analogs (pramlintide)	X (mild)	X
• DPP-4 inhibitors (sitagliptin, vildagliptin, linagliptin, saxagliptin, alogliptin)	X (mild)	X
Insulin:		
• Bolus (premeal) insulins (lispro, lispro u200, aspart, glulisine, regular)		X
• Basal (background) insulins (glargine, glargine u300, detemir, NPH, Ultralente, insulin degludec)	X	X (mild)
• Premixed insulins (NPH/regular—70/30; NPH/lispro—75/25 or 50/50; NPH/aspart—70/30; degludec/aspart—70/30)	X	X

Note: Generic names of medications are given in the table. For the trade names and manufacturers of the drugs listed in this table, refer to chapters 17 and 20.

they accurate? Are contributors to the glucose result consistent (ie, food intake, physical activity, dosing of medication, stress/illness)? Are at least 3 days of blood glucose checks taken at the same time of day to spot a trend? Are activities, food, feelings, and unusual events recorded?

Table 18.10 lists questions to consider when analyzing blood glucose data. The timing of the blood glucose check provides insight as to where to direct efforts or make changes (see Table 18.11).

The process of reviewing glucose data can be made easier by encouraging persons to record the data in a logbook or with a smartphone app, with the monitoring time and results recorded in linear and vertical fashion, or to download the data utilizing available software. An example is shown in the sample blood glucose record in Figure 18.2. In this example logbook, the 3 fasting blood glucose checks are within target range, but the post-breakfast blood glucose values are all out of range; no food records were available. Prior to making medication recommendations, the composition of the breakfast meal needs to be determined, and additional pre- and post-breakfast blood glucose checks need to be taken. The individual may find that small changes in the breakfast meal will result in in-target post-breakfast blood glucoses. Only 1 pre-dinner blood glucose is available and it is out of range; no conclusions can be drawn from one blood glucose number. Additional pre-dinner checks should be obtained to see if there is a trend. Also, only one in-target pre-lunch blood glucose value is recorded. One cannot assume from just one blood glucose number that pre-lunch blood glucoses are within target range, either. Regarding the Friday post-dinner blood glucose of 65, the individual revealed that he felt "shaky." He checked his blood glucose and treated himself for hypoglycemia. Hypoglycemia needs to be treated when it occurs. However, if blood glucose data reveal a trend for hypoglycemia, preventive action needs to be taken to reduce further episodes.

Being aware of the factors that raise or lower blood glucose is key to interpreting blood glucose results, taking action, and/or modifying lifestyle behaviors (see Table 18.12).

Postprandial Glucose Postprandial monitoring is an essential part of diabetes self-management and has gained more attention in recent years. In general, a measurement of plasma glucose 1 to 2 hours after the start of the meal provides a reasonable assessment of postprandial glycemia. Dietitians implementing MNT find assessing

TABLE 18.10 Framework for Interpreting Blood Glucose Records

	Sample Questions to Consider			
Step	*Food Plan*	*Physical Activity*	*Medications*	*Other*
1. Obtain sufficient data.	• Is a food plan being followed? • Are carbohydrates counted correctly? • If no food data, determine if there are any barriers to the individual completing this task.	• Is a physical activity plan being followed? • If no physical activity data, determine if there are any barriers to the individual logging or engaging in exercise.	• Are medications taken as prescribed? • If medication dose not available, determine how the information could be obtained?	• Are reasons for out-of-target glucoses noted? • If low glucoses are noted, how are they treated? How often do they occur and when? • Are more blood glucose checks needed? If so, when are they needed? • Can the individual offer insight into schedule or lifestyle variations? Are there trends or fluctuations?
2. Identify all possible interpretations.	• Does the individual understand and follow the food plan? • Could meals be spaced more appropriately? • Is it important that meals be consistent in size and composition? • Are regular snacks eaten or even necessary?	• Has there been a change in physical activity? • Is physical activity irregular?	• If medication is taken, is the individual taking the prescribed dose and at the correct time? • Are the medications expired? • Does the diabetes medication provide adequate or inadequate coverage at meal times?	• Are monitoring supplies in date? • Has the individual verified accuracy of the meter by using control solution that is not expired? • Has the individual's operation of the meter been observed for any concerns?
3. Collaborate with individual to integrate data and make personalized recommendations.	• Could changes be made to the food plan or timing of intake to make it easier to follow? • Are carbohydrate amounts noted? Does the individual understand how to count carbohydrates? • Could changes be made to carbohydrate amounts or timing to make the plan easier to follow?	• Could physical activity be more regular, increased, or decreased?	• Could the medication plan be adjusted or simplified? • Could a different type or amount be taken at a different time?	• What changes would the individual be willing to make? • Should the target glucose goals be changed? • What personal goals does the individual have for his or her life that would affect diabetes management?

Source: Adapted from MA Powers, *Handbook of Diabetes Medical Nutrition Therapy* (Rockville, Md: Aspen Publishers, 1996).

TABLE 18.11 Information Provided by Timing of Blood Glucose Check

Time of Blood Glucose Checks	*Information Provided*
Fasting	Assesses overnight effect of meds: • If fasting is higher than bedtime—possible nocturnal hypoglycemia or dawn effect
Premeal	Assesses basal insulin therapy needs
Postmeal	Assesses adequacy of premeal medications (rapid- or short-acting insulin, orals) in light of meal eaten • If not taking medications—assesses effect of meal
Bedtime	Assesses the effect of evening meal and basal therapy needs
Random	Can help determine if presenting symptoms are due to blood glucose fluctuations (hypoglycemic event)

Target range 70–130 mg/dL fasting and premeal, <180 at 2 hours postmeal

	Pre-breakfast	Post-breakfast	Pre-lunch	Post-lunch	Pre-dinner	Post-dinner	Bedtime
Monday	128	256			188		
Tuesday	114	248					
Wednesday	118	212	122				
Thursday							
Friday						65	
Saturday							

FIGURE 18.2 **Sample SMBG Record**

TABLE 18.12 Factors That May Raise or Lower Blood Glucose

Factors That May Raise Blood Glucose	*Factors That May Lower Blood Glucose*
• Inadequate insulin or oral medication dose	• Too much insulin or oral medications
• Other medications	• Other medications
• Physical activity	• Physical activity
• Stress (dehydration, etc)	• Stress
• More carbohydrate than normally consumed at that time	• Less carbohydrate than normally consumed at that time

postprandial blood glucose results particularly valuable in assessing food intake and guiding nutrition recommendations. Postprandial monitoring is effective for teaching the impact of food portions and meal composition on blood glucose levels. For example, an individual may choose a meal high in carbohydrate content and have an elevated blood glucose reading 2 hours later, whereas after eating the same foods in smaller portions, the person may find the postprandial reading to be within goal range.

Postprandial plasma glucose target goals for non-pregnant adults are listed in Table 18.7. Specific clinical conditions such as gestational diabetes or pregnancy complicated by diabetes may benefit from the measurement of blood glucose 1 hour after a meal (see chapter 24 on pregnancy).[45] There has been interest in determining the contribution of fasting and postprandial glucose increments to overall hyperglycemia. Monnier and colleagues evaluated the effect of postprandial glucose on A1C levels. They analyzed the diurnal glycemic profiles of persons with type 2 diabetes and investigated different levels of A1C. They concluded that as A1C levels approach 7%, postprandial glucose levels contribute more to the A1C level (~70%), while fasting glucose levels (30%) contribute less. The study showed that in persons with A1C in the mid-target range, the relative contribution of postprandial glucose excursions is predominant.[46]

The take-away message for the diabetes care and education specialist is that if individuals are aiming for an A1C of less than 7%, blood glucose monitoring efforts should focus on reaching postprandial glucose targets.

One of the most common barriers to postprandial monitoring is not remembering to check after a meal because there is no trigger to remind the person. With so many types of technology available today, the diabetes care and education specialist may suggest that people set the alarm feature on their watch, insulin pump, or glucose meter to sound or vibrate, program an alert message into their smartphone or tablet, or simply write a reminder in their appointment book and highlight it. Postprandial checking provides the person with diabetes information on the effect of the meal, the efficacy of the medication, and the impact of physical activity.

Diabetes Care and Education Specialists and SMBG

Successful behavior change results from the education interchange between the diabetes care and education specialist and the person with diabetes and the self-management efforts he or she implements. Diabetes care and education specialists and clinicians rely on SMBG to teach problem-solving skills, which are the essence of diabetes self-management, and complex management skills such as blood glucose pattern awareness and insulin dose adjustment. Diabetes care and education specialists use SMBG as a tool to link abstract principles of management with daily decision-making. Diabetes care and education specialists can use blood glucose results to teach the concept of post-exercise, late-onset hypoglycemia and the behaviors necessary to prevent this condition. Behavior change concerning food choices or portions is facilitated by relating the food or portion to the postprandial blood glucose result.[47,48]

For persons with type 2 diabetes who may be asymptomatic for hyperglycemia, the need for behavior change becomes personally relevant when they monitor and record blood glucose levels.

Diabetes care and education specialists use SMBG to identify and influence psychosocial adaptations. Self-monitoring of blood glucose can influence self-efficacy.[49] For example, persons with diabetes report increased confidence in their problem-solving abilities as a result of using SMBG. The act of monitoring can also have emotional consequences when an individual is confronted with an unacceptable number. This phenomenon, called *monitor talk*, can help identify psychosocial needs and direct future learning.[50] Diabetes care and education specialists discourage value judgment and replace the notion of good and bad readings with the terms *in range* or *out of range*. Reference to blood glucose tests can be replaced with the terms *checks* or *measurements* and using the glucose values as *feedback*.

Self-monitoring of blood glucose can be used to allay anxiety about hypoglycemia, especially parental anxiety, and is a critical tool for treating fear of hypoglycemia.[51] Although the influence of stress and stress management techniques on glycemic stability varies among individuals, it may be beneficial for individuals to assess their blood glucose levels during such times to determine how they respond to psychological stress.

Tables 18.13 and 18.14 summarize how blood glucose monitoring can be utilized in problem solving, which can impact all 7 of the AADE7 Self-Care Behaviors.®

The Diabetes Care and Education Specialist's Role in SMBG Utilization

"The diabetes care and education specialist has the skills and training required to instruct the person with diabetes on the goals and techniques of SMBG, and more importantly, on how to evaluate and use the data to improve glycemic control."[6] It is the job of the diabetes care and education specialist to not only explain *why* and *how* to perform SMBG but also help individuals identify barriers that may prevent them from continuing this activity and making it a habit.[52]

If the person has stopped monitoring, investigate. Common causes are emotional reactions to elevated or fluctuating readings, consistent readings within range, discomfort related to lancing the skin, emotional response to the sight of blood or skin piercing, cost, inconvenience, and the healthcare team not reviewing and using the data. As part of the assessment, simply ask, "Is it helpful?"[53]

A person may understand the value of SMBG but perceive multiple challenges to actually performing the monitoring. Barriers to SMBG were mentioned previously in this chapter. Use of the AADE7 Self-Care Behaviors® Goal Sheet (part of the AADE7 System® product) combines data in a format that the person with diabetes and the diabetes care and education specialist can use for problem solving and decision-making.

There are times when diabetes care and education specialists need to acknowledge the challenge and frustrations related to the daily management and care of diabetes. However, these individuals have the ability to influence and address these issues in a positive way without negating the difficulties. A model for doing so comes from the Appreciative Inquiry literature.[54] This model of addressing change focuses on asking positive questions that elicit a sense of power and empowerment. Many diabetes care and education specialists will understand the

TABLE 18.13 Blood Glucose Monitoring Problem-Solving Tool for the Person With Diabetes

For the Person With Diabetes . . .

Why is my blood sugar out of the target range? These things can make your blood sugar go up or down. Do you see anything that might explain your blood sugar? Are blood sugars out of range for several days at the same time?

Eating	*Physical Activity*	*Monitoring Blood Sugar*	*Taking Medication*	*Coping Skills*	*Problem Solving*	*Complications or Risks*
Blood Sugar Too High—Questions to Ask						
Ate more food? Ate out or special occasion? Snacking or nibbling on food? Drank alcohol? Type of food?	Got less exercise? Changed schedule? BG was >300 mg before starting exercise?	Missed checking? Got off schedule? Not enough blood? Hands were not clean?	Took after eating? Missed meds/ insulin? Problems drawing up insulin? Took too little? Need more oral medication? Insulin too hot/ cold?	Stressed out? Family problems? Financial problems? Depressed? Work problems?	Been sick? Got a sore? Over treated low blood sugar?	Stomach problems? Chest pain? Hard to draw up insulin with poor vision? Pregnant?
Blood Sugar Too Low—Questions to Ask						
Ate less food? Drank alcohol? Missed snack? Delayed or missed meal?	Changed schedule? Got more exercise? Exercise was more intense? BG low before exercise?	Missed checking? Got off schedule? Not enough blood? Meter/strips too hot or cold?	Problems drawing up insulin? Took too much? Need less medication? Took wrong insulin at wrong time?	Stressed out? Took extra insulin to cover high BG from stress?	Over treated high blood sugar?	Stomach problems? Kidneys are failing? Hard to draw up insulin with poor vision?

Source: Developed by Donna Tomky, MSN, RN, CNP, CDCES, FADCES and Sue Perry, PhD, CDCES for the New Mexico Department of Health, Diabetes Prevention & Control Program. Version 2006. Reprinted with permission.

examples provided in Table 18.15, yet it is common to revert to a negative focus when in a counseling session unless a concerted effort is made to focus positively. Practice and observing individual's responses will help highlight the advantages of positive questioning.

Continuous Glucose Monitoring

There have been significant technological advances in continuous glucose monitoring (CGM) recently. Results from randomized controlled trials show improved glycemic stability, reduced hypoglycemia, and improved satisfaction among persons with diabetes with effective use of CGM.[55–62] Increasingly, clinicians and diabetes care and education specialists are recommending CGM use to better understand glucose profiles and guide therapy decisions for the person with diabetes.[58,59] Due to improved sensor accuracy, the FDA has cleared most CGM device systems for nonadjunctive use. Adjunctive use means that treatment decisions must be made on confirmatory fingersticks (SMBG); nonadjunctive use means the person with diabetes can adjust therapy, including insulin dosing, based on the sensor glucose reading. This difference impacts cost and burden of care for the person with diabetes.[63] Other features such as share capacity have contributed to the growing popularity of this method of glucose monitoring. In addition, integration of CGM with insulin pumps has allowed even greater reduction in hypoglycemia through suspension of insulin during periods of low glucose or predicted low glucose.[55,56] The American Diabetes Association (ADA) recommends CGM as a management tool for children, adolescents, and adults with type 1 diabetes to decrease the risk of hypoglycemia and contribute to improved glycemic stability.[56] The American Association of Clinical Endocrinologists (AACE) and American College of Endocrinology (ACE)

TABLE 18.14 Blood Glucose Monitoring Assessment Tool for the Diabetes Care and Education

For the Diabetes Care Education Specialist . . .

More reasons to consider why an individual's blood glucoses are out of target ranges. Review several days of BG levels and look for patterns.

Eating	*Physical Activity*	*Monitoring Blood Sugar*	*Taking Medication*	*Coping Skills*	*Problem Solving*	*Complications or Risks*
Blood Sugar Too High—Questions to Ask						
Gastroparesis? Inaccurate carb counting? Snacking? Large or high-fat meal with slow digestion?	Insufficient insulin with counter-regulatory hormones release? Intense workout with elevated BG?	Integrity of strips? Meter/ technique? Data accuracy? Insufficient data? Somogyi or dawn phenomenon?	Lipohypertrophy? Timing of meds/ insulin? Absorption of meds or insulin? Insulin/pill integrity?	Stress hormones? Memory loss/ forgetfulness? Untreated psych disorder?	Recent infection? Silent infection? Oral or injection of steroids? Pubertal or growth hormones? Hyperthyroidism?	2nd or 3rd trimester of pregnancy? Recent myocardial infarction? Visual acuity? Dexterity problems? Gastroparesis?
Blood Sugar Too Low—Questions to Ask						
Decreased carb intake? Inaccurate carb counting? Alcohol consumption? High-fat meal with rapid insulin absorption, and slow digestion?	Injection site near active extremity? Timing of med or insulin in relationship to activity? Weight loss?	Data accuracy? Integrity of strips? Meter/ technique? Insufficient data?	Timing of insulin? Wrong med? Inconsistent taking of meds/ insulin? No access to medication?	Depression? Anxious? Memory loss/ forgetfulness? Untreated psych disorder?	Hypoglycemia unawareness? Missed other meds, ie, steroids? Hypothyroidism?	1st trimester of pregnancy? Gastroparesis? Visual acuity? Dexterity problems? Renal insufficiency?

Source: Developed by Donna Tomky, MSN, RN, CNP, CDCES, FADCES and Sue Perry, PhD, CDCES for the New Mexico Department of Health, Diabetes Prevention & Control Program. Version 2006. Reprinted with permission.

highlight the impact of effective CGM use on cost reduction and improved health outcomes for persons with diabetes in addition to reduced risk of hypoglycemia and improved glucose stability.[58]

How Does CGM Works?

Continuous glucose monitoring device systems generally include three components: a small, wearable sensor which is inserted subcutaneously; a transmitter which is exterior to the skin; and a receiver which displays the glucose readings. Continuous glucose monitoring uses a sensor to measure glucose in the interstitial fluid and converts it to an electronic signal which is captured by the transmitter.

Through wireless technology, the transmitter relays the information to a proprietary receiver, an approved smart device such as a smartphone or watch, or an insulin pump in the case of an integrated CGM and pump system. Through apps and cloud technology, designated "share" capacity is granted, allowing others (parents, caregivers, diabetes care and education specialists, clinicians) an opportunity to view the glucose data remotely. Continuous glucose monitoring devices may be programmed to sync with insulin delivery devices or BG meters through a "handshake" whereby two devices are programmed to search and recognize the other, confirming communication between the two devices.

Continuous glucose monitoring devices collect sensor glucose data every few minutes and can provide real-time glucose information including trending direction and rate of change, a marked improvement over the sporadic data provided by fingersticks. In addition, CGM devices may

TABLE 18.15 Positive Glucose Questioning

Instead of	*Consider*
What is the most difficult part of blood glucose monitoring?	What is the easiest part of blood glucose monitoring for you? What would make blood glucose monitoring easier for you? How would you know when you were successful with blood glucose monitoring?
Why did you forget to check in the morning?	What helps you remember to check?
Your numbers are running high in the morning; what do you think you are doing wrong?	Look how great your numbers are on these days (or times). Let's talk about what you do then.
Why aren't you checking your blood glucoses?	How important is blood glucose monitoring to you?
Why are your post-dinner blood glucoses always high?	Tell me about your dinner meal. Tell me about what happens the hour or 2 before dinner.
Why are you checking only fasting blood glucose?	Tell me what your fasting blood glucoses are telling you.
Why aren't you checking your blood glucose at least twice per day?	What part of your day would you most like to know something about your blood glucose results? How often do you think you would want to look at (check) your blood glucose results in a week?
Do you think checking your blood sugar 3 times a day is realistic?	On a scale of 1 to 10, how confident are you that you can check your blood glucose 3 times a day every day of the week? (If not confident, ask the individual if she or he would like to change the goal to one in which she or he felt confident.)

provide visual, vibratory, and/or auditory alerts for low- and high-sensor glucose levels, depending on the device features and programmable settings. Persons with diabetes benefit most from real-time data if educated in proper use of the information to adjust treatment, prevent hypoglycemia, and better understand the variables that contribute to glycemic excursions.[55] Glucose measured in the interstitial fluid may differ from blood glucose due to time lag, particularly during periods of rapid fluctuations of glucose levels, such as postmeal.[64] Continuous glucose monitoring devices may require periodic calibration using SMBG to maintain sensor accuracy while others are factory calibrated.

CGM Accuracy

CGM accuracy is typically reported using mean absolute relative deviation (MARD), an analytic statistic which describes the accuracy of glucose values spanning the range; MARD is less useful in quantifying information about outliers or accuracy by day of sensor wear.[64] However, accuracy is less of a barrier with recent advances in CGM technology producing MARD scores of <10% for many CGMs, an important threshold for insulin dosing.[58] Perceptions of accuracy with CGM use are associated with more wear time, improved quality of life and more effective utilization of the CGM technology.[65] False low glucose readings have been reported as possibly related to physical compression of the CGM sensor, such as during nighttime.[66] Studies have reported that CGM glucose levels may be falsely higher for some devices due to acetaminophen effect[64,67,68] or that various other substances may interfere with accurate CGM readings.[55,69] Although accuracy and safety associated with an implantable 90-day sensor have been demonstrated, substance interference has also been reported with implanted sensors. These substances are different than with short-term sensors.[70,71] Instruct persons with diabetes on which substances to avoid, based on the specific CGM device in use.

CGM versus SMBG

Use of CGM is associated with reduced hypoglycemia and lower A1C levels compared to blood glucose monitoring.[55–57,72–74] CGM supports a 24-hour glucose profile for analysis, education, and treatment decisions, both retrospectively and real-time, whereas SMBG provides only a few readings per day. When compared to SMBG, CGM provides up to 288 readings per day at no additional financial cost, pain, or user interactions.[64] There may be cost benefits associated with episodic use of real-time CGM for persons with diabetes not taking mealtime insulin.[75] In addition, CGM gives a more complete picture of nocturnal glucose patterns and undetected hypoglycemia. It is better than SMBG at showing the effects of food, medication, stress, and activity. CGM provides rate of change and trending information versus static glucose readings, as with SMBG. In other words, is the glucose going up, down, or holding steady, and if there is directional trending, how quickly is the glucose changing? Current technology provides trending alerts and alarms for hypoglycemia and hyperglycemia thresholds that can be individualized for the person with diabetes.

However, there is still a need for SMBG in certain circumstances. Some CGM devices require fingerstick calibration for accuracy and for treatment decisions if not cleared for nonadjunctive therapy. At the current time, FDA approval may not cover CGM use in special circumstances such as pregnancy, dialysis, or critical illness necessitating use of SMBG.[55] Nonetheless, SMBG is limited by several factors including user error, substandard equipment accuracy, static glucose readings, lack of alerts related to variability, lack of nighttime glucose data, and lower participation due to the inconvenience of fingersticks. The limited and potentially inaccurate data obtained through SMBG may result in inappropriate treatment decisions.[63,76]

Continuous glucose monitoring can provide insight into the impact of food, exercise, medications, and stress on glucose levels.[77] This can be useful for noninsulin users as well, particularly in understanding postmeal glycemic excursions, the effects of certain foods, and the utility of exercise postmeal to smooth glucose levels.[78]

Some persons with diabetes might prefer wearing a sensor in lieu of the fingersticks required with SMBG. Frequent use of CGM is associated with reduced emergency care and fear of hypoglycemia.[79] A 24-hour glucose profile over a period of several days can give a more complete picture of glucose patterns and guide small changes through use of self-management principles that can make a difference in well-being and improve glycemic stability.[80] CGM may help empower persons with diabetes to adjust lifestyle behaviors and improve self-management skills through effective use of CGM information.[66]

In summary, benefits of CGM include awareness of glycemic variability related to activity, hormone fluctuations and types of foods such as high-glycemic index or high-fat foods; alerts for impending hypoglycemia, particularly important for those with hypo unawareness; reduced fear of nocturnal hypoglycemia; awareness of glycemic patterns during and post-exercise; reassurance to persons with diabetes and caregivers that real-time glucose trend data allows mitigation of glycemic excursions; validation of treatment changes; and promotion of self-management of diabetes through effective utilization of glucose data.[78]

CGM and A1C

An A1C is a useful assessment measure applied to population health and is correlated with risk of complications. It has less utility in guiding treatment decisions and for self-management of diabetes.[76,81] Beck et al highlight the importance of individualized CGM glucose data as being a valuable tool for person-centered care. Persons with diabetes may report the same A1C but have dissimilar glucose profiles that may require different therapeutic interventions.[81]

Continuous glucose monitoring is better than A1C at giving information about hypoglycemia, hyperglycemia, and glycemic variability. Cardiovascular complications may be associated with glycemic variability.[82] An A1C can be unreliable for people with certain conditions, such as hemoglobinopathies, anemia, or pregnancy.[63] In addition, racial differences have been observed between mean glucose and A1C levels suggesting that glucose profiles provide a more accurate picture of glucose levels overall than A1C. In one study, A1C level for African Americans, on average, was 0.4 percentage points higher than that of Caucasians compared to given mean glucose concentration. In other words, A1C levels may overestimate mean glucose in black persons compared with white persons, perhaps related to racial differences in the glycation of hemoglobin. Nevertheless, use of CGM for individualized treatment helps mitigate any safety concerns related to this potential difference by race in A1C levels.[83] Overall, glycemic variability is more easily identified through retrospective analysis of CGM data that offers clinically meaningful information and informs optimal treatment decisions.[81]

Type of CGM System-Personal or Professional

Continuous glucose monitoring is prescribed for personal use or professional use. Characteristics are described in Table 18.16.

Personal CGM

The use of personal CGM offers many benefits for the person with diabetes. In addition to reduced hypoglycemia, frequent use (daily) of CGM is associated with increased time in target range and reduced hyperglycemia, contributing to improved overall glucose stability and lower A1C.[55] Personal CGM provides predictive information, useful in preventing hypoglycemia and hyperglycemia, and alert thresholds that can be adjusted to accommodate fear of hypoglycemia.[76] Continuous glucose monitoring provides easy access to glucose levels continuously, which supports and reinforces key concepts related to the impact of food,

TABLE 18.16 Characteristics of Personal versus Professional CGMs

Personal CGM	*Professional CGM*
Person with diabetes owns device	Clinic owns device
Sensor duration 7–14 days; 90 days implantable*	Short-term sensor use (3–14 days)
Option for continuous use	Time interval between CGM studies
Real-time data use	Blinded data during wear
Special features include hypo alerts, share capacity	No hypo alerts or data sharing features
Cost and reimbursement varies with insurance	Requires systematic loaner program

*Requires insertion by trained clinician

exercise, medication, and stress on glucose levels. This data may be useful in motivating the person with diabetes to make optimal changes to their eating habits and to better engage with recommended self-management practices.[84]

The ADA recommends real-time glucose monitoring for insulin users not meeting glycemic targets and notes that near-daily use offers the highest benefit.[56] AACE/ACE recommends real-time CGM for all persons with diabetes using insulin.[58] Guidelines from the Endocrine Society for persons with diabetes age 8 or older recommend real-time CGM for type 1 diabetes and short-term use of real-time CGM for type 2 diabetes if not taking meal-time insulin.[59,60] However, to use personal CGM effectively, the person with diabetes must know the basics of sensor insertion, calibration if required, and interpretation of CGM data.[66]

Research studies have established the benefit of CGM use with type 2 diabetes. In a study of adults using multiple daily injection (MDI) therapy to manage their type 2 diabetes, study participants were assigned to CGM use or usual care (SMBG) for a period of 24 weeks. The primary outcome for the research study showed that study participants using CGM had lower A1C levels compared to the control group and that this difference was clinically significant. Furthermore, secondary outcomes documented near-daily use of CGM by study end for more than 90% of those in the CGM group and high satisfaction with CGM according to surveys completed by study participants.[57] Another study assessed the efficacy of CGM use in type 2 diabetes by comparing intermittent use of CGM with usual care (SMBG) for those not on meal-time insulin. Study participants were assigned to use CGM intermittently for 12 weeks or follow usual care. Although both groups showed improved glycemic levels during the study, the CGM group had better glycemic stability overall with A1C levels dropping 1.0% for the CGM group versus 0.5% for the SMBG group at 12 weeks. Despite returning to usual care after 12 weeks of CGM use, the CGM group showed sustained improvement in glycemic levels with A1C levels down 0.8% for the CGM group versus 0.2% for the SMBG group at 52 weeks.[62]

Real-Time versus Intermittently Scanned CGM

Personal CGM is often classified as real-time CGM (rtCGM) or intermittently scanned CGM (isCGM). Real-time CGM has continuous glucose data transmitted automatically to the receiver or smart device and provides alerts and alarms.[56,63,76] Internally scanned CGM (sometimes referred to as "flash" monitoring) collects glucose data every minute but the person with diabetes must actively scan the transmitter at least every 8 hours to see the glucose data information and retain the data for future downloading and review.[76] Real-world testing of adults using a CGM device documented an average of 16 scans per day.[85] Currently, isCGM does not have an auditory alert or alarm capability.[56,63,76] Internally scanned CGM may be substituted for SMBG in adults requiring frequent glucose testing.[56,86]

Most personal CGM devices utilize a short-term sensor (7-14 days), though one manufacturer uses an implantable sensor that remains under the skin for 90 days.[63] This sensor is inserted by trained clinicians through a small incision and can be done in the office setting. The transmitter adheres to the skin directly over the implanted sensor, provides vibration alerts, serves as a power source for the sensor, and transmits data in real time to a smart device.[70] There are currently four manufacturers producing CGM devices in the United States (See Table 18.17.)

Integrated CGM and Insulin Pump Systems

The ADA recommends use of integrated CGM and insulin pump systems to improve glycemic stability and reduce risk of hypoglycemia.[56] Integrated sensor and pump systems allow visualization of sensor data on the pump screen. Some integrated systems include algorithms to automatize basal insulin doses, suspending when sensor glucose is trending low, and increasing basal insulin when sensor glucose is elevated.[55] Real-time CGMs may be part of an integrated insulin pump system or function as a stand-alone CGM device. Some rtCGM systems offer data transmission utilizing cloud storage and computing which supports remote data sharing.[63] Personal CGM systems may be integrated with smart devices or insulin pumps or may function independently utilizing a receiver. In addition, persons with diabetes may wear both a CGM and an insulin pump, but the devices are not integrated

TABLE 18.17 Characteristics of Available Personal CGM Systems

Manufacturer/Brand	*Abbott FreeStyle Libre*	*Dexcom G5*	*Dexcom G6*	*Medtronic Guardian™ 3*	*Eversense®*
Characteristics	isCGM	rtCGM	rtCGM	rtCGM	rtCGM
Calibration required?	No	Yes	No	Yes	Yes
Warm-up time, h	1 hour	2 hours	2 hours	2 hours	24 hours (at insertion)
Alarms and alerts	No	Yes	Yes	Yes	Yes
Nonadjunctive use	Yes	Yes	Yes	No	Yes
Sensor duration	14 days	7 days	10 days	7 days	90 days
Integrates with insulin pump	No	Yes	Yes	Yes	No
Smart device interoperability	Yes	Yes	Yes	Yes	Yes
Approved for children	No	Yes	Yes	Yes	No
Data share capacity	Yes	Yes	Yes	Yes	Yes

Adapted from Sources: SV Edelman, et al, "Clinical implications of real time and intermittently scanned continuous glucose monitoring," *Diabetes Care*. 41(11)(2018):2265-74.

AADE Practice Paper: The Diabetes Educator Role in Continuous Glucose Monitoring, 2018.

AL Peters, et al, "Advances in glucose monitoring and automated insulin delivery: supplement to endocrine society clinical practice guidelines," *Journal of the Endocrine Society*. 2(11)(2018):1214–25.

and do not communicate with one another. In this case, data must be downloaded from both the CGM and the insulin pump, resulting in 2 separate reports rather than 1 integrated data report.[78]

Recent advancements in integrated CGM and insulin pump systems allow for continuous insulin basal rate dosing adjustments that coincide with programmed target glucose settings.[60] Sometimes called sensor-augmented pump therapy or hybrid closed-loop therapy, these systems can improve glucose stability without increasing risk for hypoglycemia or severe hyperglycemia and offer additional benefit for those at high risk of hypoglycemia.[56,87] Hybrid closed-loop (HCL) systems utilize integrated CGM and insulin pumps systems but employ controller algorithms to adjust basal insulin every few minutes around-the-clock.[87] Recent changes to FDA regulatory processes governing CGM devices allow expedited approval for CGMs that offer interconnectivity with other devices.[88] This change in the approval process may help speed research and development of HCL systems.

Professional CGM

Professional CGMs are prescribed for episodic use to identify glucose patterns and inform treatment decisions. Professional CGM systems are not paired with smart devices for real-time viewing nor integrated with insulin delivery devices such as pumps. These devices are approved for adjunctive use only and sensor glucose data is typically masked real time and unmasked for retrospective review by the clinician.[55]

There are 3 professional CGM systems currently available that can be prescribed for short periods of time (6-14 days) for data collection and subsequent analysis of glycemic patterns. Professional CGM diagnostics are generally conducted in blinded mode, which gives the clinician a retrospective snapshot of typical glucose fluctuations than if the person with diabetes is responding in real time to trending glucose data as with personal systems. Following the period of sensor wear, the CGM is downloaded and reports generated for analysis. Clinicians may identify problem areas and opportunities for adjusting therapy based on short-term observation of CGM data.[61]

Documentation of medication dose and timing, activity, food intake, and health events such as illness is highly recommended for the person with diabetes during professional CGM wear. This information can be correlated with glycemic patterns for even greater understanding of the impact of food, medications, and exercise on glucose levels and self-management of diabetes.[55] Intermittent use of CGM can be useful in detecting glycemic variability in type 2 diabetes. The frequency of asymptomatic hypoglycemia in individuals with medication-treated type 2 diabetes may be underappreciated.[89]

Guided review of glucose profiles can be useful to persons with diabetes to better understand the relationship between individual behaviors and glucose stability. Diabetes care and education specialists may gain a better understanding overall into the self-management practices of the person with diabetes through the discovery of discrepancies in glucose trends and medication use.[90] In addition, professional use CGM offers persons with diabetes an opportunity to try a new monitoring method before purchasing a personal use system. This is particularly helpful if there are concerns about skin sensitivity, alarm fatigue, or cost burden associated with personal use CGM.

Using the CGM Device-Operational Skills

Select Device System

Selection of the CGM device warrants review of the significant differences between systems and individualizing the choice to find the best fit for the person with diabetes. Safety considerations, preferences, and barriers to use should be addressed during the selection process.[55] Persons with diabetes may benefit from predictive alerts in preventing hypoglycemia.[91] Personal CGM may be appropriate for most persons with diabetes who are willing to wear the system consistently, particularly those with history of severe hypoglycemia, hypoglycemia unawareness, or those not meeting glucose targets.[56,59,66,78]

Real-time sharing of glucose information allows parents and caregivers to follow their child's glucose readings when apart, including nocturnal. This feature is also useful for adults who travel or live alone. Use of CGM with remote monitoring is associated with less parental fear of hypoglycemia and higher quality of life measures.[92] Continuous glucose monitoring use in type 2 diabetes guides therapeutic decisions and encompasses the principles of diabetes self-management.[78,93] Internally scanned CGM may be helpful for persons with diabetes who have difficulty performing SMBG due to limitations in manual dexterity.[63]

Device selection includes assessment of hypoglycemia risk and subsequent need for alerts and alarms, willingness to calibrate, cost of CGM system, sensor type and duration, ease of use, desire for remote sharing of data, and whether there is a need for interoperability and/or integration with other devices such as insulin pumps.[76] It is vital that diabetes care and education specialists be facile with the various CGM systems so that the person with diabetes can receive appropriate guidance for successful use.[78] (See Table 18.18.)

TABLE 18.18 Considerations for Device Selection for Personal CGM

Real-Time CGM	*Intermittently Scanned CGM*
Intensive insulin regimen (insulin pump or multiple daily injections (MDI)	Use as an educational tool
Increased risk of hypoglycemia	Not requiring or desiring alarm/alert features
Fear of hypoglycemia	Willing to scan frequently
Athletes or those with hectic lifestyles	Low risk of hypoglycemia but want more glucose data
Person with diabetes desires tighter glucose stability	Cost prohibitive to use rtCGM
Young children or others desiring data share option	Person with diabetes prefers in lieu of SMBG

Source: Adapted from P Adolfsson, CG Parkin, A Thomas, LG Krinelke, "Selecting the appropriate continuous glucose monitoring system—a practical approach," *Eur Endocrinol.* 14(1)(2018):24-29.

Special Populations

Pediatrics The ADA recommends real-time CGM in children and adolescents with type 1 diabetes as a useful tool for improving glycemic management and reducing the risk of hypoglycemia, regardless of the method of insulin delivery. Observance and near-daily use are important for successful use of the CGM system.[56] Special consideration should be given if the child is lean and/or wearing a pump as sensor sites may be limited. Athletes may have challenges with sensor adhesion, although there are products available for improved adhesion.[76] Away from home, calibration and sensor integrity issues can present additional challenges.[78] Barrier products can help reduce skin sensitivity.[76] A remote share feature is available with some devices, which is highly desirable for parents of children with type 1 diabetes as it affords them the opportunity to monitor their child's glucose levels in real time. Thus, CGM technology is increasingly more common in the pediatric population, requiring education and support for community caregivers in schools, day care facilities, and camps.[55]

Elderly Real-time CGM may be useful for older persons living alone, particularly if there is concern related to hypo-unawareness or other medical issues that impact glucose levels. Assess for cognitive or dexterity issues that may impact the individual's ability to fully utilize the CGM system.[78] Remote viewing is important for elderly individuals, too.

Pregnancy Use of CGM in pregnancy can provide information, in addition to SMBG, for nocturnal glycemic patterns as well as postprandial glucose levels and is useful as a teaching tool.[66,94] Findings from a study show that CGM use is associated with more time in glucose target range, less time in hyperglycemia, and better health outcomes for infants and has been useful in documenting glucose patterns during pregnancy for women with type 1 and type 2 diabetes.[95,96] The ADA recommendations suggest that real-time CGM use in pregnant women with type 1 diabetes may improve A1C levels and neonatal outcomes.[56]

Inpatient Use Continuous glucose monitoring may be useful in the recognition and prevention of hypoglycemia in the inpatient setting; however, there are many technological barriers which may impact accuracy of sensor readings including substance interference, calibration requirements, and certain physiologic conditions.[97] Other challenges include sensor site selection, prep and insertion, charging of the transmitter, and maintenance of sensor integrity and connectivity between the sensor, transmitter, and receiver.[97]

Cost and Reimbursement There are considerable cost differences between professional and personal CGM and between personal CGM devices. Because reimbursement varies, coverage should be verified before initiating CGM use. Prior authorization may be required. Currently, CGM costs are reimbursed for type 1 diabetes <age 65 by most commercial insurance. Medicare covers "therapeutic CGM" which replaces fingersticks for persons with diabetes using insulin.[98]

Clinicians can bill for training and interpretation of CGM data although billing codes and requirements may differ depending on state law, CMS guidelines, and insurance requirements. The CGM reports including glycemic patterns and treatment recommendations can be reviewed with the person with diabetes in a clinic visit or through a telehealth exchange if reimbursable.[55]

Sensor Insertion and Calibration CGM device manufacturers may provide training and certification for diabetes care and education specialists and clinicians that include proper sensor insertion, maintenance and cleaning of equipment, and contraindications regarding CGM use. Educate the person with diabetes on the difference between interstitial glucose and blood glucose readings and measures which enhance sensor accuracy such as proper sensor calibration and technique including optimal timing and frequency of calibration, preferred sites for sensor placement, and sensor insertion technique.[55,80] Accuracy matters and sensor insertion technique and use should be monitored periodically including initially.

Preferred sites for sensor placement vary by device with some devices approved for sensor wear on the back of the arm or abdomen or both. The person with diabetes may have individual preferences for sensor placement that include different (non-approved) sites, but these sites may have been approved by their clinician for "off-label" use. Sensor insertion technique including skin prep, charging of the transmitter, and proper taping should be part of the instruction including teach back observation.[67,80] Instruct the person with diabetes to take care when bathing and dressing to avoid inadvertently dislodging the sensor, especially if worn on the back of the arm. Sensors should not be placed in areas of skin fold, natural bend or where there is tension on the surrounding skin. It is helpful to avoid sites where clothing or belts might impede adherence or comfort. Troubleshooting topics for CGM site problems include optimal site placement, optimizing adherence of the sensor, and minimizing skin sensitivity. Use of skin adhesives and clear film dressings can be helpful. To enhance adhesion of a sensor, exercise and bathing should be avoided immediately after sensor placement. Skin sensitivity can be addressed by changing the sensor location or by use of barrier products under the sensor tape.[55] However, care must be taken to allow a place for the sensor to be inserted without passing through the barrier product. Longer sensor wear may require education on skin care if sensitivity or adherence issues arise.[76]

Instruction should include review of calibration requirements, if calibration is required or allowed, including timing and technique for accurate calibration using proper SMBG technique. There may be a sensor glucose lag time of 5 to 15 minutes behind blood glucose, particularly if glucose levels are changing quickly. Calibration is best performed at recommended intervals during periods of glucose stability rather than fluctuation such as post-meal.[64] The person with diabetes should be educated on proper care of the transmitter that may include frequent charging and tips for transmitter attachment that are specific to the device. Individualized alert settings including rate of change should be set and reviewed with the person. Be sure the person with diabetes can see and hear alerts and alarms. Teach family members and caregivers as appropriate. Remind individuals that successful use of CGM requires near-daily use of rtCGM.[67]

Safety and Contraindications Package inserts should be reviewed with the person with diabetes for contraindications such as medication interference which could impact accuracy of sensor glucose readings.[55] The diabetes care and education specialist should instruct persons regarding CGM manufacturers' recommendations during procedures that involve radiation exposure and magnetic resonance imaging.[80] Contraindications generally include avoidance of hot tubs for CGM devices.[55] Instruct the person with diabetes about the importance of working with the CGM system to ensure optimal functioning and accuracy including ways to effectively troubleshoot technology issues such as with use of the CGM device proprietary Web site and helpline.

The person with diabetes may note sensor integrity issues on the first day of the sensor after the warm-up period and during the last day of use. Extended use of sensors beyond the recommended time frame is not recommended as accuracy could be impaired.[64,76,78] Extending sensor use should be discouraged, particularly if approved for nonadjunctive use. In situations of automatized insulin delivery, as with the hybrid closed-loop system, sensor integrity is of paramount importance.

Identifying Barriers to CGM The person with diabetes needs access to trained, supportive diabetes care and education specialists for successful utilization of CGM. Potential barriers to CGM use include unrealistic expectations about what CGM can do, aggressive treatment of hyperglycemia, over-reliance on CGM alarms to alert if hypoglycemia, alarm fatigue contributing to underutilization of CGM or blocked safety alert system, skin sensitivity or adhesion problems, body-image concerns, limited area for sensor insertion, particularly for pump users and children, cost of personal use CGM, fear of pain, unsure of utility or accuracy of technology, and data overload if lacking clinical guidance for effective use of CGM information.[55,78,98] Barriers to CGM use are summarized by category and described in detail in Table 18.19.

The person with diabetes may note skin sensitivity with rashes and itching, CGM transmission problems, particularly at night, and lack of adhesion with sensors falling off before end of sensor life possibly due to

TABLE 18.19 Potential Barriers to CGM Use

Type of Potential Barrier	*Description*	*Possible Solution*
Diabetes Care Team	Lack of trained staff, internal system firewalls, data overload, change burnout, unfamiliar glucose reports	Identify expert staff to form CGM task force Include healthcare tech support representative from your facility Attend device training sessions Review educational and interpretative tools for CGM
Financial	Start-up costs, ongoing sensor cost, excessive paperwork with prior authorization, clinic and/or reluctance of the individual to invest in new technology	Become familiar with private and government insurance coverage requirements for CGM Consider initial and ongoing out-of-pocket costs for device Explore assistance programs
Physical	Skin sensitivity, adhesion issues, lack of dexterity for sensor insertion, impaired vision or hearing, lack of available sites for sensor insertion (small child, insulin pump wearer,) medication use with potential interference in accuracy, exercise or activity limitations	Individualize device selection to mitigate these barriers by increasing options for site selection, considering physical limitations, lifestyle behaviors, and medical needs
Emotional	Body image, pain with insertion, reluctant to wear sensor, burden of CGM technology, prone to overtreatment of glucose readings	Individualize device selection to address site preference and minimize insertion pain Consider willingness to wear CGM on continuous versus episodic basis Assess potential for increased anxiety or overreaction to glucose data
Cognitive, health literacy, numeracy and technology skills	Difficulty with execution of CGM operational skills due to cognitive or learning challenges Unable to understand effective use of CGM information	Individualize device selection to address cognitive or learning barriers Consider episodic, professional CGM or isCGM Ensure accurate technique through teach back observation

(continued)

TABLE 18.19 Potential Barriers to CGM Use (continued)

Type of Potential Barrier	*Description*	*Possible Solution*
Convenience	Hassle factor of continuous sensor wear, alert/alarm fatigue, sensor changes, calibration schedule, sensor integrity issues, transmission/receiver problems, extra training time, access to data	Individualize device selection to address convenience barriers Consider episodic professional CGM or isCGM Opt for data display options that are user friendly with smart device receivers Set low and high alerts to minimize nuisance alarms and modify over time if needed
Safety	Contraindications such as X-rays, MRIs Potential accuracy issues related to lag time, medication interference, or sensor integrity Warm-up time without sensor data, nonadjunctive use	Educate individual about contraindications and medication interference SMBG during warm-up period or if lack of confidence in CGM accuracy Remote data sharing

Sources: SV Edelman, et al, "Clinical implications of real time and intermittently scanned continuous glucose monitoring," *Diabetes Care.* 41(11)(2018):2265-74.

AADE Practice Paper: The Diabetes Educator Role in Continuous Glucose Monitoring, 2018.

ADA: Diabetes Technology: Standards of Medical Care in Diabetes—2019. American Diabetes Association. *Diabetes Care.* 42(Supplement 1)(2019):S71-80.

VA Fonseca, G Grunberger, H Anhalf, et al, "Continuous glucose monitoring: a consensus conference of the American Association of Clinical Endocrinologists and American College of Endocrinology," *Endocr Pract.* 22(8)(2016):1008-21.

AL Peters, AJ Ahmann, T Battelino, et al, "Diabetes technology continuous subcutaneous insulin infusion therapy and continuous glucose monitoring in adults: an Endocrine Society clinical practice guideline," *J Clin Endocrinol Metab.* 101(11)(2016):3922-37.

AL Peters, et al, "Advances in glucose monitoring and automated insulin delivery: supplement to Endocrine Society clinical practice guidelines," *Journal of the Endocrine Society.* 2(11)(2018):1214-25.

DC Klonoff, D Ahn, A Drincic, "Continuous glucose monitoring: a review of the technology and clinical use," *Diabetes Res Clin Pract.* 133(2017):178-92.

WH Polonsky, D Hessler, "Perceived accuracy in continuous glucose monitoring: understanding the impact on patients," *J Diabetes Sci Technol.* 9(2)(2015):339-41.

P Adolfsson, CG Parkin, A Thomas, LG Krinelke, "Selecting the appropriate continuous glucose monitoring system--a practical approach," *Eur Endocrinol.* 14(1)(2018):24-9.

sweating. Heightened risk of skin sensitivity, particularly for children, may be related to longer sensor wear time, increased exposure to adhesives, and diminished skin barrier. These skin reactions may become progressively more pronounced with repeat use.[99] There are products for improved adhesion such as skin gels and tape, and there are also barrier products to reduce sensitivity.[76]

Due to alarm fatigue, the person with diabetes may turn off the CGM alerts. Tailored settings and gradual adjustments to these settings may help prevent or decrease alarm burnout.[76] Additionally, calibration requirements may impact cost and burden of care for the person with diabetes. Some CGMs are factory calibrated but others require minimum twice-daily calibration.[63] Overall, there has been increased use in CGM technology with improved accuracy, wearability, and lower cost to the user.[58]

Using the CGM Device-Interpretation Skills

Interpreting Real-Time CGM Results-Understanding Trending

Understanding trending information is necessary for effective use of rtCGM.[67] Generally, a horizontal arrow means glucose is constant. Up arrow(s) indicate rising glucose levels and rate of change. Down arrow(s) address falling glucose levels and how rapidly the change is predicted to occur. The rate of change arrows differs by CGM system (brand), and it is important to train the person with diabetes accordingly.[100]

Various methods have been identified for using CGM trending data for insulin dose adjustments in type 1 diabetes; however, the clinician should individualize the recommendations based on patient factors and differences between CGM systems.[67,100] Use trend arrows to fine-tune management in addition to the dosage prescribed based on current glucose reading, individualized target glucose range, insulin-to-carb ratio, and sensitivity factor. Further fine-tuning of insulin dose based on trend arrows considers the direction of the trend arrow and the rate of change. Use of CGM trend arrows in adjusting insulin doses requires numeracy competency to perform additional insulin dose calculations beyond the usual criterion.[67,100] Effective utilization of rtCGM trending data requires understanding the concepts related to anticipated glucose levels and appropriate actions for trending glucose levels utilizing a 30-minute window for anticipated glucose rather than adjustments based on static glucose data.[101]

Consider more conservative adjustments before, during, and post-exercise, and for frail or older adults, to reduce the risk of hypoglycemia. Clinicians must take an individualized approach to insulin adjustments based on trending arrows including establishing a plan for illness management with CGM.[100] Respond to trending arrows within 2 to 4 hours postmeal but avoid stacking insulin. Educate persons with diabetes to observe, monitor more frequently, check ketones, confirm with fingerstick if unsure, or treat rapidly trending down arrows proactively with carbs.[67] Suggest avoiding correction dose too close to last bolus, waiting at least 2 hours to reduce the risk of hypoglycemia from insulin stacking.[101] Insulin dose calculations incorporate anticipated glucose levels based on trending information in addition to other dosing criteria such as insulin-to-carb ratio and correction factor for static glucose. It is recommended to adjust for variables such as exercise, insulin on board, or meal composition.[101]

Diabetes care and education specialists must instruct on real-time use of CGM data including direction and speed of glucose trends, proactive avoidance of hypoglycemia, and reflection on potential causes of hyperglycemia such as illness or insufficient insulin due to late or missed bolus, mismatched insulin-to-carbohydrate dose, or interruption of insulin delivery. The diabetes care and education specialist should ensure that the person with diabetes understands concepts related to safe use of CGM including insulin action times and insulin on board. Education includes key concepts related to minimizing variability and increasing time in target range.[55] The availability of continuous glucose data invites manual titration of glucose levels, particularly for pump wearers, through frequent adjustments of insulin doses, "insulin stacking," and overtreatment of hypoglycemia.[80] Teach persons with diabetes how to safely utilize real-time sensor glucose trend data. More monitoring may be necessary if trending up and action may be necessary if trend is persistent such as taking correction insulin or checking pump site. A downward trend may require frequent monitoring and additional carbohydrates to avoid hypoglycemia.[78] Alerts should be tailored to individual needs, including high and low alerts, snooze settings, rate of change, and predictive alerts.[55] The role of the diabetes care and education specialist includes educating the person with diabetes on real-time use of CGM data as well as retrospective interpretation of CGM data utilizing pattern management to guide therapeutic decisions.[55]

Interpreting Retrospective CGM Results Utilizing Glucose Pattern Management

Understanding CGM Metrics Diabetes care and education specialists should be familiar with the metrics of the CGM and how to interpret the data. Table 18.20 describes the CGM metrics.

Data Sufficiency Measures The optimal minimum measurement time for collection and analysis of CGM data, representative of a 3-month time period, has been determined to be at least 14 days.[61,102] Recent clinical use recommendations suggest that data sufficiency is adequate with at least 70% wear over a 14-day period.[103]

Time in Range, Time Below Range, and Time Above Range Time in range (TIR) metric refers to the percent time CGM data is in the target range of 70 to 180 mg/dl. At least 70% time in range has been suggested as representing a clinically useful interpretation of this metric.[103] Individualization of TIR may be appropriate for pregnancy and older or high-risk persons with diabetes.

Time below range (TBR) is defined as percent time between 54 to 69 mg/dL for Level 1 hypoglycemia or percent time less than 54 mg/dL for Level 2 hypoglycemia.[103] Recommendation parameters related to TBR include less than 4% time for Level 1 hypoglycemia and less than 1% time for Level 2 hypoglycemia.[103]

Time above range (TAR) is defined as percent time between 181 to 250 mg/dL for Level 1 hyperglycemia and percent time greater than 250 mg/dL for Level 2 hyperglycemia. Recommendation parameters related to TAR include less than 25% time for Level 1 hyperglycemia and less than 5% time for Level 2 hyperglycemia.[103]

Average Glucose and Glucose Variability Continuous glucose monitoring offers the actual average (mean) glucose over the designated time interval.[63] Glucose variability metrics describe oscillations of glucose levels. The recommended measure for glucose variability is the percent coefficient of variation (CV) which is a statistic that

TABLE 18.20 Metrics for Continuous Glucose Monitoring

CGM Measure	*Parameter*	*Optimal Target*	*Notes*
Data Sufficiency	14 days; at least 70% wear time	≥70% wear time	Higher wear time associated with pattern reliability**
Average Glucose	Mean sensor glucose: mg/dL	Individualized target	Correlates with A1C; not correlated with variability
Glucose Management Index (GMI)	% calculated from mean sensor glucose	Match A1C target	GMI replaces eA1C
Time in Range (TIR)*	% TIR: 70–180 mg/dL	≥70% Individualized target*	Individualize targets to minimize hypoglycemia and maximize TIR*
Time below Range [TBR]*	Level 1: % 54–69 mg/dL Level 2: % <54 mg/dL	Level 1: <4%* Level 2: <1%* Individualized target*	Assess clinical significance; may require immediate action
Time above Range [TAR]*	Level 1: % 181–250 mg/dL Level 2: % >250 mg/dL	Level 1: <25%* Level 2: <5%* Individualized target*	Assess clinical significance; may require immediate action
Glucose Variability (CV)	≤36% Stable** >36% Unstable**	≤36% CV	Coefficient of Variation; Statistic includes standard deviation but minimizes correlation with mean glucose.
Data Visualization			Use of Ambulatory Glucose Profile (AGP)

*Adjusted targets suggested for pregnancy and older or high-risk persons with diabetes

**Adapted from sources:

ADA: Diabetes Technology: Standards of Medical Care in Diabetes—2019. American Diabetes Association. *Diabetes Care*. Jan 2019, 42 (Supplement 1) S71-80.

VA Fonseca, G Grunberger, H Anhalt, et al, "Continuous glucose monitoring: a consensus conference of the American Association of Clinical Endrocrinologist and American College of Endocrinology," *Endocr Pract*. 22(8)(2016):1008-21.

IB Hirsch, T Battelino, AL Peters, JJ Chamberlain, G Aleppo, RM Bergenstal. *Role of Continuous Glucose Monitoring in Diabetes Treatment*. Arlington, Va., American Diabetes Association, 2018.

T Battelini, et al, "Clinical targets for continuous glucose monitoring data interpretation: recommendations from the international consensus on time in range," *Diabetes Care*. Published Ahead of Print, published online June 8, 2019. https://doi.org/10.2337/dci19-0028

RM Bergenstal, et al, "Glucose management indicator (GMI): a new team for estimating A1C from continuous glucose monitoring," *Diabetes Care*. 41(8)(2019):1593-1603.

T Danne, et al, "International consensus on use of continuous glucose monitoring," *Diabetes Care*. 40(2017):1631-40.

Agiostratidou G, Anhalt H, Ball D, et al. Standardizing Clinically Meaningful Outcome Measures Beyond HbA1c for Type 1 Diabetes: A Consensus Report of the American Association of Clinical Endocrinologists, the American Association of Diabetes Educators, the American Diabetes Association, the Endocrine Society, JDRF International, The Leona M. and Harry B. Helmsley Charitable Trust, the Pediatric Endocrine Society, and the T1D Exchange. *Diabetes Care*. 40(12)(2017):1622-30.

LA Wright, IB Hirsch. "Metrics beyond hemoglobin A1C in diabetes management: time in range, hypoglycemia, and other parameters." *Diabetes Technol Ther*. 2017;19:S16-26.

measures standard deviation but minimizes correlation with mean glucose. A clinically useful threshold of less than 36% coefficient of variation has been recommended, which represents glycemic stability.[100,103]

Glucose Management Indicator (GMI) The glucose management indicator (GMI) metric provides information about overall glucose stability, similar to the A1C. It replaces estimated A1C (eA1C) that was used to convert mean glucose from SMBG or CGM to an estimate of laboratory A1C result that many found confusing and at times inaccurate. As a result, recommendation has been made to replace eA1C with GMI and the formula for obtaining GMI has been revised.[56,103,104] The formula for calculating GMI is (%)=3.31+0.02392 X [mean glucose in mg/dL] although diabetes care and education specialists may prefer to access a computational calculator for GMI at www.jaeb.org/gmi and www.AGPreport.org/agp/links.[104]

Understanding CGM Reports

Retrospective analysis of CGM data refers to glucose pattern analysis and review of CGM metrics. Standardized reports with graphic display or cues are available to help with data interpretation and diabetes management.[56] Although CGM devices have proprietary software for data analysis, most include a standardized 1-page version of the Ambulatory Glucose Profile (AGP).[56,76] (See Figure 18.3.) Standardized glucose analysis and visual report may contribute to increased utilization of CGM technology.[105] Interpretation of retrospective glucose data is less intuitive and suggests a need for educational support from the diabetes care team.[61,77,84] Asking the person with diabetes to look at

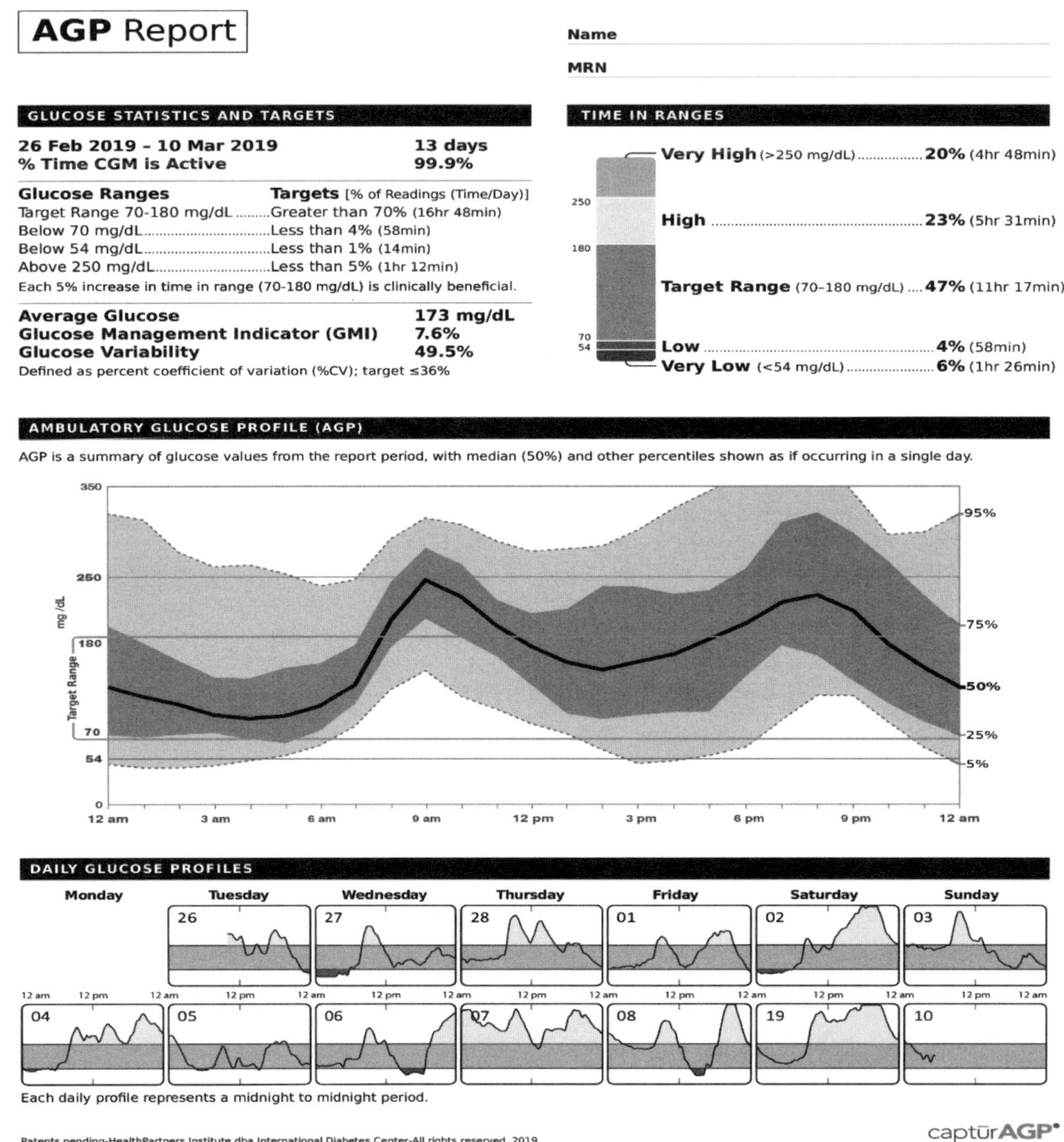

FIGURE 18.3 Standard Glucose Report-AGP

Source: International Diabetes Center. CGM AGP Report (Continuous Glucose Monitor (cited 24 Jan 2020) On the Internet at: http://www.agpreport.org/agp/agpreports. Used with permission.

the picture that represents a snapshot view of several days of glucose data can be very informative and useful for guided decision making.[82,93]

When interpreting CGM reports such as the AGP:

- Review the summary statistics to ensure data sufficiency is adequate (see Table 18.20).
- Address safety first by noting patterns of hypoglycemia, particularly overnight.
- Assess for periods of hyperglycemia overnight and pre- and postmeal.
- Finally, look for areas of significant variability that may offer insight into contributing factors such as medication timing, food choices, exercise, or alcohol use.[93,100,106]

The person with diabetes should be instructed to record when extra food is taken to avoid hypoglycemia. This information is important for clinicians doing retrospective analysis of CGM data without the benefit of food logs as patterns of hypoglycemia may be masked by proactively treating downward trending glucose levels.[78]

Role of the Diabetes Care and Education Specialist With CGM

Diabetes care and education specialists play a key role in the discussion of CGM use and product choice. Rarely does one product meet all the needs of every person. Diabetes care and education specialists can provide individuals considering, or initiating, CGM with the following:[78]

- An unbiased review of available CGM systems
- Setting appropriate expectations for CGM use
- Education regarding insulin activity and the "turnaround time" for glucose levels to respond (to potentially avoid overly aggressive therapy adjustments)
- Utilizing the person's own downloads at each clinic visit to teach the "thought process" of data analysis to empower the individual to successfully manage his or her blood glucose
- Managing sensitivity to device adhesive, or increasing device adhesion
- Additional support to older individuals and caregivers who are not confident in their use of technology but may benefit from CGM

Robust education, training, and support are necessary for effective use of CGM and diabetes care and education specialists must exhibit and maintain expertise in the education and use of this technology.[4] Understanding benefits and barriers to CGM use affords the diabetes care and education specialist an opportunity to help personalize device selection that supports successful use of CGM technology. Diabetes care and education specialists play a significant role by facilitating effective utilization of CGM and advanced technologies in self-management of diabetes.

- Take advantage of what is unique about CGM. Use trending information and multiple glucose readings to suggest treatment changes and lifestyle adjustments in response to glucose information.
- Downloading CGM data in the clinic setting and accessing data via remote viewing are essential skills/functions and critical for education related to pattern management.[2]
- Become knowledgeable about CGM metrics and skilled at interpreting CGM reports such as the AGP.
- Be familiar with processes related to billing/coding, reimbursement and coverage of CGM devices and supplies.

Data Management for SMBG or CGM

A variety of data management systems are available to help extract and view data from glucose monitoring meters and CGM devices. Data can be downloaded from monitoring meters/devices via computer connections using cables, or wirelessly using Bluetooth or cellular technology and smart devices. Data can be reported in a variety of ways, including a logbook of numbers, plotted graphs, pie charts, and an aggregated report.[105] This visual review and summarization can advance the interpretation of glucose data so that therapies can be best matched to each individual. Glucose data may be used to provide guidance on medication therapy and in making recommendations regarding food intake and physical activity. Some meter and all CGM devices have the capability to input information about food and activity. The goal of such systems is to support pattern review and decision making about therapeutic interventions related to food, activity, medications, and stress.

Manufacturers of glucose monitoring devices provide information about compatible, proprietary software on their Web sites. Data aggregation platforms, such as Glooko or Tidepool, can extract data from a variety of devices and consolidate the information into 1 report. Additionally, these platforms and individual device manufacturers offer the same data reports for devices, including more features that promote improved data interpretation.[105] Real-time CGM devices may allow interoperability with insulin pumps, smart pens, and data aggregation software.[76]

Use of telemedicine can be an effective method for improving glycemic stability. Emerging technologies such as CGM support the use of telemedicine, providing opportunity for effective interaction with healthcare teams and increased access to specialty health care, particularly in rural or underserved areas.[56] Systems that transfer real-time glucose data to healthcare providers are available, and additional systems are under development. However, there are concerns related to privacy issues with remote sharing of CGM data such as with automatic download.[98] Such systems need to comply with the Health Insurance Portability and Accountability Act and legal regulations governing patient information. It is expected that the use of technology to improve the care of persons with diabetes will rapidly expand and be more widely available in the upcoming years. Diabetes care and education specialists significantly contribute to the person with diabetes' ability to interpret data for his or her own care and can be at the forefront of utilizing new technologies to improve diabetes care and outcomes. A valuable one-stop technology resource for ADCES members is Danatech (Diabetes Advanced Network Access), where diabetes care and education specialists can become familiar with the many technology options that can be recommended and utilized in diabetes care.[107]

Other Glucose Monitoring Methods and Measurements

Noninvasive Monitoring

Noninvasive monitoring involves measuring the concentration of glucose in the blood without puncturing the skin to obtain a drop of blood. There are no FDA-approved noninvasive methods for measuring glucose in the blood at this time. However, there is ongoing research in this area (eg, contact lens, skin patches, and saliva testing).

1,5-Anhydroglucitrol Blood Test (GlycoMark™)

The 1,5-Anhydroglucitrol (1,5-AG) blood test, more commonly known as the GlycoMark™ test, measures a glucose-like sugar called 1,5-AG found in most foods and provides insight about short-term glycemic management and glycemic excursions, particularly for individuals with an A1C below 8%. Neither an A1C nor occasional blood glucose monitoring captures the frequency of blood glucose excursions (ie, glucose variability). Glucose variability has been identified as a determinant of microvascular complications. The test assesses the amount of time over a 2-week period that glucose exceeds the renal threshold (>180 mg/dL [>10 mmol/L]), which correlates with the ADA "peak" postprandial blood glucose target. During times when blood glucose is well managed, most of the 1,5-AG is reabsorbed in the renal proximal tubules and the 1,5-AG levels stay high. In people without diabetes, the median 1,5-AG is above 20 ug/mL. During times of hyperglycemia, the excess glucose blocks the reabsorption of 1,5-AG and is excreted in the urine. Whenever the blood glucose is over 180 mg/dL (>10 mmol/L), the body loses 1,5-AG. The more often the glucose spikes, the lower the 1,5-AG results will be. In the first instance, the 1,5-AG value would be low, and in the latter instance it would be high. Knowing whether you are trying to address postmeal glucose peaks or an overall elevated glucose would help guide more appropriate therapy. The validity of the test is limited by stage 4 or 5 kidney disease, advanced liver disease, and pregnancy. Additionally, acarbose and sodium-glucose co-transporter 2 inhibitors may cause a low 1,5-AG value. Additional information can be found at http://www.glycomark.com.

Fructosamine Measurement

Glycosylated serum (fructosamine), a glycated serum protein test, measures glycemic management over the past 2 to 3 weeks. Fructosamine values are used in short-term follow-up of interventions that have been recently implemented to lower blood glucose or when there is a discrepancy between A1C level and the individual's reported blood glucose readings.

Urine Testing

Urine testing was the original method of monitoring glycemic management and continues to be used in some underdeveloped countries where blood glucose meters are not available. However, since the advent of blood glucose monitoring, urine testing is no longer recommended in the United States. This is because urine testing provides retrospective information and does not reflect current blood glucose. Some individuals may, however, still use urine testing due to very limited financial resources or because they are adamant in their refusal to do an invasive testing procedure.

Urine testing for glucose has several distinct disadvantages:

- It will not detect hypoglycemia.
- It is limited to testing for elevated glucose levels.
- Elevated renal thresholds—that is, blood glucose >180 mg/dL (>10 mmol/L)—that occur with age will give false negative results.
- Renal thresholds may be low in pregnancy.
- It gives a delayed picture of what is happening in the blood, so is not indicated in flexible insulin therapy.

- False results (negative or positive) may occur with ingestion of certain medications (cephalosporins, large amounts of ascorbic acid).

Ketone Tests

Ketones are produced in the body when someone is severely depleted of carbohydrate or has inadequate insulin levels. The level of ketones can be measured in the blood or urine. The most accurate measurement of metabolic status is to measure 3-B-hydroxybutyrate in the blood. Currently, there are only 2 home blood ketone testing meters, the Precision Xtra® and NovaMax®. Urine ketone tests measure acetoacetate and are done with a test strip. The level of acetoacetate in the urine is influenced by one's hydration level and may lag a couple hours behind the blood ketone levels. Thus, urine ketone tests are not reliable for diagnosing or monitoring treatment of ketoacidosis.[108]

Situations where it is important to monitor whether ketones are present include illness, consistently elevated blood glucose levels ≥250 mg/dL (13.9 mmol/L) with type 1 diabetes,[109] infections, and pregnancy. Ketones should be routinely checked during illness by all individuals with diabetes. Individuals with type 2 diabetes can become ketotic during severe stress precipitated by infections or trauma.[110] For those using an insulin pump, ketonuria or ketonemia in the presence of hyperglycemia may indicate failure of the insulin delivery system.

Diabetes education regarding checking for ketones should include the reason why ketone spillage would occur, due to lack of adequate insulin and the body burning its own fat, of which ketones are a by-product. Teaching must also make clear that during ketone spillage, fluid replacement—as well as carbohydrate replacement—is very important. Insulin users must be taught that they should continue taking their insulin and that additional insulin is often required to treat the accompanying hyperglycemia.

See also the sections on ketone testing in chapter 8 and chapter 14.

Long-Term Monitoring of Metabolic Management

A1C Measurement

An A1C, which is expressed as a percentage of hemoglobin that is glycated, is the most widely accepted assay of glycemic management. The term *A1C* is the current preferred term in the United States, evolving from hemoglobin A1C and HbA1c. A1C, the most abundant minor hemoglobin component in the red blood cell, increases in proportion to the blood glucose level over the preceding 3 to 4 months. Glycosylation occurs as glucose in the plasma attaches itself to the hemoglobin component of the red blood cell; this process is irreversible. Because the red blood cell has a life span of 90 to 120 days, the measurement of A1C reflects the blood glucose concentration over that period of time. The more glycosylation that occurs, the higher the value. It is important to note that the National Glycohemoglobin Standardization Program (NGSP) sought to standardize worldwide the assays that were used in the Diabetes Control and Complications Trial (DCCT), which established the relationship between A1C level and risk for developing long-term complications of diabetes. A1C measures long-term glycemic management, is the standard for guiding therapy, and is considered the surrogate for the risk of complications.[111,112] Until recently, the A1C did not reflect the average blood glucose but the weighted mean over a period of time.

Because A1C is expressed as a percentage (%) of hemoglobin that is glycated, and day-to-day glucose monitoring is expressed as milligrams per deciliter (mg/dL) or millimoles per liter (mmol/L), this can be a source of confusion for both the individual and the healthcare professional. The International Federation of Clinical Chemistry (IFCC) sought to develop a global standardization that expressed long-term glycemic management (A1C) and average glucose in the same units (ie, in the same units of glucose measurements reported in self-monitoring and laboratory reports). The results of the A1C–Derived Average Glucose (ADAG) study provided the IFCC with the data to determine the relationship between A1C and average glucose, and a simple linear relationship between average glucose and A1C levels was developed. The correlation between A1C and average glucose was 0.92.[113,114] The estimated average glucose (eAG) as it relates to A1C value can be obtained by the following formula (an online calculator is available at http://professional.diabetes.org/eAG):

$$\text{eAG (mg/dL)} = (28.7 \times \text{A1C}) - 46.7$$

For example, an A1C of 8% = (28.7 × 8) = 229.6; 229.6 – 46.7 = 182.9 (183) mg/dL. Table 18.21 lists the correlation between A1C levels and eAG levels based on data from the ADAG study. Using this table to explain the connection between the A1C and glucose meter values can make it easier for individuals to interpret both values.

It is important to discuss with individuals that both finger-stick checks and an A1C are important to give day-to-day and longer-term pictures of glycemic stability. The

A1C indicates mean plasma glucose over the last 90 days, providing a long-term view of blood glucose management. However, individual glucose excursions and glycemic variability cannot be determined from an A1C value. Additionally, A1C doesn't provide day-to-day or immediate feedback on the following variables: food eaten, exercise plan, and medications taken. Self-monitoring of blood glucose results provide real-time feedback on glucose management and, when performed premeal and postmeal, can detect glucose excursions. Self-monitoring of blood glucose provides tangible information which can be used to change behavior in order to improve glycemic management. Self-monitoring of blood glucose requires training and education in order to be utilized successfully.[115]

Frequency of A1C Monitoring

Regular measurements of A1C permit timely detection of departures from the target range. In the absence of well-controlled studies that suggest a definite glucose monitoring protocol, both the ADA and the AACE suggest performing an A1C at least once or twice a year for persons with a history of stable glycemic stability, and at least quarterly for those whose therapy has changed or who are not meeting glycemic targets.[42] Many facilities use point-of-care A1C, which allows for timely decisions on therapy changes. Additionally, this provides the opportunity to directly address therapy changes during the visit with the individual and allows for discussion on glycemic goals. At-home A1C kits are also available. Most products are certified by the NGSP. Insurance reimbursement varies with the insurance plan and the type of product.

A1C Targets

It is recommended that glycemic targets be individualized for each person with diabetes. The DCCT conclusively demonstrated, however, that the risk of retinopathy, nephropathy, and neuropathy in individuals with type 1 diabetes is reduced by intensive treatment plans, as compared with conventional treatment plans.[116] These benefits were observed with an average A1C of 7.2% (normal range being 4.0% to 6.0%) in the intensively treated group. The reduction in risk of these complications correlated continuously with the reduction in A1C produced by intensive therapy. In the epidemiologic analysis of the UK Prospective Diabetes Study data, the risk for occurrence of microvascular and macrovascular complications was shown to increase at A1C values of 6.5% or more.[117]

Table 18.7 lists the glycemic goals established by the ADA and the AACE. For the person with diabetes, an A1C result within the nondiabetic reference range may reflect frequent hypoglycemia and requires further evaluation.

In 2010, the ADA added to its diagnostic criteria that an A1C of ≥6.5% can also be used as a diagnostic criterion for diabetes. The A1C should be performed in a laboratory that is NGSP certified and standardized to the DCCT assay.

A1C can be used as a teaching tool as well as a marker of metabolic status. If an individual monitors only fasting blood glucose levels and finds values in the normal range but has an A1C result of 9.8% (normal range being 4.0% to 6.0%), the diabetes care and education specialist can encourage this individual to monitor at other times of the day (especially postprandial readings) to uncover periods of elevated blood glucose and identify factors that may be associated with the elevated results.

Summary

The management of diabetes is multifaceted. Successful diabetes management requires monitoring multiple aspects of the disease, in addition to glucose management, in order to reduce complications of the disease and improve quality of life.

The success of glucose monitoring is dependent on its utilization by individuals and their healthcare providers in taking action to improve glucose management. This requires that the diabetes care and education specialist teach not only the operational skills of SMBG and CGM but also the interpretive skills. Glucose monitoring should be personalized and embedded in a diabetes management plan.

Focus on Education: Pearls for Practice

Teaching Strategies

Demonstrate empathy for the additional work of individuals embracing this tool. Monitoring the many aspects of diabetes management can be an overwhelming task, even for the most dedicated and goal-directed individuals with diabetes. At clinic appointments and outpatient visits, recognize and acknowledge the work that those you are serving have done in checking and recording blood glucose levels.

Teach not just how but why. The diabetes care and education specialist's job is to teach those with diabetes not only the how of using a glucose monitoring device but also the why so individuals with the disease are empowered to use the knowledge gained to make healthy, informed choices in their food intake, exercise, medication adjustments, and sick-day and stress management.

Be aware of the words used to describe monitoring. *Testing* may be interpreted as passing or failing. Terms such as *monitor*, *check*, or *measure* are value neutral and may be more acceptable to individuals. *Good* or *bad* glucose values may subconsciously be viewed as personal value judgments; instead, consider using *above or below target* or *above or below range*.

Use appreciative inquiry techniques when questioning individuals about their monitoring habits. The goal is to ask questions in a positive way (see Table 18.16).

Facilitate goal setting. Consider what data will best serve the individual in making informed decisions about diabetes management and obtaining a specific, yet big-picture view of his or her glycemic management.

Messages for Persons With Diabetes

Make the data work for you. Glucose monitoring is a tool that puts diabetes management in your hands, with some assistance by others. Take advantage of the technology available to make informed decisions and improve your glucose management

Try something different. Use glucose monitoring (SMBG or CGM) to determine what happens when you are more or less active or try a new restaurant.

Know your numbers. Have a clear idea of what your glucose targets are. Discuss with your healthcare team what is right for you.

Monitor progress. Keep track of your laboratory values, glucose profiles, and other elements of diabetes care. Observing progress or trends will give you more accurate assessment of your condition and self-management efforts.

Health Literacy

Self-monitoring of blood glucose frequency is not independently associated with health literacy.[118] Individuals can be taught to monitor their blood glucose no matter what their health literacy is. The important issue is to make sure that the results are used to improve glycemic management. Persons with diabetes need to learn to use the numbers to adjust lifestyle or medications. Other research indicates that persons with limited health literacy show similar or better improvement in self-management behaviors compared with those with adequate health literacy after DSME.[119]

Self-monitoring is not just about numbers. Numeracy is defined as the ability to understand and use numbers and math skills in daily life. Individuals might not understand the meaning of the numbers if they are not familiar with quantitative description terms such as the following: *small*, *decrease*, *weight*, *reduce*, and *chance*.[120]

Everyone can benefit from low health literacy education methods. Everyone appreciates when information is simple, practical, and usable. When providing education, consider the following strategies for low literacy:

- Introduce one concept at a time. Use one strategy per sentence. Make sure the concept is comprehended and then add additional applications. Instead of "If you have hypoglycemia, which is classified when your glucose is 70 mg/dL or below, have 2 to 5 glucose tablets, ½ cup (4 oz) of fruit juice, or ½ cup of a regular soft drink to raise your blood glucose," say, "Your blood glucose is considered too low when it is lower than 70 mg/dL." Then pause and ask, "What would you do if your blood glucose got that low?" Add additional concepts, one step at a time. Evaluate comprehension and actual applications of the information.
- Demonstrate/illustrate the information. You can draw a picture, use analogies, show physical representations of quantity, encourage individuals to create their own images, use vivid language, and teach with stories. Even drawing images on the white board when you explain the concepts can provide more time to think through the process and its applications (this is much more effective than briefly showing them complex pictures of complex processes).

Focus on Practice

Self-monitoring of glucose is considered a therapeutic intervention only when the results are interpreted and appropriate interventions adjusted. Create opportunities to work with individuals to review glucose results or profiles and provide specific feedback and recommendations. Evaluate the effectiveness of the corresponding recommendations/adjustments.

System integration of glucose monitoring into care delivery. All healthcare team members involved in diabetes care need to agree on methods, targets, and support methods for glucose monitoring. Trend management systems can allow for data tracking and guide decision making.

Clinical information systems need to work together. The platforms that help integrate data from a wide range of systems will allow for healthcare professionals to offer efficient services. Healthcare professionals need to be able to access and share information quickly in order to work more efficiently and make better decisions.

References

1. Powers MA, Bardsley J, Cypress M, et al. Diabetes self-management education and support in type 2 diabetes: a joint position statement of the American Diabetes Association, the American Association of Diabetes Educators, and the Academy of Nutrition and Dietetics. Diabetes Educ. 2015;41(4):417-30.
2. Peeples M, Mulcahy K, Tomky D, Weaver T; National Diabetes Education Outcomes System (NDEOS). The conceptual framework of the National Diabetes Education Outcomes System (NDEOS). Diabetes Educ. 2001;27:547-62.
3. Beck J, Greenwood D; 2017 National standards for diabetes self-management and support. Diabetes Educ. 2017; 43(5):449-64.
4. American Diabetes Association. Standards of medical care in diabetes—2019. Diabetes Care 2019;42(Suppl 1).
5. AACE/ACE glucose monitoring consensus statement. Endocr Pract. 2016;22(2):239.
6. American Association of Diabetes Educators. The American Association of Diabetes Educators position statement: self-monitoring of blood glucose using glucose meters in the management of type 2 diabetes. Issued 2014 Dec 3. On the Internet at: https://www.diabeteseducator.org/docs/default-source/default-document-library/self-monitoring-of-blood-glucose-using-glucose-meters-in-the-management-of-type-2-diabetes.pdf?sfvrsn=0.
7. Mulcahy K, Maryniuk M, Peeples M, et al. Diabetes self-management education core outcomes measures. Diabetes Educ. 2003;29:768-88.
8. Centers for Medicare & Medicaid Services. Current Medicare coverage of diabetes supplies. MLN matters number SE18011. Released Aug 16, 2018 (cited 2019 June 11). On the Internet at: https://www.cms.gov/Outreach-and-Education/Medicare-Learning-Network-MLN/MLNMattersArticles/Downloads/SE18011.pdf.
9. Centers for Medicare & Medicaid Services. DMPOS competitive bidding- home (cited 2019 June 10). On the Internet at: https://www.cms.gov/Medicare/Medicare-Fee-for-Service-Payment/DMEPOSCompetitiveBid/index.html.
10. Centers for Medicare & Medicaid Services. Durable medical equipment, prosthetics, orthotics, and supplies competitive bidding program: temporary gap period (cited 2019 June 10). On the Internet at: https://www.cms.gov/Outreach-and-Education/Outreach/Partnerships/Downloads/DMEPOS-Temporary-Gap-Period-Fact-Sheet.pdf.
11. AADE. "glucose monitoring resources" (cited 2019 May 29). On the Internet at: https://www.diabeteseducator.org/practice/educator-tools/diabetes-management-tools/self-monitoring-of-blood-glucose.
12. Heinemann L. (Analytical) accuracy of blood glucose meters and patients: how do they come together? J Diabetes Sci Technol. 2013;7:1-3.
13. Lajara R, Magwire ML. Accuracy considerations for self-monitoring of blood glucose: practical tools for primary care physicians. Prac Diabet. 2013;32(2):6-24.
14. International Organization for Standardization. ISO/FDIS 15197:2013: in vitro diagnostic test systems—requirements for blood-glucose monitoring systems for self-testing in managing diabetes mellitus. Geneva, Switzerland: International Organization for Standardization; 2013.
15. International Organization for Standardization. ISO 15197: 2003: in vitro diagnostic test systems—requirements for blood-glucose monitoring systems for self-testing in managing diabetes mellitus. Geneva, Switzerland: International Organization for Standardization; 2003.
16. Klonoff DC, Parkes JL, Kovatchev BP, Kerr D, Bevier WC, Brazg RL, Christiansen M, Bailey TS, Nichols JH, Kohn MA. Investigation of the accuracy of 18 marketed blood glucose monitors. Diabetes Care. 2018,Aug;41(8):1681-88.
17. FDA. 510(k) No: K161790 (cited 2019 May 30). On the Internet at: https://www.fda.gov/medical-devices/510k-clearances/may-2017-510k-clearances.
18. Transportation Security Administration. TSA shares tips for travelers with disabilities, medical devices, medical conditions.

Nov 15, 2016 (cited 2019 June 10). On the Internet at: https://www.tsa.gov/news/releases/2016/11/15/tsa-shares-tips-travelers-disabilities-medical-devices-medical-conditions.

19. Peragallo-Dittko V. The lowdown on lancets and lancing devices. Diabetes Self Manag. 1999;16(3):64-71.

20. Peragallo-Dittko V. How accurate is your meter? Diabetes Self Manag. 2000;17(5):78-85.

21. Jungheim K, Koschinsky T. Risky delay of hypoglycemia detection by glucose monitoring at the arm (letter). Diabetes Care. 2001;24:1303-6.

22. Bartos BJ, Cleary MJ, Kleinbeck C, Petzinger RA, Whittington A, Williams AS. Diabetes and disabilities: assistive tools, services and information. Diabetes Educ. 2008;34(4):600-5.

23. Harris MI, Crowe CC, Howie LJ. Self-monitoring of blood glucose by adults with diabetes in the United States population. Diabetes Care. 1993;16:1116-23.

24. Austin MM. The two skill sets of self-monitoring of blood glucose education: the operation and the interpretive. Diabetes Spectr. 2013 May;26(2):83-90.

25. Cypress M, Tomky D. Using self-monitoring of blood glucose in noninsulin-treated type 2 diabetes. Diabetes Spectr. 2013 May;26(2):102-6.

26. AADE. AADE tip sheet: glucose monitoring - expert recommendation.2019 (cited 2019 June 7). On the Internet at: https://www.diabeteseducator.org/docs/default-source/living-with-diabetes/tip-sheets/blood-glucose-monitoring/expertrecommendations-final9049dc36a05f68739c53ff0000b8561d.pdf?sfvrsn=10.

27. Shiraiwa T, Takahara M, Kaneto H, et al. Efficacy of occasional self-monitoring of postprandial blood glucose levels in type 2 diabetic patients without insulin therapy. Diabetes Res Clin Pract. 2010;90(3):e91-2.

28. Polonsky WH, Fisher L, Schikman CH, et al. Structured self-monitoring of blood glucose significantly reduces A1C levels in poorly controlled, noninsulin-treated type 2 diabetes: results from the Structured Testing Program study. Diabetes Care. 2011; 34(2):262-7.

29. Kempf K, Kruse J, Martin S. ROSSO-in-praxi: a self-monitoring of blood glucose-structured 12 week lifestyle intervention significantly improves glucometabolic control of patients with type 2 diabetes mellitus. Diabetes Technol Ther. 2010;12(7):547-53.

30. Franciosi M, Lucisano G, Pellegrini F, et al; ROSES Study Group. ROSES: role of self-monitoring of blood glucose and intensive education in patients with type 2 diabetes not receiving insulin. A pilot randomized clinical trial. Diabet Med. 2011; 28(7):789-96.

31. Schwedes U, Siebolds M, Mertes G. Meal-related structured self-monitoring of blood glucose: effect on diabetes control in non-insulin treated type 2 diabetic patients. Diabetes Care. 2002;25:1928-32.

32. Zhang D, Katznelson L, Ming L. Postprandial glucose monitoring further improved glycemia, lipids, and weight in persons with type 2 diabetes mellitus who had already reached hemoglobin A1C goal. J Diabetes Sci Technol. 2012;6(2):289-93.

33. McAndrew LM, Napolitano MA, Pogach LM, et al. The impact of self-monitoring of blood glucose on a behavioral weight loss intervention of patients with type 2 diabetes. Diabetes Educ. 2013;39(3):397-405.

34. Miller KM, Beck RW, Bergenstal RM, et al. Exchange Clinic Network. Evidence of a strong association between frequency of self monitoring of blood glucose and hemoglobin A1C levels in T1D Exchange clinic registry participants. Diabetes Care. 2013;36:2009-14.

35. Ziegler R, Heidtmann B, Hilgard D, Hofer S, Rosenbauer J, Holl R. DPV-Wiss-Initiative. Frequency of SMBG correlates with HbA1c and acute complications in children and adolescents with type 1 diabetes. Pediatr Diabetes. 2011;12(1):11-17.

36. Barnett AH, Krentz AJ, Strojek K, et al. The efficacy of self-monitoring of blood glucose in the management of patients with type 2 diabetes treated with a gliclazide modified release-based regimen. A multi-centre, randomized, parallel-group, 6-month evaluation (DINAMIC 1 study). Diabetes Obes Metab. 2008; 10(12):1239-47.

37. International Diabetes Federation. Guideline: self-monitoring of blood glucose in non-insulin treated type 2 diabetes. Brussels, Belgium; 2009. On the Internet at: http://www.idf.org/webdata/docs/SMBG_EN2.pdf.

38. Type 2 Diabetes BASICS Curriculum Guide. 4th ed. Minneapolis, Minn: International Diabetes Center; 2014. On the Internet at: http://www.internationaldiabetescenter.com.

39. Bosi E, Scavini M, Ceriello A, et al. Intensive structured self-monitoring of blood glucose and glycemic control in noninsulin-treated type 2 diabetes: the PRISMA randomized trial. Diabetes Care. 2013;36(10):2887-94. Epub 2013 Jun 4.

40. Duran A. Benefits of self-monitoring blood glucose in the management of new-onset type 2 diabetes mellitus: the St Carlos study, a prospective randomized clinic-based interventional study with parallel groups. J Diabetes. 2010;2(3):203-11.

41. Klonoff D, Blonde L, Cembrowski G, et al. Consensus report: the current role of self-monitoring of blood in non-insulin-treated type 2 diabetes. J Diabetes Sci Technol. 2011;5(6):1529-48.

42. Blood Glucose Pattern Control: A Guide for People Who Use Insulin. 3rd ed. Minneapolis, Minn: International Diabetes Center at Park Nicollet; 2008. On the Internet at: http://www.idcpublishing.com/Blood-Glucose-Pattern-Control/productinfo/2058-816 A/.

43. Powers M, Davidson J, Bergenstal R. Glucose pattern management teaches glycemia-related problem-solving skills in a diabetes self-management education program. Diabetes Spectr. 2013;26(2):91-7.

44. American Association of Clinical Endocrinologists. Medical Guidelines for Clinical Practice for Developing a Diabetes Comprehensive Care Plan. Endocr Pract. 2015 Apr;21(Suppl 1):1-87.

45. American Diabetes Association. Postprandial blood glucose (consensus statement). Diabetes Care. 2001;24:775-8.

46. Monnier L, Lapinski H, Colette C. Contributions of fasting and postprandial plasma glucose increments to the overall diurnal hyperglycemia of type 2 diabetic patients. Diabetes Care. 2003; 26(3):881-5.

47. Babione L. SMBG: the underused nutrition counseling tool in diabetes management. Diabetes Spectr. 1994;7:196-7.

48. Ahern JA, Gatcomb PM, Held NA, Petit WA Jr, Tamborlane WV. Exaggerated hyperglycemia after a pizza meal in well-controlled diabetes. Diabetes Care. 1993;16:578-80.

49. Rubin RR, Peyrot M, Saudek CD. The effect of a diabetes education program incorporating coping skills training on emotional well-being and diabetes self-efficacy. Diabetes Educ. 1993;19:210-4.

50. Price MJ. Qualitative analysis of the patient-provider interactions: the patient's perspective. Diabetes Educ. 1989;15: 144-8.

51. Cox DJ, Irvine A, Gonder-Frederick L, Nowacek G, Butterfield J. Fear of hypoglycemia: quantification, validation and utilization. Diabetes Care. 1987;10:617-21.

52. Austin MM. A call for standardized SMBG education. Endocr Today. 2009 Apr;7(6):24.

53. American Association of Diabetes Educators. Module 5: Monitoring. In: Diabetes Education Curriculum: Guiding Patients to Successful Self-Management. 2nd ed. Chicago: American Association of Diabetes Educators; 2015:171-209.

54. Hammond SA. The Thin Book of Appreciative Inquiry. 2nd ed. Bend, Ore: Thin Book Publishing Co.

55. AADE Practice Paper: The Diabetes Educator Role in Continuous Glucose Monitoring, 2018.

56. ADA: Diabetes Technology: *Standards of Medical Care in Diabetes—2019.* American Diabetes Association. Diabetes Care Jan 2019, 42(Suppl 1):S71-80.

57. Beck RW, Riddlesworth TD, Ruedy K, et al. Continuous glucose monitoring versus usual care in patients with type 2 diabetes receiving multiple daily insulin injections: a randomized trial. Ann Intern Med. 2017; 167:365-74.

58. Fonseca VA, Grunberger G, Anhalt H, et al. Continuous glucose monitoring: a consensus conference of The American Association of Clinical Endocrinologists and American College of Endocrinology. Endocr Pract. 2016;22(8):1008-21.

59. Peters AL, Ahmann AJ, Battelino T, et al. Diabetes technology-continuous subcutaneous insulin infusion therapy and continuous glucose monitoring in adults: an Endocrine Society clinical practice guideline. J Clin Endocrinol Metab. 2016;101(11):3922-37.

60. Peters AL, et al. Advances in glucose monitoring and automated insulin delivery: supplement to Endocrine Society clinical practice guidelines. J Endocr Soc. 2018;2(11);1214-25.

61. Rodbard D. Continuous glucose monitoring: a review of recent studies demonstrating improved glycemic outcomes. Diabetes Technol Ther. 2017;19(S3):S25-37.

62. Vigersky RA et al. Short- and long-term effects of real-time continuous glucose monitoring in patients with type 2 diabetes. Diabetes Care. 2011;35,1.

63. Edelman SV, et al. Clinical implications of real-time and intermittently scanned continuous glucose monitoring. Diabetes Care. 2018 Nov; 41(11):2265-74.

64. Klonoff DC, Ahn D, Drincic A. Continuous glucose monitoring: a review of the technology and clinical use. Diabetes Res Clin Pract 2017;133:178-92.

65. Polonsky WH, Hessler D. Perceived accuracy in continuous glucose monitoring: understanding the impact on patients. J Diabetes Sci Technol. 9(2):339–41.

66. Bailey TS, Grunberger G, Bode BW, et al. American Association of Clinical Endocrinologists and American College of Endocrinology 2016 outpatient glucose monitoring consensus statement. Endocr Pract. 2016;22(2):231-61.

67. Allepo G, et al. A practical approach to using trend arrows on the Dexcom G5 CGM system for the management of adults with diabetes. J Endocr Soc. 2017;1:1445-60.

68. Maahs DM, DeSalvo D, Pyle L, et al. Effect of acetaminophen on CGM glucose in an outpatient setting. Diabetes Care. 2015;38(10):e158–9.

69. Basu A, Slama,MQ, Nicholson WT, et al. (2017). Continuous glucose monitor interference with commonly prescribed medications: a pilot study. J Diabetes Sci Technol. 11(5), 936-41.

70. Christiansen MP, Klaff LJ, Brazg R, et al. A prospective multicenter evaluation of the accuracy of a novel implanted continuous glucose sensor: PRECISE II. Diabetes Technol Ther. 2018;20:197-206.

71. Lorenz C, et al. Interference assessment of various endogenous and exogenous substances on the performance of the eversense long-term implantable continuous glucose monitoring system. Diabetes Technol. Ther. 2018;20:5, 344-52.

72. Beck RW, Riddlesworth T, Ruedy K, et al. Effect of continuous glucose monitoring on glycemic control in adults with type 1 diabetes using insulin injections: the DIAMOND randomized clinical trial. JAMA. 2017;317(4):371-8.

73. Bolinder J, Antuna R, Geelhoed-Duijvestijn P, Kröger J, Weitgasser R. Novel glucose-sensing technology and hypoglycaemia in type 1 diabetes: a multicentre, non-masked, randomised controlled trial. Lancet. 2016;388(10057):2254-63.

74. van Beers CA, et al. Continuous glucose monitoring for patients with type 1 diabetes and impaired awareness of hypoglycemia (IN CONTROL): a randomised, open-label, crossover trial. Lancet Diabetes Endocrinology. 2016;4(11):893-902.

75. Fonda SJ, Graham C, Munakata J, Powers JM, Price D, & Vigersky RA. The cost-effectiveness of real-time continuous glucose monitoring (RT-CGM) in type 2 diabetes. J Diabetes Sci Technol. 2016;10(4):898-904.

76. Adolfsson P, Parkin CG, Thomas A, Krinelke LG. Selecting the appropriate continuous glucose monitoring system - a practical approach. Eur Endocrinol. 2018;14(1):24-9.

77. Vigersky R, Shrivastav M. Role of continuous glucose monitoring for type 2 in diabetes management and research. J Diabetes Complicat. 2017;31(1):280-7.

78. American Association of Diabetes Educators. American Association of Diabetes Educators white paper: Best practices for managing and educating patients through the use of continuous glucose monitoring (CGM), 2015.

79. Chamberlain JJ, et al. Impact of frequent and persistent use of continuous glucose monitoring (CGM) on hypoglycemia fear, frequency of emergency medical treatment, and SMBG frequency after one year. J Diabetes Sci Technol. 2015;10(2):383-8.

80. American Association of Diabetes Educators. American Association of Diabetes Educators practice paper: continuous subcutaneous insulin infusion (CSII) without and with sensor integration, 2018.

81. Beck RW, Connor CG, Mullen DM, Wesley DM, Bergenstal RM. the fallacy of average: how using HbA_{1c} alone to assess glycemic control can be misleading. Diabetes Care. 2017;40(8):994-9.

82. Hirsch IB. Glycemic variability and diabetes complications: does it matter? Of course it does! Diabetes Care. 2015;38:1610-4.

83. Bergenstal RM, Gal RL, Connor CG, et al. Racial differences in the relationship of glucose concentrations and hemoglobin A1c levels. Ann Intern Med. 2017;167:95–102.

84. Lawton J, Blackburn M, Allen J, et al. Patients' and caregivers' experiences of using continuous glucose monitoring to support diabetes self-management: qualitative study. BMC Endocr Disord. 2018;18(1).

85. Dunn TC, Xu Y, Hayter G, Ajjan RA. Real-world flash glucose monitoring patterns and associations between self-monitoring frequency and glycaemic measures: a European analysis of over 60 million glucose tests. Diabetes Res Clin Pract. 2018;137: 37-46.

86. Haak T, Hanaire H, Ajjan R, Hermanns N, Riveline JP, Rayman G. Flash glucose-sensing technology as a replacement for blood glucose monitoring for the management of insulin-treated type 2 diabetes: a multicenter, open-label randomized controlled trial. Diabetes Ther. 2017;8(1):55-73.

87. Garg SK, Weinzimer SA, Tamborlane WV, et al. Glucose outcomes with the in-home use of a hybrid closed-loop insulin delivery system in adolescents and adults with type 1 diabetes. Diabetes Technol Ther. 2017;19:155-63.

88. U.S. Department of Health and Human Services FaDA. FDA authorizes first fully interoperable continuous glucose monitoring system, streamlines review pathway for similar devices. March 27, 2018.

89. Gehlaut RR, Dogbey GY, Schwartz FL, Marling CR, Shubrook JH. Hypoglycemia in type 2 diabetes–more common than you think: a continuous glucose monitoring study. J Diabetes Sci Technol. 2015;9(5):999-1005.

90. Oliveira A. et al. Use of continuous glucose monitoring as an educational tool in the primary care setting. Diabetes Spectrum. 2013 May;26(2):120-3.

91. Puhr S, et al. Real-world hypoglycemia avoidance with a continuous glucose monitoring system's predictive low glucose alert. Diabetes Technol. Ther. 2019;21:4,155-8.

92. Burckhardt MA, et al. The use of continuous glucose monitoring with remote monitoring improves psychosocial measures in parents of children with type 1 diabetes: a randomized crossover trial. Diabetes Care. Dec 2018;41(12):2641-3.

93. Carlson AL, Mullen DM, & Bergenstal RM. Clinical use of continuous glucose monitoring in adults with type 2 diabetes. Diabetes Technol. Ther. 2017;19(S2):S-4.

94. Yamamoto JM, Murphy HR. Emerging technologies for the management of type 1 diabetes in pregnancy. Curr Diab Rep. 2018;18(1):4.

95. Feig DS, Donovan LE, Corcoy R, et al. Continuous glucose monitoring in pregnant women with type 1 diabetes (CONCEPTT): a multicentre international randomised controlled trial. Lancet 2017;390:2347-59.

96. Murphy HR, Rayman G, Duffield K, et al. Changes in the glycemic profiles of women with type 1 and type 2 diabetes during pregnancy. Diabetes Care. 2007;30:2785-91.

97. Wallia A, Umpierrez GE, Rushakoff RJ, et al. Consensus Statement on inpatient use of continuous glucose monitoring. J Diabetes Sci Technol. 2017;11(5):1036-44.

98. Petrie JR, Peters AL, Bergenstal RM, et al. Improving the clinical value and utility of CGM systems: issues and recommendations. A joint statement of the European Association for the Study of Diabetes and the American Diabetes Association Diabetes Technology Working Group. Diabetologia. 2017;60:2319.

99. Heinemann L, & Kamann S. Adhesives Used for diabetes medical devices: a neglected risk with serious consequences? J Diabetes Sci Technol. 2016;10(6):1211-15.

100. Hirsch IB, Battelino T, Peters AL, Chamberlain JJ, Aleppo G, Bergenstal RM. Role of Continuous Glucose Monitoring in Diabetes Treatment. Arlington, Va., American Diabetes Association, 2018.

101. Pettus J, Edelman SV. Recommendations for using real-time continuous glucose monitoring (rtCGM) data for insulin adjustments in type 1 diabetes. J Diabetes Sci Technol. 2016;11(1):138-47.

102. Riddlesworth TD, Beck RW, Gal RL, et al. Optimal sampling duration for continuous glucose monitoring to determine long-term glycemic control. Diabetes Technol Ther. 2018 Apr;20(4):314-6.

103. Battelino T, et al. Clinical targets for continuous glucose monitoring data interpretation: recommendations from the international consensus on time in range. Diabetes Care. Published Ahead of Print, published online June 8, 2019. https://doi.org/10.2337/dci19-0028.

104. Bergenstal, RM et al. Glucose management indicator (GMI): a new term for estimating A1C from continuous glucose monitoring. Diabetes Care. 2018 Nov;41(11):2275-80.

105. Bergenstal RM, Ahmann AJ, Bailey T, et al. Recommendations for standardizing glucose reporting and analysis to optimize clinical decision making in diabetes: the ambulatory glucose profile (AGP). Diabetes Technol Ther. 2013 Mar:198-211.

106. Scheiner G. CGM retrospective data analysis. Diabetes Technol Ther. 2016;18(S2):S2-22.

107. AADE: DANA (cited 2019 June 10). On the Internet at: https://www.diabeteseducator.org/news/aade-blog/aade-blog-details/press-releases/2018/08/06/aade-s-dana-one-stop-healthcare-technology-resource-for-diabetes-educators.

108. American Diabetes Association. Hyperglycemic crises in diabetes. Diabetes Care. 2004;27(Suppl 1):S94-102.

109. American Diabetes Association. Tests of glycemia in diabetes: clinical practice recommendations. Diabetes Care. 2004; 27(Suppl 1):S91-3.

110. Fajans SS. Classification and diagnosis of diabetes. In: Porte D Jr, Sherwin RS, eds. Ellenberg and Rifkin's Diabetes Mellitus: Theory and Practice. 5th ed. Stamford, Conn: Appleton and Lang; 1997:357-72.

111. Diabetes Control and Complications Trial Research Group. The effect of intensive diabetes treatment on the development and progression of long-term complications in insulin-dependent diabetes mellitus: Diabetes Control and Complications Trial. N Engl J Med. 1993;329:978-86.

112. DCCT Research Group. The association between glycaemic exposure and long-term diabetic complications in the Diabetes Control and Complications Trial. Diabetes. 1995;44:968-83.

113. Consensus Committee. Consensus statement on the worldwide standardization of the hemoglobin A1C measurement: the American Diabetes Association for the Study of Diabetes, International Federation of Clinical Chemistry and Laboratory Medicine, and the International Diabetes Federation. Diabetes Care. 2007;30:2394-9.

114. Nathan DM, Kuenen J, Borg R, Zheng H, Schoenfeld D, Heine R; A1C-Derived Average Glucose (ADAG) Study Group. Translating the A1C assay into estimated average glucose values. Diabetes Care. 2008;31(8):1-6.

115. Saudek CD, Derr RI, Kalvani RR. Assessing glycaemia in diabetes using self-monitoring blood glucose and hemoglobin A1C. JAMA. 2006;295:188-97.

116. Boland E, Monsod T, Delucia M, et al. Limitations of conventional methods of self monitoring of blood glucose. Diabetes Care. 2001;24(11):858-62.

117. Stratton IM, Adler AI, Neil HA, et al. Association of glycaemia with macrovascular and microvascular complications of type 2 diabetes (UKPDS 35): prospective observational study. BMJ. 2000;321:405-12.

118. Mbaezue N, Mayberry R, Gazmararian J, Quarshie A, Ivonye C, Heisler M. The impact of health literacy on self-monitoring of blood glucose in patients with diabetes receiving care in an inner-city hospital. J Natl Med Assoc. 2010 Jan;102(1):5-9.

119. Kim S, Love F, Quistberg DA, Shea JA. Association of health literacy with self-management behavior in patients with diabetes. Diabetes Care. 2004 Dec;27:2980-2.

120. Cavanaugh K, Huizinga MM, Wallston KA, et al. Association of numeracy and diabetes control. Ann Intern Med. 2008;148: 737-46.

C H A P T E R 1 9

Therapy Intensification: Technology and Pattern Management

Debbie Hinnen, APN, BC-ADM, CDCES, FAAN, FADCES
Jennifer De Groot, MSN, APN, FNP-BC, CDCES

Key Concepts

- Pattern management is an important strategy to facilitate therapy intensification and promote self-management.
- A diabetes care and education specialist's coaching for self-care skills and problem solving is a necessary prerequisite for pattern management.
- Glucose data is necessary for pattern management. Continuous glucose monitoring is emerging as the standard of care.
- For persons with diabetes, self-monitoring of blood glucose (SMBG) at representative times is needed to interpret the relationships and effect that food, physical activity, and finally medication have on glycemic stability.
- Understanding the benefits, risks, and limitations of intensive therapy is extremely important in counseling and assisting persons with diabetes in the use of multiple daily injections and continuous subcutaneous insulin infusion (CSII).
- Not all persons with diabetes are good candidates for CSII. A detailed assessment of individual characteristics, resources, problem-solving skills, and self-care behaviors is needed.
- Pump therapy is a tool for insulin delivery providing precision that mimics physiologic insulin patterns.
- Problem-solving skills with intensive insulin therapy prior to and during pump therapy are critical to using an insulin pump safely and effectively.
- Pump therapy requires a healthcare team that is knowledgeable about the technology. Professionals involved in the care of individuals using pumps must keep pace with rapidly advancing technological enhancements and developments.
- Understanding obstacles and the needs of special populations is important for intensive insulin therapy and the continuum of care.

Introduction

Attaining glucose goals is a journey, not a destination. Intensifying therapy through use of pattern management is the map for the ongoing process of navigating the terrain. Today the itinerary focuses on increasing the amount of "Time in Range," intensifying therapy with newer mediations and using CGM, pumps and technology to improve glucose values. This is an important goal of diabetes care and education. Decades ago, this was done by studying urine glucose logs; negative, +1, +2…; then A1C and self-monitoring of glucose emerged. Diabetes care and education specialists and persons with diabetes huddled over numbers written in logbooks or sometimes on the back of envelopes. Today continuous glucose monitoring is emerging as the gold standard for obtaining and organizing glucose data. Consensus work to standardize the data reports is making the "review" easier. The analysis of glucose monitoring data continues to be the critical teaching tool to problem solve and intensify therapy and thus increase time in range and ultimately overall glycemic stability. Persons with diabetes are empowered with tools that increase their independence. However, helping people with diabetes become self-sufficient and independent is a complex endeavor. This lifelong challenge and journey work best when the person with diabetes engages in their management decisions, involves their partners, and continuously works with a team of diabetes experts. This chapter will discuss strategies to implement pattern management and ongoing intensification of therapies for people with diabetes. Diabetes self-management may start with finger sticks for glucose monitoring to titrate oral agents and injectables, then progress to insulin injections or insulin pumps and glucose sensor use. Through it all, analyzing and acting on glucose patterns is the critical element for improving independence and glycemic stability. This is pattern management.

Strategies to Promote Good Outcomes

Improving outcomes for diabetes and its co-morbid conditions is a complicated undertaking. American Diabetes Association (ADA) with the European Association of the Study of Diabetes (EASD) and the American College of Clinical Endocrinology (AACE) have developed guidelines to help improve the quality of care for people with diabetes.[1,2] These guidelines also help ensure that all people with diabetes receive standard and uniform care. Pay for performance criteria incentivizes providers to improve outcomes.

Therapeutic, or clinical inertia, is a problem frequently identified as a common reason goals are not met. Clinical inertia is the failure to intensify therapy when indicated. Clinical inertia occurs in many settings, and it is attributed to provider's lack of taking action.[3]

Many strategies have been implemented and evaluated to increase provider's likelihood of intensifying therapy. Process measures in clinical practice settings have been demonstrated to increase providers' therapy adjustments, thus improving outcomes. Initiation of stepwise pharmacologic strategies, use of protocols, proactive reminders, consistent follow-up procedures, and use of clinical information systems to improve the individual's engagement with his or her therapy regimen are some effective strategies.[4,5,6,7] Decision support reminders that provide specific recommendations for management at each visit and computer-generated provider specific feedback on performance has demonstrated improved frequency with which providers intensified therapy.[8]

Clinical inertia is influenced by the person with diabetes as well. Persons with diabetes struggle with lifestyle management, access issues, understanding the complexities of diabetes, and probably most critically, failing to see themselves as partners in their own care. For instance, if engagement with the medication regimen is not maintained and the provider's recommendations are not implemented, for whatever reason, outcomes will not be improved. Poor self-management behavior by the person with diabetes increases therapeutic clinical inertia. If education, engagement in new technology and nurse involvement are present, clinical inertia appears to be less common.[8,9] Diabetes self-management and individual engagement begin with educating and empowering persons with diabetes to make adjustments in their own treatment plan. This includes adjustments in medication doses, physical activity, and eating habits. Diabetes self-management is critical to attaining metabolic stability and preventing complications of diabetes.[10]

Pattern Management: Taking a Proactive Approach to Diabetes Management

Pattern management for the diabetes care and education specialist is the analysis of glucose data in a systematic approach "to organize, sort, and process blood glucose (BG) data that links to individual self-care behaviors and reveals trends or patterns."[11] It is utilized to determine targeted strategies and therapies through shared decision making with the person with diabetes (PWD) with the intent to normalize glucose levels and thus improve time in range.[12] It involves looking not only at blood glucose values but also at food intake, activity, insulin doses, illness, and other factors that can contribute to changes in blood glucose values.

Glucose monitoring is the primary data tool for pattern recognition and managing multiple self-care behaviors. This is a comprehensive approach to blood glucose management that includes all aspects of current diabetes therapy.[13,14] Although the requirement behind pattern management is blood glucose monitoring, continuous glucose monitoring (CGM) has moved the focus beyond self-blood glucose monitoring (SMBG). Diabetes care and educations specialists, providers, and persons with diabetes alike must start with an understanding of what and how glucose data applies to basic steps of pattern management.[11,13] Using pattern management techniques during every encounter with persons with diabetes helps to provide impetus to intensify therapy and promote independence in self-management.

In addition, pattern management analysis provides a way for the person with diabetes to look at their blood glucose records in relationship to food, activity, stress, and medication and implement logical independent changes.[11,13] Although pattern management tends to be used more frequently in those treated with insulin, persons with all types of diabetes can benefit from pattern management to adjust other aspect of self-care behaviors.

The frequency and timing of testing must be individualized, with consideration given to individual's safety, the prescribed medication regimen, optimal glycemic goals, the individual's willingness to test, and resources available to cover the testing supplies needed.[13–19]

Attributes for Effective for Pattern Management

Generally, there are four attributes that a person with diabetes needs to possess for effective pattern management. These skill areas improve the likelihood of successful pattern management. These include cognitive function, health literacy and numeracy, comprehensive diabetes knowledge with self-care skills and behaviors, and problem-solving skills.

Cognitive function has been studied in T1 and T2 diabetes, suggesting there may be a relationship to diabetes.[20] In T1, learning and memory do not appear to be affected. In T2, impaired information processing, working memory, and attention during acute hyperglycemia may be affected. In older persons with diabetes, mental health examinations suggest there may be less involvement in self-care, specifically SMBG.

However, cognitive impairment was found not to adversely affect diabetes self-management in a study with uncomplicated type 2 diabetes in older adults.[20]

Health literacy, especially numeracy, is required when asking persons with diabetes to read and process numbers (BG results).[21] The National Adult Literacy Survey (NALS) revealed ~90 million adult Americans scored at the Level 1 or 2, the lowest of 5 levels when asked to find information and numbers and perform a calculation. Representing glucose data in user-friendly formats is important to all users of data but finding the best format for individuals with low literacy may be especially important.

Comprehensive diabetes knowledge and self-care skills are a critical foundation for all people with diabetes, especially people who are Independent with diabetes management. The AADE7®: healthy coping, healthy eating, physical activity, taking medications, monitoring, reducing risks, and problem solving serve as a foundation to build advanced skills.[22] Using a variety of interactive teaching and learning strategies enhances the individual's understanding and skill development for pattern management.

One of the most valuable skills to facilitate pattern management is problem solving. Reviewing blood glucose records with the person while using interactive questioning will enhance the person's understanding. Practicing and rehearsing for anticipated problems or circumstances enhances the individual's self-efficacy and helps demonstrate progress in self-problem-solving abilities.

Facilitating Pattern Management for Intensifying Therapy

Pattern management requires work, concentration, and commitment by both the diabetes care and education specialist and the person with diabetes to identify trends for intensifying therapy. Small and incremental steps move the process forward. The diabetes care and education specialist acts as a change agent in facilitating desired behavior change. The following interventions are required:

- Explaining the purpose, strategies, and value of pattern management for intensifying therapy to achieve blood glucose goals.
- Motivating the persons with diabetes to become an active participant in their care. People generally are more motivated if they feel confident in their abilities.[22]
- Negotiating individualized blood glucose goals that include his or her own personal belief system. Current acceptable targets by the American Diabetes Association[1] and American College of Endocrinology[2] are as shown in Table 19.1. Individualization of A1C goals is essential and based on assessment of hypoglycemia risk, life expectancy, duration of diabetes, co-morbid conditions, vascular complications, disease duration, and potentially modifiable issues of the individual's attitudes, motivation, self-care skills, resources and support. Supporting frequent interaction between the person with diabetes and the diabetes care team by using technology such as cloud, telephone, fax, e-mail, portals, and an on-call system to discuss glucose patterns between visits.
- Identifying support systems to provide emotional and clinical management support.

Develop processes and protocols in your facility for implementing and documenting pattern management strategies. Glucose data review and shared decision making may be completed by team members that are not providers.

Intensifying therapy starts with setting A1C goals. These should be individualized. Providers and diabetes care education specialists have an opportunity to influence motivation, education, and family support. With support and education, A1C goals may be able to be set closer to euglycemic targets and thus reduce long-term complications. Figure 19.1 indicates criteria to be considered when

TABLE 19.1 Recommendations for Glycemic Control

American Diabetes Association (ADA) and American College of Endocrinology (ACE) Recommendations for Glycemic Control by Age Group					
Values by Age	*Before Meals*	*2 Hour Postmeal*	*Bedtime*	*A1C*	*Rationale*
Non-diabetes	<100	<140	<110	<5.7–6.4%	Non-diabetes range
Adults (non-pregnant)					
ADA	80–130mg	≤180 (1–1.5 hr PP)	100–140	<7.0%	Risk of microvascular disease
AACE/ACE	≤110	≤140		<6.5%	Risk of macrovascular disease
Children, Adolescents & Young Adults					
Adolescents & Young Adults (13–19 years)[23]	90–130	**	90–150	<7.5%	Risk of hypoglycemia Developmental & psychological issues
School Age (6–12 yrs)	90–180	**	100–180	<7.5%	Risks for hypoglycemia and relatively low risk of complication prior to puberty
Toddler & Preschoolers (<6 years)	100–180	**	110–200	7.5–8.5%	High risk and vulnerability to hypoglycemia
Older Adults[24]	90–130 90–150 100–150	**	90–150 100–180 110–210	7.5% 8.0% 8.5%	Healthy Complex Very complex, poor health

**Key concepts in setting glycemic goals for children, adolescents, adults with limited life expectancy, and geriatric individuals with diabetes:

1. Goals should be individualized, and lower, more relaxed goals may be reasonable based on benefit-risk assessment.
2. Blood glucose goals should be higher for individuals with frequent hypoglycemia or hypoglycemia unawareness.
3. Postprandial blood glucose values should be measured to titrate prandial insulin, determine the need for medications to stimulate insulin release in T2, and when there is a disparity between preprandiol blood glucose values and A1C levels.
4. A lower goal (<7.0%) is reasonable if it can be achieved without excessive hypoglycemia.[25]

Meters use a drop of whole blood on the test strip but give a result in plasma glucose level. A meter that provides plasma glucose levels will have results that are closer to the laboratory's results. When whole blood is measured, then glucose results are 10% to 15% lower than plasma glucose values.

working with a person with diabetes to individualize his or her A1C goal.

> Higher A1C doesn't protect against hypoglycemia.[154] Glycemic variability is likely more responsible for severe hypoglycemia.[26]

Therapies: Initiating and Advancing Therapy in Type 2 Diabetes

We can now treat diabetes, not just *chase* blood sugars. Understanding the metabolic defects of type 2 helps facilitate targeted medication management. The specific actions of each class of medication directly impact the defects of the disease.[28] See chapter 17, Table 17.2, for the mechanisms of action of oral and noninsulin injectable medications used the management of type 2 diabetes.

Based on extensive evidence, the American Association of Clinical Endocrinologists recommends using the glycemic algorithm in Figure 19.2.[2] Intensifying therapy can be more consistent and less overwhelming for providers if they follow the sequence and confirm medication choices based on formulary preferences. The ADA guidelines are similar with additional empahsis on cardiovascular benefits, renal function, cost, hypoglycemia, and

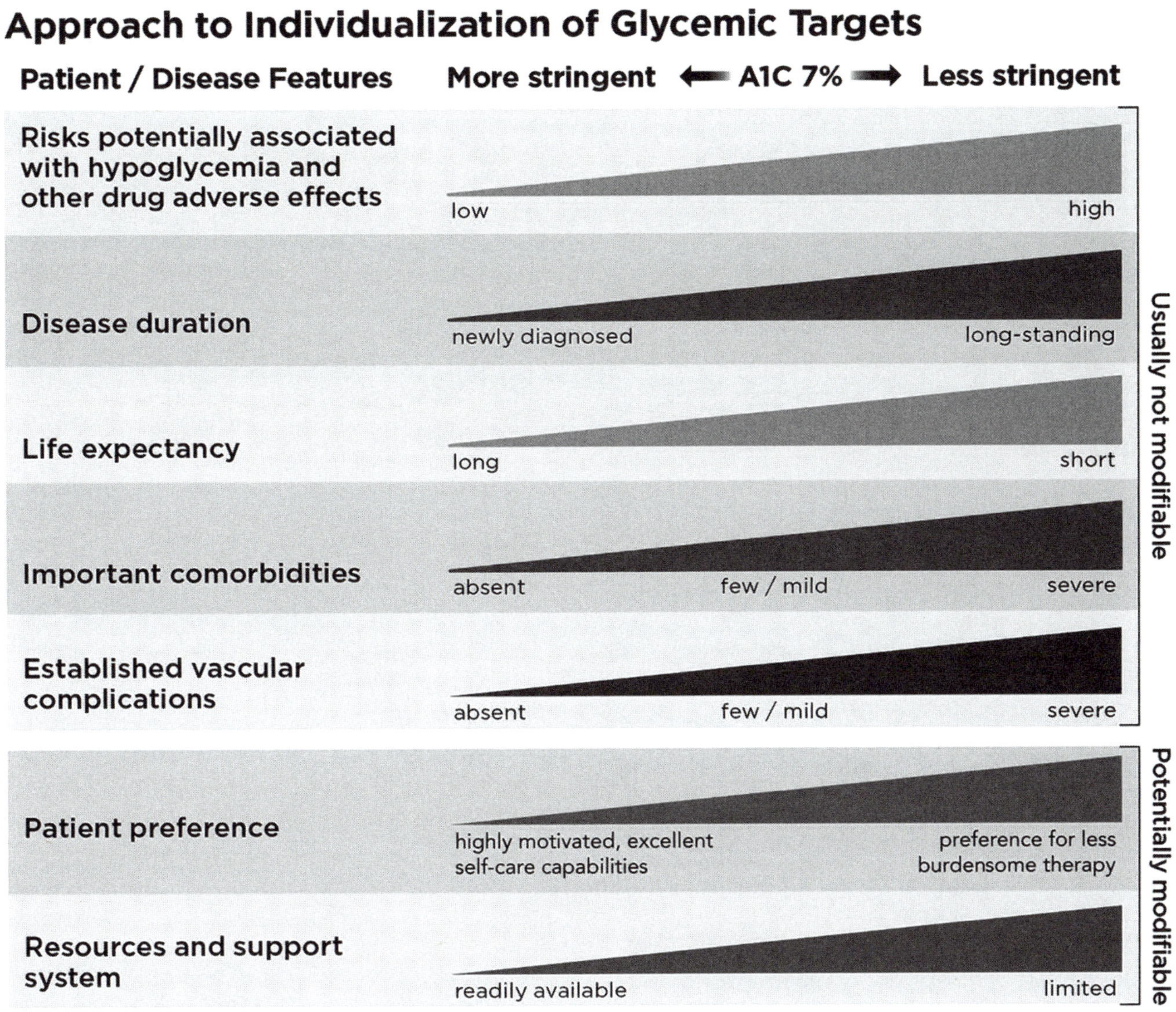

Approach to Individualization of Glycemic Targets

Patient / Disease Features — **More stringent ⟵ A1C 7% ⟶ Less stringent**

Patient / Disease Features	More stringent		Less stringent	
Risks potentially associated with hypoglycemia and other drug adverse effects	low		high	Usually not modifiable
Disease duration	newly diagnosed		long-standing	Usually not modifiable
Life expectancy	long		short	Usually not modifiable
Important comorbidities	absent	few / mild	severe	Usually not modifiable
Established vascular complications	absent	few / mild	severe	Usually not modifiable
Patient preference	highly motivated, excellent self-care capabilities		preference for less burdensome therapy	Potentially modifiable
Resources and support system	readily available		limited	Potentially modifiable

FIGURE 19.1 **Individualizing Glycemic Targets**

Source: American Diabetes Association Diabetes Care. 42(Supplement 1)(2019):S61-70. https://doi.org/10.2337/dc19-S006.

weight issues imbedded into the algorithm graph. Both organizations support therapeutic choices based on current evidence and individualizing therapy.[1]

Discussing the class of drug, mechanism of action, risk and benefit, and adverse events with the person with diabetes, verifying formulary coverage with a formulary look up tool, eg, coverage search (MMIT), Fingertip formulary, Finder, and verifying coverage and cost with the pharmacy increases the individual's initiation and engagement with the medication therapy regimen.[27]

Initial therapy in type 2 commonly is metformin.[1,2] Metformin XR 500 mg is the same cost as the 500 mg immediate release and dramatically reduces the risk of gastrointestinal problems. This dosage also is able to be titrated weekly to further reduce risk of adverse events and increase likelihood of engagement and maintenance with the medication regimen. If stability is not attained and maintenance in 3 months, guidelines recommend a GLP1-RA be initiated. SGLT2 inhibitors are recommended as the third therapy.[1,2] ADA recommends consideration for agents with proven cardiovascular risk reduction with PWD with atherosclerotic cardiovascular disease (ASCVD). Weight gain and risk of hypoglycemia are further considerations supporting use of GLP1-RA and SGLT2s.

In T2DM, basal insulin may be needed as well. If A1C is over 9% to 10%, insulin may be needed initially to

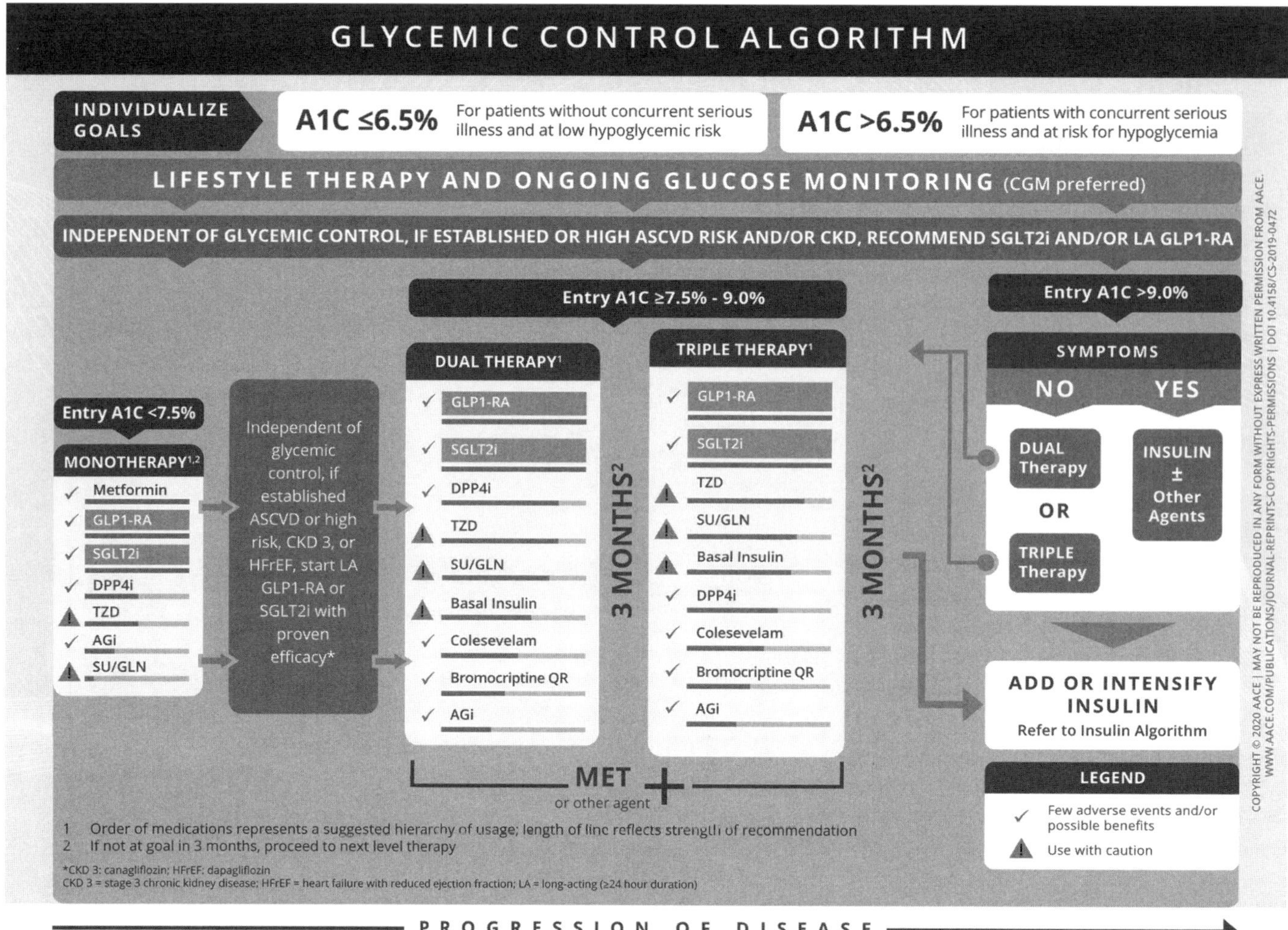

FIGURE 19.2 AACE/ACE Type 2 Glycemic Control Algorithm

Source: Reproduced with permission of American Association of Clinical Endocrinologists and American College of Endocrinology. Garber AJ, Handelsman Y, Grunberger G, et al. Consensus Statement by The American Association of Clinical Endocrinologists and American College of Endocrinology on The Comprehensive Type 2 Diabetes Management Algorithm – *2020 Executive Summary*. Endocrine Practice Vol 26, Number 1 Jan 2020 Page137.

resolve glucotoxicity. However, GLP is recommended as first injectable, if glucose/A1C is not extremely elevated. Sulfonylureas and TZDs are recommended with caution. Generic SU's would be indicated for cost reasons only, with glimepiride being most renal friendly. Glyburide is on the Beers criteria, so should not be used in the elderly.[29]

Inherent in optimization of therapies is the need for self-monitoring of blood glucose (SMBG) or CGM. This critical tool enables people to modify lifestyle behavior, adjust medication therapy, and develop a better understanding of their disease.[30] Self-management of blood glucose is clearly indicated for management of persons with type 1 diabetes and persons with type 2 diabetes on insulin and during pregnancy,[30–32] However, SMBG use in persons with type 2 diabetes not on insulin has received mixed reviews.[33,34] However, after reviewing current evidence, the International Diabetes Federation and the International SMBG Working Group developed practical recommendations for the use of SMBG in noninsulin-treated type 2 diabetes.[35,36] The recommendation continues to support the use of SMBG in all individuals with diabetes, recognizing it as a tool for guiding treatment and for its potential to actively involve individuals in managing their diabetes.

The time to monitor blood glucose is an intensely debated issue among experts. There are potentially 7 points within a 24-hour glucose profile including pre-meals, postmeals, and at bedtime.[37–38] Monnier et al found the contribution of fasting plasma glucose measurements approached 70% of overall glucose mean as A1C neared 10%. It was also found that *postprandrial* glucose contributes about 70% to the overall glucose profile when the A1C value drops below 8.4%.[39] Both monitoring and targeting pre- and postprandrial blood glucose treatment depends on A1C and individualized assessment of the individual's glycemic goals. Therefore, targeting fasting plasma glucose and overall glucose lowering is more beneficial when hemoglobin A1C results are very high, while targeting postprandial glucose is necessary when A1C results are closer to 8%. To reach glycemic targets, postprandial glucose must be addressed.[40] See chapter 18 for more information on the timing of blood glucose checks.

Continuous glucose monitoring (CGM) is evolving as a broad-based monitoring tool, arguably for all PWD. SMBG and CGM, however, should be recommended only when it is intended to promote healthy self-care behaviors and/or when both the individual with diabetes and the provider/diabetes care and education specialist are prepared to interpret the results and make appropriate adjustments in treatment based on the data.[36] Recommending SMBG/CGM, with appropriate testing instructions and collaborative data analysis provides a tool to facilitate glycemic management and the individual's involvement in problem solving and decision making.[41,42] Finally, in interpreting glucose results education and counseling programs that encourage active engagement of persons with diabetes, building self-efficacy in self-management, emphasizing behavioral strategies, and promoting engagement with treatment recommendations are associated with positive outcomes.[25,41–42] Used appropriately, glucose monitoring provides specific data for the persons with diabetes and providers to enable more timely clinical adjustments than A1C, thus improving outcomes. Similar glucose data can be displayed in very different ways, including handwritten glucose logs, report downloaded from glucose meters, or CGM tracings. See chapter 18 for more information glucose data logs and reports.

Often blood glucose records are the end results of self-care behavior, which is multi-factorial. Behavior change is the measurable outcome of diabetes self-management education (DSME/S).[25] The intent for the diabetes care and education specialist is to facilitate change with the individual for best clinical and health outcomes. For this to occur one must assess the individual's current behavior, identify appropriate intervention(s), negotiate achievable goals with the individual, and follow up to evaluate the plan. Reviewing glucose results at every visit to identify patterns of recurring problems or progress is the basis of pattern management leading to intensifying therapy. Using AADE7 Self-Care Behaviors® as a framework for reviewing results is helpful.

Another important aspect of diabetes education is identification of barriers that get in the way of monitoring blood glucose. Some barriers cited are lack of knowledge and skills, burden of treatment, health beliefs (perceived need and lack of treatment efficacy), emotional factors, depression, lack of coping resources, and financial, literacy, and numeracy skills.[25]

Methodology for Interpreting Glucose Results: Further Considerations

A systematic approach is central to the plan of care for persons with diabetes. Five basic steps guide the diabetes care and education specialist or and healthcare provider in interpreting glucose results:

1. Consider guidelines and establish individual blood glucose targets
2. Gather and organize blood glucose (BG) data
3. Find patterns by detecting trends and consider causes
4. Identify realistic changes and strategies for bringing blood glucose back to target ranges
5. Develop a shared decision plan of action including setting goals with actionable steps and follow-up assessment[13]

Make one change at a time so the result can be easily evaluated.

Effective pattern management process requires records with the following information:

1. BG results: At least 3 to 4 days of glucose records, meter download or CGM report.
2. Food: Type, quantity, and timing of food eaten
3. Physical activity: Any physical activity that occurred
4. Events: Any other event that could affect blood glucose values
5. Medications: Type, amount, and time taken[13]

Finding patterns by detecting trends and considering causes is the biggest challenge during the visit. Identifying and preventing hypoglycemia is the first priority. Not being distracted by outliers in glucose levels is important. Circling very high glucose values and focusing on indiscretions is demoralizing for persons with diabetes.

In all cases, the provider/diabetes care and education specialist must identify desired changes and consider realistic strategies for bringing blood glucose back to target ranges. Deciding on a shared plan of action should include setting realistic goals with the individual by optimizing therapies.

Asking the person with diabetes what they learned by reviewing their glucose records empowers them to make independent decisions and take action. They often have ideas in mind for implementation.

Frequent follow-up after initiating changes is important to maintain momentum

This case exemplifies a common sequence of intensification and approximate timing of needed changes. People with T2DM may indeed require insulin, but may find newer medications to manage postprandial glucose with minimal need for mealtime insulin.[43]

Progressive loss of B-cells requires the addition of exogenous insulin to maintain glycemic stability.[43] Studies are in support of adding basal insulin to oral agents/injectables.[44–46]

Case: Meet Sarah

Sarah is a 55 year-old caucasian female with type 2 diabetes for 2 years. She has been seeing her primary care provider who prescribed Metformin 500 mg bid when she was diagnosed. She met with the dietitian for an hour when she was initially diagnosed. Now her primary care provider is reporting that with her A1C at 7.9%, it is time to "do something." Sarah is 64 inches tall and weighs 226 lbs. Her kidney and liver studies are normal. Blood pressure is treated with an ACE inhibitor and she is on a statin.

Her friend went to a diabetes education program and reported that she learned a lot and was encouraged about her diabetes management. Sarah asked her provider if she could go as well. She would like to have some help losing weight. The provider agrees.

At the initial assessment:

1. The dietitian calculated the basal energy expenditure (BEE) and using the Harris Benedict equation recommended a 1400 calorie meal plan for weight loss. Consistent carbohydrate was suggested for meals at 2 to 3 servings per meal. Weekly activity goals of 30 minutes of walking most days was discussed.
2. The PharmD student taught her to use a glucose meter and when she did her BG test with the new meter, the level was 218 mg ~3 hours after her lunch.
3. The advanced practice nurse reviewed some of the medications to help improve BG levels after meals but asked Sarah to test fasting and 2 hours after meals for 3 days per week. She agreed to bring BG records to class.

At the first week of class, Sarah's levels were reviewed before class and all were above target, using American Association of Clinical Endocrinologists (AACE) guidelines:

In every diabetes-related visit, there are 4 questions that a diabetes care and education specialist should evaluate for patterns and therapy intensification:

1. What does the A1C result tell you?
2. What does the history tell you?
3. What do the glucose records tell you? Look for patterns and trends.
   - Is there hypoglycemia?
   - Are there BG levels elevated at the same time each day?
   - What are the factors that contribute to those specific BGs that are out of range?
     - —Evaluate food from the previous meal, and activity first. Then consider medication.
4. What's your approach/intervention for intensifying therapy?

In Sarah's case after reviewing BG levels, she and the nurse agreed that she:

1. Focus on implementing tips from the first class covering healthy eating, portion management, label reading, and other nutrition information.
2. Upgrade and maximize to Metformin ER 500 mg, 2 tabs with breakfast and supper. Due to it slower release, extended release reduces the risk of GI problems and 500 mg tabs are very affordable per GoodRx.org, cash price.

	Fasting	*2 Hours After Breakfast*	*2 Hours After Lunch*	*2 Hours After Dinner*
Mon	146	187	196	202
Tues	155	179	188	212
Fri	148	209	193	199

Case: The Second Week of Sarah's Class

Sarah implemented what she learned about healthy eating, changed to Metformin XR and increased the dose and her BG levels at the second week of class improved to:

	Fasting	*2 Hours After Breakfast*	*2 Hours After Lunch*	*2 Hours After Dinner*
Tues	122	176	188	194
Thurs	108	184	177	186
Sat	109	192	168	182

Even though there was improvement, especially in her fasting levels, Sarah's BG levels were still above target. The nurse certified diabetes care and education specialist (CDCES) talked the second week of class about the metabolic defects of diabetes and the medications that fix the problems. Sarah was interested in a once-a-week GLP1 RA. The advanced practice nurse (APN) called Sarah's primary provider to discuss her BG levels and possible medication change. Choosing medications to treat diabetes should be based on evidence-based guidelines as well as access. The APN used coverage search. MMIT,[27] a formulary look-up tool, to determine which by Sarah's insurance. She had samples and offered to help initiate the once-weekly injection.

Sarah's Next Steps

1. By implementing careful eating and exercise, Sarah's fasting BG improved to near normal, but postprandial levels were still above target (Goal: <140 mg ~2 hours after meals). A medication that "nudged the pancreas" and helped with weight loss was indicated. The sulfonylureas, meglitinides, or incretins would all improve after meal blood glucose levels. Sulfonylureas and meglitinides are less expensive but increase the chances of weight gain and hypoglycemia. Sitagliptin (Januvia®) Linagliptin (Tradjenta), and saxagliptin (Onglyza™) would likely help with postmeal glucose levels and were weight neutral, but would only offer about 0.5 to 0.6% A1C reduction. Sarah was anxious for some help with weight loss, she did not have financial restrictions, and had already practiced injections with saline at the second diabetes education class. Sarah and the advanced practice nurse agreed that she would be a good candidate for once weekly GLP1. Dulaglitide (Trulicity), Exenatide ER (Bydureon B-Cise), and Semaglutide (Ozempic) were reviewed. Her primary care physician verified there was no Medullary Endocrine Neoplasia (MEN), Medullary Thyroid Carcinoma (MTC), or prior history of pancreatitis and asked the advanced practice nurse to help her initiate the injection.
2. Sarah took the initial injection with the supervision of the APN. She was instructed to eat slowly and watch for feelings of fullness and then STOP eating. Additionally, reducing fat and spicy food for a few weeks might lessen the risk of nausea. If problems occurred with nausea/queasiness, Sarah was advised that these should resolve in a few weeks. She agrees she could "Power through" if this occurred. The starter kit instructions were reviewed with Sarah. She was able to use the co-pay card from the company to assist with the out of pocket costs. She also wanted to go to the Web site for more information. Lastly, she was coached to do BG levels fasting and 2 hours after meals just 1 to 2 days/week to verify improvement in glucose levels. She was relieved to learn that her risk of hypoglycemia was minimal. Frequency of glucose monitoring with this regimen is less intense and not as the risk of hypoglycemia is minimal.
3. Sarah was advised to bring BG levels to week 3 class for review and continue her Metformin ER 500 mg, 2 tabs with breakfast and supper.

At the third week of class, Sarah's BG levels were improving slightly.

	Fasting	*2 Hours After Breakfast*	*2 Hours After Lunch*	*2 Hours After Dinner*
Tues	107	169	187	196 mg
Weds	105	150	166	180
Thurs	99 mg	165	151	163

When reviewing the BG levels with the advanced practice nurse 2 weeks later, Sarah shared that she had no problem giving the injections, but did probably overeat a bit. She was a bit queasy, but reduced the amount she ate at meals. Sarah reported she continued feeling full, was eating less, and had 1 lb weight loss on her home scales. Her BG levels were much better. She had no problem getting her prescription from her pharmacy. She was very pleased with her improved BG levels and reported that she wasn't thinking about food all day.

Next Steps

Sarah completed the classes and returned to her primary care provider for ongoing care and support. At her review class *1 year later*, Sarah reported that her BG levels were in target most of the time, her A1C was 6.2%, she was exercising about 45 minutes most days, and that she had lost nearly 15 lbs. She participated in the local support group meetings several times a year. She was testing glucose 3 days/month with near normal results.

(continued)

Case: The Second Week of Sarah's Class (continued)

Two years later Sarah was referred to the APN for clinical management. Her A1C was 8.1%.

She reported she had had surgery last year with a long recovery. She was not able to exercise as consistently.

Her glucose levels for the past month averaged:

	Fasting	*2 hrs after Breakfast*	*2 hrs after Lunch*	*2 hours after Dinner*
3–4 days/mo	182	216	224	241

Sarah was interested in improving her glucose levels and A1C. She heard about the pills that pushed sugar out the urine but was worried about the lawyer ads she saw on TV. The sodium glucose transporter 2s were discussed, their mechanism of action, possible adverse events, and benefits. Canagliflozin (Invokana), Empagliflozin (Jardiance), Dapagliflozin (Farxiga), and Ertugliflozin (Steglatro) were searched on the formulary look-up tool for best insurance coverage. After completing a comprehensive foot exam, blood pressure, and lab work, Sarah decided since she hadn't had a history of yeast infections, she would try this class of pills. As advised, she drank an extra glass of water every day and saw blood sugars improve in the first week. She shared the glucose levels from her Bluetooth meter with the APN after week 3 and continued the SGLT2 inhibitor pills. Sarah also had a refresher diabetes self-management education class and met with the registered dietitian (RD).

At her follow-up in 3 months, Sarah reported eating healthier and had begun to swim 2x/week. A1C was 6.7% and average glucose levels were:

	Fasting	*2 hrs After Breakfast*	*2 hrs After Lunch*	*2 hrs After Dinner*
3–4 days/mo	122 mg	138 mg	126 mg	148 mg

Sarah and the APN discussed continuous glucose monitors at the follow-up visit as well. With the low risk of hypoglycemia and A1C in target, Sarah declined the sensors for now.

Five years later Sarah had a referral to the advanced practice nurse from her primary care provider. She had developed asthma, been started on steroids, and had lost her husband. She reported that even though she was eating carefully and exercising, her blood glucose levels remained high.

Sarah's A1C was 9.6% and BG levels for the past month averaged as follows:

	Fasting	*2 Hours After Breakfast*	*2 Hours After Lunch*	*2 Hours After Dinner*
Avg 3–4 days/wk	189	246 mg	223 mg	255 mg

She reported an occasional 300 mg reading after a large meal.

Sarah realized that her pancreas was probably not making enough insulin. The advanced practice nurse agreed. The C-Peptide test confirmed low endogenous insulin being produced. Sarah agreed to begin insulin.

Sarah weighed 181 lbs. She was started on long-acting basal insulin at 18u (0.2u/kg or ~10% of body weight). Sarah decided to take her insulin at 10p. Sarah was provided with a sample insulin pen, instructions on use and advice to test BG every day, fasting, and 2 hours after meals 3 days/week. The fasting BG would provide the primary report on the long-acting "basal" insulin, while the BG after meals would let her know if her GLP weekly injection and SGLT2 pill were still helping manage glucose levels after meals.

Sarah was advised to increase her long-acting insulin by 2 u every 3 days until her fasting BG was 100 mg. On Sarah's 1 week follow-up phone visit she was taking 22u/day. Her BG record was:

	Fasting	*2 Hours After Breakfast*	*2 Hours After Lunch*	*2 Hours After Dinner*
Mon	166 mg	202 mg	215 mg	219 mg
Tues	159 mg			
Weds	155 mg			
Thurs	148 mg	176 mg	188 mg	199 mg
Fri	135 mg			
Sat	129 mg			
Sun	124 mg	160 mg	162 mg	174 mg
Mon	122 mg			

Sarah was showing definite improvement in BG levels. Her fasting's were nearing the 100 mg target. She had increased her long-acting insulin to 22 u at 10p. When she and the advanced practice nurse discussed the other BG levels, the numbers were all above target, and results after her evening meal were consistently the highest. However, the glucose excursion was not more than 50 mg from pre-meal, so this was considered acceptable.

Case: The Second Week of Sarah's Class (continued)

In another 2 weeks Sarah's long-acting insulin dose was 32u and her glucose record was as follows:

	Fasting	*2 hrs After Breakfast*	*2 hrs After Lunch*	*2 hrs After Dinner*
Tuesday	119 mg	149 mg	145 mg	167 mg
Wednesday	115 mg			
Thursday	111 mg			
Friday	108 mg	133 mg	131 mg	149 mg
Saturday	103 mg			
Sunday	101 mg			
Monday	97 mg	129 mg	127 mg	140 mg

Sarah reported that the evening meal was her largest. Sarah advised that she was being very consistent with carbohydrate and felt like she was doing very well. The APN agreed.

Three years later, Sarah had an A1C of 7.2%. She was healthy and vibrant but wanted her A1C below 7%. The advanced practice nurse reviewed the time action of mealtime insulins. They agreed Sarah should start a mealtime (prandial) insulin with her largest meal of the day if she were going out to eat or having a high-carbohydrate meal.

Sarah agreed to begin 4 u of rapid acting insulin about 15 minutes before her evening meal.

She also wanted to discuss the glucose sensor that the APN had introduced some time ago. Sarah was prescribed a sensor and brought it to her next visit to get help with the set-up.

At her next appointment in 1 week the average BG numbers were as follows:

	Fasting	*2 Hours After Breakfast*	*2 Hours After Lunch*	*2 Hours After Dinner*	
Mon	122 mg	153 mg	155 mg	166 mg	
Tues	115 mg	152 mg	144 mg	142 mg	
Weds	112 mg	148 mg	140 mg	139 mg	4u Out to eat
Thurs	109 mg	142 mg	139 mg	142 mg	
Fri	111 mg	138 mg	141 mg	124 mg	4u Out to eat
Sat	108 mg	137 mg	135 mg	133 mg	
Sun	107 mg	147 mg	145 mg	142 mg	

As Sarah and the advanced practice nurse reviewed her BG levels, they agreed that the fasting, after breakfast, and lunch numbers were essentially in the normal range. On the days Sarah went out to eat and took 4 u meal insulin, the after-dinner numbers were in target range. If needed further down the road, the next step of intensification would be to increase the evening meal dose ~1 u/d until the after-dinner numbers were <140 mg. Sarah reported she felt comfortable adjusting the doses herself.

Basal insulin can be initiated in type 2 in various ways. Protocols for second generation basals have been evaluated using 10 u/d or 0.2u/kg/d. Titration is based on checking fasting BG and increasing basal dose 2u every 3 days until FBG is 70 to 110 mg.[47] A simpler alternative is to increase basal 1 u/day until the FBG is <100 mg.[48–50] An initial dose closer to the kilogram calculation is begun by basing the starting dose on 10% of the total body weight. This is an even simpler method and doesn't require a calculator.[13] This mathematical short cut starts the individual with a dose more realistic than 10 u/d. Ultra-long basals, Glargine U300 (Toujeo), and Degludec (Tresiba) require 3 to 4 days to reach steady state, so should not be titrated any more often than 3 to 7 days. (See Figure 19.3.)

People with diabetes should be coached on insulin titration and if able, should be empowered to make their own careful adjustments.

"Permission" to adjust insulin doses independently of the provider/diabetes care and education specialist should be encouraged whenever possible.

Education of persons with diabetes regarding self-titration leads to improved glycemic stability.[2] Studies demonstrate that a person with diabetes' titration competence is comparable to the provider, even with ultra-long basal insulins.[53–58] When advising on basal titration, provide a maximum dose to which the individual will work up. "Over-basalization" is a common mistake with providers who don't realize the necessity or have comfort with treating postprandial glucose.

The person with diabetes "owns" their diabetes. The role of the provider and the diabetes care and education specialist is to help the person with diabetes be independent and self-sufficient.

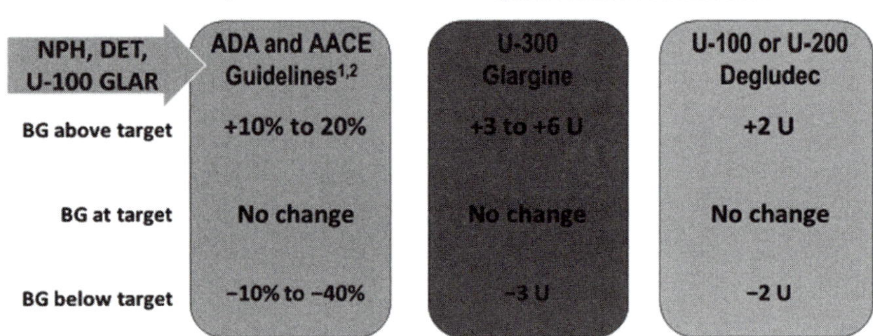

Titrating Newer Basal Insulins: Guidelines and Evidence
General Guidelines for Any Basal Insulin 1,2
Specific Guidelines for Newer Insulins 47, 48
NPH, DET, U-100 GLAR
ADA and AACE Guidelines1,2
U-300 Glargine
U-100 or U-200 Degludec
BG above target
+10% to 20%
+3 to +6 U
+2 U
BG at target
No change
No change
No change
BG below target
−10% to −40%
−3 U
−2 U
Compute average FBG from 2 to 3 previous measurements 47,48
Titrate weekly or no more frequently than every 3 to 4 days47,48

FIGURE 19.3 Titrating New Basal Insulins: Guidelines and Evidence

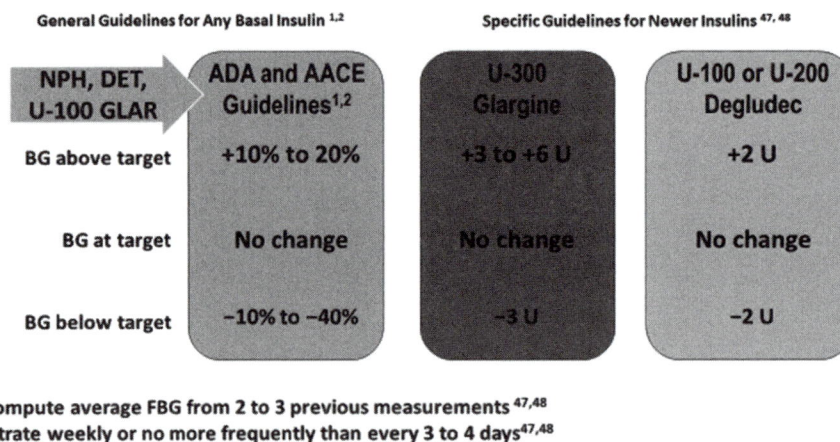

Even though individuals may be adjusting their own insulin, some therapeutic changes require prescriber involvement. Whether SMBG handwritten diary or CGM printout, identifying patterns drives changes. Hopefully, the person with diabetes is empowered to initiate a call to the provider when their resources are exhausted.

A variety of choices exist for MDI; however, a common regimen, sometimes referred to as the "poor man's pump," is to use a long-acting basal insulin, usually once a day, with injections of rapid-acting (lispro, aspart, or glulisine) insulin when eating carbohydrates. The injections coinciding with food are administered at least twice a day or several times more during the day, depending on the individual's eating schedule. When implementing pattern management and troubleshooting frequent, unpredictable glycemic fluctuations, this may indicate the need to look beyond diet and exercise. Evaluate for alcohol intake, injection site hypertrophies, or technical issues with insulin delivery.

Prandial insulin should be dosed in people with type 2 diabetes based on individual sensitivities and amount of calories and carbohydrate ingested. Considerations for initial dosing vary from 4 to 10 u/meal or 0.1 u to 0.15 u/kg/meal based on which meal is the largest.[1,59–60]

If both basal and prandial insulin is initiated, the prandial should cover about 50% of the total daily dose. Meal doses could be divided among the three meals: Breakfast 30% to 40%, lunch ~30%, and dinner ~30% to 40%.

Intensifying therapy and adjusting doses should include considerations for titrating based on patterns in BG. The type of dosing should include not only scheduled dosing, but supplemental dosing and insulin adjustments for other occasions.[59–60]

Additional injections, referred to as correction boluses, may become necessary if the blood glucose value is too high, in which case an injection of rapid-acting insulin is needed to lower the blood glucose to the target level. Some individuals may prefer using regular insulin (also known as short-acting insulin) for the correction and meal bolus dose. This insulin (Novolin R) is available without prescription at many pharmacies. Check GoodRx.org for local pricing.

Intensifying therapy in type 1 diabetes uses similar principles. Treatment originates with multiple daily injections because endogenous insulin is nearly all depleted by the time of diagnosis. Treatment may advance to pumps and continuous glucose monitoring. This progression often happens more quickly in this population.

Principles Pump Delivery

Since the first insulin pumps in 1978, insulin pump therapy has gained popularity. There were an estimated 500,000 pump users in the United States. In 2016 and pump use is considered to be a multi-billion dollar industry worldwide.[61] Pump therapy is a realistic alternative for intensive insulin delivery in both pediatric and adult populations, including older adults.[62,63,64] Insulin pumps have allowed persons with diabetes who desire intensive insulin management and can be successful in self-management to achieve as close to euglycemia as possible with no increased weight gain and minimal hypoglycemia.[65,114]

Both MDI and CSII are designed to more closely mimic pancreatic function. For optimal glycemic stability, insulin delivery should closely simulate the "normal" pattern of insulin secretion (shown in Figure 19.4). As shown in Figure 19.5, continuous or "basal" insulin levels are thus required throughout the day to cover hepatic glucose output and glucose disposal in the fasting state, while brief increases in insulin levels ("boluses") are needed to coincide with ingestion of food or meals.[62,63]

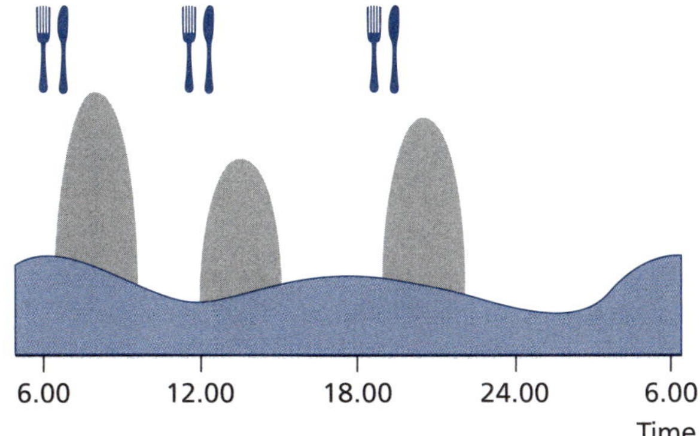

FIGURE 19.4 Insulin Secretion in Persons Without Diabetes

Source: D Tomky, Continuous subcutaneous insulin infusion (insulin pump therapy). In: Complete Nurses Guide to Diabetes Care. AB Childs, M Cypress, G Spollett, eds. American Diabetes Association: Alexandria, VA; 2005:262. Reprinted with permission from the American Diabetes Association.

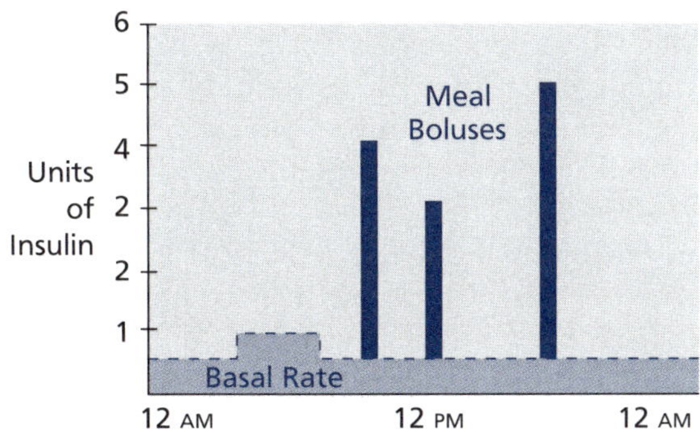

FIGURE 19.5 Pump Insulin Delivery

Source: D Tomky, Continuous subcutaneous insulin infusion (insulin pump therapy). In: *Complete Nurses Guide to Diabetes Care*. Childs AB, Cypress M, Spollett G, eds. American Diabetes Association: Alexandria, VA; 2005:262. Reprinted with permission from the American Diabetes Association.

Emerging continuous glucose monitoring (CGM) sensor technology is making insulin intensification more achievable and safer for people with T1 and T2 diabetes.

> Insulin pump therapy has been available for over 40 years. Although an "artificial pancreas" is still not commercially available, technology is advancing rapidly.

Benefits and Limitations: MDI and Pump Therapy

Multiple Daily Injections: Benefits

MDI more closely mimics normal insulin secretion than conventional therapy, ie, NPH and regular insulin that were used commonly in the 1980s. MDI with second generation basals, ie, determir and glargine and rapid-acting meal time insulins given before meals, provides for more dietary flexibility. With this therapy, the individual can calculate bolus insulin based on food intake.

Second generation basal insulins, ie, glargine (lantus, basaglar) and detemir (Levemir) offer less hypoglycemia overnight than conventional therapy, and the person is not forced to eat when not hungry to prevent hypoglycemia at peak times of insulin, ie, NPH.

Another MDI option is available. Ultra-long basal insulins have a flatter profile, less hypoglycemia and longer duration, allowing some flexibility in daily dosing times.[66–70] The ultra-long basal insulin is titrated based on patterns of fasting glucose using the same principles already described.

With use of these basal insulins, mealtime insulin is given whenever the person eats regardless of timing.

Connected Pens

The connected pen is a sophisticated option for persons with diabetes on MDI. When used in conjunction with the newer basal insulins, many features of traditional pump therapy are achieved. The connected pen uses rapid-acting insulin cartridges and is accompanied by a Bluetooth device. The device, the In-Pen,[71] is able to track insulin on board, calculate bolus doses, and remind the individual to take basal insulin. Continuous glucose monitoring and connected pen data can be integrated via phone apps. Although manual injections are still required, 32-gauge, 4mm needles are much less intrusive than previous needles and the cost comparison versus a pump and monthly supplies is dramatically less.

Multiple Daily Injections: Limitations

Basal insulin is given once or twice a day and is a steady amount of insulin. It cannot be quickly changed for exercise or other activities that may require more or less basal coverage. Frequent and multiple injections of insulin may be difficult to fit into an individual's lifestyle. While the time action is longer and flatter, there is still a modest peak and variability from day to day. Ultra-long basals have less variability and are only given once a day. However, when combined with up to 3 mealtime injections, it would still add up to 4 injections per day. People who struggle with numeracy or vision problems may have difficulty calculating and safely injecting.

Insulin Pump Therapy: Benefits

Evidence shows that using pump therapy to maintain normal or near-normal glycemia can improve health and reduce hypoglycemia and the long-term complications of diabetes.[72–74]

Pumps only use short- or rapid-acting insulin that provide more predictable physiologic delivery of insulin. Dosing of insulin is precisely delivered within one-hundredth of a unit. Insulin absorption is more predictable from a continuous insulin depot. Dawn phenomenon effects are easier to manage; a variable basal rate can be set to accommodate fluctuations in insulin requirements overnight. Basal rates can be quickly changed to accommodate growth spurts in children or increased insulin needs during pregnancy, menstrual cycle fluctuations, stress, illness, and/or physical activity. Unpredictable eating habits and low insulin requirements in very young children with type 1 diabetes make insulin pump therapy a safer option.[75–78]

Pump therapy can help reduce the frequency and severity of hypoglycemia.[62] Some pumps, combined with CGM, offer an improved safety profile by monitoring patterns and automatically reducing the basal rate during periods of low physiological requirements, which can minimize nocturnal or daytime hypoglycemia. Additionally, using a temporary basal rate that meets the increased or decreased short-term physiologic needs can accommodate for sick days or anticipated physical activity.

One of the unique features of CSII is the ability to preprogram changes in basal insulin delivery.[62] This feature is especially useful during the night when insulin pharmacokinetics and the dawn phenomenon may change basal insulin requirements.

Insulin pump therapy offers the person with diabetes an improvement in lifestyle flexibility and satisfaction by allowing meals and snacks to be customized to fit the individual's schedule and preferences in timing, size of meal, and type of food. Using insulin to carbohydrate ratios (ICR) to count carbohydrates is one method of matching appropriate amounts of insulin in bolus doses to intake of food. Although initial improved glycemia may promote weight gain if there is no alteration in caloric intake, weight loss may be achieved more easily in motivated individuals. Another benefit of a pump is the ability to tailor insulin needs to changes in schedules related to travel or work.

In MDI, a long-acting insulin analog, such as glargine (Lantus®) or detemir (Levemir®), Glargine U300 (Toujeo), or Degludec (Tresiba) is used as a basal insulin analog, and a rapid-acting insulin is given before meals or when carbohydrates are ingested.

In pump therapy, rapid-acting insulin is predominantly used. Basal and bolus doses are preprogrammed by the wearer and delivered through a small portable device that is designed to give doses precisely calculated for an individual's requirements.

Insulin Pump Therapy: Limitations

Risks and limitations of pump therapy must be fully understood by the wearer, family or support person, and healthcare team. Insulin pumps are not for everyone, and the person using a pump must maintain a high degree of motivation before and after pump initiation.[79] The person must be willing to maintain consistent and frequent self-monitoring of blood glucose or use CGM. Some people with diabetes struggle with self-care behaviors and applying appropriate problem-solving skills. Being connected to a pump is a constant reminder of having diabetes. Technical or mechanical failure is possible and if not corrected quickly can lead to diabetic ketoacidosis within a few hours in individuals with type 1 diabetes. Skin irritations and infections are possible, although these are avoidable with proper technique, including skin care and site rotation. Some populations, such as children or people who are visually impaired, may require assistance from a caregiver.

Many healthcare professionals are unfamiliar with pump therapy and may not provide the needed training and support. The cost of insulin pumps is often $6,000 to $8,000 and supplies (not including blood glucose monitoring supplies) cost more than $300 per month. Insurance companies typically cover 80% of pump expenses, and coverage varies from state to state and plan to plan. Reimbursement for diabetes education to support the individual also varies.

Contraindications to Pump Therapy

Individuals who have unrealistic expectations that pump therapy automatically will manage their diabetes are not appropriate candidates for CSII. Severe depression or other serious behavioral health disorders may impede self-management skills and prevent the person from paying attention to details that are critical to successful pump therapy. A history of poor self-care behaviors and health-care practices, such as failure to perform SMBG, keep appointments, give inconsistent insulin doses, or inappropriately apply problem-solving skills, is a predictor of poor outcomes.[80] Lack of financial resources for initiating and maintaining pump therapy are additional problems.

How Pumps Work

An insulin pump is a small, battery-operated mechanical device that delivers rapid-acting insulin via very small catheter into the subcutaneous tissue. It contains a reservoir with a syringe or pod that is filled with rapid-acting insulin. The standard pump reservoir attaches to a plastic tube, called an infusion set. At the end of the infusion set is a detachable 25- or 27-gauge needle or soft Teflon® catheter. The catheter (via needle) is inserted into the subcutaneous tissue and stays in place with self-adhesive tape or a bio-occlusive dressing. Pod pumps eliminate tubing with a built-in insulin reservoir, angled infusion set, automated inserter, pumping mechanism, and power supply. It is linked to a wireless handheld personalized diabetes manager similar to a personal digital assistant (PDA) or can be viewed via device that resembles a phone. The person wearing the insulin pump operates the device. Every 48 to 72 hours, the pump wearer changes the infusion site or pod, using aseptic technique. If forgetting the controller, the pump continues to deliver basal insulin.

Initially, insulin pumps weighed just under 1 pound and allowed simple delivery of basal and bolus insulin. Current models weigh as little as 1.2 oz and can be worn discretely under clothing or on a belt. Pumps contain miniature computers that provide an array of basal and bolus functions for more accurate calculations. Several pumps now connect via infrared ports to blood glucose monitors or CGMs to program insulin delivery. This enables direct download of blood glucose data to facilitate more accurate and easy bolus calculations. Pumps also connect to computers or handheld devices so that insulin doses and blood glucose levels can be reviewed. Pump companies are partnering with CGM companies to offer integrated glucose information with insulin delivery. Glucose data can be "shared" allowing parents, adult children, and others to assist with monitoring and adjustments remotely. Availability of these results allows the healthcare professional and wearer to analyze the data for pattern recognition to intensify diabetes management.

Other features include tracking the amount of "insulin on board," ie, the amount of insulin that is still active in the tissues from previous carbohydrate-based insulin boluses or correction boluses. Other advanced features offered by pumps include site change reminders, blood glucose and missed bolus alerts, calculation of food bolus based on preset insulin-to-carbohydrate ratios (also known as insulin to carb ratios or ICRs), alerts to recheck blood glucose (BG) if previous level was below or above target, pre-programmed temp basal rates for exercise, etc, and preprogrammed insulin sensitivity factors (ISFs) that allow for accurate calculation of required boluses to correct elevated BG. Insulin can be delivered in increments as small as 0.025units and also have a setting for maximum bolus amount. Some pumps include a food database that can be individualized for commonly consumed foods. Over time, pumps are getting smarter, but currently the wearer in some cases can deliver insulin based on the CGM data. Others still need to perform self-monitoring of blood glucose (SMBG) and make appropriate decisions based on that information. Currently one pump doubles as a CGM receiver eliminating paraphernalia for the person with diabetes to carry.

Sensor Augmented Pump Therapy and Hypoglycemia Suspend

Glucose sensors and insulin pumps are being combined into one system, allowing integration of glucose data and insulin delivery. The glucose sensor measures interstitial glucose, transmitting that to the CGM receiver which displays data on the paired pump device screen. This then integrates the glucose data into the pump settings. STAR 3, a randomized controlled trial found better A1Cs in children and adolescents likely due to easy access to CGM data on the pump allowing for quicker response to high and low glucose levels consequently reducing glycemic variability.[81,82,83]

Low glucose suspend technology proactively stops insulin delivery based on CGM data of actual or anticipated hypoglycemia. Predictive low glucose suspend systems automatically suspend insulin 30 minutes before hypoglycemia is likely to occur. This has had a 50% to 80% reduction on nocturnal hypoglycemia and a 31% to 50% reduction in hypoglycemia overall.[63,85–87]

Closed Loop Delivery Is the ultimate goal of pump therapy. This automated insulin system includes a pump and integrated CGM that evaluates glucose patterns and automatically adjusts basal insulin based on patterns observed. The hybrid closed loop system works off an algorithm and operates in auto mode when the CGM is active and calibrated. This system is available as Minimed 670G (Medtronic), and now similar features are offered in Control IQ (Tandem). These systems reduce A1C, hypoglycemia, variability, and increase time in range.[88–94,83]

Simplified pump technology has been available. Several companies are delevoping patch pumps. It is primarily for people with type 2 diabetes. Available as small disposable "patch" pumps, they are able to deliver a set basal based on total daily dose and bolus button for meal delivery.[95–97]

Evidence versus Practice: Candidate Attributes for Pump Success

Prerequisite Skills and Experience

Pumps are considered safe and effective for a variety of populations; however, changing directly to pump therapy without previous experience using intensified insulin therapy (ie, MDI) is inappropriate.

Individuals with unrealistic expectations of CSII therapy can be identified with an established screening protocol.[82]

Individuals interested in using pump therapy first need to learn and develop a variety of skills. Pump failure will require managing diabetes with MDI therapy. The following are important to master as prerequisites to pump therapy:

- Comprehensive diabetes education
- Frequent blood glucose monitoring and record keeping
- Carbohydrate counting
- Calculating bolus insulin
- Problem solving through interpretation of blood glucose pattern
- Adjusting insulin for special situations, eg, change in physical activity, menses, illness, etc
- Problem solving for hypoglycemia and hyperglycemia prevention and treatment

Only individuals who have mastered these skills should be considered for insulin pump therapy. Note also that these are just the prerequisites; other skills need to be taught and developed.[79]

Clinical Indications for Insulin Pump Therapy

The Association of Diabetes Care and Education Specialists (ADCES)–formerly the American Association of Diabetes Educators (AADE)–and the American Diabetes Association (ADA) position statements highlight clinical indications and desirable traits in selecting CSII (hopefuls.)[74,81] A letter of medical necessity requires identification of some of these items to justify insurance coverage. Careful selection of pump candidates is very important for safety and success. Lifestyle indicators, such as erratic schedule, varied work shifts, frequent travel, and the need for flexibility, further support the clinical indicators.[62,79]

Desired Traits

Motivation, cognitive abilities, technical stills, and financial resources are necessities for success with pumps. Specific details in each area are listed in Table 19.2.

TABLE 19.2 Criteria for Insulin Pump Use[76]

Medical/Metabolic Indications	*Cognitive/Psychomotor Criteria*
Suboptimal glycemic management Wide blood glucose excursions Dawn phenomenon with elevated fasting blood glucose levels Frequent severe hypoglycemia Nocturnal hypoglycemia Pregnant or planning contraception Variable daily schedule not well managed with injections Insulin sensitivity and requires low doses of insulin	Has sound rationale for pursuing and realistic expectation of CSII therapy Learns technical and cognitive components of the pump Applies appropriate problem-solving skills to troubleshoot hyper/hypoglycemia events and sick days Is able to match carbohydrate with insulin using carbohydrate-counting skills Modifies treatment plan upon outcome evaluation
Motivational Ability	*Technical/Physical Ability*
Performs frequent blood glucose monitoring as a lifetime behavior Complies with recommendations for safe insulin pump use Pays attention to details as to the insulin regimen and needed adjustments Anticipates insulin needs as situations changes	Performs blood glucose monitoring accurately and frequently, greater than 4 to 6 times daily Performs the technical components of insulin pump use or has necessary support if visually impaired Free from serious disease that would impair technical performance Provider observes set change technique and site rotation on a regular basis
Financial Resources	
Adequate financial resources to cover initial and ongoing costs of CSII therapy	

Source: D Tomky, Continuous subcutaneous insulin infusion (insulin pump therapy). In: *Complete Nurses Guide to Diabetes Care*. AB Childs, M Cypress, C Spollett, eds. American Diabetes Association: Alexandria, VA. 2017;427.

Importance of Experienced, Multidisciplinary Team

One of the important considerations for successful pump therapy is using a team for education, training, and treatment that is both multidisciplinary and familiar with insulin pump therapy.[74,79,80] Ideally, insulin pump therapy should be prescribed, implemented, and followed by a skilled diabetes care team that is familiar with the therapy and capable of supporting the person with diabetes 24 hours a day, 7 days a week.[81] Ongoing clinical follow-up is required to be every 3 months for supply reimbursement for Medicare recipients.[98–100]

Comprehensive Education Before Pump Initiation

All people with diabetes should be offered comprehensive diabetes education. People considering pump therapy need to be competent with all aspects of self-care, particularly meal planning, adjustments for exercise, hypo and hyperglycemia, and problem solving.

Healthy Eating

Core competence in diabetes medical nutrition therapy (MNT) is essential for successful implementation of intensified insulin therapy. To maximize the benefits and minimize the risks associated with intensive therapy, the pump wearer needs knowledge of meal planning and the ability to plan meals, modify food choices, and determine insulin doses.

Many meal planning methods have been evaluated including healthy food choices based on the food pyramid, exchange lists, carbohydrate counting, total calories, and total available glucose.[102] The common practice is for persons with diabetes to count total carbohydrate grams when dosing for meals with pump therapy.,[101,102]

Recent studies had demonstrated the need to account for protein in postprandial glycemic levels.[102–104]

The amount of carbohydrate/calories in the meal helps determine the mealtime bolus dose of insulin. In general the glycemic index, fiber, fat, and caloric content of the meal have less effect on the bolus insulin doses.[102] Research has provided evidence that matching insulin to the amount of carbohydrate intake, known as using an ICR, is effective for pump use.[62,105]

Carbohydrate-Counting Skills

Carbohydrate counting can be taught in levels:[101–107]

- Basic carbohydrate counting includes learning to read labels, being consistent with carbohydrate amounts, timing, and consistency for meals and snacks.

Advanced Carbohydrate-Counting Skills Advanced skills training teaches the person using MDI or CSII how to use ICRs to match short-acting or rapid-acting insulin to carbohydrate consumption.[107]

> Managing total calorie intake is necessary to prevent weight gain.

Carb Budgeting: Or Dosing Insulin Based on Carbohydrate Servings or Total Calories

Some people are more comfortable using the carbohydrate choice method as an indicator of how much insulin to take for meals or snacks. The carbohydrate choice method is similar to the method discussed above, since 1 carbohydrate choice is the amount of food containing 15 g of carbohydrate.

Clinicians and diabetes care and education specialists are also teaching persons with diabetes to dose insulin based on calories, calorie points, exchanges, and total calories. This is especially important for people trying to lose or not gain weight.

> There is not just 1 way to do insulin dosing. Diabetes care and education specialists need to adapt to the clinical and educational level of each individual.

A fixed meal carbohydrate amount with a fixed insulin dose is also possible with pump therapy. A small meal may be 15 grams of carb, ie, salad. A medium meal may be 30 to 45 grams of carb, ie, the usual meal. A large meal may be when the person goes out to eat or has a known high-carb meal like pasta. The insulin dose settings are preset, then adjusted based on postprandial glucose reading compared to food logs and carb assessments. This simplification allows individuals with numeracy problems to experience pump therapy.

Accounting for the delayed glycemic effect of protein may be needed as well.[103,104,106]

Challenges in Meal Bolusing

Avoiding Weight Gain. The temptation to eat anything and everything since insulin can be given to "cover the carbs" and provide good glucose stability is something to be avoided. With improvement of glycemic levels, weight gain may happen whether using MDI or pump therapy. Insulin is an anabolic storage hormone and will store calories as fat.

Adjusting for Fat, Fiber High-fat meals can cause a delay in gastric emptying and, therefore, problems in unpredictable food absorption. Persons with diabetes eating high-fat foods may require an adjustment in their bolus insulin amount or in the timing of their mealtime insulin to avoid early postprandial hypoglycemia and later hyperglycemia Similarly, dietary fiber is not usually digested. Some individuals may also notice their own unique responses to certain carbohydrate foods and may need to adjust their bolus doses accordingly.[107]

Carbohydrate counting is not a perfect system; it presents many challenges and concerns.[96] Keeping a food record is initially challenging, and maintaining ongoing food records can be burdensome. Monitoring blood glucose before and after meals can be challenging, but such monitoring is necessary and proven effective for identifying the appropriate dose of insulin to achieve and maintain euglycemia. Still, carbohydrate counting offers several advantages. It provides a more precise method of matching food and mealtime insulin, allows flexibility in meal planning, improves blood glucose management, and is empowering to those who use it. Understanding the need to adjust insulin for meal sizes, individualizing premeal and postmeal blood glucose targets, using pattern management skills, and calculating bolus and basal insulin doses is helpful for people with diabetes to be successful with healthy eating behaviors.[107]

There are now many carbohydrate/calorie-counting resources available online, apps for smartphones and as software programs for PDAs, and as small reference books.

Correction Bolus and Insulin Sensitivity Factor (ISF)

An important and advanced skill is using both the insulin-to-carbohydrate ratio (ICR) and the insulin sensitivity factor (ISF) for correction bolus. Correction-dose insulin therapy is an important adjunct to the scheduled insulin that is usually given before meals.[105] The ISF is used to calculate the amount of insulin needed to bring the blood glucose level into target range and is used as a correction or supplemental amount of insulin when glucose levels are too high Calculating the ISF also helps the individual make adjustments for special situations. Both the ICR, which is based on matching the rapid-acting insulin to the carbohydrate/calorie content of food to be eaten, and the ISF need to be individualized. Smart pumps have dose calculators built in to assist with accurate dosing of both the ICR and correction bolus.

Determining Insulin-to-Carbohydrate Ratios (ICR)

The insulin-to-carbohydrate ratio (ICR) is commonly used to calculate meal time insulin dosing. For individuals with type 2 diabetes not on an insulin pump, data suggests a simplified algorithm is effective for dosing.

For pump therapy, mealtime dosing is based on the principle that 1 unit of rapid-acting insulin is needed to cover or match a specified amount of carbohydrate/calories. The ratio is determined by the individual's sensitivity to insulin. An adult who is not obese may have an ICR of 1 unit of insulin to "cover or match" 10 g to 15 g of carbohydrate. The ratio can vary from toddlers (who are typically very sensitive to insulin) requiring 1 unit of rapid-acting insulin for every 30 g of carbohydrate to overweight adults requiring 1 unit of rapid-acting insulin for every 5 g of carbohydrate consumed.

There are different approaches and methods for determining the ICR for an individual (see Table 19.3 for starting adult dose calculations). Bolus or mealtime insulin doses can be based on the total number of grams of carbohydrate to be eaten or on the total number of grams of carbohydrate or choices consumed at a meal. In calculating a meal bolus, insulin dose is based on the total amount of grams of carbohydrate to be eaten.[105,107]

Being Active

Whether on an insulin pump or MDI, individuals who increase physical activity often have a decreased need for insulin.[108] Improved insulin sensitivity and glucose transport occur with exercise and increase the risk of hypoglycemia.[102,108] Consistent physical activity contributes to changes in body composition and extended glycemic benefit for 24 hours more or less. The hormonal response to an episode of increased physical activity depends on the degree of diabetes stability, insulin dose, time and content of last meal, fitness level, and type of activity performed.[101]

The type of insulin adjustment depends on when the person is going to engage in physical activity relative to his or her mealtime boluses. In MDI, the person may need to anticipate the physical activity and decrease the basal insulin. If the physical activity will occur within 3 hours after the premeal bolus, then that bolus can be adjusted.

For pump users, if physical activity will be between meals, then the basal rate needs adjusting. Some parameters are given below:[99]

- Light Activities. For light activities, a 10% to 20% reduction in insulin requirements 1 hour preceding and 1 hour after the activity
- Activities of Moderate Intensity and Short Duration (1 to 2 hours) of activity. Activities such as tennis, brisk walking, running, or biking require a 30% to 50% reduction in basal for the 1 hour preceding and the 1 hour after the activity, in addition to the duration of the activity itself.

TABLE 19.3 Starting T1 and T2 Adult Pump Dosage Calculations

Basal Rate Calculations	
Generally, a single basal rate is recommended; multiple basal rates are sometimes programmed initially based on individualized requirements (eg, prednisone doses or well-documented, distinct dawn phenomenon)	
Method 1:	1. Determine TDD* of insulin with injections; reduce by 25%–30% 2. Divide TDD by 50% = total basal dose in units 3. Divide total basal dose by 24 hours = starting basal rate (unit/hour)
Method 2:	1. Multiply 0.5 × individual's weight (kg) = TDD, then reduce by 20%–25% 2. Divide TDD by 50% = total basal dose in units 3. Divide total basal dose by 24 hours = starting basal rate (unit/hour)
Method 3:	Optimally managed basal-bolus MDI individuals may convert total dosage of glargine divided by 24 hours = starting basal rate (unit/hour) *Note:* Reducing by 10%–15% for the first 24 hours allows for "wash out" of glargine
Bolus Calculations	
Method 1:	TDD is divided into 450 or 500 to determine how many grams of carbohydrate are covered by 1 unit of insulin *Example:* 500 ÷ 50 unit/day (TDD) = 1 unit per 10 g of carbohydrate
Method 2:	1. Based on weight and TDD 2. 2.8 × weight (lb) ÷ TDD = ICR
Method 3:	Optimally managed basal-bolus MDI individuals may convert from previous ICR
Correction Bolus Calculations or Insulin Sensitivity Factor	
Method:	1. Determine the correction dose for elevated glucose levels to determine the mg/dL that 1 unit of insulin decreases the blood glucose value 2. Divide 1700 by the TDD (range 1600–2200)[83,98] *Example:* 1700 ÷ TDD = insulin sensitivity factor

*TDD is the total daily dose

Sources: JR Walsh, Pumping Insulin: Everything for Success on an Insulin Pump and CGM. 2017 Torrey Pines Press, San Diego.

Bruce W. Bode, William V. Tamborlane & Paul C. Davidson (2002) Insulin pump therapy in the 21st century, *Postgraduate Medicine*, 111:5, 69-77, DOI: 10.3810/pgm.2002.05.1200.

H Wolpert, Smart Pumping: A Practical Approach to Mastering the Insulin Pump. (Alexandria, VA: American Diabetes Association, 2002).

S Owen, "Pediatric pumps: barriers and breakthroughs," *Diabetes Educ.* 32(2006):29S-38S.

- Isometric Exercises. Isometric exercises such as weightlifting usually require no adjustment.
- Prolonged Activity. Prolonged activity requires a sustained reduction for the duration of activity and may require extended reduction hours afterward, to avoid nocturnal hypoglycemia.

Pump wearers are advised not to remove the pump during exercise; however, temp basal should be considered. Insulin deficiency will likely occur after a maximum of 2 hours of being disconcerted from the pump. To prevent hypoglycemia during a short workout, consider reducing the premeal bolus for pre-meal exercise, lowering overnight basal by 10% to 20% following late afternoon/evening activity or consuming quickly absorbable carbohydrates just before the workout. Monitoring blood glucose before and after exercise is vital to understanding individual responses.[102,108]

Focused testing: Glucose testing before and after exercise allows decisions to be made about the need for insulin adjustment or increased snacks. Testing in pairs can be achieved with CGM as well[45]

Hypoglycemia

Hypoglycemia is the main side effect of insulin, regardless of delivery method. Insulin pump therapy does not seem to have any higher rate of hypoglycemia than MDI.

Pickup and Keen's review of 25 years of CSII results found the incidence of hypoglycemia to be 30% to 60% less in insulin pump therapy compared to MDI.[110] Initial reports of severe hypoglycemia may have been due to unfamiliarity with tight management of blood glucose levels.[111] The decrease in severe hypoglycemia may be due to better pharmacokinetic delivery of insulin and better understanding that lower insulin requirements are needed at the time of pump initiation.[112]

Type 1 Diabetes: Keep glucagon (Inhaled powder -BAQSIMI, auto injector or 1-mg injectable kit) available for care partners to treat severe low blood sugars defined as cognitive or physical impairment requiring assistance.

Type 1 and Type 2 Diabetes: Consider a brief (30-minute) use of alternate basal or pump suspension for milder low blood sugar.

Intensive insulin therapy can pose a threat of severe hypoglycemia resulting in loss of consciousness. Not everyone gets warning signs of low blood glucose (hypoglycemia unawareness); therefore, reinforcing frequent blood glucose monitoring (especially before driving or when operating equipment) to individuals following an intensive insulin regimen is essential.

Frequent blood glucose monitoring or CGM is necessary to safely use a pump. The individual must be instructed to always check their blood glucose before giving insulin. Persons with diabetes need to be taught and reminded to carry rapidly absorbable carbohydrate at all times, to treat hypoglycemia if and when it occurs. Family, friends, and co-workers must be educated and trained to recognize hypoglycemia and administer glucagon via injection or nasal powder (Baqsimi) when appropriate.

Pump Initiation

Initiating pump therapy is almost exclusively done in an outpatient setting. Content for insulin pump therapy and follow-up should include:

- Initial Training. Most of the training on the technical aspects of using the new, improved pump systems can be accomplished in 1 or 2, 90- to 120-minute outpatient visits.[85] This training may be completed by the pump trainer or clinic diabetes care and education specialist.
- Best practice is to initiate CGM before the pump. This allows CGM data to be utilized for pump settings.
- Starting the pump with a "saline start" also allows people to increase comfort with button pushing and set changes, reducing the fear of making mistakes that lead to wide swings in glucose levels.[109]

- Resources and checklists for detailed training topics are available from the insulin pump manufacturers.
- www.medtronicdiabetes.com
- www.tandemdiabetes.com
- www.myomnipod.com

- Clinical Follow-Up.
- Clinical follow-up consists of having individuals continue CGM or monitor blood glucose levels 4 times a day (including 3 AM) and report results to the provider daily for the first few days via fax, email, portal, cloud, or phone. These visits should review blood glucoses, insulin doses, and carbohydrate amounts.

  Follow-up can be extended to once or twice a week after the first set change. When normal blood glucose levels are achieved, follow-up visits may be 1 to 2 months. The diabetes care and education specialist or provider providing dietary, pump dosing adjustment, and technical support may be scheduled in 3 months and as needed thereafter.[113, 114, 115]
- Medical Management Follow-Up. A follow-up visit for medical management of the diabetes is also scheduled in 2 to 4 weeks, and once the individual's condition is stable, visits are scheduled on a quarterly basis.
- Every Visit. At each visit, a healthcare professional should review hypoglycemia troubleshooting, hyperglycemia and ketoacidosis prevention, sick day management, site rotation, and all other self-care behaviors as needed. Downloading/uploading the pump data is critical for reviewing pump use. In addition to observing patterns, the pump data provides critical information on frequency of bolusing, over-correcting, entering "fake" carbs, overriding bolus recommendations, site changes, and confirming all settings. This information yields a true picture of how the pump is being used by the individual.

The Anti GAD 65 antibody is positive in approximately 80% of individuals with type 1 and latent autoimmune diabetes in adults (LADA). The test can be run alone to confirm a diagnosis.[116]

Case—Meet Max: T1DM

Max is a 20-year-old male who was admitted to the hospital in diabetic ketoacidosis (DKA). Three days prior to his admission, he was misdiagnosed with type 2 diabetes. His kidney, liver, and blood pressure results were within normal limits. Due to his classic clinical presentation of a 30-lb weight loss in 6 weeks, a hemoglobin A1C of 11%, polyuria, and polydipsia, an autoantibody panel was ordered. Max's results confirmed a diagnosis of type 1 diabetes.

Autoantibody Panel	*Reference Range*	*Result*
Insulin Autoantibody (mIAA) (draw prior to insulin therapy)	-0.2–0.010	0.019 (false positive because individual has been on insulin)
GADA	0.0–20 DK	45 DK
IA-2 Autoantibodies	0.0–5 DK	344 DK
ZNT8RW (Zinc) Antibodies	-0.2–0.02	0.012 Barbara Davis Center, Denver, CO

During Hospitalization

Max actively engaged in hands-on education with the certified diabetes care and education specialist nurse and registered dietitian at the hospital. As a college math major, he caught on very quickly to his diabetes daily routine. He verbalized understanding of blood glucose monitoring times, target goals, hypo- and hyperglycemia and mindful eating. Prior to discharge he was able to accurately count carbohydrates, calculate his insulin doses, and give himself injections via insulin pen. The hospital diabetes care and education specialist contacted Max's primary care provider to obtain a referral for comprehensive outpatient diabetes education.

Max's long-acting insulin dose was titrated during his hospital stay to achieve a fasting glucose between 80 to 130 mg/dL.

Rapid or regular insulin is necessary to cover carbohydrates at meals for persons with type 1 diabetes. To calculate an insulin to carbohydrate ratio (ICR), the individual's total daily insulin dose is divided into 450. This will determine how many grams of carbohydrate are covered by 1 unit of insulin. See Table 19.3.

Rapid or regular insulin may also be needed to correct or decrease an elevated glucose level. To determine the mg/dL that 1 unit of insulin decreases the blood glucose value, divide 1,700 by the total daily insulin dose. See Table 19.3 This is also known as the insulin sensitivity factor (ISF).

Hospital Discharge Orders

Long-acting insulin titrated to 28 units at bedtime

Rapid acting insulin to cover carbohydrates at meals 1 unit for every 10 g of carbohydrate

Rapid-acting insulin for correction before meals 1 unit for every 50 mg/dL >130 mg/dL

Check blood sugars before meals and at bedtime.

Initial Outpatient Visit

Max has been home from the hospital for 3 days. He was referred to the Advanced Practice Nurse (APN), CDCES for outpatient diabetes education and case management. At the start of the visit, he reports that his blood sugars have been "really high" in the morning. He notes that he is not eating in the middle of the night. Max's meter was downloaded for review (see below).

He has been taking all insulin doses as recommended and eating around 40 to 50 g of carbohydrate per meal. Glucose goals were determined by the provider at the hospital to be 80 to 130 mg/dL before meals.[1] The APN and Max agreed with these glucose goals and set safe bedtime goals as well (100-140 mg/dL). In addition, they discussed an A1C target of less than 7% without significant hypoglycemia.

Glucose Log Fasting and Premeal Target 80–130

Day	*Fasting*	*Before Lunch*	*Before Dinner*	*Before Bedtime*
Monday	197	118	120	115
Tuesday	201	128	125	120
Wednesday	226	123	130	118
Thursday	190			

A pattern of elevated fasting glucose was identified from the data. Other glucose values are in target. The APN completed a hypoglycemia assessment and reinforced signs and symptoms as well as treatment options for hypoglycemia. The APN also discussed the possibility of nocturnal hypoglycemia with rebound hyperglycemia and the need for Max to check some 3 AM blood sugars over the weekend.

He is highly motivated, engaged in his diabetes, and understands hypo- and hyperglycemia.

He is scheduled to start classes for comprehensive education next week.

A hypoglycemia assessment including symptoms, frequency, treatment, and prevention is important at every visit.

Dawn and Somogyi Phenomenon

Most commonly, a marked rise in blood glucose concentration from bedtime to dawn is a result of the "dawn phenomenon.[117,118] The hormonal basis for the dawn phenomenon is thought to be due mainly to overnight growth hormone (GH) secretion and cortisol and increased insulin clearance.[117]

Rarely, high morning glucose is due to the Somogyi phenomenon, a theoretical rebound from hypoglycemia late at night or in the early morning, which is thought to be due to an exaggerated counterregulatory response. The existence of this phenomenon is debated. It is unlikely to be a common cause, in that most individuals with diabetes remain hypoglycemic once nighttime glucose levels decline.[118]

Use of CGM may allow clarification of puzzlingly elevated morning glucose levels.

The APN requested that Max upload his blood sugars from his Bluetooth meter and contact her in 3 days to discuss.

Phone call check in Report

Day	*3AM*	*Treatment*	*15 Min Later*	*Fasting*	*Before Lunch*	*Before Dinner*	*Before Bedtime*
Friday	50	15 grams	88	85	100	106	116
Saturday	53	15 grams	90	108	118	125	120
Sunday	58	15 grams	98	115	128	119	115

The APN coached Max to decrease his long-acting insulin dose by 10%, from 28 units at bedtime down to 25 units at bedtime. Self-titration was discussed, and Max was comfortable with adjustments. He brought copies of his meter downloads to his education classes for review, and he has been doing well since the change.

When titrating insulin for an individual newly diagnosed and new to insulin, close follow-up is important.

Next Visit – 2 Months Later

Max presents to the clinic with a Hgb A1C of 7.2%. Since his last visit, he celebrated his 21st birthday and joined a type 1 diabetes community group. He has completed comprehensive education and attended 1:1 session with the certified diabetes care and education specialist in the clinic. He has mastered carbohydrate counting and adjusting insulin doses for his lifestyle. Today, he would like to discuss continuous glucose monitoring and insulin pump therapy. Max is educationally prepared to begin continuous glucose monitoring. He has adequate insurance coverage and stellar math and technology skills. The glucose transmitter and sensors were ordered. Max met with the CDCES nurse in the clinic for more specific training and insertion. He felt very comfortable with sensor startup, insertion, and changes.

Max has generated codes for the APN CDCES to view his CGM data online. According to the report, Max's sensor wear is 89% and he is in target 90% of the time. He has 0% very low glucose and 0.3% in the low range. See chapter 18 for CGM data interpretation.

When reviewing daily CGM profiles, the APN noticed a pattern of elevated glucose occurring on Saturday evenings. Max explained that since turning 21, he has been enjoying a couple of beers with his friends on Saturday nights.

Alcohol

Per ADA guidelines, men with adequate diabetes stability can have up to 2 drinks per day. The concern is drinking excess amounts. Alcohol in excess may cause blood glucose to spike at the time of consumption, but 5 to 6 hours later, the hypoglycemia effect of the alcohol is seen. While alcohol is being detoxified in the liver, the liver's ability to release glycogen stores to rescue a person from severe hypoglycemia is impaired.[1]

Max was coached to have a protein snack at bedtime if he is drinking. If he drinks in excess, he will have an alternate basal pattern with a reduction of 20% in the basal rate during the night.

Visit 3

Since his last visit, Max has gained 6 months experience and become an expert with MDI and adjustments. His

AGP from his sensor reports 98.5% sensor wear, 90.1% in target range, and 0% low and very low. His hemoglobin A1C is 6.4%.

Max is the ideal candidate for insulin pump therapy. He would like flexibility with his hectic work and school schedule, and he is highly motivated and engaged. He accurately counts and doses for carbohydrates and is able to problem solve. He understands how to switch from pump therapy back to MDI in case of a pump failure. After thoroughly reviewing tutorials and insulin pumps online, Max has selected the tubeless POD system for convenience. Features were discussed and confirmed. The APN completed a certificate of medical necessity (CMN) letter and ordered Max's POD and personal diabetes manager (PDM). Max completed all pump training for the POD with the certified pump trainer.

The APN calculated the appropriate doses to be programmed into the PDM. After the pump trainer walked Max through the PDM set-up and all settings were programmed, he inserted his first POD with the trainer. He was instructed to call with any issues. Max sent codes via email daily for the APN to upload and review his CGM data. He followed up with the APN 3 days later for his next change. The APN contacted Max via telephone 1 week later for follow-up. His AGP was reviewed. He continues to remain in target range >90% of the time with 0% low blood sugars.

When insulin pump rates and settings are evaluated and adjusted at follow-up visits, be sure the individual/caregiver enters the changes and the diabetes care and education specialist/provider confirms them during the visit. Information on adjusting basal rates is in Table 19.3.

Visit 4

Max has been on insulin pump therapy for 3 months. His hemoglobin A1C is 6.3%. He has noticed that eating pizza causes a delayed rise in his sugars that occasionally lasts into the next morning. The APN CDCES coached Max on the research of using his extended bolus feature to deliver 50% of the bolus at the start of the meal and the other 50% over an 8-hour period.[119] A demonstration of this was done in clinic.

The APN encouraged Max to continue to use his smartphone app resources and food library on his PDM for accurate carbohydrate counting, and to keep notes on certain foods when he sees spikes. She also discussed the effect of fiber and fat on glucose and experimenting with the extended bolus feature to achieve targets. Hypoglycemia signs, symptoms, and treatment were also reinforced.

Telephone call

Max has decided to start hiking with his friends after school on Wednesdays. He has asked the APN to review his Wednesday CGM reports.

Max is experiencing hypoglycemia during his hikes around 6 PM and 1 to 4 hours after exercise as well. The APN reviewed temporary basal rates with Max and walked through this with him over the phone. A reduction in basal 1 to 2 hours before, during, and after exercise was recommended. The APN reminded Max to check his blood sugars before driving. She also reminded him to show his friends how to use nasal glucagon in case of an emergency and to bring this along with fast-acting carbohydrates on his hikes.

Max's case is an example of the common progression and best practice of therapy intensification. Individuals with type 1 diabetes have to start on MDI due to endogenous insulin depletion, and often progress to glucose sensor and finally pump technology.

Individuals who are independent with self-management should be encouraged to experiment to achieve target glucose levels.

Fine-Tuning Basal and Bolus Ratios

- Basal and bolus doses are adjusted according to SMBG measurements taken fasting, before meals, 2 hours after meals, at bedtime, at midnight, and at 3 AM.
- The basal rate is increased or decreased by 0.1 or 10% unit per hour to keep the premeal and overnight blood glucose levels within a 50 mg glucose excursion from baseline. Newer pumps offer 0.005 unit per hour increments that may be ideal to fine-tune basal doses.
- If the glucose level raises more than 50 mg/dL (1.7 mmol/L) from the 3 AM measurement to the prebreakfast measurement, a second basal rate is added for 4 to 6 hours, starting 2 to 3 hours before the usual breakfast time. This basal rate may be 10% to 50% more than the first basal rate, although basal rate adjustments can vary from 10% to 100% depending on the rise in the glucose.[105]
- Testing the overnight basal rate requires the individual to eat an early meal and avoid snacking 3 to 4 hours before retiring for bed. SMBG measurements at midnight, 3 AM, 6 AM, and before breakfast can provide information to determine if further basal refinement is needed.

- Asking the individual to fast during a scheduled meal with frequent (hourly) SMBG measurements helps further fine-tune daytime basal rates. However, missing multiple meals changes basal insulin requirements and is not recommended.
- Adjusting bolus ratios depends on accuracy in carbohydrate counting and matching bolus insulin. The ideal method is for the individual to accurately measure carbohydrate for the selected mealtime and engage in the same activity for several days. The desired 2-hour postmeal rise of blood glucose is less than 50 mg/dL or ideally less than 140 to 180 mg/dL.
- ICRs can vary throughout the day. For example, a individual's ratio can be 1:10 at breakfast, 1:12 at lunch, and 1:8 at dinner.
- Pumps are equipped with varying bolus features. Carbohydrates are covered by a normal or standard bolus (delivered immediately). An extended, or square wave, bolus is delivered over a length of time chosen by the individual. A combination, or dual wave, bolus combines the normal and extended bolus. Type of bolus can vary based on the amount of carbohydrate or fat and gastric emptying; this is not readily measured and relies on individual experience.

Some pump manufacturers have software programs that allow a wealth of information about basal and bolus doses to be downloaded. Such information clearly shows the family and healthcare provider how the pump is being used at all times.

Special Situations

Hyperglycemia and Diabetic Ketoacidosis

Since pumps use rapid- or short-acting insulin, this puts persons with diabetes at greater risk for development of DKA, if more than a few hours interruption of insulin infusion occurs. Elevated blood glucoses can occur for numerous reasons, including infection, illness, stress, menstrual cycle, pump battery failure, infusion set or catheter occlusion, leaking connection, inadequate or missed meal bolus, or poor absorption of insulin from site.[79] Individual education about how to detect and treat high blood glucose is key in preventing DKA.[84] Persons with diabetes should be instructed to check urine ketones with unexplained hyperglycemia or if experiencing nausea or flu-like symptoms. When hyperglycemia is present, the checklist in Table 19.4 will quickly review possible explanations and assist with responding promptly to correct the problems.[79,]

TABLE 19.4 Problem Solving: Possible Causes for Hyperglycemia With Insulin Pump Therapy[76]
Red, tender, and swollen catheter site
Leakage, breakage, or kinking of tubing
Battery failure
Empty reservoir or cartridge
Improper positioning of reservoir or piston rod
Improper basal rate programming
Air in tubing
Illness
Menstrual cycle fluctuations
Omitted bolus or improper amount given
Ineffective insulin (expired date, exposure to heat or cold)
Crimped catheter or needle not penetrating skin
Change in usual routine
Suspect site not absorbing if no other apparent reason for high blood glucose
BEWARE! Any of these can occur even though the site was recently changed.

Source: D Tomky, Diabetes Technologies. In: *Complete Nurses Guide to Diabetes Care*. AB Childs, M Cypress, G Spollett, eds. (Alexandria, Va: American Diabetes Association, 2017) 430.

Individuals using CSII need to be taught *5 important steps* for detecting, treating, and preventing DKA. If blood glucose levels remain elevated after a correction dose is given, the individual should follow these steps:[99]

1. Check urine or blood for ketones.
   —If positive, give supplemental insulin with a conventional insulin syringe.
   —If negative ketones but blood glucose continues to be elevated, check for pump malfunction.
2. Correct known problems immediately.
3. Change the site, using a new reservoir or cartridge, infusion set, and catheter. Check glucose in 1 hour, if not beginning to come down, switch to MDI.
4. Contact the healthcare provider if unable to resolve problems within 2 to 3 hours or if nausea, vomiting, heavy deep breathing, Kussmaul respirations.

Always encourage hydration with sugar-free fluids, have persons with diabetes repeat BG in 2 to 3 hours. If glucose remains over 250 mg/dl consider continuing an increased temporary basal rate.

The individual should have back-up supplies, including ketone strips, batteries, infusion sets, rapid and long-acting insulin vials and/or pens, syringes, or pen needles, and copy of current pump setting—these should always be available.

If the pump malfunctions, the person with diabetes may need to return to MDI until the pump can be replaced (contact pump manufacturer immediately to facilitate timely replacement).

Evidence shows that with proper education and attention to details, the frequency of ketoacidosis is less on insulin pump therapy as injection therapy.[62] Problem-solving skills should be in place prior to initiating pump therapy, including knowing when and how to correct high blood glucoses. Supplemental insulin can now be preprogrammed within the pump to accurately adjust doses of insulin. The correction bolus or insulin sensitivity factor is derived from the previously discussed formula. Individuals still are required to check capillary blood glucoses for direct entry from the meter to the pump or input of the result into the pump by the individual. Pumps track active insulin which helps prevent the individual from frequently bolusing to correct elevated blood glucose. Catheter occlusion or pump malfunction is often responsible for elevated glucose if illness is not present. Urine/plasma ketone prescriptions are essential supplies for those on insulin pumps.

The diabetes care education specialist should always inspect the individual's subcutaneous tissue during follow-up visits to check for lipohypertrophy and poor absorption.

Problem Solving for Sick Days

In the event that someone is ill and not eating, the body still requires insulin to counteract increases in glucose and ketone production by the liver due to increased secretion of stress hormones (cortisol, glucagon, growth hormone, epinephrine/norepinephrine).

Never suspend insulin delivery or disconnect a pump when a person with diabetes is ill. Being ill can put individuals at risk for developing DKA; therefore, it is very important to advise individuals to check for ketones and monitor blood sugar every 2 to 4 hours around-the-clock, even if the blood sugar is in normal range.

Temporary basal rate increases are particularly useful in treating hyperglycemia due to intercurrent illness or use of steroids. During these times, individuals often need reminding to maintain adequate fluid intake with salted broth, water, or noncaloric beverages. If liquid carbohydrates are used for fluid replacement, appropriate boluses must be given. Often, bolus ratios need to be temporarily increased, as does the basal rate until the condition is resolved. When blood glucoses are within target range, and nausea and ketones are present, the individual needs to sip on carbohydrate-containing beverages and give appropriate boluses based on ICR to eliminate ketones.[79] Gradually start liquids (sugar free if blood sugar >150, with sugar if <150); begin with 1 tablespoon every few minutes. Persons with diabetes are often reluctant to use additional carbohydrates in this situation, but to reverse ketosis both insulin and carbohydrates are necessary.

Moderate and/or large ketones, persistent nausea, low blood sugar with nausea and/or vomiting, and any signs or symptoms of DKA such as abdominal pain, chest pain, altered consciousness, deep breathing; Kussmaul respirations, require emergency treatment.[13,79]

Insulin Stacking

Most people want to see their glucose level in their target range quickly; they may not wait long enough for the insulin to work before taking additional injections or corrections. The effect of the insulins overlap is a phenomenon referred to as *stacking*. When persons with diabetes are having extreme highs and lows, frequency of corrections, entering fake carbs, or overrides should be investigated. This may be contributing to insulin stacking.

Diabetes care and education specialists should anticipate insulin stacking and caution persons with diabetes to be patient and let the insulin work for several hours to avoid frequent repeated bolus/injections that overcorrect glucose levels that often result in hypoglycemia.

Hospitalization

The American Diabetes Association (ADA), the Association of Diabetes Care and Education Specialists (ADCES), and the American Association of Clinical Endocrinologists (AACE) advocate allowing persons with diabetes who are physically and mentally able to continue to use their insulin pumps when hospitalized. Policies and procedures must be in place to allow the PWD to continue to utilize CSII treatment. This will maximize safety and document self-management of medications.[1,121–127]

In persons with diabetes who continued pump use during hospitalization, several studies document significantly fewer episodes of severe hyperglycemia (glucose >350 mg/dl) and hypoglycemia (glucose <40 mg/dl) or no difference in frequency of hupo- or hyper glycemia.[125]

However, hypoglycemia accounts for more hospitalizations than hyperglycemia.[127]

Reasons for not continuing the insulin pump while in the hospital would include;

- Impaired level of consciousness
- Critical illness requiring intensive care
- Psychiatric illness that interferes with an individual's ability to self-manage diabetes or risk of suicide
- DKA or hyperosmolar hyperglycemic state (HHS)
- Refusal or unwillingness to participate in self-care
- Lack of pump supplies
- Lack of trained healthcare providers and diabetes care education specialists[125]

If the person with diabetes is well managed on insulin pump therapy, then basal rates should be adequate to maintain euglycemia during surgery of less than 2 hours.[121,122] Recommendations for glycemic goals during hospitalization are fasting/premeal <140 mg/dl and random glucose <180 mg/dl[1]. Monitoring glucose every 30 to 60 minutes will indicate when basal settings should be adjusted.

BG <100 mg/dl	Hold basal infusion rate
BG 101-140 mg/dl	Decrease basal rate by 25%
BG 141-180 mg/dl	Maintain basal rate
BG 181-220 mg/dl	Increase basal rate by 25%
BG >220 mg/dl	Increase basal rate by 25% to 50% and 2 to 4 u bolus correction 128

If the pump is to be worn during surgery, the individual must be instructed to insert a new catheter 12 to 24 hours in advance to establish adequate infusion of insulin. The catheter should be inserted in a site away from the planned surgical field and the tubing or pod secured with additional tape. Persons with diabetes should be prepared to provide their own pump supplies during their stay.

When transitioning to IV insulin do not stop the pump until IV insulin is initiated. When transitioning to long-acting basal insulin, initiate basal insulin 1 to 2 hours before stopping the pump.

Site Changes

Pumps remind wearers of routine site changes and indeed some force site change. One way to help persons with diabetes remember site change every 48 to 72 hours is to advise them to initiate their pump setting that reminds them to change their pump site. Older pumps without this feature may require smartphone reminders or hang a calendar in the bathroom to mark site-change days. Individuals should also be advised to avoid overfilling the pump cartridge or reservoir; this prevents the individual from wearing the pump until it literally runs out of insulin.

Infection at the site may occur if the site use is extended. Filling the reservoir without changing the site may save supplies but increase the risk of infection at the site.

Quality of Life

Pump use has demonstrated improvement in diabetes management, reduction in severe hypoglycemia, and improvement in quality of life for adults and children with T1DM and T2DM.[129–133] CGM data also supports improvement in quality of life measures related to diabetes, ie, diabetes distress and hypoglycemia fear in T1DM.[134,135]

Persons with diabetes who have switched from MDI to CSII have shown that when there are reductions in A1C and hypoglycemia, individuals generally report increased treatment satisfaction and improved quality of life.[131] Regardless of screening appropriately, the desire to discontinue CSII may occur. Individuals do "burn out" with chronic illness and need to be frequently assessed for depression or coping difficulty with self-care behaviors. If CSII adds to the individual's distress level or unhealthy coping puts the individual at risk for acute complications, then providing a temporary holiday from the pump may be warranted. After a year or 2 some individuals on pumps have deteriorating glycemic stability and require a "refresher course" and reevaluation of goals.

Switching Back to Injection Therapy

There are many reasons a person may need to "switch" back to injection therapy. Pump failure, lack of supplies, behavioral/suicidal issues all may necessitate managing diabetes with injections. The easiest way to switch back to injections from CSII is by converting the pump's total daily basal rate to a long-acting basal insulin such as glargine (Lantus®) or levemir (detemir) and adding 10%.[113,114,79] These insulins do not require 3 to 4 days to reach steady state as the ultra-long basal insulins do. With the use of glargine or levemir, mealtime injections of rapid-acting insulin can be given at the pump premeal bolus rates by syringe or pen. Correction doses are continued as set in the pump; if no long-acting insulin is immediately available, a rapid-acting insulin will need to be taken every 2 to 3 hours. Make the calculation based on the basal rate. For example: if off the pump for 2 hours × if 1.0 unit per hour basal rate = 2 u should be given to cover the time disconnected.

If the pump fails and the individual has to give insulin by injection, be sure to provide basal insulin coverage with long-acting insulin 1 to 2 times/day or rapid-acting insulin every 3 to 4 hours.

Always carry a syringe or insulin pen

Reducing Risks

Pregnancy

Pump therapy is an effective means of managing diabetes during pregnancy. Maternal A1C levels are better with pumps than MDI, but outcomes are comparable. Pregnant individuals using CSII, as a group, achieve comparable stability to those using MDI.[136–140] Continuous subcutaneous insulin infusion is a viable option for motivated and capable individuals who fail to achieve optimal levels with MDI. Keep in mind that the potential risk of DKA with interrupted insulin flow is not tolerated in pregnancy and must be carefully considered before starting this kind of therapy in a woman with type 1 diabetes. Several studies concluded that fetal prognosis is not overall significantly different with an insulin pump compared with intensified conventional therapy. Higher birth weight, neonatal hypoglycemia, and maternal hypertension have been documented with pump therapy.[138] The benefit-to-risk ratio of CSII must be assessed and result in a tailored prescription that is based on individual needs. Preferably, this option is discussed before conception, as planned pregnancy is a main prognostic factor. Diabetes duration and complications remain key factors for the prognosis for best pregnancy outcomes.

Absolute requirements for CSII therapy to be successful in pregnancy are education, motivation by an experienced team, and preconception counseling.[136–140]

Gastric Motility Gastroparesis occurs when gastric motility is slowed from autonomic neuropathy, medications such as tricyclic antidepressants, opioids, anticholinergics, or pramlintide, or high-fat meals. Rapid-acting insulin is often mismatched with food digestion. Human insulin by injection, given just before the meal may more closely mirror the postmeal glycemic rise. With this insulin given at the time of eating, the 30-minute onset and peak action at around 2 to 3 hours may allow for glucose absorption from the gut to occur. Alternatively, rapid acting insulin injected *after* the meal is another approach to "delay" the insulin to try to account for delayed emptying. With pump therapy, using an extended bolus or combination bolus allows for a slower delivery of rapid-acting insulin that can more closely match reduced gastric motility.

Even more specific insulin administration might be possible with pump therapy. With glucose sensors with low glucose alerts and low glucose suspend safety is improved. People with autonomic neuropathy may also experience hypoglycemic unawareness. Therefore, being able to suspend insulin or initiate a temporary basal may prevent severe hypoglycemia.[141]

Often pump wearers notice high-fat meals, ie, pizza, cause problems with blood glucoses, usually resulting in an elevated fasting glucose. Jones et al's research evaluated insulin pump dosing and postprandial glycemia following a pizza meal using the continuous glucose monitoring system. Their results showed that using a 50% immediate release and 50% extended release bolus delivered over an 8-hour period following a pizza meal provided significantly less postprandial hyperglycemia in the late postprandial period (8-12 hours) with no increased risk of hypoglycemia.[119]

Travel Traveling is not as cumbersome for people with diabetes as it once was. However, it is important for the person with diabetes to familiarize themselves with the Transportation Security Associations and Federal Aviation Administration guidelines.

Travel through times zones is a challenge for individuals on insulin, whether MDI or pump users. The insulin pump clock may need to be changed. Adjust the pump clock to the arrival time zone when reaching your destination. Nighttime basal rates may need to be adjusted based on when the person will be sleeping. Travel on the lowest basal rate to prevent hypoglycemia. Correction doses can be given if needed. Persons with diabetes should try to keep their basal injections on their home time. So, if they are taking lantus or Levemir in the evening, it may be taken in the morning, if they are crossing multiple time zones. Likewise, Toujeo or Tresiba if taken in the morning could be taken in the evening to be similar to what they were doing at home.

Mealtime bolus or injections can be moved to match the meals regardless of the time zones.

If travel includes increased exercise and walking, proactively reduce basal settings by 10% to 20%. Increased exercise improves insulin sensitivity and so bolus doses may need to be adjusted as well.

When packing supplies, bring 2 times more pump supplies and insulin than usual for the length of time traveling. Be sure to have long-acting insulin and syringes or pens. Pack all supplies in carry-on luggage. While insulin is stable out of the refrigerator for at least 30 days, do not

TABLE 19.5 Emergency Pump Supplies
Glucose meter and monitoring supplies including back-up battery and control solution
Ketone test strips (preferably individually foil-wrapped)
Pump supplies: insulin, reservoirs, infusion sets, batteries, site preparation supplies
Back-up insulin syringe or pen with needles
Carbohydrates to treat hypoglycemia and glucagon emergency kit in case of severe hypoglycemia
Written record of basal rates and an alternative insulin injection regimen if pump fails
Emergency contact numbers for pump manufacturer, physician, diabetes care and education specialist, and family member to contact in an emergency

allow supplies/insulin to get too hot (over 86 degrees) or freeze.

The pump and sensors (whether they are being worn or are extra supplies) *should not* go through the X-ray machines or full-body scanners. Metal detectors will likely not disrupt pump functioning. Even though pumps are expected to function during air travel, some have airplane mode.[13] See Table 19.5 to review a list of emergency pump supplies.

Special Populations Using Pump Therapy

Older Adults

In older subjects with insulin-treated type 2 diabetes, both CSII and MDI achieved excellent glycemic stability with good safety and individual satisfaction.[113,114] Pump therapy in older adults may be more efficacious, safe, and useful (Lepore)[143,71] When paired with a glucose sensor, it offers safety features regarding hypoglycemia mitigation, siren alarms for treating hypoglycemia, and low glucose suspend. Hypoglycemia contributes to more hospitalization costs than hyperglycemia.[127] Hypoglycemia is of particular concern for seniors. Conversely, ensuring continuous insulin delivery may preclude extreme hyperglycemia, requiring emergent treatment.

All previously discussed screening criteria would apply to any selected population. Goals of therapy should, as usual, be individualized, eg, addressing the individual's living situation, family caregiver support, and comorbid conditions. If individuals are overwhelmed with operating the pump, changing sites or converting to MDI when needed, they may not be candidates for this technology. All persons with diabetes, type 1 or 2, requesting benefits from Medicare for pump therapy must prove to be insulinopenic by requesting verification of complete absence of insulin production, C-Peptide <10%.[52,142] Private insurance coverage varies from plan to plan.

Type 2 Diabetes

Experience with insulin pump therapy in persons with type 2 diabetes is growing and encouraging.[134,135,144–150] Investigators have confirmed the benefits of pump therapy for type 2 diabetes with similar clinical indicators issues as those with T1DM.[62,134,135,144–147] Differences in the pathophysiology of type 1 and type 2 diabetes affect pump selection. Certain features better suit the needs of those with type 2 diabetes. People with type 2 diabetes often have higher insulin needs due to insulin resistance, so reservoir capacity and frequency for refilling it are a concern. Concentrated insulins (Humulin R U500 and Lispro U200) utilized in pumps, while off label, help address this issue. Other key concerns for the persons with type 2 diabetes, as compared to those with type 1, are needs for a higher basal rate, larger premeal boluses, and battery life.[147,79]

In general, adult candidates are individuals searching for a more flexible treatment plan who are unable to achieve optimal stability with injection regimens, either related to unpredictable and varying schedules and activity levels or who have noted limitations in management when using multiple daily injections.

Specific candidates are individuals who, despite frequent blood sugar monitoring and consistent and appropriate insulin administration, may have absolute insulin deficiency, frequent hypoglycemia, or hypoglycemia unawareness or experience erratic glucose swings.

Pediatric Population

Current evidence indicates CSII is safe and an effective method of insulin delivery in young children, especially those with highly motivated parents.[111,134,135,144–153] Observational studies, registry data, and meta-analysis suggest glycemic management is improved with CSII.[111,152–153] Reduction in hypoglycemia, DKA risk, complications, ie, retinopathy and peripheral neuropathy, and improved treatment satisfaction and quality of life compared to MDI make CSII safe and effective in children with T1 diabetes.[155–158] For children under 7, pump therapy is often preferred.[159,62] Table 19.6 indicates starting pediatric dosing calculations.

Not surprisingly, when it is important to be like everyone else, wearing a pump is sometimes a barrier for children

TABLE 19.6 Starting Pediatric Dosing Calculations*

Basal and Bolus Calculations for Pediatric Population
1. Determine how much insulin to use in the pump by averaging the total units of insulin used per day for 2 weeks. Decrease by 20% for hypoglycemia, by 10% for euglycemia, and make no reduction for hyperglycemia for children.
2. Divide the total dosage in half: 50% for basal and 50% bolus.
3. Divide the portion for bolus by 3. Divide the portion for basal by 24 to determine the hourly basal rate.
4. Check midnight and 3 AM blood glucose levels for 2 weeks before pump placement for evidence of night or early-morning abnormalities of glycemia. For hypoglycemia, reduce the nighttime basal rate by 10%. For hyperglycemia, increase the 3 AM by 10%.
5. Determine the insulin:carb ratio. (Divide 450 or 500 rule by the total units per day to determine the number of grams of carbohydrate for 1 unit of insulin.)
6. Determine the correction dose for elevated glucose levels. (Divide *1,700 the total units of insulin per day to determine the mg/dL that 1 unit of insulin decreases the blood glucose value.) *Range to use varies from 1,600–2,200[197,198]

*Children's Hospital Los Angeles methods (Kaufman et al, 2001.)

Sources: M Phillip, T Battelino, H Rodriguez, T Danne, K Kaufman for the Consensus forum participants, "Use of insulin pump therapy in the pediatric age group: consensus statement from the European Society for Paediatric Endocrinology, the Lawson Wilkins Pediatric Endocrine Society, and the International Society for Pediatric and Adolescent Diabetes, endorsed by the American Diabetes Association and the European Association for the Study of Diabetes," *Diabetes Care*. 30(2007):1653-62.

G Scheiner, R Sobel, DE Smith, et al, "Insulin pump therapy: guidelines for successful outcomes," *Diabetes Educa.* 35(2009):29S-41S.

BW Bode, WV Tamborlane, PC Davidson, "Insulin pump therapy in the 21st century," *Postgrad Med.* 11(5)(2002):69-78.

FR Kaufman, M Halvorson, S Carpenter, et al, "Pump therapy for children: weighing the risks and benefits: view 2: insulin pump therapy in young children with diabetes," *Diabetes Spectrum*. 14(2)(2001):84-89.

and adolescents. The potential interference with activities and sports and physical discomfort also provide resistance from young people. As with other populations, pediatric populations should have appropriate child/parent selection criteria. Standardized methodology and protocols for initiating, following, and supporting children with diabetes and their families are important. This requires expert staff sufficient to be on call, to provide ongoing teaching and support.

Diabetes care and education specialists and providers need to develop non-judgmental assessments of adolescents for potential insulin omission for weight control.

Summary

Intensifying therapy by utilizing pattern management and technology provides a systematic approach to diabetes clinical management. Intensification of therapy begins with lifestyle coaching, maximizing metformin, adding other oral or injectable medications to treat the glucose patterns identified. Intensive insulin therapy, whether achieved through MDI or CSII therapy, can be a safe and effective therapeutic tool. The diabetes provider and diabetes care and education specialist have an opportunity and some would say responsibility to facilitate behavior change and inspire motivation in capable individuals with diabetes. Selection of appropriate candidates and helping fine-tune their skills is one of the most important factors in determining whether an individual will be successful. Extensive preparation through self-management training can reduce discontinuation rates.

Pump preparation for potential candidates must include their ability to follow an intensive regimen of blood glucose monitoring or use of CGM, MDI, carbohydrate/calorie counting, and problem solving before being considered for insulin pump therapy. The training and ongoing support by an experienced pump team is critical to achieving desired learning, behavioral, and clinical outcomes. Diabetes care and education specialists today must lead the way with technology adoption and training of persons with diabetes and peers.

Focus on Education

Teaching Strategies

Using the AADE7 Self-Care Behaviors® provides a conceptual framework for assessing and applying interventions related to use of insulin pump therapy.

Successful intensive insulin therapy. Preparation is the key. The professional skills required are in-depth knowledge of blood sugar interpretation (patterns), pump equipment and functions, the calculation and use of correction factors, onboard insulin, and carbohydrate counting. Discussion, demonstration, and role-playing strategies enhance the individual's understanding. Wearing a pump for several days, or using saline injections, and testing blood sugars with meal and activity plans in mind is useful to "get a feel" for the demands of this regimen.

Candidate screening and selection. Advance review and assessment of potential candidates (using Table 20.9) during educational events and clinic visits, problem-solving using MDI, follow-up visits, and phone interventions offer opportunities for teaching. This sets up experiential learning and practice time. Establishing the time and personal commitment to intensive therapy as a part of clinical, educational practice is critical.

Real-time continuous glucose monitoring enables insulin pump therapy wearers to review trends and patterns.

Teaching pattern management skills in reviewing glucose results is critical to success. Implementing CGM for safety requires consistent wearing of the device on a daily basis. Strategies for adjustments are similar to other pattern management skills. The challenge to date has been getting the data organized for systematic review.

Do one thing at a time. Don't overwhelm persons with diabetes with too many changes at once.

Use teaching materials that allow the individuals to calculate and figure out the process of adjusting his/her therapy. You can provide immediate feedback and evaluate comprehension.

Use technology, devices and therapy that eventually will not only improve the person with diabetes' metabolic stability but their satisfaction with daily care. Individuals often know what they want, but not what it takes to get there. Understanding cost-benefits before making changes to therapy impacts starting and continuing therapy.

Pattern management needs to be carefully reviewed. Evaluate its relationship to food, activity, stress, and finally medication. Shared decision-making helps move ownership of diabetes to the person with diabetes.

Intensifying therapy and dose adjusting is based on patterns in blood glucose. Dosing includes scheduled dosing and supplemental adjustments for special situations.

Evaluate prerequisite skills and experiences. The following are needed before considering pump therapy: frequent blood glucose monitoring and record keeping or CGM, experience and skill with MDI, carbohydrate counting, calculating bolus insulin, problem solving through interpretation of blood glucose pattern, adjusting insulin for special situations, problem solving for hypoglycemia, and hyperglycemia prevention and treatment.

Review the clinical indications for insulin pump therapy, blood glucose monitoring, intensive medication/insulin therapy, carbohydrate counting, and other elements of intensifying therapy. The position statements by ADCES and ADA include specific indications for practice. Stay updated with the revisions.

Messages for Persons With Diabetes

Benefits and risks. Take time to investigate all the facts about the benefits, risk, and limitations of intensifying insulin, whether considering a new intensive insulin treatment plan using multiple daily injection or an insulin infusion pump. Read information and ask questions. Think about what signs and symptoms to look for if the blood sugar patterns are not at target. Persons using intensive therapy need to be able to recognize, treat, and prevent very low or elevated blood glucose.

Realistic expectations. Recognize that this approach may require new skills, more intense observation of food intake and activity expenditure, and medication adjustments. Accepting the self-care and informed decision making that are needed with this therapy could be new and a bit overwhelming. Plan to experiment and discuss options with others, including the healthcare team.

Problem solving. Advancing diabetes care strategies require that the individual pay close attention to his or her blood glucose trends and adjusting insulin accordingly. Initially, the individual might need to create a very controlled environment with minimal variations. Once the individual learns how to achieve optimal blood glucose levels under regular circumstances, he or she will be able to adjust it to different situations. The person with diabetes must learn how to manage his or her blood glucose levels in order to manipulate the therapy to meet his or her lifestyle needs.

Health Literacy and Gaining Commitment

Health literacy refers to the ability to read and understand written information, the ability to process numbers (numeracy), and the ability to navigate the healthcare system. It is not enough to just provide information. Make sure the person with diabetes actually knows what to do with it. Create a follow-up mechanism where you can review the therapy, what is working well versus what is not working as desired. This will allow you to provide an immediate feedback, troubleshoot, and advance treatment accordingly. Ask the person with diabetes: "What is the most difficult thing for you . . .?," "What do you think needs to be done to make it work better?" Many times, individuals know the solutions to their problems but need the diabetes care and education specialist to confirm that they are accurate or right about their strategy.

Evaluate the individual's comprehension by asking them to "teach back" to you. Ask, "What are you going to do when X happens . . .?" or "What would you do differently in response to. . . ." or "Why do you think it is important for you to do this . . .?"

Most individuals forget up to 80% of what their clinician tells them as soon as they leave the office, and nearly 50% of what they do remember is recalled incorrectly.[151] Allow individuals to explain to you how they will perform each task and how they will apply the information learned to real daily events. Record the ideas for an easy and practical reference. Simple handouts are customized to each individual and can be easily accessed for reference.

The process of learning brings together cognitive, emotional, and environmental influences for acquiring knowledge, skills, and values.[152] People often can verbalize what needs to be done and how they can do it. However, they also need to be able to actually do it. Assess their confidence, readiness, and ability to do specific tasks. You can use scaling to quantify the progress: "On a scale of 1 to 10, with 1 as not ready and 10 as ready, how ready/willing/able are you to do . . .?"

Focus on Practice

Providers/diabetes care and education specialists need to discuss discipline-specific guidelines/state scope of practice with their medical director(s) or diabetes team. Identify what the expectations are and who is responsible for what part of care.

The multidisciplinary approach. Pattern management and corresponding therapy advancement requires a team of skilled diabetes care professionals who know the devices, medications/insulin symptom management, and clinical care necessary to manage their specific population of persons with diabetes. The system designed to provide intensive diabetes management therapy needs to support individuals 24 hours a day, 7 days a week. Individuals need to know where and how to get the support when they need it when they need it.

Continue to advance your knowledge and skills. Intensifying therapy for persons with diabetes means intensifying your skills and knowledge as well. In addition to formal learning, learn from persons with diabetes. They will teach you what it really takes to implement the recommended therapy.

References

1. American Diabetes Association. Standards of medical care in diabetes, 2019. Diabetes Care. 2019;42(Suppl 1).
2. Garber AJ, Abrahamson MJ, Barzilay JI, et al. Consensus statement by the American Association of Clinical Endocrinologists and American College of Endocrinology on the comprehensive type 2 diabetes management algorithm—2019 executive summary. Endocr Pract: Off J Am Coll Endocr Am Assoc Clin Endocrinologists. 25(1):69.
3. van Bruggen R, Gorter K, Stolk R, Klungel O, Rutten G. Clinical inertia in general practice: widespread and related to the outcome of diabetes care. Fam Pract. 2009;26(6):428-36. doi:10.1093/fampra/cmp053.
4. Scheen AJ. New therapeutic approaches in type 2 diabetes. Acta Clinica Belgica. 2008;63(6):402-7. doi:10.1179/acb.2008.083.
5. Joy SV. Clinical pearls and strategies to optimize patient outcomes. Diabetes Educ. 2008;34(3_suppl):54S-59S. doi:10.1177/0145721708319233.
6. Trujillo JM, Barsky EE, Greenwood BC, et al. Improving glycemic control in medical inpatients: A pilot study. J Hosp Med. 2008;3(1):55-63. doi:10.1002/jhm.263.
7. Boyle PJ, Zrebiec J. Impact of therapeutic advances on hypoglycaemia in type 2 diabetes. Diabetes/Metab Res Rev. 2008:24(4):257-85. doi:10.1002/dmrr.795.
8. Okemah J, Peng J, Quiñones M. Addressing clinical inertia in type 2 diabetes mellitus: a review. Adv Ther. 2018;35(11):1735-45.
9. Khunti K, Gomes MB, Pocock S, et al. Therapeutic inertia in the treatment of hyperglycaemia in patients with

type 2 diabetes: a systematic review. Diabetes Obes Metab. 2018;20(2):427-37. doi:10.1111/dom.13088

10. Beck J, Greenwood DA, Blanton L, et al. 2017 national standards for diabetes self-management education and support. Diabetes Educ. 2019;45(1):34-49. doi:10.1177/0145721718820941.

11. Tomky D. Deciphering the blood glucose puzzle with pattern management skills. In: Weinger K, Carver C, eds. Educating Your Patient With Diabetes. New York, NY: Humana Press; 2009.

12. American Association of Diabetes Educators. AADE guidelines for the practice of diabetes self-management education and training (DSME/T). Diabetes Educator. 2009;35(3 suppl): 85S-107S. doi:10.1177/0145721709352436.

13. Hinnen D, Guthrie DR. Self-management practices: problem solving. In: Childs B, ed. Complete Nurse's Guide to Diabetes Care. American Diabetes Association; 2017:109-31.

14. Hinnen D, Childs B, Guthrie DW, et al. Combating clinical inertia with pattern management. In: Mensing C, ed. The Art and Science of Diabetes Self-Management Education: A Desk Reference for Healthcare Professionals. 1st ed. Chicago, IL: American Association of Diabetes Education; 2006.

15. Bergenstal RM, Gavin JR; Global Consensus Conference on Glucose Monitoring Panel. The role of self-monitoring of blood glucose in the care of people with diabetes: Report of a global consensus conference. Am J Med. 2005;118(9):1-6. doi:10.1016/j.amjmed.2005.07.055

16. Polonsky WH, Fisher L, Schikman CH, et al. Structured self-monitoring of blood glucose significantly reduces A1C levels in poorly controlled, noninsulin-treated type 2 diabetes: Results from the structured testing program study. Diabetes Care. 2011;34(2):262-7. doi:10.2337/dc10-1732.

17. Polonsky W, Fisher L, Schikman C, et al. The value of episodic, intensive blood glucose monitoring in non-insulin treated persons with type 2 diabetes: design of the structured testing program (STeP) study, a cluster-randomised, clinical trial [NCT00674986]. BMC Family Pract. 2010;11(1):11-37. doi:10.1186/1471-2296-11-37.

18. Fisher L, Polonsky WH, Parkin CG, Jelsovsky Z, Petersen B, Wagner RS. The impact of structured blood glucose testing on attitudes toward self-management among poorly controlled, insulin-naïve patients with type 2 diabetes. Diabetes Res Clin Pract. 2011;2012;96(2):149-55. doi:10.1016/j.diabres.2011.12.016.

19. International Diabetes Federation, 2009. http://www.idf.org/idf-guideline-self-monitoring-blood glucose-non-insulin-treated-type-2-diabetes.

20. Pelimanni E, Jehkonen M. Type 2 diabetes and cognitive functions in middle age: A meta-analysis. J Int Neuropsychol Soc.: JINS. 2018;2019;25(2):1-229. doi:10.1017/S1355617718001042.

21. Mann B, Ycaza Singh S, Dabas R, Davoudi D, Osvath J. Evaluation of effects of health literacy, numeracy skills, and English proficiency on health outcomes in the population of people with diabetes. Clin Diabetes. 2019;37(2):172-5. https://doi.org/10.2337/cd18-0068.

22. Association of Diabetes Care and Education Specialists (ADCES). An effective model of diabetes care and education: revising the AADE7 self-care behaviors®. Published online ahead of print, Feb 2020. Diabetes Educ. doi: https://doi.org/10.1177/0145721719894903.

23. American Diabetes Association. Children and adolescents: Standards of medical care in diabetes—2019. Diabetes Care. 2019;42(1):S148.

24. Kirkman MS, Briscoe VJ, Clark N, et al. Diabetes in older adults. Diabetes Care. 2012;35(12):2650-64. doi:10.2337/dc12-1801.

25. O'Hara MC, Hynes L, O'Donnell M, et al; The Irish Type 1 Diabetes Young Adult Study Group. A systematic review of interventions to improve outcomes for young adults with type 1 diabetes. Diabetic Med. 2017;34(6):753-69. doi:10.1111/dme.13276.

26. Lipska KJ, Warton EM, Huang ES, et al. HbA1c and risk of severe hypoglycemia in type 2 diabetes: The diabetes and aging study. Diabetes Care. 2013;36(11):3535-42. doi:10.2337/dc13-0610.

27. MMIT Formulary Look Up Tool. https://www.formularylookup.com/. Accessed Aug. 30, 2019.

28. Adapted from DeFronzo RA. Diabetes. 2009;58(4):773-95.

29. 2019 American Geriatrics Society Beers Criteria® Update Expert Panel. American geriatrics society 2019 updated AGS beers criteria® for potentially inappropriate medication use in older adults: 2019 AGS BEERS CRITERIA® UPDATE EXPERT PANEL. J Am Geriatr Soc. 2019;67(4):674-94. doi:10.1111/jgs.15767.

30. Gallwitz B. Implications of postprandial glucose and weight control in people with type 2 diabetes: understanding and implementing the international diabetes federation guidelines. Diabetes Care. 2009;32 Suppl 2(11):S322-5. doi:10.2337/dc09-S331.

31. Austin MM, Haas L, Johnson T. Self-monitoring of blood glucose: benefits and utilization. Diabetes Educ. 2006;32(6): 835-37.

32. International Diabetes Federation. IDF Clinical Guidelines Task Force: Global guideline for type 2 diabetes. Brussels, Belgium: International Diabetes Federation: 2006.

33. Farmer AJ, Wade AN, French DP, et al.; DiGEM Trial Group. Blood glucose self-monitoring in type 2 diabetes: a randomised controlled trial. Health Technol Assess (Winchester, England). 2009;13(15):iii-iv. doi:10.3310/hta13150.

34. Davidson MB, Castellanos M, Kain D, et al. The effect of self-monitoring of blood glucose concentration on glycated hemoglobin levels in diabetic patient not taking insulin: a blinded, randomized trial. Am J Med. 2005;118(4):422-5.

35. International Diabetes Federation, International SMBG working Group. Self-monitoring of blood glucose in diabetes:

appraisal of available data and defining perspectives. Brussels, Belgium: International Diabetes Federation; 2008.

36. Klonoff DC, Blonde L, Cembrowski G, et al.; Coalition for Clinical Research-Self-Monitoring of Blood Glucose Scientific Board. Consensus report: the current role of self-monitoring of blood glucose in non-insulin-treated type 2 diabetes. J Diabetes Sci Technol. 2011;5(6):1529-48. doi:10.1177/193229681100500630.

37. Service FJ, O'Brien PC. Influence of glycemic variables on hemoglobin A1c. Endocr Pract: Off J Am Coll Endocr Am Assoc Clin Endocrinologists. 2007;13(4), 350.

38. McCarter RJ, Hempe JM, Chalew SA. Mean blood glucose and biological variation have greater influence on HbA1c levels than glucose instability: an analysis of data from the diabetes control and complications trial. Diabetes Care. 2006;29(2):352-5. doi:10.2337/diacare.29.02.06.dc05-1594.

39. Monnier L, Lapinski H, Colette C. Contributions of fasting and postprandial plasma glucose increments to the overall diurnal hyperglycemia of type 2 diabetic patients: variations with increasing levels of HbA1c. Diabetes Care. 2003;26(3):881-5. doi:10.2337/diacare.26.3.881.

40. Schrot RJ. Targeting plasma glucose: preprandial versus postprandial. Clin Diabetes. 2004;22(4):169-72. doi:10.2337/diaclin.22.4.169.

41. Parkin CG, Hinnen D, Campbell RK, Geil P, Tetrick DL, Polonsky WH. Effective use of paired testing in type 2 diabetes. Diabetes Educ. 2009;35(6):915-27. doi:10.1177/0145721709347601.

42. Polonsky WH, Fisher L, Schikman CH, et al. Structured self-monitoring of blood glucose significantly reduces A1C levels in poorly controlled, noninsulin-treated type 2 diabetes: results from the structured testing program study. Diabetes Care. 2011;34(2):262-7. doi:10.2337/dc10-1732.

43. DeFronzo RA, Bonadonna RC, Ferrannini E. Pathogenesis of NIDDM. A balanced overview. Diabetes Care. 1992;15:318-68.

44. Yki-Jarvinen H, Dressler A, Ziemen M. Less nocturnal hypoglycemia and better post-dinner glucose control with bedtime insulin glargine compared with bedtime NPH insulin during insulin combination therapy in type 2 diabetes. Diabetes Care. 2000;23:1130-6.

45. Maiorino MI, et al. Insulin and Glucagon-Like Peptide 1 Receptor Agonist Combination Therapy in Type 2 Diabetes: A Systematic Review and Meta-analysis of Randomized Controlled Trials. Diabetes Care. 2017;40:614-24.

46. Wysham C, et al. Safety and efficacy of a glucagon-like peptide-1 receptor agonist added to basal insulin therapy versus basal insulin with or without a rapid-acting insulin in patients with type 2 diabetes: results of a meta-analysis. Postgrad Med. 2017;129:436-45.

47. Nathan DM, Buse, JB, Davidson, MB, et al. Medical management of hyperglycemia in type 2 diabetes: a consensus algorithm for the initiation and adjustment of therapy: a consensus statement of the American Diabetes Association and the European Association for the Study of Diabetes Diabetes Care. 2009;32(1):193-203.

48. Gerstein HC, Yale JF, Harris SB, et al. A randomized trial of adding insulin glargine vs. avoidance of insulin in people with type 2 diabetes on either no oral glucose-lowering agents or submaximal doses of metformin and/or sulphonylureas. The Canadian INSIGHT (Implementing New Strategies with Insulin Glargine for Hyperglycaemia Treatment) Study. Diabet Med. 2006;23:736-42.

49. Riddle MC, Rosenstock J, Gerich J. The treat-to-target trial: randomized addition of glargine or human NPH insulin to oral therapy of type 2 diabetic patients. Diabetes Care. 2003;26:3080-5.

50. Mooradian AD, Bernbaum M, Albert SG. Narrative review: a rational approach to starting insulin therapy. Ann Intern Med. 2006;145(2):125.

51. Yki-Järvinen H, Bergenstal R, Ziemen M, et al.; EDITION 2 Study Investigators. New insulin glargine 300 units/mL versus glargine 100 units/mL in people with type 2 diabetes using oral agents and basal insulin: glucose control and hypoglycemia in a 6-month randomized controlled trial (EDITION 2). Diabetes Care, 2014;37(12):3235-43. doi:10.2337/dc14-0990.

52. Vora J, et al. Clinical use of insulin degludec. Diabetes Res Clin Pract. 2015;109:19-31.

53. Davies M, Lavalle-González F, Storms F, Gomis R; AT.LANTUS Study Group. A trial comparing Lantus algorithms to achieve normal blood glucose targets in subjects with uncontrolled blood sugar with type 2 diabetes mellitus (AT-LANTUS). Diabetes Obes Metab. 2008;10(5):387-99.

54. Meneghini L[1], Koenen C, Weng W, Selam JL. The usage of a simplified self-titration dosing guideline (303 Algorithm) for insulin detemir in patients with type 2 diabetes–results of the randomized, controlled PREDICTIVE 303 study. Diabetes Obes Metab. 2007 Nov;9(6):902-13.

55. Riddle MC[1], Rosenstock J, Vlajnic A, Gao L. Randomized, 1-year comparison of three ways to initiate and advance insulin for type 2 diabetes: twice-daily premixed insulin versus basal insulin with either basal-plus one prandial insulin or basal-bolus up to three prandial injections. Diabetes Obes Metab. 2014 May;16(5):396-40.

56. Edelman SV, Liu R, Johnson J, Glass LC. Response to comment on edelman et al. AUTONOMY: the first randomized trial comparing two patient-driven approaches to initiate and titrate prandial insulin lispro in type 2 diabetes. Diabetes Care. 2014;37(12):e263-4. doi:10.2337/dc14-1900.

57. Bode B, Chaykin L, Sussman A, et al. Efficacy and safety of insulin Degludec 200 U/mL and insulin Degludec 100 U/mL in patients with type 2 diabetes (Begin: Compare). Endocr Pract. 2014;20(8):785-91.

58. Russell-Jones D, Pouwer F, Khunti K. Identification of barriers to insulin therapy and approaches to overcoming them. Diabetes Obes Metab. 2019 Mar 8.

59. Unger J, Tenzer-Iglesias P, Brunton S. Initiating and intensifying therapy in type 2 diabetes: managing the progressive nature of the disease. J Fam Pract. 2008;57(10):S17.

60. Leahy JL. Basal-prandial insulin therapy: scientific concept review and application. Am J Med Sci. 2006;332(1):24.

61. Businesswire.com. The North America Insulin Pump Market Prospect, Share, Development, Growth and Demand Forecast to 2022. https://www.researchandmarkets.com/research/r243bn/north_america. Accessed Aug. 30, 2019.

62. American Diabetes Association. Diabetes technology: standards of medical care in diabetes—2918. Diabetes Care. 2019;42(Suppl 1):S71-80. August 30, 2019.

63. Berget C, Messer L, Forlenza G. A clinical overview of insulin pump therapy for the management of diabetes: past, present and future of intensive therapy. Diabetes Spectrum. Summer 2019;194-205.

64. Miller KM, Foster NC, Beck RW, et al.; TID Exchange Clinic Network. Current state of type 1 diabetes treatment in the U.S.: updated data from the T1D exchange clinic registry. Diabetes Care. 2015;38:971-8.

65. American Association of Diabetes Educators. Education for continuous subcutaneous insulin infusion pump users (position statement). Diabetes Educ. 2003;29(1):97-9.

66. Heise T, Nosek L, Biilmann Rønn B. Lower within-subject variability of insulin detemir in comparison to NPH insulin and insulin glargine in people with type 1 diabetes. Diabetes. 2004;53:1614-20.

67. Becker RH, Nowotny I, Teichert L, et al. Long-term safety and efficacy of insulin degludec in the management of type 2 diabetes. Diabetes, Metabolic Syndrome and Obesity. 2015;8:483–93.

68. Wysham C, Bhargava A, Chaykin L, et al. Effect of insulin degludec vs insulin glargine U100 on hypoglycemia in patients with type 2 diabetes. The SWITCH 2 Randomized Clinical Trial. JAMA. 2017;318:45-56.

69. Marso SP, McGuire DK, Zinman B, et al.; DEVOTE Study Group. Efficacy and safety of degludec versus glargine in type 2 diabetes. N Engl J Med. 2017;377(8):723-32. doi:10.1056/NEJMoa1615692.

70. Diez-Fernandez A, Cavero-Redondo I, Moreno-Fernández J, et al. Effectiveness of insulin glargine U-300 versus insulin glargine U-100 on nocturnal hypoglycemia and glycemic control in type 1 and type 2 diabetes: a systematic review and meta-analysis. et al. Acta Diabetol. 2019;56:355-64.

71. https://www.companionmedical.com/InPen. In-Pen. Accessed Aug. 31, 2019.

72. Burckhardt M, Smith GJ, Cooper MN, Jones TW, Davis EA. Real-world outcomes of insulin pump compared to injection therapy in a population-based sample of children with type 1 diabetes. Pediatr Diabetes. 2018;19(8):1459-66. doi:10.1111/pedi.12754.

73. Mameli C, Scaramuzza AE, Ho J, Cardona-Hernandez R, Suarez-Ortega L, Zuccotti GV. A 7-year follow-up retrospective, international, multicenter study of insulin pump therapy in children and adolescents with type 1 diabetes. Acta Diabetologica. 2014;51(2):205-10. doi:10.1007/s00592-013-0481-y.

74. Brorsson AL, Viklund G, Örtqvist E, Lindholm Olinder A. Does treatment with an insulin pump improve glycaemic control in children and adolescents with type 1 diabetes? A retrospective case–control study. Pediatr Diabetes. 2015;16(7):546-53. doi:10.1111/pedi.12209.

75. Weinzimer SA, Swan KL, Sikes KA, Ahern JH. Emerging evidence for the use of insulin pump therapy in infants, toddlers, and preschool-aged children with type 1 diabetes. Pediatric Diabetes. 2006;7(s4):15-19. doi:10.1111/j.1399-543X.2006.00172.x.

76. Alsaleh FM, Smith FJ, Taylor KM. Experiences of children/young people and their parents, using insulin pump therapy for the management of type 1 diabetes: qualitative review: experiences of using insulin pumps. J Clin Pharm Ther. 2012;37(2):140-7. doi:10.1111/j.1365-2710.2011.01283.x.

77. Retnakaran R, Hochman J, DeVries JH, et al. Continuous subcutaneous insulin infusion versus multiple daily injections: the impact of baseline A1c. Diabetes Care. 2004;27(11):2590-6. doi:10.2337/diacare.27.11.2590.

78. Pańkowska E, Błazik M, Dziechciarz P, Szypowska A, Szajewska H. Continuous subcutaneous insulin infusion vs. multiple daily injections in children with type 1 diabetes: a systematic review and meta-analysis of randomized control trials. Pediatric Diabetes. 2009;10(1):52-8. doi:10.1111/j.1399-5448.2008.00440.x.

79. Tomky D. Diabetes technologies. In: Childs B, ed. Complete Nurse's Guide to Diabetes Care. American Diabetes Association. 2017;422-36.

80. Beck RW, Riddlesworth TD, Ruedy KJ, et al.; DIAMOND Study Group. Effect of initiating use of an insulin pump in adults with type 1 diabetes using multiple daily insulin injections and continuous glucose monitoring (DIAMOND): a multicentre, randomised controlled trial. The Lancet Diabetes Endocrinol. 2017;5(9):700.

81. Gómez AM, Marín Carrillo LF, Muñoz Velandia OM, et al. Long-term efficacy and safety of sensor augmented insulin pump therapy with low-glucose suspend feature in patients with type 1 diabetes. Diabetes Technol Ther. 2017;19(2):109.

82. Bergenstal RM, Tamborlane WV, Ahmann A, et al. Effectiveness of sensor-augmented insulin-pump therapy in type 1 diabetes. N Engl J Med. 2010;363:311-20.

83. Grunberger G, Handelsman Y, Bloomgarden Z, et al. American Association of Clinical Endocrinologists and American College of Endocrinology 2018 position statement on integration of insulin pumps and continuous glucose monitoring in patient with diabetes mellitus. Endocr Pract. 2018;24(3):302-8.

84. Slover RH, Welsh JB, Criego A, et al. Effectiveness of sensor-augmented pump therapy in children and adolescents with type 1 diabetes in the STAR 3 study. Pediatric Diabetes. 2012;13(1):6-11. doi:10.1111/j.1399-5448.2011.00793.x.

85. Buckingham BA, Raghinaru D, Cameron F, et al. Predictive low-glucose insulin suspension reduces duration of nocturnal hypoglycemia in children without increasing ketosis. Diabetes Care. 2015;38:1197-04.

86. Forlenza GP, Li Z, Buckingham BA, et al. Predictive low-glucose suspend reduces hypoglycemia in adults, adolescents, and children with type 1 diabetes in an at-home randomized crossover study: results of the PROLOG trial. Diabetes Care. 2018;41(10):2155-61. doi:10.2337/dc18-0771.

87. Abraham MB, Nicholas JA, Smith GJ, et al.; on behalf of the PLGM Study Group. Reduction in hypoglycemia with the predictive low-glucose management system: a long-term randomized controlled trial in adolescents with type 1 diabetes. Diabetes Care. 2017;2018;41(2):303-10. doi:10.2337/dc17-1604.

88. Forlenza GP, Cameron FM, Ly TT, et al. Fully closed-loop multiple model probabilistic predictive controller artificial pancreas performance in adolescents and adults in a supervised hotel setting. Diabetes Technol Ther. 2018;20:335-43.

89. Zisser H, Renard E, Kovatchev B, et al.; Control to Range Study Group. Multicenter closed-loop insulin delivery study points to challenges for keeping blood glucose in a safe range by a control algorithm in adults and adolescents with type 1 diabetes from various sites. Diabetes Technol Ther. 2014;16(10):613.

90. Buckingham BA, Forlenza GP, Pinsker JE, et al. Safety and feasibility of the OmniPod hybrid closed-loop system in adult, adolescent, and pediatric patients with type 1 diabetes using a personalized model predictive control algorithm. Diabetes Technol Ther. 2018;20(4):257.

91. Brown S, Raghinaru D, Emory E, Kovatchev B. First look at control-IQ: a new-generation automated insulin delivery system. Diabetes Care. 2018;41(12):2634-6. doi:10.2337/dc18-1249.

92. Weisman A, Bai J, Cardinez M, Kramer CK, Perkins BA. (2017). Effect of artificial pancreas systems on glycaemic control in patients with type 1 diabetes: a systematic review and meta-analysis of outpatient randomised controlled trials. The Lancet. Diabetes Endocrinol. 2017;5(7):501.

93. Garg SK, Weinzimer SA, Tamborlane WV, et al. Glucose outcomes with the in-home use of a hybrid closed-loop insulin delivery system in adolescents and adults with type 1 diabetes. Diabetes Technol Ther. 2017;19(3):155.

94. Pinsker JE, Li Z, Buckingham BA, et al. Exceptional usability of tandem t:Slim X2 with basal-IQ predictive low-glucose suspend (PLGS)—The PROLOG study. Diabetes. 2018; 67(Supplement 1):86. doi:10.2337/db18-86-LB.

95. Lilly LC, Mader JK, Warner J. Developing a simple 3-day insulin delivery device to meet the needs of people with type 2 diabetes. J Diabetes Sci Technol. 2019;13(1):11-19. doi:10.1177/1932296818807223.

96. Hermanns N, Lilly LC, Mader JK, et al. Novel simple insulin delivery device reduces barriers to insulin therapy in type 2 diabetes: results from a pilot study. J Diabetes Sci Technol. 2015;9(3):581-7. doi:10.1177/1932296815570709.

97. Mader JK, Lilly LC, Aberer F, et al. Improved glycaemic control and treatment satisfaction with a simple wearable 3-day insulin delivery device among people with type 2 diabetes. Diabetic Med. 2018;35(10):1448-56. doi:10.1111/dme.13708.

98. American Diabetes Association. 12. Children and adolescents: standards of medical care in diabetes-2018. Diabetes Care. 2018;41(Suppl 1):S126-36. doi:10.2337/dc18-S012.

99. Sherr JL, Tauschmann M, Battelino T, et al. ISPAD clinical practice consensus guidelines 2018: diabetes technologies. Pediatric Diabetes. 2018;19(S27);302-25. doi:10.1111/pedi.12731.

100. Peters AL, Ahmann AJ, Battelino T, et al. Diabetes Technology—Continuous subcutaneous insulin infusion therapy and continuous glucose monitoring in adults: an endocrine society clinical practice guideline. J Clin Endocrinol Metab. 2016;101(11):3922-37. doi:10.1210/jc.2016-2534.

101. Tascini G, Berioli MG, Cerquiglini L, et al. Carbohydrate counting in children and adolescents with type 1 diabetes. Nutrients. 2018;10(1):109. doi:10.3390/nu10010109.

102. Lifestyle management: standards of medical care in diabetes–2019. Diabetes Care. 2019;42(1):S46.

103. Bell KJ, Smart CE, Steil GM, Brand-Miller JC, King B, Wolpert HA. Impact of fat, protein, and glycemic index on postprandial glucose control in type 1 diabetes: implications for intensive diabetes management in the continuous glucose monitoring era. Diabetes Care. 2015;38(6):1008-15. doi:10.2337/dc15-0100.

104. Bell KJ, Toschi E, Steil GM, Wolpert HA. Optimized mealtime insulin dosing for fat and protein in type 1 diabetes: application of a model-based approach to derive insulin doses for open-loop diabetes management. Diabetes Care. 2016;39(9):1631-4. doi:10.2337/dc15-2855.

105. Deeb A, Al Hajeri A, Alhmoudi I, Nagelkerke N. Accurate carbohydrate counting is an important determinant of postprandial glycemia in children and adolescents with type 1 diabetes on insulin pump therapy. J Diabetes Sci Technol. 2017;11(4):753-8. doi:10.1177/1932296816679850.

106. Paterson MA, Smart CEM, Lopez PE, et al. Increasing the protein quantity in a meal results in dose-dependent effects on postprandial glucose levels in individuals with type 1 diabetes mellitus. Diabetic Med. 2017;34(6):851-4. doi:10.1111/dme.13347.

107. Maryniuk MD, Evert A, Rizzotto JA. Evidence and implementation of medical nutrition therapy in persons with diabetes. In: Rodriguez-Saldana J, ed. The Diabetes Textbook. Springer, Cham.; 2019. https://doi.org/10.1007/978-3-030-11815-0_30.

108. Riddell M, Gallen I, et al. Exercise management in type 1 diabetes: a consensus statement. The Lancet. Diabetes Endocrinol. 2017;5(5):377-90.

109. Pickup JC, Keen H, Parsons JA, et al. Continuous subcutaneous insulin infusion: an approach to achieving normoglycaemia. BMJ. 1978;1(6107):204-7.

110. Diabetes Control and Complications Trial Research Group. The effect of intensive treatment of diabetes on the development and progression of long-term complications in insulin-dependent-diabetes mellitus. New Engl J Med. 1993;329;997-86.

111. Karges B, Schwandt A, Heidtmann B, et al. Association of insulin pump therapy vs insulin injection therapy with severe hypoglycemia, ketoacidosis, and glycemic control among children, adolescents, and young adults with type 1 diabetes. JAMA. 2017;318:1358-66.

112. Bode BW, Tamborlane WV, Davidson PC. Insulin pump therapy in the 21st century: strategies for successful use in adults, adolescents, and children with diabetes. Postgrad Med. 2002;111(5):69-78.

113. McCrea DL. A primer on insulin pump therapy for health care providers. Nurs Clin North Am. 2017;52(4):553-64. doi:10.1016/j.cnur.2017.07.005.

114. Walsh J, Roberts R. Pumping insulin: everything for success on an insulin pump and CGM. Torrey Pines Press, San Diego, CA; 2017.

115. Pickup J, Reznik Y, Sutton A. Glycaemic control during continuous subcutaneous insulin infusion vs multiple daily insulin injections in type 2 diabetes: individual patient data meta-analysis and meta-regression of randomised controlled trials. Diabetes Care. 2017;40(5):715-22.

116. Towns R, Pietropaolo M. (2011). GAD65 autoantibodies and its role as biomarker of type 1 diabetes and latent autoimmune diabetes in adults (LADA). Drugs Future. 2011;36(11):847.

117. Schmidt MI, Hadji-Georgopoulos A, Rendell M, et al. The dawn phenomenon, an early morning glucose rise: implications for diabetic intraday blood glucose variation. Diabetes Care. 1981;4(6):579-85.

118. Graveling AJ, Frier BM. (2017). The risks of nocturnal hypoglycaemia in insulin-treated diabetes. Diabetes Res Clin Pract. 2017;133:30-39. doi:10.1016/j.diabres.2017.08.012.

119. Jones SM, Quarry JL, Caldwell-McMillan M, Mauger DT, Gabbay RA. Optimal insulin pump dosing and postprandial glycemia following a pizza meal using the continuous glucose monitoring system. Diabetes Technol Ther. 2005; 7(2):233.

120. Hirsch IB, Bode BW, Garg S, et al.; for the Insulin Aspart CSII/MDI Comparison Study Group. Continuous subcutaneous insulin infusion (CSII) of insulin aspart versus multiple daily injection of insulin Aspart/Insulin glargine in type 1 diabetic patients previously treated with CSII. Diabetes Care. 2005;28(3):533-8. doi:10.2337/diacare.28.3.533.

121. Umpirrez G, Klonoff D. Diabetes technology update: use of insulin pumps and continuous glucose monitoring in the hospital. Diabetes Care. 2018;41:1579-89. https://doi.org/10.2337/dci18-0002.

122. Grunberger G, Bailey TS, Cohen AJ, et al.; AACE Insulin Pump Management Task Force. Statement by the American Association of Clinical Endocrinologists consensus panel on insulin pump management. Endocr Pract: Off J Am Coll Endocr Am Assoc Clin Endocrinologists. 2010;16(5):746.

123. American Association of Diabetes Educators. Role of the diabetes educator in inpatient diabetes management. Diabetes Educ. 2019;45(1):60-65. doi:10.1177/0145721718820944.

124. Cook CB, Beer KA, Seifert KM, Boyle ME, Mackey PA, Castro JC. Transitioning insulin pump therapy from the outpatient to the inpatient setting: a review of 6 years' experience with 253 cases. J Diabetes Sci Technol. 2012;6(5):995-1002. doi:10.1177/193229681200600502.

125. Kannan S, Satra A, Calogeras E, Lock P, Lansang MC. Insulin pump patient characteristics and glucose control in the hospitalized setting. J Diabetes Sci Technol. 2014;8(3):473-8. doi:10.1177/1932296814522809.

126. Orchard TJ, Nathan DM, Zinman B, et al.; Writing Group for the DCCT/EDIC Research Group. Association between 7 years of intensive treatment of type 1 diabetes and long-term mortality. JAMA. 2015;313(1):45-53. doi:10.1001/jama.2014.16107.

127. Lipska KJ, Ross JS, Wang Y, et al. National Trends in US Hospital Admissions for Hyperglycemia and Hypoglycemia Among Medicare Beneficiaries, 1999 to 2011. *JAMA Intern Med.* 2014;174(7):1116-24. doi:10.1001/jamainternmed.2014.1824.

128. Bruttomesso D, Bonomo M, Costa S, et al.; Italian Group for Continuous Subcutaneous Insulin Infusion in Pregnancy. Type 1 diabetes control and pregnancy outcomes in women treated with continuous subcutaneous insulin infusion (CSII) or with insulin glargine and multiple daily injections of rapid-acting insulin analogues (glargine-MDI). Diabetes Metab. 2011;37:426-31.

129. Reddy M, Godsland I.F, Barnard K.D, Herrero P, Georgiou P, Thomson H, . . . Oliver N.S. Glycemic variability and its impact on quality of life in adults with type 1 diabetes. Journal of Diabetes Science and Technology, 2015, 2016;10(1), 60-6. doi:10.1177/1932296815601440

130. Cooke D, Bond R, Lawton J, Rankin D, Heller, S, Clark M, . . . for the U.K. NIHR DAFNE Study Group. Structured type 1 diabetes education delivered within routine care: impact on glycemic control and diabetes-specific quality of life. Diabetes Care. 2013;36(2), 270-2. doi:10.2337/dc12-0080

131. Polonsky W, Ruedy K, Hessler D, Beck R; for the DAMOND Study Group. The impact of continuous glucose monitoring on markers of quality of life in adults with type 1 diabetes: further findings from the DIAMOND randomized clinical trial. Diabetes Care. 2017 Jun;40(6):736-41. https://doi.org/10.2337/dc17-0133.

132. Barendse S, Singh H, Frier BM, Speight J. The impact of hypoglycaemia on quality of life and related patient-reported outcomes in type 2 diabetes: a narrative review: Hypoglycaemia QoL type 2 DM review. Diabetic Med. 2012;29(3): 293-302. doi:10.1111/j.1464-5491.2011.03416.x.

133. Speight J, Reaney MD, Barnard KD. Not all roads lead to Rome–a review of quality of life measurement in adults with

diabetes. Diabetic Med.: J Brit Diabetic Assoc. 2009;26(4): 315-27. doi:10.1111/j.1464-5491.2009.02682.x.

134. Herman WH, Ilag LL, Johnson SL, et al. A clinical trial of continuous subcutaneous insulin infusion versus multiple daily injections in older adults with type 2 diabetes. Diabetes Care. 2005;28(7):1568-73.

135. Bergenstal R, Peryot M, Dreon D. Implementation of basal bolus therapy in type 2 diabetes: a randomized controlled trial comparing bolus insulin delivery using an insulin patch with an insulin pen. Diabetes Technol Ther. 2019 May;21(5):273-85.

136. Kallas-Koeman MM, Kong JM, Klinke JA, et al. Insulin pump use in pregnancy is associated with lower HbA1c without increasing the rate of severe hypoglycaemia or diabetic ketoacidosis in women with type 1 diabetes. Diabetologia. 2014;57(4):681-9. doi:10.1007/s00125-014-3163-6.

137. Farrar D, Tuffnell DJ, West J, West HM. Continuous subcutaneous insulin infusion versus multiple daily injections of insulin for pregnant women with diabetes. Cochrane Database System Rev. 2016;(6):CD005542-CD005542. doi:10.1002/14651858.CD005542.pub3.

138. Ranasinghe PD, Maruthur, NM, Nicholson WK, et al. Comparative effectiveness of continuous subcutaneous insulin infusion using insulin analogs and multiple daily injections in pregnant women with diabetes mellitus: A systematic review and meta-analysis. J Women's Health. 2015;24(3):237-49. doi:10.1089/jwh.2014.4939.

139. Ringholm L, Damm P, Mathiesen ER. Improving pregnancy outcomes in women with diabetes mellitus: modern management. Nat Rev Endocrinol. 2019 Jul;15(7):406-16.

140. McCance DR. Diabetes in pregnancy review. Best Pract Res Clin Obstet Gynaecol. 2015 Jul;29(5):685-99.

141. Krishnasamy S, Abell TL. Diabetic gastroparesis: principles and current trends in management. Diabetes Ther. 2018; 9(Suppl 1):1-42. doi:10.1007/s13300-018-0454-9.

142. CMS.gov Decision Memo for Insulin Pump: C-Peptide Levels as a Criterion for Use (CAG-00092R). December 17, 2004.

143. CMS.gov. Decision Memo for Insulin Infusion Pump (CAG-00041N). August 26, 1999. IDF Global Guideline for Managing Older People with Type 2 Diabetes, 2013.

144. Reznik Y, Joubert M. The OPT2MISE Study—a review of the major findings and clinical implications. Eur Endocrinol. 2015 Aug;11(2):70-4.

145. Pickup JC. Insulin pumps. Diabetes Technol Ther. 2017 Feb;19(S1):S19-26.

146. Millstein R, Becerra NM, Shubrook JH. Insulin pumps: beyond basal-bolus. Cleve Clin J Med. 2015 Dec;82(12):835-42.

147. Edelman SV, Bode BW, Bailey TS, et al. Insulin pump therapy in patients with type 2 diabetes safely improved glycemic control using a simple insulin dosing regimen. Diabetes Technol Ther. 2010;12:627-33.

148. Vigersky RA, Huang S, Cordero TL, et al.; OpT2mise Study Group. Improved HbA1c, total daily insulin dose, and treatment satisfaction with insulin pump therapy compares to multiple daily injections in patients with type 2 diabetes irrespective of baseline C-peptide levels. Endocr Pract. 2018;24:446-52.

149. Aronson R, Reznik Y, Conget I, et al.; OpT2mise Study Group. Sustained efficacy of insulin pump therapy compared with multiple daily injections in type 2 diabetes: 12-month data from the OpT2mise randomized trial. Diabetes Obes Metab. 2016;18:500-7.

150. Reznik Y, Cohen O, Aronson R, et al.; OpT2mise Study Group. Insulin pump treatment compared with multiple daily injections for treatment of type 2 diabetes (OpT2mise): a randomized open-label controlled trial. Lancet. 2014;384:1265-72.

151. Yeh H-C, Brown TT, Maruthur N, et al. Comparative effectiveness and safety of methods of insulin delivery and glucose monitoring for diabetes mellitus: a systematic review and meta-analysis. Ann Intern Med. 2012;157:336-47.

152. Sherr JL, Hermann JM, Campbell F, et al.; T1D Exchange Clinic Network, the DPV Initiative, and the National Paediatric Diabetes Audit and the Royal College of Paediatrics and Child Health registries. Use of insulin pump therapy in children and adolescents with type 1 diabetes and its impact on metabolic control: comparison of results from three large, transatlantic paediatric registries. Diabetologia. 2016;59:87-91.

153. Jeitler K, Horvath K, Berghold A, et al. Continuous subcutaneous insulin infusion versus multiple daily insulin injections in patients with diabetes mellitus: systematic review and meta-analysis. Diabetologia 2008;51:941–51.

154. Haynes A, Hermann JM, Miller KM, et al. Severe hypoglycemia rates are not associated with HbA1c: a cross-sectional analysis of 3 contemporary pediatric diabetes registry databases. Pediatr Diabetes. 2017;18:643-50.

155. Pickup JC, Sutton AJ. Severe hypoglycaemia and glycaemic control in type 1 diabetes: meta-analysis of multiple daily insulin injections compared with continuous subcutaneous insulin infusion. Diabet Med. 2008;25:765-74.

156. Maahs DM, Hermann JM, Holman N, et al.; National Paediatric Diabetes Audit and the Royal College of Paediatrics and Child Health, the DPV. Initiative, and the T1D Exchange Clinic Network. Rates of diabetic ketoacidosis: international comparison with 49,859 pediatric patients with type 1 diabetes from England, Wales, the U.S., Austria, and Germany. Diabetes Care. 2015;38:1876-82.

157. Zabeen B, Craig ME, Virk SA, et al. Insulin pump therapy is associated with lower rates of retinopathy and peripheral nerve abnormality. PLoS One. 2016;11:e0153033.

158. Opipari-Arrigan L, Fredericks EM, Burkhart N, Dale L, Hodge M, Foster C. Continuous subcutaneous insulin infusion benefits quality of life in preschool-age children with type 1 diabetes mellitus. Pediatr Diabetes. 2007;8:377-83.

159. Sundberg F, Barnard K, Cato A, et al. ISPAD Guidelines. Managing diabetes in preschool children. Pediatr Diabetes. 2017;18:499-517.

CHAPTER 20

Pharmacotherapy: Dyslipidemia and Hypertension in Persons With Diabetes

John D. Bucheit, PharmD, BCACP, CDCES
Dave L. Dixon, PharmD, BCACP, BCPS, CDCES, CLS, FACC, FCCP

Key Concepts

- Pharmacotherapy for management of dyslipidemia and hypertension in persons with diabetes is complex and continually evolving.
- When developing strategies for managing diabetes, equal emphasis should be given to dyslipidemia and hypertension to reduce the burden of cardiovascular disease. These need to be treated as aggressively as hyperglycemia.
- Treatment strategies for dyslipidemia and hypertension may require combination therapies that provide different mechanisms of action to obtain optimal lipid and blood pressure levels.
- Patients on multiple medications should be monitored frequently for adverse events and possible drug or food interactions.
- Patient education should include the importance of medication adherence, medication safety, proper dosing, and timing medications for optimum effect.

Introduction

Atherosclerotic cardiovascular disease (ASCVD) is the leading cause of morbidity and mortality for people with diabetes. Atherosclerotic cardiovascular disease includes acute coronary syndromes, a history of myocardial infarction (MI), stable or unstable angina, coronary revascularization, stroke, transient ischemic attack, and peripheral arterial disease.[1]

Death due to ASCVD is 2 to 4 times higher in those with diabetes compared with those without diabetes.[2] This is partly due to the coexistence of hypertension and dyslipidemia, both of which are independent risk factors for ASCVD by themselves. Managing hypertension and dyslipidemia in persons with diabetes is an effective strategy to mitigate the risk of ASCVD.

Persons with diabetes who have an MI are likely to have an increased risk of death from that MI. Results from one Finnish study showed that the 1-year mortality rate following an MI was higher in men and women with diabetes (44% and 37%, respectively) compared with those without diabetes (33% and 20%).[3] A Swedish study examined patients hospitalized for an MI who had not been diagnosed with type 2 diabetes and found that one third had prediabetes and one third had newly diagnosed diabetes.[4,5] Additionally, complications from cardiovascular disease contribute significantly to overall healthcare expenditures in people with diabetes.[1]

Therefore, prioritizing and treating ASCVD risk factors in people with diabetes is crucial. When developing strategies for managing diabetes, equal emphasis must be given to dyslipidemia and hypertension, and they should be treated as aggressively as hyperglycemia.

Common Dyslipidemia Patterns in Persons With Diabetes

Triglycerides (TGs) and cholesterol are water-insoluble lipids derived from dietary sources (exogenous system) and hepatic synthesis (endogenous system). Lipoproteins, other than TGs and cholesterol, are involved in these systems and include very low-density lipoproteins (VLDL), low-density lipoproteins (LDL-C), and high-density lipoproteins (HDL-C).[6] Figure 20.1 depicts the exogenous and endogenous lipid transport system.

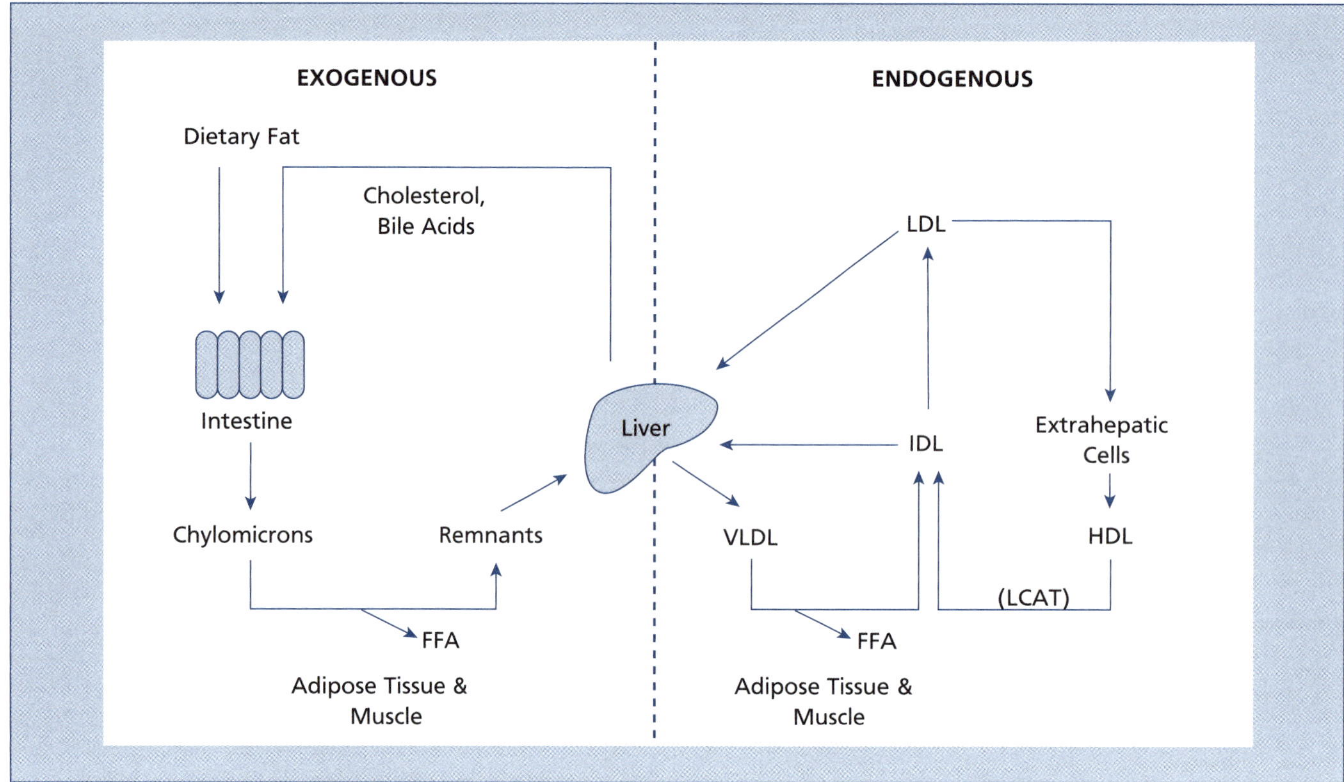

FIGURE 20.1 **Exogenous and Endogenous Lipid Transport System**

Dyslipidemia in persons with diabetes is typically composed of elevated TGs and decreased HDL-C, with LDL-C elevations comparable to those of persons without diabetes. However, the particle size of the LDL-C in persons with diabetes tends to be smaller and denser, which can increase atherogenicity.[6]

The small, dense LDL-C particles often seen with diabetes raise the risk for heart disease.

The abnormalities in the small, dense LDL-C composition are partially due to hypertriglyceridemia and are associated with a threefold increased risk of coronary heart disease (CHD).[7] This increased risk is caused by the particles' ability to enter blood vessel walls more easily than the normal, large, and less dense LDL-C particles; thus, endothelial function is impaired and susceptibility to thrombosis increases.[8]

However, serum LDL-C may be less predictive of CHD risk than other measurements. Therefore, non-HDL-C (calculated as total cholesterol [TC] – HDL-C) has been recommended as an alternative to LDL-C because of data suggesting it may be a better predictor of CHD risk than LDL-C.[9] Furthermore, non-HDL-C represents an individual's entire atherogenic lipoprotein burden and is easily measured during a non-fasting state.

Elevated TGs are a key contributor to low HDL-C.

Elevated TG levels can result from 2 abnormalities: overproduction of VLDL and impaired lipolysis of TGs. Persons with type 2 diabetes overproduce TG-rich VLDL, a result of elevated free fatty acid levels, hyperglycemia, obesity, and insulin resistance.[10] Impaired lipolysis of VLDL TGs is thought to be due to a reduction in lipoprotein lipase activity.[10]

HDL-C is the major lipoprotein responsible for removing excess cholesterol from peripheral tissues, which is known as reverse cholesterol transport. Therefore, suboptimal levels of HDL-C can result in increases in TGs, VLDL, and LDL-C.[6] Low levels of HDL-C is a known risk factor for CHD; however, studies involving medications that raise HDL-C have not been shown to reduce ASCVD risk.[11–13]

Cardiovascular Risk Assessment

The aim of conducting an accurate ASCVD risk assessment is to identify those individuals with accelerated atherosclerosis who are at high risk for ASCVD and ASCVD-related mortality. As previously stated, diabetes is associated with a high degree of ASCVD risk that is due to more than hyperglycemia alone. The total risk borne by a person with diabetes results from the combination of metabolic risk factors (eg, hypertension, low HDL-C, high TGs, obesity), degree of hyperglycemia, time since diabetes diagnosis, and presence of microvascular complications. Thus, it is necessary to assess a person's individual cardiovascular risk to establish the need for lipid-lowering therapy.[14]

In 2013, the American College of Cardiology/American Heart Association (ACC/AHA) Cholesterol Guideline introduced the ASCVD Risk Estimator, which offers several advantages over the traditionally used Framing Risk Score (FRS).[14] First, the ASCVD Risk Estimator is based on race- and gender-specific pooled cohort equations developed from several large, diverse modern cohort studies. Additionally, the output is broader, as an ASCVD event is defined as CHD death, nonfatal myocardial infarction, or fatal or nonfatal stroke. The ASCVD Risk Estimator can estimate the 10-year risk for a first ASCVD event in African-American and white men and women between ages 40 and 79. Because persons with diabetes are already deemed to be at increased risk, the 10-year risk assessment is used to inform the decision regarding intensity of statin therapy rather than whether to initiate statin therapy.[14]

In 2018, the ASCVD Risk Estimator Plus was released, which allows clinicians to project for potential benefit of risk-lowering interventions (eg, statins, aspirin, smoking cessation) as well as the ability to track an individual's change in ASCVD risk over time.[9] The ASCVD Risk Estimator Plus does not include all potential factors associated with increased ASCVD risk. These "risk-enhancing factors" include family history of premature ASCVD, defined as having a first-degree relative that had a CHD event before age 55 (men) or age 65 (women); primary hypercholesterolemia (LDL-C 160-189 mg/dL), metabolic syndrome, chronic kidney disease, chronic inflammatory conditions (ie, psoriasis, rheumatoid arthritis, human immunodeficiency virus), history of premature menopause, preeclampsia, gestational diabetes, South Asian ancestry, or presence of select lipid/biomarkers (TG ≥175 mg/dL, high-sensitivity C-reactive protein ≥2 mg/L, lipoprotein(a) ≥50 mg/dL or ≥125 mmol/L, apolipoprotein B ≥130 mg/dL, or ankle-brachial index <0.9).[9] The presence of any one of these factors warrants revising an individual's risk assessment upward.

In summary, current guidelines continue to support that individuals with diabetes are at higher ASCVD risk than those without diabetes, and the majority would benefit from statin therapy. However, ASCVD risk is not equal among all persons with diabetes, so individualized ASCVD risk assessment is necessary to inform treatment decisions.

Treatment: Management of Dyslipidemia in Persons With Diabetes

Current guidelines for managing dyslipidemia recommend a "risk-based" approach that emphasizes use moderate-high intensity statin therapy to reduce LDL-C by at least 30% (≥50% in higher risk patients) from baseline.[9] The 2018 ACC/AHA Cholesterol Guideline recommends statin therapy for the following groups who are most likely to benefit from statin therapy: (1) secondary prevention of ASCVD, (2) severe hypercholesterolemia (LDL ≥190 mg/dL), (3) type 1 and type 2 diabetes, and (4) primary prevention. For purposes of this chapter, we will focus on the recommendations aimed at individuals with diabetes.[9]

Given the extensive body of evidence supporting the benefit of statins in persons with diabetes, the 2018 ACC/AHA Cholesterol Guideline recommends moderate-intensity statin therapy to reduce LDL-C by 30% to 49% in all individuals between 40 and 75 years of age.[9] A 10-year ASCVD risk score may be calculated to help stratify ASCVD risk but is not required before initiating statin therapy. Moderate-intensity statin therapy may be considered in younger patients between age 20 and 39 years if they have a longstanding history of diabetes or presence of microvascular complications (eg, retinopathy, nephropathy). As for patients ≥75 years of age, statin therapy may be considered but only after a clinician-patient discussion of the risks and benefits. Individuals with diabetes and ≥1 ASCVD risk factors (eg, hypertension, tobacco use) should receive high-intensity statin therapy to reduce LDL-C by ≥50%. Additionally, ezetimibe may be added to maximally tolerated statin to ensure an LDL-C reduction of ≥50% in those with a 10-year ASCVD risk ≥20%. The ACC/AHA do not recommend PCSK9 inhibitors in patients with diabetes that have not had an ASCVD event; however, PCSK9 inhibitors may be considered in patients who have an LDL-C ≥70 mg/dL despite taking maximally tolerated statin and ezetimibe. Calculating the 10-year ASCVD risk is unwarranted in individuals with diabetes who have had an ASCVD event, as they are already considered to be at very high risk and should receive high-intensity statin therapy. It remains important to obtain a lipid panel 4 to 12 weeks after statin initiation to ensure the desired percent reduction in LDL-C is achieved. This is evident by a study showing that slightly less than half of patients receiving rosuvastatin 20 mg daily experienced a ≥50% reduction in LDL-C and were found to be at increased ASCVD risk compared to those who achieved the anticipated ≥50% reduction in LDL-C.[15] Once stable, routine lipid monitoring every 3 to 12 months is useful to ensure adherence.

The 2020 American Diabetes Association (ADA) Standards of Care also provide recommendations for managing dyslipidemia in persons with diabetes.[1] One major difference is that the ADA relies more on the ASCVD Risk Estimator to guide statin intensity. Like ACC/AHA, the ADA recommends moderate-intensity statin therapy in all adults ≥40 years of age; however, the ADA recommends high-intensity statin therapy if the 10-year ASCVD risk is ≥20%, regardless of age. Moderate-intensity statin therapy may be considered in adults <40 years of age and with a 10-year ASCVD risk <20% if they have multiple ASCVD risk factors. The ADA also recommends adding either ezetimibe or a PCSK9 inhibitor in patients with established ASCVD who have an LDL-C ≥70 mg/dL despite maximally tolerated statin, regardless of age.

Despite minor differences between the guidelines, there is general agreement that statin therapy is a major component of comprehensive diabetes care and the primary approach to reduce ASCVD risk. A summary of the basic tenets of the guidelines is available in Table 20.1. Readers are encouraged to review each of these guidelines in greater detail at their own discretion based on the needs of their individual patients.

Each of the guidelines agrees, in principle, that lifestyle modification, including medical nutrition therapy (MNT), physical activity, and smoking cessation, should always be a standard treatment of dyslipidemia in addition to pharmacotherapy.[1,9]

Standard Treatment

Dyslipidemia—Lifestyle modification, including MNT, physical activity, and smoking cessation, should always be a standard treatment of dyslipidemia in addition to pharmacotherapy.

Children and Adolescents

Children with diabetes should be screened and monitored for dyslipidemia beginning at age 10 after glucose stability has been established; see the ADA Standards of Care for specific recommendations.[1] The initial management approach should consist of optimizing glucose levels and MNT, but statin therapy may be initiated in children ≥10 years of age who have either an LDL-C level >160 mg/dL or an LDL-C level >130 mg/dL plus at least 1 ASCVD risk factor. An LDL-C Level of >100 mg/dl is considered acceptable in children.[1]

TABLE 20.1 Synopsis of Recommendations for Managing Dyslipidemia in Persons With Diabetes

Characteristic	*Goal*	*Treatment Recommendation*
Diabetes plus any of the following: • Clinical ASCVD • 10-year ASCVD risk >20% • Multiple ASCVD risk factors*	≥50% reduction in LDL-C	High-intensity statin‡ Consider adding ezetimibe if LDL-C remains ≥70 (non-HDL-C ≥100) or desired ≥50% reduction is not achieved on maximally tolerated statin • Ezetimibe generally preferred over PCSK9 inhibitors due to cost and ease of use
Diabetes plus any of the following: • No clinical ASCVD • 10-year ASCVD risk <20% • No ASCVD risk factors*	30 to 49% reduction in LDL-C	Moderate-intensity statin‡ Consider high-intensity statin if desired 30% to 49% reduction is not achieved Consider non-statin therapies in patients unable to tolerate moderate-intensity statin

*ASCVD risk factors include LDL-C >100, hypertension, premature ASCVD, low HDL-C, smoking, overweight, and obesity.

‡A lesser intensity statin may be used in those >75 years of age and those at risk for, or with a prior history of, statin-associated adverse effects.

Sources: American Diabetes Association, "Standards of medical care in diabetes—2020". *Diabetes Care*. (2020):43(Suppl 1):S111-134. Grundy SM, Stone NJ, Bailey AL, et al, "2018 AHA/ACC/AACVPR/AAPA/ABC/ACPM/ADA/AGS/APhA/ASPC/NLA/PCNA Guideline on the Management of Blood Cholesterol: Executive Summary: A Report of the American College of Cardiology/American Heart Association Task Force on Clinical Practice Guidelines, *J Am Coll Cardiol*. (2018). doi: https://doi.org/10.1016/j.jacc.2018.11.003.

Case: An African American With Type 2 Diabetes and Hypertension

DC is a 58-year-old African-American male who was diagnosed with type 2 diabetes 2 years ago. He presented at the clinic for a follow-up visit (from his appointment 2 weeks earlier) to review the results of his lipid panel.

Past Medical History

- Seasonal allergic rhinitis
- Obesity
- Type 2 diabetes

Family History

- Father: history of MI, deceased at age 59
- Mother: history of type 2 diabetes, hypertension, deceased at age 72

Social History

- (+) tobacco
- (–) illicit drug use
- (+) alcohol (socially)

Vital Signs

- Blood pressure: 136/82 mm Hg (Last visit: 128/76 mm Hg)
- Heart rate: 76
- Respiratory rate: 14

Physical Exam

- Height: 70 in
- Weight: 235 lb
- Body mass index: 34 kg/m^2
- Waist circumference: 43 in

Current Medications

- Metformin (Glucophage®) 2000 mg daily
- Multivitamin daily
- Aspirin 81 mg daily
- Fexofenadine (Allegra®) 60 mg twice daily as needed

Adherence to Pharmacologic Therapy

DC picks up most of his medications every 30 days at his pharmacy. However, pharmacy records indicate he purchases his metformin every 45 days. Initially, DC denied missing doses, but upon further interviewing, he admitted to forgetting occasional doses of medications because he "does not like to take too many pills."

Laboratory Data

- TC: 235 mg/dL (13.04 mmol/L)
- LDL-C: 143 mg/dL (7.94 mmol/L)
- TGs: 287 mg/dL (15.93 mmol/L)
- HDL-C: 35 mg/dL (1.94 mmol/L)
- Non-HDL-C: 200 mg/dL (11.01 mmol/L)
- Fasting blood glucose: 155 mg/dL (8.60 mmol/L)
- A1C: 7.1%
- Liver function test:
  - Aspartate aminotransferase (AST): 16 U/L (reference range: 10–42)
  - Alanine aminotransferase (ALT): 12 U/L (reference range: 10–40)

Assessment

DC has diabetes and is >40 years of age suggesting he would benefit from statin therapy. He has several ASCVD risk factors (age >45 years old, smoker, low HDL-C, metabolic syndrome), which strongly suggests he would benefit from statin therapy. Although he has not previously been diagnosed with hypertension, his blood pressure will need to be monitored at later visits since his blood pressure is 136/82 mmHg today.

His 10-year ASCVD risk is 28.8%, suggesting he would benefit from *high-intensity* statin therapy to reduce his LDL-C by ≥50%. DC does have elevated TGs and low HDL-C; however, these are not current targets of therapy, as the primary goal is to reduce his atherogenic lipoprotein burden (LDL-C and non-HDL-C) with statin therapy based on the evidence to support this approach.

Table 20.2 lists statins according to dosing intensity. Both atorvastatin 40 to 80 mg/d (Lipitor®, Pfizer) and rosuvastatin (Crestor®, Astra Zeneca) 20–40 mg/d are reasonable options as they are generically available and taken once daily, day or night. If non-statin therapy is warranted due to the inability to tolerate a high-intensity statin or as an add-on to achieve a ≥50% decrease in LDL-C, combination therapy (eg, Vytorin®) might be preferred given DC's preference to keep his pill burden low.

The case study progresses throughout the chapter. Considerations for the risk of ASCVD need to be addressed as well as appropriate treatment options for dyslipidemia and hypertension with diabetes. Furthermore, smoking cessation should be offered at every encounter and resources provided to ensure success given this is a major preventable risk factor for ASCVD.

TABLE 20.2 Guideline Recommendations on Statin Dosing Intensity

High-Intensity Statin (>50% Reduction in LDL-C)	*Moderate-Intensity Statin (30–50% Reduction in LDL-C)*
Atorvastatin, 40–80 mg daily Rosuvastatin, 20–40 mg daily	Atorvastatin, 10–20 mg daily Rosuvastatin, 5–10 mg daily Simvastatin, 20–40 mg daily Pitavastatin (Livalo, Kowa), 2–4 mg daily Lovastatin, 40 mg daily Pravastatin, 40–80 mg daily Fluvastatin XL, 80 mg daily Fluvastatin, 40 mg twice daily

Key: LDL-C = low-density lipoprotein cholesterol; XL = extended-release.

Sources: Grundy SM, Stone NJ, Bailey AL, et al, "2018 AHA/ACC/AACVPR/AAPA/ABC/ACPM/ADA/AGS/APhA/ASPC/NLA/PCNA Guideline on the Management of Blood Cholesterol: Executive Summary: A Report of the American College of Cardiology/American Heart Association Task Force on Clinical Practice Guidelines," *J Am Coll Cardiol.* (2018). doi: https://doi.org/10.1016/j.jacc.2018.11.003.

Pharmacotherapy: Dyslipidemia in Persons With Diabetes

There are currently 7 classes of lipid-lowering agents prescribed in the treatment of dyslipidemia:

- HMG-CoA reductase inhibitors (statins)
- Selective intestinal absorption inhibitors
- Proprotein convertase subtilisin/kexin type 9 (PCSK9) inhibitors
- Fibric acid derivatives (fibrates)
- Omega-3 fatty acids
- Bile acid resins
- Niacin

Plant stanols and sterols, although not considered pharmacotherapy, may also play a role in the management of dyslipidemia; see chapter 16, on nutrition therapy, for more information.

HMG-CoA Reductase Inhibitors (Statins)

HMG-CoA reductase inhibitors, commonly referred to as statins, are the most widely used lipid-lowering agent and often the first choice for treatment of dyslipidemia in persons with diabetes.[1,9] Their primary lipoprotein effect is in lowering LDL-C and non-HDL-C, with secondary beneficial effects of decreased TGs and increased HDL-C. Additionally, statins may increase the buoyancy or particle size of LDL-C, thereby reducing the amount of small, dense LDL-C in circulation.[7,8]

HMG-CoA Reductase Inhibitors (Statins): Dosage Information

Drug	*Trade Name*	*Common Dose*	*Common Frequency*
Atorvastatin	Lipitor®	10–80 mg	Once daily
Fluvastatin	Lescol®	20–40 mg	Once or twice daily
	Lescol® XL	80 mg	Once daily
Lovastatin	Mevacor®	10–40 mg	Once or twice daily
	Altoprev®	10–60 mg extended-release	Once daily
Pitavastatin	Livalo®	1–4 mg	Once daily
Pravastatin	Pravachol®	10–80 mg	Once daily
Rosuvastatin	Crestor®	5–40 mg	Once daily
Simvastatin	Zocor®	10–40 mg	Once daily

Mechanism of Action

Statins primarily reduce LDL-C by competitively inhibiting HMG-CoA reductase, the enzyme that converts HMG-CoA to melvalonate in the hepatic synthesis of cholesterol, resulting in reduced endogenous cholesterol. Statins will reduce but not totally block cholesterol synthesis. The decreased endogenous cholesterol production activates LDL-C receptor synthesis, resulting in enhanced clearance of circulating LDL-C particles.[6]

Dosing

Statins are generally administered once daily. Because of their short half-life, lovastatin, fluvastatin, pravastatin, and simvastatin should be taken in the evening to coincide with nighttime cholesterol synthesis.[16] Atorvastatin, rosuvastatin, and pitavastatin may be taken at any time of day. The dosage is based on the desired statin intensity according to an individual's risk.[9] Low-intensity doses are only appropriate for those patients unable to tolerate moderate- or high-intensity doses; for individuals at higher risk of adverse effects due to unavoidable drug-drug interactions; and Asian populations, who are known to have a greater response to statin therapy than other groups.[9] Table 20.2 stratifies statins by dose intensity and ability to lower LDL-C according to current guidelines.

Pregnancy, Precautions, and Contraindications

Statins are contraindicated in pregnancy and in women who are breastfeeding; they should be used cautiously in those with significantly impaired renal or hepatic function.[9]

Adverse Effects

Statins are generally well tolerated with minimal adverse effects, especially with appropriate monitoring. However, several statin-associated side effects involving the musculoskeletal, metabolic, liver, neurological, and other systems have been reported.[9,17]

Statin-associated muscle symptoms (SAMS) are the most commonly reported adverse effect, with reports ranging from 10% to 25% of those on statin therapy.[17] Muscle pain, stiffness, and/or achiness often develop bilaterally and involve large muscle groups (eg, thighs, back), while cramping is unilateral and involves smaller muscles in the hands and/or feet. Terms used to describe SAMS vary and include *myopathy*, *myositis*, and *myalgia*. Interestingly, SAMS can occur in those with normal creatine kinase (CK) levels, while some individuals can have elevated CK levels but no muscle symptoms. Rarely (0.1% of statin users), patients develop rhabdomyolysis, which is evident by a CK greater than 10 times the upper limit of normal and symptoms of fever, nausea, tachycardia, and dark colored urine.[17] SAMS are most common with high-intensity statin therapy, concomitant use of drugs that interact with statins, those of advanced age, the female gender, lower body mass index, alcohol use, and regular exercisers. Therefore, instruct patients to report any experience of muscle weakness, tenderness, pain, or fever.

Vitamin D status may be considered a modifiable risk factor for muscle-related adverse effects of statins, and supplementation of vitamin D (particularly when ≤20 ng/mL) may improve statin tolerance.

Statins have also been associated with causing new-onset diabetes (as reported in the JUPITER Study).[17] Several meta-analyses including several statin trials observed a small but statistically significant increase in the risk of new-onset diabetes in statin users.[17] However, a post-hoc analysis of the JUPITER study found that new-onset diabetes developed only in those individuals enrolled in the trial who had at least 1 risk factor for diabetes.[18] Furthermore, rosuvastatin 20 mg daily prevented 3 ASCVD events for every new case of diabetes. Thus, the benefit of statin therapy exceeded the diabetes risk in those at high risk of developing diabetes. Mechanisms for statin-associated diabetes are unclear. It appears that there is merely an "association" but no definitive evidence that statins "cause" or "worsen" diabetes.[9]

Significant elevations of liver enzymes can occur and are more common during the first 12 weeks of therapy.[19] Statin therapy should be discontinued when liver enzymes exceed 3 times the upper limit of normal. Of note, there have been few reports of statins directly causing liver failure.[19] While measuring liver enzymes before statin initiation and after any dose increase is reasonable, there are currently no recommendations to routinely monitor liver enzymes.[9]

Drug Interactions

Most statins are metabolized through multiple complex mechanisms that primarily involve the cytochrome P-450 pathway in the liver.[20] However, the degree to which statins are involved with specific enzymes varies, and intestinal transports also contribute to the metabolism of statins. Inhibitors of CYP3A4 and/or CYP2C9 decrease statin metabolism and increase serum statin levels and the risk for adverse effects. Contrarily, inducers would increase statin metabolism and reduce statin efficacy.

Concurrent medications and foods that are also metabolized through this system (such as grapefruit juice) should be used cautiously and patients should be monitored for increased levels and adverse reactions. Monitoring adverse effects and lipid profiles can help identify the potential impact of drug-drug interactions and reduce the risk of toxicity. The reader is encouraged to review the FDA package insert for each statin for specific guidance on dosing with specific interacting drugs.[20] Table 20.3 lists common drugs that interact with statins (Note: This is not a comprehensive list).

Monitoring

A baseline lipid profile, liver function, and renal function tests should be conducted prior to initiating statin therapy. Monitor lipid profiles every 4 to 12 weeks after starting statin therapy or changing the dose or drug.[9] Once stable, lipid profiles should be obtained every 3 to 12 months to assess patient adherence. This is extremely important as statin discontinuation rates are high, even in those who have been discharged after a myocardial infarction.[21] Furthermore, less than half of patients will take their statin ≥80% of time.[21] Routine liver function monitoring after statin initiation is currently not recommended unless patients develop symptoms suggesting liver toxicity.[9] Measuring CK levels before initiating statin therapy may assist in identifying SAMS, but evidence supporting the routine use of CK levels is limited.[9]

TABLE 20.3 Statin Use: Selected Interactions Between Cytochrome P-450 Isoenzymes and Common Drugs

Isoenzyme	*Substrate*	*Inhibitor*	*Inducer*
CYP3A4	Amlodipine (Norvasc®)	Clarithromycin (Biaxin®)	Carbamazepine (Tegretol®)
	Atorvastatin (Lipitor®)	Diltiazem (Cardizem®)	Dexamethasone (Decadron®)
	Diltiazem (Cardizem®)	Cyclosporine	Phenytoin (Dilantin®)
	Felodipine (Plendil®)	Erythromycin	Primidone (Mysoline®)
	Lovastatin (Mevacor®)	Fluconazole (Diflucan®)	Rifampin
	Nifedipine (Procardia)	Fluoxetine (Prozac®)	
	Simvastatin (Zocor®)	Grapefruit juice	
	Verapamil (Calan®)	Ketoconazole (Nizoral®)	
	R-Warfarin (Coumadin®)	Miconazole	
		Norfloxin (Noroxin®)	
		Protease inhibitors	
		Verapemil (Calan®)	
		Zafirlukast (Accolate®)	
CYP2C9	**Fluvastatin (Lescol®)**	Amiodarone (Cordarone®)	Carbamazepine (Tegretol®)
	Losartan (Cozaar®)	Cimetidine (Tagamet®)	Phenytoin (Dilantin®)
	Rosuvastatin (Crestor®)	Fluconazole (Diflucan®)	Rifampin
	S-Warfarin (Coumadin®)	Fluoxetine (Prozac®)	
		Fluvastatin (Lescol®)	
		Isoniazid	
		Ketoconazole (Nizoral®)	
		Metronidazole (Flagyl®)	
		Nateglitinide (Starlix®)	
		Omeprazole (Prilosec®)	
		Sertraline (Zoloft®)	
		Zafirlukast (Accolate®)	

Note: Drugs in bold are statins.

Sources: TA Jacobson, "NLA Task Force on statin safety—2014 update," *J Clin Lipidol* 8, Suppl 3 (2014): S1–4; R Talbert, "Dyslipidemia," in JT DiPiro, RL Talbert, GC Yee, et al, eds, *Pharmacotherapy: A Pathophysiologic Approach,* 8th ed. (New York: McGraw-Hill, 2011), 365–88.

Instructions

Statins can be taken with or without food in most cases. Educate patients on the signs and symptoms of SAMS, such as persistent bilateral muscle pain, stiffness, or weakness. Patients should disclose all medications, prescribed and over the counter, to their healthcare provider to reduce the risk of potential drug interactions with statins. Caution patients on consuming large amounts of grapefruit juice (more than 8 oz per day).

Selective Intestinal Absorption Inhibitors

The primary effect of selective intestinal absorption inhibitors is observed in the reduction of LDL-C and non-HDL-C; however, slight decreases in TGs and increases in HDL-C may also be noticed. Selective intestinal absorption inhibitors are used in combination with statins for dyslipidemia in persons with diabetes to enhance the lowering of LDL-C and reduce the burden of mortality and morbidity in high-risk patients with ASCVD.[9,22]

Mechanism of Action

Selective intestinal absorption inhibitors reduce cholesterol by selectively inhibiting its absorption from the small intestine. This results in a decreased delivery of cholesterol to the liver and a reduction of hepatic cholesterol stores, with an overall lowering of cholesterol, primarily LDL-C.[6]

Selective Intestinal Absorption Inhibitors: Dosage Information

Drug	*Trade Name*	*Common Dose*	*Common Frequency*
Ezetimibe	Zetia®	10 mg	Once daily
Ezetimibe/ Simvastatin	Vytorin®	10/10 mg 10/20 mg 10/40 mg	Once daily

Dosing

Both the initial and maintenance dosage is 10 mg once daily and may be used in conjunction with statins or bile acid resins. A combination product, ezetimibe/simvastatin (Vytorin®), is also available.

Pregnancy, Precautions, and Contraindications

Ezetimibe (Zetia®, Merck) is listed as Pregnancy Category C and should be avoided to reduce risks. Caution should be used in persons with hepatic dysfunction.[6]

Adverse Effects

Ezetimibe is generally well tolerated with minimal adverse effects. Common complaints are gastrointestinal issues, such as diarrhea and abdominal pain, as well as back pain, arthralgia, and sinusitis.[23]

Drug Interactions

Bile acid resins may interfere with absorption. Therefore, ezetimibe should be administered 1 hour before or 4 hours after the bile acid resins if used concurrently.[23]

Monitoring

A baseline lipid profile and liver function tests are reasonable prior to initiating therapy. When used concurrently with statins, liver enzymes should be monitored prior to and when clinically indicated thereafter. When used concurrently with fenofibrate, monitor for signs and symptoms of cholelithiasis.[23]

Instructions

Tablets can be taken with or without food. Statins can be taken at the same time as ezetimibe; however, bile acid resins must be separated, either 1 hour after or 4 hours before ezetimibe.

Proprotein Convertase Subtilisin/Kexin Type 9 (PCSK9) Inhibitors

The primary effect of PCSK9 inhibitors is observed in the reduction of LDL-C and non-HDL-C; however, slight decreases in TGs and increases in HDL-C may also be observed. PCSK9 inhibitors are generally only indicated for use in patients with familial hypercholesterolemia or patients with clinical ASCVD that require additional LDL-C lowering despite maximally tolerated statin.[9,24] While PCSK9 inhibitors are recommended as add-on therapy to statins, it is reasonable to use these agents in patients who are unable to tolerant statin therapy in the presence of familial hypercholesterolemia or clinical ASCVD.[9]

Mechanism of Action

PCSK9 is an enzyme that binds to the LDL receptor, preventing it from being recycled back to the surface of the hepatocyte. Thus, fewer LDL receptors are present on the surface of the hepatocyte to bring in LDL-C for degradation in the liver. PCSK9 inhibitors are monoclonal antibodies that bind to PCSK9 allowing the LDL-R to be recycled back to the surface of the hepatocyte, resulting in decreased levels of LDL-C.[25]

PCSK9 Inhibitors: Dosage Information

Drug	*Trade Name*	*Common Dose*	*Common Frequency*
Alirocumab	Praluent®	75–150 mg	Every 2 weeks
Evolocumab	Repatha®	140 mg 420 mg	Every 2 weeks Once monthly (use three 140-mg syringes)

Dosing

The recommended starting dose for alirocumab is 75 mg every 2 weeks. If additional LDL-C lowering is desired, the dose may be increased to 150 mg every 2 weeks. Evolocumab can be given as 140 mg every 2 weeks or 420 mg (3 syringes given at 1 time) once monthly. Both agents can be used in combination with a maximally tolerated statin.[23]

Pregnancy, Precautions, and Contraindications

There are no data available regarding the use of PCSK9 inhibitors during pregnancy. PCSK9 inhibitors should not be given to patients with a history of an allergic reaction to these agents.

Adverse Effects

PCSK9 inhibitors are generally well tolerated, with the most common adverse effect being injection site reactions. Other reported adverse effects include nasopharyngitis, influenza, and upper respiratory infections.[23]

Drug Interactions

There are no known clinically meaningful drug-drug interactions.

Monitoring

A baseline lipid profile should be conducted prior to initiating therapy and then repeated in 4 to 8 weeks.

Instructions

PCSK9 inhibitors can be administered using a single-use prefilled auto-injector or single-use prefilled syringe. Refrigeration is necessary until use, except for the evolocumab auto-injector, which is stable at room temperature for up to 30 days. After removing from the refrigerator, allow 30 minutes for the medication to warm before injecting; this will minimize discomfort. If an injection is missed and it has been less than 7 days, administer the missed dose and continue the same schedule.[23]

Fibric Acid Derivatives (Fibrates)

Fibrates exert their lipoprotein-lowering effects on TGs, with an additional benefit of increasing HDL-C and decreasing non-HDL-C. These agents are more commonly prescribed when elevations in fasting TGs ≥ 500 mg/dL are present. Although previously used concomitantly with statin therapy, fibrates are no longer indicated for use in combination with statins, considering the benefit does not seem to outweigh the risks.[9,26] There are data, however, showing that fenofibrate slows the progression of retinopathy in persons with diabetes.[1]

Mechanism of Action

Fibrates are most effective for decreasing VLDL and TG levels while raising HDL-C levels.[6] Although the mechanism of action is not clear, these agents can increase lipoprotein lipase, resulting in the breakdown of VLDL. Fibrates also decrease hepatic VLDL synthesis while enhancing the removal of TG-rich lipoproteins.

Fibrates: Dosage Information

Drug	*Trade Name*	*Common Dose*	*Common Frequency*
Fenofibrate	Tricor® Antara® Fenoglide® Lipofen® Lofibra® Triglide®	48–145 mg	Once daily
Gemfibrozil	Lopid®	600 mg	Twice daily

Dosing

Fibrates are generally administered once or twice daily, often prior to or with a meal. The dosage depends on the percentage of TG lowering needed to achieve normal levels of TG. However, initial therapy commonly starts with a low dose and can be titrated up every 4 to 8 weeks as necessary to reach the optimal or maximum dosage and to minimize adverse effects.[23]

Pregnancy, Precautions, and Contraindications

Fibrates are listed as Pregnancy Category C and should be avoided to reduce risks.[23] Caution and lower dosages should be used for patients with renal dysfunction and for the older adult. Preexisting gallbladder disease, hepatic dysfunction, and severe renal dysfunction are contraindications.[23]

Adverse Effects

Fibrates are generally well tolerated with minimal adverse reactions. Common adverse effects are gastrointestinal and include indigestion, nausea, diarrhea, flatulence, and abdominal pain. Rare adverse effects that have been reported are rash, fever, weight gain, muscle weakness, drowsiness, decreased potassium levels, anemia, and low white blood cell count. Myopathy and rhabdomyolysis have been seen in monotherapy but are more common in conjunction with statin therapy.[23]

Drug Interactions

Fibrates are highly protein bound and can increase the adverse reactions of medications that are also highly protein bound. Common protein-bound medications include warfarin, sulfonylureas, and meglitinides.[23]

Bile acid resins may impair absorption. Fibrates should be administered 1 hour before or 4 hours after the bile acid resins.

Monitoring

A lipid profile and liver enzymes should be measured prior to initiating fibrate therapy and as clinically warranted. Discontinue treatment when liver enzymes are greater than 3 times the upper limit of normal. Complete blood cell counts should also be monitored periodically during the first year of therapy. Monitor for hematologic changes such as decreased hemoglobin and hematocrit, thrombocytopenia, and neutropenia.[23] Renal function should also be evaluated at baseline, at 3 months, and every 6 months thereafter.[23] If concurrent therapy includes statins, sulfonylureas, warfarin, or bile acid resins, close monitoring for enhanced adverse reactions is warranted, especially for hypoglycemia and increased international normalized ratio (INR).[23,27]

Instructions

Gemfibrozil (Lopid®, Pfizer) should be taken 30 minutes prior to a meal. Fenofibrate (Tricor®, AbbVie, Inc) can be administered without regard to meals. Patients should be educated on the signs and symptoms of myopathy, such as persistent muscle or joint pain.

Omega-3 Fatty Acids

Lower TGs is the primary effect observed with omega-3 fatty acids, which include eicosapentaenoic acid (EPA) and docosahexaenoic acid (DHA). A dose-related increase in LDL-C levels has also been observed with omega-3-acid ethyl esters (Lovaza®) and omega carboxylic acids (Epanova®). However, 1 formulation of omega-3 fatty acids, icosapent ethyl (Vascepa®), contains only EPA and does not appear to increase LDL-C.[23]

Mechanism of Action

Omega-3 fatty acids are effective at lowering elevated TGs through a reduction in hepatic VLDL production. Omega-3 fatty acids reduce the quantity of free fatty acids available for TG synthesis, subsequently lowering VLDL synthesis and increasing lipoprotein lipase activity, which results in TG clearance.[6,28]

Dosing

The total daily dose of omega-3 fatty acids is generally 2 g to 4 g given in divided doses. Omega-3 fatty acids should be taken with food to minimize gastrointestinal adverse effects.[23]

Omega-3 Fatty Acids: Dosage Information

Drug	*Trade Name*	*Common Dose*	*Common Frequency*
Omega-3-acid ethyl esters	Lovaza®	2 g	Twice daily
Icosapent ethyl	Vascepa®	2 g	Twice daily
Omega carboxylic acids	Epanova®	1–2 g	Twice daily

Pregnancy, Precautions, and Contraindications

There are no adequate studies with pregnant women; therefore, omega-3 fatty acids should be avoided during pregnancy. Caution should be used in persons with renal or hepatic dysfunction, older adult patients, and those at high risk of hemorrhage. Avoid use in those with a fish allergy.[23]

Adverse Effects

Common adverse effects are dizziness and gastrointestinal effects, such as dyspepsia, nausea, and abdominal pain. Rare adverse effects of headache, pruritis, and hyperglycemia have been reported.[23]

Drug Interactions

Omega-3 fatty acids may decrease the production of thromboxane A_2, resulting in an increase in bleeding time, which may be problematic in those taking antiplatelets or anticoagulants.[23]

Monitoring

A baseline lipid profile should be performed prior to initiating omega-3 fatty acids therapy and repeated as clinically warranted.

Instructions

Omega-3 fatty acids should be taken with food to minimize adverse effects.

Bile Acid Resins

The primary lipoprotein affected by bile acid resins is LDL-C and non-HDL-C, with a secondary effect of a modest increase in HDL-C. Bile acid resins are not commonly prescribed in the treatment of dyslipidemia. They can induce severe hypertriglyceridemia when fasting TGs are ≥300 mg/dL, which is more commonly seen in persons with diabetes.[9] However, it should be noted that bile acid resins also modestly improve glycemic stability in persons with diabetes and may be used as adjunct therapy in select persons with diabetes.[1]

Mechanism of Action

Bile acid resins bind to bile acids in the intestinal lumen, thereby decreasing cholesterol production. They also inhibit enterohepatic circulation of bile acids and increase elimination of fecal acidic steroids, resulting in a decrease in LDL-C.[6,23]

Bile acid resins may increase TGs due to increased production of VLDL from the upregulation of cholesterol synthesis.

Bile Acid Resins: Dosage Information

Drug	*Trade Name*	*Common Dose*	*Common Frequency*
Cholestyramine	Questran®	4–16 g per day	1-g tablets, powder (1 scoop = 4 g)
Colesevelam	Welchol®	3.8–4.5 g per day	625-mg tablets
Colestipol	Colestid®	2–16 g per day	1-g tablets, powder (1 scoop = 5 g)

Dosing

Bile acid resins are available as a tablet and as a powder for dilution. Dosing can be once or twice daily. A low dose is recommended for initial therapy and can be titrated up every 4 to 8 weeks as necessary to reach optimal or maximum dose.[23]

Pregnancy, Precautions, and Contraindications

The safety of bile acid resins in pregnancy varies with the different agents. Colesevelam is listed as Pregnancy Category B, indicating no evidence of risk in humans, whereas cholestyramine and colestipol are listed as Category C, indicating risk cannot be ruled out.[23]

Bile acid resins are contraindicated when the TG level is ≥300 mg/dL and in primary biliary cirrhosis.

Caution should be used in persons with renal insufficiency, volume depletion, and chronic constipation. Bowel and biliary obstructions are contraindications.[23]

Adverse Effects

The adverse effects reported with bile acid resins are mostly gastrointestinal in nature, due to the lack of systemic absorption. The most common complaints are headache, unpalatable taste, nausea, bloating, flatulence, and constipation.[23]

Drug Interactions

Bile acid resins can bind to other medications, resulting in decreased absorption and clinically significant drug interactions. Therefore, it is recommended to separate bile acid resins from other medications by administering the other medications 1 hour before or 4 hours after the bile acid resins.[23]

Prolonged use of bile acid resins may result in decreased absorption of fat-soluble vitamins and folic acid.[23]

Monitoring

A baseline lipid profile with a follow-up at 4 to 6 weeks for efficacy is recommended for bile acid resins. This medication is not systemically absorbed and is considered safe overall, except, as noted above, in cases of high TGs. Electrolytes should be routinely checked, as imbalances have been reported. Prolonged use of bile acid resins may produce hyperchloremic acidosis. Due to the gastrointestinal discomfort associated with bile acid resins, the person with diabetes' monitoring engagement should be reviewed at each visit.

Instructions

Tablets should be swallowed whole and taken with plenty of liquid. Powder packets must be thoroughly diluted in liquid prior to consuming. Bile acid resins should be taken separately from other medications, either 1 hour after or 4 hours before.

Niacin

The primary lipoprotein effect of niacin is an increase in HDL-C, with a modest reduction in TGs and LDL-C. Niacin has been used historically in combination with statin therapy to maximize LDL-C lowering and improve HDL-C levels. However, recent data suggest this combination has no additional benefit and the risks may outweigh the potential benefit.[11,12] Thus, it is no longer recommended to use combined statin and niacin therapy.[9] The concept of raising serum HDL-C levels with drug therapy to reduce ASCVD risk has generally fallen out of favor. Niacin does remain an alternative for those individuals unable to tolerate statin therapy.

Mechanism of Action

Niacin reduces the catabolism of HDL and selectively decreases the excretion of HDL apo-A-1, stimulating reverse cholesterol transport in hepatic cells.[6,23] Additionally, niacin reduces hepatic VLDL production, resulting in a reduction of LDL-C, thereby lowering TG and LDL-C levels.

Niacin: Dosage Information

Drug	*Trade Name*	*Common Dose*	*Common Frequency*
Niacin sustained release	Niaspan®	500–1000 mg	Once daily
Nicotinic acid immediate release	Niacin®	100–1000 mg	1–3 times daily
Nicotinic acid sustained release	Slo-Niacin®	250 mg	Once or twice daily

Dosing

Niacin is available in immediate-release, sustained-release, and extended-release doses; these formulations should not be interchanged.

Immediate-release nicotinic acid is often preferred over sustained release for initial treatment, due to unfavorable adverse drug effects. Therapy should be started with small doses and titrated up as necessary and tolerable. Doses as low as 100 mg 3 times daily can be gradually increased to the maximum dose of 3 g per day in divided doses.[23]

Sustained-release nicotinic acid can be initiated at 250 mg twice daily and titrated up as tolerated to a maximum dose of 2 g per day, administered in a single or divided dose. Single doses can be given at bedtime with a low-fat snack.[23]

Pregnancy, Precautions, and Contraindications

Niacin is listed as Pregnancy Category C and should be avoided to reduce risks.[23]

Caution should be used in persons with preexisting gout, heavy alcohol use, or renal dysfunction.

Liver dysfunction, active peptic ulcer disease, and arterial bleeding are contraindications.

Adverse Effects

The adverse effects of niacin can be a limitation to its use. Common effects include headache; hypotension; and gastrointestinal discomfort, such as nausea, vomiting, and diarrhea; as well as the more notorious dermatological reactions of flushing, pruritis, and rash.[11,23] Flushing typically decreases with continuous use and can be reduced by taking niacin with meals. Aspirin taken once daily, 30 minutes prior to the niacin dose, can also minimize flushing.[23]

Patients on large doses of niacin, greater than 2 g per day, may be at increased risk of hepatotoxic effects. Significant elevation of liver enzymes can occur. Discontinue treatment when liver enzymes are greater than 3 times the upper limit of normal.[23]

Drug Interactions

Niacin is known to inhibit the release of insulin from the beta cell, resulting in hyperglycemia. This is especially notable in those newly diagnosed with type 2 diabetes and in those with prediabetes, in whom beta-cell production of insulin has not been diminished or exhausted.

Alcohol and hot drinks can increase flushing and pruritis effects. Rhabdomyolysis may occur when used in combination with statins.[23]

Monitoring

A baseline lipid profile, liver function, uric acid, and blood glucose levels should be performed prior to initiating niacin therapy and repeated at 6-week intervals while adjusting the dosage. Lipid profiles should be reviewed at 3- to 6-month intervals. Blood glucose levels should be monitored regularly, especially in those newly diagnosed or with prediabetes. Liver enzymes should also be monitored at 12-week intervals during the first year of treatment.[23]

Instructions

Niacin should be taken 30 minutes after an aspirin or with a low-fat snack to minimize flushing effects. Advise patients to avoid taking niacin with hot beverages or alcohol. Blood glucose levels need to be monitored to identify glycemic elevations. Educate patients on the signs and symptoms of myopathy, such as persistent muscle or joint pain, especially if they are concurrently on a statin.

Combination Therapies

Although statins are highly effective therapies for reducing LDL-C and ASCVD risk, there remains a high degree of risk for recurrent ASCVD events in many patients.[9] Therefore, non-statin therapies that have been shown to further reduce ASCVD risk when used in combination with maximally tolerated statin therapy are preferred over other non-statin agents.

Ezetimibe can provide up to an additional 25% reduction in LDL-C when combined with statin therapy and has been shown to also reduce ASCVD risk in patients with clinical ASCVD. The IMPROVE-IT study, a large randomized controlled trial that compared the combination of ezetimibe and simvastatin with simvastatin alone, was the first study to show a reduction in ASCVD events with combination therapy in patients after an acute coronary syndrome.[22] Most importantly, the benefit was more robust in those with diabetes. Ezetimibe is generically available, well tolerated, and easy to administer as it is orally administered once daily. Thus, ezetimibe is generally favored over other non-statins in patients needing additional LDL-C lowering.[9] In the rare event that a patient does not tolerate ezetimibe, a bile acid resin may be considered if the TG level is <300 mg/dL since bile acid resins can increase TGs.

Another option for patients requiring additional reduction in LDL-C are the PCSK9 inhibitors, alirocumab and evolocumab. When combined with statin therapy, these therapies can reduce LDL-C by up to an additional 60%.[9] Furthermore, the FOURIER[29] and ODYSSEY OUTCOMES[30] trials both demonstrated that evolocumab and alirocumab, respectively, reduce the risk of recurrent ASCVD events in high-risk patients with clinical ASCVD. Subgroup analyses have also suggested that patients with diabetes also benefit from these therapies. The main limitation to using PCSK9 inhibitors is cost as their original wholesale price was nearly $15,000/year, but this has recently been reduced to less than $6,000/year.[9,31] Although the value of PCSK9 inhibitors is improving, this class should generally be reserved for those unable to achieve an LDL-C below 70 mg/dL on maximally tolerated statin and ezetimibe.[9] The subcutaneous administration may also be a barrier for some patients.

In addition to lowering LDL-C, there has been considerable interest in using combination therapies in patients who also have elevated TG levels.[28] Until recently, nonstatin therapy had not convincingly been shown to reduce ASCVD risk when used in combination with statin therapy. The REDUCE-IT study demonstrated that adding 4 g per day of icosapent ethyl (Vascepa®), a high-dose prescription only omega-3 fatty acid, to statin therapy significantly reduced ASCVD events and cardiovascular-related death when compared to statin therapy alone.[32] Participants in this trial had to have a TG level between 150 and 499 mg/dL and an LDL-C between 41 and 100 mg/dL. Although this study was not published until after the 2018 AHA/ACC Cholesterol Guideline was released, the ADA updated their 2019 recommendations to include that icosapent ethyl should be considered in patients with ASCVD or other ASCVD risk factors on maximally tolerated statin with controlled LDL-C, but elevated triglycerides.[33]

Fibrates are not routinely recommended due to the lack of outcomes data showing the addition of a fibrate to a statin reduces ASCVD risk. However, fibrates may be considered in patients with very high TG levels, especially if >1000 mg/dL, to reduce the risk of acute pancreatitis.[9,28] Fenofibrate is preferred over gemfibrozil since it is less likely to increase the risk of SAMS compared to gemfibrozil.

Considerations for Managing Dyslipidemia in Persons with Diabetes

Treatment goals and strategies for dyslipidemia must be given equal emphasis and be as aggressive as those developed for hyperglycemia.

Primary Target

The primary lipoprotein target remains LDL-C; however, the indication to treat is not based solely on an individual's serum level of LDL-C but also ASCVD risk. Considering the burden of ASCVD risk observed in persons with diabetes, most will benefit from LDL-C lowering. Moderate-intensity statin therapy is indicated in nearly all individuals with diabetes, while high-intensity statins are reserved for those with clinical ASCVD or who have multiple ASCVD risk factors. Less emphasis is placed, however, on modifying levels of TG and HDL-C with drug therapy to achieve a desired level due to a lack of evidence to support such an approach. Combination therapy should be reserved for high-risk patients unable to achieve desired treatment goals or are unable to tolerate the recommended statin intensity.

Adding a medication to an existing regimen requires behavior change by the patient. Thus, the person's readiness to change, conviction, and confidence levels require assessment. This should be addressed when combination therapy is being considered, as some patients may not be willing to deal with the extra pill burden, additional costs, and risk for adverse effects. Any consideration of adding drug therapy to reduce ASCVD risk should involve a clinician-patient discussion of the risks and benefits.[9]

First-Line Therapy

Statins remain the initial drug of choice for persons with diabetes. In patients unable to tolerate any statin, nonstatin therapies shown to further reduce ASCVD risk (eg, ezetimibe, PCSK9 inhibitors, icosapent ethyl) may be considered as reasonable alternatives. Two or more lipid-lowering agents may be necessary for some patients.

Lipid profiles, adverse effects, as well as management by the persons with diabetes must be routinely monitored.

Hypertension

Blood pressure is the product of cardiac output (CO) and total peripheral resistance (TPR), where CO is the result of stroke volume and heart rate. The pathophysiology of hypertension in most people is a multifactorial process that occurs due to the body's inability to maintain the homeostasis between CO and TPR.[34]

Two important systems exist that work to maintain normal blood pressure: the autonomic nervous system and the renin-angiotensin-aldosterone system (RAAS).[34] Evidence suggests that the RAAS is part of the multifactorial progression of diabetes, CVD, and renal disease. Through RAAS inhibition, blood pressure is reduced and albuminuria can be reversed. Studies have also shown that RAAS inhibition can decrease ASCVD and slow progression of diabetes.[35,36]

Renin-Angiotensin-Aldosterone System

Understanding of the RAAS has evolved over the decades and continues to do so. The RAAS regulates the balance of fluid volume, electrolytes, and blood volume in the body. Changes in the RAAS result in changes in vascular tone and sympathetic nervous system activity.

Stimulation of the RAAS leads to vasoconstriction, sodium retention, smooth muscle proliferation, and increased antidiuretic hormone in the vasculature.[37–39] In the kidney, activation of the RAAS is associated with intraglomerular hypertension, a precursor of proteinuria. Endothelial cells line the glomerulus as well as the blood vessels and function as the gatekeeper for cardiovascular and renal systems.[38,39] Abnormal RAAS activity can impair endothelium-dependent vasodilation in persons with type 2 diabetes, resulting in decreased acetylcholine stimulation and enhanced oxidative stress.[38,39] These changes lead to insulin resistance, endothelial dysfunction, and microalbuminuria.

To briefly review, the RAAS begins with a release of renin, an enzyme synthesized in the kidney, in response to changes within or outside the kidney. Renin then acts on angiotensinogen, a hepatic peptide, to create angiotensin-I (AT-I). Angiotensin-converting enzyme (ACE), located in the pulmonary and vascular endothelium, converts AT-I to angiotensin-II (AT-II).[37–39] Angiotensin-converting enzyme converts approximately 30% of circulating AT-I to AT-II. Other enzymes, such as chymase, tonin, and cathepsin-G, are responsible for the remaining 70% of AT-II production.[39,40] This peptide, AT-II, binds to AT-I receptors, which are primarily in vascular and myocardial tissue, to increase vasoconstriction, sympathetic activity, and aldosterone secretion. These increases result in peripheral vascular resistance, vasoconstriction and increased heart rate, and fluid retention, respectively, which contribute to the development of hypertension.[38–40] Figure 20.2 summarizes this process.

Diagnosis: Hypertension

The 2017 multi-society guideline, led by the AHA and ACC, provided a comprehensive, evidence-based guideline for diagnosing and classifying patients with hypertension.[41] A major update in this guideline was the change in how blood pressure is classified.

Blood pressure is now classified into 4 stages: normal, elevated blood pressure (previously names prehypertension), stage 1 hypertension, and stage 2 hypertension.[41] Those with stage 1 hypertension should have their 10-year ASCVD risk calculated, and if the 10-year ASCVD risk is ≥10%, antihypertensive therapy plus lifestyle interventions should be considered. For those with a 10-year ASCVD risk <10%, only lifestyle interventions are appropriate. In patients with stage 1 hypertension who have clinical ASCVD, antihypertensive therapy is warranted and ASCVD risk calculation is unnecessary. Table 20.4 lists the criteria for each stage and Figure 20.3 provides a summary of treatment recommendations.

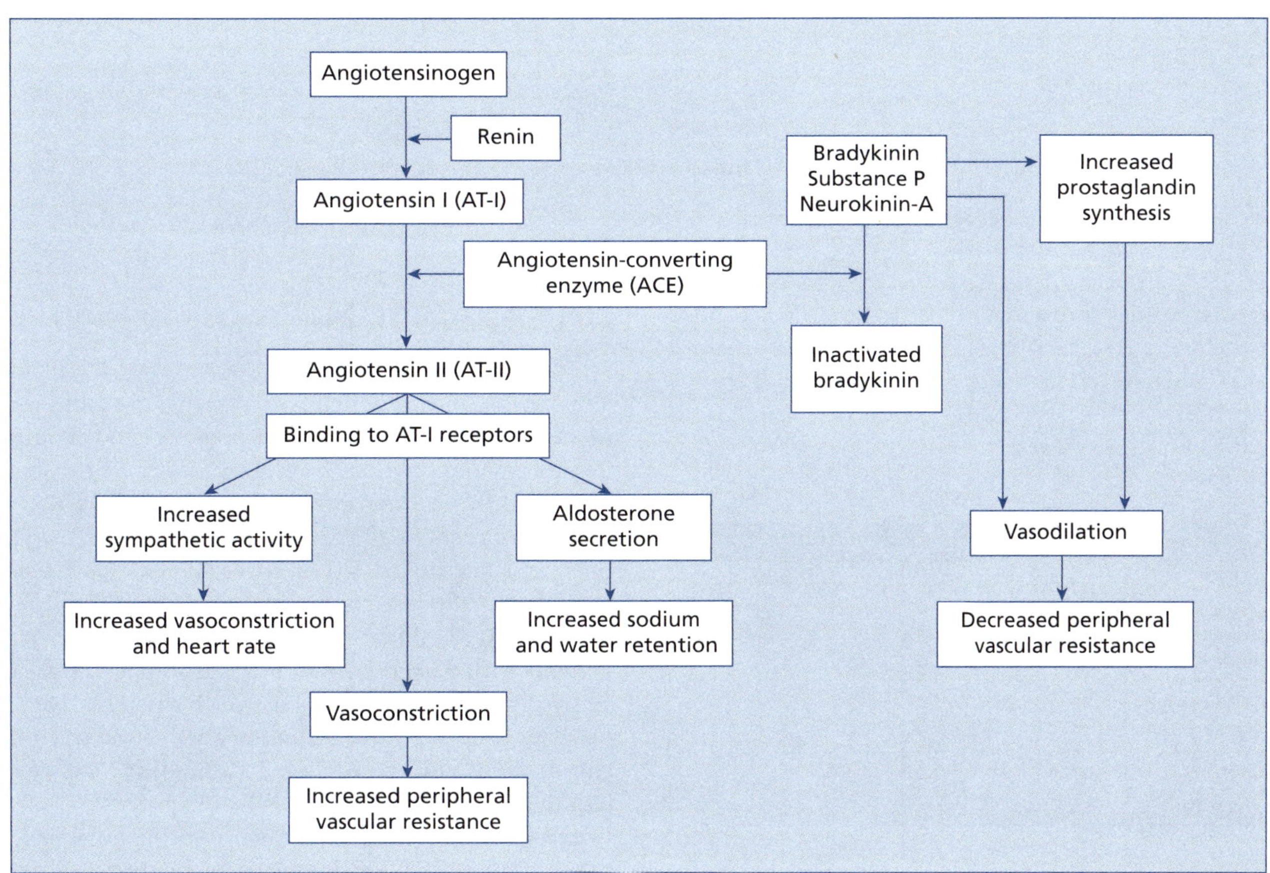

FIGURE 20.2 **Renin-Angiotensin-Aldosterone System**

Sources: BL Carter, JJ Saseen, "Hypertension," in JT Dipiro, RL Talbert, GC Yee, GR Matzke, BG Wells, LM Posey, eds, *Pharmacotherapy: A Pathophysiologic Approach*, 6th ed. (New York: McGraw-Hill, 2005), 185–218; BL Carter, "Management of Essential Hypertension," in *Pharmacotherapy Self-Assessment Program Book 1: Cardiovascular I*, 4th ed. (Kansas City, Mo: American College of Clinical Pharmacy, 2001), 1–39; EJ Jacobsen, "Hypertension: update on use of angiotensin II receptor blockers," *Geriatrics* 56, no. 2 (2001): 25–8.

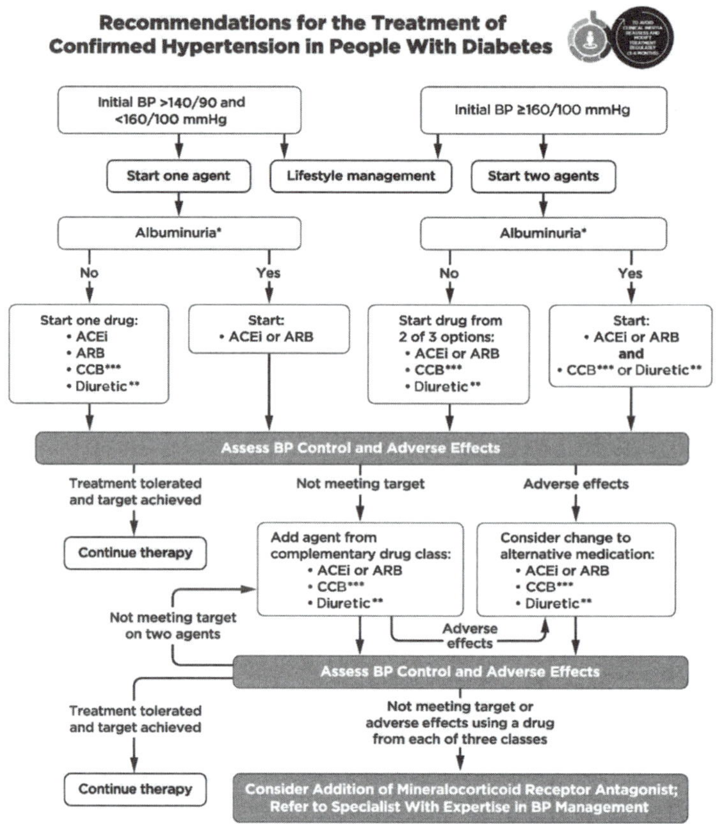

FIGURE 20.3 **Recommendations for the Treatment of Confirmed Hypertension in People with Diabetes**

Sources: American Diabetes Association, "Standards of medical care in diabetes—2020," *Diabetes Care.* 43, Suppl 1 (2020): S111-134.

Diagnosis and classification of hypertension is determined from the average of ≥2 blood pressure readings obtained from ≥2 separate clinic visits; it is measured using an appropriately sized cuff with the person in a seated position, after a ≥5-minute rest.[41]

TABLE 20.4 Classification of Hypertension in Adults

Stage	*Systolic Pressure (mm Hg)*	*Diastolic Pressure (mm Hg)*
Normal	<120 *and*	<80
Elevated blood pressure	120–129 *and*	<80
Stage 1 hypertension	130–139 *or*	80–89
Stage 2 hypertension	≥140 *or*	≥90

Source: Whelton PK, Carey RM, Aronow WS, et al, "2017 ACC/AHA/AAPA/ABC/ACPM/AGS/APhA/ASH/ASPC/NMA/PCNA Guideline for the Prevention, Detection, Evaluation, and Management of High Blood Pressure in Adults," *J Am Coll Cardiol.* 71 (2018)(19):127–248.

2017 AHA/ACC Multi-Society High Blood Pressure Guideline

This guideline redefined hypertension and recommended vastly different blood pressure goals compared to previous guidelines. A primary driver of this change was SPRINT, a randomized controlled study that randomized patients ≥50 years of age with hypertension and other risk factors to either an intensive blood pressure goal of <120/80 mmHg or a standard blood pressure goal of <140/90 mmHg.[42] Importantly, this study excluded patients with diabetes. The study was stopped early due to an overwhelming benefit observed in the intensive blood pressure control group, including a reduction in all-cause and cardiovascular mortality, and incident cases of heart failure. Serious adverse effects (eg, hypotension, electrolyte abnormalities, acute kidney injury), however, were more common in the intensive blood pressure control group. Given the variation in methods used to measure blood pressure in SPRINT compared to routine clinical practice, the guideline writing committee settled on a blood pressure goal of <130/80 mmHg for all patients with hypertension, including those with diabetes.[41]

Although SPRINT did not directly inform what the blood pressure goal should be in patients with diabetes, additional analyses have helped address this issue. The ACCORD-BP trial did specifically look at intensive versus standard blood pressure management in a diabetes population; however, there was no difference in outcomes between the two groups.[43] This was largely attributed to the study likely not enrolling enough patients to show a difference. After SPRINT was published, a post-hoc subgroup analysis of the ACCORD-BP trial was performed that included only those with diabetes who had a 10-year risk score of ≥10%.[44] Intensive blood pressure management reduced cardiovascular outcomes compared to standard blood pressure management, suggesting those with diabetes and additional cardiovascular risk factors benefit from more intensive blood pressure lowering compared to lower risk patients without additional cardiovascular risk factors. Meta-analyses of randomized controlled trials evaluating blood pressure targets for patients with diabetes have found similar results.[41]

Hypertension Goal – Guideline Comparison

ADA Standards of Care 2020[1]

In adults with diabetes, the recommended blood pressure goal is based on the individual's cardiovascular risk. If the 10-year ASCVD risk exceeds 15%, the recommended blood pressure goal is <130/80 mmHg; however, if the 10-year ASCVD risk is <15%, the recommended blood pressure goal is <140/90 mmHg.[1]

2017 AHA/ACC Multi-Society High Blood Pressure Guideline[41]

This guideline also recommends ASCVD risk assessment in all patients with diabetes and hypertension; however, the writing committee also believes that the majority of patients with diabetes will have a 10-year ASCVD risk ≥10%. Thus, placing patients with diabetes at high risk of ASCVD warranting a more intensive blood pressure goal of <130/80 mmHg.

Treatment strategies for hypertension often require combination therapy that targets different mechanisms to obtain optimal levels in blood pressure.

Children and Adolescents

Updated guidelines on the diagnosis and management of hypertension in pediatric patients was published in 2017.[45] This guideline reiterates that having hypertension in childhood greatly increases the likelihood of hypertension in adulthood. Like the adult guidelines, the term "prehypertension" was replaced with "elevated blood pressure" and new normative blood pressure tables were developed according to age, sex, and height percentile. Blood pressure should be measured at every routine visit beginning at 3 years of age, and those children noted to have elevated blood pressure or hypertension should have their blood pressure repeated and confirmed on 3 separate days.[45] Ambulatory blood pressure monitoring is also highly recommended to confirm a diagnosis of hypertension. Hypertension in childhood is defined as an average systolic or diastolic blood pressure ≥95th percentile for age, sex, and height percentile.

Treatment in Children and Adolescents

Lifestyle modifications are key in managing hypertension in this population; however, pharmacotherapy should not be withheld if blood pressure remains elevated after lifestyle modifications or if the hypertension is associated with diabetes or chronic kidney disease. Optimal blood pressure in these patients is <90th percentile for age, sex, and height percentile, or <130/80 mmHg in adolescents ≥13 years of age.[45]

Like most adults with diabetes, the pharmacologic treatment of hypertension should begin with an angiotensin-converting enzyme inhibitor (ACEI) or angiotensin receptor blocker (ARB). Long-acting calcium channel blockers and thiazide diuretics may be considered if single drug therapy is not sufficient to achieve optimal blood pressure. Reproduction counseling may be necessary in females of childbearing age because of teratogenicity associated with ACEIs and ARBs.

Pharmacotherapy: Hypertension

Lifestyle modification should always be a standard treatment of hypertension in addition to pharmacotherapy. Medical nutrition therapy, increased activity, moderation of alcohol consumption, and modest weight reduction can have beneficial effects on blood pressure.[41] See chapter 16's discussion of the role of nutrition therapy in hypertension prevention and management.

Classes of Antihypertensive Agents

Many classes of antihypertensive agents target different mechanisms in the treatment of hypertension (see Table 20.5).[41] However, several classes are preferred and traditionally used as first-line therapy because of their blood pressure–lowering and/or renal-protection effects in people with diabetes.[1,41] The benefit of medications that target the RAAS is their ability to delay the progression of albuminuria and chronic kidney disease; however, evidence in those without albuminuria at baseline and the African-American population is limited. As such, an ACEI or ARB is recommended as first-line therapy only in individuals with albuminuria.[1] For all other adults with diabetes, first-line therapies include ACEIs, ARBs, thiazides, and calcium channel blockers. Other drug classes (eg, beta-blockers) may be preferred first-line therapies in the setting of other comorbidities (eg, heart failure).[1]

Standard Treatment

Hypertension—Standard treatment of hypertension includes pharmacotherapy plus lifestyle modifications: MNT, increased activity, moderation of alcohol consumption, and modest weight reduction.

TABLE 20.5 Classes of Antihypertensive Medications

Classes
Angiotensin-converting enzyme inhibitors
Angiotensin II receptor blockers
α1-Receptor blockers
β-Blockers
Combined α- and β-receptor blockers
Calcium channel blockers
Central-acting α-adrenergic agonists
Direct Renin Inhibitors
Diuretics
Thiazide
Loop
Potassium-sparing
Carbonic anhydrase inhibitors
Vasodilators

Note: Classes listed in bold are preferred in persons with diabetes who have albuminuria.

Diuretics

Diuretics are clinically classified based on their mechanism and/or site of action. There are 4 types: thiazide-type, loop, potassium-sparing, and carbonic anhydrase inhibitors. Carbonic anhydrase inhibitors, however, are not used in the treatment of essential hypertension. Baseline renal function and serum potassium are important factors in determining the initial choice of diuretic.

Thiazide-Type Diuretics

Thiazide-type diuretics remain as options for first-line therapy for uncomplicated hypertension and in persons with concomitant diabetes, especially African Americans.[41] Hydrochlorothiazide (HCTZ) is the most frequently prescribed diuretic for the treatment of hypertension alone. In fact, many hypertensive drugs have HCTZ coformulations, in which HCTZ is combined with a drug from the same or another class, such as an ACEI or an ARB. Some examples of coformulations include Hyzaar® (ARB with HCTZ; Merck), Prinizide® (ACEI with HCTZ; Merck), and Aldactazide® (potassium-sparing diuretic with HCTZ; Pfizer).

Chlorthalidone is another thiazide-type diuretic that has been used more in recent years. In fact, a combination product, Edarbyclor® (Takeda), is now available that includes an ARB (azilsartan) and chlorthalidone. The reason for this change is that several landmark clinical trials used chlorthalidone-based regimens instead of HCTZ.[41] Chlorthalidone is also more potent than HCTZ and provides better 24-hour blood pressure stability. However, these characteristics of chlorthalidone increase the potential for electrolyte abnormalities, especially hypokalemia.

Thiazide diuretics are also used when treating hypertension with compelling indications. They can be used as monotherapy and in combination in the management of heart failure, recurrent stroke prevention, and diabetes and in individuals at high ASCVD risk.[41]

Potassium-Sparing Diuretics: Dosage Information

Drug	*Trade Name*	*Common Dose*	*Common Frequency*
Amiloride	Midamor®	5–10 mg	Once daily
Triamterene	Dyrenium®	37.5–75 mg	Once daily
Spironolactone	Aldactone®	25–50 mg	Once or twice daily
Eplerenone	Inspra®	50 mg	Once or twice daily

Loop Diuretics

Loop diuretics are often employed when the person's glomerular filtration rate (GFR) falls below 30 mL per minute or the person needs greater diuresis due to another disease state (eg, heart failure). Thiazide-type diuretics (except metolazone) are relatively ineffective when GFR falls below 30 mL per minute. Reduced GFR allows more opportunity for sodium and water reabsorption to occur.[34]

Potassium-Sparing Diuretics

As their name implies, potassium-sparing diuretics prevent the loss of potassium that commonly occurs with fluid loss, thus resulting in a net gain in serum potassium levels. Potassium-sparing diuretics are combined with a thiazide-type diuretic to balance serum potassium.[34] Individually, amiloride and triamterene do little to lower blood pressure. Aldosterone antagonists, however, are effective at lowering blood pressure and should be considered in those individuals failing to reach a blood pressure goal of <130/80 mm Hg on ≥3 other antihypertensives.[41,46]

Loop Diuretics: Dosage Information			
Drug	*Trade Name*	*Common Dose*	*Common Frequency*
Furosemide	Lasix®	20–40 mg	Once or twice daily
Torsemide	Demadex®	5–10 mg	Once daily
Bumetanide	Bumex®	0.5–2 mg	Once or twice daily

Mechanisms of Action

The various types of diuretics exert their effects on different areas of the kidney. Thiazide-type diuretics inhibit the Na^+/Cl^- symporter on the distal convoluted tubule of the nephron, whereas loop diuretics inhibit the $Na^+/K^+/2Cl^-$ symporter on the ascending limb of the loop of Henle.[34,37] These inhibitions increase the urinary excretion of sodium, chloride, potassium, and water. Initially, the decrease in blood pressure from diuretics is due to a decreased cardiac output because of decreased blood volume. With chronic use, the blood pressure reduction is not a result of diuresis. Cardiac output normalizes, and the blood pressure reduction becomes a result of decreased peripheral vascular resistance.[34,37]

The mechanism of potassium-sparing diuretics is more complicated. Potassium-sparing diuretics inhibit the absorption of Na^+ and the excretion of K^+ in the principal cells of the late distal tubule and collecting duct.[34] Amiloride and triamterene inhibit the luminal Na^+ channels of the principal cell. Spironolactone and eplerenone are antagonists at aldosterone receptors on the principal cell.[34]

Dosing

Diuretics are generally taken once daily in the morning. The rationale for morning dosing is that people prefer to deal with the increased frequency of urination from diuretics during the day rather than during the night. However, some potassium-sparing and loop diuretics may require twice daily dosing to maintain sufficient diuresis for conditions other than hypertension (eg, heart failure).[23] A low dose is recommended for the initial therapy and can be titrated up if necessary. When solely treating hypertension, high doses have not shown any additional benefit of further decreasing blood pressure when compared with low doses.[47]

Pregnancy, Precautions, and Contraindications

Diuretic safety in pregnancy varies with the different agents. Most are Category C, where risk cannot be ruled out; however, HCTZ, torsemide, eplerenone, indapamide, and metolazone are listed as Category B, indicating there is no evidence of risk in humans. The ADA standards recommend against the use of chronic diuretic management because it is associated with restricted maternal plasma volume and decreased perfusion, potentially causing birth defects.[1] Reference to the packet insert of the individual diuretic is always recommended.

Caution should be used when treating persons with preexisting gout or uric acid stone disease, severe renal impairment, hepatic dysfunction, or electrolyte imbalances.[41]

Thiazide-type diuretics (except metolazone) should be used with caution in persons with a known hypersensitivity to sulfonamides. The absolute risk of cross-sensitivity in a sulfa-allergic patient is not well established. However, extreme caution is advised in patients with a documented allergic reaction.[23]

The sodium-glucose co-transporter 2 (SGLT2) inhibitors also reduce blood pressure and act as an osmotic diuretic.[1] Thus, patients receiving both diuretics and SGLT2 inhibitors should be monitored closely to ensure adequate volume status and to avoid hypotension.

Adverse Effects

Adverse effects associated with diuretics, such as hypokalemia, hypomagnesemia, hyperuricemia, hyperglycemia, hyperlipidemia, and hyper/hypocalcemia, are often associated with changes in serum electrolytes. Signs and symptoms of these imbalances are muscle cramps, fatigue, dizziness, and cardiac arrthymias.[23] Other common adverse effects include headache, photosensitivity, dry mouth, taste alterations, nausea, vomiting, impotence, and orthostatic hypotension.[23]

Drug Interactions

Since diuretics increase the excretion of sodium and potassium, many drug interactions stem from changes in electrolytes. Significant interactions include nonsteroidal anti-inflammatory drugs (NSAIDs), which can decrease the antihypertensive efficacy of diuretics.[46] Diuretics can substantially increase lithium levels by decreasing lithium's elimination; therefore, lithium levels should be monitored 5 to 7 days after starting or discontinuing a diuretic.[23] Also, high sodium intake can decrease the effectiveness of diuretics.

Thiazide diuretics are known to inhibit the release of insulin from the beta cell, resulting in hyperglycemia. This is especially notable in persons newly diagnosed with type 2 diabetes or with prediabetes, where beta-cell production of insulin has not been diminished or exhausted. In general, this disease interaction is clinically insignificant at lower doses, such as less than 25 mg of HCTZ daily.[48]

Monitoring

Baseline blood pressure, serum electrolytes, uric acid, glucose, and lipids should be measured prior to initiating therapy and periodically thereafter. Potassium and magnesium supplementation may be required in some patients.[41] When diuretics are combined with other antihypertensive agents, monitoring for hypotension is warranted.

Instructions

Diuretics should be taken in the morning, with or without food. Intake of foods high in potassium, such as bananas or strawberries, can help maintain adequate potassium levels. Blood pressure must be monitored daily to identify elevations and patterns. Blood glucose levels need to be monitored to identify possible glycemic elevations from the diuretic. Patients should be educated on signs and symptoms of hypokalemia, such as muscle cramps and fatigue. To avoid episodes of orthostatic hypotension, patients should be reminded to rise slowly from lying or seated positions.

Angiotensin-Converting Enzyme Inhibitors

An ACEI is traditionally used as first-line or preferred therapy for hypertension and renal protection in persons with diabetes.[35,37,39] An ACEI can delay the progression of albuminuria, but is less efficacious in reducing blood pressure when used as single agents in African-Americans. There are also no studies showing ACEI improve renal outcomes in diabetes patients without albuminuria.

Angiotensin-converting enzyme inhibitors are also beneficial in the treatment of hypertension with compelling indications, such as heart failure, post-myocardial infarction, recurrent stroke prevention, and chronic kidney disease.[35]

Angiotensin-Converting Enzyme Inhibitors: Dosage Information

Drug	*Trade Name*	*Common Dose*	*Common Frequency*
Benazepril	Lotensin®	10–40 mg	Once daily
Captopril	Capoten®	12.5–50 mg	2 or 3 times daily
Enalapril	Vasotec®	2.5–20 mg	Once or twice daily
Fosinopril	Monopril®	10–40 mg	Once daily
Lisinopril	Prinivil® Zestril®	10–40 mg	Once daily
Moexipril	Univasc®	7.5–30 mg	Once daily
Perindopril	Aceon®	4–8 mg	Once daily
Quinapril	Accupril®	10–80 mg	Once daily
Ramipril	Altace®	2.5–20 mg	Once daily
Trandolapril	Mavik®	1–4 mg	Once daily

Mechanism of Action

Angiotensin-converting enzyme inhibitors inhibit the formation of AT-II by blocking the conversion of AT-I to AT-II. Additionally, ACEI block the action of kinase, the enzyme that converts bradykinin, substance P, and neurokinin-A to inactive ingredients, thereby increasing their concentrations. The increase in bradykinin stimulates the release of nitric oxide, a vasodilator.[35,37,39]

Dosing

Angiotensin-converting enzyme inhibitors are generally administered 1 to 3 times daily, with or without food. Once-daily dosing can be in the morning or evening, based on patient preference and adverse effects such as drowsiness. However, taking the medication at the same time every day is important. The presence of food may affect the absorption of captopril and moexipril, and dosing prior to a meal may be warranted.[23] Adding a thiazide diuretic is usually more beneficial at lowering blood pressure than increasing to the maximum dosage of the ACEI.[41] Angiotensin-converting enzyme inhibitors are often co-formulated with low-dose HCTZ (6.25-25 mg) to enhance blood pressure reduction and improve the person with diabetes' medicaton taking.

Pregnancy, Precautions, and Contraindications

Angiotensin-converting enzyme inhibitors are contraindicated during pregnancy. Use in the second or third trimester can lead to fetal injury or death.

Angiotensin-converting enzyme inhibitors are also contraindicated in persons with bilateral renal artery stenosis or unilateral stenosis of a single, functional kidney. They cause dilation of the efferent arteriole in the renal circulation, which can substantially reduce GFR and result in acute renal failure.

Caution should be used in patients with a history of renal and/or hepatic dysfunction, angioedema, heart failure, and hyperkalemia.[47]

In African-American patients, ACEIs are often less effective at lowering blood pressure due to low renin levels common to this ethnic group.[49] Coadministration of thiazide diuretics is often sufficient to overcome the low renin levels and return observed blood pressure lowering with ACEIs to that of the general population. African Americans are also more likely to experience angioedema and should be appropriately counseled prior to initiating therapy.

Adverse Effects

Overall, ACEIs are well tolerated with few side effects, especially if monitored appropriately. The most common adverse effect, and often the reason for discontinuation of ACEIs, is cough. This adverse effect is primarily due to the increase in bradykinin activity that increases prostaglandin synthesis and is more commonly observed in African and Asian Americans.[41]

Other adverse effects commonly associated with ACEIs include fatigue, headache, dizziness, drowsiness, hyperkalemia, acute hypotension, and gastrointestinal problems, such as diarrhea, nausea, and vomiting. Skin rash, taste disturbances, angioedema, and hematologic effects, such as neutropenia and agranulocytosis, have also been reported.[23]

Drug Interactions

Concurrent use of NSAIDs, potassium-sparing diuretics, and potassium supplements may increase potassium levels significantly. Angiotensin-converting enzyme inhibitors can increase lithium levels, due to decreased fluid volume and loss of sodium ions; therefore, close monitoring of lithium levels is recommended.[23]

Monitoring

Blood pressure, serum electrolytes, and renal function should ideally be measured at baseline and 10 to 14 days after initiating treatment. Monthly follow-up, however, is recommended by most practice guidelines and is likely more practical in routine clinical practice.

Changes in renal function can occur with the use of ACEIs; this is more common in patients with preexisting renal dysfunction. Kidney function should be closely monitored throughout treatment and especially during dose titration. Discontinuation of the ACEI is not always necessary, provided the patient is being monitored and assessed closely.[41]

Instructions

Angiotensin-converting enzyme inhibitors should be taken at the same time each day. If the patient experiences drowsiness or dizziness, taking the medication in the evening can minimize these effects when the patient is awake. Monitor blood pressure daily to identify elevations and patterns. Patients who develop a persistent cough within the first few months of initial therapy should discuss this with their healthcare provider at their next clinic visit. To avoid episodes of orthostatic hypotension, patients should be reminded to rise slowly from lying or seated positions.

Angiotensin Receptor Blockers

Angiotensin receptor blockers can be beneficial for persons with diabetes because these medications lower blood pressure and have nephroprotective and cardioprotective effects.[1] Angiotensin receptor blockers are traditionally prescribed when ACEI therapies are not tolerated; however, ARBs are now considered an alternative to ACEI therapy for initial blood pressure lowering.[1,41] Similar to ACEIs, ARBs may have reduced efficacy when used as single agents in African-Americans; however, ARBs may be better tolerated since they are less likely to cause cough or angioedema.[41] Additional compelling indications for which ARBs are used as monotherapy or in combination include heart failure and chronic kidney disease.[41] Despite their compelling evidence in monotherapy, combination ACEI and ARB therapy is not recommended in patients with diabetes.[1]

Mechanism of Action

Angiotensin receptor blockers inhibit AT-II release by blocking the AT-I receptor, causing a reduction in AT-II mediated effects, including aldosterone secretion, vasoconstriction, and sympathetic activity.[34,39]

Angiotensin Receptor Blockers: Dosage Information

Drug	*Trade Name*	*Common Dose*	*Common Frequency*
Azilsartan	Edarbi®	40–80 mg	Once daily
Candesartan	Atacand®	8–32 mg	Once daily
Eprosartan	Teveten®	600 mg	Once daily
Irbesartan	Avapro®	150–300 mg	Once daily
Losartan	Cozaar®	25–100 mg	Once daily
Olmesartan	Benicar®	20–40 mg	Once daily
Telmisartan	Micardis®	20–80 mg	Once daily
Valsartan	Diovan®	80–320 mg	Once daily*

*Dose divided and given 2 times daily if patient also has heart failure.

Dosing

Angiotensin receptor blockers are generally administered once daily and can be dosed in the morning or evening, based on patient preference and adverse effects such as drowsiness. However, taking the medication at the same time every day is important. Initial therapy often starts with a low dose and can be titrated up as tolerated. Adding a thiazide diuretic is usually more beneficial at lowering blood pressure than increasing the dosage of ARBs.[41]

Angiotensin receptor blockers are often co-formulated with low-dose HCTZ (6.25-25 mg) to enhance blood pressure reduction and improve the person with diabetes' medicaton taking.

Pregnancy, Precautions, and Contraindications

Angiotensin receptor blockers are listed as Pregnancy Category C for the first trimester of pregnancy and Category D for the second and third trimesters; therefore, ARBs should be avoided in pregnancy.

They are also contraindicated in persons with bilateral renal artery stenosis or unilateral stenosis of a single functional kidney.[23] Caution should be used in persons with renal and/or hepatic dysfunction, angioedema, and/or heart failure.

Adverse Effects

Angiotensin receptor blockers are generally well tolerated with minimal side effects. Common adverse effects associated with this class of antihypertensive agents include dizziness, drowsiness, diarrhea, dyspepsia, hyperkalemia, headache, and upper respiratory complaints, such as infection, pharyngitis, rhinitis, and cough. However, the frequency of cough associated with ARBs is significantly less than that with ACEIs.[41]

Drug Interactions

Concurrent use of potassium-sparing diuretics, potassium supplements, or salt substitutes may increase serum potassium levels significantly. Increases in serum creatinine in persons with heart failure have also been reported. Angiotensin receptor blockers can increase lithium levels due to decreased fluid volume and loss of sodium ions; therefore, close monitoring of lithium levels is recommended.[23]

Monitoring

Similar to ACEIs, blood pressure, serum electrolytes, and renal function should ideally be measured at baseline and 10 to 14 days after initiating treatment. Monthly follow-up, however, is recommended by most practice guidelines and is likely more practical in routine clinical practice.

Changes in renal function can occur with the use of ARBs; this is more common in patients with preexisting renal dysfunction. Kidney function should be closely monitored throughout treatment and especially during dose titration. Discontinuation of the ARB is not always necessary, provided the patient is being monitored and assessed closely.[41]

Instructions

Angiotensin receptor blockers should be taken at the same time each day. If the patient experiences drowsiness or dizziness, taking the medication in the evening can minimize these effects when the patient is awake. Blood pressure needs to be monitored daily to identify elevations and patterns. To avoid episodes of orthostatic hypotension, patients should be reminded to rise slowly from lying or seated positions.

Direct Renin Inhibitors

Direct renin inhibitors (DRIs) lower blood pressure and have renal-protective benefits in people with diabetes. Despite these benefits, their place in therapy remains unclear following publication of results from the Aliskiren Trial in Type 2 Diabetes Using Cardiovascular and Renal Disease Endpoints Including 12 Month Safety Follow-up Off-treatment (ALTITUDE).[50] This study compared the effects of aliskiren versus placebo when added to ARBs or ACEIs. The trial was stopped prematurely due to lack of benefit with the aliskiren combination and an increase in adverse events that included nonfatal stroke, renal complications, hyperkalemia, and hypotension. The FDA-approved labeling for aliskiren was subsequently changed in 2012 to warn against using aliskiren in combination with ARBs or ACEIs for people with diabetes or decreased kidney function.

Mechanism of Action

Direct renin inhibitors block RAAS at the point of activation to inhibit the conversion of angiotensinogen to AT-1, thereby reducing plasma renin activity and lowering blood pressure.[51]

Direct Renin Inhibitors: Dosage Information

Drug	*Trade Name*	*Common Dose*	*Common Frequency*
Aliskiren	Tekturna®	150–300 mg	Once daily

Dosing

Direct renin inhibitors are taken once daily, and though they can be taken with or without food, high-fat meals may decrease absorption. Initial therapy often starts with a low dose and can be titrated up as tolerated. The addition of an ARB or thiazide diuretic has been shown to be beneficial in lowering blood pressure. Direct renin inhibitors are combined with HCTZ (12.5–25 mg), amlodipine, and valsartan to enhance blood pressure reduction and improve the person with medicaton taking.[51]

Pregnancy, Precautions, and Contraindications

Direct renin inhibitors are contraindicated during pregnancy and should be discontinued as soon as pregnancy is detected. Use in the first, second, or third trimester can lead to fetal injury, as DRIs act directly on the RAAS.[51]

Caution should be used in patients with moderate to severe renal dysfunction or with a history of or currently on dialysis. Additionally, volume and sodium depletion should be reviewed and corrected prior to starting therapy and closely monitored if needed. Coadministration with potassium-sparing diuretics or potassium supplements should be avoided if possible.[51]

Use of DRIs (alone or in combination with ACEIs or ARBs) in people with diabetes has been associated with increased risk of renal impairment, hypotension, and hyperkalemia. Furthermore, DRIs are contraindicated in people with diabetes who are also taking an ACEI or ARB.[51]

Adverse Effects

Direct renin inhibitors are well tolerated and have minimal adverse effects. They may produce a cough because of the increase in bradykinin, but it is notably less frequent than that produced by ACEIs. Diarrhea, dizziness, drowsiness, headache, rash, edema, elevated uric acid levels, and hypotension have been reported.[51]

Drug Interactions

Aliskiren is metabolized in the liver by the cytochrome P-450 3A4 isoenzyme. Concurrent medications that are also metabolized through this system should be used cautiously, and aliskiren should be monitored for increased or decreased levels and risk of adverse reactions. Agents that have demonstrated notable increases in aliskiren include atorvastatin, ketoconazole, cyclosporine, and verapamil. Decreases in aliskiren levels were noted with irbesartan.[51]

Monitoring

As with other RAAS blood pressure–lowering agents, blood pressure, serum electrolytes, and renal function should be measured at baseline and 10 to 14 days after initiating DRI treatment.

Instructions

Direct renin inhibitors should be taken daily and as close to the same time as possible. Though DRIs can be taken with or without food, they should not be taken with a high-fat meal. If drowsiness occurs, aliskiren can be taken in the evening. Patients should monitor their blood pressure regularly. For the most part, DRIs are well tolerated in terms of adverse effects; however, patients should immediately report any swelling of the face, lips, tongue, throat, arms, or legs, or of the whole body, as angioedema is a rare adverse effect that can happen at any time while taking aliskiren.[51]

Beta-Blockers

Beta-blockers are commonly prescribed as an addition to an existing hypertension treatment plan for persons with diabetes. They are traditionally not first-line or preferred treatment for persons with diabetes, but they may be a second or third option. Beta-blockers are beneficial for persons with ASCVD. In addition to reducing hypertension, beta-blockers are indicated for persons at high risk of coronary disease and for prevention of a second MI and heart failure.

Beta 1–Selective Receptor Blockers: Dosage Information

Drug	*Trade Name*	*Common Dose*	*Common Frequency*	*Lipid Solubility*
Acebutolol*	Sectral®*	200–400 mg	Twice daily	Low
Atenolol	Tenormin®	25–100 mg	Once daily	Low
Betaxolol	Kerlone®	5–20 mg	Once daily	Low
Bisoprolol	Zebeta®	2.5–10 mg	Once daily	Low
Metoprolol tartrate	Lopressor®	25–50 mg	Once or twice daily	Moderate
Metoprolol succinate	Toprol XL®	25–100 mg	Once daily	Moderate
Nebivolol	Bystolic®	2.5–40 mg	Once daily	High

*Agents with intrinsic sympathomimetic activity.

Nonselective Beta-Receptor Blockers: Dosage Information

Drug	*Trade Name*	*Common Dose*	*Common Frequency*	*Lipid Solubility*
Nadolol	Corgard®	40–120 mg	Once daily	Low
Penbutolol*	Levatol®*	20 mg	Once daily	High
Pindolol*	Visken®*	5–20 mg	Twice daily	Low
Propanolol	Inderal®	40–120 mg	Twice daily	High
Propanolol extended release	Inderal LA®	80–160 mg	Once daily	High
Timolol	Blocadren®	10–30 mg	Twice daily	Low to moderate

*Agents with intrinsic sympathomimetic activity.

Combined Alpha- and Beta-Receptor Blockers: Dosage Information			
Drug	*Trade Name*	*Common Dose*	*Common Frequency*
Carvedilol	Coreg®	6.25–25 mg	Twice daily
Labetalol	Normodyne®	100–300 mg	Twice daily

Mechanism of Action

There are 2 main types of beta-receptors in human physiology: beta 1 and beta 2. Receptors are located on the heart, where activation causes an increase in heart rate, contractility, and conduction velocity. Blockade of these receptors reduces cardiac output.[34]

Beta-receptors also have a wide range of functions in the body outside the heart. Activation of beta 1 receptors located in the juxtaglomerular cells of the kidney affects the RAAS by stimulating the release of renin. Activation of beta 2 receptors in the liver increases hepatic-mediated glucose output.[23] Activation of beta 2 receptors in the lungs induces bronchodilation.[23]

As for differences with beta-blocker drugs, some are beta 1–receptor selective and preferentially inhibit the beta 1 receptor. Others are nonselective and inhibit both beta 1 and beta 2 receptors with equal affinity. It is important to remember that when higher doses of a beta 1–selective blocker are given, selectivity diminishes.[34] Beta-receptor blockers also differ in lipid solubility. Highly lipid-soluble beta-receptor blockers cross the blood brain barrier (BBB) readily and increase the risk of adverse effects to the central nervous system (CNS). Some beta-blockers also have intrinsic sympathomimetic activity (ISA). Intrinsic sympathomimetic activity beta-blockers act as a partial agonist at beta-receptors while blocking physiological beta-agonists such as epinephrine. The net effect is some preservation of beta-receptor function and a potential decrease in side effects.[34] These agents are used infrequently, however, due to inferior clinical trial data in post-MI patients.[54]

Dosing

Beta-blockers are administered once or twice daily and given without regard to meals. If drowsiness is experienced, daily doses can be given in the evening to minimize this adverse effect when the patient is awake. However, administration should occur at a consistent time. Initial therapy often starts with a low dose and can be titrated up as tolerated.

Pregnancy, Precautions, and Contraindications

Most beta-blockers are classified as Pregnancy Category C; however, there is reasonable data demonstrating that labetalol is generally safe to use in pregnancy.[23] Atenolol is classified as Pregnancy Category D. Atenolol crosses the placental barrier and has resulted in the birth of infants small for their gestational age.

Beta-blockers are contraindicated in persons with sinus bradycardia.[23] Nonselective beta-blockers are contraindicated in persons with asthma, due to the blockade of beta 2–mediated bronchodilation.[23]

Beta 1–selective agents should be used cautiously and with the lowest possible dose.[23] Additionally, beta-blockers must be used with caution in older adults who have preexisting ventricular dysfunction.[23]

Persons with diabetes must also exercise caution when using beta-blockers. Beta-blockers may inhibit the release of insulin from the pancreas, resulting in increased blood glucose levels in persons with type 2 diabetes. Additionally, all beta-blockers have the potential to mask hypoglycemic-induced tachycardia, which can decrease the individual's awareness of hypoglycemia.[23,41] Dizziness and sweating induced by hypoglycemia are typically unaffected by beta-blockers.[23,34]

Adverse Effects

Common adverse effects associated with this class of antihypertensive agents are CNS-related, such as sedation, dizziness, drowsiness, lightheadedness, fatigue, and headache. Other notable adverse effects include bradycardia, hypotension, depression, and sexual dysfunction, especially in older adults. Gastrointestinal effects of constipation, diarrhea, and nausea have been reported but are less frequent.[23]

Drug Interactions

Beta-blockers have additive effects with nondihydropyridine calcium channel blockers (CCBs) (diltiazem and verapamil), amiodarone, and digoxin.[23] Concurrent use of these agents may cause heart block; therefore, extreme caution should be used when combining these agents. Typically, persons taking beta-blockers need to be tapered off the drug and should not abruptly discontinue.[23,34] Diphenhydramine and hydrochloroquine may increase the plasma concentrations of some beta-blockers through inhibition of the cytochrome P-450 isoenzyme CYP2D6, resulting in enhanced adverse effects including hypotension.[23] Nonsteroidal anti-inflammatory drugs may decrease the antihypertensive effects of beta-blockers.[46]

Monitoring

Baseline blood pressure, heart rate, lipid profile, and blood glucose levels should be conducted. Since beta-blockers can decrease heart rate, patients should have their heart rate assessed at each clinician visit. Symptomatic bradycardia (heart rate <60 beats per minute) may require dose adjustment or discontinuation. Beta-blockers also have the potential to increase total cholesterol, LDL-C, and TGs and decrease HDL-C, although these effects are transient and usually of little clinical significance.[52] Nevertheless, serum lipids should be monitored regularly, especially when coadministered with other agents that increase serum lipids, such as thiazide diuretics.[52] Blood glucose levels should be monitored regularly, especially in those newly diagnosed with diabetes or with prediabetes.

Instructions

Educate patients not to stop beta-blockers abruptly, unless directed by their healthcare provider. Abrupt withdrawal could lead to increased blood pressure and worsening of preexisting angina and possibly lead to MI. Monitor blood pressure and heart rate daily to identify changes, elevations, and patterns. Encourage people with diabetes to monitor their blood glucose levels more frequently. Educate patients on the signs and symptoms of hypotension and worsening heart failure, such as edema and difficulty in breathing during activity.

Calcium Channel Blockers

Calcium channel blockers may be used as first-line therapy for lowering blood pressure in persons with diabetes, especially African Americans. In practice, amlodipine is generally prescribed due to its antihypertensive effect and low toxicity. Furthermore, the ACCOMPLISH trial illustrated that ACEI plus CCB therapy may be superior to ACEI plus thiazide therapy in reducing cardiovascular events.[53] Non-dihydropyridine CCB's antiproteinuric effects may also be useful in patients who do not tolerate ACEIs or ARB therapy, but have diabetes-related kidney disease and albuminuria.[1]

Non-Dihydropyridine CCBs: Dosage Information

Drug	*Trade Name*	*Common Dose*	*Common Frequency*
Diltiazem sustained release	Cardizem SR®	60–180 mg	Twice daily
Diltiazem extended release	Cardizem CD® Tiazac® Cardizem LA®	120–360 mg	Once daily
Verapamil immediate release	Calan®	40–80 mg	Three times daily
Verapamil sustained release	Calan SR®	120–360 mg	Once daily
Verapamil extended release	Covera-HS® Verelan PM®	120–360 mg 100–300 mg	Once daily

Mechanism of Action

Calcium channel blockers are classified into non-dihydropyridine or dihydropyridine, based on their chemical structure. Calcium channel blockers block the L-type calcium channel, which results in vasodilation. Non-dihydropyridine CCBs primarily cause vasodilation within coronary vessels and have a more depressive effect on cardiac conduction. Thus, blood pressure reduction is due to decreased CO.[34] Dihydropyridine CCBs primarily cause vasodilation in the vascular smooth muscle. Thus, blood pressure reduction is due to decreased TPR.[34]

Dosing

Calcium channel blockers are dosed 1 to 3 times daily and can be taken with food to minimize adverse effects. Dose initially at the low range and titrate up every 2 weeks based on patient tolerance, blood pressure, and heart rate. The immediate-release dosage forms are rarely used for treating hypertension. Once-daily formulations are dosed in the morning, except verapamil extended-release products, which are dosed at bedtime.[64]

Dihydropyridine CCBs: Dosage Information			
Drug	*Trade Name*	*Common Dose*	*Common Frequency*
Amlodipine	Norvasc®	2.5–10 mg	Once daily
Felodipine	Plendil®	2.5–20 mg	Once daily
Isradipine controlled release	DynaCirc CR®	5–10 mg	Once daily
Nicardipine sustained release	Cardene SR®	30–60 mg	Twice daily
Nifedipine long-acting	Adalat® CC Procardia XL®	30–60 mg	Once daily
Nisoldipine	Sular®	10–40 mg	Once daily

Dihydropyridine CCBs are dosed once daily and can be given without regard to time of day. However, administration should be at a consistent time. Dose initially at the low range and titrate up gradually based on patient tolerance, blood pressure, and heart rate.

Pregnancy, Precautions, and Contraindications

All CCBs are Pregnancy Category C and should be avoided unless the benefit outweighs the risk.

Calcium channel blockers are also contraindicated in persons with sick sinus syndrome or a heart block, without a pacemaker. Non-dihydropyridine CCBs, specifically, are contraindicated in persons with heart failure. Caution should be used in persons with renal and/or hepatic dysfunction.[23]

Adverse Effects

Calcium channel blockers have a wide range of adverse effects, which can include headache, dizziness, nausea, dyspepsia, flushing, and constipation. Non-dihydropyridine CCBs are associated with cardiac adverse effects including cardiac conduction abnormalities and bradycardia, which are typically found in persons with preexisting cardiac conditions. Dihydropyridine CCBs have adverse effects related to their relaxing of vascular tone. Peripheral edema occurs more frequently with these agents; however, all CCBs have the potential to cause peripheral edema.[23]

Drug Interactions

Most CCB drug interactions stem from the cytochrome P-450 enzyme system. All inducers and inhibitors of the CYP3A4 isoenzyme affect the metabolism of CCBs, thereby delaying or enhancing their elimination from the body and resulting in increased or decreased CCB concentration.[64] Concurrent medications and foods that are also metabolized through this system (such as grapefruit juice) should be used cautiously, and patients should be monitored for increased levels and adverse reactions. Additionally, amlodipine, diltiazem, and verapamil can inhibit other CYP3A4 substrates, such as simvastatin, lovastatin, and theophylline.[23] Monitoring adverse effects and blood pressure can help identify potential drug interactions and reduce the risk of toxicity. See Table 20.3 for a list of common drugs that interact with CCBs.

Concurrent use of diuretics, beta-blockers, and ACEIs may increase risk of hypotension. Additive effects may occur with agents that affect cardiac contractility.[23,34]

Monitoring

Blood pressure, heart rate, liver enzymes, and cardiac function should be measured at baseline and periodically throughout treatment, especially when titrating doses of CCBs and/or other medications metabolized by the cytochrome P-450 system.[23] Monitor for heart failure, edema, angina, and changes in heart rate.

Instructions

Calcium channel blockers should be taken at the same time each day. For once-daily dosed CCBs, persons with diabetes can take the medication in the evening if they experience drowsiness or dizziness. Taking CCBs with meals can minimize gastrointestinal adverse effects and can often increase engagement with medicaton taking. Monitor blood pressure daily to identify changes, elevations, and patterns. Educate patients on the signs and symptoms of heart failure, such as edema and shortness of breath at rest or during activity.

Case—Part 2: An African American With Type 2 Diabetes and Hypertension

DC was asked to return to the clinic in 1 month to reevaluate his blood pressure. Particularly concerning to DC's healthcare team was his elevated risk for ASCVD and how hypertension contributes to this risk. DC reports tolerating atorvastatin (40 mg) started at his previous visit, but now he is concerned about his blood pressure. DC started checking his blood pressure at home on a device he borrowed from his friend. He stated that over the last 2 weeks, his systolic blood pressure ranged from 130 to 138 mm Hg and his diastolic blood pressure was usually in the upper 80s.

Case—Part 2: An African American With Type 2 Diabetes and Hypertension (continued)

Vital Signs

- Blood pressure: 138/80 mm Hg (Last visit: 136/82 mmHg)
- Heart rate: 74
- Respiratory rate: 15

Current Medications

- Metformin (Glucophage®) 2000 mg daily
- Multivitamin daily
- Aspirin 81 mg daily
- Fexofenadine (Allegra®) 60 mg twice daily as needed
- Atorvastatin (Lipitor®) 40 mg daily

Laboratory Data

- Na+: 138 mEq/L
- K+: 4.1 mEq/L
- BUN: 12 mg/dL
- Scr: 0.95 mg/dL
- Glucose: 135 mg/dL
- Urine to creatinine ratio: 352 mg/g (severely elevated albuminuria)

Diagnosis and Plan

This is DC's second visit with elevated blood pressure readings and his home readings provide further confirmation that he has stage 1 hypertension. Given he has multiple ASCVD risk factors (age >45 years old, smoker, low HDL-C, metabolic syndrome), albuminuria, and his 10-year ASCVD risk is well over 10%, antihypertensive therapy is warranted, and his blood pressure goal should be <130/80 mmHg.

There are 4 first-line antihypertensive classes to consider for DC (ACE or ARB, thiazide, or CCB). Similar to goal setting, pharmacologic choices should be individualized. Prior to choosing a blood pressure medication, renal function, potassium, and presence of albuminuria should be evaluated. DC's labs show that his kidney function and potassium would tolerate any of the 4 classes of antihypertensives, although the presence of albuminuria is an early risk indicator for both cardiovascular and kidney disease. Comorbid hypertension and severely increased albuminuria make an ACEI or ARB the proper choice for DC due to their nephroprotective effects. Both ACEI and ARBs are generically available. Lisinopril 10 mg once daily is a reasonable choice for DC given its widely available and inexpensive. If additional antihypertensive therapy is warranted, combination therapy should be considered given the patient's preference to keep his pill burden low.

DC should be brought back to clinic in 1 month to follow up on his blood pressure and to monitor his kidney function and potassium levels. He should be advised to continue monitoring his blood pressure at home and to follow a heart healthy lifestyle that is low in sodium. Smoking cessation should be discussed extensively as this would significantly decrease his blood pressure.

Alpha 1–Receptor Blockers

Although indicated for the treatment of hypertension, alpha 1–receptor blockers are infrequently prescribed for this indication, especially in persons with diabetes. They are most beneficial in persons with benign prostatic hyperplasia (BPH). Alpha-receptor blockers can be a treatment option for persons with both diabetes and BPH.

Mechanism of Action

The alpha 1–receptor blockers inhibit the binding of norepinephrine to vascular alpha 1 receptors. Activation of the alpha 1 receptor by norepinephrine leads to vasoconstriction, resulting in an increase in TPR. In addition, inhibition of the alpha 1 receptor in the prostate causes a decrease in urethral resistance and improvement in symptoms in persons with BPH.[23]

Dosing

The alpha 1–receptor blockers are preferably dosed at bedtime to minimize the risk of postural hypertension often observed within hours after administration. Initial therapy often starts with a low dose and can be titrated up as tolerated.[23,34]

Alpha 1–Receptor Blockers: Dosage Information

Drug	*Trade Name*	*Common Dose*	*Common Frequency*
Doxazosin	Cardura®	1–16 mg	Once daily
Prazosin	Minipress®	1–5 mg	2 or 3 times daily
Terazosin	Hytrin®	1–10 mg	Once or twice daily

Pregnancy, Precautions, and Contraindications

All alpha 1–receptor blockers are classified as Pregnancy Category C and should be avoided unless the benefit outweighs the risk. Animal studies indicated possible risk, and no human studies exist.

Adverse Effects

Adverse effects commonly associated with alpha 1–receptor blockers include fatigue, malaise, dizziness, shortness of breath, hypotension, edema, and weight gain. Blurred vision, palpitations, and sexual dysfunction have also been reported. Thrombocytopenia has been observed in patients on terazosin.[23]

Drug Interactions

The alpha 1–receptor blockers have relatively few drug interactions. Alcohol increases the risk of hypotension with these agents, and coadministration of verapamil increases the serum concentrations of prazosin and terazosin. Concurrent use of other antihypertensive agents with alpha 1–receptor blockers may increase the risk of hypotension.[23]

Monitoring

Monitor blood pressure and heart rate at baseline and frequently after initiating treatment. If antihypertensive agents are added, assess the patient for first-dose syncope and postural hypotension.[67] Syncope is managed by having the patient lie down, rest, and receive supportive care as necessary. Syncope may be prevented by starting with a low dose and increasing slowly. Dizziness and lightheadedness are more common than loss of consciousness.[67] Interruptions in therapy increase the risk; thus, persons with diabetes who do not consistently monitor are poor candidates for this drug.

Instructions

Educate patients that alpha 1–receptor blockers have the potential to cause syncope and postural hypotension. Alcohol, exercise, long periods of standing, and hot weather can increase the risk.[34] Educate patients and their families on the management of syncope in case it occurs. Advise patients to avoid driving or operating machinery after the first dose, an increase in dose, or the addition of another antihypertensive agent until they can tolerate treatment. Lastly, advise male patients to go immediately to the emergency room if they experience a prolonged erection lasting 4 hours or more.

Central-Acting Alpha-Adrenergic Agonists

Although indicated for the treatment of hypertension, central-acting alpha-adrenergic agonists are rarely prescribed for this indication, especially in persons with diabetes.

Mechanism of Action

Central-acting alpha-adrenergic agonists stimulate alpha 2 receptors in the brain, inhibiting the production of serotonin, dopamine, norepinephrine, and epinephrine. This inhibition results in a decrease in heart rate and TPR.[23]

Central-Acting Alpha-Adrenergic Agonists: Dosage Information

Drug	*Trade Name*	*Common Dose*	*Common Frequency*
Clonidine tablets	Catapres®	0.1–0.8 mg	Twice daily
Clonidine patch	Catapres-TTS®	0.1- to 0.3-mg per day patch	Once weekly
Methyldopa	Aldomet®	250–1000 mg	2 or 3 times daily

Dosing

Central-acting alpha-adrenergic agonists are available in either tablets or a transdermal patch. Tablets are taken in daily divided doses, preferably at consistent times. Patches are applied once weekly.[23] When methyldopa is administered with any other antihypertensive agent, other than thiazide-type diuretics, limit the initial dose to no more than 500 mg per day in divided doses.[23]

Pregnancy, Precautions, and Contraindications

Clonidine is classified as Pregnancy Category C and should be avoided.[23] Methyldopa is Pregnancy Category B and is a preferred therapy in pregnancy. It is converted to alpha-methylnorepinephrine, a natural by-product of catecholamine breakdown. There are no documented fetal adverse effects despite wide use, and it does not reduce maternal cardiac or fetal blood flow.[23] Although it can be used during pregnancy, methyldopa presents with many adverse effects to the mother that often lead to discontinuation (see adverse effects below).

The use of a monoamine oxidase inhibitor (MAOI) is contraindicated in persons taking methyldopa. Central-acting alpha-adrenergic agonists are contraindicated in persons with severe coronary insufficiency, recent MI, cerebrovascular disease, and renal or hepatic dysfunction.[34,41]

Adverse Effects

Although methyldopa can be used in pregnancy, it presents with many adverse effects to the mother and to the general patient. These include nausea, vomiting, constipation, dry mouth, and CNS-related effects, such as sedation, weakness, nervousness, dizziness, and drowsiness. Hypotension, blood dyscrasia, sexual dysfunction, and hair thinning, or loss have also been reported.[68,70]

Drug Interactions

The use of an MAOI is contraindicated in persons taking methyldopa. Although the mechanism is unknown, there are numerous reports of hypertensive crisis in persons taking both medications.[68,69]

Iron can decrease the absorption of methyldopa by up to 66%. Therefore, iron should be separated by at least 2 hours from methyldopa administration.[68] Methyldopa also increases the risk of lithium toxicity, even in the presence of normal lithium levels. Monitor for signs and symptoms of lithium toxicity, such as lethargy and muscle weakness.[70] Patients should also exercise caution when taking entacapone (Comtan®, Novartis) and methyldopa. Entacapone is a catechol-O-methyltransferase (COMT) inhibitor, and methyldopa is metabolized by COMT.[70]

The over-the-counter drug products pseudoephedrine and ma huang (ephedra, ephedrine) can increase blood pressure. This is greatly enhanced for persons taking methyldopa and clonidine.[68–70] Tricyclic antidepressants—eg, amitriptyline (Elavil®) and imipramine (Janimine®, Tofranil®)—may antagonize central alpha 2 receptors. Use clonidine and methyldopa with caution when combined with beta-blockers, since withdrawal of these agents has led to life-threatening increases in blood pressure.[68–70]

Monitoring

Monitor blood pressure and heart rate at baseline and frequently after initiating treatment. Monitor patients for signs of depression at follow-up visits. Clinicians who wish to discontinue a central-acting alpha-adrenergic agonist should taper the dose gradually over 2 to 4 days to prevent withdrawal.[68–70] Monitor for tachycardia, rebound hypertension, nausea, vomiting, and flushing. Patients on methyldopa should also undergo liver function testing at periodic intervals.[68]

Instructions

Educate patients to never abruptly discontinue their medication and to review the signs and symptoms of withdrawal. Since these agents affect catecholamine and aldosterone levels, remind persons with diabetes to monitor blood glucose levels more frequently, as greater fluctuation can occur.[68–70] Drowsiness is common, so until the medication is tolerated, patients should exercise caution when driving or operating heavy machinery.[68] Dry mouth can occur during the first 2 weeks of therapy. Ice chips, hard candy, or chewing gum can minimize problems with dry mouth.[68] The clonidine patch should be applied every 7 days on a hairless part of the upper arm or torso. Educate patients to apply the adhesive overlay over the system for proper adhesion. Advise patients taking methyldopa that their urine may darken in color after exposure to air.[69]

Considerations in Hypertension Therapy in Persons With Diabetes

Treatment goals and strategies for hypertension in persons with diabetes must be given equal emphasis and be as aggressive as those developed for hyperglycemia. Most likely, 2 or more antihypertensive agents will be necessary to lower blood pressure and maintain it at a goal of <130/80 mmHg (or <140/90 mm Hg in low-risk patients).[1,41] Combination therapy is recommended for all patients with stage 2 hypertension (blood pressure ≥140/90 mmHg and > or = 20/10 mmHg away from goal). Thiazide diuretics are commonly used as adjunct therapy because of their synergistic effect with RAAS inhibiting therapies. Due to these synergistic effects, they are commonly marketed in ACEI or ARB/thiazide combinations. Dihydropyridine calcium channel blockers (eg, amlodipine) may be considered as well. Monthly follow-up and astute monitoring of blood pressure, at clinic and at home, is necessary to achieve and maintain adequate blood pressure levels.

Managing hypertension in older adults can be challenging given their increased sensitivity to orthostatic hypotension. Monitoring blood pressure outside of the clinic is even more important in older adults to rule out the possibility of white coat hypertension. White coat hypertension is characterized by elevated blood pressure readings in the clinic office and normal readings outside of the office. It is more common in older adults. Older adults also should be monitored for hypotension. While a blood pressure goal of <130/80 mm Hg may be appropriate for some older adults, a more lenient goal may be necessary for those who have dementia, short life expectancy (<6 months), or who live in an older adult care home.[41] Older adults are more likely to take multiple medications, making pill burden and medication costs key considerations in this group. Thus, blood pressure goals and the aggressiveness of treatment with antihypertensives must be individualized.

Treatment resistant hypertension is defined as the inability to maintain blood pressure levels on ≥3 antihypertensive agents from ≥3 drug classes.[46] In these persons with diabetes engagement with drug therapy and lifestyle modifications should be addressed before modifying drug therapy, as well as ruling out secondary causes of hypertension (eg, hyperaldosteronism). If the patient is on hydrochlorothiazide, switching to a long-acting thiazide diuretic (eg, chlorthalidone) should be considered. If this deems ineffective, a mineralocorticoid receptor antagonist (eg, spironolactone) should be considered; however, potassium levels and renal function must be closely monitored. Other antihypertensive drug classes (eg, beta-blockers, alpha-1 receptor blockers) may also be used in select patients. Referral to a hypertension specialist should also be considered.

A patient-centered approach is warranted to ensure the patient can manage the additional pill burden and expense, as well as tolerate additional antihypertensive therapy. When using multiple antihypertensives for hypertension in persons with diabetes, engagement with medicaton taking must be reviewed at each patient visit. Adding medication to existing regimens requires behavior change on the part of the patient; thus, the person's readiness to change, conviction, and confidence levels require assessment. Use of combination medications can be beneficial for individuals who are reluctant to take more medication, thus improving adherence and reducing costs to the patient.

Focus on Education

Teaching Strategies

Patient education should include medication safety, proper dosing, and timing medications for optimum effect.

Acknowledge the need for lifestyle change. Lifestyle modification, including MNT, physical activity, and smoking cessation, should always be a standard treatment of dyslipidemia in addition to pharmacotherapy.

Dosing starts low and increases as tolerated and needed. Initiation of medication therapy is an important change in treatment and health management. Titration of medications to achieve targets is essential for effective and comprehensive diabetes care management.

Combining medications. Combination therapy with medications possessing different mechanisms of action may be necessary to treat dyslipidemia and hypertension. Describe each medication's unique function and effect.

Resisting medications. Adding medication to existing regimens is a behavior change. Readiness to change, conviction, and confidence levels affect engagement with the regimen. Discuss and plan for accommodation into existing lifestyle. Identify and help diminish barriers to effective pharmacotherapy.

Messages for Patients

Treatment goals. Identify target goals for dyslipidemia and hypertension, and be as aggressive with these goals as you are with your blood glucose goals. Be certain you are aware of the target blood levels your healthcare team identifies for lipids, blood pressure, and blood glucose.

Consistency. Work with the healthcare team and pharmacist to keep them informed of all the medications you are taking (prescription and over the counter). Always carry a list of current medications and know their interactions and side effects. Never abruptly discontinue a medication; be aware of the signs and symptoms of withdrawal. Have a list of resources to call if you have any questions.

Therapeutic lifestyle changes. Healthy eating, physical activity, and stress management are part of your cardiovascular well-being and will help you manage your hypertension and blood lipids.

Health Literacy

Numerous barriers may exist to prevent patients from properly using their medications. They might include financial constraints, cultural beliefs, and limited educational attainment. Asking probing questions can help you explore those possibilities and address them accordingly.

Inadequate health literacy may lead to an increase in medication errors. Medication error is the most common medical mistake. Two thirds of US adults 60 years of age and older have inadequate or marginal literacy skills. Eighty-one percent of patients 60 years of age and older at a public hospital could not read or understand basic materials such as prescription labels.[54]

Patients with low literacy may misunderstand the warning labels on their medication. One of many studies indicated that patients with low literacy skills demonstrated a lower rate of correct interpretation of the 8 most commonly used prescription drug warning labels than did those with higher literacy skills. Multiple-step instructions, reading difficulty of text, the use of icons, the use of color, and the lack of message clarity were common causes of label misinterpretation.[55]

The design and layout of medication handouts can make navigation problematic. Consider the following when developing or using medication handouts:

- Use short, familiar words.
- Use short sentences.
- Use short headings that stand out.
- Use a large type size.
- Use capital and lowercase letters rather than all capital letters.
- Bold, highlight, or enlarge font of content most important to the patient.
- Do not use abbreviations that are not easily referenced.
- Leave plenty of white space.
- Use bullet points to organize lists.
- Use a 3-step rule; multistep instructions are rarely understood.
- Involve your patients in the design of reference/teaching materials.
- Clarify the purpose of the handout as the information for decision-making.

Health numeracy can negatively impact medication taking. Health numeracy is defined as "the degree to which individuals have the capacity to access, process, interpret, communicate, and act on numerical, quantitative, graphical, biostatistical, and probabilistic health information needed to make effective health decisions."[56] Even the most knowledgeable person is at risk of misusing/misinterpreting the numbers and consequently not taking his or her medications as intended. Ask your patients to bring their medications to the office, and ask what kind of system they have in place to know when and how to take those medications. Ask your patients to answer the following questions in their own words: "What is this medication for?" "Why do you need to take this medication?" "How do you remind yourself to take this medication?" "How often do you skip doses of this medication?" Normalize some predicted nonengagement behaviors by asking persons with diabetes whether they are exemplifying them. Address the difference between trade names and generic names, as this can be confusing for many.

Provide patients with some useful strategies to accurately track medicaton taking behaviors. Strategies could include keeping medicine bottles in the same container with color-coded tops, using colors/rubber bands to mark their medications, or using medication dispensers with daily compartments, among others. Support your patients in establishing good communication with their pharmacist. Explain that the pharmacist is part of their diabetes care team and can educate them not only about medications but on how to take them and what to do if they cannot take them.

Focus on Practice

Dyslipidemia and hypertension management are part of the chronic care model. Patients with chronic conditions like dyslipidemia and hypertension need support, as well as information, to become effective managers of their health. An effective decision support mechanism, a delivery system design, a clinical information system, organization of health care, and community support are part of delivering effective care.

Quality assurance. To improve the quality of care, its structure, process, and outcomes need to be evaluated. Follow evidence-based guidelines to optimize resource utilization as well as improve the management and outcome of care for persons with diabetes and hypertension/dyslipidemia. Advance clinicians' knowledge and adherence to current evidence-based pharmacotherapy guidelines and delivery systems.

Create a system for effective behavioral interventions. Strategies include developing prompts and reminder systems, identifying a potential relapse into old behavior, setting appropriate and realistic goals, simplifying regimens to once or twice daily, using opportunities to model behavior, and reinforcing positive behaviors.

References

1. American Diabetes Association. Standards of medical care in diabetes—2020. Diabetes Care. 2020;43(Suppl 1):S111-134.
2. Mozaffarian D, Benjamin EJ, Go AS, et al. Heart disease and stroke statistics—2016 update: a report from the American Heart Association. Circulation. 2016 Jan 26;133(4):e38-360. Epub 2015 Dec 16.
3. Kapur A, De Palma R. Mortality after myocardial infarction in patients with diabetes mellitus. Heart. 2007;93(12):1504-6.
4. Haffner SM, Lehto S, Rönnemaa T, et al. Mortality from coronary heart disease in subjects with type 2 diabetes and in nondiabetic subjects with and without prior myocardial infarction. N Engl J Med. 1998;339(4):229-34.
5. Norhammar A, Tenerz A, Nilsson G, et al. Glucose metabolism in patients with acute myocardial infarction and no previous diagnosis of diabetes mellitus: a prospective study. Lancet. 2002;359(9324):2140-4.
6. Talbert RL. Dyslipidemia. In: DiPiro JT, Talbert RL, Yee GC, Matzke GR, Wells BG, Posey LM, eds. Pharmacotherapy: A Pathophysiologic Approach. 8th ed. New York: McGraw-Hill; 2011:365-88.
7. Lamarche B, Lemieux I, Després JP. The small, dense LDL phenotype and the risk of coronary heart disease: epidemiology, patho-physiology and therapeutic aspects. Diabetes Metab. 1999;25(3):199-211.
8. Tribble DL, Holl LG, Wood PD, Krauss RM. Variations in oxidative susceptibility among six low density lipoprotein subfractions of differing density and particle size. Atherosclerosis. 1992;93(3):189-99.
9. Grundy SM, Stone NJ, Bailey AL, et al. 2018 AHA/ACC/AACVPR/AAPA/ABC/ACPM/ADA/AGS/APhA/ASPC/NLA/PCNA Guideline on the Management of Blood Cholesterol: Executive Summary: A Report of the American College of Cardiology/American Heart Association Task Force on Clinical Practice Guidelines. J Am Coll Cardiol. 2018. doi: https://doi.org/10.1016/j.jacc.2018.11.003.
10. Dallinga-Thie GM, Kroon J, Borén J, Chapman MJ. Triglyceride-rich lipoproteins and remnants: targets for therapy? Curr Cardiol Rep. 2016;18(7):67.
11. Boden WE, Probstfield JL, Anderson T, et al; AIM-HIGH Investigators. Niacin in patients with low HDL cholesterol levels receiving intensive statin therapy. N Engl J Med. 2011;365(24):2255-67.
12. The HPS2-THRIVE Collaborative Group. Effects of extended-release niacin with laropiprant in high-risk patients. N Engl J Med. 2014;371(3):203-12.
13. Schwartz GG, Olsson AG, Abt M, et al. Effects of dalcetrapib in patients with a recent acute coronary syndrome. N Engl J Med. 2012;367(22):2089-99.
14. Goff DC, Lloyd-Jones DM, Bennett G, et al. 2013 ACC/AHA guideline on the assessment of cardiovascular risk: a report of the American College of Cardiology/American Heart Association Task Force on Practice Guidelines. Circulation. 2013;129:S49-73.
15. Ridker PM, Mora S, Rose L. Percent reduction in LDL cholesterol following high-intensity statin therapy: potential implications for guidelines and for the prescription of emerging lipid-lowering agents. Eur Heart J. 2016;37:1373-9.
16. Awad K, Serban MC, Penson P, et al. Effects of morning vs evening statin administration on lipid profile: a systematic review and meta-analysis. 2017;11(4):972-85.
17. Thompson PD, Panza G, Zaleski A, Taylor B. Statin-associated side effects. J Am Coll Cardiol. 2016;67(20):2395-410.
18. Ridker PM, Pradhan A, MacFadyen JG, Libby P, Glynn RJ. Cardiovascular benefits and diabetes risks of statin therapy in primary prevention: an analysis from the JUPITER trial. Lancet. 2012;380(9841):565-71.
19. Bays H, Cohen DE, Chalasani N, et al; The National Lipid Association's Statin Safety Task Force. An assessment by the Statin Liver Safety Task Force: 2014 update. J Clin Lipidol. 2014;8 Suppl 3:S47-57.
20. Jacobson TA. NLA Task Force on Statin Safety—2014 update. J Clin Lipidol. 2014;8 Suppl 3:S1-4.
21. Boothill JN, Colantonio LD, Chen L, et al. Statin discontinuation, reinitation, and persistence patterns among Medicare beneficiaries after myocardial infarction: a cohort study. Circ Cardiovasc Qual Outcomes. 2017;10:e003626.
22. Cannon CP, Blazing MA, Giugliano RP, et al. Ezetimibe added to statin therapy after acute coronary syndromes. N Engl J Med. 2015;372:2387-97.
23. Lexi-Comp® Online. Hudson, Ohio.
24. Dixon DL, Pamulapati LG, Bucheit, JD, et al. Curr Atheroscler Rep (2019) 21: 16. https://doi.org/10.1007/s11883-019-0778-6.
25. Dixon DL, Trankle C, Buckley L, et al. A review of PCSK9 inhibition and its effects beyond LDL receptors. J Clin Lipidol. 2016;10(5):1073–80.
26. Wendling P. FDA pulls approval of niacin, fibrate in combo with statins. Medscape (cited 2016 June 3). On the Internet at: http://www.medscape.com/viewarticle/862022.
27. Dixon DL, Williams VG. Interaction between gemfibrozil and warfarin: case report and review of the literature. Pharmacother. 2009;29(6):744-8.
28. Kelly MS, Beavers C, Bucheit JD, et al. Pharmacologic approaches for the management of patients with moderately elevated triglycerides (150-499 mg/dL). J Clin Lipidol. 2017;11:872-9.
29. Sabatine MS, Giugliano RP, Keech AC, et al. Evolocumab and clinical outcomes in patients with cardiovascular disease. N Engl J Med. 2017;376:1713-22.
30. Schwartz GG, Szarek SM, Bhat DL, et al. Alirocumab and cardiovascular outcomes after acute coronary syndrome. N Engl J Med. 2018;379(22):2097-2107.

31. Robinson JG, Jayanna MB, Brown AS, et al. Enhancing the value of PCSK9 monoclonal antibodies by identifying patients most likely to benefit. J Clin Lipidol. 2019; DOI: https://doi.org/10.1016/j.jacl.2019.05.005

32. Bhatt DL, Steg PG, Miller M, et al. Cardiovascular risk reduction with icosapent ethyl for hypertriglyceridemia. N Engl J Med. 2019;380:11-22.

33. American Diabetes Association. Cardiovascular disease and risk management: standards of medical care in diabetes—2020. Diabetes Care. 2020;43(Suppl 1):S111-134.

34. Saseen J, McLaughlin E. Hypertension. In: Dipiro JT, Talbert RL, Yee GC, Matzke GR, Wells BG, Posey LM, eds. Pharmacotherapy: A Pathophysiologic Approach. 7th ed. New York: McGraw-Hill; 2008:101-36.

35. Sowers JR, Haffner SM. Treatment of cardiovascular and renal risk factors in the diabetic hypertensive. Hypertension. 2002;40:781-8.

36. Higashi Y, Sasaki S, Nakagawa K, et al. Endothelial function and oxidative stress in renovascular hypertension. N Engl J Med. 2002;346:1954-62.

37. Atlas S. The renin-angiotensin aldosterone system. J Manag Care Pharm. 2007;13(8) Supp S-b:S9-20.

38. Jacobsen EJ. Hypertension: update on use of angiotensin II receptor blockers. Geriatrics. 2001;56(2):25-8.

39. Ramahi TM. Expanded role for ARBs in cardiovascular and renal disease. Postgrad Med. 2001;109(4):115-22.

40. Willenheimer R, Dahlof B, Rydberg E, et al. AT-1 receptor blockers in hypertension and heart failure: clinical experience and future directions. Eur Heart J. 1999;20(14):997-1008.

41. Whelton PK, Carey RM, Aronow WS, et al. 2017 ACC/AHA/AAPA/ABC/ACPM/AGS/APhA/ASH/ASPC/NMA/PCNA Guideline for the Prevention, Detection, Evaluation, and Management of High Blood Pressure in Adults: Executive Summary: A Report of the American College of Cardiology/American Heart Association Task Force on Clinical Practice Guidelines. Hypertension. 2018;71(6):1269-1324.

42. SPRINT Research Group. A randomized trial of intensive versus standard blood-pressure control. N Engl J Med. 2015;373(22):2103-16.

43. The ACCORD Study Group. Effects of intensive blood-pressure control in type 2 diabetes mellitus. N Engl J Med. 2010;362:1575-85.

44. Buckley LF, Dixon DL, Wohlford GF 4th, et al. Intensive versus standard blood pressure control in SPRINT-eligible participants of ACCORD-BP. Diabetes Care. 2017;40(12):1733-8.

45. Flynn JT, Kaelber DC, Baker-Smith CM, et al. Clinical practice guideline for screening and management of high blood pressure in children and adolescents. Pediatrics. 2017;140:e20171904.

46. Carey RM, Calhoun DA, Bakris GL, et al. Resistant hypertension: detection, evaluation, and management: a Scientific Statement from the American Heart Association. Hypertension. 2018;72:e53-e90.

47. Black HR. The evolution of low-dose diuretic therapy: the lessons from clinical trials. Am J Med. 1996;101(3A):47S-52S.

48. Siegel D, Saliba P, Haffner S. Glucose and insulin levels during diuretic therapy in hypertensive men. Hypertension. 1994;236 pt 1:688-94.

49. Williams SF, Nicholas SB, Vaziri ND, et al. African Americans, hypertension and the renin angiotensin system. World J Cardiol. 2014;6(9):878-89.

50. Parving HH, Brenner BM, McMurray JJ, et al; for the ALTITUDE Investigators. Cardiorenal end points in a trial of aliskiren for type 2 diabetes. N Engl J Med. 2012;367:2204-13.

51. Tekturna [package insert]. East Hanover, NJ: Novartis Pharmaceuticals Corporation; 2007.

52. Lakshman MR, Reda DJ, Materson BJ, et al. Diuretics and beta-blockers do not have adverse effects at 1 year on plasma lipid and lipoprotein profiles in men with hypertension. Department of Veterans Affairs Cooperative Study Group on Antihypertensive Agents. Arch Intern Med. 1999;159(6):551-8.

53. Jamerson K, Weber M, Bakris G, et al. Benazapril plus amlodipine or hydrochlorothiazide for hypertension in high-risk patients (ACCOMPLISH). N Engl J Med. 2008;359:2417-28.

54. Williams MV, Parker RM, Baker DW, et al. Inadequate functional health literacy among patients at two public hospitals. JAMA. 1995;274(21):1677-82.

55. Wolf MS, Davis TC, Tilson HH, Bass III PF, Parker RM. Misunderstanding of prescription drug warning labels among patients with low literacy. Am J Health Syst Pharm. 2006;63(11):1048-55.

56. Golbeck AL, Ahlers-Schmidt CR, Paschal AM, et al. A definition and operational framework for health numeracy. Am J Prev Med. 2005;29(4):375-6.

CHAPTER 21

Dietary Supplements and Diabetes: A Focus on Complementary Health Approaches

Skye McKennon, PharmD, BCPS
Jennifer Danielson, PharmD, MBA, CDCES

Key Concepts

- Dietary supplements may include botanical, nonbotanical, and other products such as different herbs or foods and are part of biologically based practices included in complementary health approaches. *Complementary and alternative medicine* (CAM) is the more familiar term used to describe biologically based practices and will be used in this chapter.
- The Dietary Supplement Health and Education Act (DSHEA) of 1994 provides a specific definition of dietary supplements.
- Many persons with diabetes use dietary supplements to lower blood glucose or treat diabetes-related comorbidities.
- There are several reasons for concern with the use of dietary supplements.
- Dietary supplements contain various pharmacologically active ingredients with varying theorized mechanisms of action.
- Dietary supplements may produce side effects and drug interactions.
- Diabetes care and education specialists must have a clear understanding of dietary supplements to provide unbiased, nonjudgmental information to persons with diabetes.
- Evidence-based references should be used to answer questions about dietary supplements.

Introduction

This chapter reviews information about dietary supplements, a part of biologically based practices that individuals may use to treat diabetes and its comorbidities. With the emerging focus on personalized health care, many individuals, including those with diabetes, have had an increased interest in using dietary supplements. The article "Complementary, Alternative, or Integrative Health: What's in a Name?," published by the National Institutes of Health (NIH) National Center for Complementary and Integrative Health (NCCIH), explains the difference between *complementary* and *alternative*. According to the NCCIH, a nonmainstream practice used *together with* conventional medicine is considered *complementary*, and a nonmainstream practice used *instead of* conventional medicine is considered *alternative*. Furthermore, the NCCIH states *integrative* health care brings complementary and conventional health approaches together in a coordinated manner. The NCCIH uses the term *complementary health approaches* when referring to nonmainstream practices and *integrative health* when incorporating complementary approaches into mainstream health care. The NCCIH states there are 2 types of complementary health approaches—natural products and mind and body practices:[1]

- Natural products—herbs, vitamins and minerals, and probiotics
- Mind and body practices—yoga, chiropractic and osteopathic manipulation, meditation, massage therapy, acupuncture, relaxation techniques, Tai Chi, Qigong, healing touch, hypnotherapy, and movement therapies

Other modalities do not fall into either of these categories, including Ayurveda, traditional Chinese medicine, naturopathy, and traditional healers. Table 21.1 provides an overview of definitions relevant to complementary health approaches.

TABLE 21.1 Definitions of Terms Relevant to Complementary Health Approaches

Term	*Definition*
Alternative Medicine	Nonmainstream practice used *instead of* conventional medicine
Complementary Health Approaches	Nonmainstream practices
Complementary Medicine	Nonmainstream practice used *together with* conventional medicine
Dietary Supplement	A product taken by mouth that contains a "dietary ingredient" (vitamin, mineral, herb or other botanical, amino acid, or other substance) intended to supplement the diet
Integrative Health	Complementary approaches being incorporated into mainstream health care
Integrative Medicine	Medicine that brings complementary and conventional health approaches together in a coordinated fashion
Natural Products	Herbs, vitamins and minerals, and probiotics
Mind and Body Practices	Yoga, chiropractic and osteopathic manipulation, meditation, massage therapy, acupuncture, relaxation techniques, Tai Chi, Qigong, healing touch, hypnotherapy, and movement therapies

Case: Person With Diabetes Inquires About Dietary Supplements

ME, a 69-year-old woman with type 2 diabetes, hypertension, hyperlipidemia, hypothyroidism, and depression, is seen for diabetes education.

- ME is taking a combination of glipizide and metformin (Metaglip®, Bristol-Myers Squibb) for diabetes; a combination of losartan and HCTZ for hypertension (Hyzaar®, Merck); rosuvastatin (Crestor®, AstraZeneca) for hyperlipidemia; levothyroxine (Synthroid®, Abbott), and duloxetine (Cymbalta®, Eli Lilly) for depression and mild neuropathy.
- She has heard that some dietary supplements may be useful for diabetes and for her other diseases. These include ginger, cinnamon, fenugreek, ginseng, and chromium. She has also heard that garlic may be useful for hypertension and hyperlipidemia, and St John's wort may be useful for depression. She is experiencing muscle aches with the rosuvastatin and is wondering if a supplement will help alleviate the pain. She also wonders about using turmeric for her knee pain due to osteoarthritis as well as for the diabetes.

ME is also concerned about taking so many prescription products. She is hopeful that she may be able to discontinue some of these drugs and substitute them with "natural" products that have no side effects and are more holistic. She asks her diabetes care and education specialist to help select some products that may be better alternatives to all the drugs she has to take.

- What products mentioned by ME may be useful? Which ones should be avoided?
- What other "natural" products may ME or another person with diabetes consider taking for diabetes or diabetes-related conditions?
- What sources of information may be useful for a diabetes care and education specialist to answer the questions ME has raised?

This chapter will help diabetes care and education specialists answer some of the questions raised in this case. Diabetes care and education specialists must be knowledgeable about products that individuals may consider for diabetes or related conditions.

Dietary Supplement Health and Education Act (DHSEA) of 1994

Dietary supplement use is part of biologically based practices. Prior to 1994, these products were classified as either foods or drugs. In 1994, Congress passed the DSHEA. This legislation created a separate category for botanicals and other products that classifies them as dietary supplements.[2] DSHEA defines dietary supplements as products taken orally that contain one or more dietary ingredient (including vitamins, minerals, herbs or other botanicals, amino acids, and certain other substances) that are intended to supplement the diet.[3] Supplements are thus considered foods and are excluded from the same stringent approval process required for drugs. Under the DSHEA, supplements do not require proof of safety and effectiveness prior to going to market.

Standards of "purity and potency" are the responsibility of manufacturers. Problems with adulteration and contaminants have posed serious threats.[4] A possible solution is to use standardized products since standardization guarantees that each dose provides a consistent level of the active ingredient. However, standardized extracts may not contain all of the therapeutic ingredients found in the natural product.

When enacted, the DSHEA required that good manufacturing practices (GMPs) be established. In 2007, the Food and Drug Administration (FDA) issued a final rule on proposed changes to GMP dietary supplement standards.[5] This rule mandated that products be manufactured without adulterants or impurities and be labeled accurately.

Dietary supplement manufacturers must comply with certain labeling requirements.[6] Labels must list the following: product name as well as the word *dietary supplement*; net content quantity; manufacturer's, packer's, or distributor's name and place of business; and directions for use. The label must also include a "supplement facts panel" that lists the serving size; dietary ingredients; nondietary or inactive ingredients such as fillers, artificial colors, or flavors; amount per serving size; percent daily value (if established); and whether the product is a proprietary blend (a manufacturer exclusive blend).

Products fall under one of three types of product claims: health claims, nutrient content claims, or structure and function claims. This allows dietary supplement manufacturers to make claims regarding the ability to maintain "structure and function" of the body, but not regarding diagnosis, treatment, cure, or prevention of disease. For instance, a manufacturer may claim that a product "maintains a healthy prostate" but may not state that the product "treats benign prostatic hyperplasia."[6] If a manufacturer makes a claim that the product affects body structure or function, the label must include the following statement: "This statement has not been evaluated by the Food and Drug Administration (FDA). This product is not intended to diagnose, treat, cure, or prevent any disease." An example of a supplement label may be found on the Web site of the Council for Responsible Nutrition (https://www.fda.gov/media/99158/download).

The Dietary Supplement and Non-Prescription Drug Consumer Protection Act (Public Law 109–462) was a critical sentinel legislative event.[7] This legislation requires reporting of serious adverse events to the FDA based on specific information received from the public. Individuals and clinicians are encouraged to report supplement-related adverse outcomes to the FDA.[8] Since persons with diabetes and healthcare providers are not required to report these events, there may be underreporting of adverse outcomes. Nevertheless, over half of Class 1 drug recalls (those that may result in serious harm or even death) from 2004 to 2012 were of supplements.[9] The September 2016 issue of *Consumer Reports* on vitamins and supplements stated that more than 6,300 serious adverse events were reported to the FDA between 2007 and 2012, and 92 deaths occurred.[10] A *New England Journal of Medicine* report estimated over 23,000 annual emergency room visits secondary to adverse events attributed to dietary supplements.[11]

Testing of Dietary Supplements

Resources are now available that enable consumers and healthcare professionals to verify the accuracy and purity of ingredients listed on the label of a dietary supplement. However, no available resources evaluate product efficacy.

Some organizations have established certification programs for dietary supplements. US Pharmacopeia (USP) has a program called the Dietary Supplement Verification Program (DSVP).[12] A product showing the "USP-verified" mark on the label indicates the product's ingredients are accurate, the product is pure and will dissolve properly, and the product has been manufactured using GMPs. The USP Web site lists manufacturers that have gone through the evaluation process. NSF International also verifies products for label and content accuracy, checks the product for purity and for contaminants, and audits the manufacturing process for GMP compliance.[13] Consumer Lab (CL) also tests supplements for accuracy of ingredient identity, content, and purity.[14] The CL seal of approval is licensed for manufactured products that pass the review. Product names that have failed the review are available only to subscribers. The Natural Products Association also has a GMP program.[15]

Evaluating Claims Made by Manufacturers of Dietary Supplements

Diabetes care and education specialists need to be aware of deceptive marketing tactics used by manufacturers to promote their products. Diabetes care and education specialists may instruct individuals to check the FDA's MedWatch Web site (http://www.fda.gov/medwatch) for information regarding products that may contain adulterants, such as steroids. Three categories of supplements that may be problematic include body building, sexual performance, and weight loss. For example, numerous weight-loss products have been found to contain prescription weight-loss drugs.[16] Diabetes care and education specialists may refer individuals to the FDA's "Health Fraud Scams – Be Smart, Be Aware, Be Careful Video" where diabetes is highlighted.[17] Another FDA consumer health information alert has also highlighted the need to be cautious with supplements for diabetes that make astonishing claims such as "protects your eyes, kidneys, and blood vessels from damage," or it is an "effective treatment to relieve all symptoms of diabetes," or "replaces your diabetes medicine."[18] The FDA Web site (http://www.fda.gov) also has safety alerts and advisories for false advertising and MedWatch safety alerts for safety recalls and labeling concerns.

Examples of phrases with misleading claims listed in the *Handbook of Nonprescription Drugs* include the following:[19]

- Lists disease states or hints that the product may be used to treat conditions normally treated with prescriptions
- States that the product has similar efficacy (or may be used as an alternative) to prescription or nonprescription drugs
- Lists a wide variety of unrelated clinical conditions ("works for everything") that the product may treat
- States only benefits of the product (and not harmful side effects)
- Neglects to provide other critical information on the label, such as expiration date, lot number, or contact information for the manufacturing company
- Uses "pseudo-medical" terminology such as *detoxify*, *purify*, or *breakthrough treatment*
- Uses terms such as *revolutionary therapy* or *miraculous discovery* or other statements that indicate the product is superior to prescriptions
- Suggests the product is more expensive because it works so well
- Provides personal testimonials as proof of efficacy
- Promises rapid relief of a health condition
- Promises superiority over conventional medicine
- Seller offers a money-back guarantee, but changes locations frequently
- Suggests that drug manufacturers and clinicians are collaborating to delude consumers and discourage them from using healthier supplement options

Resources

The FDA Center for Food Safety and Applied Nutrition Web site helps individuals evaluate information about dietary supplements. Healthcare professionals can read and direct persons to the center's articles on supplements.[20,21] The Web site includes points to consider, such as these:

- Check with a healthcare provider before using a supplement.
- Understand that some supplements may interact with prescription or over-the-counter medicines.
- Be aware that supplements can have unwanted effects during surgery.
- Know how to report adverse effects of dietary supplements.
- Know how to search the Internet for information on dietary supplements, such as finding out who operates the site, the purpose of the site, information source and references, and whether the information is current.

The National Center for Complementary and Integrative Health, a division of the National Institutes of health, offers fact sheets on certain herbals and dietary supplements (https://nccih.nih.gov/health/herbsataglance.htm). The fact sheets contain information on common names of products, evidence (if available), side effects, and safety.[22]

The following information is helpful when counseling people on the use of dietary supplements:[18,23]

- Always discuss supplement use with all healthcare providers—such as your diabetes care and education specialist and all medical prescribers—so that they may add the supplements you are taking to your medication list.
- Purchase products that have a quality seal on the label, such as the USP's DSVP or the NSF mark, or products that match content claims assessed by CL.
- Purchase products from reputable companies that have a reputation to uphold. Manufacturers that also produce prescription or nonprescription medications are more likely to have GMPs in place. Some examples are American Home Products or drugstore chain store brands or pharmaceutical companies that manufacture both prescription and supplement products (eg, Pfizer).
- Continue to use the same brand and formulation. Consider that variability may exist between different product lots. Read the label carefully and do

not exceed the recommended dose. Do not select a product that lacks dosing recommendations, lot numbers, expiration dates, or contact information for the manufacturer. Do not share the product with others.

- Be cautious about product use in children, pregnant or lactating women, and older adults.
- Do not combine a supplement with alcohol or drugs that have sedative properties.
- Consider that a supplement may result in side effects or interact with other medications or supplements. Be especially wary of combining a supplement with blood-thinning drugs.
- Due to possible adverse events or drug interactions, discontinue a supplement 2 weeks before surgery.
- Do not substitute a dietary supplement for a prescription drug.
- Consider that the term *natural* does not mean devoid of side effects or other potential problems.
- Do not expect unrealistic results—if it sounds too good to be true, it probably is.
- Do not substitute a supplement for a healthy diet, physical activity, or proper rest.
- Track the effectiveness of the product by keeping a log of blood glucose, A1C, blood pressure, and lipids.

Who Uses Complementary Health Approaches and Why

There are no consistently performed surveys that track how many persons take supplements and thus there are varying statistics. The Council for Responsible Nutrition conducted a survey that found that between 69 and 78% of US adults take dietary supplements. This translates to approximately $35 billion in annual spending.[24]

Complementary Health Approach Use Amongst Persons With Diabetes

The diabetes care and education specialist must be aware that many individuals use CAM, and there are numerous surveys describing CAM use. Data from the 2012 National Health Interview survey indicate 26.2% of adults with diabetes use CAM.[25] Another survey indicated that persons with diabetes are 1.6 times more likely than persons without diabetes to use CAM.[26]

In one survey of adults with diabetes, 67% were using some type of vitamin or supplement.[27] A different survey found that herbs and vitamins were used by 81.9% of persons with diabetes, and that product use varied among different ethnic groups. A review of medication histories of 459 individuals with diabetes indicated that 55% use a supplement on a daily basis.[28] A survey of parents found that 18% were administering CAM to their children with type 1 diabetes, and modalities included homeopathy, modified diet, and supplements such as aloe vera and cinnamon.[29]

Complementary Health Approaches and Older Adults

One-quarter of older adults with diabetes utilize complementary health approaches.[30] Of these older adults, 62.8% utilize herbal therapies specifically. Chiropractic (23.9%), massage (14.7%), acupuncture (10.2%), and yoga (5.2%) were the other most popular therapies used.[30] In particular, managing older adults with diabetes that utilize complementary health approaches may present unique challenges. Older adult persons with diabetes are more likely to have chronic medical conditions as well as diabetes complications. Furthermore, polypharmacy increases with age, and older adults are more likely to use multiple medications.[31]

CAM and Supplement Use Amongst Various Ethnic Groups

Certain ethnic groups may be more likely to use supplements—these include Hispanic, Asian, and Native American populations. A survey of CAM use in 806 individuals with diabetes belonging to different ethnic minorities found that 84.1% of African Americans, 85.6% of Hispanics, 77.8% of Native Americans, 79.6% of Asians, and 66.1% of Pacific Islanders or other minorities used supplements for diabetes.[32] One study found Whites used CAM in addition to their diabetes medications more frequently than Mexican American persons with diabetes. However, Mexican American persons with diabetes were more likely to use CAM instead of their diabetes medications than non-Hispanic Whites.[33]

Reasons Persons With Diabetes Utilize Complementary Health Approaches

Reasons for use of complementary health approaches in persons with diabetes vary. One study sites overall wellness (28% of users), treatment of diabetes (15%), or a combination of the two (57%).[25] Increased medication and provider visit costs may prompt individuals to seek more easily accessible products.[28] Other factors may include a desire to avoid adverse effects of conventional medications since supplements are viewed as "natural," the limited efficacy of traditional medications to "cure" diseases, and the ever-powerful influence of friends, coworkers, and possibly the media that suggests supplement use.[34]

Diabetes severity and duration may influence supplement use. The National Health Interview Survey (2002 and 2007) suggested that persons with more severe diabetes had nearly twice the odds of using CAM. Severity was based on a count of measures such as 5 or more years since diagnosis, use of insulin or oral hypoglycemic agents, and at least 1 functional limitation secondary to the diabetes, as well as 3 known diabetes complications. Those with diabetes duration greater than 10 years had a 66% higher CAM use compared with those whose diabetes duration was less than 10 years.[35] Contrary to previous years, the number of persons with diabetes that report use of supplements to providers has increased.[36]

Reasons for Concern Regarding Use of CAM

There are a number of reasons for concern with dietary supplement use that diabetes care and education specialists need to convey to persons with diabetes. Table 21.2 summarizes these concerns, with details provided in the paragraphs that follow.

Side Effects and Drug Interactions

Potential side effects and drug interactions of dietary supplements are two critical issues that must be considered. Although the percentage of persons with diabetes that inform their provider they are using supplements has increased to 75%,[36] there may still be issues with determining whether any unusual side effects are due to a supplement or whether drug interactions may occur. The primary reason cited for not informing a provider about supplement use was that the individual was not asked about use of supplements.[36] An individual may experience a side effect that the provider attributes to another medication. Since persons with diabetes take several medications, concomitant use of dietary supplements may result in toxicity secondary to exaggerated or subtherapeutic effects of medications. Individuals may concomitantly take several different supplements, and the potential for interactions with conventional medications may dramatically increase. For instance, a person may be taking garlic along with fenugreek, and the potential for bleeding reactions secondary to the intrinsic antiplatelet activity of these agents may result in an additive danger to the individual.

TABLE 21.2 Reasons for Concern With Dietary Supplement Use
• Potential side effects
• Drug interactions
• Lack of proven effectiveness
• Product variability
• Lack of product standardization
• Possibility of contamination
• Possibility of misidentification
• Delay in using more effective interventions
• Additional costs for medical care

Product Variability

Product variability is another reason for concern. Products are available as capsules, tablets, powders, or liquid forms that are water or alcohol based. The quality of botanical products depends on what part of the plant was used, how it was grown and stored, length of storage, processing technique, and how the extract was prepared.[37,38] There may also be variability in doses and consistency of reported ingredients.[39] Lead contamination in some products has been reported.[40]

Lack of Standardization

Standardization should guarantee consistency between different lots as well as stability of the active ingredients. However, standardization is not a simple process, because the active constituents are unknown for many agents. A product that is standardized for certain markers may show consistency, but the marker may not be the active ingredient. Pharmacologic action may be due to additive or synergistic effects of several ingredients, but individual ingredients found separately may not have the same activity as the whole plant.[41] Active constituents in extracts or dried botanicals may vary due to differences in geographic location or soil, exposure to sunlight or rainfall, harvest time, and methods of drying, storage, and processing. These variables may affect pharmacologic activity.[42]

"Other Ingredient" Concerns

Other cautions involve potential misidentification, mislabeling, possible addition of unnatural toxic substances such as heavy metals and steroids, or contamination with microbes, pesticides, fumigants, and radioactive products.[16,43] As another example, herbal products for diabetes have been found to contain undeclared medications that resulted in hypoglycemic reactions and lactic acidosis.[44]

Increased Costs

Another concern is possible increased indirect costs because individuals may substitute ineffective therapies for proven medications or delay treatment and thus have needless problems. Costs may include hospitalizations, acute problems (such as ketoacidosis or acute hyperglycemia), or complications such as retinopathy.[45] Other costs include decreased work productivity or ability to function in social or occupational settings. Treatment of adverse events and emergency department visits may add to increased costs.[12]

Points for Education

Discuss with interested individuals how dietary supplements are subject to variability, may or may not have standardized ingredients, or may be vulnerable to product contamination or substitution with unwanted ingredients. All of these factors make the individual vulnerable to potential side effects, drug interactions, and possible increased costs.

Review of Dietary Supplements

Persons with diabetes may inquire most often about products to achieve two main goals: lowering blood glucose and decreasing the complications of diabetes. Not all products proposed for these uses can be recommended as safe supplements, therapies, or foods, as this part of the chapter will show. The sections that follow describe characteristics of (1) botanical and nonbotanical products used to lower blood glucose and (2) botanical and nonbotanical products used to treat diabetes complications. Tables 21.5 and 21.6 provide specific information regarding each entity's name, chemical constituents, mechanism of action, side effects, and drug interactions.

In previous editions, these tables had provided a classification for efficacy available through a Web site called Natural Standard, which is no longer available. Natural Standard and the Natural Medicines Comprehensive Database have merged, and the new Web site is Natural Medicines.[46] The new Web site no longer provides an evidence grade since the previous classification did not address product safety. Natural Medicines now provides comparative effectiveness charts for disease states (Tables 21.3 and 21.4). In Tables 21.5 and 21.6, the new classification system will replace the nomenclature previously used.

TABLE 21.3 Effectiveness Categories From Natural Medicines

- "Effective"—Evidence is consistent with passing a review by a rigorous process that has achieved a high level of reliable clinical evidence, such as passing a review by the FDA or Health Canada.
- "Likely effective"—There is highly reliable clinical evidence, usually by support from randomized clinical trials or meta-analysis involving hundreds to thousands of patients.
- "Possibly effective"—Evidence is supported by one or more randomized clinical trials or a meta-analysis with low to moderate risk of bias and moderate to high level of validity.
- "Possibly ineffective"—There is evidence showing negative results, but it may be limited by quantity, quality, or contradictory findings.
- "Likely ineffective"—There is highly reliable evidence showing ineffectiveness for use for a specific indication from consistently negative outcomes without significant evidence to the contrary. Trials may involve several hundred patients.
- "Ineffective"—There is highly reliable evidence that shows ineffectiveness for use for a specific indication. Trials may involve several hundreds to thousands of patients. Use is not recommended.
- "Insufficient reliable evidence to rate"—There is insufficient reliable evidence to provide an effectiveness rating.

Source: "Natural Medicines" (cited 2019 June 4), on the Internet at: https://naturalmedicines.therapeuticresearch.com.

TABLE 21.4 Safety Categories From Natural Medicines

- "Likely safe"—There is highly reliable evidence demonstrating the product is safe if used appropriately. Usually there is a high level of reliable clinical evidence, such as passing a review by the FDA or Health Canada.
- "Possibly safe"—There is some clinical evidence supporting safe use if used appropriately. The evidence may be limited by quality, quantity, or contradictory findings. Usually there is not enough high-quality evidence to recommend the product for most persons.
- "Possibly unsafe"—There is some clinical evidence showing safety concerns or adverse outcomes. However, the evidence may be limited by quality, quantity, or contradictory findings. Patients should be discouraged from taking a product with this rating.
- "Likely unsafe"—There is highly reliable evidence showing negative safety issues or adverse outcomes. Patients are discouraged from taking products with this rating. Data are available from multiple randomized trials, meta-analysis, or large-scale post-marketing surveillance.
- "Unsafe"—There is highly reliable evidence that shows safety issues or adverse outcomes. Patients should be discouraged from taking products with this rating. Safety data are available from randomized clinical trials or meta-analysis or post-marketing surveillance. Data are gathered from studies in several hundred to several thousand patients. Trials adequately evaluate and report safety and adverse outcomes, and studies consistently show problems without valid evidence to the contrary.
- "Insufficient evidence"—There is insufficient reliable evidence to provide an adequate safety rating.

Source: "Natural Medicines" (cited 2019 June 4), on the Internet at: https://naturalmedicines.therapeuticresearch.com.

Botanical and Nonbotanical Products Used to Lower Blood Glucose

Persons with diabetes may have heard about the following products for use in lowering blood glucose. Not all are safe or effective. Each is discussed in detail in the paragraphs that follow. The diabetes care and education specialist should note that these are only a few agents and that many other products have been reputed to lower blood glucose levels. Although there are hundreds of studies, only those thought to be most relevant to understand the place in therapy of the individual agents have been included in this chapter.

- Aloe
- Berberine
- Bitter melon
- Chromium
- Cinnamon
- Fenugreek
- Flaxseed
- Ginger
- Ginseng
- Gymnema
- Honey
- Milk thistle
- Nopal
- Probiotics
- Psyllium fiber
- Turmeric
- Vinegar

Information regarding chemical constituents, mechanism of action, side effects, and drug interactions for each of these products is found in Table 21.5. Each of these 17 products is reviewed separately following Table 21.5.

Aloe

Aloe (*Aloe vera L*) is a desert plant with a cactus-like appearance that belongs to the family *Liliaceae*.[46–49] Aloe gel is the clear substance extracted from the leaf core after the main stalk has been removed. Aloe gel is used topically for burns, sunburn, wound healing, moisturizing, and other skin problems, including psoriasis and seborrhea. It has also been used orally to enhance the immune system and to treat asthma, diabetes, and hyperlipidemia.[46,49,50] While aloe is mostly a benign agent, in some instances it is of questionable safety.[46–49] Another plant component, dried aloe leaf juice, was a former ingredient in nonprescription laxative formulations.[46,49]

Recent studies comparing aloe to placebo given over 8 to 12 weeks have shown potential for small but statistically significant results on glucose reduction. For example, a 2-month randomized controlled study compared aloe gel in 30 persons with type 2 diabetes on oral medications (sulfonylureas and metformin) with placebo in another 30 persons with type 2 diabetes.[51] A1C declined by 0.7 percentage points (from 7.3% to 6.6%) in the aloe group compared with a 0.5 percentage point increase (from 7.3% to 7.8%) in the placebo group ($P = 0.036$). Fasting glucose also decreased significantly from 173 to 168 mg/dL (9.6 to 9.3 mmol/L) in the aloe vera group versus an increase of 185 to 191 mg/dL (10.2 to 10.6 mmol/L) in the placebo group ($P = 0.036$). Although low-density lipoprotein (LDL)[52] and triglycerides decreased, the results were not significant. Another trial in 90 persons with diabetes lasting 12 weeks showed small but statistically significant reductions ($P < 0.01$) in fasting glucose, total cholesterol, triglycerides, and LDL.[53] In this controlled trial, subjects were given nutrition education in addition to aloe, and the best results were seen in those who received education.

A 2016 meta-analysis evaluated the impact of aloe vera in persons with diabetes.[54] A decrease in fasting glucose was reported in 9 trials, and a decrease in A1C was reported in 5 trials. Fasting glucose decreased 46.6 mg/dL (2.6 mmol/L) in 283 individuals ($P < 0.0001$), and A1C decreased 1.05% in 89 persons ($P = 0.004$). Another systematic review including aloe given along with contemporary antidiabetic medications is now under way.[55]

An emerging use of aloe is for prediabetes. One study compared 2 doses of aloe vera with placebo for 8 weeks in 72 individuals with prediabetes.[56] Fasting glucose decreased significantly by 4 and 7 mg/dL (0.22 and 0.38 mmol/L, respectively) with both doses ($P = 0.002$ and $P < 0.001$, respectively). A1C decreased by 0.2% with the lower dose and 0.4% with the higher dose ($P = 0.042$ and $P = 0.011$, respectively). Lipids also improved with decreases in LDL ($P < 0.001$ and $P = 0.01$, respectively). In another study comparing 2 doses of aloe complex per day with placebo, fasting glucose decreased by 3 mg/dL ($P = 0.02$) and weight decreased by 1 kg ($P = 0.05$) after 8 weeks of treatment.[57] A systematic review and meta-analysis of randomized controlled trials evaluated aloe in prediabetes and type 2 diabetes.[58] The analysis included 8 randomized controlled trials—3 in prediabetes and 5 in type 2 diabetes. In the prediabetes trials, fasting glucose declined slightly but significantly (4 mg/dL [0.22 mmol/L] decrease; $P < 0.0001$). However, A1C did not decrease in prediabetes. In the diabetes trials, fasting glucose and A1C declined significantly by 21 mg/dL (1.17 mmol/L; $P = 0.05$) and 1% ($P = 0.01$), respectively. A second review published that same year confirmed these findings.[59]

Summary

Doses of aloe are variable, ranging from 50 to 600 mg per day of aloe gel.[46,51] In 2 studies, 15 mL twice daily of aloe leaf gel was used.[47] Aloe gel contains acemannan, a polysaccharide that is high in fiber and may slow or prevent glucose absorption.[46] However, aloe juice contains cathartics, and there is concern that there may be inadvertent inclusion of these components in aloe products. Aloe is used as capsules, tablets, or liquids. Many Hispanics use aloe in shakes and smoothies (the Spanish word for aloe is *sábila*). A case report of prolonged bleeding when used with the anesthetic agent sevoflurane warrants discontinuation 2 weeks before surgery.[49] Cases of acute hepatitis and thyroid dysfunction have been reported.[48] Although studies have shown some benefit, there is insufficient evidence for use of aloe as an oral product in diabetes or prediabetes. Short-term use has decreased fasting glucose, triglycerides, LDL, and A1C. However, supplementation is not recommended, especially due to the potential contamination with cathartic ingredients and problems with fluid and electrolyte disturbances, particularly potassium.

Berberine

Berberine is an isoquinoline alkaloid extracted from many different plants, such as the Chinese herb *Coptis chinensis [Huanglian or French]*, goldenseal, tree turmeric, European barberry, and others. It was found to lower glucose when it was used to treat bacterial diarrhea in persons with diabetes.[46] Besides lowering glucose it also has been shown to have lipid- and blood pressure–lowering effects.[46,59–68]

Evidence

Berberine was compared with placebo in a 3-month study in 116 persons with newly diagnosed type 2 diabetes mellitus (T2DM) and hyperlipidemia.[64] There was a significant decrease in A1C and in fasting and postprandial glucose in the berberine group compared with placebo ($P < 0.0001$ for each parameter). A1C decreased from 7.5% to 6.6% in the berberine group and from 7.6% to 7.3% in the placebo group. There were also significant decreases favoring berberine in LDL cholesterol ($P < 0.0001$), weight ($P = 0.034$), and systolic blood pressure ($P = 0.038$).

A different randomized study evaluated 97 persons with T2DM for 2 months.[63] Of these, 50 were randomized to berberine, 26 to metformin, and 21 to rosiglitazone. Fasting glucose and A1C decreased significantly from baseline in all 3 groups ($P < 0.001$ for berberine and metformin; $P < 0.01$ for rosiglitazone). A1C decreased from 8.3% to 6.8% in the berberine group, 9.4% to 7.2% in the metformin group, and 8.3% to 6.8% in the rosiglitazone group. Triglycerides decreased significantly only in the berberine group ($P < 0.01$).

Another randomized controlled trial evaluated 2 groups with T2DM—one group was newly diagnosed and the other was poorly controlled.[65] The newly diagnosed group took berberine or metformin for 3 months. In both groups there was a significant decline from baseline in A1C, fasting glucose, and postprandial glucose ($P <$ 0.01 compared with baseline). A1C decreased from 9.5% to 7.5% in the berberine group and from 9.2% to 7.7% in the metformin group. Fasting glucose also decreased in both groups. The authors did not provide a statistical analysis of the comparison between berberine and metformin, but the numbers were very similar. Persons with diabetes in the poorly managed group continued their medications (oral agents or insulin), and berberine was added for 3 months. A1C decreased from 8.1% to 7.3%, and fasting and postprandial glucose also decreased. The decreases were all statistically significant ($P < 0.001$ for all 3 parameters).

In a meta-analysis comprising 14 randomized controlled trials and 1068 persons, berberine was significantly more effective than placebo, as effective as metformin or sulfonylureas or glitazones, and was also effective when combined with glucose-lowering agents.[69] A more recent meta-analysis of 27 studies in 2,569 persons also evaluated effects on diabetes (17 trials), lipids (6 trials), and blood pressure (4 trials).[62] This analysis corroborated the benefit of berberine for diabetes, hyperlipidemia, and hypertension. In addition, the analysis also found that the combination of berberine with oral agents (for diabetes, hyperlipidemia, or hypertension) was more effective than the individual oral agents as monotherapy for those disease states.

Summary

Berberine may work in a variety of ways. The main side effects are abdominal upset and constipation.[46,50,69] However, it should not be used by pregnant women due to possible uterine contractions or in lactating women or infants, because it may result in fatal kernicterus.[46] Caution is warranted when used with other agents because berberine may inhibit certain cytochrome P450 enzymes (CYP3A4, 2C9, 2D6) and thus increase levels of drugs metabolized by these enzymes (eg, cyclosporine, certain statins, some calcium channel blockers, warfarin, and certain antihypertensives and psychiatric medications).[46] Berberine (in combination with oral diabetes agents) is now being studied in combination with milk thistle, a different glucose-lowering supplement, and this combination has been found to have greater benefit for A1C lowering than berberine alone.[70] Berberine is one of the more promising supplements that may benefit persons with diabetes since it not only works for lowering glucose but also has lipid- and blood pressure–lowering effects. Doses used in studies have been 500 mg 2 to 3 times daily.

Bitter Melon

Bitter melon (*Momordica charantia*)—also known as bitter gourd, bitter apple, bitter cucumber, karolla, and karela—is a vegetable cultivated in tropical areas, including India, Asia, South America, and Africa. A member of the melon family, bitter melon is yellow-orange, resembles a gherkin, and is bitter but edible.[46] Bitter melon has been used in a variety of diseases, including diabetes, cancer, HIV, and psoriasis.[46,71]

Evidence

Most studies of bitter melon in humans involve few patients, are of short duration, and provide only vague details of the study design, including blinding and randomization. Multiple studies have now been conducted in individuals with prediabetes and diabetes (type 1 and 2) with varying results.[72] Results from various studies have shown that there are responders as well as nonresponders. The first randomized, double-blind, placebo-controlled study was conducted in 40 adults with newly diagnosed or poorly controlled type 2 diabetes; both groups showed a slight nonsignificant decrease in A1C.[73] A 4-week randomized, double-blind, active-control trial compared 3 different doses of bitter melon with metformin in 123 persons with newly diagnosed type 2 diabetes.[74] Metformin and the highest dose of bitter melon decreased fructosamine significantly, although metformin showed a greater lowering. The difference between treatments was not significant. A 16-week parallel, randomized, double-blind, placebo-controlled trial was conducted in 19 persons assigned to 6.26 mg per day of bitter melon and 19 persons assigned to placebo.[75] A1C in those receiving bitter melon declined significantly by 0.5 percentage points, from 7.47% at baseline to 6.97% at endpoint ($P = 0.001$); as compared to the placebo group (0.2%, from 7.32% at baseline to 7.12% at endpoint ($P = 0.153$). The difference between bitter melon and placebo was significant ($P =$ 0.044). A 10-week randomized parallel group trial in 95 persons recently diagnosed with type 2 diabetes was conducted.[71] Two groups were randomized to 2 or 4 g per day of bitter melon (Group I and Group II, respectively), and the third group (Group III) was randomized to 2.5 mg per day of glibenclamide (glyburide, a sulfonylurea) for 10 weeks. Group I had a decrease from 8.25% at baseline to 7.4% at endpoint ($P < 0.05$), Group II decreased from 8.3% to 7.15% ($P < 0.02$), and Group III decreased from 8.45% to 6.9% ($P < 0.005$). There was no statistically significant difference between the three groups.

The most recent studies of bitter melon's effect on glucose are in prediabetes. A randomized placebo-controlled, single-blind study in 52 individuals with prediabetes suggested that bitter melon 2.5 g daily over 8 weeks may significantly reduce fasting plasma glucose up to 5 mg/dL.[76] Another randomized, placebo-controlled, double-blinded study in 114 individuals with prediabetes found that taking 2 g bitter melon daily not only produced a statistically significant reduction in fasting plasma glucose and A1C but also reduced risk (47%) of progression to diabetes.[77] Lastly, bitter melon extract has been shown in a relatively small yet randomized, placebo-controlled double-blinded study of 42 individuals with metabolic syndrome to significantly lower LDL (P = 0.02). No effect was seen on weight, body mass index, blood pressure, total cholesterol, or glucose in this study.[78]

Multiple systematic reviews and meta-analyses have been conducted on the effects of bitter melon in diabetes management. The first Cochrane review of randomized controlled trials comparing bitter melon with placebo or other controls in 479 persons reported that there is insufficient evidence to support its use.[79] Another meta-analysis including 4 randomized controlled trials for a total of 208 persons with type 2 diabetes confirmed bitter melon supplementation lacked effectiveness in lowering A1C or fasting plasma glucose.[80] A third meta-analysis which included 10 studies for a total of 1045 persons found that bitter melon reduced fasting plasma glucose and A1C in both diabetes and prediabetes; however, the evidence was rated as low quality and thus further research was deemed necessary before confidence in its use was warranted.[72]

Summary

Dosage forms for bitter melon include juice, powder, vegetable pulp suspensions, and extract.[46] The dose of bitter melon is 2 to 4 g per day.[46] Some sources recommend eating 1 small unripe melon daily or drinking 50 to 100 mL of fresh juice daily with food.[81] Bitter melon contains a variety of ingredients that may produce hypoglycemic effects and affect glucose uptake.[46,50,59,81–83] Bitter melon may inhibit enzymes involved in glucose production and glucose oxidation, which may be of importance in persons of Mediterranean ancestry.[46,50,81] Medical supervision is always necessary when using bitter melon, due to the possibility of adverse effects, especially in certain populations, such as those of Mediterranean ancestry, women of childbearing age,[81] or those with melon allergies.[46] Studies evaluating the role of bitter melon supplements continue to be done, and it is unknown which dosage forms are the most appropriate. The overall evidence does not justify its use; however, it is important to acknowledge that many persons throughout the world consume it as a vegetable as part of their diet.

Chromium

Chromium is a trace element found in certain foods such as brewer's yeast, oysters, mushrooms, liver, potatoes, beef, cheese, and fresh vegetables.[46] Chromium has been studied in type 1 and type 2 diabetes, gestational diabetes, impaired glucose tolerance, and hyperlipidemia.[46] Chromium has also been studied for weight loss. Increased chromium levels with supplementation is not the factor that improves hyperglycemia. The concept of chromium responders versus nonresponders has been suggested. Responders are more likely to have higher baseline fasting glucose and A1C and be more insulin resistant than nonresponders.

Chromium deficiency may occur if a person is on total parenteral nutrition (TPN), during pregnancy, or if the person has a poor diet, high glucose intake, or poor glucose management. Currently, no evidence shows that chromium deficiency rates in persons with diabetes are different from those of the general population. The Food and Nutrition Board of the Institute of Medicine (IOM) determined there was not sufficient evidence to set an estimated average requirement for chromium. An adequate intake was set based on estimated mean intakes. The adequate intake for young men is 35 mcg per day (30 mcg per day for those aged 51 and older) and 25 mcg per day for young women (20 mcg per day for those aged 51 and older). Because few serious adverse effects are reported from excess intake of chromium from food, no tolerable upper level was established. Since there is no accurate assay for body chromium stores, it is difficult to determine when an individual has chromium deficiency and whether supplementation is effective.

Evidence

Positive effects of chromium have been shown in persons with type 1 or type 2 diabetes, gestational diabetes, polycystic ovarian syndrome (PCOS),[84] and impaired glucose tolerance.[46,85–92] Multiple meta-analyses have shown variable benefits for diabetes and hyperlipidemia.[93–96] Recent studies have shown variable results for the benefits of chromium on glucose management in type 2 diabetes and other metabolic markers such as weight maintenance. One study of 200 mcg of chromium picolinate twice daily in 73 elderly person with diabetes showed a significant reduction in A1C (8.2%-7.7%, P = 0.01).[87] Another study of 1,000 mcg chromium daily in 39 persons was found to reduce weight gain associated with sulfonylurea use.[89] However, a third study in 56 persons over 90 days found no difference in glucose metabolism, body mass index, or insulin sensitivity for daily doses of 50 mcg or 200 mcg as compared to placebo.[97] The longest study to date was a randomized, placebo-controlled, single-blind trial in 71 persons taking 300 mcg chromium picolinate twice daily over 4 months.[91] A1C was significantly reduced in both the control and intervention groups (P = 0.001), but those taking chromium saw a greater decrease (-1.9%, P = 0.015). Both fasting and postprandial glucose also decreased significantly, while no change in lipids was seen.[91]

Chromium picolinate has been combined with biotin, a water-soluble B vitamin that plays a role in carbohydrate and lipid metabolism and enhances the effect of chromium on glucose disposal and lipid metabolism.[98] A 90-day randomized, double-blind, placebo-controlled study demonstrated improved glycemic levels with a combination of chromium and biotin in people with type 2 diabetes.[99] Mean A1C declined by 0.54% from a baseline of 8.73% in the chromium group and by 0.34% from a baseline of 8.46% in the placebo group (P = 0.03 vs. placebo). Mean fasting glucose also decreased significantly in the chromium group. Chromium has also been used in combination with vitamins C and E with limited success in reducing oxidative stress, which also has beneficial effects on glucose metabolism.[100]

In 40 persons with newly diagnosed T2DM, half were randomized to 9 g of a brewer's yeast extract containing 42 mcg of chromium, and the other half were randomized to placebo.[101] After 3 months, A1C decreased from 9.5% to 6.86% in the chromium group ($P < 0.001$), fasting glucose and LDL declined significantly ($P < 0.001$), and triglycerides also decreased significantly. The placebo group had slight, nonsignificant decreases in these clinical values.[101] Another study randomized 15 persons to have chromium-enriched yeast whole wheat bread and another 15 to whole wheat bread without chromium.[102] After 12 weeks, A1C decreased from 6.9% to 6.3% (P < 0.05) in the chromium group, as well as significant reductions in other parameters (fasting glucose, BMI, and blood pressure).

Multiple systematic reviews and meta-analyses have been conducted for the effects of chromium supplementation on glucose metabolism. The first analysis identified a total of 41 studies with 1,138 total subjects taking a variety of formulations and doses of chromium between 8 weeks to 4 months.[93] When pooled, the results produced an estimated decrease in A1C of 0.6% (95% CI -0.9 to -0.2) in the 18 studies that measured it. However, the overall quality of the studies included was low.[93] No significant changes were found for LDL, triglycerides, or HDL. The second analysis included 25 randomized controlled trials evaluating efficacy and safety of chromium monosupplementation, or in combination with biotin (2 trials), or with vitamins C and E (1 trial) versus placebo for diabetes treatment.[94] There were 1,284 persons with diabetes in the 22 trials involved in monosupplementation. The trials lasted from 4 to 24 weeks. In the 14 trials that assessed A1C, the decrease was 0.55% (P = 0.001), and in the 24 studies that evaluated fasting glucose, the decrease was 20.7 mg/dL (1.15 mmol/L; P = 0.001) versus placebo. Chromium monosupplementation lowered triglycerides by 26.6 mg/dL (0.30 mmol/L; P = 0.002) and high-density lipoprotein (HDL) increased 4.6 mg/dL (0.115 mmol/L; P = 0.01). Decreases in total and LDL cholesterol were not significant. A third pooled analysis, including 28 studies lasting 7 to 24 weeks and a total of 1,295 persons with diabetes, found similar results: significant reductions in A1C (–0.54%; 95% CI, –0.82, –0.25; P = 0.0002), fasting glucose, and triglycerides.[96] No change in LDL, blood pressure, or body mass index was detected. An analysis of additional trials reviewing various formulations of chromium, including brewer's yeast, reported no effect on A1C lowering and marginal but significant decreases in fasting plasma glucose (19.23 mg/dL [1.07 mmol/L]; 95% CI, –35.3, –3.16).[103] The most rigorous meta-analysis of 20 trials established clinically meaningful treatment goals (reduction in fasting glucose to <130 mg/dL and A1C to <7% or a decrease of at least 0.5%).[95] In this analysis, only 5 studies reached the goal for fasting glucose and only 3 reached the goal for A1C. Based on these results, the authors concluded the studies are not of high enough quality to produce clinically relevant confidence in the effects of chromium in treatment of type 2 diabetes.[95]

Summary

The typical dose of chromium ranges from 200 mcg to 1,000 mcg per day.[46] Short-term dose-related responses have been shown, and doses up to 1,000 mcg per day for 64 months have not shown adverse effects.[88] However, more study is needed. Results from chromium research are not conclusive, particularly in light of the lack of information regarding the most appropriate biomarkers for chromium or the most appropriate formulation. If used, the picolinate salt appears to be the most appropriate form due to superior bioavailability. Although chromium supplementation has shown both positive and negative results, there is evidence that it may help lower A1C and fasting glucose. However, many experts believe that until there is an appropriate assay to determine chromium body stores and thus ascertain whether deficiency exists, supplementation will remain controversial.

Cinnamon

Cinnamon (*Cinnamomum cassia*) comes from an evergreen tree that grows in tropical climates. The tree's aromatic bark is removed in short lengths and dried.[46] Cinnamon has been used in both type 1 diabetes and type 2 diabetes, in prediabetes, and for gastrointestinal (GI) complaints such as dyspepsia and flatulence. Cinnamon is a popular flavoring agent in different foods and beverages.[46,50,59] There are several species of cinnamon, including *C. cassia* and *C. zeylanicam* (often referred to as "true cinnamon"), but the *cassia* species has been the most studied in humans.[104]

Evidence

Numerous studies have evaluated cinnamon for diabetes, and while some studies have shown efficacy, others have not shown a benefit.[105–113] There are no large long-term randomized controlled trials. The first meta-analysis of 5 randomized controlled trials in 282 persons found that A1C does not decrease, although potential benefits in individual studies included decreases in fasting glucose and lipids.[109] A subsequent review included 6 trials using cinnamon for 40 days to 4 months, 5 of which showed significant reduction in glucose markers and 2 did not.[104] The most recent review included 11 randomized controlled trials, all of which reported reduction in fasting glucose and modest decrease in A1C.[114] However, only 4 of the trials achieved clinically relevant goals of fasting glucose <130 mg/dL or A1C <7%.[114] A Cochrane Database review evaluated 10 randomized controlled studies of 577 persons and reported that evidence to support cinnamon use is insufficient and that there was no statistically significant difference in A1C with a mean difference of only –0.06%.[115] A different meta-analysis of 10 clinical trials of 543 individuals reported that cinnamon significantly improved fasting glucose by 24.6 mg/dL (1.36 mmol/L), improved fasting lipids, and slightly although nonsignificantly decreased A1C in short-term studies.[116]

Recent studies continue to report conflicting results. A randomized placebo-controlled study evaluated a standardized aqueous cinnamon extract in 173 persons with hyperglycemia.[117] At a dose of 250 mg twice daily for 2 months, fasting and 2-hour postprandial glucose declined significantly in the cinnamon group. Fasting glucose decreased from 159.3 mg/dL (8.85 mmol/L) to 147.4 mg/dL (8.19 mmol/L) ($P < 0.005$). The 2-hour postprandial glucose decreased from 271.6 mg/dL (15.09 mmol/L) to 239.4 mg/dL (13.3 mmol/L) ($P < 0.0001$). Fructosamine also declined significantly ($P < 0.05$). A smaller study in 58 persons with type 2 diabetes showed that 2 g daily decreased A1C by only 0.36%, but this was significant.[106] A smaller study in 44 persons with type 2 diabetes over 8 weeks showed cinnamon 3,000 mg/day was not associated with a decrease in A1C.[118] The most recent randomized controlled trial in 116 individuals with metabolic syndrome taking 3,000 mg/day cinnamon for 16 weeks showed significant reductions in fasting glucose, A1C, waist circumference, and body mass index.[119]

Summary

Cinnamon is thought to work by a variety of mechanisms. Cinnamon has been found to decrease fasting glucose, total cholesterol, LDL, and triglycerides in some studies, but even when results are significant there may be substantial heterogeneity, making individual results for patients difficult to determine. A1C lowering has not been consistently significant. Long-term safety has been questioned, due to possible coumarin content in some species and subsequent hepatotoxicity. Doses used have ranged from 1 to 6 g per day in divided doses.[46] It is unknown whether the most appropriate form is the whole powdered spice (possibly a combination of different types of cinnamon) or an aqueous extract.[112] Overall, cinnamon used as a food is safe, and even though there are conflicting results there continues to be great interest in its use for diabetes and prediabetes.

Fenugreek

Fenugreek (*Trigonella foenum-graecum*) is a member of the *Leguminosae* family, along with other plants such as chickpeas, peanuts, and green peas. The plant grows in India, Egypt, and other parts of the Middle East and has been used for centuries as a cooking spice and flavoring agent and for various other purposes.[46,50,59] The seed has been used medicinally to treat diabetes, constipation, and hyperlipidemia. Fenugreek has also been used postpartum with a substance called jaggery to promote lactation, although there is scant evidence for this use.

Evidence

There are few human studies on fenugreek. Most are short-term involving few patients and do not adequately report details. Few if any recent studies have been published. A 10-day study in 10 persons with type 1 diabetes reported a decrease in fasting glucose and lipids.[120] A 6-month trial evaluated 60 persons with inadequately managed type 2 diabetes.[121] Twice-daily fenugreek powder decreased fasting and postprandial glucose, and A1C decreased from 9.6% to 8.4% after 8 weeks.[121] In a 2-month study in 25 persons with newly diagnosed type 2 diabetes, a hydroalcoholic fenugreek seed extract improved "area under the curve" blood glucose, insulin levels, hypertriglyceridemia, and HDL cholesterol.[122] Fenugreek, at a dose of 6.3 g daily, in combination with sulfonylureas, has been shown to decrease A1C from a baseline of 8.02% to 6.56% after 12 weeks of use in 69 persons with type 2 diabetes.[123]

Another small trial showed that when 10 g per day of powdered fenugreek seeds was first soaked in hot water and then later consumed, fasting glucose and triglycerides decreased significantly but there was no significant reduction in A1C.[124]

A meta-analysis evaluated 10 clinical controlled trials in 278 individuals with study duration ranging from 10 to 84 days.[125] The study design was heterogeneous and various dosage forms were used. Some used fenugreek included in chapati bread (unleavened bread); others used fenugreek capsules. Doses ranged from 1 to 100 g daily, and trials were of parallel design or crossover trials. The comparison was with placebo in 6 studies, unspecified in 1, and with chapati bread without fenugreek in 3 studies. All 10 studies evaluated fasting glucose, which showed a decrease of 17.3 mg/dL (0.96 mmol/L, P = 0.001). Two-hour postprandial glucose was evaluated in 7 trials and showed a decrease of 39.4 mg/dL (2.19 mmol/L, P < 0.001). In the 3 trials that evaluated A1C, there was a decrease of 0.85% (P = 0.009). Another meta-analysis included 12 trials in 1,173 individuals with type 2 diabetes or prediabetes for treatment periods ranging from 1 week to 3 years (median treatment time 60 days).[126] Pooled results showed fenugreek significantly reduced fasting glucose ~15 mg/dL (P = 0.002). Seven of the studies measured A1C, which when pooled showed a significant reduction of −1.16% (P = 00001). Changes in lipids (triglycerides, LDL, and HDL) were incremental.[126] Both meta-analyses reported that the studies on fenugreek are small and some of low quality.

Summary

Although fenugreek has been categorized by the FDA as generally recognized as safe (GRAS), the quality of studies evaluating this agent is suboptimal. Fenugreek contains a variety of saponins and glycosides, and the seeds contain hydroxyisoleucine and a variety of alkaloids.[46,127] Fenugreek also has coumarin-like ingredients and other components that may affect carbohydrate absorption and glucose transport.[46,127] Most side effects are uncomfortable GI effects.[46] Pregnant women should avoid fenugreek since uterine contractions may occur. Fenugreek has been used as a galactogogue, and since it may appear in breast milk, it could potentially adversely affect the breastfeeding infant. Individuals taking antiplatelet agents should avoid fenugreek. Hence, fenugreek has limited overall safety. The recommended dose is variable, although a typical dose is 10 to 15 g per day (as a single dose or divided with meals) or 1 g per day of a hydroalcoholic extract.[46,122] As with all supplements, medical supervision is warranted with fenugreek use, especially in women of childbearing age and persons who are on anticoagulants.

Flaxseed

Flaxseed (*Linum usitassimum*) is a grain that is rich in soluble fiber and contains alpha-linolenic acid (a plant omega-3 fatty acid) and lignans (a phytoestrogen).[46,128] Flaxseed (in various forms such as whole seed, ground seed, or flaxseed oil) is a popular product consumed by many individuals with and without diabetes primarily for cardiovascular disease protection and for a variety of maladies such as constipation and diarrhea. A major plant lignan in flaxseed is secoisolariciresinol diglucoside (SDG).[46,129] Although flaxseed consumption increases omega-3 fatty acids in plasma and red blood cells, the alpha-linolenic acid in flaxseed does not have the same physiological effects as the omega-3 fatty acids in fish oil.[130] In diabetes and prediabetes, flaxseed is used for glucose lowering[46,129,131,132] as well as for hyperlipidemia,[46,128,132] inflammation,[46,133] and hypertension.[130,134] Postmenopausal women may use flaxseed for menopausal symptoms such as hot flashes because the lignans in flaxseed are phytoestrogens with a mixed profile of estrogenic and anti-estrogenic effects.[46]

Evidence

In an evaluation of flaxseed on diabetes outcomes, 73 persons with type 2 diabetes took a flaxseed derivative or placebo for 12 weeks, and after an 8-week washout were then crossed over to the other group.[129] The main benefit was a very modest but statistically significant decrease in A1C (decrease of 0.1%; P = 0.01). Another open-label study evaluated 10 g per day of flaxseed in 18 persons with type 2 diabetes compared with 11 persons on placebo for 1 month.[131] A1C decreased 0.59 percentage points, from 8.75% to 8.16%, in the flaxseed group (P = 0.009 versus baseline) and increased 0.1% in the placebo group. Fasting glucose decreased 28.9 mg/dL (1.6 mmol/L) in the flaxseed group (P = 0.02 vs. baseline) but increased slightly in the placebo group. Triglycerides and LDL cholesterol also decreased significantly in the flaxseed group (P = 0.02 for triglycerides and P = 0.02 vs. baseline for LDL). A recent meta-analysis on the effects of flaxseed on measures of blood glucose control identified 25 studies for which data could be pooled.[135] Results showed that flaxseed did not significantly affect A1C. Subgroup analysis stratified results according to the type of flaxseed used. A significant reduction in blood glucose was found for whole flaxseed but not for flaxseed oil or lignan.[135]

In a randomized, placebo-controlled trial in 60 persons with gestational diabetes, a dose of 1,000 mg omega-3 fatty acids from flax seed oil plus 400IU vitamin E was found to modestly but statistically significantly decrease fasting glucose and other markers of glucose metabolism over a 6-week period, but no difference in lipids was detected.[136] In a randomized crossover study, 25 overweight or obese individuals with prediabetes were randomized to 2 different doses of flaxseed or placebo.[132] After 12 weeks, individuals had a 2-week washout and were crossed over to another group. Fasting glucose decreased significantly in patients on the lower dose of flaxseed ($P = 0.021$). There were no significant changes in inflammatory markers.[132]

Lipid-lowering effects were evaluated in a meta-analysis of 28 trials in 1,381 individuals.[137] A variety of flaxseed product types were used. In the flaxseed groups, total cholesterol decreased nonsignificantly by 3.867 mg/dL (0.10 mmol/L, $P = 0.06$), but LDL cholesterol decreased significantly by 3.09 mg/dL (0.08 mmol/L, $P = 0.04$). Women had greater decreases than men for total cholesterol (9.2 mg/dL [0.24 mmol/L], $P < 0.0001$; 3.48 mg/dL [0.09 mmol/L], $P = 0.21$, respectively). However, there was substantial heterogeneity in the studies. A systematic review and meta-analysis corroborated the lack of impact on lipid and inflammatory markers.[133]

Flaxseed was administered to hypertensive patients with peripheral arterial disease (PAD) to determine the impact on blood pressure in a randomized controlled trial.[130] Systolic blood pressure decreased from 143.3 to 136.2 mm Hg ($P = 0.04$) in the flaxseed group and increased in the placebo group. Diastolic pressure decreased from 77 to 71.8 mm Hg in the flaxseed group ($P = 0.004$) and remained the same in the placebo group.

Summary

Flaxseed is a very popular product used by individuals to lower glucose, lipids, and hypertension. The mechanism of action is varied, and the fiber it contains helps decrease not only glucose absorption and postprandial glucose but also lipids and blood pressure.[46] Studies of flaxseed have shown mixed results, and study limitations include small numbers of patients, limited duration of use, and modest benefit. The fiber content promotes satiety, and thus there is interest in possibly helping promote weight loss.[46] Patients should be cautioned regarding use of raw or unripe flaxseed due to possible toxic cyanide ingredients.[46]

Ginger

Ginger comes from the tuberous root of a perennial plant (*Zingiber officinale, Amomum zingiber*).[46] Ginger is used as a culinary spice and medicinally for a variety of ailments but most often is used as a remedy for nausea/vomiting and motion sickness.[46]

Evidence

Ginger has been studied for its effects in type 2 diabetes both in formulated doses as well as effects of dietary intake. Trials evaluating the use of ginger in measurable doses are summarized in 2 recent meta-analyses.[138,139] The first systematic review and meta-analysis included 12 randomized, controlled trials lasting 6 to 12 weeks in length for doses of 1 to 3 g ginger per day.[139] Results suggest that ginger is potentially effective as A1C was shown in 4 studies to be statistically significantly reduced up to 1% ($P = 0.001$, 95% CI –1.56 to –0.44). A statistically significant reduction in mean fasting glucose (up to –21 mg/dL) was found when pooling data from 6 studies. Other markers of metabolic syndrome (LDL, total cholesterol, HDL) were also found to be slightly improved. No change in BMI was detected.[139]

The most recent meta-analysis focused on trials reporting fasting glucose and/or A1C results only, which included 8 of the 12 trials that the first analysis included.[138] The dose of ginger in these studies was higher on average than the previous meta-analysis (2-4 g per day). Data from a total of 245 subjects were pooled to evaluate change in fasting glucose, which was found to produce no significant difference. Data from a total of 215 subjects were assessed to show an improvement in A1C –0.46% (95% CI, 0.09, 0.84; $P = 0.02$).[138]

Summary

The results from multiple studies suggest that ginger may have some modest effect on overall glucose stability when taken long-term, but may not produce reductions in fasting glucose when taken for less than 3 months.[138] Doses closer to 3 g per day are likely to be needed to produce beneficial effects.[46] When taken at these larger doses side effects such as bloating, flatulence, and diarrhea could potentially be more likely to occur.

Ginseng

Two main ginseng products are used in diabetes: Asian or Korean ginseng (*Panax ginseng*) and American ginseng (*Panax quinquefolius L.*). The root is the part used.[46,140] Asian and American ginseng belong to the plant family *Araliaceae* and the genus *Panax*. Ginseng has been described as an adaptogen, an agent that may increase resistance to adverse influences such as infection and stress.[46,140] Individuals use ginseng to enhance physical or psychomotor performance and cognitive function, and for immunomodulation, infections, sexual dysfunction, and diabetes.[46,140] Overall, ginseng is a popular product used for diabetes and other purposes because of a variety of pharmacologic effects.[46,140,141]

Evidence

Ginseng has been studied extensively for a variety of uses. Several studies have focused on diabetes.[140,142–145]

In persons with newly diagnosed type 2 diabetes, 100 mg or 200 mg of ginseng daily was compared with placebo. Although baseline values for glucose and A1C levels were not stated, lower endpoint A1C values were reported.[144] The endpoint A1C level in the 200-mg ginseng group was 6%, and A1C was 6.5% in both the 100-mg and placebo groups. Hence, there may have been an issue with the accuracy of diagnosis or the study population. In two other studies, American ginseng was reported to acutely lower postprandial glucose levels when persons with diabetes were given a 25-g OGTT.[142,143] In a double-blind crossover trial, Asian ginseng improved erectile dysfunction, which may be of importance to men with diabetes.[140]

One double-blind, randomized, placebo-controlled crossover study in 19 persons with type 2 diabetes found that 6 g per day of Asian ginseng for 12 weeks did not decrease A1C, but the persons with diabetes were at target A1C at baseline.[146] However, some OGTT indices improved, such as peak plasma glucose and peak plasma insulin. Also, fasting insulin sensitivity increased significantly. A different randomized, placebo-controlled, double-blind crossover study evaluated 2.2 g per day of Asian ginseng given for 4 weeks to 20 persons with type 2 diabetes.[147] Fasting glucose decreased slightly, but significantly, and insulin resistance also improved. A different study in 15 overweight or obese subjects (with impaired glucose tolerance or newly diagnosed type 2 diabetes) found that administration for 30 days of ginseng root extract 8 g per day, ginsenoside Re, or placebo did not improve beta cell function or insulin sensitivity.[145]

Two systematic reviews evaluated Asian ginseng for various medical disorders and found that results are promising for glucose metabolism and immune response moderation but that further studies are needed.[141,148] The review by Shergis et al emphasized that studies use a variety of preparations, and this may be problematic.[148] Shistar et al also noted that inconsistencies in inclusion criteria for each study may lead to much different outcomes.[141] A third systematic review by Gui et al noted no significant difference in regard to A1C lowering, but did find an improvement in fasting glucose and postprandial insulin levels.[149] A fourth meta-analysis including 17 trials looked at the effect of ginseng on blood pressure and found no significant change after 4 weeks of treatment.[150]

Summary

Ginseng is a complex product that contains several ginsenosides with varying effects on blood pressure and the central nervous system.[46] Some estimates indicate that 6 million Americans use ginseng regularly for a variety of therapeutic reasons, including increased energy.[46] Although ginseng is used for a variety of reasons, it has been studied in type 2 diabetes.[46,140,143] The 2 main types of ginseng used for diabetes are Asian and American. Asian ginseng is dosed at 200 mg per day.[46,144] American ginseng is dosed at 3 g per day, right before and up to 2 hours before a meal.[46,142,143] Other forms of ginseng used include fresh and dried roots, extracts, solutions, sodas, teas, and cosmetics. Length of use should be limited to 3 months, due to concerns about hormone-like effects.[46] There has been inconsistency between the actual amount of active ginsenosides contained in ginseng products and the amount stated on the label.[151] Although ginseng may provide some benefits to persons with diabetes, it is difficult to know the appropriate form and dose, and there are a variety of side effects and drug interactions.

Gymnema

A member of the milkweed family, gymnema (*Gymnema sylvestre* R. Br.) is a woody climbing plant that is found in the tropical forests of India (where it is known as *gurmar*) and also in Africa.[46] Gymnema leaf has been used for centuries to treat diabetes and has a unique history of research and use.[152–155]

Evidence

There are only a few human studies of gymnema. Trials conducted in persons with type 1 diabetes and in persons with type 2 diabetes reported decreases in levels of A1C, fasting blood glucose, and lipids.[153,156,157] Most of these studies did not report important details of study design, such as blinding and randomization. A study evaluating gymnema sylvestre in type 2 diabetes noted a decrease in fasting glucose through 30 days, but this effect was not sustained at day 40.[158] In a study in type 1 diabetes, 27 subjects were followed for 6 to 30 months.[153] A1C declined from 12.8% at baseline to 9.5% after 6 to 8 months ($P < 0.001$). At the end of 30 months, only 6 individuals remained, and mean A1C was 8.2% (P values not reported).[153] In a study of 22 individuals with type 2 diabetes, A1C declined from 11.9% to 8.5% ($P < 0.001$) after 18 to 20 months. Fasting glucose and lipids also decreased.[156]

An open-label study evaluated 500 mg per day of gymnema or placebo for 3 months in 58 persons with type 2 diabetes.[154] A total of 39 people took gymnema and 19 people took either placebo or no supplement. A1C decreased approximately 1 percentage point in the gymnema group (9.6% to 8.6%; exact P not provided, but the authors stated it was significant). Fasting glucose also decreased significantly ($P < 0.005$). Postmeal glucose also declined (exact P not provided, but authors stated it was significant). There was even a small decrease in systolic blood pressure ($P < 0.005$).[154] Another article reported that 500 mg twice daily of an aqueous extract of gymnema leaf for 60 days in 11 persons with diabetes reduced mean fasting glucose ($P < 0.005$) and postprandial glucose ($P < 0.02$).[155] Another study in 32 individuals with type 2 diabetes taking 1 g of gymnema sylvestre for 30 days showed a reduction in fasting glucose and LDL, but it is not clear if randomization and blinding were conducted.[158] The most recent randomized, placebo-controlled trial in 24 individuals studied gymnema 600 mg per day versus placebo.[157] After 12 weeks body weight was 3 kg lower (P = 0.02) and body mass index was lower (30.4 vs. 31.2, P = 0.02) in the intervention group as compared to placebo. Markers of glucose and lipid metabolism were unaffected.

One systematic review of gymnema in obesity and diabetes management was published in 2014. This review concluded that while gymnema has antidiabetic properties, additional human studies are needed to assess both antidiabetic benefits and changes to lipid accumulation.[159]

Summary

Gymnema has limited efficacy data in humans, although there are ongoing studies. Gymnema has been studied for up to 2 years in type 1 diabetes and type 2 diabetes. The gymnemosides may help stimulate glucose uptake and utilization as well as stimulate beta cell function.[46] Some have speculated that gymnema may help treat obesity since it binds to the same taste buds where sugar binds and thus may help curb sugar cravings.[153] Typical doses are 400 mg per day, standardized to contain 24% gymnemic acids, although new aqueous extract forms are emerging.[46,155] The product should not be used without medical supervision, because of potential hypoglycemia and a case report of hepatitis.[160] Doses of secretagogues may have to be adjusted if gymnema is used. Safety of gymnema may be a concern when combined with other diabetes medications.

Honey

Honey as a potential alternative treatment of diabetes mellitus represents a complex recommendation. This sweet food is high in sugar and would typically be limited in a diabetic diet.[161] Honey, which is produced by bees from plant nectar, contains approximately 38% fructose and 31% glucose.[162,163] In addition to sugars, honey also contains proteins, amino acids, fatty acids, vitamins, and various enzymes.[162,164] While honey has long been recognized for its antibacterial activity, its use in the treatment of diabetes mellitus likely relates to the ability to scavenge reactive oxygen species.[164,165] While the mechanism of glucose lowering by honey is still unknown, this antioxidant effect may also lead to additional benefits, including reduced levels of triglycerides and increased HDL cholesterol.[165] Honey preparations containing higher amounts of fructose compared with glucose demonstrate better improvement in glycemic levels. Thus, the fructose to glucose ratio in honey preparations should be taken into account when assessing their blood-sugar-lowering effect.[46,165] Properties of honey also make it a potentially dangerous alternative medication, as honey made from poisonous plants can also be poisonous. Honey made from rhododendrons, for example, contains grayanotoxin, which may lead to cardiovascular adverse effects.[46] Additionally, honey can be contaminated with microorganisms and dust. While most contamination will not survive, spore-forming organisms associated with botulism may remain. Medical grade honey, or Medihoney, has low risk for bacterial spores, as any remaining spores have been irradiated by gamma rays.[46]

Evidence

Human studies regarding the benefits of honey in diabetes mellitus are limited; however, its use is supported by data from the use of honey in diabetic rodents.[166] Data to support honey in the treatment of diabetes mellitus in humans have been limited, with the studies only lasting between 8 and 12 weeks.[46] Nazir et al evaluated the effects of honey on an OGTT, comparing 30 g of honey, 75 g of honey, and 75 g of glucose. This open-label study evaluated 97 adults with type 2 diabetes and noted that mean rise in blood glucose values was substantially higher in the 75-g glucose group when compared with values from the 2 honey groups ($P < 0.001$). A small percentage of those in the 30-g honey group (10.7%) also noted decreased blood glucose from baseline when measured at 2 hours.[167] This study illustrated that there is a lower glycemic response to honey, which can result in a smaller rise in plasma blood glucose following ingestion of honey, compared with the response to oral glucose. This further illustrates the potential for honey to have a lowering effect on plasma blood glucose.[167]

Abdulrhman et al assessed the effect of honey consumption (0.5 mL/kg per day) in persons with type 1 diabetes when compared with a control group. This study evaluated the dietary intervention after 12 weeks and noted a decrease in both fasting plasma glucose (–21 vs. –0.08 mg/dL [1.16 mmol/L vs. 0.0044 mmol/L], $P = 0.001$) and 2-hour postprandial plasma glucose (–13 vs. –0.77 mg/dL [0.72 mmol/L vs. 0.042 mmol/L], P –.031) in the group randomized to honey consumption.[168,169] However, not all studies thus far have shown positive results. Bahrami et al evaluated the effects of honey in 40 people with type 2 diabetes. This study noted no significant difference in fasting blood glucose and actually showed an increase in A1C in the honey group at 8 weeks.[170]

Summary

Use of honey has been proposed to have a lowering effect on plasma blood glucose.[167–169] Risks of using honey are minimal,[46] but emphasis must be placed on the fructose and glucose content of honey, as this may have a detrimental effect on HbA1C.[170] The typical dose of honey consumption is 1 to 2.5 g or 0.5 mL/kg per day for 8 to 12 weeks.[46,168,169] Data to support the use of honey in the treatment of diabetes mellitus are conflicting and support cautious use of honey as a complementary alternative medicine. Overall, honey is likely safe to use, and further studies are needed to validate the findings of the previously mentioned studies.

Milk Thistle

Milk thistle (*Silybum marianum*) is a member of the aster family (*Asteraceae* or *Compositae*), which also includes daisies and thistles.[46,171] Milk thistle has been used extensively for various hepatic disorders and for nonalcoholic steatohepatitis.[172,173] It is used for uterine complaints and stimulating menstrual flow. In Europe, it is also used as a vegetable. Chemical constituents are found in the fruit, seeds, and leaves of the plant.

Evidence

Studies of milk thistle in persons with type 2 diabetes have included those on insulin or oral agents. One study in 40 persons showed 140 mg of milk thistle taken 3 times daily for 45 days reduced fasting glucose, serum insulin, and triglycerides by 11%, 14%, and 23%, respectively.[174] In a randomized open-label trial in a small number of persons with type 2 diabetes and cirrhosis, a number of benefits were reported, including improved glucose and liver function and lower insulin requirements.[175] In another small study of persons with cirrhosis, 10 persons on silymarin plus insulin treatment were compared with 10 persons on insulin plus L-ornithine and L-aspartate.[176] Certain liver function tests improved and mean random glucose decreased significantly in the silymarin group ($P < 0.001$).[176] In a small, 4-month double-blind trial in persons on oral agents for diabetes, A1C declined significantly from 7.8% at baseline to 6.8%.[177] A different study showed that milk thistle added to oral agents also resulted in a decreased A1C from 8.9% at baseline to 7.45%.[178]

A unique emerging role is decreased proteinuria when silymarin is added to angiotensin-converting enzyme (ACE) inhibitors in persons with diabetes. A 3-month randomized, double-blind, placebo-controlled trial of 60 persons with proteinuria and at maximum doses of renin angiotensin system inhibitors evaluated the impact on proteinuria and inflammatory markers.[179] Half were assigned to 420 mg per day of silymarin and half to placebo. Urinary albumin to creatinine ratio (UACR) decreased significantly in the silymarin group. Serum malondialdehyde levels (a marker for oxidative stress) and urinary tumor necrosis factor-α (TNF-α) also decreased significantly.[179] The theorized protective mechanism is that silymarin decreases oxidative stress and inflammation.

Studies have also evaluated a combination of berberine extract with milk thistle and noted the combination was more effective than berberine alone in reducing A1C in persons with type 2 diabetes.[70] Two additional studies found that a fixed dose of this combination significantly reduced fasting glucose and LDL over 90 days and A1C over 1 year.[68,70] A separate study in 85 persons with type 1 diabetes taking this combination over 6 months found that milk thistle and berberine together decreased A1C significantly.[180] Persons taking this combination supplement also used less insulin at meal times than those taking placebo.[180]

Summary

Use of milk thistle has been proposed in diabetes to diminish insulin resistance.[175] Side effects include GI upset and possible allergies to members of the daisy family.[46,171] Milk thistle may have estrogenic effects, so women with breast or uterine cancer should avoid its use.[46] However, milk thistle may increase the clearance of exogenously administered estrogens.[46] Milk thistle may inhibit certain isoenzymes and thus increase serum concentrations of warfarin.[46] Beneficial drug interactions include the attenuation of hepatotoxicity of liver toxic drugs.[171] The typical dose of milk thistle for liver disease is 200 mg 3 times daily. Milk thistle is often standardized to contain 70% silymarin (140 mg of silymarin). Since phosphatidylcholine enhances oral absorption, preparations containing this ingredient may be dosed at 100 mg per day.[171] Doses differ from those used in clinical studies, which ranged from 280 to 800 mg per day. Overall, milk thistle may be safe to use, and more information is emerging.

Nopal

Nopal (*Opuntia streptacantha*), also known as prickly pear, is a member of the cactus family.[46] Multiple species are known as *Opuntia*, including *Opuntia megacantha*, *Opuntia ficus indica*, and *Opuntia fuliginosa*. Research has focused on *Opuntia streptacantha Lemaire* to lower blood glucose. Nopal originated as a food source in Mexico; the stems, flowers, and fruit are used. Leaves and stems are also used to treat diabetes and hyperlipidemia.[46] Many publications regarding its use are emerging.[46,181–185]

Evidence

Most trials with nopal have been small and published in Spanish only, although abstracts are available in English. In 2 small trials in persons with type 2 diabetes, the acute glucose responses of nopal, water, and zucchini or nopal and water were compared.[186,187] A decrease in the postprandial glucose response from nopal was noted. One small study showed that when added to traditional Mexican breakfasts (chilaquiles, burritos, quesadillas), nopal significantly decreased the area under the curve for blood glucose response.[183,188]

A 200-mg capsule consisting of a mixture of the cladode and fruit skin extract has been studied in a randomized placebo-controlled trial in 29 persons with prediabetes.[184] Persons with diabetes underwent 2 different OGTT challenges—1 without nopal to determine baseline values and 1 administered 30 minutes after 2 capsules were administered. Glucose values decreased significantly ($P < 0.05$) when the nopal was administered acutely before the OGTT. Half of the persons with diabetes also took 1 capsule daily of the supplement and half took placebo for 16 weeks. Glucose declined in both groups, but there was no difference in results between the supplement and placebo.[184]

Summary

Nopal may help lower blood glucose when cooked or taken as a supplement.[46] Nopal is a very popular food, and many Hispanics use it in smoothies and shakes. Nopal may decrease carbohydrate absorption due to the soluble fiber and pectin content.[46] There is speculation that high concentrations of trivalent chromium in the cactus pad may be responsible for improved glucose metabolism.[185] Major side effects are related to GI upset.[46,181] A possible side effect is hypoglycemia when taken in combination with sulfonylureas and metformin, based on a case report.[182,186]

The dose used is 100 to 500 g of broiled nopal stems taken with meals.[46] However, ideal doses and the optimal preparation have not been established, and standardized capsule forms are emerging. Nopal is a high-fiber, low-calorie functional food that may be useful for diabetes and hyperlipidemia, and persons with diabetes should be cautioned regarding hypoglycemia if they are on a secretagogue.

Probiotics

Millions of microbes in the gut constitute what is known as the human microbiota.[189,190] The role of the human microbiota is being researched and evaluated in different disease states such as obesity,[191,192] insulin resistance, and diabetes.[193] Altered gut microbiota may correlate with suppression of beneficial incretins such as GLP-1, increased inflammation, increased triglyceride production,[194] inhibition of insulin signaling, and energy changes.[195] Thus, changes in microbiota may be associated with inflammation, obesity, and possibly diabetes.

Evidence

Most available evidence suggests changes in microbiota in diabetes. Most published literature on microbiota in the setting of diabetes are reviews, not experimental trials. Recently, a study found that gut microbiota changes may help identify persons who are at risk for diabetes.[196] An evaluation of 36 individuals with and without T2DM found that certain gram-negative bacteria are found in persons with diabetes.[197] In one small 4-week study, 45 males with type 2 diabetes and either impaired glucose tolerance or normal glucose tolerance were randomized to receive treatment with a probiotic or placebo; after 4 weeks, probiotics enhanced insulin sensitivity.[198] Another study in 238 pregnant women randomized to intensive dietary counseling plus probiotics, intensive dietary counseling plus placebo, or standardized dietary counseling found that probiotic use resulted in fewer cases of gestational diabetes.[199] A systematic review looking at probiotic use in diabetes identified 7 randomized, placebo controlled trials and 13 other experimental studies related to probiotic use and metabolic control.[200] Products containing Lactobacillus and Bifidobacterium were the most commonly used and studied. However, results from analyses of these studies showed conflicting results on probiotic effect on metabolic markers, oxidative stress, inflammation, and incretin production.[200]

Summary

Studies suggest that persons with diabetes have an altered microbiome, and this may start with changes that are correlated with obesity and insulin resistance.[201] The theoretical mechanisms are that probiotics release beneficial organic and free fatty acids that act against pathogenic microbes associated with obesity and insulin resistance, and also that probiotics may enhance incretin effects, decrease inflammation, and enhance insulin sensitivity.[189,190,202] Another potential cause for changes in gut microbiota is use of metformin, a common drug used in diabetes.[196,203] However, probiotic supplementation is not without adverse effects, and problems may occur. For example, increased mortality in persons with pancreatitis who were given probiotics has been reported.[204] Other effects have included GI upset, constipation, possible microbe migration from the digestive tract into the bloodstream, and transfer of antibiotic resistance to pathogenic bacteria.[189] In immunocompromised patients, infections may occur.[189]

Drug interactions may occur with different agents. With antibiotics or antifungals, the probiotic benefit may be diminished.[189,202] Antibiotics should be administered separately from probiotics by at least 2 hours.[189] Caution should be exercised in persons on immunosuppressants since the probiotic may cause an infection.[189] There are many unknowns, such as what is the most appropriate probiotic or combination of probiotics to use for specific diseases, what is the most appropriate form since they are available in various formulations (yogurt, powders, supplements, etc.), and should prebiotics be used instead—these are nondigestible food constituents that help the host organism stimulate growth or activity of gut bacteria[205] and have been shown to enhance incretin secretion in animals.[206] It is important for individuals to learn how to read a probiotic label for information such as the strain, expiration dates, dosing, and storage.[207] It's also important to know that testing of some products found that product content often varies from what is stated on the label, per the testing laboratory CL.[38] Studies that research the impact of probiotics in persons with diabetes are emerging, and studies that find an improvement are not definitive. More research is needed, and evidence of long-term benefit on morbidity and mortality is absent.

Psyllium Fiber

Psyllium, also known as black psyllium, dietary fiber, or soluble fiber, comes from an herb commonly used as a laxative for constipation and to reduce the risk of elevated cholesterol on cardiovascular health.[46] Manufactured dosage forms include many commercially available fiber supplements often marked for bowel regularity and as an adjunct to treatment for high cholesterol. A diet high in fiber is generally known as beneficial for heart health; however, few studies definitively demonstrate the effectiveness of over-the-counter products in these conditions. The FDA requires over-the-counter products containing psyllium to carry a warning that they should be taken with a full glass of water or liquid to reduce risk of choking.[46]

Evidence

A few, yet growing number of studies have evaluated the effect of psyllium on glucose levels. The most recent randomized trial of psyllium (soluble fiber) evaluated effects on blood glucose, cholesterol, and blood pressure in 36 persons with type 2 diabetes.[208] Subjects were given 10.5 g/day psyllium or placebo for 8 weeks. Fasting glucose was reduced by 43 mg/dL ($P < 0.001$), triglycerides decreased by 37 mg/dL ($P = 0.001$), and systolic blood pressure fell by 7 mmHg ($P = 0.001$) as compared to placebo.[208] Two additional trials looked at glycemic effect of psyllium on persons with constipation and type 2 diabetes. In a single-blind, randomized controlled trial 51 persons with diabetes received either 10 g psyllium or placebo for 12 weeks.[209] Fasting plasma glucose decreased by 13 mg/dL (P = 0.04), and A1C fell by –1.7% ($P = 0.002$) as compared to placebo. Cholesterol, triglycerides and constipation also improved.[209] Another single-blind, randomized trial compared psyllium or flaxseed to placebo in 77 persons with type 2 diabetes and constipation.[210] Results found that 10 g psyllium daily lowered fasting glucose by 19.7 mg/dL as compared to placebo ($P = 0.004$). Psyllium decreased A1C by 0.8% while flaxseed lowered it by 0.7%, giving them equivalent effectiveness. Constipation in both intervention groups improved.[210]

The first published systematic review found 6 single-meal postprandial studies and 4 multi-week studies conducted in persons with type 2 diabetes.[211] In these studies, the most common dose was 5 g per meal per day. When data were pooled, the mean summary effect on fasting glucose was a significant decrease of –37 mg/dL ($P = 0.001$) as compared to control. Mean summary effect on A1C was a decrease of –0.97% (P = 0.048) as compared to control.[211] An umbrella meta-analysis of the effect of dietary fiber intake on type 2 diabetes included 16 meta-analyses comparing high versus low fiber intake.[212] Results showed that high fiber intake produced a statistically significant reduction in relative risk (RR = 0.81–0.85) of type 2 diabetes.[212] The most recent systematic review and meta-analysis evaluated psyllium's effect on cholesterol alone.[213] This analysis included the Cochrane Database and yielded 28 trials for inclusion (n = 1924). Psyllium (median dose 10.2g/day) significantly decreased LDL by 5 to 10 mg/dL effectively reducing cardiovascular risk.[213]

Summary

Psyllium is widely available and generally safe when taken with sufficient water or fluids.[46] It is a common supplement used to increase fiber intake, which is known to improve lipid profiles and reduce cardiovascular risk. Psyllium may also have modest effects on glucose levels in type 2 diabetes.[211,212] It is well tolerated but can cause flatulence and bloating. These effects are usually transient. When taken without enough fluids, psyllium can cause esophageal or intestinal obstruction.[46] Inhaling psyllium powder (such as when preparing psyllium for administration) can cause allergic reactions.

Turmeric

Turmeric is a popular culinary spice used for both flavor and color in curry powder, perfumes, mustards, butters, and cheeses.[46] Turmeric is included in the ginger family and has long been used in Chinese and Ayurvedic traditional medicine for its potential hypoglycemic effect.[214] Curcumin is derived from the root of turmeric and is thought to be the major constituent and likely active ingredient.[214] The first published case report demonstrated the potential for the use of turmeric in glucose lowering.[215]

Evidence

Chuengsamarn et al assessed the efficacy of curcumin in delaying the development of type 2 diabetes in the prediabetic population in 2 different studies.[216,217] The most recent randomized, double-blinded, placebo-controlled trial included 240 individuals with prediabetes.[217] After 9 months, curcumin intervention significantly lowered the number of prediabetic individuals who went on to develop type 2 diabetes. No individuals in the curcumin group had an A1C rise above 6.5%, and an overall lowering in A1C was noted when compared with the placebo group (A1C 5.6% vs. 6.02%, $P < 0.01$).[217] Another study to evaluate curcuminoid effect in type 2 diabetes supports a significant decrease in fasting plasma glucose ($P < 0.01$) and A1C ($P = 0.031$).[218] This randomized, double-blind, placebo-controlled trial compared curcuminoid capsules 150 mg by mouth twice daily with placebo. The effect on A1C was modest (decrease by about 0.75%) but was improved after intervention, whereas the placebo group actually saw a rise in A1C. This study was concluded after 3 months and does not give the long-term effectiveness and safety of turmeric.[218] Another study in 100 persons with type 2 diabetes taking 500 mg/day curcumin plus piperine 5 mg/day for 3 months showed a statistically significant decrease in glucose ($P = 0.048$) and reduction in A1C in the intervention group as compared with the controls (–0.9% versus –0.2%, $P = 0.001$).[219] A review of 9 studies assessing effect of curcumin use over 11 days to 12 weeks (average 4 weeks) showed that curcumin supplementation may exert beneficial effects on glucose and lipid metabolism.[220]

Summary

Turmeric, and its main constituent curcumin, is likely safe to use in individuals with prediabetes and type 2 diabetes. Turmeric is generally well tolerated but may have adverse GI effects including dyspepsia, diarrhea, gastroesophageal reflux, nausea, and vomiting.[46] The World Health Organization Expert Committee on Food Additives (JECFA) approved curcumin as a food additive in ranges of 5 to 500 mg/kg. The mechanism by which curcumin leads to improved blood glucose is unknown but likely relates to an effect on insulin resistance.[218] While the studies to prove benefit in humans with T2DM are limited, there is evidence to support curcumin use for the treatment of many diabetic complications, including liver disorders, diabetic neuropathy, and diabetic nephropathy.[214]

Vinegar

Vinegar is a byproduct of fermentation—often of beer, wine, or cider. Vinegar is comprised of a acetic acid and citric acid, often along with pectin and various vitamins and minerals, depending on the fermentation source.[46] The FDA defines any item labeled as "vinegar" to contain 4 g of acetic acid per 100 mL.[221] Vinegar, especially apple cider vinegar (a byproduct of fermentation of apple cider), is consumed as a food and used medicinally. Use of vinegar for medicinal purposes is not novel—it is reported Hippocrates and Civil War soldiers utilized it for antibiotic and general health purposes.[46] In the 1820s, vinegar was used for weight loss. More recently, the role of vinegar in glucose lowering has been explored.[221] Vinegar is traditionally available in liquid form and can be purchased from many grocery stores. However, tablet and capsule formulations are also available.

Evidence

A systematic review of 12 studies (n = 278) sought to determine the impact of various vinegars on short- and long-term glucose parameters in persons with diabetes. Secondary outcomes included fasting plasma insulin and postprandial insulin. Most studies included in the review used apple cider vinegar, with several using white vinegar. Fasting glucose was –0.80 mmol/L (–14.4 mg/dL) lower in the vinegar group ($P < 0.05$) compared to control. HbA1C was also lower (-0.39%) in the vinegar group (95% CI; -0.59, -0.18). Postprandial glucose was significantly lower ($P < 0.05$) at 30 minutes in the vinegar group (-0.88 mmol/L [–15.6 mg/dL]), but there was no difference at 60, 90, or 120 minutes. Fasting plasma insulin was not different between groups.[222]

A different meta-analysis studied the impact of vinegar intake with a meal on postprandial glucose response. Eleven studies (n = 204) were included utilizing a variety of vinegar types (apple cider, wine vinegar, grape vinegar, and white vinegar). The pooled analysis revealed a statistically significant reduction in glucose "area under the curve" in vinegar users (SMD = –0.60; 95% CI, –1.08, –0.11, $P = 0.01$). This effect remained ($P < 0.001$, $P = 0.002$) when subgroup analyses examined patients with (–0.74) and without diabetes (–0.46). Apple cider vinegar and white vinegar demonstrated significantly ($P < 0.001$) lower glucose AUC (–0.90 and –0.64, respectively). Eight studies in the analysis reported insulin AUC. Vinegar consumption significantly reduced mean insulin AUC compared to placebo (SMD = –1.30; 95% CI, –1.98, –0.62; $P < 0.001$).[223]

A randomized trial examined the impact of apple cider vinegar on body weight and metabolic profiles in overweight or obese individuals on a restricted calorie diet (n = 39). Participants were randomized to apple cider vinegar (30 mL per day) with a calorie restricted diet or a calorie restricted diet alone for 12 weeks. BMI, hip circumference, visceral adiposity index, and appetite score were all significantly lower in the apple cider vinegar group compared to control ($P < 0.05$). Triglycerides were lower in the treatment group ($P = 0.001$); HDL-C was higher ($P = 0.0049$). Significant reduction in appetite was found in the apple cider vinegar users ($P = 0.04$).[224]

Summary

Use of vinegar has been proposed to lower glucose and improve weight and metabolic parameters in those with and without insulin resistance.[222–224] Reported side effects of oral ingestion include acid reflux, eructation, flatulence, and changes in bowel activity.[225] One case of hypokalemia, hypereninemia, and osteoporosis has been published.[226] Reports of chemical burns with topical apple cider vinegar application have also been reported.[227,228] Vinegar may delay gastric emptying (and worsen gastroparesis in patents with type 1 diabetes) and decrease carbohydrate absorption.[221] Vinegar may potentiate the effects of glucose lowering agents. Studied doses of vinegar include 30 mL daily (often split into two 15 mL doses) and 20 grams daily.[46] Overall, vinegar may be a promising dietary supplement for persons with diabetes; however, further studies are needed to validate the findings of the discussed evidence.

TABLE 21.5 Botanical and Nonbotanical Products Used to Lower Blood Glucose

Product	*Chemical Constituents*	*Mechanism of Action*	*Side Effects and Drug Interactions*
Aloe Effectivencss rating:[46] • "Likely effective" Safety rating:[46] • "Possibly safe"	Various ingredients:[46,47,50] • Aloe gel contains acemannan (polysaccharide similar to guar gum and glycoprotein) • Aloeresin A • Phenolic and saponin contents	Various mechanisms:[46,48–50] • Fiber may delay or prevent glucose absorption • Aloeresin may have possible alpha-glucosidase inhibition • Decreased insulin resistance • Acemannan possibly decreases inflammation • Acemannan possibly stimulates benefit through gut microbiota through production of short chain fatty acids	Side effects: • Acute hepatitis • Thyroid dysfunction[48] Drug interactions: • Possible hypoglycemia if combined with secretagogues[46] • Intraoperative blood loss in surgery patients where sevoflurane was used[49] Safety rating in special populations:[46] • Pregnancy: "Possibly unsafe" • Lactation: "Possibly unsafe" • Children: "Possibly safe" Advise against use in these populations Use with caution in patients with liver disease[308]
Berberine Effectiveness rating:[46] • "Possibly effective" Safety rating:[46] • "Possibly safe"	Isoquinoline alkaloid[46,50,59–61]	Various mechanisms:[46,50,59–61] • Enhances glucose-stimulated insulin secretion • Increased insulin receptor expression	Side effects:[46,50,69] • Abdominal upset, constipation • Kernicterus • May stimulate uterine contractions

(continued)

TABLE 21.5 Botanical and Nonbotanical Products Used to Lower Blood Glucose (continued)

Product	*Chemical Constituents*	*Mechanism of Action*	*Side Effects and Drug Interactions*
		• Glucose transporter type 4 (GLUT4) translocation • Alpha-glucosidase inhibition • Enhanced adenosine monophosphate-activated protein kinase (AMPK) • Glucagon-like peptide-1 (GLP-1) activity • Peroxisome proliferator-activated receptor (PPAR) gamma receptor activation • Stimulates gut microbiota • Upregulates LDL receptors	Drug interactions:[39] • Increased levels of drugs metabolized by CYP3A4 (cyclosporine, certain statins, and calcium channel blockers) • Increased levels of drugs metabolized by CYP2C9 (warfarin, losartan), thus additive anticoagulant activity with warfarin or additive hypotension with losartan • Increased levels of drugs metabolized by CYP2D6 (metoprolol, certain tricyclic antidepressants, tramadol) • Additive hypoglycemia if combined with secretagogues • Additive hypotension if combined with antihypertensives • Additive central nervous system (CNS) depression if combined with CNS depressants Safety rating in special populations:[46] • Pregnancy: "Likely unsafe" • Lactation: "Likely unsafe" • Children: "Likely unsafe" Advise against use in these populations Use with caution in patients with kidney disease[309]
Bitter melon Effectiveness rating:[46] • "Insufficient reliable evidence to rate" Safety rating:[46] • "Possibly safe"	Various ingredients:[46,81] • Momordin • Charantin • Polypeptide-P • Vicine	Various mechanisms:[46,50,59,81–83] • Hypoglycemic action • Tissue glucose uptake; glycogen synthesis • Inhibition of enzymes involved in glucose production • Enhanced glucose oxidation of glucose-6-phosphate-dehydrogenase (G6PDH) pathway • AMPK pathway activation • Alpha-glucosidase inhibition • PPAR gamma receptor activation • GLUT4 translocation	Side effects:[46,50,81] • Gastrointestinal (GI) discomfort • Hypoglycemic coma • Favism • Hemolytic anemia in persons with G6PDH deficiency • Contains known abortifacients (a and b momorcharin) • Seeds have produced vomiting, death in children Drug interactions:[46] • Hypoglycemia when used with sulfonylureas Safety rating in special populations:[46] • Pregnancy: "Likely unsafe"

(continued)

TABLE 21.5 Botanical and Nonbotanical Products Used to Lower Blood Glucose (continued)

Product	*Chemical Constituents*	*Mechanism of Action*	*Side Effects and Drug Interactions*
			• Lactation: "Insufficient reliable information available" • Children: No information available on safety Advise against use in these populations Use with caution in patients with kidney disease[309]
Chromium Effectiveness rating:[46] • "Possibly effective" Safety rating:[46] • Short-term use: "Likely safe" • Long-term use: "Possibly safe"	Trivalent chromium[46,88]	Various mechanisms:[46,88] • May enhance cellular effects of insulin • May increase the number of insulin receptors • May increase insulin binding or insulin activation • Lipid metabolism modulation in peripheral tissues • Increased tyrosine kinase activity at insulin receptor • GLUT4 translocation • Increased AMPK activity • Inhibits acetyl-coenzyme A carboxylase, resulting in decreased malonyl coenzyme A	Side effects:[46,88,310] • Related to excessive intake: renal toxicity or possibly hemorrhage with or without shock • Potential liver toxicity Drug interactions: • May decrease blood glucose if used with secretagogues Safety rating in special populations:[46] • Pregnancy: "Possibly safe" • Lactation: "Possibly safe" • Children: "Possibly safe"
Cinnamon Effectiveness rating:[46] • "Possibly effective" Safety rating:[46] • Short-term use: "Likely safe" • Long-term use at high doses: "Possibly unsafe"	Procyanidin type-A polymers[46]	Various mechanisms:[46,50] • Increased insulin sensitivity and action • Increased insulin receptor phosphorylation and improved insulin signaling • Increased cell/tissue glucose uptake • Promotes glycogen synthesis • Alpha-glucosidase inhibition • Peroxisome proliferator-activated receptor activation • May help delay gastric emptying and reduce excess postprandial glucose and triglyceride levels • GLUT4 translocation	Side effects:[46] • No side effects reported; may cause irritation or dermatitis if used topically • High coumarin content in certain species or products may result in hepatotoxicity, per animal models • Prolonged use of large amounts may theoretically result in hepatotoxicity in persons susceptible to or with preexisting liver disease Drug interactions:[46] • May decrease blood glucose if used with secretagogues • Due to a coumarin ingredient, it may theoretically result in bleeding if combined with anticoagulants

(continued)

TABLE 21.5 Botanical and Nonbotanical Products Used to Lower Blood Glucose (continued)

Product	*Chemical Constituents*	*Mechanism of Action*	*Side Effects and Drug Interactions*
		• AMPK activation • GLP-1 activity	Safety rating in special populations:[46] • Pregnancy: "Insufficient reliable information available" • Lactation: "Insufficient reliable information available" • Children: "Possibly safe" Advise against use in these populations
Fenugreek Effectiveness rating:[46] • "Possibly effective" Safety rating:[46] • In foods: "Likely safe" • In medicinal amounts up to 6 months: "Possibly safe"	Various ingredients:[46,50,59] • Saponins • Glycosides • Seeds contain: –alkaloids (including trigonelline) –4-hydroxyisoleucine –fenugreekine	Various mechanisms:[46,50] • Delayed gastric emptying • Slowed carbohydrate absorption • Glucose transport inhibition • Increases insulin receptors • Improved peripheral glucose utilization • Possible stimulation of glucose-dependent insulin secretion	Side effects:[46,59] • Diarrhea, gas • Uterine contractions • Allergic reactions • Body odor or urine smell similar to that of sweet maple syrup Drug interactions:[46,311] • Possible hypoglycemia if combined with secretagogues • May increase the anticoagulant effects of warfarin or herbs with anticoagulant activity (boldo, garlic, ginger) • Decreased effect of theophylline by decreasing its serum concentrations • Its high fiber content may affect gastrointestinal transit, thus slowing down absorption, including that of other drugs. Therefore, medications should be administered 2 hours apart from fenugreek. Safety rating in special populations:[46] • Pregnancy: "Likely unsafe" (avoid using) • Lactation: "Possibly safe" • Children: "Possibly unsafe" Advise against use in pregnancy and children
Flaxseed Effectiveness rating:[46] • "Possibly ineffective" Safety rating:[46] • Ground flaxseed: "Likely safe"	Various ingredients:[46,128] • Lignans • Soluble fiber in seed and oil • Insoluble fiber	Various mechanisms:[46] • Soluble fiber slows gastric emptying • Decreased glucose absorption and postprandial glucose • May reduce cholesterol by reducing platelet aggregation	Side effects:[46,128] • GI upset and bloating • Flax hypersensitivity • Uncooked flaxseed contains cyanogenic glycosides, which may be a problem if large quantities are consumed

(continued)

TABLE 21.5 Botanical and Nonbotanical Products Used to Lower Blood Glucose (continued)			
Product	*Chemical Constituents*	*Mechanism of Action*	*Side Effects and Drug Interactions*
• Flaxseed lignan extract: "Possibly safe" • Raw/unripe flaxseed: "Possibly unsafe"	• Alpha-linolenic acid, a plant omega-3 fatty acid	• Fiber in flaxseed increases fecal bile acid elimination • Modulation of 7 α–hydroxylase and acyl CoA cholesterol transferase • Decreased production of proinflammatory eicosanoids • For hypertension: alteration of circulating oxylipins	Drug interactions:[46] • Bleeding if combined with warfarin • Possible hypoglycemia if combined with secretagogues • Possible hypotension if combined with antihypertensives • Possible additive estrogenic or antiestrogenic effect with estrogens • May decrease absorption of certain medications, such as acetaminophen or furosemide • Antibiotics may affect the efficacy of flaxseed Safety rating in special populations:[46] • Pregnancy: "Possibly unsafe" • Lactation: "Insufficient reliable evidence available" • Children: No information available on safety Advise against use in these populations Use with caution in patients with kidney disease[309]
Ginger Effectiveness rating:[46] • "Possibly ineffective" Safety rating:[46] • "Likely safe"	Various ingredients:[46] • Gingerol • Gingerdione • Shagaol • Sesquiterpene and monoterpene oils	Various mechanisms:[46] • Stimulates insulin release which raises insulin levels in the blood Decrease serum cholesterol and triglycerides	Side effects:[46] • Abdominal discomfort: belching, nausea, heartburn • Oral numbness or throat burning • Diarrhea • Drowsiness • Hives, flushing, rash Drug interactions:[46] • Bleeding if combined with warfarin, nifedipine • Possible hypoglycemia if combined with secretagogues • May increase absorption of metronidazole Safety rating in special populations:[46] • Pregnancy: "Possibly safe" • Lactation: "Insufficient reliable evidence available" • Children: "Possibly safe"

(continued)

TABLE 21.5 Botanical and Nonbotanical Products Used to Lower Blood Glucose (continued)

Product	*Chemical Constituents*	*Mechanism of Action*	*Side Effects and Drug Interactions*
Ginseng *American Ginseng* Effectiveness rating:[46] • "Possibly effective" Safety rating:[46] • "Likely safe" *Panax Ginseng* Effectiveness rating:[46] • "Insufficient reliable evidence to rate" Safety rating:[46] • "Likely safe" when used orally and short term • "Possibly unsafe" when used orally and long term	Ginsenosides[46]	Various mechanisms:[46] • May decrease carbohydrate absorption in portal circulation • May decrease glucose transport and uptake • Modulation of insulin secretion	Side effects:[46,140] • Insomnia, headache, restlessness • Increased blood pressure or heart rate • Mastalgia • Mood changes, nervousness Drug interactions:[46,140] • Decreased warfarin, diuretic effectiveness with Panax ginseng • Additive estrogenic effects with a combination of estrogens and Panax ginseng • Possible increased effects of certain analgesics and antidepressants • Possible additive hypoglycemia with secretagogues Safety rating in special populations:[46] • Pregnancy: "Possibly unsafe" • Lactation: "Insufficient reliable evidence available" • Children: American ginseng—"Possibly safe," orally and short term; Panax ginseng—"Likely unsafe"
Gymnema Effectiveness rating:[46] • "Insufficient reliable evidence to rate" Safety rating:[46] • "Possibly safe"	Various ingredients:[46] • Gymnemosides • Saponins • Stigmasterol • Amino acid derivatives –betaine –choline –trimethylamine	Various mechanisms:[46] • Impairs ability to discriminate "sweet" taste • Increases enzymes promoting glucose uptake • May stimulate beta cells • May increase beta cell numbers • May stimulate insulin release	Side effects:[46,160] • May cause hypoglycemia • Hepatitis Drug interactions:[46] • Possible hypoglycemia if combined with secretagogues Safety rating in special populations:[46] • Pregnancy: "Insufficient reliable evidence available" • Lactation: "Insufficient reliable evidence available" • Children: No information available on safety (avoid use)
Honey Effectiveness rating:[46] • "Possibly effective" Safety rating:[46] • "Likely safe"	Various ingredients:[46,163] • Fructose • Glucose • Fatty acids	Various mechanisms:[46,165,312] • Scavenge reactive oxygen species and meliorate oxidative stress, which may play a role in pancreatic beta-cell dysfunction	Side effects:[46] • Allergic reactions • Potential for botulism poisoning (typically in infants and children)

(continued)

TABLE 21.5 Botanical and Nonbotanical Products Used to Lower Blood Glucose (continued)

Product	*Chemical Constituents*	*Mechanism of Action*	*Side Effects and Drug Interactions*
• "Likely unsafe" if honey is produced from nectar of rhododendrons	• Proteins • Amino acids	• Prolonged gastric emptying leading to slower rate of intestinal absorption of fructose • Stimulate insulin secretion from enhanced intestinal fructose absorption	Drug interactions:[46] • Additive effects of anticoagulant/antiplatelet drugs. May increase time to clotting through inhibition of platelet aggregation. Safety rating in special populations:[46] • Pregnancy: "Likely safe" • Lactation: "Likely safe" • Children: "Likely safe" over 12 months of age
Milk thistle Effectiveness rating:[46] • "Possibly effective" Safety rating:[46] • "Likely safe"	Various ingredients:[171,313] • Silymarin, containing silybin, silychristine, and silidianin	Various mechanisms:[46,171,313] • Decreased insulin resistance • Peroxisome proliferator-activated receptor-gamma (PPARγ) agonist properties • Reduced oxidative stress on pancreatic beta cells • Other anti-inflammatory and immunomodulating effects	Side effects:[46,171] • Diarrhea, weakness, sweating • Possible allergic reactions including itching, rash, eczema, or anaphylaxis if also allergic to ragweed, marigolds, daisies, or chrysanthemums • May have estrogenic effects, so women with breast or uterine cancer should avoid its use Drug interactions:[46,171] • May increase warfarin concentrations and decrease levels of exogenously administered estrogens • Beneficial interactions with hepatotoxic agents such as acetaminophen, antipsychotics, and alcohol Safety rating in special populations:[46] • Pregnancy: "Insufficient reliable evidence available" • Lactation: "Insufficient reliable evidence available" • Children: No information available on safety[309] Use with caution in patients with kidney disease[309]
Nopal Effectiveness rating:[46] • "Possibly effective" Safety rating:[46] • "Likely safe" orally as a food	Various ingredients:[46] • Mucopolysaccharide fibers • Pectin	Various mechanisms:[46,187,314] • Slows carbohydrate absorption • Decreases lipid absorption	Side effects:[46,181,187] • Diarrhea, nausea, abdominal fullness • Increased stool volume Drug interactions:[46,182] • Potential hypoglycemia when combined with oral glucose-lowering agents

(continued)

TABLE 21.5 Botanical and Nonbotanical Products Used to Lower Blood Glucose (continued)

Product	*Chemical Constituents*	*Mechanism of Action*	*Side Effects and Drug Interactions*
• "Possibly safe" when leaf or stem extracts are used		• Possibly increases insulin sensitivity • Action on alpha-glucosidase	Safety rating in special populations:[46] • Pregnancy: "Insufficient reliable evidence available" • Lactation: "Insufficient reliable evidence available" • Children: No information available on safety (avoid use)
Probiotics Effectiveness rating:[46] • No evidence grade assigned Safety rating:[46] • "Possibly safe" up to 6 months	Numerous species:[189,202] Examples: • Lactobacillus species • Bifidobacterium species • *Streptococcus thermophilus* • *Saccharomyces boulardii*	Theoretical:[189,202] • Release of beneficial organic and free fatty acids that act against pathogenic microbes • Possible enhanced incretin action • Decreased inflammation • Decreased insulin resistance	Side effects:[189] • GI upset • Constipation • Possible systemic infections Drug interactions:[189] • Antibiotics, antifungals: decreased probiotic effects • Immunosuppressants (cyclosporine, methotrexate, etc): weakened state may lead to infections due to probiotic microbes Safety rating in special populations:[46] • Pregnancy: "Insufficient reliable evidence available" • Lactation: "Insufficient reliable evidence available" • Children: No information available on safety (avoid use)
Psyllium Effectiveness rating:[46] • "Insufficient reliable evidence to rate" Safety rating:[46] • "Likely safe when taken with adequate water"	Various soluble polysaccharides:[46] • D-xylose • L-arabinose • Rhamnose • Galacturinic acid	Various mechanisms:[46] • Slow carbohydrate absorption Reduce insulin release postprandially	Side effects:[46] • Flatulence and bloating • Allergic reactions if inhaled Drug interactions:[46] • Possible hypoglycemia if combined with other medications for diabetes • Reduction in effect of carbamazepine, digoxin, and lithium when taken together • Can reduce absorption in general of other drugs from the GI tract Safety rating in special populations:[46] • Pregnancy: "Likely safe" • Lactation: "Likely safe" Children: No information available on safety (avoid use)

(continued)

TABLE 21.5 Botanical and Nonbotanical Products Used to Lower Blood Glucose (continued)

Product	*Chemical Constituents*	*Mechanism of Action*	*Side Effects and Drug Interactions*
Turmeric Effectiveness rating:[46] • "Insufficient reliable evidence to rate" Safety rating:[46] • "Likely safe" orally or topically	Various ingredients:[46] • Curcumin • Curcumine • Curcumae • Curcuminoids	Various mechanisms:[46,214,218] • Induction of PPARγ • Activation of liver enzymes associated with glycolysis, gluconeogenesis, and lipid metabolism • Decrease in serum free fatty acids	Side effects:[46] • GI upset • Diarrhea • Possible increased bleeding risk Drug interactions:[46] • Potential increased bleeding risk when combined with anticoagulants/antiplatelets Safety rating in special populations:[46] • Pregnancy: "Likely safe" when used in food amounts; "Likely unsafe" when used in medicinal amounts • Lactation: "Likely safe" when used in food amounts; "Insufficient reliable evidence available" when used in medicinal amounts • Children: No information available on safety (avoid use) Use with caution in patients with kidney disease[309]
Vinegar Effectiveness rating:[46] • "Insufficient reliable evidence to rate" Safety rating:[46] • "Likely safe" when used orally and in food amounts • "Possibly safe" when used orally and appropriately for short-term medicinal purposes • "Possibly unsafe" topically	Various ingredients:[46,221,315] • All vinegar contains acetic acid • Apple cider vinegar contains acetic acid, citric acid, and polyphenolic compounds	Various mechanisms:[46,221,225] • Insulin sensitizer • Delay of gastric emptying • Acetic acid may suppress disaccharidsase activity • Decrease carbohydrate absorption	Side effects: • GI issues (acid reflux, eructation, flatulence, and changes in bowel activity)[225] • Hypokalemia[226] • Chemical burns with topical use[227,228] Drug interactions:[46] • Possible hypoglycemia if combined with glucose lowering agents Safety rating in special populations:[46] • Pregnancy: "Insufficient reliable information available" • Lactation: "Insufficient reliable information available" • Children: "Insufficient reliable information available" Advise against use in these populations

Botanical and Nonbotanical Products Used to Treat Diabetes Complications

Complications of diabetes may be devastating and disrupting to individuals' lives. Many use supplements to try to prevent or treat complications. Persons with diabetes may inquire about the following products for use in decreasing diabetes complications. Not all are safe or effective, and only a few products have been highlighted, although numerous other products are available that persons with diabetes may use. Each is discussed separately in the paragraphs that follow.

- Alpha-lipoic acid
- Benfotiamine
- Bilberry
- Coenzyme Q10
- Fish oil
- Garlic
- Red yeast rice
- St John's wort

Information regarding chemical constituents, mechanism of action, side effects, and drug interactions for these products is found in Table 21.6. Each of these 8 products is reviewed separately following Table 21.6.

Alpha-Lipoic Acid

Alpha-lipoic acid (ALA), a vitamin-like substance also known as thioctic acid, is a disulfide compound that is synthesized in the liver. Foods containing ALA include greens such as spinach and broccoli, potatoes, yams, carrots, and red and organ meat.[46] Alpha-lipoic acid functions as a cofactor in enzyme complexes such as pyruvate dehydrogenase and assists in the conversion of pyruvic acid to acetyl-coenzyme A in oxidative glucose metabolism.[229] Alpha-lipoic acid is readily converted to the reduced form, dihydrolipoic acid (DHLA). Both ALA and DHLA are potent antioxidants.[46] Alpha-lipoic acid may increase insulin sensitivity.[230] Since ALA may decrease oxidative stress (caused by increased blood glucose), it may potentially help minimize symptoms of neuropathy. There is also evidence to suggest ALA is associated with weight loss.[46]

Evidence

A meta-analysis of 15 randomized controlled trials in persons with diabetic peripheral neuropathy analyzed safety and efficacy of intravenous ALA treatment. The treatment group in all trials received intravenous ALA at 300 to 600 mg daily for 2 to 4 weeks. Nine of the included trials (n = 651) investigated efficacy. In these trials, ALA was compared with placebo, ginkgo biloba leaves injection, methylcobalamin, or vitamin B1. The meta-analysis determined treatment with ALA was superior for improved efficacy ($P < 0.05$, odds ratio [OR] = 4.03). Ten trials (n = 754) investigated median motor nerve conduction velocity (MNCV); treatment with ALA increased MNCV by a weighted mean difference (WMD) of 4.63 ($P < 0.05$). Median sensory nerve conduction velocity (SNCV) was assessed in 10 trials (n = 754) and a significant beneficial improvement was associated with ALA (WMD = 3.17, 95% CI; 1.75 to 4.59). The most common adverse effect reported in ALA users was stomach upset; however, not all studies included in the meta-analysis reported adverse effects.[231]

Another meta-analysis of 1,258 persons in trials who used IV ALA or placebo (ALADIN I and III trials, the NATHAN II and SYDNEY trials) found that 52.7% of patients on ALA versus 36.9% on placebo had improved total symptom scores. Patients treated with ALA showed a relative improvement of total symptom scores of 24.1% compared with placebo ($P < 0.05$). Treatment-emergent adverse effects occurred more frequently with ALA compared with placebo (92.6% and 90.2%, respectively). Serious adverse effects were also more common in the ALA group (38.1% vs. 28.0%); however, there was no statistical difference compared with placebo in terms of cardiovascular disorders, cerebrovascular disorders, infection, inflicted injuries, and death.[232,233]

To determine the impact of ALA on anthropometric parameters, a meta-analysis of 12 place-controlled studies was conducted. The authors found ALA supplementation reduced body weight statistically significantly compared to placebo (–0.69 kg; 95% CI, –1.27, –0.10). Body mass index (BMI) was also significantly lower (–0.38 kg/m2) in the ALA group (95% CI, –0.53, –0.24). There was no significant change in waist circumference.[234] Another meta-analysis of 11 randomized, double-blind, placebo-controlled studies was conducted to determine the impact of ALA on weight and BMI. There were 534 patients included in the meta-analysis that received ALA and 413 that received placebo. The doses of ALA ranged from 300 to 1,800 mg daily. Mean weight loss in the ALA group was 1.27 kg greater than the placebo group (95% CI, –2.29 to –0.25). BMI was significantly lower in the ALA group compared to placebo (–0.43 kg/m2 [95% CI, –0.82 to –0.03]). Three of the included studies reported adverse effects. Gastrointestinal effects were the most common (stomach upset, nausea) followed by dermatological (urticaria). No severe adverse effects were reported.[235]

A randomized controlled trial (n = 60) investigated the influence of ALA on body weight, total cholesterol, triglycerides, and glucose levels in metformin-treated persons with type 2 diabetes mellitus. At the end of 20 weeks, the treatment group receiving 600 mg daily of ALA had significantly lower body mass indexes (29.1 ± 0.57 m^2 versus 31.17 ± 0.74 m^2) and triglyceride concentrations (214.16 ± 22.12 mg/dL [2.42 ± 0.25 mmol/L] vs. 284.07 ± 24.78 mg/dL [3.21 ± 0.28 mmol/L]). There was no significant difference in cholesterol or glucose between the treatment and control groups.[236]

Summary

Alpha-lipoic acid is a much-studied agent that may potentially help with peripheral neuropathy. No serious side effects have been reported, even though it has been used intravenously and in long-term trials. The SYDNEY 2 trial showed that although pain improved significantly, paresthesias and numbness did not.[237] Decreases in A1C levels have been significant in some trials,[238–240] but insignificant in others.[241,242] Typical doses of oral ALA are 600 to 1200 mg per day.[46] Although ALA has been used for decades in Germany, long-term trials are necessary to determine whether ALA slows the progression of neuropathy versus only improving the neuropathy symptoms. Overall, studies have confirmed that ALA may improve numbness, pain, burning, and prickly sensations to the feet and legs. Newer evidence suggests ALA may have a role in weight reduction and triglyceride lowering.[235,236] Although the American Diabetes Association (ADA) does not recommend use of unproven therapies, ALA has a long track record of proven benefit and is a relatively safe agent to use.

Benfotiamine

Persons with neuropathy may have thiamine deficiency. Different neurological disorders, including diabetes and alcohol-related neuropathy, have been treated with vitamin B1 (thiamine). However, thiamine is not well absorbed, and high doses are needed for successful treatment. Benfotiamine, a fat-soluble form of thiamine, provides much higher blood and tissue levels and thus may be a more effective form.[243] Benfotiamine may be useful in persons with microvascular complications.[243,244] Another name for these vitamins is allithiamines, because they are found in the *Allium* vegetable family (which includes garlic, onions, shallots, and leeks). Other foods containing thiamine include whole grain cereals and breads and certain meats.[243]

Evidence

Several clinical trials have evaluated benfotiamine for microvascular complications. Some studies are open-label, and others are randomized controlled trials. One open-label 6-week study of persons with T1DM or T2DM with painful neuropathy looked at different doses of benfotiamine in combination with B vitamins (n = 36).[245] Although all groups had beneficial effects, the best results were reported in those patients taking the highest dose ($P < 0.01$ for all parameters compared with baseline). A different 3-month open-label study in persons with type 1 diabetes or type 2 diabetes evaluated benfotiamine plus other B vitamins or only B vitamins.[246] The benfotiamine group had better results for neuropathic pain ($P < 0.001$), and vibration perception threshold also improved.

A 3-week randomized pilot study in 40 persons with type 1 diabetes or type 2 diabetes evaluated benfotiamine or placebo 4 times daily for neuropathy. Painful neuropathy symptoms improved significantly ($P < 0.05$).[247] A 6-week randomized controlled trial evaluated 133 persons with type 1 diabetes or type 2 diabetes. Neuropathy symptom scores improved in the benfotiamine group.[248] A 12-week randomized, double-blind, placebo-controlled trial evaluated varying doses of benfotiamine plus vitamins B6 and B12 in 24 persons with type 1 diabetes or type 2 diabetes. The benfotiamine group had improved vibration perception threshold scores in the metacarpal and metatarsal nerves (although the results were not significant), and improved nerve conduction velocity scores in the peroneal nerve ($P = 0.006$) but not the median nerve.[249]

Results are not always positive. A 24-month randomized trial in 67 persons with T1DM found no benefit with benfotiamine for peripheral nerve function.[250] However, other researchers have questioned the results of this study.[251] One study aimed to investigate whether benfotiamine prevented postprandial endothelial dysfunction in patients with T2DM. This randomized, double-blind, placebo-controlled, crossover study showed no difference between patients treated with benfotiamine and those who took placebo. However, a subgroup of patients with the highest endothelial dysfunction showed improvement with benfotiamine treatment.[252]

Summary

Benfotiamine is a promising fat-soluble form of vitamin B1 for diabetes complications and has been evaluated in both type 1 diabetes and type 2 diabetes. Although highly studied for neuropathy, it has also been studied for retinopathy[244] and nephropathy.[252,253] It enhances activity of certain enzymes that may inhibit major pathways involved in vascular damage.[243] It may also block hyperglycemia-induced activation of pro-inflammatory transcription factors.[244] It may even diminish or correct cell damage by normalizing cell division rates and decreasing apoptosis.[243]

Several medications deplete thiamine levels, including metformin.[46] The dose used for diabetes is 300 to 600 mg daily, administered in divided doses (eg, 100 or 150 mg 3 times a day).[245–248,250,251] Benfotiamine is also found in combination with other B vitamins and ALA. Its role in treating microvascular complications of diabetes is promising, and overall it is a safe agent to use.

Bilberry

Bilberry, otherwise known as European blueberry, belongs to the *Vaccinium* family (which also includes blueberries, cranberries, and lingonberries).[254] It is thought the fruit and the leaf contain biologically active components. Tannins, anthocyanin constituents, polyphenols (such as resveratrol), flavonoids (such as quercetin), and chromium have all been identified in bilberry.[255,256]

Evidence

An open-label trial of 140 participants studied the impact of a proprietary extract of bilberry in retinal vasculopathies. Patients received standard care (n = 38), 160 mg daily of the proprietary bilberry extract (n = 47), or 160 mg daily of a generic bilberry extract (n = 55). After six months, both bilberry groups had significant improvements compared to standard care for dot and blot retinal hemorrhage, hard exudates, arteriolar vasoconstriction, and atherosclerosis ($P < 0.05$). The proprietary bilberry extract also demonstrated significantly lower edema, capillary microaneurisms, soft exudates, and arteriovenous crossing ($P < 0.05$). Snellen chart scores for edema and blurring were also lower in the bilberry groups compared to placebo ($P < 0.05$).[254]

Perossini and colleagues conducted a double-blind, placebo-controlled study to ascertain the effect of bilberry anthocyanosides on retinopathy of diabetes. Participants received either bilberry 160 mg twice daily or placebo for 1 month. After 1 month, the placebo persons with diabetes were crossed over to bilberry for an additional month. Moderate improvements were found in ophthalmoscopy and fluorangiographic findings.[257]

Summary

Visual health remains a concern for persons with diabetes. Bilberry is a botanical agent used to treat retinopathy. Bilberry's medicinal properties are thought to result from anthocyanins and polyphenols, as well as flavonoids and chromium.[255,256] Studied doses for retinopathy include 160 mg once or twice daily.[254,257] Bilberry may also lower glucose so use in persons with diabetes should be closely monitored by a healthcare provider. Anti-platelet activity has also been reported so use with anticoagulants is not advised.[46] While initial evidence for use of bilberry in retinopathy is promising, more robust study is needed to verify initial results.

Coenzyme Q10

Coenzyme Q10 (CoQ10)—also known as ubiquinone because it is found in almost all human cells[46,258,259]—is a lipid-soluble vitamin-like substance that is thought to be deficient in many diseases, including diabetes.[260,261] Humans synthesize CoQ10, and it is highly concentrated in the heart, brain, liver, kidneys, and pancreas. Dietary sources include beef, poultry, and broccoli; dietary supplements are manufactured via beet and sugarcane fermentation.[46] Human CoQ10 levels decline with age and with certain cardiovascular diseases (heart failure, hypertension, and other diseases such as Parkinson's).[260] CoQ10 has been used to treat a variety of cardiovascular diseases that are common in persons with diabetes, although there is evidence that it may also help improve glucose.[262] It is widely used to offset the body's decreased CoQ10 levels secondary to statin us and is used for other disease states, such as Parkinson's disease.[46]

Evidence

CoQ10 has been evaluated extensively. A meta-analysis was conducted to assess the effect of CoQ10 on hypertension. Twelve studies were included (n = 362) and the primary endpoint was blood pressure. CoQ10 administration significantly reduced systolic (–16.57 mm Hg, $P < 0.001$) and diastolic blood pressure (–8.19 mm Hg, $P < 0.001$). Placebo did not have a significant effect on blood pressure. The doses used in the trials varied from 34 mg CoQ10 daily up to 225 mg daily. A robust discussion of side effects was not included.[263]

Two studies of CoQ10 use demonstrated a significant decrease in blood pressure, although blood pressure was still higher than the target goals in persons with diabetes.[264,265] The subjects were thought to have insulin resistance, and mean baseline glucose decreased in the CoQ10 group after 8 weeks ($P < .05$).[265]

One study showed that compared with placebo, CoQ10 did not have statistically significant reductions in 24-hour blood pressure in patients with metabolic syndrome. However, there were significant decreases in daytime diastolic pressures. CoQ10 was well tolerated without any clinically significant adverse effects.[266]

A meta-analysis of 7 randomized, placebo-controlled trials (n = 356) was conducted to determine the impact of CoQ10 on glycemic levels, lipid parameters, and blood pressure in patients with diabetes. Seven of the trials included patients with type 2 diabetes; one trial included patients with type 1 diabetes. CoQ10 did not appear to significantly impact glycemic levels, LDL-C, HDL-C, or blood pressure. Triglycerides, however, were significantly reduced by 4.7 mg/dL (0.26 mmol/L) with CoQ10 use ($P = 0.02$). Total cholesterol was also lower, −8.1 mg/dL (0.45 mmol/L) in the CoQ10 group ($P = 0.02$).[267]

A meta-analysis in heart failure showed improved ejection fraction and a slight improvement in New York Heart Association (NYHA) functional class.[268] However, there were few studies, and many trials were older publications where patients were not on agents that are now commonly used to treat heart failure. In combination with selenium, CoQ10 has shown decreased cardiovascular mortality.[269]

Summary

CoQ10 is a highly used product, both by persons with diabetes and by persons without diabetes. One unique reason for use is that statins decrease serum CoQ10 concentrations, and it has been theorized that myopathy may then ensue. However, this benefit has not been conclusively shown.[258] One of the biggest concerns is use by persons who are on the anticoagulant warfarin, since CoQ10 has a structure similar to vitamin K and may thus result in breakthrough thromboembolism.[258] CoQ10 has been used for a variety of disorders, and although blood pressure may decrease significantly, endpoint values are still higher than advocated for persons with diabetes. In persons with type 1 diabetes or type 2 diabetes, CoQ10 supplementation has shown neutral to slightly improved effects on fasting glucose and A1C. One of the main reasons it is used in diabetes is because of its improvement of endothelial dysfunction.[270] The doses are variable and for hypertension and other cardiovascular diseases, the dose has ranged from 34 to 225 mg daily, although up to 600 mg daily has been used. The dose for diabetes has ranged from 100 to 200 mg daily.[263,265,271–273] Although there is much enthusiasm for CoQ10, and long-term use has not shown harm, further studies are needed to determine its place in treatment.

Fish Oil (Omega-3 Fatty Acids)

Omega-3 fatty acids are essential polyunsaturated fats found in plant and marine sources. Notable omega-3 fatty acids include eicosapentaenoic acid (EPA), docosahexaenoic acid (DHA), and alpha-linolenic acid (ALA). EPA and DHA are found in marine sources—in particular, salmon, lake trout, mackerel, sturgeon, herring, tuna, sardines, and their oils.[46] Other sources of EPA and DHA include various strains of algae.[274] Many plant-based sources of omega-3 fatty acids contain ALA (such as flaxseed, walnut, canola, olive, soybean, and chia). Humans are capable of converting ALA to EPA and DHA, however conversion is inefficient (less than 8%) and varies throughout life.[275,276] Therefore, EPA and DHA (as opposed to ALA) are typically consumed to supplement appreciable quantities of omega-3 fatty acids. Fish oil is one of the most commonly used non-vitamin/non-mineral dietary supplements in the US, with nearly 8% of adults admitting to use within the last month.[277] Fish oil is primarily used for hypertriglyceridemia, dyslipidemia, prevention of coronary heart disease, hypertension, mood disorders, rheumatoid arthritis, and dermatologic conditions.[46]

Evidence

Numerous studies have assessed fish oil for cardiovascular disease. In 2018, a meta-analysis was published that aimed to assess the association of omega-3 fatty acids with the risk of cardiovascular events. Ten randomized clinical trials (n = 77,917) were included. Of patients included, 35% had a diagnosis of diabetes and 66.4% had a prior history of cardiovascular disease. Omega-3 fatty acid consumption had no significant associations with coronary heart disease death, nonfatal myocardial infarction, coronary heart disease, or major cardiovascular events.[278] However, the results of this meta-analysis are questioned by experts citing lack of therapeutic dosing and short study duration.[279]

In 2019, multicenter, randomized, controlled, double-blinded trial was published that studied the cardiovascular effects of EPA on patients with established cardiovascular disease or with diabetes and other cardiovascular risk factors. All enrolled patients (n = 8179) were currently on statin therapy and had fasting triglycerides of 135 to 499 mg/dL (1.53 to 5.63 mmol/L) and LDL-C of 41 to 100 mg/dL (1.06 to 2.59 mmol/L). Patients received 2 grams of EPA twice daily or placebo and were followed for 4.9 years. The primary endpoint, a composite of cardiovascular death, nonfatal myocardial infarction, nonfatal stroke, coronary revascularization, or unstable angina, occurred in 17.2% of those using EPA and 22.0% of the placebo group ($P < 0.001$). The secondary endpoint—a composite of cardiovascular death, nonfatal myocardial infarction, or nonfatal stroke—occurred in 11.2% of the EPA group and 14.8% in the placebo group ($P = 0.03$). However, more patients in the EPA group were hospitalized for atrial fibrillation or flutter (3.1% compared to 2.1%, $P = 0.004$). There was no difference in serious bleeding between the groups.[280]

The impact of fish oil on triglyceride lowering has been extensively studied. A meta-analysis of 21 studies evaluated the effects of fish oil and alpha-linolenic acid on serum cardiovascular disease measurements. Fish oil consumption decreased triglycerides on average by 27 mg/dL (0.306 mmol/L, $P < 0.0001$), increased HDL by 1.6 mg/dL (0.04 mmol/L, $P = 0.0003$), and increased LDL by 6 mg/dL (0.156 mmol/L, $P = 0.0006$). There was no significant difference in total cholesterol or hemoglobin A1C. Alpha-linolenic acid did not have a significant impact on any measurements.[281]

Summary

Fish oil has a variety of therapeutic effects that may benefit cardiovascular disease, including antithrombotic, anti-inflammatory effects, and cardiac cell membrane stabilization. Fish oil contains EPA and DHA. Many clinicians are unclear as to the amounts of EPA and DHA that dietary supplements should contain. One prescription product, Lovaza®,[282] contains approximately 1 g of EPA and DHA (465 mg and 375 mg, respectively) per capsule and is dosed at 1 to 4 capsules daily, depending on triglyceride level.[282] Another prescription product (Vascepa®, Amarin),[283] contains an ethyl ester of EPA only (500 to 1000 mg per capsule) and is dosed at 4 grams daily.[283] Many OTC supplements contain 200 to 500 mg of EPA plus DHA per capsule, and thus patients may need to take as many as 12 to 16 capsules daily to obtain the amount equivalent to the prescription product. Newer dietary supplements are more concentrated and liquid and gummy options are available. Persons taking supplements should look for the total amount of EPA and DHA, not just total fish oil. In a 2017 publication, the American Heart Association (AHA) stated omega-3 fatty acid treatment is reasonable in patients with prevalent CHD to prevent future CVD events. The AHA does not recommend treatment for patients with diabetes and prediabetes to prevent CHD; however, there was lack of expert consensus.[284] Although recent research shows conflicting evidence regarding supplementation with fish oil, it's important to note that perhaps the benefit of fish oil was not seen because patients were already taking medications that lower risk, such as statins, ACE inhibitors, and aspirin. It's also important to remember that the AHA and the ADA recommend 2 weekly servings of fatty fish, such as salmon or mackerel.[46,285]

Garlic

Garlic (*Allium sativa*), a member of the lily family, has been used in cooking for thousands of years.[46] Garlic is used for hyperlipidemia, hypertension, cancer prevention, and antibacterial activity.[46,286] The name *Allium* is derived from the Celtic word "all," which means "burning." Highly valued in ancient Egypt and ancient Chinese medicine, garlic has a rich history of thousands of years of medicinal use.[286,287] Garlic has been reported to be helpful for diabetes.[46]

Evidence

Several studies have evaluated the impact of garlic on dyslipidemia and blood pressure. A meta-analysis of 14 studies sought to determine the effect of garlic on improving lipids. Total cholesterol (SMD = –22.7 mg/dL [–1.26 mmol/L]) and LDL-C (SMD = –19.3 mg/dL [–1.07 mmol/L]) decreased significantly with garlic use compared to placebo ($P < 0.05$). HDL-C increased significantly (SMD = 9.0 mg/dL [0.50 mmol/L], $P < 0.05$), but significance did not withstand the removal of several studies from the meta-analysis. There was no difference in triglycerides.[288]

A different meta-analysis of randomized controlled trials reviewed the effect of garlic on serum lipid concentrations. Compared with placebo, the garlic treatment groups decreased total cholesterol (WMD –10.8 mg/dL [0.279 mmol/L], $P = 0.001$) and triglycerides (WMD –5.0 mg/dL [0.056 mmol/L], $P < 0.001$). There was no difference between garlic and placebo for LDL-C, HDL-C, and apolipoprotein B.[289]

The impact of garlic on blood pressure was examined by meta-analysis of 10 trials (n = 401) in patients with elevated systolic blood pressure and those without elevations. Garlic significantly reduced systolic blood pressure compared with placebo in patients with baseline systolic elevation. There was no difference in systolic blood pressure in patients without elevated systolic pressure.[290]

A 12-week single-blind, placebo-controlled trial evaluated garlic use in 70 persons with type 2 diabetes and newly diagnosed hyperlipidemia. Several lipid values decreased significantly. Total cholesterol and LDL decreased, and HDL increased.[291] The same group of researchers conducted a 24-week randomized, single-blind, placebo-controlled study that compared a combination of garlic plus metformin in 30 persons with type 2 diabetes with metformin only in 30 persons with diabetes. Fasting glucose decreased in the combination group ($P < 0.005$). LDL-C and triglycerides decreased slightly ($P < 0.005$ for both).[292]

Garlic was studied in an open-label 12-week study in combination with metformin in 30 persons with type 2 diabetes and compared with 30 persons with diabetes who took only metformin. Although A1C decreased slightly from 7.48% to 7.05%, the change was not significant. However, fasting blood glucose, postmeal glucose, and cholesterol decreases were significant in the garlic plus metformin group ($P < 0.001$ for fasting and postprandial; $P < 0.05$ for LDL).[293]

A 6-year follow-up study investigated the correlation between consumption of allium vegetables (garlic and onion) on the incidence of CVD, HTN, chronic kidney disease (CKD), and type 2 diabetes. This study included adult men and women that completed a validated food frequency questionnaire (n = 3642). Higher habitual intake of allium vegetables was associated with a 64% reduced risk of CVD outcomes (hazard ratio = 0.36; 95% CI, 0.18, 0.71). The incidence of CKD was 32% lower in participants that consumed high amounts of allium (hazard ratio = 0.69; 95% CI 0.46, 0.98). There was no statistically significant difference in HTN development (hazard ratio = 0.74; 95% CI, −0.54, 1.00) or the risk of type 2 diabetes. However, triglycerides were significantly lower and creatinine clearance significantly higher in those that consumed high amounts of allium vegetables ($P = 0.01$ for both).[294]

Summary

Garlic contains the sulfur-based chemical constituent alliin, which must be converted to the active form, allicin, by the enzyme alliinase. This reaction occurs when the garlic bulb is chewed or crushed. Commercial preparations of garlic usually contain alliin, not allicin or ajoene. Conversion requires alliinase, which is unstable in stomach acids. Dried garlic preparations may be effective if the product is enteric-coated to prevent gastric acid breakdown and permit release in the small intestine. Thus, dried garlic preparations should be enteric-coated to prevent breakdown by stomach acids.[46]

Animal studies suggest that garlic may decrease glucose concentrations and increase insulin sensitivity.[295] However, human studies have mixed results.[292,293,296] Garlic may also inhibit formation of the advanced glycation end products that contribute to microvascular disease (studies suggests aged garlic has more potent activity compared to fresh).[297,298] In hyperlipidemia and hypertension studies, garlic extracts (600 to 1,200 mg per day in divided doses) have been used. For diabetes, 500 to 900 mg daily has been used. Fresh garlic is effective, and the appropriate amount is approximately 1 clove daily (containing approximately 1% alliin).[46] Garlic demonstrates one of the important controversies regarding supplements—varying results are shown in different studies, and the most appropriate dose and form are not known. Garlic is a very popular product, and it is estimated that up to half of patients with hypertension take garlic in varying forms. A Cochrane Review that evaluated the impact of garlic in hypertensive patients reported that garlic decreases blood pressure, but there is insufficient evidence to determine the effect on reducing cardiovascular morbidity and mortality.[299] It is important that diabetes care and education specialists instruct individuals that antiplatelet activity is a serious potential problem and that the person may experience bleeding reactions, especially if using drugs or CAM therapies with antiplatelet properties. As a food, garlic is safe; however, when used as a supplement, very close monitoring is required due to the potential for bleeding reactions.

Red Yeast Rice

Red yeast rice (RYR) is the product of rice fermented with a specific type of yeast, *Monascus purpureus*. It is also known by several other names, including "xuezhikang." Red yeast rice contains several compounds, called the monacolins, that inhibit cholesterol synthesis. One specific monacolin, monacolin K or mevinolin, is a potent inhibitor of 3-hydroxy-3-methylglutaryl-coenzyme A (HMG-CoA) reductase, a key enzyme in cholesterol synthesis. Red yeast rice is used for hyperlipidemia.[46,300]

Evidence

The effectiveness of RYR in reducing cholesterol levels has been evaluated in meta-analyses. One analysis utilized data from 93 randomized controlled trials (n = 9625) using 3 different RYR preparations. Compared with placebo, there was a statistically significant reduction in total cholesterol (WMD −38.7 mg/dL [1 mmol/L], $P < 0.05$), LDL-C (WMD −28.2 mg/dL [0.73 mmol/L], $P < 0.05$), and triglycerides (WMD −15.9 mg/dL [0.18 mmol/L], $P < 0.05$). High-density lipoprotein concentrations increased significantly (WMD 5.8 mg/dL [0.145 mmol/L], $P < 0.05$).[301]

A 6-month randomized placebo-controlled trial evaluated 1.8 g twice daily of RYR and placebo in 62 persons who had previously discontinued statin therapy due to myalgia. Total and LDL-C cholesterol were assessed at 12 and 24 weeks, and both decreased significantly in the RYR group ($P < 0.001$ and $P = 0.016$ at 12 and 24 weeks for total cholesterol; $P < 0.001$ and $P = 0.011$ at 12 and 24 weeks for LDL). Triglycerides and HDL-C were similar in the 2 groups at baseline and endpoint.[302]

A study done in China evaluated 300 mg of RYR twice daily in 4870 persons with previous myocardial infarction over an average 4.5-year period. The primary endpoint was a major coronary event, including nonfatal myocardial infarction and death. Frequency of the primary endpoint was 5.7% and 10.4% in the RYR and placebo groups, respectively, and was significantly lower in the RYR group ($P < 0.001$).[303]

Summary

Red yeast rice is a product used to treat hyperlipidemia. The typical dose is 600 mg to 1.2 g twice daily, although doses as high as 1.8 g twice daily have been used.[46,302] A typical dose contains approximately 6 to 7 mg of lovastatin, a conventional statin. Of note, the FDA considers any RYR product containing statin to be illegal.[46] Studies show that commercially available RYR preparations contain no, small, or significant concentrations of statins.[301]

Although information on RYR is emerging, individuals may experience side effects and drug interactions similar to those of statins. If not appropriately manufactured, RYR may contain an inadvertent nephrotoxic, citrine. The diabetes care and education specialist should counsel persons that use of this product requires extreme caution, and a healthcare provider must closely monitor not only the efficacy but side effects and drug interactions.[46]

St John's Wort

St John's wort (*Hypericum perforatum*) is a perennial that grows throughout the United States, Canada, and Europe. The bright yellow flowers bloom in late June, and the flowering top is used in the product. St John's wort (SJW) has been used for many different disorders as well as to treat a variety of psychiatric disorders, including depression and anxiety.[46] Many persons with diabetes have depression, and some clinicians consider this a complication of diabetes.

Evidence

Many published studies have evaluated SJW for depression, and it has been compared with placebo and conventional antidepressants, with varying results. The Cochrane Review assessed randomized controlled studies evaluating SJW for major depression.[304] A total of 5,489 persons were assessed in 29 studies. Results indicated that SJW is equivalent to conventional antidepressants (tri- or tetracyclic antidepressants and selective serotonin reuptake inhibitors) and superior to placebo. A unique finding is that SJW has fewer side effects than conventional antidepressants. The review found that trials performed in German-speaking countries found more favorable results.

Summary

St John's wort is a unique botanical product that has been used for centuries to treat depression, although studies show it may be useful only for mild to moderate depression. Two of the chemical constituents, hypericin and hyperforin, have been used as standardized extracts, but some researchers believe the constituents most likely to produce antidepressant effects are hyperforin, adhyperforin, and other related compounds. These compounds modulate different neurotransmitters including serotonin, norepinephrine, and dopamine. The serotonergic effects may be the major antidepressant activity. St John's wort use may have significant consequences because of the potential for serious drug interactions. It is a CYP450 enzyme inducer of important drugs that persons with diabetes may be using, such as certain statins, calcium channel blockers, angiotensin receptor blockers, oral contraceptives, warfarin, and cyclosporine. It may also reduce serum concentrations of digoxin and interact adversely with serotonergic drugs (such as fluoxetine, sertraline, or paroxetine) or narcotics and result in toxicity. Doses used are 300 to 600 mg 3 times daily. Standardized extracts used in studies include 0.3% hypericin and the hyperforin-stabilized version of this extract.[46] Persons with diabetes should always inform their healthcare providers if they are taking SJW, particularly because of the potential for drug interactions with medications they may be using. Persons with diabetes should be informed that SJW may reduce serum concentrations of certain drugs to subtherapeutic levels. Conversely, persons with diabetes should also be informed that abrupt discontinuation may result in dangerously increased serum concentrations of drugs that normally have lower concentrations during coadministration. Use of SJW has been banned in certain countries, due to the potential for drug interactions. St John's wort may not be considered a safe agent to use in diabetes because of the potential harm if it lowers serum concentrations of medications critical for diabetes or its comorbidities. Moreover, if a person is depressed, use of a traditional antidepressant should be encouraged.

TABLE 21.6 Botanical and Nonbotanical Products Used to Treat Diabetes Complications

Product	*Chemical Constituents*	*Mechanism of Action*	*Side Effects and Drug Interactions*
Alpha-lipoic acid Effectiveness rating:[46] • "Possibly effective" for peripheral neuropathy, diabetes, and weight loss Safety rating:[46] • "Possibly safe"	Disulfide compound synthesized in the liver[46]	Various mechanisms:[46,229,230] • Increased insulin sensitivity • Functions as antioxidant to: scavenge free radicals regenerate endogenous antioxidants (vitamins C and E, glutathione) • Has metal chelating activity • May stimulate glucose transporter systems	Side effects:[46,232] • May cause GI upset • Possible skin allergies • Decreased triiodothyronine levels • Possible heart rate and rhythm disturbances • Toxicity with high doses in persons with thiamine deficiency Drug interactions:[46] • May be bound by antacids if given at the same time • May decrease the effectiveness of thyroid hormone • Possible hypoglycemia if combined with secretagogues Safety rating in special populations:[46] • Pregnancy: "Possibly safe" (insufficient reliable evidence in large quantities) • Lactation: "Insufficient reliable evidence available" (avoid use) • Children: "Possibly unsafe" (avoid use) Advise against use in these populations
Benfotiamine Effectiveness rating:[46] • "Possibly effective" for peripheral neuropathy Safety rating:[46] • "Likely safe"	Fat-soluble form of thiamine[243]	Various mechanisms:[243,244] Enhances transketolase activity and may thus inhibit 3 pathways involved in vascular damage: – Diacylglycerol-protein kinase C pathway – Advanced glycation end product formation pathway – Hexosamine pathway	Side effect:[243] • Possible skin rashes Drug interactions:[46] • Several drugs may deplete thiamine body stores (metformin, antibiotics, oral contraceptives, diuretics, phenytoin, some chemotherapy agents) • Some supplements may decrease thiamine activity or deplete thiamine (betel nuts, horsetail) Safety rating in special populations:[46] • Pregnancy: "Likely safe" • Lactation: "Likely safe" (Insufficient reliable information in larger amounts) • Children: No information available on safety (avoid use)

(continued)

TABLE 21.6 Botanical and Nonbotanical Products Used to Treat Diabetes Complications (continued)

Product	*Chemical Constituents*	*Mechanism of Action*	*Side Effects and Drug Interactions*
Bilberry Effectiveness rating:[46] • "Possibly effective" for chronic venous insufficiency and retinopathy • "Possibly ineffective" for night vision • "Insufficient reliable evidence to rate" for diabetes, impaired glucose tolerance, hypertension, and weight loss Safety rating:[46] • "Likely safe" when used orally and in food amounts • "Possibly safe" when used orally and appropriately • "Possibly unsafe" when the leaves are used for orally in high doses or for prolonged use	Various ingredients:[46,316] • Anthocyanins • Polyphenols • Flavonoids • Chromium	Various mechanisms:[46,316] • Antioxidant • Lowers intraocular pressure • Improves ocular blood flow • Inhibits prostacyclin synthesis • Anti-platelet activity	Side effects:[46,317] • Dyspepsia • Flatulence • Nausea • Heartburn • Dark blue-black tongue and feces with sieved bilberries or concentrated bilberry juice Drug interactions:[46] • Possible hypoglycemia if combined with glucose lowering agents • Increased risk of bleeding when used with anticoagulants • Decreased efficacy of erlotinib Safety rating in special populations:[46] • Pregnancy: "Insufficient reliable information available" • Lactation: "Insufficient reliable information available" • Children: "Insufficient reliable information available" Advise against use in these populations
CoQ10 Effectiveness rating:[46] • "Possibly effective" for heart failure, hypertension, and diabetic neuropathy • "Insufficient reliable evidence" for diabetes Safety rating:[46] • "Likely safe"	10-carbon side chain with structure similar to vitamin K[46,258]	Various mechanisms:[46,258] • Antioxidant • Membrane stabilizer • Cofactor in metabolism in adenosine triphosphate production and oxidative respiration • Increased glycerol-3-phosphate dehydrogenase activity, thus improving glucose-stimulated insulin secretion	Side effects:[46,259] • GI upset • No serious effects with long-term use Drug interactions:[46] • Theoretical additive hypoglycemia if combined with secretagogues • May antagonize effects of warfarin and decrease international normalized ratio • Statins may lower CoQ10 levels • Theoretical additive hypotension with antihypertensives • Decreased doxorubicin cardiotoxicity (CoQ10 may also decrease effectiveness of doxorubicin)

(continued)

TABLE 21.6 Botanical and Nonbotanical Products Used to Treat Diabetes Complications (continued)

Product	*Chemical Constituents*	*Mechanism of Action*	*Side Effects and Drug Interactions*
			Safety rating in special populations:[46] • Pregnancy: "Possibly safe" (used starting at 20 weeks gestation until term) • Lactation: "Insufficient reliable evidence available" (avoid use) • Children: "Possibly safe" (with medical supervision)
Fish oil Effectiveness rating:[46] • "Effective" for hypertriglyceridemia • "Possibly effective" for secondary prevention of cardiac events in heart failure, hypertension • "Likely ineffective" for diabetes • "Insufficient evidence" for diabetic nephropathy Safety rating:[46] • "Likely safe" • "Possibly unsafe" if fish oil from dietary sources is used in large amounts	Various ingredients:[46,318] • Omega-3 fatty acids • Eicosapentaenoic acid (EPA) • Docosahexaenoic acid (DHA)	Various mechanisms:[46,318] • Antithrombotic • Anti-inflammatory due to arachidonic acid cascade inhibition • Inhibits interleukin-1 and tumor necrosis factor-alpha • Decreases secretion and increases clearance of very low-density lipoproteins (VLDL) • Alters metabolism of adhesion molecules (vascular cell adhesion molecule-1, e-selectin, intercellular adhesion molecule-1)	Side effects:[46,318,319] • Fishy aftertaste • GI upset • Halitosis • Increases mercury or polychlorinated biphenyls • Doses > 3 g per day may increase glucose • High doses may increase nonatherogenic LDL particles Drug interactions:[46,318,319] • Bleeding if high doses taken with antiplatelet agents • Possible hypoglycemia if combined with secretagogues • Possible additive effects with antihypertensives or statins • Decreases hypertensive effects of cyclosporine Safety rating in special populations:[46] • Pregnancy: "Likely safe" • Lactation: "Likely safe" • Children: "Possibly safe" In all these populations: "Possibly unsafe" if fish oil from dietary sources is used in large amounts
Garlic Effectiveness rating:[46] • "Possibly effective" for atherosclerosis, diabetes, hyperlipidemia, and hypertension Safety rating:[46] • "Likely safe" (orally and appropriately)	Various ingredients:[46,287] • Alliin Must be converted to allicin (active form) by the enzyme alliinase • Ajoene (formed by acid-catalyzed reaction from 2 allicin molecules) • Allylpropyl disulfide	Various mechanisms:[46,287] • Antioxidant activity • Allicin may increase levels of catylase and glutathione peroxidase activity	Side effects:[46,287] • Increases GI upset • Bleeding reactions • Halitosis • Body odor Drug interactions:[46,287] • Additive antiplatelet effects when combined with drugs or complementary products having antiplatelet properties

(continued)

TABLE 21.6 Botanical and Nonbotanical Products Used to Treat Diabetes Complications (continued)

Product	*Chemical Constituents*	*Mechanism of Action*	*Side Effects and Drug Interactions*
		• Ajoene decreases the activity of factors needed for lipid synthesis by reducing the thiol group in coenzyme A and HMG CoA reductase and by oxidizing NADPH • Ajoene has antiplatelet activity and interferes with thromboxane synthesis and decreases platelet activity • Allopropyl disulfide may decrease blood glucose and increase insulin • Increased serum insulin and improved hepatic glycogen storage	• May induce CYP450 3A4, thus decreasing serum concentrations of many drugs (oral contraceptives, certain calcium channel blockers, angiotensin receptor blockers, certain statins, macrolides, certain anticonvulsants, and cyclosporine) • May increase concentrations of acetaminophen, ethanol, and other drugs Safety rating in special populations:[46] • Pregnancy: "Likely safe" • Lactation: "Possibly unsafe" • Children: "Possibly safe" (orally and appropriately) In all these populations: "Possibly unsafe" orally in large amounts greater than foods Use with caution in patients with kidney disease (contains potassium)[309]
Red yeast rice Effectiveness rating:[46] • "Likely effective" for hyperlipidemia • "Possibly effective" for cardiovascular disease • "Insufficient evidence" for diabetes Safety rating:[46] • "Possibly safe" (orally and appropriately)	Various ingredients:[46,300] • Monacolin K • Hydroxy acids • Other ingredients – beta sitosterol – stigmasterol – campesterol – isoflavones – saponins	HMG-CoA reductase inhibition[46,300]	Side effects:[46,300] • GI upset • Increased liver function enzymes • Myalgia • Allergies • Inadvertent citrinin content may cause nephrotoxicity Drug interactions:[46,300] • Possible increased effects with CYP450 3A4 inhibitors (macrolides, azole antifungals, nefazodone, protease inhibitors) • Possible myopathy if used with gemfibrozil or niacin (may lead to rhabdomyolysis) • May decrease CoQ10 levels Safety rating in special populations:[46] • Pregnancy: "Likely unsafe" • Lactation: "Insufficient reliable information" • Children: No information available on safety Avoid using in all these populations Use with caution in patients with liver disease[308]

(continued)

TABLE 21.6 Botanical and Nonbotanical Products Used to Treat Diabetes Complications (continued)

Product	*Chemical Constituents*	*Mechanism of Action*	*Side Effects and Drug Interactions*
St John's wort Effectiveness rating:[46] • "Likely effective" for depression • "Possibly ineffective" for neuropathy Safety rating:[46] • "Likely safe" (orally and appropriately) • "Possibly unsafe" in large doses	Various ingredients:[46] • Hypericin • Hyperforin	Serotonergic activity as well as possible effects on other neurotransmitters[46]	Side effects:[46] • Phototoxicity • Gastrointestinal upset, anxiety • Increased thyroid-stimulating hormone • Withdrawal symptoms when discontinued abruptly Drug interactions:[46] • Induces metabolism of certain drugs metabolized by CYP3A4, thereby decreasing their serum concentrations (certain antihypertensives, certain statins, oral contraceptives, cyclosporine, protease inhibitors); also induces CYP2C9, thereby decreasing serum concentrations of warfarin • Glycoprotein modulation, thereby decreasing serum concentrations of digoxin • Serotonin syndrome if combined with serotonergic drugs such as paroxetine or fluoxetine Safety rating in special populations:[46] • Pregnancy: "Possibly unsafe" • Lactation: "Possibly unsafe" • Children: "Possibly safe" (orally and appropriately)

Case Wrap-up

All of the dietary supplements (biologically based practices) that ME has heard about—cinnamon, ginger, fenugreek, ginseng, chromium, and possibly turmeric—may have an effect on lowering blood glucose.

Regarding the specific products, these comments can be made:

- ME may be advised that cinnamon may be used in her foods (for instance, in cereal or oatmeal), or if she prefers, as an aqueous extract.
- The other products, particularly fenugreek and ginger, may produce side effects such as hypoglycemia and interact with the sulfonylurea that she is taking, which may further increase her risk of hypoglycemia. Fenugreek also may produce allergic reactions and adverse GI effects.
- Ginger may produce modest effect on glucose levels if taken long-term, but ME would need to take doses up to 3 g/day to see any effect. At this dose she may experience abdominal discomfort, diarrhea, or even drowsiness.
- Chromium may be a relatively benign agent and may help as an insulin sensitizer, although there are still unknown consequences with long-term use.
- Ginseng may cause edema, increase blood pressure, and produce anxiety.
- St John's wort may lower serum concentrations of the statin and result in subtherapeutic effect. In combination with the antidepressant, St John's wort may result in serotonin syndrome.
- The turmeric may help with her diabetes and knee osteoarthritis.

Other Products: More Information

There are hundreds of other products that have been used for diabetes or its complications. Books for both clinicians[305] and consumers[306] provide brief summaries of many products.

The diabetes care and education specialist is directed to the statement by the ADA on unproven therapies, which acknowledges the widespread use of alternative therapies and the need for cautious evaluation of these products. The ADA also states there is no clear evidence of benefit from "herbal or nonherbal (ie, vitamin or mineral) supplementation for people with diabetes without underlying deficiencies."[161] The ADA also suggests that healthcare providers should ask persons with diabetes whether they are taking any supplements.[307] Thus, a clinician would be able to evaluate the potential for side effects or interactions between supplements and conventional medications. Diabetes care and education specialists who want more information in this area can check the FDA's Web site for consumer tips on using supplements[2,20,21] and the Natural Medicines Web site.[46] Major research continues on CAM therapies, such as determining the role of honey or turmeric for diabetes. Diabetes care and education specialists can keep current by checking the NIH Web site for information on different studies.[1,6,41] Other valuable sources of information include the Cochrane Reviews, a database of systematic reviews (http://www.cochrane.org), and AltMedDex (published by Micromedex, Inc.).

Self-Care Implications

Persons with diabetes need to be made aware that if dietary supplements are used, self-care behaviors should include the following:

- Consider that the dietary supplement may have no impact whatsoever on blood glucose or A1C levels; seek to evaluate results in a defined time period.
- Inform healthcare provider of products used so appropriate monitoring will be done.
- Closely monitor products' effect(s) on blood glucose and A1C levels.

The diabetes care and education specialist needs to make the person with diabetes aware of the AADE7 Self-Care Behaviors® and remind the person with diabetes of the following:

- Healthy eating—Learn about foods that affect blood glucose, blood pressure, or lipids and remember that supplements do not replace healthy foods. Some foods or nutrients, such as calcium, may bind to supplements. Foods that are high in fiber have been found to decrease glucose, and the use of psyllium fiber may help lower glucose, postprandial glucose, and lipids.
- Physical activity—Persons should continue to maintain a regimen of regularly scheduled physical activity. Physical activity has been shown to decrease insulin resistance and possibly decrease insulin dose.
- Monitoring—To assess the impact of supplements on blood glucose, it is important to check glucose levels. Other monitoring that is important is the impact of supplements on blood pressure or lipids. Monitoring may need to be increased due to additive effects on glucose or hypoglycemia or lack of efficacy.
- Taking medication—It's important that supplements not be used in place of regularly scheduled medications for diabetes, blood pressure, or lipids or for other conditions, such as depression. There may be interactions between supplements and diabetes medications or supplement–disease state interactions.
- Problem solving—If a person does not feel well, it may be because of adverse effects caused by supplements. Or if a person's blood glucose levels or other clinical endpoints change (blood pressure or lipids), it's important to consider that supplements may adversely affect these parameters, and it's important to troubleshoot what is occurring.
- Healthy coping—Learning how to adapt to difficult situations, including the ups and downs of diabetes, is an important lesson for everyone with diabetes. It's important to remember that supplements will not replace creative coping skills or cure depression or anxiety.
- Reducing risks—Regardless of how beneficial a supplement may be, it's important to remember that evidence-based information resulting from long-term clinical trials has indicated that the best way to reduce risks is to manage blood glucose levels, blood pressure, and lipids.

Implications for Special Populations

Certain groups should be closely monitored if the decision is made to try supplements. These groups include vulnerable individuals such as children, older adults, and pregnant or lactating women. For several supplements discussed in this chapter, the Natural Medicines website advises against use by pregnant or lactating women as well as children. Recognizing that older adults are a vulnerable group that may use supplements, the FDA has a page on its Web site to help guide older consumers on the use of supplements.[21] Individuals who also have other serious diseases, such as lupus, multiple sclerosis, or cancer, are especially vulnerable, and supplements should only be used in consultation with the person's medical provider.

Other Products

There are many other products that persons with diabetes may be tempted to use. For instance, many persons are treated for depression with selective serotonin reuptake inhibitors (SSRIs), such as fluoxetine and sertraline, which may cause them to have difficulty sleeping. If a person with diabetes is also taking ginseng, he or she may have more problems with anxiety and difficulty sleeping. Persons with diabetes may decide on their own to add a "natural product" such as St John's wort, which may result in serotonin syndrome, due to serotonin excess (melatonin may also be used for insomnia). Agents such as valerian or kava may be used to alleviate anxiety related to serotonin syndrome. There are intrinsic problems in that these agents may result in polypharmacy or interact with prescription sedative-hypnotic medications or with alcohol. Furthermore, kava has the potential for hepatotoxicity and may interact with agents such as statins or glitazones and result in additive toxicity.

Summary

Dietary supplements are not approved for treatment of diabetes, but they may contain biologically active ingredients that may have a benefit in diabetes treatment. However, it is important to note that many have side effects or may interact in adverse ways with other concurrent disease states or with prescription products the individual is taking. For instance, although ginseng may benefit postprandial glucose values, it may also increase blood pressure and attenuate the antihypertensive effects of blood pressure medications the person is taking. Another equally important issue is that some of the products may have contaminants or subtherapeutic or supratherapeutic amounts of the active ingredients. But strides are being made in this area with different verification programs and with use of standardized extracts. Caution regarding potential supplement-drug interactions is always warranted. Just because an interaction is not listed does not mean that a supplement may be safely combined with medications—it may be that an interaction is not known because it has not yet been reported. For instance, although St John's wort has been used for thousands of years, the interaction noting that it decreases serum concentrations of many important medications such as cyclosporine (to prevent organ transplant rejection) was not known until the 1990s.

Those working on the diabetes care team must bear in mind that persons with diabetes are more prone to use biologically based practices, including dietary supplements, than other persons. Those involved in diabetes care and education should not turn their backs on the use of these products. The healthcare beliefs of persons with diabetes must be acknowledged and respected if they decide to use these products. Diabetes care and education specialists must collaborate with persons with diabetes so that all aspects of their care may be improved.

Focus on Education

Teaching Strategies

Complementary health approaches (herbs, vitamins, foods, and dietary supplements) are frequently used among people with diabetes in an attempt to manage metabolic markers and symptoms. In some cases, complementary health approaches are used as a stand-alone approach and considered alternative medicine.

Be respectful of people's use of complementary health approaches and preferences. The diabetes care and education specialist's initial reaction to a person with diabetes using herbs, vitamins, or dietary supplements can either make or break the whole perception on conventional medicine and the diabetes care and education specialist's credibility. The person with diabetes might not come back to see the diabetes care and education specialist or may choose to withhold sharing this information with the diabetes care and education specialist and others in the future. That is why it is important for the diabetes care and education specialist to examine his or her professional CAM health belief system first. How the diabetes care and education specialist reacts and what he or she says can influence the effectiveness of recommendations and subsequent treatment. Discrediting someone's beliefs may negatively impact the relationship.

Support persons with diabetes' efforts at self-care. Individuals who use dietary supplements are likely to be very actively involved in their own health care—congratulate them for their initiative. Be aware, however, that many individuals are reluctant to inform their healthcare providers of dietary supplement use. Diabetes care and education specialists should (1) work in partnership with persons with diabetes to encourage open communication about biologically based practices, (2) provide safety and efficacy information about supplements, and discourage use of dangerous or ineffective products and those for which there is little evidence of efficacy. Evaluate health literacy by assessing person with diabetes' analytical and decision-making skills, along with the ability to apply these skills to health situations.

Ask the right questions to assess the person with diabetes' use of supplements and belief system. The right questions will reflect genuine interest in the person with diabetes' life and treatment, and will not sound offensive. If you notice resistance in the person with diabetes' answer, you may not have asked the right question:

- What supplements or medications do you take that your doctor did not give you a prescription for?
- What do you hope to achieve by using this supplement? How does this medication/supplement help you?
- How do you monitor the effects of this medication so you know it does what it is supposed to do?

Explore the individual's conviction level in taking supplements or using alternative medicine. You can ask the following:

- On a scale from 1 to 10, how confident are you that this medication will do better than the one recommended to you?
- On a scale from 1 to 10, how willing are you to explore other options?
- What can I do to help you explore other (safer, more effective, etc) options?

Be a knowledgeable resource. Remain nonjudgmental and provide evidence-based information. Examine evidence on what herbs, vitamins, foods, and dietary supplements work versus those that do not work and those that are still under investigation. This will help persons with diabetes incorporate what works into their treatment regimen.

- Document the use of specific products and why taken (beliefs, financial reasons, knowledge, attitude, etc), along with the person with diabetes' willingness to modify and progress in making changes.
- Respect individuals' choices for doing what they believe is right.
- Provide other options to achieve the desired outcomes that are safer, more effective, or more appropriate.
- Allow the individual to examine the options and decide if willing to change or modify.
- Use evidence-based approaches in medical care (use biologically based therapies with strong efficacy) and in counseling.

Follow up with the usage and therapeutic impact of the complementary health approaches. Identify the person with diabetes' goals. A key role of diabetes care and education specialists is to keep records of the effects and evaluate the impact on diabetes care. Assess a person with diabetes' attitude to change or modify or eliminate its usage (if needed).

Help persons with diabetes share information about their use of supplements with other providers. Use a multidisciplinary team approach. Explain why and how a physician, pharmacist, dietitian, and other providers can assist a person with diabetes in achieving his or her biologically based therapeutic goals. For example, a pharmacist can help the person with diabetes keep a medication history, check for drug interactions, and provide information on supplement potency/quality and expectations. A dietitian can review the meal plan to incorporate therapeutic foods that will positively impact the metabolic goals. The physician can evaluate the effectiveness of the therapy and adjust accordingly.

Messages for People with Diabetes

Consider the following when using complementary health approaches:

- Healthcare professional's knowledge about biologically based practices
- Safety, including side effects and possibility of drug or disease interactions
- Glucose-lowering capacity
- Better options
- Risks of not meeting glucose level targets by delaying appropriate therapy
- Starting with one new product at a time and monitoring outcomes
- Evaluating the effect
- Sharing information with healthcare team

Consider the financial implications of supplement use. Many individuals may decide to stop filling their prescriptions and opt to use supplements, thinking they may be safer, be less expensive, and have more benefits. Hence, all of the issues concerning documentation of use become extremely critical.

References

1. Health, N.C.f.C.a.I. Complementary, alternative, or integrative health: What's in a name? 2017. https://nccih.nih.gov/health/integrative-health. Cited June 7, 2018.
2. Administration, U.F.a.D. FDA 101: Dietary Supplements. Updated July 15, 2015.
3. National Institutes of Health, N.C.f.C.a.I.H. Complementary, alternative, or integrative health: What's in a name? https://nccih.nih.gov/health/integrative-health. Updated July 1, 2018.
4. Timbo BB, Chirtel SJ, Ihrie J, et al. Dietary supplement adverse event report data From the FDA fCenter for Food Safety and Applied Nutrition Adverse Event Reporting System (CAERS), 2004-2013. Ann Pharmacother. 2018;52(5):431-8.
5. Administration, U.F.a.D. Current good manufacturing practices (CGMPs) for dietary supplements. 2007 2015 August 10; 72: 34752-958. https://www.fda.gov/food/current-good-manufacturing-practices-cgmps/current-good-manufacturing-practices-cgmps-dietary-supplements.
6. National Institutes of Health, O.o.D.S. Dietary supplements: Background information. https://ods.od.nih.gov/factsheets/dietarysupplements-healthprofessional/. Last reviewed June 24, 2011.
7. Administration, U.F.a.D. Dietary Supplement and Non-Prescription Drug Consumer Protection Act. Pub L. No. 109-462. 109th Congress. https://www.congress.gov/109/plaws/publ462/PLAW 109publ462.pdf. December 22, 2006.
8. Administration, U.F.a.D. How to report a problem with dietary supplements. https://www.fda.gov/food/dietary-supplements/how-report-problem-dietary-supplements. Last reviewed Sept 21, 2018.
9. Harel Z, Harel S, Waid R, Mamdani M, Bell CM. The frequency and characteristics of dietary supplement recalls in the United States. JAMA Intern Med. 2013;173:926-8.
10. Interlandi J. Supplements can make you sick. https://www.consumerreports.org/vitamins-supplements/supplements-can-make-you-sick/. September 2016.
11. Geller AI, Shehab N, Weidle NJ, et al. Emergency department visits for adverse events related to dietary supplements. N Engl J Med. 2015;373(16):1531-40.
12. Convention, U.S.P. USP Verication Services. 2019. http://www.usp.org/usp-verification-services.
13. Organization., N.I.-T.P.H.a.S. Dietary supplement ingredients and finished product testing—quality and safety assurance. http://www.nsf.org/services/by-industry/dietary-supplements/dietary-supplements-testing.
14. ConsumberLab.com. 2019. http://www.consumerlab.com/.
15. Association, N.P. NPA GMP certification program. 2019. https://www.npanational.org/certifications/npa-gmp-certification-program/.
16. Brown AC. An overview of herb and dietary supplement efficacy, safety and government regulations in the United States with suggested improvements. Part 1 of 5 series. Food Chem Toxicol. 2017;107(Pt A):449-71.
17. Administration, U.S.F.a.D. Health Fraud Scams—Be Smart, Be Aware, Be Careful Video. 2011. YouTube.
18. Information, F.C.H. Beware of illegally sold diabetes treatments. https://www.fda.gov/consumers/consumer-updates/beware-illegally-marketed-diabetes-treatments. November 5, 2017.
19. Krinsky DL, Ferreri SP, Hemstreet Brian, et al. Handbook of Nonprescription Drugs: An Interactive Approach to Self-Care. 19th ed. Nonprescription drugs. Washington, DC: American Pharmacists Association; 2018.
20. Administration, U.F.a.D. Tips for dietary supplements users: making informed decisions and evaluating information. http://www.fda.gov/Food/DietarySupplements/UsingDietarySupplements/ucm110567.htm. February 23, 2018.
21. Administration, U.F.a.D. Tips for older dietary supplement users. http://www.fda.gov/Food/DietarySupplements/UsingDietarySupplements/UCM110493.htm. November 29, 2017.
22. National Center for Complementary and Integrative Health. Herbs at a glance. https://nccih.nih.gov/health/herbsataglance.htm. Updated June 20, 2019.
23. Tsourounis C, Dennehy C. Introduction to dietary supplements. In Handbook of Nonprescription Drugs: an Interactive Approach to Self-Care. 18th ed. Washington, DC: D.A.P.A.; 2015.
24. Nutrition, C.f.R. 2018 CRN Consumer Survey on Dietary Supplements. 2018.
25. Rhee TG, Westberg SM, Harris IM. Complementary and alternative medicine in US adults with diabetes: reasons for use and perceived benefits. J Diabetes. 2018;10(4):310-19.
26. Egede LE, Ye X, Zheng D, et al. The prevalence and pattern of complementary and alternative medicine use in individuals with diabetes. Diabetes Care. 2002;25(2):324-9.
27. Garrow D, Egede LE. Association between complementary and alternative medicine use, preventive care practices, and use of conventional medical services among adults with diabetes. Diabetes Care. 2006;29(1):15-9.
28. Odegard PS, Janci MM, Foeppel, MP, et al. Prevalence and correlates of dietary supplement use in individuals with diabetes mellitus at an academic diabetes care clinic. Diabetes Educ. 2011;37(3):419-25.
29. Dannemann K, Hecker W, Haberland H, et al. Use of complementary and alternative medicine in children with type 1 diabetes mellitus—prevalence, patterns of use, and costs. Pediatr Diabetes. 2008;9(3 Pt 1):228-35.
30. Rhee T, Westberg S, Harris I. Use of complementary and alternative medicine in older adults with diabetes. Diabetes Care. 2018;41(6):E95.

31. Peron EP, Ogbonna KC, Donohoe KL. Antidiabetic medications and polypharmacy. Clin Geriatr Med. 2015;31(1):17-27, vii.

32. Villa-Caballero L, Morello CM, Chynoweth ME, et al. Ethnic differences in complementary and alternative medicine use among patients with diabetes. Complement Ther Med. 2010;18(6):241-8.

33. Nguyen H, Sorkin DH, Billimek John, et al. Complementary and alternative medicine (CAM) use among non-Hispanic white, Mexican American, and Vietnamese American patients with type 2 diabetes. J Health Care Poor Underserved. 2014;25(4):1941-55.

34. Palinkas LA, Kabongo ML; N. San Diego Unified Practice Research in Family Medicine. The use of complementary and alternative medicine by primary care patients. A SURF*NET study. J Fam Pract. 2000; 49(12):1121-30.

35. Nahin RL, Byrd-Clark D, Stussman BJ, et al. Disease severity is associated with the use of complementary medicine to treat or manage type-2 diabetes: data from the 2002 and 2007 National Health Interview Survey. BMC Complement Altern Med. 2012;12:193.

36. Jou J, Johnson PJ. Nondisclosure of complementary and alternative medicine use to primary care physicians: Findings from the 2012 National Health Interview Survey. JAMA Intern Med. 2016;176(4):545-6.

37. Ekor M. The growing use of herbal medicines: issues relating to adverse reactions and challenges in monitoring safety. Frontiers Pharmacol. 2014;4:177.

38. Boullata JI, Nace AM. Safety issues with herbal medicine. Pharmacotherapy. 2000;20(3):257-69.

39. Garrard J, Harms S, Eberly LE, et al. Variations in product choices of frequently purchased herbs: caveat emptor. Arch Intern Med. 2003;163(19):2290-5.

40. Beigel Y, Ostfeld I, Schoenfeld N. Clinical problem-solving. A leading question. N Engl J Med. 1998;339(12):827-30.

41. National Institutes of Health, O.o.D.S. *Botanical dietary supplements: background information.* https://ods.od.nih.gov/factsheets/BotanicalBackground-HealthProfessional/- h4. June 24, 2011. Cited May 16, 2019.

42. Firenzuoli F, Gori L. Herbal medicine today: clinical and research issues. Evid Based Complement Alternat Med. 2007;4(Suppl 1):37-40.

43. Gyamfi ET. Metals and metalloids in traditional medicines (Ayurvedic medicines, nutraceuticals and traditional Chinese medicines). Environ Sci Pollut Res. 2019.

44. Ching CK, Lam YH, Chan AY, et al. Adulteration of herbal antidiabetic products with undeclared pharmaceuticals: a case series in Hong Kong. Br J Clin Pharmacol. 2012;73(5):795-800.

45. Gill GV, Redmond S, Garratt F, et al. Diabetes and alternative medicine: cause for concern. Diabet Med. 1994;11(2):210-3.

46. Natural Medicines [database on the Internet]. Somerville (MA): Therapeutic Research Center; 2020. Available from: https://naturalmedicines.therapeuticresearch.com.

47. Pothuraju R, Sharma RK, Onteru SK, et al. Hypoglycemic and hypolipidemic effects of aloe vera extract preparations: a review. Phytother Res. 2016;30(2):200-7.

48. Ngo MQ, Nguyen NN, Shah SA. Oral aloe vera for treatment of diabetes mellitus and dyslipidemia. Am J Health Syst Pharm. 2010;67(21):1804, 1806, 1808 passim.

49. Lee A, Chui PT, Aun CS, et al. Possible interaction between sevoflurane and Aloe vera. Ann Pharmacother. 2004;38(10):1651-4.

50. Chang CL, Lin Y, Bartolome AP, et al. Herbal therapies for type 2 diabetes mellitus: chemistry, biology, and potential application of selected plants and compounds. Evid Based Complement Alternat Med. 2013: 378657.

51. Huseini HF, Kianbakht S, Hajiaghaee R, et al. Anti-hyperglycemic and anti-hypercholesterolemic effects of Aloe vera leaf gel in hyperlipidemic type 2 diabetic patients: a randomized double-blind placebo-controlled clinical trial. Planta Med. 2012;78(4):311-6.

52. Services, U.S.F.a.W. List of States and Tribes with Approved Export Programs for Furbearers, Alligators, and Ginseng. 2017.

53. Choudhary M, Kochhar A, Sangha J. Hypoglycemic and hypolipidemic effect of Aloe vera L. in non-insulin dependent diabetics. J Food Sci Technol. 2014;51(1):90-6.

54. Dick WR, Fletcher EA, Shah SA. Reduction of fasting blood glucose and hemoglobin A1c using oral aloe vera: a meta-analysis. J Altern Complement Med. 2016;22(6):450-7.

55. Kaur N, Fernandez R, Sim J. Effect of Aloe vera on glycemic outcomes in patients with diabetes mellitus: a systematic review protocol. JBI Database System Rev Implement Rep. 2017;15(9):2300-06.

56. Alinejad-Mofrad S, Foadoddini M, Saadatjoo SA, et al. Improvement of glucose and lipid profile status with Aloe vera in pre-diabetic subjects: a randomized controlled-trial. J Diabetes Metab Disord. 2015;14:22.

57. Choi HC, Kim SJ, Son KY, et al. Metabolic effects of aloe vera gel complex in obese prediabetes and early non-treated diabetic patients: randomized controlled trial. Nutrition. 2013;29(9):1110-4.

58. Suksomboon N, Poolsup N, Punthanitisarn S. Effect of Aloe vera on glycaemic control in prediabetes and type 2 diabetes: a systematic review and meta-analysis. J Clin Pharm Ther. 2016;41(2):180-8.

59. Rios JL, Francini F, Schinella GR. Natural products for the treatment of type 2 diabetes mellitus. Planta Med. 2015;81(12-13):975-94.

60. Pirillo A, Catapano AL. Berberine, a plant alkaloid with lipid- and glucose-lowering properties: from in vitro evidence to clinical studies. Atherosclerosis. 2015;243(2):449-61.

61. Li Z, GY-N., Jiang J-D, Kong W-J. Antioxidant and anti-inflammatory activities of berberine in the treatment of diabetes mellitus. Evid Based Complement Alternat Med. 2014; Article ID 289264. http://dx.doi.org/10.1155/2014/289264. Cited May 14, 2016.

62. Lan J, Zhao Y, Dong F, et al. Meta-analysis of the effect and safety of berberine in the treatment of type 2 diabetes mellitus, hyperlipemia and hypertension. J Ethnopharmacol. 2015;161:69-81.

63. Zhang H, Wei J, Xue R, et al. Berberine lowers blood glucose in type 2 diabetes mellitus patients through increasing insulin receptor expression. Metabolism. 2010;59(2):285-92.

64. Zhang Y, Li X, Zou D, et al. Treatment of type 2 diabetes and dyslipidemia with the natural plant alkaloid berberine. J Clin Endocrinol Metab. 2008;93(7):2559-65.

65. Yin J, Xing H, Ye J. Efficacy of berberine in patients with type 2 diabetes mellitus. Metabolism. 2008;57(5):712-7.

66. Memon MA, Khan RN, Riaz S, et al. Methylglyoxal and insulin resistance in berberine-treated type 2 diabetic patients. J Res Med Sci. 2018;23:110.

67. Derosa G, D'Angelo A, Romano D, et al. Effects of a combination of Berberis aristata, Silybum marianum and monacolin on lipid profile in subjects at low cardiovascular risk; a double-blind, randomized, placebo-controlled trial. Int J Mol Sci. 2017;18(2):343.

68. Di Pierro F, Bellone I, Rapacioli G, et al. Clinical role of a fixed combination of standardized Berberis aristata and Silybum marianum extracts in diabetic and hypercholesterolemic patients intolerant to statins. Diabetes Metab Syndr Obes. 2015;8:89-96.

69. Dong H, Wang N, Zhao L, et al. Berberine in the treatment of type 2 diabetes mellitus: a systemic review and meta-analysis. Evid Based Complement Alternat Med. 2012;2012:591654.

70. Di Pierro F, Putignano P, Villanova N, et al. Preliminary study about the possible glycemic clinical advantage in using a fixed combination of Berberis aristata and Silybum marianum standardized extracts versus only Berberis aristata in patients with type 2 diabetes. Clin Pharmacol. 2013;5:167-74.

71. Rahman IU, KR, Rahman KU, Bashsir M. Lower hypoglycemic but higher antiatherogenic effects of bitter melon than glibenclamide in type 2 diabetic patients. Nutr J. 2015;14(13): p. http://nutritionj.com/content/14/1/13. Cited May 14, 2016.

72. Peter EL, Kasali FM, Deyno S, et al. Momordica charantia L. lowers elevated glycaemia in type 2 diabetes mellitus patients: Systematic review and meta-analysis. J Ethnopharmacol. 2019;231:311-24.

73. Dans AM, Villarruz MV, Jimeno CA, et al. The effect of Momordica charantia capsule preparation on glycemic control in type 2 diabetes mellitus needs further studies. J Clin Epidemiol. 2007;60(6):554-9.

74. Fuangchan A, Sonthisombat P, Seubnukarn T, et al. Hypoglycemic effect of bitter melon compared with metformin in newly diagnosed type 2 diabetes patients. J Ethnopharmacol. 2011;134(2):422-8.

75. Trakoon-osot W, Sotanaphun U, Phanacet P, et al. Pilot study: hypoglycemic and antiglycation activities of bitter melon (Momordica charantia L.) in type 2 diabetic patients. J Pharm Res. 2013;6:859-64.

76. Krawinkel MB, Ludwig C, Swai ME, et al. Bitter gourd reduces elevated fasting plasma glucose levels in an intervention study among prediabetics in Tanzania. J Ethnopharmacol. 2018;216:1-7.

77. Nakanekar A, Kohli K, Tatke P. Ayurvedic polyherbal combination (PDBT) for prediabetes: A randomized double blind placebo controlled study. J Ayurveda Integr Med. 2019;10(4):284-9.

78. Kinoshita H, Ogata Y. Effect of bitter melon extracts on lipid levels in Japanese subjects: a randomized controlled study. Evid Based Complement Alternat Med. 2018;2018:4915784.

79. Ooi CP, Yassin Z, Hamid TA. Momordica charantia for type 2 diabetes mellitus. Cochrane Database Syst Rev. 2012;(8):CD007845.

80. Yin RV, Lee NC, Hirpara H, et al. The effect of bitter melon (Mormordica charantia) in patients with diabetes mellitus: a systematic review and meta-analysis. Nutr Diabetes. 2014;4:e145.

81. Basch E, Gabardi S, Ulbricht C. Bitter melon (Momordica charantia): a review of efficacy and safety. Am J Health Syst Pharm. 2003;60(4):356-9.

82. Tan MJ, Ye JM, Turner N, et al. Antidiabetic activities of triterpenoids isolated from bitter melon associated with activation of the AMPK pathway. Chem Biol. 2008;15(3):263-73.

83. Nhiem NX, Kiem PV, Minh CV, et al. alpha-Glucosidase inhibition properties of cucurbitane-type triterpene glycosides from the fruits of Momordica charantia. Chem Pharm Bull (Tokyo). 2010;58(5):720-4.

84. Heshmati J, Omani-Samani R, Vesali S, et al. The effects of supplementation with chromium on insulin resistance indices in women with polycystic ovarian syndrome: a systematic review and meta-analysis of randomized clinical trials. Horm Metab Res. 2018;50(3):193-200.

85. Lee NA, Reasner CA. Beneficial effect of chromium supplementation on serum triglyceride levels in NIDDM. Diabetes Care. 1994;17(12):1449-52.

86. Anderson RA, Cheng N, Bryden NA, et al. Elevated intakes of supplemental chromium improve glucose and insulin variables in individuals with type 2 diabetes. Diabetes. 1997;46(11):1786-91.

87. Rabinovitz H, Friedensohn A, Leibovitz A, et al. Effect of chromium supplementation on blood glucose and lipid levels in type 2 diabetes mellitus elderly patients. Int J Vitam Nutr Res. 2004;74(3):178-82.

88. Cefalu WT, Hu FB. Role of chromium in human health and in diabetes. Diabetes Care. 2004;27(11):2741-51.

89. Martin J, Wang ZQ, Zhang XH, et al. Chromium picolinate supplementation attenuates body weight gain and increases insulin sensitivity in subjects with type 2 diabetes. Diabetes Care. 2006;29(8):1826-32.

90. Wang ZQ, Qin J, Martin J, et al. Phenotype of subjects with type 2 diabetes mellitus may determine clinical response to chromium supplementation. Metabolism. 2007;56(12):1652-5.

91. Paiva AN, Lima JG, Medeiros AC, et al. Beneficial effects of oral chromium picolinate supplementation on glycemic control in patients with type 2 diabetes: a randomized clinical study. J Trace Elem Med Biol. 2015;32:66-72.

92. Jovanovic L, Gutieerez M, Peterson CM. Chromium supplementation of women with gestational diabetes mellitus. J Trace Elem Exp Med. 1999;12:91-107.

93. Balk EM, Tatsioni A, Lichtenstein AH, et al. Effect of chromium supplementation on glucose metabolism and lipids: a systematic review of randomized controlled trials. Diabetes Care. 2007;30(8):2154-63.

94. Suksomboon N, Poolsup N, Yuwanakorn A. Systematic review and meta-analysis of the efficacy and safety of chromium supplementation in diabetes. J Clin Pharm Ther. 2014;39(3):292-306.

95. Costello RB, Dwyer JT, Bailey RL. Chromium supplements for glycemic control in type 2 diabetes: limited evidence of effectiveness. Nutr Rev. 2016;74(7):455-68.

96. Huang H, Chen G, Dong Y, et al. Chromium supplementation for adjuvant treatment of type 2 diabetes mellitus: results from a pooled analysis. Mol Nutr Food Res. 2018;62(1).

97. Guimaraes MM, Carvalho AC, Silva MS. Effect of chromium supplementation on the glucose homeostasis and anthropometry of type 2 diabetic patients: Double blind, randomized clinical trial: Chromium, glucose homeostasis and anthropometry. J Trace Elem Med Biol. 2016;36:65-72.

98. Althuis MD, Jordan NE, Ludington EA, et al. Glucose and insulin responses to dietary chromium supplements: a meta-analysis. Am J Clin Nutr. 2002;76(1):148-55.

99. Albarracin CA, Fuqua BC, Evans JL, et al. Chromium picolinate and biotin combination improves glucose metabolism in treated, uncontrolled overweight to obese patients with type 2 diabetes. Diabetes Metab Res Rev. 2008;24(1):41-51.

100. Lai MH. Antioxidant effects and insulin resistance improvement of chromium combined with vitamin C and e supplementation for type 2 diabetes mellitus. J Clin Biochem Nutr. 2008;43(3):191-8.

101. Yin RV, Phung OJ. Effect of chromium supplementation on glycated hemoglobin and fasting plasma glucose in patients with diabetes mellitus. Nutr J. 2015;14:14.

102. Yanni AE, Stamataki NS, Konstantopoulos P, et al. Controlling type-2 diabetes by inclusion of Cr-enriched yeast bread in the daily dietary pattern: a randomized clinical trial. Eur J Nutr. 2018;57(1):259-67.

103. Sharma S, Agrawal RP, Choudhary M, et al. Beneficial effect of chromium supplementation on glucose, HbA1C and lipid variables in individuals with newly onset type-2 diabetes. J Trace Elem Med Biol. 2011;25(3):149-53.

104. Medagama AB. The glycaemic outcomes of Cinnamon, a review of the experimental evidence and clinical trials. Nutr J. 2015;14:108.

105. Crawford P. Effectiveness of cinnamon for lowering hemoglobin A1C in patients with type 2 diabetes: a randomized, controlled trial. J Am Board Fam Med. 2009;22(5):507-12.

106. Akilen R, Tsiami A, Devendra D, et al. Glycated haemoglobin and blood pressure-lowering effect of cinnamon in multiethnic Type 2 diabetic patients in the UK: a randomized, placebo-controlled, double-blind clinical trial. Diabet Med. 2010;27(10):1159-67.

107. Lu T, Sheng H, Wu J, et al. Cinnamon extract improves fasting blood glucose and glycosylated hemoglobin level in Chinese patients with type 2 diabetes. Nutr Res. 2012;32(6):408-12.

108. Vanschoonbeek K, Thomassen BJ, Senden JM, et al. Cinnamon supplementation does not improve glycemic control in postmenopausal type 2 diabetes patients. J Nutr. 2006;136(4):977-80.

109. Baker WL, Gutierrez-Williams G, White CM, et al. Effect of cinnamon on glucose control and lipid parameters. Diabetes Care. 2008;31(1):41-3.

110. Blevins SM, Leyva MJ, Brown J, et al. Effect of cinnamon on glucose and lipid levels in non insulin-dependent type 2 diabetes. Diabetes Care. 2007;30(9):2236-7.

111. Kirkham S, Akilen R, Sharma S, et al. The potential of cinnamon to reduce blood glucose levels in patients with type 2 diabetes and insulin resistance. Diabetes Obes Metab. 2009;11(12):1100-13.

112. Rafehi H, Ververis K, Karagiannis TC. Controversies surrounding the clinical potential of cinnamon for the management of diabetes. Diabetes Obes Metab. 2012;14(6):493-9.

113. Wainstein J, Stern N, Heller S, et al. Dietary cinnamon supplementation and changes in systolic blood pressure in subjects with type 2 diabetes. J Med Food. 2011;14(12):1505-10.

114. Costello RB, Dwyer JT, Saldanha L, et al. Do cinnamon supplements have a role in glycemic control in type 2 diabetes? A narrative review. J Acad Nutr Diet. 2016;116(11):1794-1802.

115. Leach MJ, Kumar S. Cinnamon for diabetes mellitus. Cochrane Database Syst Rev. 2012;9:CD007170.

116. Allen RW, Schwartzman E, Baker WL, et al. Cinnamon use in type 2 diabetes: an updated systematic review and meta-analysis. Ann Fam Med. 2013;11(5):452-9.

117. Anderson RA, Broadhurst CL, Polansky MM, et al. Isolation and characterization of polyphenol type-A polymers from cinnamon with insulin-like biological activity. J Agric Food Chem. 2004;52(1):65-70.

118. Talaei B, Amouzegar A, Sahranavard S, et al. Effects of cinnamon consumption on glycemic indicators, advanced glycation end products, and antioxidant status in type 2 diabetic patients. Nutrients. 2017;9(9).

119. Gupta Jain S, Puri S, Misra A, et al. Effect of oral cinnamon intervention on metabolic profile and body composition of Asian Indians with metabolic syndrome: a randomized double-blind control trial. Lipids Health Dis. 2017;16(1):113.

120. Sharma RD, Raghuram TC, Rao NS. Effect of fenugreek seeds on blood glucose and serum lipids in type I diabetes. Eur J Clin Nutr. 1990;44(4):301-6.

121. Sharma RD, Sarkar A, Hazra DK, et al. Use of fenugreek seed powder in the management of non-insulin-depdendent daibetes mellitus. Nutr Res. 1996;16:1331-9.

122. Gupta A, Gupta R, Lal B. Effect of Trigonella foenum-graecum (fenugreek) seeds on glycaemic control and insulin resistance in type 2 diabetes mellitus: a double blind placebo controlled study. J Assoc Physicians India. 2001;49:1057-61.

123. Lu FR, Shen L, Qin Y, et al. Clinical observation on trigonella foenum-graecum L. total saponins in combination with sulfonylureas in the treatment of type 2 diabetes mellitus. Chin J Integr Med. 2008;14(1):56-60.

124. Kassaian N, Azadbakht L, Forghani B, et al. Effect of fenugreek seeds on blood glucose and lipid profiles in type 2 diabetic patients. Int J Vitam Nutr Res. 2009;79(1):34-9.

125. Neelakantan N, Narayanan M, de Souza RJ, et al. Effect of fenugreek (Trigonella foenum-graecum L.) intake on glycemia: a meta-analysis of clinical trials. Nutr J. 2014;13:7.

126. Gong J, Fang K, Dong H, et al. Effect of fenugreek on hyperglycaemia and hyperlipidemia in diabetes and prediabetes: a meta-analysis. J Ethnopharmacol. 2016;194:260-68.

127. Vijayakumar MV, Singh S, Chhipa RR, et al. The hypoglycaemic activity of fenugreek seed extract is mediated through the stimulation of an insulin signalling pathway. Br J Pharmacol. 2005;146(1):41-8.

128. Bloedon LT, Szapary PO. Flaxseed and cardiovascular risk. Nutr Rev. 2004;62(1):18-27.

129. Pan A, Sun J, Chen Y, et al. Effects of a flaxseed-derived lignan supplement in type 2 diabetic patients: a randomized, double-blind, cross-over trial. PLoS One. 2007;2(11):e1148.

130. Rodriguez-Leyva D, Dupasquier CM, McCullough R, et al. The cardiovascular effects of flaxseed and its omega-3 fatty acid, alpha-linolenic acid. Can J Cardiol. 2010;26(9):489-96.

131. Mani UV, Mani I, Biswas M, et al. An open-label study on the effect of flax seed powder (Linum usitatissimum) supplementation in the management of diabetes mellitus. J Diet Suppl. 2011;8(3):257-65.

132. Hutchins AM, Brown BD, Cunnane SC, et al. Daily flaxseed consumption improves glycemic control in obese men and women with pre-diabetes: a randomized study. Nutr Res. 2013;33(5):367-75.

133. Ren GY, Chen CY, Chen GC, et al. Effect of flaxseed intervention on inflammatory marker C-reactive protein: a systematic review and meta-analysis of randomized controlled trials. Nutrients. 2016;8(3).

134. Caligiuri SP, Aukema HM, Ravandi A, et al. Flaxseed consumption reduces blood pressure in patients with hypertension by altering circulating oxylipins via an alpha-linolenic acid-induced inhibition of soluble epoxide hydrolase. Hypertension. 2014;64(1):53-9.

135. Mohammadi-Sartang M, Sohrabi Z, Barati-Boldaji R, et al. Flaxseed supplementation on glucose control and insulin sensitivity: a systematic review and meta-analysis of 25 randomized, placebo-controlled trials. Nutr Rev. 2018;76(2):125-39.

136. Taghizadeh M, Jamilian M, Mazloomi M, et al. A randomized-controlled clinical trial investigating the effect of omega-3 fatty acids and vitamin E co-supplementation on markers of insulin metabolism and lipid profiles in gestational diabetes. J Clin Lipidol. 2016;10(2):386-93.

137. Pan A, Yu D, Demark-Wahnefried W, et al. Meta-analysis of the effects of flaxseed interventions on blood lipids. Am J Clin Nutr. 2009;90(2):288-97.

138. Huang FY, Deng T, Meng LX, et al. Dietary ginger as a traditional therapy for blood sugar control in patients with type 2 diabetes mellitus: a systematic review and meta-analysis. Medicine (Baltimore). 2019;98(13):e15054.

139. Zhu J, Chen H, Song Z, et al. Effects of ginger (Zingiber officinale Roscoe) on type 2 diabetes mellitus and components of the metabolic syndrome: a systematic review and meta-analysis of randomized controlled trials. Evid Based Complement Alternat Med. 2018;2018:5692962.

140. Kiefer D, Pantuso T. Panax ginseng. Am Fam Physician. 2003;68(8):1539-42.

141. Shishtar E, Sievenpiper JL, Djedovic V, et al. The effect of ginseng (the genus panax) on glycemic control: a systematic review and meta-analysis of randomized controlled clinical trials. PLoS One. 2014;9(9):e107391.

142. Vuksan V, Sievenpiper JL, Djedovic V, et al. American ginseng (Panax quinquefolius L) reduces postprandial glycemia in nondiabetic subjects and subjects with type 2 diabetes mellitus. Arch Intern Med. 2000;160(7):1009-13.

143. Vuksan V, Stavro MP, Sievenpiper JL, et al. Similar postprandial glycemic reductions with escalation of dose and administration time of American ginseng in type 2 diabetes. Diabetes Care. 2000;23(9):1221-6.

144. Sotaniemi EA, Haapakoski E, Rautio A. Ginseng therapy in non-insulin-dependent diabetic patients. Diabetes Care. 1995;18(10):1373-5.

145. Reeds DN, Patterson BW, Okunade A, et al. Ginseng and ginsenoside Re do not improve beta-cell function or insulin sensitivity in overweight and obese subjects with impaired glucose tolerance or diabetes. Diabetes Care. 2011;34(5):1071-6.

146. Vuksan V, Sung MK, Sievenpiper JL, et al. Korean red ginseng (Panax ginseng) improves glucose and insulin regulation in well-controlled, type 2 diabetes: results of a randomized, double-blind, placebo-controlled study of efficacy and safety. Nutr Metab Cardiovasc Dis. 2008;18(1):46-56.

147. Ma SW, Benzie IF, Chu TT, et al. Effect of Panax ginseng supplementation on biomarkers of glucose tolerance, antioxidant status and oxidative stress in type 2 diabetic subjects: results of a placebo-controlled human intervention trial. Diabetes Obes Metab. 2008;10(11):1125-7.

148. Shergis JL, Zhang AL, Zhou W, et al. Panax ginseng in randomised controlled trials: a systematic review. Phytother Res. 2013;27(7):949-65.

149. Gui QF, Xu ZR, Xu KY, et al. The efficacy of ginseng-related therapies in type 2 diabetes mellitus: an updated systematic review and meta-analysis. Medicine (Baltimore). 2016;95(6):e2584.

150. Komishon AM, Shishtar E, Ha V, et al. The effect of ginseng (genus Panax) on blood pressure: a systematic review and meta-analysis of randomized controlled clinical trials. J Hum Hypertens. 2016;30(10):619-26.

151. Harkey MR, Henderson GL, Gershwin ME, et al. Variability in commercial ginseng products: an analysis of 25 preparations. Am J Clin Nutr. 2001;73(6):1101-6.

152. Kanetkar P, Singhal R, Kamat M. Gymnema sylvestre: a memoir. J Clin Biochem Nutr. 2007;41(2):77-81.

153. Shanmugasundaram ER, Rajeswari G, Baskaran K, et al. Use of Gymnema sylvestre leaf extract in the control of blood glucose in insulin-dependent diabetes mellitus. J Ethnopharmacol. 1990;30(3):281-94.

154. Kumar SN, Mani UV, Mani I. An open label study on the supplementation of Gymnema sylvestre in type 2 diabetics. J Diet Suppl. 2010;7(3):273-82.

155. Al-Romaiyan A, Liu B, Asare-Anane H, et al. A novel Gymnema sylvestre extract stimulates insulin secretion from human islets in vivo and in vitro. Phytother Res. 2010;24(9):1370-6.

156. Baskaran K, Kizar Ahamath B, Radha Shanmugasundaram K, et al. Antidiabetic effect of a leaf extract from Gymnema sylvestre in non-insulin-dependent diabetes mellitus patients. J Ethnopharmacol. 1990;30(3):295-300.

157. Zuniga LY, Gonzalez-Ortiz M, Martinez-Abundis E. Effect of Gymnema sylvestre administration on metabolic syndrome, insulin sensitivity, and insulin secretion. J Med Food. 2017;20(8):750-4.

158. Li Y, Zheng M, Zhai X, et al. Effect of Gymnema sylvestre, Citrullus colcynthis and Artemisia absinthium on blood glucose and lipid profile in diabetic human. Acta Pol Pharm. 2015;72(5):981-5.

159. Pothuraju R, Sharma RK, Chagalamarri J, et al. A systematic review of Gymnema sylvestre in obesity and diabetes management. J Sci Food Agric. 2014;94(5):834-40.

160. Shiyovich A, Sztarkier I, Nesher L. Toxic hepatitis induced by Gymnema sylvestre, a natural remedy for type 2 diabetes mellitus. Am J Med Sci. 2010;340(6):514-7.

161. American Diabetes Association. Lifestyle management: Standards of medical care in diabetes-2019. Diabetes Care. 2019;42(Suppl 1):S46-60.

162. Cianciosi D, Forbes-Hernandez TY, Afrin S, et al. Phenolic compounds in honey and their associated health benefits: a review. Molecules. 2018;23(9).

163. Gheldof N, Wang XH, Engeseth NJ. Identification and quantification of antioxidant components of honeys from various floral sources. J Agric Food Chem. 2002;50(21):5870-7.

164. Samarghandian S, Farkhondeh T, Samini F. Honey and health: a review of recent clinical research. Pharmacognosy Res. 2017;9(2):121-7.

165. Erejuwa OO. Effect of honey in diabetes mellitus: matters arising. J Diabetes Metab Disord. 2014;13(1):23.

166. Arabmoazzen S, Sarkaki A, Saki G, et al. Antidiabetic effect of honey feeding in noise induced hyperglycemic rat: involvement of oxidative stress. Iran J Basic Med Sci. 2015;18(8):745-51.

167. Nazir L, Samad F, Haroon W, et al. Comparison of glycaemic response to honey and glucose in type 2 diabetes. J Pak Med Assoc. 2014;64(1):69-71.

168. Abdulrhman M, El Hefnawy M, Ali R, et al. Effects of honey, sucrose and glucose on blood glucose and C-peptide in patients with type 1 diabetes mellitus. Complement Ther Clin Pract. 2013;19(1):15-9.

169. Abdulrhman MM, El-Hefnawy MH, Aly RH, et al. Metabolic effects of honey in type 1 diabetes mellitus: a randomized crossover pilot study. J Med Food. 2013;16(1):66-72.

170. Bahrami M, Ataie-Jafari A, Hosseini S, et al. Effects of natural honey consumption in diabetic patients: an 8-week randomized clinical trial. Int J Food Sci Nutr. 2009;60(7):618-26.

171. Pepping J. Milk thistle: Silybum marianum. Am J Health Syst Pharm. 1999;56(12):1195-7.

172. Flora K, Hahn M, Rosen H, et al. Milk thistle (Silybum marianum) for the therapy of liver disease. Am J Gastroenterol. 1998;93(2):139-43.

173. Medina J, Fernandez-Salazar LI, Garcia-Buey L, et al. Approach to the pathogenesis and treatment of nonalcoholic steatohepatitis. Diabetes Care. 2004;27(8):2057-66.

174. Ebrahimpour-Koujan S, Gargari BP, Mobasseri M, et al. Lower glycemic indices and lipid profile among type 2 diabetes mellitus patients who received novel dose of Silybum marianum (L.) Gaertn. (silymarin) extract supplement: A Triple-blinded randomized controlled clinical trial. Phytomedicine. 2018;44:39-44.

175. Velussi M, Cernigoi AM, De Monte A, et al. Long-term (12 months) treatment with an anti-oxidant drug (silymarin) is effective on hyperinsulinemia, exogenous insulin need and malondialdehyde levels in cirrhotic diabetic patients. J Hepatol. 1997;26(4):871-9.

176. Jose MA, Abraham A, Narmadha MP. Effect of silymarin in diabetes mellitus patients with liver diseases. J Pharmacol Pharmacother. 2011;2(4):287-9.

177. Huseini HF, Larijani B, Heshmat R, et al. The efficacy of Silybum marianum (L.) Gaertn. (silymarin) in the treatment of type II diabetes: a randomized, double-blind, placebo-controlled, clinical trial. Phytother Res. 2006;20(12):1036-9.

178. Hussain SA. Silymarin as an adjunct to glibenclamide therapy improves long-term and postprandial glycemic control and body mass index in type 2 diabetes. J Med Food. 2007;10(3):543-7.

179. Fallahzadeh MK, Dormanesh B, Sagheb MM, et al. Effect of addition of silymarin to renin-angiotensin system inhibitors on proteinuria in type 2 diabetic patients with overt nephropathy: a randomized, double-blind, placebo-controlled trial. Am J Kidney Dis. 2012;60(6):896-903.

180. Derosa G, D'Angelo A, Maffioli P. The role of a fixed Berberis aristata/Silybum marianum combination in the treatment of type 1 diabetes mellitus. Clin Nutr. 2016;35(5):1091-5.

181. Rayburn K, Martinez R, Escobedo M, Wright F, Farias M. Glycemic effects of various species of nopal (Opuntia sp) in type 2 diabetes mellitus. Texas J Rural Health. 1998;26:68-76.

182. Sobieraj DM, Freyer CW. Probable hypoglycemic adverse drug reaction associated with prickly pear cactus, glipizide, and metformin in a patient with type 2 diabetes mellitus. Ann Pharmacother. 2010;44(7-8):1334-7.

183. Bacardi-Gascon M, Duenas-Mena D, Jimenez-Cruz A. Lowering effect on postprandial glycemic response of nopales added to Mexican breakfasts. Diabetes Care. 2007;30(5):1264-5.

184. Godard MP, Ewing BA, Pischel I, et al. Acute blood glucose lowering effects and long-term safety of OpunDia supplementation in pre-diabetic males and females. J Ethnopharmacol. 2010;130(3):631-4.

185. Diaz-Medina EM, M.-H.D., Rodriguez-Rodriguez EM, Diaz-Romero C. Chromium (III) in cactus pad and its possible role in the antihyperglycemic activity. J Funct Foods. 2012;4:311-4.

186. Frati AC, Gordillo BE, Altamirano P, et al. Acute hypoglycemic effect of Opuntia streptacantha Lemaire in NIDDM. Diabetes Care. 1990;13(4):455-6.

187. Frati-Munari AC, Gordillo, BE, Altamirano P, Ariza CR. Hypoglycemic effect of opuntia streptacantha lemaire in NIDDM. Diabetes Care. 1998;11:63-6.

188. López-Romero P, Pichardo-Ontiveros E, Avila-Nava A, et al. The effect of nopal (Opuntia ficus indica) on postprandial blood glucose, incretins, and antioxidant activity in Mexican patients with type 2 diabetes after consumption of two different composition breakfasts. J Acad Nutr Diet. 2014;114(11):1811-8.

189. Williams NT. Probiotics. Am J Health Syst Pharm. 2010;67(6):449-58.

190. Musso G, Gambino R, Cassader M. Obesity, diabetes, and gut microbiota: the hygiene hypothesis expanded? Diabetes Care. 2010;33(10):2277-84.

191. Turnbaugh PJ, Ley RE, Mahowald MA, et al. An obesity-associated gut microbiome with increased capacity for energy harvest. Nature. 2006;444(7122):1027-31.

192. Turnbaugh PJ, Hamady M, Yatsunenko T, et al. A core gut microbiome in obese and lean twins. Nature. 2009;457(7228):480-4.

193. Qin J, Li Y, Cai Z, et al. A metagenome-wide association study of gut microbiota in type 2 diabetes. Nature. 2012; 490(7418):55-60.

194. Baggio LL, Drucker DJ. Biology of incretins: GLP-1 and GIP. Gastroenterology. 2007;132(6):2131-57.

195. Cani PD, Possemiers S, Van de Wiele T, et al. Changes in gut microbiota control inflammation in obese mice through a mechanism involving GLP-2-driven improvement of gut permeability. Gut. 2009;58(8):1091-103.

196. Karlsson FH, Tremaroli V, Nookaew I, et al. Gut metagenome in European women with normal, impaired and diabetic glucose control. Nature. 2013;498(7452):99-103.

197. Larsen N, Vogensen FK, van den Berg FW, et al. Gut microbiota in human adults with type 2 diabetes differs from non-diabetic adults. PLoS One. 2010;5(2):e9085.

198. Andreasen AS, Larsen N, Pedersen-Skovsgaard T, et al. Effects of Lactobacillus acidophilus NCFM on insulin sensitivity and the systemic inflammatory response in human subjects. Br J Nutr. 2010;104(12):1831-8.

199. Luoto R, Laitinen K, Nermes M, et al. Impact of maternal probiotic-supplemented dietary counselling on pregnancy outcome and prenatal and postnatal growth: a double-blind, placebo-controlled study. Br J Nutr. 2010;103(12):1792-9.

200. Bordalo Tonucci L, Dos Santos KM, De Luces Fortes Ferreira CL, et al. Gut microbiota and probiotics: Focus on diabetes mellitus. Crit Rev Food Sci Nutr. 2017;57(11):2296-309.

201. Brunkwall L, Orho-Melander M. The gut microbiome as a target for prevention and treatment of hyperglycaemia in type 2 diabetes: from current human evidence to future possibilities. Diabetologia. 2017;60(6):943-51.

202. Diamant M, Blaak EE, de Vos WM. Do nutrient-gut-microbiota interactions play a role in human obesity, insulin resistance and type 2 diabetes? Obes Rev. 2011;12(4):272-81.

203. Forslund K, Hildebrand F, Nielsen T, et al. Disentangling type 2 diabetes and metformin treatment signatures in the human gut microbiota. Nature. 2015;528(7581):262-6.

204. Besselink MG, van Santvoort HC, Buskens E, et al. Probiotic prophylaxis in predicted severe acute pancreatitis: a randomised, double-blind, placebo-controlled trial. Lancet. 2008;371(9613):651-9.

205. Gibson GR, Roberfroid MB. Dietary modulation of the human colonic microbiota: introducing the concept of prebiotics. J Nutr. 1995;125(6):1401-12.

206. Cani PD, Dewever C, Delzenne NM. Inulin-type fructans modulate gastrointestinal peptides involved in appetite regulation (glucagon-like peptide-1 and ghrelin) in rats. Br J Nutr. 2004;92(3):521-6.

207. Prebiotics, I.S.A.f.P.a. Probiotics a Consumer Guide to Making Smart Choices. https://4cau4jsaler1zglkq3wnmje1-wpengine.netdna-ssl.com/wp-content/uploads/2015/10/Consumer-Guidelines-probiotic.pdf. 2015. Cited June 3, 2019.

208. Abutair AS, Naser IA, Hamed AT. The effect of soluble fiber supplementation on metabolic syndrome profile among newly diagnosed type 2 diabetes patients. Clin Nutr Res. 2018;7(1):31-9.

209. Noureddin S, Mohsen J, Payman A. Effects of psyllium vs. placebo on constipation, weight, glycemia, and lipids: a randomized trial in patients with type 2 diabetes and chronic constipation. Complement Ther Med. 2018;40:1-7.

210. Soltanian N, Janghorbani M. Effect of flaxseed or psyllium vs. placebo on management of constipation, weight, glycemia, and lipids: a randomized trial in constipated patients with type 2 diabetes. Clin Nutr ESPEN. 2019;29:41-8.

211. Gibb RD, McRorie JW, Jr., Russell DA, et al. Psyllium fiber improves glycemic control proportional to loss of glycemic control: a meta-analysis of data in euglycemic subjects, patients at risk of type 2 diabetes mellitus, and patients being treated for type 2 diabetes mellitus. Am J Clin Nutr. 2015;102(6):1604-14.

212. McRae MP. Dietary fiber intake and type 2 diabetes mellitus: an umbrella review of meta-analyses. J Chiropr Med. 2018;17(1):44-53.

213. Jovanovski E, Yashpal S, Komishon A, et al. Effect of psyllium (Plantago ovata) fiber on LDL cholesterol and alternative lipid targets, non-HDL cholesterol and apolipoprotein B: a systematic review and meta-analysis of randomized controlled trials. Am J Clin Nutr. 2018;108(5):922-32.

214. Zhang DW, et al. Curcumin and diabetes: a systematic review. Evid Based Complement Alternat Med. 2013;2013:636053.

215. Srinivasan M. Effect of curcumin on blood sugar as seen in a diabetic subject. Indian J Med Sci. 1972;26(4):269-70.

216. Chuengsamarn S, Rattanamongkolgul S, Luechapudiporn R, et al. Curcumin extract for prevention of type 2 diabetes. Diabetes Care. 2012;35(11):2121-7.

217. Chuengsamarn S, Rattanamongkolgul S, Phonrat B, et al. Reduction of atherogenic risk in patients with type 2 diabetes by curcuminoid extract: a randomized controlled trial. J Nutr Biochem. 2014;25(2):144-50.

218. Na LX, Li Y, Pan HZ, et al. Curcuminoids exert glucose-lowering effect in type 2 diabetes by decreasing serum free fatty acids: a double-blind, placebo-controlled trial. Mol Nutr Food Res. 2013;57(9):1569-77.

219. Panahi Y, Khalili N, Sahebi E, et al. Effects of curcuminoids plus piperine on glycemic, hepatic and inflammatory biomarkers in patients with type 2 diabetes mellitus: a randomized double-blind placebo-controlled trial. Drug Res (Stuttg). 2018;68(7):403-9.

220. Mantzorou M, Pavlidou E, Vasios G, et al. Effects of curcumin consumption on human chronic diseases: A narrative review of the most recent clinical data. Phytother Res. 2018;32(6):957-75.

221. Kohn JB. Is vinegar an effective treatment for glycemic control or weight loss? J Acad Nutr Diet. 2015;115(7):1188.

222. Siddiqui FJ, Assam PN, de Souza NN, et al. Diabetes control: is vinegar a promising candidate to help achieve targets? J Evid Based Integr Med. 2018;23:2156587217753004.

223. Shishehbor F, Mansoori A, Shirani F. Vinegar consumption can attenuate postprandial glucose and insulin responses; a systematic review and meta-analysis of clinical trials. Diabetes Res Clin Pract. 2017;127:1-9.

224. Sadat Khezri SS, Atoosa; Hosseinzadeh, Nima; Amiri, Zohreh, Beneficial effects of Apple Cider Vinegar on weight management, Visceral Adiposity Index and lipid profile in overweight or obese subjects receiving restricted calorie diet: a randomized clinical trial. J Functional Foods. 2018;43:95-102.

225. Johnston CS, White AM, Kent SM. A preliminary evaluation of the safety and tolerance of medicinally ingested vinegar in individuals with type 2 diabetes. J Med Food. 2008;11(1):179-83.

226. Lhotta K, Hofle G, Gasser R, et al. Hypokalemia, hyperreninemia and osteoporosis in a patient ingesting large amounts of cider vinegar. Nephron. 1998;80(2):242-3.

227. Feldstein S, Afshar M, Krakowski AC. Chemical burn from vinegar following an internet-based protocol for self-removal of Nevi. J Clin Aesthet Dermatol. 2015;8(6):50.

228. Bunick CG, Lott JP, Warren CB, et al. Chemical burn from topical apple cider vinegar. J Am Acad Dermatol. 2012;67(4):e143-4.

229. Nichols T. Alpha-lipoic acid: biological effects and clinical implications. Altern Med Rev. 1997;2:177-83.

230. Evans JL, Goldfine ID. Alpha-lipoic acid: a multifunctional antioxidant that improves insulin sensitivity in patients with type 2 diabetes. Diabetes Technol Ther. 2000;2(3):401-13.

231. Han T, Bai J, Liu W, et al. A systematic review and meta-analysis of alpha-lipoic acid in the treatment of diabetic peripheral neuropathy. Eur J Endocrinol. 2012;167(4):465-71.

232. Ziegler D, Low PA, Litchy WJ, et al. Efficacy and safety of antioxidant treatment with alpha-lipoic acid over 4 years in diabetic polyneuropathy: the NATHAN 1 trial. Diabetes Care. 2011;34(9):2054-60.

233. Ziegler D, Nowak H, Kempler P, et al. Treatment of symptomatic diabetic polyneuropathy with the antioxidant alpha-lipoic acid: a meta-analysis. Diabet Med. 2004;21(2):114-21.

234. Namazi N, Larijani B, Azadbakht L. Alpha-lipoic acid supplement in obesity treatment: A systematic review and meta-analysis of clinical trials. Clin Nutr. 2018;37(2):419-28.

235. Kucukgoncu S, Zhou E, Lucas KB, et al. Alpha-lipoic acid (ALA) as a supplementation for weight loss: results from a meta-analysis of randomized controlled trials. Obes Rev. 2017;18(5):594-601.

236. Okanovic A, Prnjavorac B, Jusufovic E, et al. Alpha-lipoic acid reduces body weight and regulates triglycerides in obese patients with diabetes mellitus. Med Glas (Zenica). 2015;12(2):122-7.

237. Ziegler D, Ametov A, Barinov A, et al. Oral treatment with alpha-lipoic acid improves symptomatic diabetic neuropathy: the SYDNEY 2 trial. Diabetes Care. 2006;29:2365-70.

238. Porasuphatana S, Suddee S, Nartnampong A, et al. Glycemic and oxidative status of patients with type 2 diabetes mellitus following oral administration of alpha-lipoic acid: a randomized double-blinded placebo-controlled study. Asia Pac J Clin Nutr. 2012;21(1):12-21.

239. Ansar H, Mazloom Z, Kazemi F, et al. Effect of alpha-lipoic acid on blood glucose, insulin resistance and glutathione peroxidase of type 2 diabetic patients. Saudi Med J. 2011;32(6):584-8.

240. Volchegorskii IA, Rassokhina LM, Koliadich MI, et al. [Comparative study of alpha-lipoic acid and mexidol effects on affective status, cognitive functions and quality of life in diabetes mellitus patients]. Eksp Klin Farmakol. 2011;74(11):17-23.

241. Haritoglou C, Gerss J, Hammes HP, et al. Alpha-lipoic acid for the prevention of diabetic macular edema. Ophthalmologica. 2011;226(3):127-37.

242. Lukaszuk J, Schultz T, Prawitz A, Hofmann E. R-alpha lipoic acid effect on HBA1c in type-2 diabetics. J Complementary Integrative Med. 2009;6(1):1-14.

243. Head K. Benfotiamine. Altern Med Rev. 2006;11:238-42.

244. Hammes HP, Du X, Edelstein D, et al. Benfotiamine blocks three major pathways of hyperglycemic damage and prevents experimental diabetic retinopathy. Nat Med. 2003;9(3):294-9.

245. Winkler G, Pal B, Nagybeganyi E, et al. Effectiveness of different benfotiamine dosage regimens in the treatment of painful diabetic neuropathy. Arzneimittelforschung. 1999;49(3):220-4.

246. Simeonov S, Pavlova M, Mitkov M, et al. Therapeutic efficacy of "Milgamma" in patients with painful diabetic neuropathy. Folia Med (Plovdiv). 1997;39(4):5-10.

247. Haupt E, Ledermann H, Kopcke W. Benfotiamine in the treatment of diabetic polyneuropathy–a three-week randomized, controlled pilot study (BEDIP study). Int J Clin Pharmacol Ther. 2005;43(2):71-7.

248. Stracke H, Gaus W, Achenbach U, et al. Benfotiamine in diabetic polyneuropathy (BENDIP): results of a randomised, double blind, placebo-controlled clinical study. Exp Clin Endocrinol Diabetes. 2008;116(10):600-5.

249. Stracke H, Lindemann A, Federlin K. A benfotiamine-vitamin B combination in treatment of diabetic polyneuropathy. Exp Clin Endocrinol Diabetes. 1996;104(4):311-6.

250. Fraser DA, Diep LM, Hovden IA, et al. The effects of long-term oral benfotiamine supplementation on peripheral nerve function and inflammatory markers in patients with type 1 diabetes: a 24-month, double-blind, randomized, placebo-controlled trial. Diabetes Care. 2012;35(5):1095-7.

251. Ziegler D, Tesfaye S, Kempler P. Comment on: Fraser et al. The effects of long-term oral benfotiamine supplementation on peripheral nerve function and inflammatory markers in patients with type 1 diabetes: a 24-month, double-blind, randomized, placebo-controlled trial. Diabetes Care. 2012;35:1095-1097. Diabetes Care. 2012;35(11):e79; author reply e80.

252. Stirban A, Pop A, Tschoepe D. A randomized, double-blind, crossover, placebo-controlled trial of 6 weeks benfotiamine treatment on postprandial vascular function and variables of autonomic nerve function in Type 2 diabetes. Diabet Med. 2013;30(10):1204-8.

253. Alkhalaf A, Klooster A, van Oeveren W, et al. A double-blind, randomized, placebo-controlled clinical trial on benfotiamine treatment in patients with diabetic nephropathy. Diabetes Care. 2010;33(7):1598-1601.

254. Gizzi C, Belcaro G, Gizzi G, et al. Bilberry extracts are not created equal: the role of non anthocyanin fraction. Discovering the "dark side of the force" in a preliminary study. Eur Rev Med Pharmacol Sci. 2016;20(11):2418-24.

255. Fraisse D, Carnat A, Lamaison JL. [Polyphenolic composition of the leaf of bilberry]. Ann Pharm Fr. 1996;54(6):280-3.

256. Erlund I, Marniemi J, Hakala P, et al. Consumption of black currants, lingonberries and bilberries increases serum quercetin concentrations. Eur J Clin Nutr. 2003;57(1):37-42.

257. Perossini M, GG, Chiellini S, Siravo D. Diabetic and hypertensive retinopathy therapy with Vaccinium myrtillus anthocyanosides (Tegens): double blind placebo controlled clinical trial. Annali di Ottalmaologia e Clinica Oculistica. 1987;113:1173-90.

258. Bonakdar RA, Guarneri E. Coenzyme Q10. Am Fam Physician. 2005;72(6):1065-70.

259. Langsjoen PH, Langsjoen PH, Folkers K. Long-term efficacy and safety of coenzyme Q10 therapy for idiopathic dilated cardiomyopathy. Am J Cardiol. 1990;65(7):521-3.

260. Pepping J. Coenzyme Q10. Am J Health Syst Pharm. 1999;56(6):519-21.

261. Villalba JM, Parrado C, Santos-Gonzalez M, et al. Therapeutic use of coenzyme Q10 and coenzyme Q10-related compounds and formulations. Expert Opin Investig Drugs. 2010;19(4):535-54.

262. Gaby A. The role of coenzyme Q10 in clinical medicine: part II. Cardiovascular disease, hypertension, diabetes mellitus, and infertilit. Alt Med Rev. 1996;1:168-75.

263. Rosenfeldt FL, Haas SJ, Krum H, et al. Coenzyme Q10 in the treatment of hypertension: a meta-analysis of the clinical trials. J Hum Hypertens. 2007;21(4):297-306.

264. Langsjoen P, Langsjoen P, Willis R, et al. Treatment of essential hypertension with coenzyme Q10. Mol Aspects Med. 1994;15 Suppl:S265-72.

265. Singh RB, Niaz MA, Rastogi SS, et al. Effect of hydrosoluble coenzyme Q10 on blood pressures and insulin resistance in hypertensive patients with coronary artery disease. J Hum Hypertens. 1999;13(3):203-8.

266. Young JM, Florkowski CM, Molyneux SL, et al. A randomized, double-blind, placebo-controlled crossover study of coenzyme Q10 therapy in hypertensive patients with the metabolic syndrome. Am J Hypertens. 2012;25(2):261-70.

267. Suksomboon N, Poolsup N, Juanak N. Effects of coenzyme Q10 supplementation on metabolic profile in diabetes: a systematic review and meta-analysis. J Clin Pharm Ther. 2015;40(4):413-8.

268. Fotino AD, Thompson-Paul AM, Bazzano LA. Effect of coenzyme Q(1)(0) supplementation on heart failure: a meta-analysis. Am J Clin Nutr. 2013;97(2):268-75.

269. Alehagen U, Johansson P, Bjornstedt M, et al. Cardiovascular mortality and N-terminal-proBNP reduced after combined selenium and coenzyme Q10 supplementation: a 5-year prospective randomized double-blind placebo-controlled trial among elderly Swedish citizens. Int J Cardiol. 2013;167(5):1860-6.

270. Hamilton SJ, Chew GT, Watts GF. Coenzyme Q10 improves endothelial dysfunction in statin-treated type 2 diabetic patients. Diabetes Care. 2009;32(5):810-2.

271. Henriksen JE, Andersen CB, Hother-Nielsen O, et al. Impact of ubiquinone (coenzyme Q10) treatment on glycaemic control, insulin requirement and well-being in patients with Type 1 diabetes mellitus. Diabet Med. 1999;16(4):312-8.

272. Eriksson JG, Forsen TJ, Mortensen SA, et al. The effect of coenzyme Q10 administration on metabolic control in patients with type 2 diabetes mellitus. Biofactors. 1999;9(2-4):315-8.

273. Hodgson JM, Watts GF, Playford DA, et al. Coenzyme Q10 improves blood pressure and glycaemic control: a controlled trial in subjects with type 2 diabetes. Eur J Clin Nutr. 2002;56(11):1137-42.

274. Napier JA, Usher S, Haslam RP, et al. Transgenic plants as a sustainable, terrestrial source of fish oils. Eur J Lipid Sci Technol. 2015;117(9):1317-24.

275. Burdge GC, Wootton SA. Conversion of alpha-linolenic acid to eicosapentaenoic, docosapentaenoic and docosahexaenoic acids in young women. Br J Nutr. 2002;88(4):411-20.

276. Burdge GC, Jones AE, Wootton SA. Eicosapentaenoic and docosapentaenoic acids are the principal products of alpha-linolenic acid metabolism in young men. Br J Nutr. 2002;88(4):355-63.

277. Clarke TC, Black LI, Stussman BJ, et al. Trends in the use of complementary health approaches among adults: United States, 2002-2012. Natl Health Stat Report. 2015;(79):1-16.

278. Aung T, Halsey J, Kromhout D, et al. Associations of omega-3 fatty acid supplement use with cardiovascular disease risks: meta-analysis of 10 trials involving 77917 individuals. JAMA Cardiol. 2018;3(3):225-34.

279. Nodari S, Butler J, Temporelli PL. Questioning the associations of omega-3 fatty acid supplement use with cardiovascular disease risks. JAMA Cardiol. 2018;3(8):781.

280. Bhatt DL, Steg PG, Miller M, et al. Cardiovascular risk reduction with icosapent ethyl for hypertriglyceridemia. N Engl J Med. 2019;380(1):11-22.

281. Balk EM, Lichtenstein AH, Chung M, et al. Effects of omega-3 fatty acids on serum markers of cardiovascular disease risk: a systematic review. Atherosclerosis. 2006;189(1):19-30.

282. Lovaza [product information]. Research Triangle Park, N.G.P., 2019.

283. Vascepa [product information]. Bedminster, N.A.P. and 2016.

284. Siscovick DS, Barringer TA, Fretts AM, et al. Omega-3 polyunsaturated fatty acid (fish oil) supplementation and the prevention of clinical cardiovascular disease: a science advisory from the American Heart Association. Circulation. 2017;135(15):e867-84.

285. Rimm EB, Appel LJ, Chiuve SE, et al. Seafood long-chain n-3 polyunsaturated fatty acids and cardiovascular disease: a science advisory from the American Heart Association. Circulation. 2018;138(1):e35-e47.

286. Bayan L, Koulivand PH, Gorji A. Garlic: a review of potential therapeutic effects. Avicenna J Phytomed. 2014;4(1):1-14.

287. Tattelman E. Health effects of garlic. Am Fam Physician. 2005;72(1):103-6.

288. Sun YE, Wang W, Qin J. Anti-hyperlipidemia of garlic by reducing the level of total cholesterol and low-density lipoprotein: A meta-analysis. Medicine (Baltimore). 2018;97(18):e0255.

289. Zeng T, Guo FF, Zhang CL, et al. A meta-analysis of randomized, double-blind, placebo-controlled trials for the effects of garlic on serum lipid profiles. J Sci Food Agric. 2012;92(9):1892-902.

290. Reinhart KM, Coleman CI, Teevan C, et al. Effects of garlic on blood pressure in patients with and without systolic hypertension: a meta-analysis. Ann Pharmacother. 2008;42(12):1766-71.

291. Ashraf R, Aamir K, Shaikh AR, et al. Effects of garlic on dyslipidemia in patients with type 2 diabetes mellitus. J Ayub Med Coll Abbottabad. 2005;17(3):60-4.

292. Ashraf R, Khan RA, Ashraf I. Garlic (Allium sativum) supplementation with standard antidiabetic agent provides better diabetic control in type 2 diabetes patients. Pak J Pharm Sci. 2011;24(4):565-70.

293. Kumar R, Chhatwal S, Arora S, et al. Antihyperglycemic, antihyperlipidemic, anti-inflammatory and adenosine deaminase-lowering effects of garlic in patients with type 2 diabetes mellitus with obesity. Diabetes Metab Syndr Obes. 2013;6:49-56.

294. Bahadoran Z, Mirmiran P, Momenan AA, et al. Allium vegetable intakes and the incidence of cardiovascular disease, hypertension, chronic kidney disease, and type 2 diabetes in adults: a longitudinal follow-up study. J Hypertens. 2017;35(9):1909-16.

295. Augusti KT, Sheela CG. Antiperoxide effect of S-allyl cysteine sulfoxide, an insulin secretagogue, in diabetic rats. Experientia. 1996;52(2):115-20.

296. Sobenin IA, Andrianova IV, Demidova ON, et al. Lipid-lowering effects of time-released garlic powder tablets in double-blinded placebo-controlled randomized study. J Atheroscler Thromb. 2008;15(6):334-8.

297. Ahmad MS, Ahmed N. Antiglycation properties of aged garlic extract: possible role in prevention of diabetic complications. J Nutr. 2006;136(3 Suppl):796S-799S.

298. Elosta A, Slevin M, Rahman K, et al. Aged garlic has more potent antiglycation and antioxidant properties compared to fresh garlic extract in vitro. Sci Rep. 2017;7:39613.

299. Stabler SN, Tejani AM, Huynh F, et al. Garlic for the prevention of cardiovascular morbidity and mortality in hypertensive patients. Cochrane Database Syst Rev. 2012;8:CD007653.

300. Monascus purpureus (red yeast rice). Altern Med Rev. 2004;9:208-10.

301. Liu J, Zhang J, Shi Y, et al. Chinese red yeast rice (Monascus purpureus) for primary hyperlipidemia: a meta-analysis of randomized controlled trials. Chin Med. 2006;1:4.

302. Becker DJ, Gordon RY, Halbert SC, et al. Red yeast rice for dyslipidemia in statin-intolerant patients: a randomized trial. Ann Intern Med, 2009. 150(12): p. 830-9, W147-9.

303. Lu Z, Kou W, Du B, et al. Effect of Xuezhikang, an extract from red yeast Chinese rice, on coronary events in a Chinese population with previous myocardial infarction. Am J Cardiol. 2008;101(12):1689-93.

304. Linde K, Berner MM, Kriston L. St John's wort for major depression. Cochrane Database Syst Rev. 2008;(4):CD000448.

305. Shane-McWhorter L. Complementary & Alternative Medicine (CAM) Supplement Use in People with Diabetes: A Clinician's Guide, A.D. Association, Editor. Washington, DC; 2007.

306. Shane-McWhorter L. The American Diabetes Association Guide to Herbals and Natural Supplements: From Aloe to Zinc, A.D. Association, Editor. Washington, DC; 2009.

307. Association AD. Unproven therapies (Position Statement). Diabetes Care. 2004;27Suppl1:S135.

308. Injury., N.I.o.H.L.C.a.R.I.o.D. I.L. Herbal and Dietary Supplements 2019.

309. Foundation NK. Herbal supplements and kidney disease. 2019.

310. Lanca S, Alves A, Vieira AI, et al. Chromium-induced toxic hepatitis. Eur J Intern Med. 2002;13(8):518-20.

311. Lambert JP, Cormier J. Potential interaction between warfarin and boldo-fenugreek. Pharmacotherapy. 2001;21(4):509-12.

312. Erejuwa OO, Sulaiman SA, Wahab MS. Honey—a novel antidiabetic agent. Int J Biol Sci. 2012;8(6):913-34.

313. Kazazis C, Evangelopoulos AA, Kollas A, Vallianou NG. The therapeutic potential of milk thistle in diabetes. Rev Dieab Stud. 2014;11(2):167-74.

314. Becerra-Jimenez J, Andrade-Cetto A. Effect of Opuntia streptacantha Lem. on alpha-glucosidase activity. J Ethnopharmacol. 2012;139(2):493-6.

315. Denis MC, Furtos A, Dudonne S, et al. Apple peel polyphenols and their beneficial actions on oxidative stress and inflammation. PLoS One. 2013;8(1):e53725.

316. Chu W, CS, Lau RAW. Bilberry (Vaccinium myrtillus L.), in Herbal Medicine: Biomolecular and Clinical Aspects. W.-G.S. Benzie IFF, Editor. Boca Raton, FL: CRC Press/Taylor & Francis; 2011.

317. Biedermann L, Mwinyi J, Scharl M, et al. Bilberry ingestion improves disease activity in mild to moderate ulcerative colitis—an open pilot study. J Crohns Colitis. 2013;7(4):271-9.

318. Nettleton JA, Katz R. n-3 long-chain polyunsaturated fatty acids in type 2 diabetes: a review. J Am Diet Assoc. 2005;105(3):428-40.

319. Kris-Etherton PM, Harris WS, Appel LJ, et al. Fish consumption, fish oil, omega-3 fatty acids, and cardiovascular disease. Circulation. 2002;106(21):2747-57.

CHAPTER 22

Complementary Health Approaches and Diabetes Care

Diana W. Guthrie, PhD, APRN, BC-ADM, DCES, FADCES, FAAN, AHN-BC (retired)
Ethel Elkins, DHSc, MHA, MA (LCSW)

Key Concepts

- Nonbiologically based practices cited by the National Center for Complementary and Integrative Health (NCCIH) include both mind-body practices and natural products.
- *Complementary and alternative medicine*, or CAM, is now generally referred to as *complementary health approaches*.
- An increasing number of persons with diabetes are using complementary health approach practices; while many of these practices could help, others could interfere with their diabetes management.
- Care should be taken in relation to type and use of complementary health approaches and their effect on blood glucose levels.
- Use of complementary health approach therapies without the knowledge of the person's diabetes care and education specialist and other healthcare professionals may lead to problems with the person's diabetes management.
- Adverse effects must be considered when using any therapy that is not supported by evidence-based references and/or the knowledge of one's healthcare professional(s).
- Education on integration of the use of complementary health approaches should lead to greater safety and efficacy of their use.
- Evidence-based references should be used to answer questions about complementary health approach practices.

Introduction

There are any number of terms used for non-mainstream healthcare including "complementary," "alternative," and "integrative." The National Center for Complementary and Integrative Health (NCCIH), a division within the National Institutes of Health (NIH), notes that the terms are continually "evolving" with the term *complementary health approaches* generally used when discussing practices and products of non-mainstream health care as used simultaneously with conventional medicine. The term *integrative health* is used when discussing practices and products which are incorporated into mainstream health care. The term *alternative health* is used when discussing non-mainstream practices used in place of conventional, mainstream medicine.[1]

The NCCIH uses the following categories to describe complementary health approaches:

1. Natural products: dietary supplements, botanicals (herbal products), vitamins, minerals, and probiotics. See Chapter 21 for a detailed discussion of this category.
2. Mind and body practices: such as meditation, Pilates, yoga, acupuncture, deep breathing, guided imagery, hypnotherapy, progressive relaxation, Qigong, and Tai Chi.
3. "Other" approaches: do not fit into the above categories and include practices within Ayurvedic medicine, Traditional Chinese Medicine (TCM), homeopathy, naturopathy and functional medicine, as well as the practices of traditional healers.

Surveys continue to note the use of complementary health approaches. These surveys are classic references for the reader to note the use of complementary health approaches and the increased out-of-pocket expense of these therapies. It should also be noted that statistics on the use and costs of complementary health approaches vary widely and there has been no consistency in the surveys completed. Numbers are based on information available by credible sources.

As reported in the July 2018 update on the NCCIH Web site, the use of complementary health approaches (in the 2012 National Health Interview Survey [NHIS]), by American adults was noted as follows:[1]

- Natural products: 17.7%
- Deep breathing: 10.9%
- Yoga/Tai Chi/Qigong: 10.1%
- Chiropractic and osteopathic manipulation: 8.4%
- Meditation: 8%
- Massage: 6.9%
- Special diets: 3.0%
- Homeopathy: 2.2%
- Progressive relaxation: 2.1%
- Guided imagery: 1.7%

Other modalities used, but at smaller percentages, were acupuncture, hypnotherapy, Feldenkrais method, Alexander technique, Pilates, Rolfing Structural Integration, and Trager psychophysical integration. The use of essential oils has become very popular and can be effective in some patients.

The complementary health questionnaire is administered every 5 years as a part of the annual NHIS that looks at the health and illness experiences of Americans. Data summarized and reported in November 2018 in the National Center for Health Statistics (NCHS) Data Briefs (No. 324 and 325) for 2017 indicate that the use of practices such as yoga, meditation and chiropractic are on the rise in both children and adults. Yoga was most prevalent with an increase of 4.8% during the reporting period of 2012 to 2017. The percentage increase in 4- to 17-year-olds using yoga during the past year was 5.3% during the same time frame.[2,3]

The definitions of *complementary*, *alternative*, and *integrative* have not changed.

Complementary Versus Alternative Versus Integrative Medicine

Complementary generally refers to using a nonmainstream approach simultaneously with conventional medicine.

Integrative care includes the use of complementary health approaches with allopathic therapies, commonly called "Western medicine" or conventional medicine.

For example, cancer treatment centers with integrative healthcare programs may offer services such as acupuncture and meditation to help manage symptoms and side effects for patients receiving conventional cancer treatments such as chemotherapy.

Alternative refers to using a nonmainstream approach in place of conventional, mainstream medicine.

True alternative medicine is not common, except in specific cultures where Western medicine or other whole-body medical systems are unknown. Most people use non-mainstream approaches along with conventional treatments. The boundaries between complementary and conventional medicine overlap and change with time. For example, guided imagery and massage, both of which were once considered complementary or alternative, are used regularly in some hospitals to help with pain management.

Use of Complementary Health Approach Therapies by People With Diabetes

Diabetes Mellitus has reached a global epidemic stage with an estimated 387 million sufferers worldwide in 2014 and is associated with astronomical healthcare costs. Moher (in Rakel)[4] notes that it is a "largely preventable" disease and that a holistic therapeutic approach can be used with persons with diabetes. For historical purposes, refer to the works of Eisenberg et al, in 1993, 1998, and 2002, as their surveys noted the increased use of complementary health approaches.[5–7]

Many complementary health approaches increase relaxation and can help individuals cope with managing diabetes. Appropriate breathing and posture lead to supporting the improved health of a variety of conditions as found in Traditional Chinese Medicine (TCM), an alternative medical system dating back thousands of years. Within the broad categories of nonbiological therapies, there are a multitude of specific practices, a few of which will be addressed in this chapter.

Concerns Regarding the Use of Complementary Health Approach Modalities

Therapies that are inappropriately used in place of traditional (conventional or Western) medicine are cause for concern. These concerns include the following, which are still true for today's population of people with diabetes:[8]

- Potential impacts on glycemic control
- Modality variability
- Lack of scientific study on effectiveness and safety
- Delay of use of more effective interventions
- Additional costs for medical care

Potential Impacts

Potential impacts to consider when a person with diabetes is using a complementary health approach include the following:

- Will the complementary health approach be used in place of conventional therapy?
- Will the complementary health approach delay the use of needed conventional therapy?
- Is the person with diabetes using complementary health approaches in consultation with their treating physician?
- Will the person with diabetes experience an increase in the occurrence of hypoglycemia or hyperglycemia if he or she uses a complementary health approach?
  —If the person becomes so relaxed that the usual level of epinephrine output is decreased, the occurrence of hypoglycemia is possible unless the diabetes medication is appropriately decreased before and/or shortly after the period of relaxation practice.
  —If the person becomes so relaxed that sleep occurs, he or she might miss consuming a projected meal or snack.
  —If the person has taken too large of a dose of diabetes medication for the previous meal, symptoms of hypoglycemia might not be noticed when the person is in a relaxed state (not usually the case, but it could happen).

Modality Variability

Modality is a term used for a method of treatment: specific or general use of a complementary health approach. Any modality may need to be adjusted as appropriate for each person. What might be useful and safe in an adult should be carefully thought out when used with a child. Specifically, therapeutic touch sessions for children should be shorter than sessions for adults. Anyone using a complementary health approach should be warned that more or increased length of use is not necessarily better. A woman who is pregnant or breastfeeding should exercise caution in the use of complementary health approaches. For example, the effect of magnet therapy on young children and in pregnancies is unknown.

Just as with the use of botanicals (see chapter 21 on biologically based practices), certain populations including children, the elderly, and pregnant or lactating women must be taught to watch for any adverse effects of using a modality. It is especially important when first starting a complementary health approach program that individuals use extra care regarding the time of day the modality is used, the length of time of use, and the intensity of use. A practitioner should be well trained in the use of said modality (for example, a massage should only be performed by a licensed or certified practitioner).

Case: The Use of Meditation While on Pump Therapy

Henry, a male who has had type 1 diabetes since childhood, is on an insulin pump with various basal insulin rates throughout the day and self-administers a variety of bolus insulin doses depending on his dietary intake. Lately he has been experiencing afternoon hypoglycemia on some, but not all, days. Varying his afternoon basal insulin only resulted in hyperglycemia 1 day and hypoglycemia the next day.

His healthcare provider asked about his lifestyle and, with some insistence, learned that Henry was participating in meditation practices in the middle of the afternoon on a few days. He is also seeing a massage therapist weekly and is considering adding some supplements, including herbs and spices in his diet. Henry is on a fixed income in his retirement and is struggling with the cost of insulin and his other medications.

Questions for consideration

- Is this use of meditation, a mind-body-based therapy, helpful or harmful?
- What herbs and spices should Henry add to his foods? Are there particular supplements that might be suggested (or not) for Henry to use?
- What could be used in its place? Should Henry stop his meditation practice, or does he just need to decrease his previous bolus of insulin or decrease his basal insulin during this time?
- Where could the diabetes care and education specialist find answers to questions that might be raised in the use of this practice (or modality)?
- What cautions should the diabetes care and education specialist/practitioner suggest to Henry as he struggles to maintain a more level blood glucose? (Think about how quickly and "how" modalities should be introduced.)

Both practitioners and persons with diabetes should be aware of the need for extra blood glucose monitoring until the effects of the treatment modality are determined. This is especially true of older adults and those persons with diabetes on multiple medications or with co-morbid conditions which might be impacted by complementary or alternative practices. Practitioners should be aware that many persons with diabetes may be seeking alternatives due to the high cost of medications. They also should caution persons with diabetes to comply with medications as prescribed.

Lack of Scientific Study

Although anecdotes on the use of complementary health approaches might be compelling, many are not evidence based. This is especially true regarding the efficacy of complementary health approaches for children. Children are not "miniature adults." Since children are not usually included in most complementary health approach studies, the results of the studies cannot be applied to them. Such modalities might be valuable as complementary therapy, but care must be taken when using a therapy alternatively—for example, using Reiki in place of a specific medication or known physical therapy practices. If Reiki were used in concert with an evidence-based practice (although Reiki is becoming more evidence based), the person would obtain safer care.

Delays Use of Conventional Medicine

If people choose complementary health approaches over conventional medicine or are not guided by their provider to seek such help when needed, the problem could become more serious and valuable time lost. For example, if a child (or adult) comes in with symptoms of high blood glucose levels or fever, what should the practitioner do? Some practitioners would immediately send them to their family doctor. Others might choose to administer the modality and then send them to their doctor—with the idea that the person would respond better to the conventional treatment after receiving their intervention. Serious and perhaps even life-threatening results could occur.

Additional Costs

If a problem becomes more serious, more time and money will be needed to reverse the situation and stabilize the patient's illness. What are the costs for complementary health approaches? A 2007 survey found that over 83 million US adults spent more than $30 billion in out-of-pocket payments for complementary health approaches, while in 2012 they spent $33.9 billion—compared to $268.6 billion in out-of-pocket expenses for traditional medicine practices (total healthcare expenditure was $2.2 trillion). Additionally, $4.2 billion was spent on massage therapists; over $4.1 billion on classes for yoga, Tai Chi, and Qigong; $3.9 billion on chiropractic or osteopathic manipulation; $3.1 billion on homeopathic practitioners; and $200,000 on relaxation techniques.[9]

The NHIS, completed in 2012 and analyzed as a part of the National Health Statistics Reports of 2016, notes that an estimated 59 million people (ages 4 and up) had at least 1 expenditure for a complementary healthcare treatment and spent more than $30.2 billion out-of-pocket. This report notes that estimates vary due to the difference in the questions asked on the NHIS in 2007 and 2012.[9]

Parents' Choice of Using Complementary Health Approaches on Their Children

We are learning more and more about the use of complementary health approaches in children, while at the same time the NCCIH notes that little is known about the effects and safety of these treatments. The US Department of Health and Health Statistics reviewed and reported on the 2007–2012 National Health Statistics Reports survey and found that not much had changed for children aged 4 to 11 and 12 to 17 who had used some form of complementary health approach during the past year, especially if their parents had also used such therapies. Parents stated the reason they selected some form of complementary health approach for their children was that traditional care (conventional care) cost more than using a complementary health approach. Natural or herbal products were most frequently used, followed by therapies including deep breathing, yoga, chiropractic or osteopathic treatment, massage, meditation, and others.

Information on the NHIS for 2017 however noted that the use of complementary approaches, specifically yoga, meditation and chiropractic in children, has risen "significantly," but the report also notes that preliminary questions on the survey varied so it is difficult to determine the precise numbers. The 2017 NHIS reported that the use of yoga increased from 3.1% to 8.4% with meditation increasing from 0.6% to 5.4% over previous survey results.[10]

It is important to note here that there is really very little research on the impact of complementary health approaches on children with diabetes. The few studies available date to the early part of the century, and each note that most research is done on adults and that the efficacy of complementary health approaches in children is not well established.[11]

Points for Education

Recognizing the variation and in general the increase in the use of complementary health approaches, a question should be included in the initial assessment about whether the individual is using any type of such therapies (along with or separate from biological therapies). The diabetes care and education specialist may need to list or describe the complementary health approaches since a person may not realize that massage, for example, is considered such a therapy. The diabetes care and education specialist should also ask whether the complementary health approach is impacting blood glucose levels, positively or negatively, or if the person has even noticed a change.

It is also important for the diabetes care and education specialist to assess the timing of the therapy practice to ascertain whether changes in blood glucose levels are occurring during the peak action of a medication or more specifically related to the complementary health approach being practiced. It must be emphasized that only 1 modality or practice be changed at a time with careful monitoring of the changes recorded. As many elders struggle with the high costs of medications, they may want to add a number of alternative treatments but should do so slowly so that the impact of each change can be evaluated.

The diabetes care and education specialist should help the person locate or evaluate a reliable therapist. Credentialing organizations exist for some complementary health approaches, but requirements vary from state to state; the credentialing process considers education, experience, and perhaps an exam before the credential can be awarded. Sources to consider are the American Holistic Nurses Association (http://www.ahna.org) and Healing Beyond Borders (https://www.healingbeyondborders.org) as well as each state's individual credentialing or professional licensing bureau. The person with diabetes should be educated to question the type of therapy or the specific practitioner on its use and ask questions about the timing of the therapy and its effect on blood glucose responses. Individuals and healthcare providers can locate certified complementary health approach therapists through the NCCIH Web site (http://nccih.nih.gov).

Before choosing a therapist, the individual should consider the following:

- Does the practitioner have experience in treating people with diabetes?
- Is the practitioner aware of current research done on the modality as it relates to diabetes?
- What is the practitioner's philosophy of care?
- What is the cost per session? Is there a charge for cancelled appointments?
- How long is the session? Will the person have to spend an extended period in the waiting room, such as when receiving more than 1 therapeutic modality, that might result in a missed meal?
- Will insurance cover any of the costs? (Insurance plans in an increasing number of states are covering massage therapy, traditional Chinese medicine, and chiropractic therapy.)
- How accessible is the practitioner's office to public transportation? Is free or validated parking available?
- What should the person expect on the first and subsequent visits?
- Most important: will the therapy interfere with the conventional treatment of diabetes, and are there any contraindications to the use of the therapy (eg, not using magnets on a pregnant woman)?

Working With Persons With Diabetes Who Are Using Complementary Health Approaches

After the first modality therapy visit, the diabetes care and education specialist should ask the person with diabetes to be aware of benefits or problems associated with the therapy (eg, most massage therapists give their clients a bottle of water and request that they keep themselves well hydrated over the next 24 hours), and what their blood glucose readings were before and after the therapy. It is also common for the massage therapist to forewarn individuals about feeling a cramp or muscle weakness rather than increased strength.

The diabetes care and education specialist also needs to know any effect the therapy might have on blood pressure. For example, deep breathing practiced 20 minutes a day may result in a slower pulse rate, lower blood pressure, and the more efficient use of less oxygen, as historically reported by Benson.[12]

Persons with diabetes should be asked to keep a log or journal of their experiences with complementary health approach therapy whether the practice is done at home on their own or done with a therapist. If the persons with diabetes cannot keep a continuous log, they should at least make notations during the few weeks of participation regarding blood glucose monitoring along with a blood pressure check (if appropriate) and any differences in feelings, emotions, or body responses. It is important that any changes, concerns, or questions be addressed with the person with diabetes in a timely manner.

Research

Observational studies have found that people who chose non-evidence-based alternative practices over conventional practices had more problems than individuals who used practices that were complementary to evidence-based practices. This section discusses some earlier work that is appropriate to the use of complementary health approaches today.

There is concern for people with diabetes who use alternative medicine. Gill et al, as far back as 1994, noted that some persons with diabetes stopped their insulin in favor of faith healing, unusual diets, or supplements of vitamins or trace elements.[13] The response, as might be expected, was that people were going into ketoacidosis. It is important to note that they were using alternative therapy rather than using these therapies as complementary therapy.

In a 2003 article, Remli and Chan wrote about 43 randomly selected people with diabetes who, through interviews and questionnaires and chart records, were found to most commonly use herbal therapy, homeopathy, and reflexology as complementary therapies. Whether using complementary therapy or conventional therapy, all these individuals "showed poorly controlled fasting blood sugar (FBS) levels." Remli and Chan's conclusion was that the effect of complementary health approach therapies on diabetes outcomes must be assessed over a longer period.[14]

From the standpoint of professionals, Hawk et al found that there was a need to train complementary health approach providers in evidence-based health promotion counseling and in effective communication with the person with diabetes' primary care provider.[15]

In another article, Miller et al found that persons with diabetes felt that their overall health was improved when using complementary health approach therapy. Thus, the authors advised the "diabetes healthcare team" to ask about such use and to oversee its safe use.[16] This group of colleagues also wanted to learn whether the use of complementary health approaches in children with diabetes correlated with healthcare beliefs, psychosocial variables, and religious beliefs of the child's parent or guardian. Seventy-five percent of the parents in the study had tried complementary health approaches. The children most commonly used faith healing or prayer while parents did the same and used chiropractic therapy, massage, and herbal teas. This appeared to lead to children who used complementary health approaches as having problems with engaging with their treatment of diabetes (ie, complementary health approach therapies were used in place of some, but not all, conventional treatments). The research concluded that there were no differences in diabetes control, healthcare beliefs, stress, or quality of life between users of complementary health approaches and nonusers.[16]

In Europe, Dannemann et al also found that the use of complementary health approaches in children was less well documented than that for adults. They found that the parents in their population did not question the use of insulin but thought that the use of complementary therapy "improved well-being and the quality of life" for their children.[17]

Bradley et al found that persons with type 2 diabetes were in favor of using naturopathic medicine more frequently, but only if naturopathic medicine practices were covered by insurance and if they were less satisfied with their present diabetes care.[18]

Review of the above literature indicates that adults will often use complementary health approaches when they are not satisfied with their conventional therapy. Eisenberg et al found that people with higher socioeconomic status were more apt to use complementary health approaches than to use conventional therapy, but this finding was not necessarily associated with the person having diabetes mellitus.[5–7]

It has been found that quality of life is improved in people with type 2 diabetes when a complementary health approach is integrated with daily care.[19] Researchers have also found that behavior toward disease management also improves.[20] Chang et al found that in people with type 2 diabetes, quality of life scores were improved when used in relation to dietary intake education and some sort of complementary intervention.[21] However, in a 2014 report by the NCCIH, it was noted that, "There is not enough scientific evidence to suggest that any dietary supplements can help prevent or manage type 2 diabetes."[22]

If a child with diabetes uses any of the complementary health approaches available, it is important that he or she carefully monitor blood glucose levels and report any "funny feelings" to a parent and healthcare professional. McCarty et al found improved quality of life scores when complementary health approaches were used in relation to dietary intake.[23]

Whole-Body Medical Systems

Ayurvedic Medicine

Ayurvedic Medicine is the "science of life" and is a primary form of health care found and practiced as one of three major medicinal systems in modern India, the other two being Siddha and Unani.[24] Diabetes is referred to as *madhumeha* in Ayurveda, meaning "sweet urine disease," and there are many suggested treatments in the Ayurvedic system including herbs and spices, meditation, and yoga. "The ancient description of this disease includes an appreciation for the fact that derangements in body tissues take place due to imbalances in metabolism. The term for this in Sanskrit is *dhatupaka janya vikruti*."[25] Patel[25] offers an excellent description of diabetes and its treatment from the Ayurvedic Medicine system on the Chopra Center Web site at https://chopra.com/articles/mind-body-approach-diabetes.

As with many other studies of Ayurvedic intervention, the conclusion of one 2015 study "warranted further research." Banerjee et al concluded that Ayurvedic medicine opened novel opportunities by integrating relaxation practices, eating practices, and meditation practices into the care of persons with diabetes. They recognized that further studies were needed, but the observational outcome of persons with diabetes participating in this coordinated type of complementary approach warrants that this intervention be strongly considered.[26]

Homeopathy

Homeopathy was developed by Samuel Hahnemann in 1796 and uses "highly diluted solutions said to hold the vibrational principle of a given remedy, which is carefully tailored after a detailed evaluation of a person's symptoms."[27] Homeopathy was once the major approach to health care. It eventually lost its place in Western medicine with the introduction of antibiotics. Although there has been concern regarding research based on related changes, whether by beliefs or alteration of symptoms, the Food and Drug Administration has not restricted its use, due to few, if any, side effects.

A recent study by Nayak et al used a total of 25 homeopathic medicines that were believed to have an effect on the nerves of the body. After 12 months, their scoring system showed significant improvement, but they determined that further controlled studies should be done to ensure that it was the intervention alone that led to the improvement.[28] An earlier study by Pomposelli et al using the quality of life reports noted that patients using homeopathic interventions reported fewer neuropathic symptoms.[29] These are poorly controlled research studies and may just indicate a Hawthorne effect. No harm was done, but were money and time wasted? Until more thorough and long-term studies can be carried out, care must be taken when such statements are made.

More information can be found at http://www.homeopathic.org/

Native American Medicine

Micozzi[24] notes the increase in the need to recognize cultural and spiritual beliefs and continued reliance on traditional practices in the treatment of illness. Various Native American tribes have different cultural practices, as noted by Villa-Caballero et al.[30] Such practices can include food and healing approaches. Herbal use depends on which plants are in the vicinity. Shaman interaction might involve gourds, feathers, herbs, songs, or dances or a combination of these.

In 2011, Shiyanbola and Nelson found that when working with a specific tribe, it was important to assess illness, perceptions, and beliefs/attitudes about having diabetes. The perspectives on healing by women of a South Dakota tribe who had diabetes is a good example. The researchers found that for study participants, (1) their belief in God was expressed in prayers for healing, (2) people had to take care of themselves to stay healthy, and (3) support from their community was important to survive.[31]

An understanding of sociocultural factors is needed when working with any population and its use of what Caucasians would consider complementary health approaches. Although education is not considered a complementary health approach, it was the intervention used with the Zuni First People Tribe. It reduced health disparities and "engaged the population in participating in their own care more effectively."[32]

There are nearly 600 American Indian/Alaska Native (AI/AN) tribes whose members' and their descendants' health is covered by the Indian Health Service (IHS), The Federal Health Program for American Indians and Alaska Natives (https://www.ihs.gov/). There are any number of health disparities but it should be noted that diabetes is one of the leading causes of death in this population. In the Disparities Fact Sheet of April 2018, it is noted that the rate of diabetes in "AI/AN" peoples is 66/100,000 as compared to 20.8/100,000 in the "U.S. All Races" number for a 3:2 ratio, making diabetes a serious concern for these peoples.[33]

"In response to the diabetes epidemic among American Indians and Alaska Natives, Congress established the SDPI (Special Diabetes Program for Indians) grant programs in 1997. This $150 million annual grant program, coordinated by IHS Division of Diabetes with guidance from the Tribal Leaders Diabetes Committee, provides funds for diabetes treatment and prevention to IHS, Tribal, and Urban Indian health programs across the United States" (https://www.ihs.gov/sdpi/). Educational offerings consider the special cultural needs and beliefs of those struggling with prevention and treatment of diabetes.[34]

Naturopathy

Naturopathy or "nature cure" has been defined as a healing concept which uses several natural means such as dietetics and botanicals taken from various disciplines. Micozzi and colleagues have described naturopathy as "an art, science, philosophy, and practice of diagnosis, treatment, and prevention of illness" using the body's self-healing processes.[24]

Oberg et al studied a naturopathic dietary intervention over a 12-week period. They found a P value = 0.02 in changes of hemoglobin A1C sufficient to warrant a full study on the use of such an approach in a larger population of subjects.[35] In 2012, Oberg et al then reported their further study using a naturopathic intervention that emphasized a person-centered approach, health promotion, and clinical counseling on wellness and prevention to promote behavior change. Study participants were individuals with type 2 diabetes who were studied for 1 year. Three themes were factored out: (1) the program was person-centered, (2) the focus was on holistic health rather than diabetes, and (3) the use of collaboration with the healthcare professional. Among other factors, these themes were effective "in promoting self-efficacy and improving clinical outcomes."[36]

Bradley et al also reported improvements in what they termed *adjunctive naturopathic care* (ANC) in Bastyr University's *Journal of the American Association of Naturopathic Physicians*, in which interventions appeared quite like those used by Oberg. Their concluding remarks indicated that they needed to determine whether ANC by itself or as part of a plan of care was responsible for the significant changes and that the Hawthorne effect was certainly possible in such studies.[37]

Osteopathic Medicine

The osteopathic approach to a person with diabetes is well reviewed by Shubrook and Johnson. They reported that osteopathic physicians see "(1) the person as a unit of body, mind, and spirit, (2) the body is capable of self-regulation, self-healing, and health maintenance, (3) structure and function are reciprocally interrelated, and (4) rational treatment is based upon an understanding of these basic principles." The article goes on to outline the actions and intentions of osteopathic care for a person with type 2 diabetes, including the forces that can either help or hinder a person's general health.[38] Shubrook and colleagues concluded that although residency programs were improving related to outcome measures for persons with diabetes, better training is needed for better performance in outcomes related to this population.[39]

Ciervo et al further clarifies the previous work of Shubrook et al in stating that the end result relates to quality care and reduced healthcare costs through the use of osteopathic intervention.[40] Selby notes that many musculoskeletal disorders are comorbid with diabetes and that osteopathic medicine takes a full-body approach to the treatment of diabetes: the body is a unit and must be treated as such.[41]

Traditional Chinese Medicine

Traditional Chinese medicine (TCM) which dates back more than 2000 years named diabetes-related symptoms as "Xiaoke disease." Although the use of Chinese herbal medicine is and has been an important part of TCM's therapeutic approach, other parts of care are reported, such as the balance of yin (the moist, cooling water element, or so-called female element) and yang (the warm, dry fire element, or so-called male element), and its part in the holistic approach used in TCM as noted by Tong et al.[42]

Diagnosis by use of the pulse and observation of the tongue is related to the quality and function of various parts of the body. Zhao et al reported on the use of Chinese medicine and found "serious adverse events including hypoglycemia, coma and death, related to 'adulteration' with the orthodox Chinese herbal medicine, errors in substitution, self-medication, overdoses and improper preparation."[43]

In a midwestern school of Chinese medicine, all treatments, such as acupressure, body movements, and acupuncture, were given in conjunction with an herbal tea called "6 flavor tea." This tea was assessed for blood glucose lowering effects. While blood glucose levels were found to be lowered, it was unclear whether this effect was due to the use of an alternative treatment or the tea. Additionally, as the tea was composed of 6 different herbs, none of which were identified, reasonable research on the source of the blood glucose lowering effect was not possible. The use of herbs needs to be closely monitored to determine whether there are any interactions with other medicine or if they are truly helpful in managing diabetes. The traditional medical approach of TCM, just as with Western medicine, continues to need much research, whether related to herbal usage or the intervention of other modalities.

Traditional Chinese medicine is well known for the use of acupuncture. Acupuncture has been used in the treatment of many health- and pain-related conditions. Tseng et al reported on its use with obese patients. In a study using laser acupuncture they found significantly improved scores "on the fullness, hunger, satiety, desire to eat, and overall well-being" for both achieving and maintaining weight loss.[44]

Mind-Body Intervention

Essential Oils

The appropriate use of essential oils can be beneficial, but care must be taken to use the right oil for the right purpose in the right strength and for the right amount of time. Aromatherapy is included in the training of nurses in the United Kingdom. To effectively use such a variety of oils, certification from qualified individuals must be obtained. "Essential oils are pharmacologically active and can be administered by different routes, according to the specific needs of the individual."[24] Our sense of smell is our most powerful "memory-holder" and Micozzi notes that several studies have shown the connection between olfactory stimulation and the brain's central pain center. Inhaling, absorbing, and even ingesting essential oils can have a major impact on the body's pain and stress and can even impact inflammation and infection.[24]

Beware, however, in the hand of the novice, the use or choice of oils or their preparation can result in toxicity that can lead to illness or even death. Malachowska et al noted that the use of essential oils for aromatherapy was helpful in decreasing the pain response but not the perception of pain when used with children participating in blood glucose testing.[45]

Art Therapy

"Art Therapy is an integrative mental health and human services profession that enriches the lives of individuals, families, and communities through active art-making, creative process, applied psychological theory, and human experience within a psychotherapeutic relationship" (American Art Therapy Association at https://arttherapy.org/about/).

Harel and colleagues studied the use of art therapy in youth who had poorly controlled type 1 diabetes. They concluded that intensive, individualized art therapy in such a population may influence and improve glycemic control.[46] A study is still needed to determine whether it was the individualized attention or the art therapy itself that resulted in better diabetes control.

Elertson and colleagues suggest that studies with youth and art therapy in relation to diabetes are limited but they worked with 4- to 17-year olds to "draw the face" of diabetes: how does it look like to live with this chronic illness? These youth were able to convey their unspoken emotions, experiences and attitudes toward their disease.[47]

Guided Imagery

Stress is a known factor in the control of diabetes. Guided imagery or visualization can have a powerful effect on the mind. Although there has not been a lot of research done, one study involving children compared the use of just background music or auditory stimuli with background music. The study found that states of relaxation were achieved more consistently when the children were guided by auditory stimuli.[48]

Hypnosis

Hypnosis is a method of education administered by a therapist qualified to work with an individual or group in a directive or permissive approach. Hypnosis can be learned by an individual to assist with decreasing pain, anxiety, and depression and general desensitization of fears and has been found to be helpful. It is important to understand the culture of the person before initiating as the use of this therapy is not considered acceptable in some cultures and may instead be harmful.

In the treatment of persons with diabetes, it can be used as calming therapy which then might allow for diabetes treatment to be more acceptable for the individual. One such study found that hypnotherapy was quite useful for dealing with phobias, such as the fear of self-injection.[49]

Combining hypnosis with other therapies has also been found to be useful. Otani found that a combination of hypnosis and mindfulness worked quite well when integrated.[50]

Mindfulness/Meditation

Mindfulness or meditation practice has come of age. Moher[3] notes that a "plethora" of research now supports the benefits of mindfulness. Over 100 randomized controlled studies were completed in 2014 alone. The NCCIH has published on YouTube (https://www.youtube.com/watch?v=Zt02r0EU8tY) information on teaching children a simple model for meditation. It is well known that mindfulness can help in the reduction of stress, decrease acting out behaviors, and can lower blood pressure and even reduces cardiovascular risk. Emotional well-being is a benefit for anyone suffering from chronic disease.

Although Loucks et al stated that further research is needed, they found the use of such a practice was associated with better glucose regulation. However, it was unclear whether mindfulness practice had a direct effect on glucose regulation or whether the effect was indirect, causing weight loss which in turn lowered blood glucose.[51]

It has been established that people who have diabetes are more prone to depression. A study by Noordali et al noted that mindfulness-based interventions were effective in decreasing depression. Although they used a computer program to teach the mindfulness practices in an effort to reduced personal contact, they noted that that long-term studies were still needed to rule out the possibility that the effect was related to the presence of others (ie, a Hawthorne effect).[52]

Consideration must also be given to family caregivers. In a review article by Li et al, the use of mindfulness-based stress reduction resulted in an improvement in psychological symptoms no matter the condition of the patient being cared for.[53]

Laughter

What about laughter?

Laughter has long been known for its healing properties. Throughout history the anecdotal literature about laughter's pain killing properties is "massive." The journalist Norman Cousins wrote on the benefits in his *Anatomy of An Illness* (1979) and Dr. Hunter "Patch" Adams is well known for his use of humor in treating his patients.[54] Humor and humor therapy has become one of the best tools we have for cognitive, emotional, and physical response to stress and illness.

Hayashi et al found that laughter is linked to gene expression related to natural killer cell activity in diabetes. They found that laughter affected the cells related to the immune responses and, therefore, has a direct impact on blood glucose levels.[55]

In the treatment of cancer patients, laughter was found to be "the best form of therapy"—anxiety, depression, and stress were decreased. Oftentimes if an intervention works for one chronic condition, there is a high probability it will work for other conditions.[56] Additionally, Micozzi[24] points out that recent studies have even found that humor can improve memory.

Pet Therapy

Mayo Clinic notes that service dogs may provide many benefits to persons with diabetes. They are able to alert patients to impending blood sugar changes (hypoglycemia or hyperglycemia), act as a brace for patients who have fallen and need support getting up, alert others if a patient becomes unresponsive and needs assistance, bring objects such as juice bottles or medications, and retrieve cell phones in case of an emergency, even dialing 911 with a special assistance device.[57]

Just as dogs, with their special abilities, are trained to warn owners of oncoming epileptic seizures, they can also be trained to warn their owners of an oncoming hypoglycemia event and as such are not only companions but also supporters of health.[58]

Prayer and Meditation

Praying to a higher being in times of stress and illness can help people achieve a greater sense of well-being. While the style of prayer may vary greatly, it is the basis of all religions. We pray for ourselves or others, out loud or silently, and in varying times and places. Synovitz and Larson[59] point to numerous studies where prayer, both by patients and for patients, has led to better outcomes. They note that skeptics believe it is pointless to "validate the supernatural" but that evidence suggests otherwise.

Prayer has been studied in a variety of cases and for a variety of situations. In a pilot study, Sacco et al studied the use of the Serenity Prayer in people with type 2 diabetes. After weeks of daily statement of the prayer, the following results were seen. Two individuals had lowered serum glucose levels while 2 individuals had increased serum glucose levels, and 4 individuals had no change. Of course, Sacco and colleagues determined that future research was needed because of this unusual outcome.[60]

Spiritual practices and religious beliefs of African Americans were highlighted in an article by Watkins et al. Their study found that the use of prayer enhances self-care behaviors, especially when there is a need and desire for behavior change.[61]

Relaxation

McGinnis et al noted that the use of biofeedback enhances relaxation in persons with type 2 diabetes and has a lasting effect even after training. They found the hemoglobin A1C was significantly decreased in those who participated in daily relaxation practice training from baseline to 3 months later.[62]

It is a given that when epinephrine levels are lower, blood glucose levels are lower. When a person is stressed, epinephrine levels are higher; it may be concluded that epinephrine levels are related to blood glucose levels. A more relaxed person has lower epinephrine output, resulting in a decrease in physiological responses that is associated with lower blood glucose levels. Blood glucose testing (biofeedback) supports the assumption that, in most instances, a lower stress level is indicative of a more relaxed state.

Mind and Body–Based Methods

Massage

The term "massage therapy" includes many techniques. The most common form of massage therapy in Western countries is called Swedish or classical massage; it is the core of most massage training programs. Other styles include sports massage, clinical massage to accomplish specific goals such as releasing muscle spasms, and massage traditions derived from Eastern cultures, such as Shiatsu and Tuina.[63]

"The extreme stress-reducing benefits of massage have raised the possibility that massage may be of benefits to people with diabetes by including the relaxation response, thereby controlling the counter-regulatory stress hormones and permitting the body to use insulin more effectively," note the authors of a 2011 article.[64]

Massage in and of itself has been questioned with regard to improvement in diabetes control. A 2012 article found that massage, versus relaxation exercises using a CD, for adult Swedish-born patients ($P = 0.05$) had limited effects on the quality of life of persons with type 2 diabetes.[65] The article's authors queried that massage might be effective if the perceived levels of stress were higher.

In 2011, Sajedi et al found that Swedish massage, as part of a daily routine, was an effective intervention to reduce blood glucose levels in children with diabetes; unknown is whether the results were due to the massage or the attention being given to an individual child.[66]

Chiropractic Medicine

Chiropractic medicine has been addressed by some as an important component of the US healthcare system. Chiropractors believe that the correction of a spinal abnormality is a critical healthcare intervention. To some, along with spinal manipulation, this appears to be related to collaborative care, although to others improvement is related to a more holistic approach to care.

In one study of older adults with back pain, the positive outcomes were more often associated with collaborative care.[67] In another study, it was noted that 80% of chiropractic physicians gave some form of nutritional counseling, which supports the notion that such chiropractors are more holistic in nature than perhaps previously thought.[68]

In Tuchin's review of the literature, it was noted that there were several problems in spinal manipulation. He concluded that appropriate use by legislated treatment needs to be considered when reporting on a particular use of a complementary health approach in the field of chiropractic medicine.[69]

Qigong/Qi Gong

The term Qigong refers to the manipulation of bioenergy or more loosely "qi work" (energy work). Qigong is an area of Chinese medicine that is similar to Tai Chi. Qigong is the name of Chinese therapeutic exercises and dietary care, and has been considered for the treatment of type 2 diabetes.

In their review of the literature, Freire and Alves found that Qigong increased C-peptide and reduced fasting blood glucose levels, along with improving insulin resistance and hemoglobin A1C.[70] Even though these authors saw such a positive outcome, a large randomized clinical trial was still needed to definitively support the use of this modality. In the study comparing Yi Ren Medical Qigong (YRMQ) with both progressive resistance training (PRT) and standard care, there were not enough subjects and not enough time for participation to make any credible conclusions in regard to the psychological effects of these approaches in people with type 2 diabetes.[71] This is an example of a potentially good study that essentially becomes lost due to a variety of factors that decrease its credibility.

Liu et al recommended "cautious review" when considering the use of Qigong and/or Tai Chi for the treatment of depression.[72] A 2016 survey reported the use of Tai Chi and Qigong for general use rather than specific treatment.[73] The Liu et al study reported in 2011 gave more supportive data for the use of Qigong, which included appropriate weight loss, increased leg strength, and less insulin resistance.[74]

Reflexology

According to Bisson,[75] reflexology is a "focused pressure" technique, generally directed toward the hands or feet. It is not considered a massage technique because there is no movement involved, though many US states require a practitioner to be licensed as a massage therapist in order to offer reflexology. Reflexology, a common practice in many places, has been studied for a range of conditions, including diabetes.

Da Silva et al in randomized, controlled, and blind clinical trial concluded that foot reflexology is helpful for people with type 2 diabetes. Fewer impairments in indicators to skin and hair were noted in the persons with diabetes who received reflexology.[76]

Tai Chi

Visitors to China's parks in the early morning may see its citizens practicing the ancient art of Tai Chi, a martial art emphasizing meditative aerobic activity and relaxation. Slow, smooth body movements help achieve a relaxed body and soul, improve balance and overall well-being.

Yan and colleagues, in a 2013 meta-analysis of Tai Chi–related effects, reported that there is not sufficient evidence to support the benefits to people with type 2 diabetes, and that larger scale studies are needed to determine long-term efficacy in spite of reduced hemoglobin A1C ($P < 0.00001$), fasting blood glucose ($P = 0.003$), and triglycerides ($P = 0.006$). No improvements were noted for total cholesterol, HDL, or other body parameters.[77] Another study found that balance improvement led to increased "ankle" proprioception.[78] Lee et al, in their review of the literature and meta-analysis, found improvement in overall health outcomes for people with type 2 diabetes who used Tai Chi.[79]

In a 2018 meta-analysis looking at 14 studies with nearly 800 participants, Chao and colleagues found that regular practice of Tai Chi had a significant impact on the overall health of persons with type 2 diabetes by promoting the metabolism of cells and tissues, promoting blood flow to the heart and improving the body's utilization of glucose, increasing target cell reactivity, improving glucose tolerance and preventing the composition of HbA1c, ultimately reducing the levels of FBG, HbA1c, and 2hPBG.[80]

Yoga

Yoga is a Sanskrit word meaning *union*, most commonly a spiritual union. The practice of yoga dates back thousands of years in the Indian tradition. It is thought that the first written teachings appeared from about 7000 BCE to 1500 AD in 4 volumes written in Sanskrit: *Rig-Veda, Yajur-Veda, Sama-Veda and Atharva-Veda.* Today's yoga practice is more about learning postures, getting exercise, and participating in meditation. In ancient times, however, yoga was a lifestyle that included eating, bathing, prayer, work, and social interactions. Yoga develops strength and flexibility and helps to manage pain, stress, depression, and can lower heart rate, blood pressure, anxiety, and offers improved physical and sexual health.[60]

Alexander et al found that yoga, as an 8-week intervention, had little effect on physical activity over time.[81] The authors recommended further research to look at behavioral health outcomes and people with type 2 diabetes. Hegde et al found that yoga can be used to reduce oxidative stress in this same population. They also found that when yoga is used in addition to standard care, body mass index (BMI) and glycemic values may be reduced.[82]

In spite of "risk bias," an article by Kumar et al concluded that yoga should be considered a complementary health approach for people with type 2 diabetes.[83] Similarly, Chimkode et al were able to document the lowering of blood glucose levels with 3 months of yoga practice.[84] In an article in the *Journal of Diabetes Research*, reviewers were cautious of the use of yoga in the type 2 diabetes population, in spite of their positive findings.[85]

Energy Therapies

Biofield Therapies

Reiki Reiki practitioners "lay hands" on their patients at specific locations and transfer energy from themselves to the patient. Micozzi[24] notes that energy modalities are thought to repattern the energy field to accelerate healing. The idea is to re-balance the patient's energy field rather than to treat or cure specific diseases.

In 2011, Bowden et al reported on a randomized controlled single-blind trial of the effect of Reiki on mood and well-being. This study was carried out on 40 university students; half of the subjects had high depression/mood scores, while the other half had low depression scores. Both groups received Reiki treatments. Those with the high depression/mood scores had significant improvement in mood as compared with the group with low scores. Since many people with diabetes have greater problems with depression, Reiki might become a useful tool to use on their behalf.[86]

Although the following 3 papers are not specifically related to diabetes care, they do reflect the use of Reiki for stress reduction and depression. Bukowski and Berardi reported on their work with children who had high stress levels, especially due to epilepsy and sleep disturbance problems. They found that the negative responses in the children appeared to be alleviated when their mothers were trained in relaxation practices.[87] Bukowski later reported, using a larger population, that there was improvement in the Perceived Stress Scale (used for measurement of change) and self-rating of improvement.[88] Joyce and Herbison then concluded that the evidence was still insufficient for the use of Reiki for the treatment of "anxiety or depression or both" for adults.[89]

In a review of PubMed articles, no paper to date has reported on the use of Reiki for those people experiencing neuropathy. Micozzi[24] addresses several studies which have been done on energy healing. Results have been mixed, with reduced anxiety, promotion of relaxation, and improvement of functional status being some of the outcomes.

Therapeutic Touch/Healing Touch Therapeutic touch (TT) or Healing touch (HT) is described as a "relaxing, nurturing, heart-centered energy therapy that uses gentle, intentional touch that assists in balancing physical, emotional, mental and spiritual well-being" as described on the Healing Beyond Borders Web site at (https://www.healingbeyondborders.org/index.php/about/what-is-healing-touch).

Although not presently listed in the newer complementary health approaches, TT or HT has been used in a variety of settings, but not specifically for people with diabetes. More often it has been used with individuals with some sort of discomfort, such as postoperative pain.

In a study by Coakley and Duffy, patients who received TT reported less pain and had documented lower cortisol levels and natural killer cells (NKCs).[90] In a review article, 5 of 7 studies, published between 1997 and 2004, were scientifically well grounded enough to conclude that TT supported a reported and documented decrease in the sensation of pain.[91]

O'Mathuna and Ashford, in their efforts to continue assessing the use of TT for the healing of acute wounds, found that even though there were a few reported cases of improvement, there was no robust evidence that TT promoted the healing of acute wounds.[92] Tabatabaee et al assessed studies completed between 1990 and 2015 and concluded that TT is useful for adult patients with cancer and therefore could also be of considerable use in supporting people with diabetes.[93]

Rindfleisch presents an excellent history as well as a summary of key systematic review, meta-analyses, and randomized clinical trials relating to clinical efficacy of human energetic therapies. Most positive results have been in some pain relief, but more research is indicated.[94]

Electromagnetic-Based Therapies

Light Therapy Micozzi[24] addresses light therapy at length, noting that there are any number of colors and "kinds" of light that can help with a variety of health problems. Seasonal affective disorder, Vitamin D deficiencies, depression, and Parkinson's disease are just a few of the ones that were mentioned. While nature and being outside is suggested as the best "light therapy" there are benefits to sitting in front of light boxes and undergoing light treatments. Laser treatments and infrared light have been explored for varying illnesses.

One study of light therapy, reported in *Diabetes Care* by Lavery et al, found that anodyne light therapy (ie, monochromatic infrared photoenergy) improved feeling in people with diabetes who had sensory neuropathy.[95] Amall et al published a paper in 2006 and later reported in a 2009 paper that the suspected nitric oxide was not responsible for this change, but that infrared light improves peripheral changes by means other than nitric oxide.[96] This could indicate that 1 type of light therapy might be more effective than another type for neuropathic treatment, but no follow-up paper was found as of this printing.

In a randomized double-blind study, light therapy was used for people who had major depression and type 2 diabetes. Light therapy was found to improve both mood and insulin sensitivity in people with type 2 diabetes.[97] A more recent look at people with diabetes and depression was inconclusive regarding whether light therapy was a viable option for a subgroup of highly insulin-resistive persons with diabetes.[98]

Magnet Therapy Micozzi[24] describes magnetic therapy as, "reportedly a safe, noninvasive method of applying magnetic fields to the body for therapeutic purposes." While the quality of research is uncertain with very few randomized controlled trials, the retail business has boomed. It is estimated that annual sales on bracelets and other magnetic items has exceeded $500 million in the United States and Canada alone with as much as $5 billion being spent worldwide.

Magnets do have their place as a form of therapy but may not be recognized as such. In addition to magnetic resonance imaging (MRI), another magnetic instrument has been introduced; magnetic resonance spectroscopy. Its place in diabetes treatment has yet to be determined. These magnets are given higher field strength and improved delineation, and thus it is likely that their use will lead to more research into the metabolic syndrome and chronic diseases such as diabetes mellitus.[99]

A literature review by Colbert et al was conducted regarding magnets applied to acupuncture points as therapy.[100] Of the 380 papers reviewed, only 50 studies met their inclusion criteria. They deduced that the use of acupuncture with magnet therapy, if properly studied, would yield some useful results in treatment of certain conditions, such as neuropathy.

Several other studies were reported but not specific to people with diabetes. Micozzi's text reports on several magnetic devices for both conventional and complementary/alternative practices.[24]

TENS Units One paper on TENS (transcutaneous electrical nerve stimulation) application and its potential in controlling blood glucose levels reported that when the TENS unit was in place, pain was decreased but the person with diabetes became hypoglycemic. In continued use of TENS, it was found that the person's insulin dosage was adjusted to half of what it previously had been to prevent hypoglycemic episodes. Khan's conclusion was that "decreased sympathetic stimulation, enhanced insulin sensitivity or altered muscle metabolism due to electrical stimulation" led to decreased blood glucose levels.[101]

Other Related Research

In a feasibility study, Mandel et al found music therapy and music-assisted relaxation improved their measured outcomes but found better but inclusive results (especially with blood pressure measurements) when diabetes self-management education was added.[102]

Which modality is responsible for the appropriately lowered and stabilized blood glucose levels? Bay and Bay studied the combination of acupressure, hypnotherapy, and transcendental meditation in 20 persons with diabetes who were provided 60- to 90-minute training sessions over 10 successive days. "Convenience sampling" of persons with type 2 diabetes who received the combination of modalities found that these individuals had lower blood glucose levels than the placebo group.[103]

Kanodia et al performed a national survey to look at the use of complementary health approaches for the treatment of back pain. Most commonly used were massage, herbal therapy, yoga, Tai Chi, Qigong, and acupuncture. All were associated with perceived benefit, but the researchers' concluding remarks indicated that further investigation was needed.[104]

A study by De Leon Rodriguez et al used biofeedback to reduce foot pressure in people with peripheral neuropathy. The study noted that personal training and knowledge resulted in less pressure on desired areas of the foot.[105] McGrady also found biofeedback useful as a complementary health approach when treating people with hypertension.[106] This study indirectly demonstrates that the biofeedback of blood glucose testing also contributes to a knowledgeable person's response to self-management and general care.

Case Wrap-Up

Henry was found to be intermittently practicing meditation in the middle of the afternoon. He reported that he felt relaxed by the end of the meditation session. Coincidentally, he was participating in this practice at about the same time as the peak action of his bolus dose of insulin self-administered before lunch.

Henry was educated to either decrease the bolus dose at the time of his previous meal or have a small snack before the time he chooses to meditate. Overall concern should be on safety first and control second, along with his quality of life and having diabetes. His meditation should contribute to an improved quality of life. It is important to ensure that he stays safe by not becoming hypoglycemic.

Conclusion

While many of these complementary health approaches need further study and exploration, it should be noted that many studies showed that persons with diabetes of varying ages and backgrounds experienced positive feelings of increased well-being when these modalities were incorporated into their daily lifestyles.

Focus on Education

Teaching Strategies

Be respectful of people's preference for and use of alternative or complementary modalities. A diabetes care and education specialist's initial reaction to a person with diabetes' use of any modality can positively or negatively affect the perception of being a caring and capable healthcare professional.

Be a knowledgeable resource on complementary health approaches and ask the right questions.

- Are you using any modalities (like . . .), including vitamins, minerals, and/or herbs?
- What do you hope to achieve by using the modality?
- How does this modality help you?
- How do you know that this modality does what it is supposed to do?

Encourage open communication about biologically based therapies, alternative medical systems, mind-body intervention, manipulative and body-based methods, energy therapies, supplements, and other modalities and discourage the use of dangerous or ineffective modalities (and products).

Assess and follow up on diabetes-related impacts and issues with complementary health approaches. Recommend that people start with one new product or modality at a time. For additional help, refer persons with diabetes to the NCCIH Web site: http://nccih.nih.gov.

Messages for Persons With Diabetes

- What is labeled as natural is not necessarily safe.
- Look for the USP mark or standardized notation on the bottle label to confirm that the product has been inspected for consistency.

- A product or modality advertised on the Internet may not always be in the best interest of the user—consult with a knowledgeable person.
- If in doubt, don't use the product or modality, especially if you have a compromised liver or kidneys.
- **Safety first.** Provide a complete list of all modalities, medicines, supplements, and/or herbs to your health professional.
- **One at a time.** Add one complementary or alternative practice into your regiment at a time to determine whether it works for you.
- **Trial period.** Unless you are suffering ill effects or have been told by your healthcare provider to stop, don't abandon your selected complementary health approach after just a few attempts or sessions. It can take a while for positive effects of a modality to become evident.

Focus on Practice

Recognize the potential value of complementary health approaches and be prepared to address them when indicated by the person with diabetes' use or interest in use.

Be prepared to help consumers identify practitioners of complementary health approaches that will meet their needs and preferences. Use the NCCIH Web site as a resource: http://nccih.nih.gov/health/decisions.

Document use of the specific products/modalities in the medical record to communicate your findings with the entire diabetes healthcare team.

Respect consumers' choices regarding the use of complementary health approaches while guiding them on safe use and any precautions they need to take.

References

1. National Center for Complementary and Integrative Health. Complementary, alternative, or integrative health: what's in a name? (updated 2018 July; cited 2019 June 1). On the Internet at: https://nccih.nih.gov/health/integrative-health.
2. Clarke RC, Barnes PM, Black LI, Stussman BJ, Nahin RL. Use of yoga, meditation, and chiropractors among U.S. adults aged 18 and over. NCHS Data Brief, no 325. Hyattsville, MD: National Center for Health Statistics. 2018.
3. Moher, M. Diabetes Mellitus. In: Rakel, D. ed. Integrative Medicine (4th ed.). Philadelphia: Elsevier; 2018:334-46.
4. Black LI, Barnes PM, Clarke TC, Stussman BJ, Nahin RL. Use of yoga, meditation, and chiropractors among U.S. children aged 4-17 years. NCHS Data Brief, no 324. Hyattsville, MD: National Center for Health Statistics. 2018.
5. Eisenberg DM, Kersaler RC, Foster C, Norlock FE, Calkins DR, Delbanco TL. Unconventional medicine in the United States: prevalence, costs and patterns of use. N Engl J Med. 1993;328(4):248-52.
6. Eisenberg DM, Davis RM, Ettner SL, et al. Trends in alternative medicine use in the United States, 1990-1997: results of a follow-up national survey. JAMA. 1998;280(18):1569-75.
7. Yeh GY, Eisenberg DM, Davis RM, Phillips RS. Use of complementary and alternative medicine among persons with diabetes mellitus: results of a national survey. Am J Public Health. 2002;92(10):1648-52.
8. Tindie HA, Davis RM, Phillips RS, Eisenberg DM. Trends in use of complementary and alternative medicine by US adults: 1997-2002. Altern Ther Health Med. 2005;11(1):42-9.
9. Nahin, RL, Barnes, PM, Stussman, BA. Expenditures on complementary health approaches: United States, 2012. Centers for Disease Control and Prevention: National Health Statistics Reports. 2016 June 22; 95. On the Internet at: https://www.cdc.gov/nchs/data/nhsr/nhsr095.pdf.
10. Black LI, Barnes PM, Clarke TC, Stussman BJ, Nahin RL. Use of yoga, meditation, and chiropractors among U.S. children aged 4-17 years. NCHS Data Brief, no 324. Hyattsville, MD: National Center for Health Statistics. 2018.
11. Haliloğlu B, Işgüven P, Yıldız M, Arslanoğlu I, Ergüven M. Complementary and alternative medicine in children with type 1 diabetes mellitus. J Clin Res Pediatr Endocrinol. 2011; 3(3):139–43. doi:10.4274/jcrpe. v3i3.27.
12. Benson H. The relaxation response: therapeutic effect. Science. 1997;278(5344):1694-5.
13. Gill GC, Redmond S, Garratt F, Pfaisey R. Diabetes and alternative medicine: cause for concern. Diabet Med. 1994;11(2):210-3.
14. Remli R, Chan SC. Use of complementary medicine among diabetes patients in a public primary care clinic in Ipoh. Med J Malaysia. 2003;58(5):688-93.

15. Hawk C, Ndetan H, Evans MW Jr. Potential role of complementary and alternative health care providers in chronic disease prevention and health promotion: an analysis of National Health Interview Survey data. Prev Med. 2012;54(1):18-22; updated 2016 Mar 31.

16. Miller JL, Cao D, Miller JG, Lipton RB. Correlates of complementary and alternative medicine (CAM) use in Chicago area children with diabetes (DM). Prim Care Diabetes. 2009;3(37):149-56.

17. Dannemann K, Hecker W, Haberland H, et al. Use of complementary and alternative medicine in children with type 1 diabetes mellitus—prevalence, patterns of use, and costs. Pediatr Diabetes. 2008;9(3):228-35.

18. Bradley R, Sherman KJ, Catz S, et al. Survey of CAM interest, self-care, and satisfaction with health care for type 2 diabetes at group health cooperative. BMC Complement Altern Med. 2011;11:121.

19. Clark TC, Black LI, Stussman BJ, Barnes PM, Nahin RL. Trends in the use of complementary health approaches among adults: United States, 2002-2012. Natl Health Stat Report. 2015 Feb 10;(79):1-16.

20. DiNardo MM, Gibson JM, Siminerio L, Morell AR, Lee ES. Complementary and alternative medicine in diabetes care. Curr Diab Rep. 2012;12(6):749-61.

21. Chang HY, Wallis M, Tiralongo E. Predictors of complementary and alternative medicine use by people with type 2 diabetes. J Adv Nurs. 2012;68(6):1256-66.

22. National Center for Complementary and Integrative Health. Diabetes and dietary supplements. (updated 2014 Nov; cited 2019 June 4). On the internet at: https://nccih.nih.gov/sites/nccam.nih.gov/files/Diabetes_11-08-2015.pdf.

23. McCarty RL, Weber WJ, Loots B, et al. Complementary and alternative medicine use and quality of life in pediatric diabetes. J Altern Complement Med. 2010;16(2):165-73.

24. Micozzi, MS. Fundamentals of complementary, alternative, and integrative medicine (6th ed.). St. Louis: Elsevier; 2019.

25. Patel, S. A mind-body approach to diabetes. The Chopra Center. 2019 (cited 2019 June 4). On the Internet at https://chopra.com/articles/mind-body-approach-diabetes.

26. Banerjee S, Debnath P, Rao PN, Tripathy TB, Adhikari A, Debnath PK. Ayurveda in changing scenario of diabetes management for developing safe and effective treatment choices for the future. J Complement Integr Med. 2015;12(2):101-10.

27. Bergquist, PE. Therapeutic Homeopathy. In: Rakel, D. ed. Integrative Medicine (4th ed.). Philadelphia: Elsevier; 2018: 1064-1080.

28. Nayak C, Oberai P, Varanasi R, et al. A prospective multi-centric open clinical trial of homeopathy in diabetic distal symmetric polyneuropathy. Homeopathy. 2013;102(2):130-8.

29. Pomposelli R, Piasere V, Andreoni C, et al. Observational study of homeopathic and conventional therapies in patients with diabetic polyneuropathy. Homeopathy. 2009;98(1):17-25.

30. Villa-Caballero L, Morello CM, Chynoweth ME, et al. Ethnic differences in complementary and alternative medicine use among patients with diabetes. Complement Ther Med. 2010;18(6):241-8.

31. Shiyanbola OO, Nelson J. Illness perceptions, beliefs in medicine and medication non-adherence among South Dakota minority with diabetes: a pilot study. S D Med. 2011;64(10):365-7.

32. Shah Vo, Carroll C, Mals R, et al. A home-based educational intervention improves patient activation measures and diabetes health indicators among Zuni Indians. PLoS One. 2015;10(5): e0125820. doi: 10.1371/journal.pone.0125820. eCollection 2015.

33. Indian Health Service. Disparities: Fact Sheet. (Updated 2018 April; Cited 2019 June 6) On the Internet at https://www.ihs.gov/newsroom/factsheets/disparities/.

34. Indian Health Service. Special Diabetes Program for Indians. (Cited 2019 June 6). On the Internet at https://www.ihs.gov/sdpi/.

35. Oberg EB, Bradley RD, Allen J, McCrory MA. CAM: naturopathic dietary interventions for patients with type 2 diabetes. Complement Ther Clin Pract. 2011;17(3):157-61.

36. Oberg EM, Bradley R, Hsu C, et al. Patient-reported experiences with first-time naturopathic care for type 2 diabetes. PloS One. 2012;7(11):485-9.

37. Bradley R, Sherman KJ, Catz S, et al. Adjunctive naturopathic care for type 2 diabetes: patient-reported and clinical outcomes after one year. BMC Complement Altern Med. 2012;12:44.

38. Shubrook JH Jr, Johnson AW. An osteopathic approach to type 2 diabetes mellitus. J Am Osteopath Assoc. 2011;111(9):531-7.

39. Shubrook JH Jr, Snow RJ, McGill SL. Effects of repeated use of the American Osteopathic Association's Clinical Assessment Program on measures of care for patients with diabetes mellitus. J Am Osteopath Assoc. 2011;111(1):13-20.

40. Ciervo CA, Shubrook JH, Grundy P. Leveraging the principles of osteopathic medicine to improve diabetes outcomes within a new era of health care reform. J Am Osteopath Assoc. 2015;115 Suppl 4:S8-19.

41. Selby, L. Empowering patients: The osteopathic approach to type 2 diabetes. The DO. 2015 August 20 (cited 2019 June 6). On the Internet at https://thedo.osteopathic.org/2015/08/empowering-patients-the-osteopathic-approach-to-type-2-diabetes/

42. Tong XL, Dong L, Chen L, Zhen Z. Treatment of diabetes using traditional Chinese medicine: past, present and future. Am J Chin Med. 2012;40(5):877-86.

43. Zhao X, Zhen Z, Guo J, et al. Assessment of the reporting quality of placebo-controlled randomized trials on the treatment of type 2 diabetes with Traditional Chinese Medicine in Mainland China: a PRISMA-compliant systematic review. Medicine (Baltimore). 2016;95(3): e2522. doi: 10.1097/MD.0000000000002522.

44. Tseng CC, Tseng A, Tseng J, Chang CH. Effect of laser acupuncture on anthropometric measurements and appetite sensations in obese subjects. Evid Based Complement Alternat Med. 2016; 2016:9365326. doi: 10.1155/2016/9365326. Epub 2016 Mar 9.

45. Malachowska B, Fendler W, Pomykala A, Suwala S, Mlynarski W. Essential oils reduce autonomous response to pain sensation during self-monitoring of blood glucose among children with diabetes. J Pediatr Endocrinol Metab. 2016;29(1):47-53.

46. Harel S, Yanai L, Brooks R, et al. The contribution of art therapy in poorly controlled youth with type 1 diabetes mellitus. J Pediatr Endocrinol Metab. 2013;26(7-8):669-73.

47. Elertson, K. M., Liesch, S. K., & Babler, E. K. (2016). The "Face" of Diabetes: insight into youths' experiences as expressed through drawing. *Journal of patient experience*, 3(2):34–38. doi: 10.1177/2374373516654771

48. Gelemter R, Lavi G, Yanai L, et al. Effect of auditory guided imagery on glucose levels and on glycemic control in children with type 1 diabetes mellitus. J Pediatr Endocrinol Metab. 2016;29(2):139-44.

49. Williamson M, Gregory C. Hypnotherapy: the salutogenic solution to dealing with phobias. Pract Midwife. 2015;18(5):35-7.

50. Otani A. Hypnosis and mindfulness: the twain finally meet. Am J Clin Hypn. 2016;58(4):383-98.

51. Loucks EB, Gilman SE, Britton WB, Gutman R, Eaton CB, Buka SL. Associations of mindfulness with glucose regulation and diabetes. Am J Health Behav. 2016;40(2):258-67.

52. Noordali F, Cumming J, Thompson JL. Effectiveness of mindfulness-based interventions on physiological and psychological complications in adults with diabetes: a systematic review. J Health Psychol. 2015 Dec 30. pii: 1359105620293.

53. Li G, Yuan H, Zhang W. The effects of mindfulness-based stress reduction for family caregivers: systematic review. Arch Psychiatr Nurs. 2016;30(2):292-9.

54. Adams, H, Micozzi, MS, Dibra, SM. In: Micozzi, MS. In: Fundamentals of complementary, alternative, and integrative medicine (6th ed.). St. Louis: Elsevier; 2019:171-87.

55. Hayashi T, Tsujii S, Iburi T, et al. Laughter up-regulates the genes related to NK cell activity in diabetes. Biomed Res. 2007;28(6):281-5.

56. Kim SH, Kim YH, Kim HJ. Laughter and stress relief in cancer patients: a pilot study. Evid Based Complement Alternat Med. 2015; 2015:864739. doi: 10.1155/2015/864739. Epub 2015 May 24.

57. Carlson, SJ. Service dogs: Should I get one if I have diabetes? Mayo Clinic. (2018 September 8: cited 2019 June 1) On the Internet at https://www.mayoclinic.org/diseases-conditions/diabetes/expert-answers/service-dogs-should-i-get-one-if-i-have-diabetes/faq-20388892.

58. Hardin DS, Anderson W, Cattet J. Dogs can be successfully trained to alert to hypoglycemia samples from patients with type 1 diabetes. Diabetes Ther. 2015;6(4):509-17.

59. Synovitz, LB, Larson, KL. Complementary and alternative medicine. Burlington, MA: Jones and Bartlett; 2013.

60. Sacco LM, Griffin MT, McNulty R, Fitzpatrick JJ. Use of the Serenity Prayer among adults with type 2 diabetes: a pilot study. Holist Nurs Pract. 2011;25(4):192-8.

61. Watkins YJ, Quinn LT, Ruggiero L, Quinn MT, Choi YK. Spiritual and religious beliefs and practices and social support's relationship to diabetes self-care activities in African Americans. Diab Educ. 2013;39(2):2331-9.

62. McGinnis RA, McGrady A, Cox SA, Grower-Dowling KA. Biofeedback-assisted relaxation in type 2 diabetes. Diabetes Care. 2005;28(8):2145-9.

63. National Center for Complementary and Integrative Health. Massage therapy: What you need to know (updated 2019 May; cited 2019 June 1). On the Internet at: https://nccih.nih.gov/health/massage/massageintroduction.htm#hed2.

64. Pandey A, Tripathi P, Pandey R, Srivatava R, Goswami S. Alternative therapies useful in the management of diabetes: a systematic review. J Pharm Bioallied Sci. 2011;3(4):504–512. doi: 10.4103/0975-7406.90103.

65. Wandell PE, Carlsson SC, Gafvels C, Andersson K, Tomkvist L. Measuring possible effect on health-related quality of life by tactile massage or relaxation in patients with type 2 diabetes. Complement Ther Med. 2012;20(1-2):8-15.

66. Sajedi F, Kashaninia Z, Hoseinzadeh S, Abedinipoor A. How effective is Swedish massage on blood glucose level in children with diabetes mellitus? Acta Med Iran. 2011;49(9):592-7.

67. Goertz CM, Salsbury SA, Vining RD, et al. Collaborative care for older adults with low back pain by family medicine physicians and doctors of chiropractic (COCOA): study protocol for a randomized controlled trial. Trials. 2013;16:14-8.

68. Seaman DR, Palombo AD. An overview of the identification and management of the metabolic syndrome in chiropractic practice. J Chiropr Med. 2014;13(3):210-9.

69. Tuchin P. A replication of the study "Adverse effects of spinal manipulation: a systematic review." Chiropr Man Therap. 2012;20(1):30.

70. Freire MD, Alves C. Therapeutic Chinese exercises (Qigong) in the treatment of type 2 diabetes mellitus: a systematic review. Diabetes Metab Syndr. 2013;7(1):56-9.

71. Putiri AL, Lovejoy LC, Gilliham S, Sassagawa M, Bradley R, Sun GC. Psychological effects of Yi Ren Medical Qigong and progressive resistance training in adults with type 2 diabetes mellitus: a randomized controlled pilot study. Altern Ther Health Med. 2012;18(1):30-4.

72. Liu X, Clark J, Siskind D, et al. A systematic review and meta-analysis of the effects of Qigong and Tai Chi for depressive symptoms. Complement Ther Med. 2015;23(4):516-34.

73. Lauche R, Wayne PM, Dobos G, Cramer H. Prevalence, patterns, and predictors of T'ai Chi and Qigong use in the United States: results of a nationally representative survey. J Altern Complement Med. 2016:22(4):336-42.

74. Liu X, Miller YD, Burton NW, Chang JH, Brown WJ. Qi-gong mind-body therapy and diabetes control. A randomized controlled trial. Am J Prev Med. 2011;41(2):152-8.

75. Bisson, DA. Reflexology. In: Fundamentals of complementary, alternative, and integrative medicine (6th ed.). St. Louis: Elsevier; 2019:261-66.

76. da Silva NC, Chaves Ede C, de Carvalho EC, Carvalho LC, Iunes DH. Foot reflexology in feet impairment of people with type 2 diabetes mellitus: randomized trial. Rev Lat Am Enfermagem. 2015;23(4):603-10.

77. Yan JH, Gu WJ, Pan L. Lack of evidence on Tai Chi-related effects in patients with type 2 diabetes mellitus: a meta-analysis. Exp Clin Endocrinol Diabetes. 2013;121(5):266-71.

78. Cavegn EI, Riskowski JL. The effects of Tai Chi on peripheral somatosensation, balance, and fitness in Hispanic older adults with type 2 diabetes: a pilot and feasibility study. Evid Based Complement Alternat Med. 2015;2015:767213. doi: 10.1155/2015/767213. Epub 2015 Oct 27.

79. Lee MS, Jun JH, Lim HJ, Lim HS. A systematic review and meta-analysis of Tai Chi for treating type 2 diabetes. Maturitas. 2015;80(1):14-23.

80. Chao M, Wang C, Dong X, Ding M. The effects of Tai Chi on type 2 diabetes mellitus: a meta-analysis. *J Diabetes Res*. 2018; 2018:7350567. Published 2018 Jul 5. doi: 10.1155/2018/7350567.

81. Alexander G, Innes KE, Bourgulgnon C, Bovbjerg VE, Kulbok P, Taylor AG. Patterns of yoga practice and physical activity following a yoga intervention for adults with or at risk for type 2 diabetes. J Phys Act Health. 2012;9(1):53-61.

82. Hegde SV, Adhikari P, Kolian S, Pinto VJ, D'Souza S, D'Souza V. Effect of 3-month yoga on oxidative stress in type 2 diabetes with or without complications: a controlled clinical trial. Diabetes Care. 2011;34(10):2208-10.

83. Kumar V, Jagannathan A, Philip M, Thulasi A, Angadi P, Ragharam N. Role of yoga for patients with type II diabetes mellitus: a systematic review and meta-analysis. Complement Ther Med. 2016;25:104-12.

84. Chimkode SM, Kumaran SD, Kanhere VV, Shivanna R. Effect of yoga on blood glucose levels in patients with type 2 diabetes mellitus. J Clin Diagn Res. 2015;9(4): CCOI-3. doi: 10.78601 /JCDR/2015/12666.5744. Epub 2015 Apr 1.

85. Innes KE, Selfe TK. Yoga for adults with type 2 diabetes: a systematic review of controlled trials. J Diabetes Res. 2016; 2016:6979370. doi: 10.1155/2016/6979370. Epub 2015 Dec 14.

86. Bowden D, Goddard L, Gruzellier J. A randomized controlled single-blind trial of the efficacy of Reiki at benefitting moods and well-being. Evid Based Complement Alternat Med. 2011; 2011:381862. doi: 10.11551/2011/381862.

87. Bukowski EL, Berardi D. Reiki brief report: using Reiki to reduce stress levels in a nine-year-old child. Explore (NY). 2014;10(4):253-5.

88. Bukowski EL. The use of self-Reiki for stress reduction and relaxation. J Integr Med. 2015;13(5):336-40.

89. Joyce J, Herbison GP. Reiki for depression and anxiety. Cochrane Database Syst Rev. 2015 Apr 3;4:CD006833. doi: 10.1002/14651858.CD006833.pub2.

90. Coakley AB, Duffy ME. The effect of therapeutic touch on postoperative patients. J Holist Nurs. 2010;28(3):193-200.

91. Monroe CM. The effects of therapeutic touch on pain. J Holist Nurs. 2009;27(2):85-92.

92. O'Mathuna DP, Ashford RL. Therapeutic touch for healing acute wounds. Cochrane Database Syst Rev. 2014 Jul 29;(7):CD002766.

93. Tabatabaee A, Tafreshi MZ, Rassouli M, Aledavood SA, Alavimajd H, Farahmand SK. Effect of therapeutic touch in patients with cancer: a literature review. Med Arch. 2016;70(2):142-7.

94. Rindfleisch, JA. Biofield Therapies. In: Rakel, D. ed. Integrative Medicine (4th ed.). Philadelphia: Elsevier; 2018:1073-80.

95. Lavery LA, Murdoch DP, Williams J, Mavery DC. Does anodyne light therapy improve peripheral neuropathy in diabetes? A double-blind, sham-controlled, randomized trial to evaluate monochromatic infrared photoenergy. Diabetes Care. 2008;31(2):316-21.

96. Amall DA, Nelson AG, Stambaugh L, et al. Pulsed infrared light therapy does not increase nitric oxide concentration in the blood of patients with type 1 and type 2 diabetes mellitus. Acta Diabetol. 2009;46(3):233-7.

97. Brouwer A, van Raalte DH, Diamant M, et al. Light therapy for better mood and insulin sensitivity in patients with major depression and type 2 diabetes: a randomized double-blind, parallel-arm trial. BMC Psychiatry. 2015;24(15):169.

98. Brouwer A, van Raalte DH, Nguyen, H-T, et al. Effects of light therapy on mood and insulin sensitivity in patients with type 2 diabetes and depression: results from a randomized placebo-controlled trial. Diabetes Care. 2019 Feb; dc181732. https://doi.org/10.2337/dc18-1732

99. Dagnellie PC, Leij-Halfwerk S. Magnetic resonance spectroscopy to study hepatic metabolism in diffuse liver disease, diabetes and cancer. World J Gastroenterol. 2010;16(13):1577-86.

100. Colbert AP, Cleaver J, Brown KA, et al. Magnets applied to acupuncture points as therapy—a literature review. Acupunct Med. 2008;26(3):160-70.

101. Khan MU. Is there a role for TENS application in the control of diabetes mellitus I insulin-dependent patients? Singapore Med J. 2012;53(1):249-50.

102. Mandel SE, Davis BA, Secic M. Effects of music therapy and music-assisted relaxation and imagery on health-related outcomes in diabetes education: a feasibility study. Diabetes Educ. 2013:39(4):568-81.

103. Bay R, Bay F. Combined therapy using acupressure therapy, hypnotherapy, and transcendental meditation versus placebo in type 2 diabetes. J Acupunct Meridian Stud. 2011;4(3);183-6.

104. Kanodia AK, Legedza AT, Davis RB, Eisenberg DM, Phillips RS. Perceived benefit of complementary and alternative medicine (CAM) for back pain: a national survey. J Am Board Fam Med. 2010;(23):354-62.

105. De Leon Rodriguez D, Allet L, Golay A, et al. Biofeedback can reduce foot pressure to a safe level and without causing new at-risk zones in patients with diabetes and peripheral neuropathy. Diabetes Metab Res Rev. 2013;29(2):139-44.

106. McGrady A. The effects of biofeedback in diabetes and essential hypertension. Cleve Clin J Med. 2010;77 Suppl 3:S68-71.

CHAPTER 23

Acute Hyperglycemia

Dace L. Trence, MD, MACE

Key Concepts

- Diabetic ketoacidosis (DKA) occurs when there is so little insulin available to transport glucose into cells that glucose accumulates in the blood, raising levels to 250 mg/dL (13.88 mmol/L) or greater (mean 475 mg/dL [26.36 mmol/L]).[1] Diabetic ketoacidosis can evolve quickly (within 24 hours), causing dehydration, ketosis, electrolyte imbalance, and acidosis. This condition requires immediate treatment.
- Hyperosmolar hyperglycemic state (HHS) occurs when hyperglycemia and dehydration slowly exacerbate each other until both are extreme. Blood glucose levels often rise to greater than 600 mg/dL, though few, if any, ketones are present. Hyperosmolar hyperglycemic state occurs primarily in undiagnosed or older adults with type 2 diabetes. Residents of long-term care facilities are at risk and should be monitored to prevent HHS. Hyperosmolar hyperglycemic state is even more life threatening than DKA.
- Chronic hyperglycemia is glucose that is persistently elevated. Everyone with diabetes experiences hyperglycemia and, to some extent, chronic hyperglycemia. How high and how often glucose levels rise over the reference range vary greatly. People with high blood glucose may not feel well, but they typically continue with their usual activities and responsibilities. Very high glucose levels are acute and serious and can evolve from chronic hyperglycemia.
- Euglycemic ketoacidosis is an increasingly recognized state associated with the use of gliflozin (SGLT-2 inhibitor) medications, when the glucose may be only minimally elevated, if at all. The development of this unusual situation is felt to be associated with concomitant dehydration and/or lack of calorie ingestion. Data from randomized studies with the use of SGLT-2 inhibitors reported low incidence of DKA in persons with T2DM ~0.07%[2,3,4]; however, the risk of ketosis and DKA is higher in persons with T1D. About 10% of persons with T1D treated with SGLT2-inhibitors develop ketosis and 5% require hospital admission for DKA.[3]

State of the Condition

Hyperglycemia is defined as blood glucose that is above the normal range of 70 to 130 mg/dL (3.88-7.21 mmol/L). In persons with diabetes, significant hyperglycemia is the objective finding of poorly managed diabetes. A gradual or abrupt decline of insulin production or availability, in conjunction with insulin resistance, contributes to elevated blood glucose levels. Stress, whether psychological or metabolic, can exacerbate insulin resistance, which in turn stimulates hepatic glucose production and further elevates blood glucose. People with diabetes may suffer long-term complications from chronic hyperglycemia as well as acute episodes of life-threatening complications with critically high glucose levels. This chapter will help the reader recognize the symptoms of acute hyperglycemia (acute stages of elevated blood glucose), understand principles of evaluation and treatment, and prevent recurrent episodes in persons with diabetes. For information on ongoing hyperglycemia, see chapters 8, 9 and 25, on monitoring, reducing risks, and cardiovascular disease (CVD).

Diabetic Ketoacidosis

Pathology

Diabetic ketoacidosis occurs more often in people with type 1 diabetes, but it can also be seen in individuals with type 2 diabetes during acute illness and/or after they have become insulin deficient.[1] Rates of DKA in youth with type 1 diabetes vary widely nationally and internationally, from 15% to 70% at diagnosis to 1% to 15% per established patient per year.[5] Diabetic ketoacidosis is the leading cause of mortality among children and young adults with type 1 diabetes mellitus (T1DM), accounting for ~50% of all deaths in this population.[1]

Overall DKA mortality recorded in the United States is <1%,[6] but a higher rate is reported among persons with diabetes aged >60 years and individuals with concomitant life-threatening illnesses.[6,7] Up to 80% of newly diagnosed children present with DKA.[8] An unexpected finding in the pediatric population has been the frequency of DKA as a presenting clinical picture in those with type 2 diabetes. In one study, DKA was seen in 59.44% of individuals with T1DM and 23.91% of individuals with type 2 diabetes mellitus (T2DM). Of those with T2DM, 58.82% had presented in DKA.[9] Diabetic ketoacidosis may also appear as an acute presentation of unrecognized T2DM, as a new diagnosis, particularly in certain ethnicities.[10–13]

Type 1 diabetes, by definition, is characterized by insulin deficiency. Treatment provides insulin in an amount designed to match what is required for glucose uptake into the cells. Available insulin and insulin delivery systems have improved tremendously but remain imperfect. Some situations, such as illness, may quickly and substantially elevate blood glucose even when good blood glucose stability has been previously maintained.[11] Other conditions, such as persistent untreated hyperglycemia, newly prescribed medications or regimen changes, and missed insulin, can also disrupt the perfect match. A recent analysis of reported precipitating DKA events among many different countries, showed that the new diagnosis of diabetes, infection, and poor engagement with the medication regimen made up the vast majority of reported DKA etiologies.[14] Anything that increases blood glucose and decreases insulin action can contribute to the development of DKA.

Ingested Glucose

Eating more food or more carbohydrates than usual, without changing insulin dosing, elevates blood glucose. This happens frequently to people who take fixed doses of insulin but do not eat fixed quantities of food. Hyperglycemia itself can stimulate hunger, leading to increased food intake. Excessive food intake alone is not sufficient to cause DKA but may cumulatively contribute to it. Two small studies of pediatric patients reported consumption of large volumes of high-calorie beverages before admission for DKA.[13,16] In type 2 diabetes, alcohol has been associated with DKA development.

Case: DKA in a Busy Woman With Type 1 Diabetes

GT is a 24-year-old female who has had type 1 diabetes since age 12. She has been using an insulin pump for 8 years and checks her blood glucose 4 to 6 times per day. She does not understand why others she meets do not take their diabetes more seriously. GT is 5 ft 8 in and 160 lb. Her latest A1C was 6.2%, and her daily glucose readings range from 50 to 200 mg/dL. She has not had any complications, and other than having diabetes, she is a healthy young adult. She is a full-time student working toward an MBA and works part-time as an accountant for a gift shop.

Precipitating Events

GT usually eats regularly, matches her premeal insulin dose to her carbohydrate intake, exercises, and sleeps 7 to 8 hours a night. Since mid-November, though, life has been chaotic as extra hours at work, end-of-semester exams, and holiday preparations converged. Some days she skipped meals, grabbed a sandwich, or snacked from the vending machine. She missed most of her scheduled times at the gym. She was tired and began drinking more coffee and diet soda to keep going. Increased commitments had disrupted her routine.

GT was eagerly awaiting her next 3-month shipment of diabetes supplies, which seemed to be delayed in the mass of holiday packages. She began testing her blood glucose less often to conserve strips and hoped the new shipment would arrive before her holiday trip to visit with family. At the end of the semester, she was flying to Maine for a quick visit with her grandparents before heading home for Christmas.

Monitoring

Evidence from an international survey of over 35,000 insulin pump users showed that good glycemic stability is correlated to frequency of blood glucose measurements of 4 or 5 or more times per day.[17] Pump users who monitored blood glucose levels 4 or more times a day achieved a lower average A1C level than persons with diabetes who monitored levels once or twice daily (7.2% versus 8%). Of person with diabetes who self-reported that they monitored blood glucose levels 5 or more times a day, 62% had an average A1C level of less than 7%.[18] The advent of continuous glucose monitoring (CGM) used with or without pump technology has further decreased DKA.[19] From the Type 1 Diabetes Exchange registry, at least 1 DKA event in the 3 months before the questionnaire was reported by 3% of participants, with the highest frequency (4%) in participants under 26 years old. Participants using an insulin pump were less likely to report experiencing a DKA event than participants using injections (2% vs. 4%; $P = 0.002$ adjusted for age, diabetes duration, sex, race/ethnicity, insurance status, CGM,

SMBG, and HbA1c). Similarly, participants using CGM had fewer DKA events than non-CGM users (1% vs. 3%; $P = 0.04$ adjusted for age, diabetes duration, sex, race/ethnicity, insurance status, pump use, and HbA1c).[20] Available technology using a pump linked to a continuous glucose sensor that can automatically suspend or increase pump insulin delivery has shown even more impact on lessening DKA episodes.[20,21]

Inadequate Insulin

Glucose levels rise directly from deficient insulin production and/or an inability to effectively use the insulin produced (insulin resistance). People with type 1 diabetes—and, to a lesser extent, people with type 2 diabetes requiring insulin—can receive inadequate insulin from poorly designed or poorly followed treatment plans. Inadequate insulin impacts other physiological functions that elevate glucose levels indirectly.

Glucose stored in the liver as glycogen is available to provide fuel between meals and during sleep. Ideally, hepatic glucose offers stored energy as needed to maintain blood glucose levels, support exercise, and provide extra fuel for extraordinary events such as surgery or fighting a grizzly bear. When adequately available, insulin turns off this hepatic glucose production and release as soon as there is sufficient glucose available to the cells.

When there is inadequate insulin, the liver keeps producing glucose, as there is no ability to sense the problem of inadequate insulin availability to promote glucose entry into cells. This process of glycogenolysis and even gluconeogenesis (the production of glucose from amino acids obtained from protein breakdown) floods the bloodstream with unwelcome sugar molecules. Multiple forms of stress (illness, trauma, menses, pregnancy, fear, worry, excitement, and other physical or emotional stressors) and some medications stimulate the counter-regulatory and stress hormones. These hormones stimulate hepatic glucose production and, at the same time, interfere with insulin effectiveness and glucose uptake in the peripheral tissues. Glucagon, secreted in response to meal ingestion, is another hormone that stimulates hepatic glucose production and exacerbates an already disruptive situation.

Ketones

A homeostatic mechanism to feed cells when glucose cannot enter cells is to break down fat (lipolysis) into glucose and ketone bodies. As the concentration of ketones increases, the kidneys via osmotic diuresis excrete both glucose and ketones. The increasing amount of water lost in the process causes dehydration. Dehydration concentrates serum glucose and further increases hyperglycemia. Increased hyperglycemia drives further dehydration.

With dehydration and the increasing accumulation of ketones in the serum, sodium and potassium (key electrolytes that impact muscle and other organ functions) are affected. Potassium is involved with regulating the heart rhythm; therefore, loss of potassium may be life threatening. Further, as potassium is imperative to facilitate insulin action, hypokalemia can inhibit the ability of provided insulin to be therapeutic.

When ketone accumulation is excessive, blood becomes too acidic to support life. Diabetic ketoacidosis can be termed mild, moderate, or severe, depending on parameters of blood glucose levels, acidity, and ketone formation.[11] Prompt treatment is essential.

Precipitating Situations

Inadequate Insulin

Numerous factors contribute to inadequate insulin. Worsening insulin resistance or suboptimal treatment plans are reasons for inadequate insulin being available. In many instances diabetes medications, particularly insulin injections, may be skipped because of psychosocial reasons, a lack of adequate planning, financial difficulty, or a person with diabetes' lack of knowledge about adequate self-management. The following are some examples:

- *Insulin omitted to manage weight:* Insulin omission can be a form of bulimia. In a study of subjects aged 11 to 25 years, 36% reported insulin misuse to manage weight.[22] The Assessing Health and Eating Among Adolescents With Diabetes survey showed 10.3% of females reported skipping insulin, and 7.4% reported taking less insulin to manage their weight.[24] Omission of or not taking adequate insulin may be the most important contributor to DKA in urban African Americans with type 2 diabetes.[24] Musey reported in his study that half of patients (50%) stopped insulin because of a reported lack of money to buy insulin from an outside pharmacy or get transportation to the hospital, 21% stopped insulin because of lack of appetite, 14% stopped insulin because of behavioral or psychological reasons, and 14% did so because they did not know how to manage diabetes on sick days.[25]
- *Psychological problems complicated by eating disorders:* May be a factor in 20% of recurrent ketoacidosis cases.[11]
- *Insulin omitted to avoid hypoglycemia, especially when home alone or during active workdays:*[12] May be seen as a self-initiated safety measure, or may

occur during illness due to the mistaken belief that insulin is not needed when eating less.

- *Insulin omitted to avoid the inconvenience or embarrassment of injecting in a public situation:* Many people feel uncomfortable injecting insulin in a restaurant or asking permission to leave their work site to do so.
- *Inadequate or poorly timed insulin due to inadequate organization:* Some people never seem to have all the supplies they need in the right place at the right time.
- *Insulin dose reduced to save money:* Many people are faced with economic challenges and are forced to choose whether they will spend their limited income on housing, food, or medicine.
- *Insulin dose reduced or omitted when ill:* Some believe they need less insulin if they eat less. Because nausea, vomiting, and stomach pain are symptoms of DKA, omitting insulin for gastrointestinal symptoms may only push glucose levels higher and make symptoms worse.
- *Insulin is outdated, improperly stored, inaccurately measured, or incorrectly injected:* Can provide a lower dose than planned.

Missing insulin doses, whether by accident or deliberately, has become more of a concern with increasing insulin costs. Intentional insulin omission was reported by more than half of respondents; regular omission was reported by 20% in a study reported by Peyrot in 2010.[27] This has become even more of an issue with the exponential rise of insulin costs in the past decade, raising concerns at the national level about the lethal consequences of either making insulin "stretch" or specifically skipping skipping doses.[28]

Excess Hepatic Glucose

Stress, whether physical, emotional, or psychological, can dramatically and acutely increase blood glucose levels. All forms of stress increase adrenal glucocorticoid production and catecholamine levels, both of which raise glucose levels through increased hepatic glucose production. This can increase the risk of DKA if there is no intervention to either decrease the instigating stress or provide compensatory insulin adjustment. The following are a few examples of situations that increase hepatic production and release glucose:

- Infection—the most common precipitating factor
- Pneumonia and urinary tract infections—account for 30% to 50% of DKA cases
- Gastrointestinal bleeding
- Cerebrovascular accident (CVA)
- Alcohol abuse
- Pancreatitis
- Myocardial infarction
- Trauma
- Pregnancy
- Drugs that affect carbohydrate metabolism (corticosteroids, thiazides, dobutamine, terbutaline, cocaine)[23]

Prevention

Preventing or at least greatly limiting the severity of DKA from causes other than acute glycemic decompensation is possible. Early recognition of hyperglycemia and appropriate treatment can prevent acute complications and reduce fatalities, which have been reduced to an overall 2% but rise with age and seriousness of concomitant disease.[26] When hyperglycemia is ignored or occurs unexpectedly, coma and even death are possible.

> **Inadequate Insulin**
>
> If an individual intentionally omits or is deprived of insulin for any reason, discussing DKA prevention may be ineffective unless underlying problems are also addressed.

Some people with diabetes purposely avoid insulin during school or work hours, and others omit insulin as a way to lose weight; disadvantaged children are more vulnerable to episodes of DKA.[29] Intentionally omitting insulin for any reason suggests there are other problems that need to be addressed before further discussing DKA prevention. Also recognized is the possible contribution of drug abuse as a risk factor for DKA. Active use of cocaine has been reported as an independent risk factor for recurrent DKA, supporting toxicology screening in persons with diabetes with recurrent DKA.[30]

Education regarding glucose self-management during illness and stress management is essential to prevent DKA. Persons with diabetes benefit from having sick-day management information reinforced over and over again during routine appointments (see Table 23.1).

Persons with diabetes should also be provided with information about possible causes and how to recognize symptoms of DKA. Identifying the cause of or risks for DKA in the individual's specific situation may help with prevention. Common contributors to acute hyperglycemia include the following:

- Relying on "how you feel" to assess glucose levels rather than testing blood glucose
- Skipping insulin/other medications when not eating

TABLE 23.1 Sick-Day Management

	Type 1 Diabetes	*Type 2 Diabetes*
Hydration	8 oz fluid per hour; type depends on glucose level (containing or not containing carbohydrates) Every third hour, consume this 8 oz as a sodium-rich choice such as bouillon	Same
Self-monitoring of blood glucose	Test every 2 to 4 hours while blood glucose is elevated or until symptoms subside	Same
Ketones	Test every 4 hours or until negative	Determine for the individual
Medication adjustments	Continue as able Adjust insulin doses to correct hyperglycemia, but do not stop or hold insulin if diagnosed as having type 1 diabetes mellitus Hold metformin during serious illness Instruct persons with diabetes to call their healthcare provider for specific instructions if they have not previously received them	Same
Food and beverage selections	Guide person with diabetes to consume 150 to 200 g carbohydrates daily, in divided doses Switch to soft foods or liquids as tolerated Provide patients a list of foods and beverages in portion sizes containing 15 g carbohydrates	Same
Contact healthcare professionals	Provide guidelines on conditions that require the person with diabetes to call: • Vomiting more than once • Diarrhea more than 5 times or for longer than 6 hours • Blood glucose levels >300 mg/dL on 2 consecutive measurements that are not responsive to increased insulin and fluids Moderate or large urine ketones or blood ketones >10.8 mg/dL (>0.6 mmol/L)	Same

- Inadequate monitoring during illness
- Not having/following a sick-day plan

Other possible causes of acute hyperglycemia include the following:

- Use of expired insulin
- Rationing insulin due to financial constraints
- Increased insulin needs during growth or hormonal spurts
- Preoccupation with other priorities and missing (or not learning to recognize) symptoms of escalating glucose levels

The more persons with diabetes understand how their medications work, the better able they are to use them to their advantage. Learning to supplement with extra insulin for high glucose levels and for ketones prepares them to handle acute situations.

Remaining attentive to the symptoms of hyperglycemia and monitoring glucose in the midst of other priorities could prevent many incidents of DKA. Finding and using resources, including knowing when to contact a physician, can ease the burden of living with diabetes.

Ultimately, information is essential, but to prevent DKA, persons with diabetes and their family require more than information. The individual must be prepared to effectively employ self-management strategies to prevent severe hyperglycemia and intervene early when at risk.

Assessing Diabetic Ketoacidosis

Signs, Symptoms, and Laboratory Indicators

The symptoms of hyperglycemia may mimic those of other diseases or conditions. Assessment of the following helps accurately diagnose the problem:

- Hyperglycemia
- Dehydration

- Electrolyte status
- Ketosis
- Acidosis
- Osmolality

The physical signs and symptoms and the laboratory findings consistent with DKA relate physiologically to one of these markers: hyperglycemia, dehydration, electrolyte imbalance, ketosis, or acidosis. Persons with diabetes can present with a spectrum of low energy to confusion, lethargy to coma, abdominal pain, polyuria, and polydipsia. Table 23.2 summarizes these markers.

Initial Evaluation Findings

- *Blood glucose:* Finger-stick blood glucose of >250 mg/dL if outpatient; serum glucose will be obtained in urgent or acute care setting
- *Urine/serum ketones:* Positive

Confirmation of Diagnosis

- *Arterial pH:* <7.3
- *Serum bicarbonate:* <16 mEq/L
- *Anion gap:* >15

Identification of Precipitating Factors

- *History and full clinical exam:* Identify precipitating etiologies; includes looking for potential sources of infection, such as perirectal abscess or cellulitis or any major stressor including emotional and physical
- *Vital signs:* Weight, blood pressure in the supine and upright positions, and pulse rate to assess hydration status
- *Laboratory evaluation:*[1] Serum electrolyte values (with calculated anion gap), blood urea nitrogen (BUN)/creatinine levels, beta-hydroxybutyric acid (or serum ketones, if not available), calcium and phosphorus concentrations, serum osmolality, complete blood cell count with differential, and electrocardiogram (EKG)
- *Additional tests, as needed:*[24] Bacterial blood cultures if infection suspected; urine analysis for urinary tract infection; chest X-ray; EKG; A1C (to identify whether DKA was an isolated event or the cumulative result of undiagnosed or poorly managed diabetes); or pregnancy (if of childbearing age)

TABLE 23.2 Markers of DKA

	Hyperglycemia	*Dehydration*	*Electrolyte Imbalance*	*Ketosis*	*Acidosis*
Physical signs	Polyuria Polydipsia Blurred vision Polyphagia Weight loss if insulin deficiency is present long enough (days to weeks) Fatigue	Decreased intravascular volume Decreased neck vein filling from below while person is lying absolutely flat Orthostatic hypotension (systolic blood pressure drop of 20 mm Hg after 1 min of standing) Poor skin turgor, seen earlier in children "Soft eyeballs": late sign of profound dehydration in adults	Muscle cramps Irregular heart rate	"Fruity" or acetone breath Nausea Vomiting Abdominal pain	Kussmaul respirations (hyperpnea)
Laboratory tests	Glucose typically >250 mg/dL	Hemoglobin Hematocrit Total protein values are often mildly elevated Creatinine Blood urea nitrogen (BUN)	Sodium: low, normal, or high Potassium: low, normal, or high Phosphorus: normal or high	Positive ketones	Low pH (<7.2) Low HCO_3 (<15 mEq/L) Low PCO (<35 mm Hg)

Additional Notes on Markers of DKA

Hyperglycemia

Elevated glucose is a marker of DKA but not a good index of the severity. Diabetic ketoacidosis does occur with lower glucose levels, especially in children, pregnant women, and persons who have been vomiting frequently.

Additionally, there have now been a large number of reports regarding euglycemic diabetic ketoacidosis in users of SGLT2 inhibitors, resulting in an FDA alert regarding the association between DKA and this drug class.[31] Euglycemic DKA associated with SGLT2 inhibitor use can occur in persons with either type 1 diabetes or type 2 diabetes.[3] But there can be other causes of euglycemic DKA, including recent use of insulin, decreased caloric intake, heavy alcohol consumption, chronic liver disease, glycogen storage disorders, and pregnancy.[32]

Persons with diabetes should be carefully and extensively counseled regarding keeping hydrated and maintaning adequate nutrition and, at a minimum, instructed to check urine or blood ketones if nauseated or if any change in well-being is noted. If moderate or large urine ketones are present, persons with diabetes should be instructed to withhold SGLT2 inhibitor use at least temporarily, to maintain vigorous hydration, and to consume carbohydrates to allow at least full-dose insulin therapy until ketones resolve. If the person with diabetes is not able to take liquids and carbohydrates liberally or self-monitor carefully, the person with diabetes should be encouraged to seek medical attention in a setting where intravenous fluids can be administered.[3]

The American Association of Clinical Endocrinologists published a position statement on SGLT2 inhibitor–associated DKA following a consensus conference in late 2015.[33]

Dehydration

Due to the severity of dehydration, the lab values listed are likely to be elevated before treatment of DKA and may auto-correct with routine treatment. Elevated creatinine or BUN after rehydration suggests further assessment for renal problems.

Electrolyte Imbalance

- *Sodium.* Dehydration causes a profound loss of total body sodium (Na^+) that serum levels cannot accurately measure. The results of testing serum sodium may appear low, normal, or high, depending on whether the sodium lost was greater than, equal to, or less than the relative amount of water lost.
- *Potassium.* Similarly, total body depletion of potassium always occurs with DKA, but lab values of serum potassium (K^+) can test low, normal, or high. As with sodium, serum potassium reflects the relative amount of water lost compared with potassium lost. Potassium may be low before treatment or fall as it enters the cells, with glucose and fluids reducing the serum concentration. The status of renal function should be ascertained before any potassium is replaced.
- *Phosphate.* Phosphate concentrations are usually high or high-normal initially and decrease with insulin therapy, sometimes markedly, to very low levels over the next day or two. Phosphate replacement remains controversial at this time, as it is believed that with rapid access to oral normal food intake, phosphate can be replaced without the need for parenteral phosphate.[11]

Ketosis

One ketone produced during DKA, acetoacetate, converts to acetone and is excreted by the lungs. Acetone has a fruity odor that may be detectable on the breath of someone in ketosis. Beta-hydroxybutyric acid is the most prevalent ketone in DKA, and measurement of this acid is the most reliable way to diagnose DKA and measure treatment progress.

Acidosis

Very deep and sometimes rapid breathing unrelated to exertion, or the inability to "catch one's breath," is a symptom of acidosis called Kussmaul respiration or hyperpnea. This form of hyperventilation is an effort to correct the metabolic acidosis by blowing off carbon dioxide.

Increased Osmolality

Mental-status changes seem to correlate best with serum osmolality and less so with the glucose level. Mental status in a person with DKA may range from alert, to obtunded, to stuporous, to coma. The changes in mentation, rather than the status itself, offer clues to diagnosis.

Other Significant Symptoms of DKA

- *Nonspecific symptoms.* Include weakness, lethargy, malaise, confusion, and headache.
- *Acute abdomen.* A common condition; marked by tenderness to palpation, diminished bowel sounds, and some muscle guarding, especially in children. Some may have more severe signs (absent bowel sounds, rebound tenderness, boardlike abdomen) that suggest a surgical emergency. These signs

can be due to profound DKA and disappear after treatment, but can present a challenge to diagnose, as appendicitis, pancreatitis, or cholecystitis can be a precipitating cause of DKA.

- *Hypotonia (poor muscle tone).* Signs that do not appear until late in the progression of DKA and suggest a poor prognosis are uncoordinated ocular movements and fixed, dilated pupils.
- *Hypothermia.* Common during DKA, making the presence of a fever a strong indicator of infection.

Symptoms of DKA That Are Probably Insignificant

- Increased amylase alone does not suggest pancreatitis. In DKA, salivary glands, not the pancreas, release most of the amylase.
- Increased white blood cells (WBCs) with DKA do not indicate infection. The differential count may be helpful with increased immature WBCs (>10% band forms), but clinical exam findings, such as fever, can supersede laboratory findings.[23]
- Mildly elevated liver function tests (LFTs) usually do not suggest liver damage and return to normal in several weeks.
- Serum creatinine can be elevated at initial evaluation. This needs to be monitored, as often the creatinine will fall as fluid replacement is initiated, but the issue as to when potassium replacement is safe requires that the creatinine be monitored closely.

Although the symptoms of poorly managed diabetes may be present for several days, the metabolic alterations typical of ketoacidosis usually occur within a short time frame (typically less than 24 hours). Occasionally, DKA may develop more acutely with no prior signs or symptoms.[8]

Treatment of DKA

The first part of this section describes treatment of moderate to severe DKA. Mild DKA is covered at the end of this section. Goals of DKA treatment, listed in Table 23.3, are discussed individually below.

Mortality for moderate to severe DKA is high.

Hospitalization may be required for appropriate treatment of DKA that is moderate to severe. Mortality remains high, even in teaching institutions. Treatment always requires supplemental fluids (first), followed by additional insulin.

Although hyperglycemia is the cause of osmotic diuresis, which leads to dehydration, the dehydration must be treated first, then the hyperglycemia—particularly when hypotension indicates potential impending circulatory collapse. Eventually, providing additional glucose is necessary to stop cellular starvation and intracerebral swelling. Treatment of DKA would not be complete without providing information and coaching to help prevent future episodes.

TABLE 23.3 Treatment Goals for DKA
1. Provide adequate fluids to rehydrate
2. Provide adequate insulin to restore and maintain normal glucose metabolism
3. Correct electrolyte abnormalities and acidosis if needed
4. Provide source of glucose when needed
5. Prevent complications
6. Provide education and follow-up for the person with diabetes and their family

Source: MB Davidson, S Schwartz, "Hyperglycemia," in MJ Franz, ed, *A Core Curriculum for Diabetes Education: Diabetes and Complications*, 5th ed (Chicago: American Association of Diabetes Educators, 2003), 27-8.

Case—Part 2: DKA Diagnosis and Identification of Precipitating Factors

The holiday commitments GT tried to meet that fall were additional stressors. Less sleep and changes in eating habits are known to stimulate counter-regulatory hormones and hepatic glucose release. With these stressors, compounded by hyperglycemia from increasingly inadequate self-management, GT was at risk for an infection.

She began to feel nauseous and noted decreasing energy. While studying for finals with her roommates, GT started to vomit and complained of stomach cramps. Her friends escorted her to the emergency department. The hospital staff suspected DKA when they learned GT had type 1 diabetes and heard about the nausea, vomiting, and abdominal pain, which were signs of ketones in her blood. The result of a finger-stick glucose reading was 350 mg/dL. Urinary ketones were large.

Diagnosis

GT's laboratory results were compatible with DKA (see Table 23.4, listing DKA, HHS, and reference range values):

- Serum glucose was 395 mg/dL.
- Serum ketones/beta-hydroxybutyric acid was positive.

Case—Part 2: DKA Diagnosis and Identification of Precipitating Factors (continued)

- Low serum bicarbonate and arterial pH confirmed acidosis.
- Previous lab work had suggested slight anemia, but hemoglobin and hematocrit were now both elevated, as were BUN and creatinine—signs of dehydration.
- Increased serum osmolality conveyed the extent to which glucose was elevated and fluids were lost.
- Sodium was slightly low, and potassium was slightly high—dehydration caused the potassium number to look higher than it was. Excess glucose can falsely lower the laboratory-determined sodium in the blood.

Identification of Precipitating Cause

To find the precipitating cause of DKA, cultures were obtained of GT's blood and urine, as was a pregnancy test. GT's blood glucose had probably been running higher than usual for several weeks as she became increasingly less focused on her diabetes self-management. GT had been unknowingly decreasing her fluid intake, and with accompanying diuresis from hyperglycemia, GT's fluid deficit was increasing over time. The hormonal changes of increasing estrogen (accompanying menses) and the stress of incident infection quickly elevated blood glucose and precipitated ketone production.

TABLE 23.4 GT's Lab Values: Comparing DKA and HHS With Reference Range

Test	*Reference Range*[1]	*DKA*[2]	*HHS*[2]
Serum glucose (mg/dL)	70–140	>250	>600
Serum osmolality (mOsm/kg)	275–295	>320	>320
Sodium bicarbonate (mEq/L)	22–26	<15	>15
Arterial pH	7.36–7.44	<7.2	>7.3
Serum beta-hydroxybutyrate (mmol/L)	0.02–0.27	>1.1 mmol/L	
Ketones	absent	moderate to large	absent to small
Increases Due to Dehydration			
BUN (mg/dL)	5–20	32	61
Serum creatinine (mg/dL)	0.7–1.2	1.1	1.4
Losses Often Masked by Dehydration			
Serum potassium (mmol/L)	3.5–5.0	4.5	3.9
Serum sodium (mmol/L)	135–145	varies, but typically low	varies, but typically above normal
Serum phosphorus (mg/dL)	2.3–4.3	varies	varies

Sources:

1. S Bakerman, "Bakerman's ABC's of Interpretive Laboratory Data," (Scottsdale, Ariz: Interpretive Laboratory Data, Inc; 2002).
2. BW Nugent, "Hyperosmolar hyperglycemic state," *Emerg Med Clin North Am.* 23(3)(2005):629-48.

Goal 1: Provide Adequate Fluids to Rehydrate

Begin fluid replacement. In all cases, adequate fluid replacement is critical to maintain circulation, expand volume, and restore renal perfusion.[1]

Initial Fluid Replacement

Initiate rapid administration of saline and reduce rate after first hour. Initial fluid replacement uses one-half normal (0.45%) or normal (0.9%) saline, depending on serum sodium and state of hydration. Avoid changes in osmolality by more than 3 mOsm per kilogram per hour.

- *For adults.* The average adult requires 1 to 2 L in the first hour, after which the perosn's status is reassessed.[1,15,23]
- *For children.* Deliver 10 to 20 mL per kilogram of body weight in the first hour. If no urination occurs, continue giving 20 mL per kilogram of body weight during the second and third hours.

Subsequent Fluid Replacement

The level of fluid replacement is monitored and adjusted based on maintenance needs, replacement requirements, and ongoing losses. The rate is adjusted to avoid fluid overload for renal and cardiac patients.

- Hyperglycemia will persist (even with appropriate insulin therapy) if fluid replacement is inadequate.
- Hydration status should typically correct within 48 hours. Several hours of hydration may be necessary before some persons are able to produce urine. If there is no urine flow after 4 hours of appropriate hydration, bladder catheterization may be warranted.

Goal 2: Provide Adequate Insulin to Restore and Maintain Normal Glucose Metabolism

All persons with DKA need insulin supplementation. Regular insulin by continuous intravenous infusion is the treatment of choice.[8]

- *Insulin type:* Regular or rapid-acting insulin offers relatively fast results in reducing glucose levels.
- *Delivery method:* Insulin delivery via intravenous infusion rather than injections offers these advantages: (1) more predictable decreases in glucose and (2) reduced risk of cerebral edema.
- *Pediatrics:* Rapid-acting insulin delivered via subcutaneous injections may be a cost-effective way to treat DKA in a pediatric population to prevent admission to the hospital.[26] Target decreases in plasma glucose of 50 to 75 mg/dL per hour.

Goal 3: Correct Electrolyte Abnormalities and Acidosis if Needed

Potassium

Total body potassium depletion is associated with DKA. All persons with diabetes with urine flow eventually need potassium repletion to avoid hypokalemia. Hypokalemia, if not treated properly, can lead to death. Prolonged hyperglycemia will be persistent in the setting of hypokalemia.

- The person is closely observed for clinically significant signs of potential hypokalemia, such as cardiac arrhythmias; serum potassium is checked periodically (ie, every 2 to 4 hours until level is stable or glucose is stable).
- Once urine output is documented, depending on the serum potassium level, 20 to 30 mEq of potassium per liter of fluid to be infused is added.[9]

Serum potassium concentration is frequently monitored, as it is essential to guide therapy. Serum potassium concentrations can drop rapidly from the initial results obtained before therapy. With increased hydration, the intravascular volume expands and renal perfusion increases renal excretion of potassium. With insulin administration, more potassium enters the cells, contributing to a drop in serum potassium while restoring total body potassium.

Phosphate

Serum phosphate (PO_4) levels are monitored. Research does not support routine supplementation with phosphate, as oral intake of food can promptly replace deficits.

Acidosis/Anion gap

Adequate insulin is continued to resolve acidosis. Acidosis takes longer to reverse than does hyperglycemia treated with insulin. The time required to resolve acidosis has not been well studied, because the serial pH measurements necessary to measure acidosis have not been done.

Sodium Bicarbonate

Treating acidosis with sodium bicarbonate ($NaHCO_3$) is controversial. It may be appropriate in special circumstances (as with acute cardiorespiratory arrest or hyperkalemia-induced cardiac arrhythmias). Caution is warranted for the following reasons:

- No clinical benefit has been documented.
- Sodium bicarbonate increases the risk for hypokalemic-induced arrhythmias because it causes potassium levels to drop so quickly.
- There is some evidence that bicarbonate increases the risk for cerebral edema.[23]

Hyperchloremic Acidosis

In hyperchloremic acidosis, bicarbonate levels plateau at approximately 15 to 20 mEq/L (15-20 mmol/L), usually 12 to 24 hours after treatment begins. At this time, chloride levels remain elevated, pH has returned to normal, and serum ketone bodies have dropped to low or absent. Expect hyperchloremic acidosis following DKA to be transient and require no treatment.

Pseudohyponatremia

To assess the severity of sodium and water deficit, serum sodium should be corrected by adding 1.6 mg/dL to the measured serum sodium for each 100 mg/dL of glucose above 100 mg/dL. An increase in serum sodium concentration in the presence of severe hyperglycemia indicates a profound degree of dehydration and water loss-often the serum sodium appears low, but with correction will be normal.[34,35]

Goal 4: Provide Source of Glucose When Needed

- When glucose reaches 250 mg/dL, 5% to 10% dextrose is added to the intravenous solution.[24] Cellular starvation perpetuates ketosis. In addition, sudden drops in glucose can be associated with cerebral edema.
- Ketosis is usually reversed in 12 to 24 hours, although occasionally urinary ketone bodies may be present for several days. If ketones persist, evaluation of adequacy of dietary intake is recommended.

Goal 5: Prevent Complications

Hypoglycemia, hypokalemia, and hyperglycemia are frequent complications of, respectively, overzealous treatment with insulin, use of bicarbonate, and inadequate insulin delivery during the transition from intravenous to subcutaneous administration. A minimum 2-hour overlap between infused insulin and initiation of subcutaneous basal insulin helps avoid gaps in insulin delivery.

A delay in diagnosis and misdiagnosis add to severity.

Identification and treatment of the initial cause of hyperglycemia as well as early intervention substantially improve clinical outcomes following DKA.

Two common errors—a delay in diagnosis and misdiagnosis—delay treatment and make the consequences of DKA worse than they need to be. The longer that treatment is delayed, the more severe the DKA episode and the more complex the treatment. Diabetic ketoacidosis is often misdiagnosed as gastroenteritis or appendicitis. Hypokalemia and cerebral edema may also go unrecognized, causing critical delays in beginning appropriate therapy for these conditions.

Most deaths occur in older persons with diabetes with medical complications other than DKA.[24] Older age and depth of coma predict mortality risk. Death is usually due to infection, arterial thrombosis, shock, or an unrecognized precipitating event that is not treated adequately. Complications such as aspiration and pulmonary edema may occur even in the most rigorously controlled treatment environment.

Cerebral Edema

Cerebral edema occurs rarely and is more common in children with DKA, yet it accounts for 90% of the deaths associated with DKA in children. Some studies question the significance of osmolality-induced injury, suggesting instead that cerebral hypoperfusion injury may be a predominant cause of cerebral edema that begins even prior to DKA treatment.[34,35] The optimal fluid type and rate of administration to treat pediatric DKA are currently under study. The Pediatric Emergency Care Applied Research Network (PECARN) is gathering data on more than 1,500 pediatric patients in DKA using 4 treatment protocols with different types and rates of fluid administration, with mental-status assessments during treatment and neurocognitive testing 3 months after DKA.[36] Cerebral edema occurs early in the course of treatment, typically in the first 24 hours and usually in the first 12 hours of treatment. The following help minimize the risks for this complication:

- Assess mental status frequently (every 1 to 2 hours), especially in children, who are more susceptible to cerebral edema than adults.
- Monitor for headache, lethargy, and mental-status changes; all are symptoms of cerebral edema.
- Suspect cerebral edema if improvement in lethargy and mental function is followed by deterioration, while metabolic status continues to improve and normalize.
- Avoid rapid drops in blood glucose (>100 mg/dL per hour), which may be a factor in the development of cerebral edema. To moderate the rate of glucose drop, add intravenous glucose to the regimen as the serum glucose level reaches about 250 mg/dL.
- If cerebral edema does occur, include IV osmotic diuretics (mannitol) and possibly high-dose glucocorticoids (dexamethasone) in the treatment.

The earlier the treatment, the better the prognosis. Treatment of cerebral edema at early stages may be beneficial, but it is usually ineffective at later stages. Once clinical symptoms (seizures, incontinence, bradycardia, respiratory arrest) appear, the mortality rate is >70%, with only 7% to 14% recovering completely.[11]

Goal 6: Provide Persons With Diabetes and Family Education and Follow-Up

After an episode of DKA, persons with diabetes and their family may be more receptive to learning how they might avoid a repeat hospitalization. A multidisciplinary team approach, including psychosocial intervention, may be needed to address concerns of persons with diabetes with recurrent episodes of DKA. See the earlier section on prevention of DKA.

Self-Care Behaviors in the Prevention of Severe Hyperglycemia

The AADE7 Self-Care Behaviors® provide a framework for prevention of severe hyperglycemia. Table 23.5 demonstrates how these behaviors can be used in the prevention of DKA. More details on fostering specific self-care behaviors are provided in chapters 4 through 10 in section 1 of this book.

TABLE 23.5 Applying Self-Care Behaviors to Prevention of DKA

AADE7 Self-Care Behaviors®	*Concept*	*Application*
Healthy Coping	Eating well, taking medications, testing BG, and using results to problem solve are difficult, never-ending aspects of self-management.	Use information, support, and encouragement to help overcome barriers that interfere with optimal prevention of DKA. Acknowledge the inevitable struggle that is part of living with diabetes. Discuss growth and hormonal spurts. Discuss inattention to signs and distractions of life. Identify resources and situations in which to seek medical attention. Consider counseling for emotional stress or depression.
Healthy Eating	Matching premeal insulin and carbohydrate to manage glucose levels. Having a sick-day plan and supplies (food and fluids).	Identify acceptable, easy-to-digest foods for sick days. Avoid an extreme carbohydrate load by limiting volume of sweetened beverages.
Being Active	Being safely active: Exercising without adequate insulin can dangerously elevate blood glucose (BG). Maintaining hydration is also important.	If glucose before exercise is high (>250 mg/dL), check for ketones. Presence of ketones indicates glucose is high due to inadequate insulin. Do not exercise until ketones are gone. To compensate for fluids lost during physical activity, drink adequately before, during, and after, especially on hot days.
Taking Medication	Exogenous insulin is essential to life for people with type 1 diabetes. Oral medications (T2DM) help improve/stabilize glucose.	Inadequate insulin dosing or poor timing of insulin action increases the risk for DKA. Omitting insulin almost guarantees it. To reduce risks for acute hyperglycemia, understand how insulin works and maintain the skills needed to take it appropriately. Everyone with type 1 diabetes needs this understanding. Persons with T2DM should be instructed to take all medications as prescribed and not to stop without PCP approval.
Monitoring	Monitoring BG and ketone levels provides feedback about the treatment plan and early warning of impending DKA.	Monitor regularly to help identify hyperglycemia before it becomes life threatening and enable early intervention and progress assessment. Increase monitoring frequency when not eating or ill. Do not rely strictly on "how you feel"—this provides an inaccurate measure of BG. Monitor to obtain accurate BG levels. Access to monitoring supplies may be a barrier to self-monitoring of BG. Address issues of concern. Assess problems with monitoring. Resistance to monitoring may have multiple causes.

TABLE 23.5 Applying Self-Care Behaviors to Prevention of DKA (continued)

AADE7 Self-Care Behaviors®	*Concept*	*Application*
Reducing Risks	Reducing the risk as well as the impact of DKA is possible. Unlike most diabetes management decisions, reducing complications from DKA treatment is primarily a provider responsibility.	Delayed treatment, excessive insulin, and inadequate insulin are common errors of treating DKA. Reduce complications with prompt diagnosis, adjusting insulin to glucose response, and beginning injected insulin before stopping IV. Discuss sick days—interventions for nausea, fever, loss of appetite; correction factors for hyperglycemia and further corrections for ketones; when to seek medical care and after-hours procedures.
Problem Solving	Applying information to individual situations so information already learned helps solve problems—avoiding initial events as well as recurrence.	Review the circumstances preceding a DKA episode. Identify precipitating factors to obtain clues to prevent another episode. Questions to reduce risk may relate to delaying exercise, limiting carbohydrate intake, monitoring blood glucose, or adjusting medication. Review factors contributing to DKA and learn to recognize signs and symptoms to prevent recurrence.

Treating Mild DKA

Some mild cases of DKA may be treated at home without hospitalization or an emergency department visit.[31] The following are parameters:

- The person with diabetes can still drink and retain oral fluids without difficulty, and
- The person with diabetes or their family can provide accurate blood glucose values and results of urine ketone tests and supplement insulin doses, and
- A knowledgeable healthcare professional is available to guide therapy over the phone.

Attention to physical symptoms, timely monitoring, and ability to adjust insulin all contribute to reducing the incidence and severity of DKA. Treatment at this stage should focus on oral hydration and supplemental insulin. Fluid intake should target 3 to 5 oz of fluids per hour; type of fluid is dependent on glucose value. The amount may be better tolerated if ingested in smaller doses every 20 to 30 minutes (or at every television commercial). If there are no contraindications (congestive heart failure, hypertension), broths containing sodium may be given, as they are more efficacious than the carbohydrate fluids and are not as likely to be voided as "free water."

Adequate Insulin to Restore and Maintain Normal Glucose Metabolism

In addition to usual insulin, provide supplemental insulin to compensate for hyperglycemia and ketosis. The amount needed depends on the person with diabetes' known sensitivity to insulin and current level of ketosis.

- *For children.* 0.25 to 0.5 units per kilogram of regular insulin every 4 to 6 hours, or rapid-acting insulin every 3 to 4 hours as needed.[1] A range for insulin replacement might be more appropriate.[38]
- *For adults.* 4 to 10 units or 10% to 20% of the usual total daily dose. Monitor frequently and adjust insulin for slow drop in glucose and resolution of ketosis.

Treatment of DKA (pre-hospital) depends on the severity of the episode, the abilities of the person with diabetes, and access to competent support. When someone with diabetes successfully treats mild DKA at home, clinical follow-up is still appropriate to reinforce information and support efforts to prevent DKA.

Problem Solving for Sick Days

Providers and persons with diabetes should not automatically assume illness or flu-like symptoms are the cause of elevated blood glucoses. Nausea, vomiting, or dehydration often heralds the onset of DKA. Persons with diabetes always need to address the areas of hydration, self-monitoring of blood glucose, ketones, medication adjustments, and food and beverage selections in the troubleshooting checklist (see Table 23.1) and then decide whether illness is causing the elevated glucoses.

For those on insulin pump therapy, temporary basal rate and/or bolus changes are particularly useful

Case—Part 3: DKA Treatment, Including Education Components

Before the laboratory results were back, the medical staff started an IV of normal saline to replace GT's fluids. Then they added regular insulin infusion at the recommended dose (0.1 units per kilogram per hour) to slowly lower blood glucose. Glucose and insulin doses were routinely entered into a flow sheet in her medical record.

- After 1 hour, glucose was 260 mg/dL. Because this drop exceeded the target rate for lowering glucose, the physician reduced the insulin drip to 0.08 units per kilogram per hour. The following were reassessed: glucose, sodium, potassium, and phosphorus. The results indicated that glucose was down to 248 mg/dL, potassium 3.9 mEq/L, sodium 135 mEq/L, and phosphate 2.5 mg/dL. The rate of IV insulin was maintained. Potassium was already being supplemented, and the lab finding was in the reference range. However, it was anticipated that potassium would drop further as GT's glucose level normalized and potassium moved intracellularly. Additional IV potassium was added in the form of potassium phosphate.
- After another hour, glucose was 214 mg/dL and urine ketones were moderate. Glucose was added to GT's IVF.
- The next day, GT's labs were much improved. Electrolytes were within the reference range, glucose ranged from 150 to 220 mg/dL, and ketones were small.

As GT talked with her nurse, she began to see what had happened in the days leading up to this DKA episode. In retrospect, she could see how, little by little, meals had become erratic and had been replaced with caffeine to help keep her going, and insulin doses had been missed. GT had not realized that her growing fatigue probably reflected her climbing glucose levels—something she would have known if she had continued to test regularly. The two reviewed sick-day guidelines and reviewed why GT's body required insulin even when she was not eating as much as usual. The diabetes resource nurse provided sample strips to support her blood glucose testing at home until the mail-order strips arrived, and a new prescription for ketone test strips was filled.

Reviewing the sick-day management principles helped GT. If GT checked her blood glucose and found that it was over 250 mg/dL, she would do a urine test for ketones. If ketones were positive, she could take her usual supplemental insulin dose to lower glucose. Because ketones increase insulin resistance, to effectively lower blood glucose, GT would need to take more supplemental insulin than usual. That information made more sense now. At initial diagnosis, GT had believed DKA would never happen to her; she now knew better.

in treating hyperglycemia due to intercurrent illness or use of steroids. During these times, persons with diabetes often need reminding to maintain adequate fluid intake with salted broth, water, or noncaloric beverages. If liquid carbohydrates are used for fluid replacement, appropriate boluses must be given. Often, bolus ratios need to be temporarily increased, as does the basal rate, until the condition is resolved. When blood glucoses are within target range, and nausea and ketones are present, the person with diabetes needs to sip on carbohydrate-containing beverages and give appropriate boluses based on insulin-to-carbohydrate ratio to eliminate ketones.[40] Persons with diabetes are often reluctant to use additional carbohydrates in this situation, but to reverse ketosis both insulin and carbohydrates are necessary.

Special Inpatient Hyperglycemia Concerns

The development of inpatient protocols for insulin delivery was spurred by awareness that previously accepted glycemic targets, the most recent data suggesting above 180 mg/dL, were associated with greater morbidity and mortality than glycemic targets of less than 180 mg/dL.[43] However, there remains some disagreement with absolute glycemic targets, with the recent recommendation of the American College of Physicians to target a blood glucose level of 140 to 200 mg/dL in SICU/MICU (surgical intensive care unit/mobile intensive care unit) patients, and with avoiding targets <140 mg/dL because hypoglycemia and associated risks are likely to increase with lower blood glucose targets.[43]

Despite several large-scale trials, absolute targets for glucose stability control remain controversial due to differences in populations studied, comorbidities, and etiologies to admitting illnesses.[44] Successful improvement in the overall care of hyperglycemic patients is not dependent on glycemic-lowering needs alone.

The Society of Hospital Medicine identified the following essential elements for inpatient hyperglycemia management[45]:

- Institutional support
- A multidisciplinary team or steering committee
- Data collection and reliable metrics
- Specific aims or goals
- Standardized insulin order sets

TABLE 23.6 Current Glycemic Targets in Hospitalized Patients

All Critically Ill Patients in Intensive Care Unit Settings	*Non-Critically Ill Patients*	*Hypoglycemia*
Blood glucose level 140–180 mg/dL (7.78–10.0 mmol/L)	Premeal: <140 mg/dL (7.78 mmol/L)	Reassess the regimen if blood glucose level is <100 mg/dL (5.56 mmol/L)
Intravenous insulin preferred	Random: <180 mg/dL (10.0 mmol/L)	Modify the regimen if blood glucose level is <70 mg/dL (3.89 mmol/L)
	Scheduled subcutaneous dosing preferred	Sliding-scale insulin discouraged

Source: ES Moghissi, MT Korytkowski, M DiNardo, et al, "American Association of Clinical Endocrinologists/American Diabetes Association consensus statement on inpatient glycemic control," *Endocr Pract* 15, no. 4 (2009): 1-17.

- Algorithms, policies, and protocols
- Comprehensive education and certification programs

The 2019 American Diabetes Association Standards of Care recommend a blood glucose target of 140 to 180 mg/dL (7.8-10.0 mmol/L) for most hospitalized patients.[46] Greater benefit may be realized at the lower end of this range. Although strong evidence is lacking, somewhat lower glucose targets may be appropriate in selected persons with diabetes, such as the surgical population in units that have shown low rates of hypoglycemia.[47,48] However, targets below 110 mg/dL (6.1 mmol/L) are no longer recommended (see Table 23.6).

The National Quality Forum has identified "serious reportable events," also called "never events," defined as "errors in medical care that are clearly identifiable, preventable, and serious in their consequences for persons with diabetes, and that indicate a real problem in the safety and credibility of a health care facility."[49] Third-party payers, including the Centers for Medicare & Medicaid Services (CMS), have begun to withhold payments for care related to these types of events. The CMS categorizes death or serious disability associated with hyperglycemia or hypoglycemia as a "never event."

Hyperosmolar Hyperglycemic Nonketotic Syndrome

A blood glucose level greater than 600 mg/dL without significant ketones characterizes hyperosmolar hyperglycemic state (HHS).[26] Hyperosmolar hyperglycemic state can occur whether or not diabetes medications are part of usual treatment.[26] Elevated blood glucose can escalate for days before it becomes a serious, acute threat.

> In HHS, extreme dehydration is the primary precipitating factor.

Extreme dehydration, more than profound insulin deficiency, is the primary precipitating factor. Profound dehydration, with subsequent hyperosmolarity and electrolyte losses, compounds the seriousness of this acute complication. Hyperosmolar hyperglycemic state occurs most frequently in undiagnosed or older adults with type 2 diabetes, but it also occurs in children and in people with type 1 diabetes. In 30% to 40% of HHS cases, HHS is the initial presentation of type 2 diabetes. While about 25% of new pediatric cases present with DKA, an estimated 4% of newly diagnosed children present with symptoms of HHS.[27]

Because HHS develops slowly (average 12 days) and does not cause the gastrointestinal pain associated with DKA, it is often overlooked or misdiagnosed.[50] Lack of treatment prolongs the osmotic diuresis secondary to hyperglycemia and worsens the clinical outlook. Due to delayed treatment as well as other medical conditions common in an older population, the mortality rate is about 15%, higher than the rate for DKA.

Pathophysiology of HHS

Hyperosmolar hyperglycemic state is similar to DKA except that insulin deficiency is less profound and dehydration plays a much more significant role. When blood glucose levels exceed 180 mg/dL, the kidneys are no longer able to reabsorb glucose. The concomitant renal water loss reduces renal perfusion and furthers dehydration. The water loss and inability to make up this water loss with oral intake causes levels of hyperglycemia and osmolarity in HHS that are more extreme than those found in DKA. The alterations in consciousness seen with HHS and the risk for morbidity are related to the degree of osmolarity.

Ketosis does not occur, because there remains some circulating insulin, although not in sufficient amounts to prevent hyperglycemia. Without significant ketone formation, related symptoms typical of DKA, like ketosis, acidosis, gastrointestinal discomfort, and Kussmaul respirations, do not occur. Without the physical discomfort of ketosis, persons with diabetes and their caregivers do not recognize a problem and the need for medical care. The mutual exacerbation of hyperglycemia and dehydration can begin with either problem (elevated glucose or inadequate fluids) and steadily escalate.

Precipitating Situations

Anything that elevates blood glucose or reduces hydration can contribute to development of HHS.

Elevated Blood Glucose

- New-onset type 2 diabetes
- Infection—a precipitating factor in 60% of cases[50]
- Surgery
- Myocardial infarction
- Gastrointestinal hemorrhage
- Uremia
- Arterial thrombosis
- Pancreatitis
- CVA
- Pulmonary embolism
- Medications that impact carbohydrate metabolism, such as glucocorticoids, thiazides, phenytoin, and beta-blockers

Decreased Water Intake and Access to Fluids

- Osmotic diuresis due to hyperglycemia—this is primary
- Fever
- Severe burns
- Diarrhea
- Peritoneal and hemodialysis
- Diuretic medications
- Hypertonic feeding
- Impaired thirst mechanism
- Inability to replace fluids may initiate dehydration

Particularly vulnerable are elderly people who must depend on others for their daily care and have difficulty communicating. Older people with impaired thirst who live alone may drink little unless prompted in some way. There are many opportunities to disrupt the development of HHS with regular monitoring and attention to those at risk.

Emphasize the importance of fluids to prevent dehydration. Situations that warrant extra care include physical activity, illness, institutionalized care settings (hospital, long-term care), forgetfulness, and aversion to drinking water or other hydrating fluids such as thickened liquids for those with swallowing difficulties.

Assessing Hyperosmolar Hyperglycemic State

Signs, Symptoms, and Laboratory Indicators

The signs and symptoms of HHS are similar to those of DKA, with some important exceptions.

The primary markers of HHS are the following:

- Severe hyperglycemia
- Profound dehydration
- Neurologic changes
- Absence of significant ketosis

Severe Hyperglycemia

Blood glucose levels in HHS are typically greater than 600 mg/dL. The reported mean glucose is greater than 1,000 mg/dL, with elevations as high as 1,500 mg/dL due to the extreme deficit of intravascular fluids.[51]

Profound Dehydration

Profound dehydration is marked by plasma osmolality greater than 320 mOsm per kilogram. Deficits of 20% to 25% of total body water or 12% to 15% of body weight may be observed. Physical symptoms include dry mucous membranes, poor skin turgor, and sunken eyes. Weakness, anorexia, leg cramps, dizziness, lethargy, and confusion may be signs of worsening hydration status. Coma affects about 20% of cases.[50]

Electrolyte losses of sodium, potassium, phosphorus, and magnesium accompany fluid losses. Sodium and potassium losses usually require supplementation, but due to their concentration from dehydration, laboratory results may initially appear high and do not represent total body loss. Blood urea nitrogen, serum creatinine, hematocrit, and many other routine blood chemistry levels may appear high but will resolve without treatment following hydration. Persistent elevations in BUN signal follow-up evaluation of renal function, and normal hematocrit when dehydrated is likely to indicate anemia. Access to medical history and information regarding usual lab results help the provider focus on the most relevant parameters.

Neurologic Changes

The neurologic changes of decreased mentation (eg, lethargy and mild confusion) are more common in HHS than in DKA and are the result of extreme dehydration. Persons with HHS may have focal neurological signs (hemisensory deficits, hemiparesis, aphasia, and seizures) that mimic a CVA. These signs will reverse completely as biochemical

Case: HHS in an Elderly Man With Type 2 Diabetes

Early in October, GT's Grandpa Joe had fallen and broken his hip while shopping. GT understood that the surgery had gone smoothly and that Grandpa was making reasonable progress with physical therapy postoperatively, but Grandma said he seemed a bit confused and slept more and more during the day. Before the fall, Grandpa had been active despite a little arthritis. He had managed his type 2 diabetes with a careful eye on what he ate and had kept his A1C less than 6%. After his fall, Joe needed the help of a senior center or outpatient therapy program so he could receive daily physical therapy. His doctor saw no reason for Grandpa to check his own blood glucose daily at home, as his granddaughter GT, who had "the serious kind" of diabetes, needed to do.

GT delayed her trip to visit her grandparents in Maine until after Christmas. When her flight arrived, Grandpa Joe was still in his physical therapy session, so she took a taxi straight there from the airport. Both grandparents welcomed her warmly and wanted to hear more about her DKA episode. As she talked, she noticed Grandpa nodding off or jumping into the conversation with comments about his "'54 Chevy." Grandma was cheery, but her face signaled her worry about Grandpa's slow recovery. GT took out her glucose meter and checked Grandpa's glucose from a finger-stick.

They were all flabbergasted when the result read "high," meaning the glucose level was too high for the meter to read it. They called the home health nurse to confirm their reading and to check on Grandpa.

Precipitating Events

It is not unusual for the stress of surgery to elevate glucose levels. Grandpa had little appetite after surgery, so his losing a little weight did not alarm anyone. In fact, he had begun to eat a little more with Grandma there with him for most meals. What no one noticed was that Grandpa was not drinking. He ate rather than drank his calories at meals and left containers of water untouched most of the day.

Slowly, Grandpa became more and more dehydrated, concentrating glucose and further increasing hyperglycemia.

status returns to normal. As in DKA, decreases in mentation best correlate with serum osmolality.

Absence of Significant Ketosis

Ketone bodies are not present in significant quantities. Starvation and dehydration may elevate serum ketones slightly. If present, gastrointestinal symptoms are usually milder than those found in DKA, and Kussmaul respirations are rare. Arterial pH greater than 7.3 mm Hg and a bicarbonate level greater than 15 mEq/L are typical of HHS.

Other Tests

Other tests are necessary to determine the precipitating cause of HHS:

- Cultures of blood, urine, and sputum
- Chest X-ray
- EKG

An EKG is used to assess cardiac status in a population at risk for cardiac complications as well as to quickly evaluate potassium status. Serial EKGs can monitor and guide potassium replacement therapy.

Treatment of HHS

Hyperosmolar hyperglycemic state requires hospitalization for appropriate and effective treatment. Treatment goals for HHS, as listed in Table 23.7, are similar to those for DKA. Each goal is discussed separately below.

Goal 1: Provide Adequate Fluids to Rehydrate

The cornerstone of treatment of HHS is to expand intravascular volume and restore renal perfusion. A guideline for fluid replacement is to infuse half of the fluid deficit over the first 12 hours and the remainder during the following 12 to 24 hours. Glucose levels may drop as much as 80 to 200 mg/dL per hour from rehydration alone.[50]

- *Elderly.* Particularly with an elderly person, care must be taken to adjust the hydration rate to the person's individual needs and consider the person's current hydration, cardiovascular, and renal status.
- *Renal insufficiency.* For people with renal insufficiency, restoring blood flow is critical; for older persons with compromised cardiovascular status, fluid loss must be replaced with saline slowly and cautiously to avoid fluid overload and congestive heart failure.

TABLE 23.7 Treatment Goals for HHS
1. Provide adequate fluids to rehydrate
2. Correct electrolyte deficits
3. Provide adequate insulin to restore and maintain normal glucose metabolism
4. Prevent complications
5. Treat underlying medical condition
6. Provide education and follow-up for a person with diabetes and their family

Source: G Umpierrez, M Koytkowski, "Diabetic emergencies—ketoacidosis, hyperglycemic hyperosmolar state and hypoglycemia," *Nat Rev Endocrinol* 12 (2016): 222-32.

- *Cardiovascular disease.* Persons with a history of CVD may require more intensive fluid status monitoring using either a noninvasive technique (eg, the IMPELLA, an FDA-approved, percutaneous ventricular assist device designed to provide a person's heart with hemodynamic support) or an invasive technique (eg, Swan-Ganz catheterization, a type of pulmonary artery catheterization procedure).

Goal 2: Correct Electrolyte Deficits

Laboratory tests provide critical information to guide replacement decisions for electrolytes.

Potassium

The EKG may provide immediate feedback regarding potassium status. Potassium replacement is similar to that required for DKA even though losses tend to be greater. However, insulin therapy needs to be withheld if initial laboratory results are less than 3.3 mEq/L, indicating profound deficiency. Potassium supplementation should be conservative until the renal function is known to be normal/improving.

Sodium

Sodium levels can be falsely low in HHS from extreme glucose concentration. The following correction provides a more accurate assessment of hydration status. Note that if the corrected sodium is high, dehydration is extreme.

$$\text{Corrected Na}^+ \text{ (mg/dL)} = \text{Reported Na}^+ \text{ (mg/dL)} + 1.6 \times (\text{glucose mg/dL} - 100)$$

Phosphorus and Magnesium

Phosphorus and magnesium laboratory results may be elevated or normal, indicating some losses with dehydration, but the levels tend to normalize without replacement therapy.

Routine Blood Work

Routine blood work is similarly elevated with dehydration. Monitor and reassess metabolic status after hydration.

Goal 3: Provide Adequate Insulin to Restore and Maintain Normal Glucose Metabolism

Hydration is essential primary treatment to lower glucose levels. Following hydration, insulin administration is usually but not always required to restore normal glycemia.

- *Insulin.* Treatment of acidosis is not part of HHS, so insulin requirements are typically not as high as those for DKA. Infuse insulin separately. Once insulin is started, do not interrupt delivery until hyperglycemia is adequately resolved.
- *Serum glucose.* Expect serum glucose to decrease 50 to 75 but no more than 100 mg/dL per hour. If serum glucose falls less than 50 mg/dL, consider whether to add or increase insulin and increase hydration. When glucose values reach acceptable levels (~300 mg/dL), reduce insulin and add 5% dextrose to infusion.[43] Monitor glucose hourly.

Goal 4: Prevent Complications

Preventing complications is important in treating HHS.

- Monitor frequently for blood pressure, fluid, electrolyte, and hourly glucose levels (hypoglycemia is unlikely because these individuals usually are very hyperglycemic—more so than individuals in DKA).
- Watch for complications of underlying atherosclerosis and consider low-dose heparin for at-risk individuals.
- Rhabdomyolysis may occur in persons with DKA and more commonly with HHS resulting in increased risk of acute kidney failure. The classic symptom triad of rhabdomyolysis includes myalgia, weakness, and dark urine, and monitoring creatine kinase concentrations every 2 to 3 his recommended for early detection.[35]
- Once insulin is started, do not interrupt delivery until euglycemia is ensured.

Goal 5: Treat Underlying Medical Condition

Treatment of the underlying medical condition(s) is critical to resolving HHS. In an elderly population, potential contributors to HHS are multiple and require thorough exploration and follow-up. It is difficult to prevent excessive fluid losses or manage hyperglycemia without identifying the source of the problem.

Goal 6: Provide Person With Diabetes and Family Education and Follow-Up

The risks for HHS include inadequate fluid intake, excessive fluid losses, and prolonged hyperglycemia. The tools to prevent or at least moderate the devastating impact of HHS are not complicated, but they require understanding and attention to daily habits. Regularly monitoring blood glucose and promptly treating mild hyperglycemia can interrupt the cycle leading to HHS before it is much of a problem.

Self-Care Behaviors in the Prevention of HHS

The AADE7 Self-Care Behaviors® provide a framework for prevention of HHS. Table 23.8 demonstrates how these behaviors can be used in the prevention of HHS. For more details on fostering specific self-care behaviors, see chapters 4 through 10 in section 1 of this book. As a priority, diabetes care and education specialists should assist individuals in avoiding HHS by encouraging hydration and identifying those at high risk.

Encourage Hydration

Encourage adequate hydration for every person with diabetes. Many people will need frequent reminders and suggestions for specific ways to include more fluids before they will be able to do so.

TABLE 23.8 Applying Self-Care Behaviors for Prevention of HHS

AADE7 Self-Care Behaviors®	*Concept*	*Application*
Healthy Coping	Eating well, taking medications, testing blood glucose, and using the results to problem solve are difficult, never-ending aspects of self-management.	Use information, support, and encouragement for caregivers as well as persons with diabetes to help prevent HHS. Identify resources and situations in which to seek medical attention.
Healthy Eating	Matching timing of food with medication and activity. Having a sick-day plan and supplies (food and fluids). Do not skip meals.	To avoid high BG, do not consume extra carbohydrate without taking extra insulin. It is easy to consume extra carbohydrate with liquids. A large soft drink at a fast-food restaurant is equal in carbohydrate to 5 slices of bread. Skipping meals can lead to overeating at a subsequent meal.
Being Active	Activity continues to lower insulin resistance and improve blood glucose (BG) levels. Be safely active at all ages. Maintain adequate hydration.	To compensate for fluids lost during physical activity, drink adequately before, during, and after physical activity, especially on hot days.
Taking Medication	If glucose goals are not met with activity and meal planning, medication is necessary.	Underuse of diabetes medication, especially reluctance to initiate insulin when needed, significantly contributes to high glucose levels.
Monitoring—Blood Glucose	Monitoring provides feedback about the treatment plan and warning of impending HHS.	Monitor regularly to help identify hyperglycemia before it becomes life threatening; this is true even for those not treated with medication, especially during illness or other stress. Monitoring allows early intervention and progress assessment. Discuss usual monitoring routine and what to do when not eating or ill. Do not rely strictly on "how you feel"—this has been shown to be an inaccurate measure of BG values. Monitor to obtain an accurate BG level. Access to monitoring supplies may present a barrier to self-monitoring of BG. Address issues of concern. Assess problems with monitoring. Resistance to monitoring may have multiple causes.

(continued)

TABLE 23.8 Applying Self-Care Behaviors for Prevention of HHS (continued)

AADE7 Self-Care Behaviors®	*Concept*	*Application*
Reducing Risks	Reducing the risk as well as the impact of HHS is possible. HHS also increases risks for many concomitant conditions.	As HHS usually occurs in an older, more vulnerable population, individualize and carefully monitor therapy for these persons to help prevent complications. Discuss sick days—interventions for nausea, fever, loss of appetite; correction factors for hyperglycemia; when to seek medical care and after-hours procedures.
Problem Solving	Applying information already learned to individual situations helps solve problems.	Review the circumstances preceding the HHS episode to look for clues to prevent another. Would a system for drinking fluids, monitoring blood glucose, or a change in medication have reduced the risk? To prevent recurrence, review signs, symptoms, and treatment.

Note: See also chapters 4 to 10 on each of these 7 behaviors in this book.

- *Living alone.* Individuals who live alone may require help devising a system for remembering to drink fluids, such as keeping fluids within reach or having someone remind the individual to drink water every 2 to 4 hours.
- *Dependent on others.* Intake of adequate fluids can be a special challenge when the individual is dependent on others (eg, older adults in a hospital or nursing home and those who cannot communicate a request for water). These individuals depend on the institution to monitor fluid intake, evaluate fluid status, and establish a plan that keeps residents adequately hydrated.

Identify High-Risk Individuals

Identify high-risk individuals and, when dealing with them, put special emphasis on the basics. Examples are (1) the elderly in nursing homes, hospitals, or other settings where dehydration may not be noticed and (2) persons being treated with glucocorticoids or other medications that may precipitate hyperglycemia. Offer information to both the person with diabetes and the person's family and caregivers. Be sure everyone involved in the care understands the rationale for having the supplies necessary to accomplish the following:

- Obtain adequate fluids.
- Monitor blood glucose regularly.
- Manage sick days that may include fever and vomiting.
- Keep sick-day supplies on hand and accessible (eg, thermometer, acceptable and easy-to-eat food and drink, contact numbers for physician and urgent care services).
- Know the signs and symptoms of HHS and the critical need for medical attention should they appear.
- Know how and when to contact the healthcare provider.

Identify Vulnerabilities

Help individuals, especially those at high risk, understand the problems that may occur, signs and symptoms, precipitating factors, and appropriate actions. Provide education to help prevent DKA and HHS.

Key Aspects of Education, Prevention, and Treatment

Education

Education is the key to preventing hyperglycemia, and the diabetes care and education specialist needs to work with the person with diabetes, as well as the members of his or her family, caregivers, and other healthcare providers. Following are the topics that should be addressed with each person or group:

For persons with diabetes:

- Sick-day management
- When to call a physician
- Medication adjustments during illness
- Need for no-calorie fluids and carbohydrate-containing fluids

For family, caregivers, and school personnel:

- Recognizing symptoms of hyperglycemia
- Knowing what to do about hyperglycemia
- Understanding the person with diabetes' sick-day plan
- When to seek medication attention
- Medications that can affect glucose levels

For primary care providers:

- Instruction for persons with diabetes for supplemental insulin during illness
- Who benefits from home blood glucose monitoring

For nursing home/hospital staff and caregivers:

- How to monitor glucose, hydration, and mentation
- How to identify at-risk persons with diabetes

Prevention

The person with diabetes needs knowledge and skills to perform the necessary actions to prevent hyperglycemic episodes.

Monitoring supplies:

- How to time monitoring when strips are limited

Hydration:

- Getting fluids when the person is not thirsty and does not like the taste

Treatment

If a person with diabetes has a hyperglycemic episode, the medical staff needs to recognize symptoms and respond quickly and appropriately.

Why infuse dextrose when blood glucose is 250 mg/dL?

- To prevent cerebral edema
- To prevent hypoglycemia

Why not give insulin when blood glucose is 600 mg/dL?

- Fluids alone can significantly decrease hyperglycemia in HHS

How to adjust sodium for elevated glucose:

- To correct for dilution from glucose when concentration is very high:[50]

$$\text{Corrected Na}^+ \text{ (mg/dL)} = \text{Reported Na}^+ \text{ (mg/dL)} + 1.6 \times (\text{glucose mg/dL} - 100)$$

Testing for ketones:

- Measure beta-hydroxybutyrate to diagnose DKA and monitor progress[11]

Case: Preventing Hyperglycemia in an Institutional Care Setting

A skilled-care facility supervisor called for advice regarding a person with type 2 diabetes of known 16-year duration. JM is an 85-year-old man who came to the skilled nursing facility after a CVA that resulted in some difficulty ambulating unassisted. He appeared fatigued and somewhat lethargic, and the symptoms seemed to have been slowly more perceptible over the past 3 days. There had been no acute change in overall well-being, but the JM just seemed to appear somewhat different from usual. The CVA also left JM with mild dysarthria, which was exacerbated when he was fatigued, making him more difficult to understand. He was seen in his primary care clinic within the last week, and a thiazide was started to target better management of hypertension. The family members who typically visited JM once a week and were very involved with his care had been out of town, so the supervisor was relying on staff reports of change in JM's behavior. Staff had not been able to speak with the family about their observations. That day, there was concern regarding JM's increasing lethargy, and a finger-stick blood glucose of 390 mg/dL was obtained.

Case Wrap-Up: Preventing Hyperglycemia in an Institutional Care Setting

Applying the principles presented in the text of this chapter, hydration would be imperative, followed by a discussion on the effects of a thiazide, a medication that can potentiate hyperglycemia.[53,54] Many commonly prescribed pharmacologic agents for treatment of diabetes comorbidities such as hypertension and dyslipidemia can potentiate hyperglycemia.[53]

Inadequate access to water or hydrating fluids is a major confounder of hyperglycemia,[55] and neurologic deficits can be a barrier to appropriate fluid intake.[56,57] The recognition of inadequate water intake can be challenging in a skilled care facility.

Additionally, many metabolic disease states common in the older population can be associated with hyperglycemia; in particular, hyperthyroidism,[58] Cushing syndrome,[58] and even hyperparathyroidism[59] can potentiate hyperglycemia that responds to treatment of the specific instigating metabolic problem.[53] Early identification of the hyperosmolar nonketotic state and prompt initiation of treatment are directly associated with survival.[60]

When to consider phosphorus supplementation:

- To avoid skeletal and cardiac muscle weakness and respiratory depression in persons with diabetes cardiac dysfunction, anemia, or respiratory depression if PO_4 <1.0 mg/dL[11]

When to consider bicarbonate supplementation:

- If pH is <6.9, although no research substantiates benefit[11]

Ketoacidosis without DKA:

- Starvation and alcoholic ketoacidosis (AKA)

Focus on Education

Teaching Strategies

Know signs and symptoms. Diabetes care and education specialists should be very familiar with signs and symptoms of hyperglycemia so they can help persons with diabetes and family recognize and intervene early.

Relate monitoring to prevention. Teaching the benefits of blood glucose monitoring can often prevent severe hyperglycemia. Monitoring recognizes low as well as high blood glucose. Teach the concept of testing.

Show how planning leads to prevention. Planning ahead is an important part of preventing hyperglycemia. This includes having proper supplies (blood glucose meter and ketone testing equipment) and not running out of them, testing and treating with insulin, and knowing when to call the healthcare provider.

Be alert for issues among adolescents and elderly adults. Teenagers or young adults with diabetes, particularly type 1 diabetes, who have recurrent DKA may be purposely omitting insulin for weight loss or attention. In elderly adults, an underlying illness, the cause of high blood glucose, dehydration, and medication taking can be a concern. Assess the person with diabetes and family for referral for counseling.

Identify high-risk situations. Identify potential high-risk situations such as the following: young adults going off to college, teenagers beginning to drive, elderly in nursing homes who may become dehydrated, and persons being treated with glucocorticoids or other medications that may precipitate hyperglycemia.

Provide a "when to call" list. Give persons with diabetes a prepared list of situations of when to call the physician. Include contact information for days, nights, and weekends. This reassures persons with diabetes that it is necessary to call if they have concerns and that calling is not a bother.

Prepare family members. Educate family members to recognize high-risk situations and intervene early enough to prevent development of severe, life-threatening hyperglycemia.

Educate emergency personnel. Offer a hyperglycemia refresher course to local emergency departments, hospital staff, paramedics, school nurses, and others in the community. Bring equipment for hands-on blood testing and ketone testing. Reinforce the need for ketone testing equipment in the home for early detection and intervention. For HHS, urge earlier identification by recognizing dehydration status, underlying illness, and potential causes.

Offer telephone care for mild DKA. In some cases in which DKA is mild and recognized early, it can be treated with insulin and oral fluids via telephone consults. Know also when this is not appropriate.

Evaluate and reeducate. Always carefully assess the reasons for a DKA or HHS occurrence so that preventive strategies can be taught and instituted.

Use situational problem solving. Identify person-specific circumstances of hyperglycemia and have a person with diabetes verbalize what he or she would do. This could involve role playing with the person with diabetes in the setting of what to do when ill, and role playing with the family members/spouse who would be providing care for an individual with diabetes who is ill. An example is a "sick-day readiness box"—what to include in the box and when to call for medical advice.

Messages for Persons With Diabetes

Ensure family, significant others, and caregivers understand what puts you at high risk. Family members and friends need to recognize high-risk situations and be able to respond with early interventions to prevent the development of severe, life-threatening hyperglycemia. Recognizing the underlying cause of high blood glucose, such as illness, insulin that may have expired or was kept improperly, or an inadequate insulin amount, is important.

Distribute handouts so others can help you. Provide family, friends, roommates, your workplace or school, and leaders of groups you participate in with informational handouts and contact information for emergency medical care. Invite family and close friends to attend education classes and clinic visits. Teach appropriate people in your life how to test your blood glucose and ketones. Remind these people, especially if you are an older adult, about the importance of getting adequate fluids.

Be reflective and proactive. Review the events that contributed to the hyperglycemia. Come up with a plan to prevent future occurrence.

Health Literacy

The diabetes care and education specialist needs to establish a health literacy level in the person with diabetes before initiating education. Explore treatment beliefs within the cultural context of illness. Identify specific herbs/teas/potions that the person with diabetes may use in treating common illnesses which could impact body temperature and/or hydration status. Some examples of these practices are:

- Comfrey tea, which contains aspirin-like compounds that could impact body temperature
- Inducing sweating for an illness, as done in certain Hispanic cultures, which potentially could add to dehydration already seen in hyperglycemic states

Determine whether the person with diabetes has someone who is familiar with obtaining finger-stick glucoses, helping inject insulin, and so on, who could help him or her when ill.[36]

Health literacy is the ability to obtain, process, and understand basic health information and services needed to make appropriate decisions. Consider 3 steps in hyperglycemia management:

- Recognize hyperglycemia. Identify actual blood glucose numbers that are considered over the desirable range. Provide examples of the actual glucose numbers instead of just indicating "above . . ."
- Process the information by identifying specific circumstances of where and how hyperglycemia occurs.
- Put meaning to the numbers by asking: What will you do when your blood glucose is . . . ?

Ask a person with diabetes to teach you about high blood glucose. Consider asking the following questions:

- How do you know you have high blood glucose (higher than you would like it to be)?
- What do you consider "high" blood glucose?
- When do you typically have high blood glucose?
- What do you do when you have high blood glucose?

Health numeracy. Many people, even those who are highly educated and literate, can have trouble understanding numbers. To communicate quantitative information such as blood glucose levels associated with hyperglycemia, focus on just one idea at a time and express it in simple sentences. The following are additional strategies to make sure that persons with diabetes understand the numbers and what they mean:

- Draw a picture showing what the low versus high level is.
- Use analogies or reference points to explain glucose levels and ranges.
- Show physical representations of glucose density and what happens in a body when hyperglycemia occurs.
- Encourage persons with diabetes to create their own images.

Teach with stories to connect high glucose to specific symptoms or events.

Focus on Practice

Examine the system of decision making on hyperglycemia management. Physicians, nurses, and quality improvement coordinators need to make hyperglycemia management protocols. Use evidence-based strategies to minimize risks and maximize cost savings and productivity.

Educate staff on hyperglycemia management protocols. Hyperglycemia management might involve exploring some common misconceptions about hyperglycemia and its corresponding interventions. Implement aggressive but achievable standards of care that involve all necessary parties.

Perform a cost-benefit analysis. Administrators and third-party payers will need to see the cost benefits that can accrue from shorter hospital stays and fewer complications when hyperglycemia is reduced.

Quality ensure your hyperglycemia management. Monitor systems and processes to ensure that the protocols are implemented within the desirable scope. Adjust practice based on findings.

References

1. Umpierrez G, Korytkowski M. Diabetes emergencies—ketoacidosis, hyperglycemic hyperosmolar state and hypoglycemia. Nat Rev Endocrinol. 2016;12:222-32.
2. Erondu N, Desai M, Ways K, Meininger G. Diabetic ketoacidosis and related events in the Canagliflozin Type 2 diabetes clinical program. Diabetes Care. 2015;38:1680-6.
3. Tang H, Li D, Wang T, Zhai S, Song Y. Effect of sodium-glucose cotransporter 2 inhibitors on diabetic ketoacidosis among patients with Type 2 Diabetes: a meta-analysis of randomized controlled trials. Diabetes Care. 2016; 39:e123-4.
4. Peters AI, Busher EO, Buse JB, et al. Euglycemic diabetic ketoacidosis: a potential complication of treatment with sodium-glucose cotransporter 2 inhibition. Diabetes Care. 2015;38:1687-93.
5. Maahs DM, Hermann JM, Holman N, et al. Rates of diabetic ketoacidosis: international comparison with 49,859 pediatric patients with type 1 diabetes from England, Wales, the U.S., Austria, and Germany. Diabetes Care. 2015;38:1883-90.
6. Centers for Disease Control and Prevention. Diabetes data and trends (online) (cited 2016 Jun 5). On the Internet at: http://www.cdc.gov/nchs/fastats/diabetes.htm.
7. Malone ML, Gennis V, Goodwin JS. Characteristics of diabetic ketoacidosis in older versus younger adults. J Am Geriatr Soc. 1992;40:1100-4.
8. Usher-Smith JA, Thompson M, Ercole A, Walter M. Variation between countries in the frequency of diabetic ketoacidosis at first presentation of type 1 diabetes in children: a systematic review. Diabetologia. 2012;55:2878-94.
9. Cakan N, Kizilbash S, Kamat D. Changing spectrum of diabetes mellitus in children: challenges with initial classification. Clin Pediatr (Phila). 2012;51:939-44.
10. Tan KC, Mackay IR, Zimmet PZ, et al. Metabolic and immunologic features of Chinese patients with atypical diabetes mellitus. Diabetes Care. 2000;23(3):335-8.
11. Kitabchi AI, Umpierrez GE, Miles JM, et al. Hyperglycemic crises in adult patients with diabetes. Diabetes Care. 2009;32:1335-43.
12. Wilson C, Krakoff J, Gohdes D. Ketoacidosis in Apache Indians with non-insulin-dependent diabetes mellitus. Arch Intern Med. 1997;157(18):2098-100.
13. Balasubramanyam A, Zern JW, Hyman DJ, et al. New profiles of diabetic ketoacidosis: type 1 vs type 2 diabetes and the effect of ethnicity. Arch Intern Med. 1999;159(19):2317-22.
14. Umpierrez G, Korytkowski M. Diabetic emergencies—Ketoacidosis, hyperglycemia hyperosmolar stat and hypoglycemia. Nat Rev Endocrinol. 2016;12:222-32.
15. McDonnell CM, Pedreira CC, Vadamalayan B, et al. Diabetic ketoacidosis, hyperosmolarity and hypernatremia: are high-carbohydrate drinks worsening initial presentation? Pediatr Diabetes. 2005 Jun;6:90-4.
16. Kershaw MJ, Newton T, Barrett TG, et al. Childhood diabetes presenting with hyperosmolar dehydration but without ketoacidosis: a report of three cases. Diabet Med. 2005;22:645-7.
17. Hammond P, Liebl A, Grunder S. International survey of insulin pump users: impact of continuous subcutaneous insulin infusion therapy on glucose control and quality of life. Prim Care Diabetes. 2007;1(3):143-6.
18. Bode BW, Tamborlane WV, Davidson PC. Insulin pump therapy in the 21st century: strategies for successful use in adults, adolescents, and children with diabetes. Postgrad Med. 2002;111(5):69-78.
19. Scaramuzza AE, Iafusco D, Rabbone I, et al. Use of integrated real-time continuous glucose monitoring/insulin pump system in children and adolescents with type 1 diabetes: a 3-year follow-up study. Diabetes Technol Ther. 2011;13:99-103.
20. Foster NC, Beck RW, Miller KM, et al.; and for the T1D Exchange Clinic Network. State of Type 1 Diabetes Management and Outcomes from the T1D Exchange 2016-2018. Diabetes Tech Ther. 2019;21:66-72.
21. Bergenstal RM, Klonoff DC, Garg SK, et al; ASPIRE In-Home Study Group. Threshold-based insulin-pump interruption for reduction of hypoglycemia. N Engl J Med. 2013;369:224-32.
22. Peveler RC, Bryden KS, Neil HA, et al. The relationship of disordered eating habits and attitudes to clinical outcomes in young adult females with type 1 diabetes. Diabetes Care. 2005;28:84-8.
23. Neumark-Sztainer D, Patterson J, Mellin A, et al. Weight control practices and disordered eating behaviors among adolescent females and males with type 1 diabetes. Diabetes Care. 2002;25:1289-96.
24. Charfen MA, Fernandez-Frackelton M. Diabetic ketoacidosis. Emerg Med Clin North Am. 2005;23:609-28.
25. Musey VC. Diabetes in urban African-Americans. I. Cessation of insulin therapy is the major precipitating cause of diabetic ketoacidosis. Diabetes Care. 1995;18:483-9.
26. Kitabchi AE, Umpierrez GE, Fischer JN, et al. Thirty years of personal experience with hyperglycemic crises: diabetic ketoacidosis and hyperglycemic hyperosmolar state. J Clin Endocrinol Metab. 2008;93:1541-52. Epub 2008 Feb 12.
27. Peyrot M, Rubin RR, Kruger DF, Travis LB. Correlates of insulin injection omission. Diabetes Care. 2010 Feb;33(2):240-5.
28. Higgs MM. The High Price of Insulin is Literally Killing People. VICE, Apr 5 2017. On the Internet at: https://www.vice.com/en_us/article/ezwwze/the-high-price-of-insulin-is-literally-killing-people-accessed 09/06/2019.
29. Agus MS, Wolfsdorf JI. Diabetic ketoacidosis in children. Pediatr Clin North Am. 2005;52:1147-63.
30. Nyenwe EA, Loganathan RS, Blum S, et al. Active use of cocaine: an independent risk factor for recurrent diabetic ketoacidosis in a city hospital. Endocr Pract. 2007;13:22-9.
31. FDA Drug Safety Communication. FDA warns that SGLT2 inhibitors for diabetes may result in a serious condition of too much acid in the blood (cited 2016 Jun 5). On the Internet

at: http://www.fda.gov/Drugs/DrugSafety/ucm446845.htm?source=govdelivery&utm_medium=email&utm_source=govdelivery.

32. Tauschmann M, Thabit H, Bally L, et al.; APCam11 Consortium. Closed loop-insulin delivery in suboptimally controlled type 1 diabetes: a multicentre, 12-week randomised trial. Lancet 2018;392:1321-9.

33. Handelsman Y, Henry RP, Bloomgarden ZT, et al. American Association of Clinical Endocrinologists and American College of Endocrinology position statement on the association of SGLT-2 inhibitors and diabetic ketoacidosis. Endocr Pract. 2016;22:753-62.

34. Modi A, Agrawal A, Morgan F. Euglycemic diabetic ketoacidosis: a review. Curr Diabetes Rev. 2017;13(3):315-21.

35. Fayfman M, Pasquel FJ, Umpierrez GE. Management of hyperglycemic crises: diabetic ketoacidosis and hyperglycemic hyperosmolar state. Med Clin North Am. 2017;101(3):587-606.

36. Glaser NS, Wootton-Gorges SL, Marcin JP, et al. Mechanism of cerebral edema in children with diabetic ketoacidosis. J Pediatr. 2004;145:164-71.

37. Glaser NS, Marcin JP, Wootton-Gorges SL, et al. Correlation of clinical and biochemical findings with diabetic ketoacidosis-related cerebral edema in children using magnetic resonance diffusion-weighted imaging. J Pediatr. 2008;153:541-6.

38. Glaser NS, Ghetti S, Casper TC, et al. Pediatric diabetic ketoacidosis, fluid therapy, and cerebral injury: the design of a factorial randomized controlled trial. Pediatr Diabetes. 2013;14(6): 435-46. Epub 2013 Mar 13.

39. Trachtenbarg DE. Diabetic ketoacidosis. Am Fam Physician. 2005;71(9):1705-14.

40. Al Hanshi S, Shann F. Insulin infused at 0.05 versus 0.1 units/kg/hr in children admitted to intensive care with diabetic ketoacidosis. Pediatr Crit Care Med. 2011;12(2):137-40.

41. Cramer JA. A systematic review of adherence with medication for diabetes. Diabetes Care. 2004;27:1218-24.

42. The NICE-SUGAR Study Investigators. Intensive versus conventional glucose control in critically ill patients. N Engl J Med. 2009;360:1283-97.

43. Qaseem A, Chou R, Humphrey LL, et al. Inpatient glycemic control: best practice advice from the Clinical Guidelines Committee of the American College of Physicians. Am J Med Qual. 2014;29(2):95-8. Epub 2013 Jun 7.

44. Van den Berghe G, Schetz M, Vlasselaers DJ, et al. Clinical review: intensive insulin therapy in critically ill patients: NICE-SUGAR or Leuven blood glucose target? J Clin Endocrinol Metab. 2009;94(9):3163-70. Epub 2009 Jun 16.

45. Schnipper JL, Magee M, Larsen K, Inzucchi SE, Maynard G; Society of Hospital Medicine Glycemic Control Task Force. Society of Hospital Medicine Glycemic Control Task Force summary: practical recommendations for assessing the impact of glycemic control efforts. J Hosp Med. 2008;3 Suppl 5:66-75.

46. American Diabetes Association. Diabetes care in the hospital: standards of medical care in diabetes—2019. Diabetes Care. 2019 Jan;42(Supplement 1):S173-81.

47. Trence DL, Kelly JL, Hirsch IB. The rationale and management of hyperglycemia for in-patients with cardiovascular disease: time for change. J Clin Endocrinol Metab. 2003;88(6):2430-7.

48. Penfold S, Gouni R, Hamilton P, et al. Immediate in-patient management of hyperglycaemia—confusion rather than consensus? QJM. 2008 Feb;101(2):87-90. Epub 2008 Jan 7.

49. Ishikawa H, Takeuchi T, Yano E. Measuring functional, communicative, and critical health literacy among diabetic patients. Diabetes Care. 2008 May;31(5):874-9. Epub 2008 Feb 25.

50. Della MT, Steinmetz L, Campos PR, et al. Subcutaneous use of a fast-acting insulin analog: an alternative treatment for pediatric patients with diabetic ketoacidosis. Diabetes Care. 2005;28:1856-61.

51. Nugent BW. Hyperosmolar hyperglycemic state. Emerg Med Clin North Am. 2005;23:629-48.

52. Kitabchi AE, Umpierrez GE, Murphy MB, et al. Management of hyperglycemic crises in patients with diabetes mellitus (technical review). Diabetes Care. 2001;224:131-53.

53. Trence DL, Hirsch IB. Hyperglycemic crises in diabetes mellitus type 2. Endocrinol Metab Clin North Am. 2001;30(4): 817-31.

54. Fonseca V, Phear DN. Hyperosmolar non-ketotic diabetic syndrome precipitated by treatment with diuretics. BMJ. 1982;284:36-7.

55. Ennis ED, Stahl E JVB, Kreisberg RA. The hyperosmolar hyperglycemic syndrome. Diabetes Rev. 1994;2(1):115-26.

56. Lorber D. Non-ketotic hypertonicity in diabetes mellitus. Med Clin North Am. 1995;79:39-52.

57. Maccario M. Neurologic dysfunction associated with nonketotic hyperglycemia. Arch Neurol. 1968;19:525-34.

58. Berelowitz M, Go EH. Non-insulin-dependent diabetes mellitus secondary to other endocrine disorders. In: LeRoith D, Taylor SI, Olefsky JM, eds. Diabetes Mellitus. Philadelphia: Lippincott-Raven Publishers; 1996:496-502.

59. Akgun S, Ertel NH. Hyperparathyroidism and coexisting diabetes mellitus: altered carbohydrate metabolism. Arch Intern Med. 1978;138(10):1500-2.

60. Wachtel TJ, Silliman RA, Lamberton P. Predisposing factors for the diabetic hyperosmolar state. Arch Intern Med. 1987; 147:499-501.

CHAPTER 24

Pregnancy With Diabetes

Diane M. Reader, RD, CDCES
Alyce Thomas, RD

Key Concepts

- Health professionals involved in the care of pregnant women with diabetes should develop an understanding of the pathophysiology of diabetes and pregnancy.
- Preconception counseling should be available to all women with preexisting diabetes and those with previous gestational diabetes and prediabetes to improve perinatal outcomes.
- Optimal blood glucose levels are associated with lower perinatal morbidity and mortality rates.
- Strategies to improve outcomes include maternal and fetal monitoring and self-management skills.
- Weight gain goals based on current recommendations from the Institute of Medicine are established at the initial prenatal visit.
- Unless contraindicated, breastfeeding is recommended for all women with preexisting or gestational diabetes.
- Women who have gestational diabetes mellitus have 7 times the risk of developing type 2 diabetes after delivery. Steps should be taken to prevent diabetes through weight management, food choices, and physical activity.

Introduction

The most prevalent medical complication in pregnancy is diabetes mellitus. Diabetes in pregnancy is divided into 2 groups:

- Women with *preexisting diabetes*, which includes type 1 diabetes and pregnancy (T1DP) and type 2 diabetes and pregnancy (T2DP)
- Women with *gestational diabetes mellitus* (GDM), which is defined as diabetes diagnosed in the second or third trimester of pregnancy that is not clearly either type 1 or type 2 diabetes.[1] This recently revised definition identifies that hyperglycemia in the first trimester is not considered GDM.

The prevalence of diabetes mellitus in women of childbearing age is reported to be from 3.1% to 6.8%, with preexisting diabetes observed in 1% to 2% of all pregnancies.[2]

Approximately 34% of pregnant women with preexisting diabetes have type 1 diabetes. In recent years, intensive insulin therapy and greater attention to diabetes self-management have resulted in better maternal glycemic management. The current perinatal mortality rate in women with preexisting diabetes is 2%, which is comparable to women without diabetes.[3]

Type 2 diabetes is associated with obesity and other comorbidities, such as hypertension. The management of type 2 diabetes during pregnancy may include changes in medications to improve glycemic stability and to decrease the risk of harm to the woman and/or fetus.

The incidence of GDM varies among populations and ethnicities, as well as with the diagnostic criteria used. In the United States, it is estimated that 6% to 7% of pregnancies are complicated by diabetes mellitus and that approximately 90% of these are GDM.[4] The rate of GDM in any community or geographic region will vary depending on multiple factors; the range is quite wide, from as low as 2% to as high as 50%.[5] More importantly, the rate is increasing, likely due to the high rates of overweight and obesity in the population of women in their childbearing years.

Glycemic stability is key to decreasing fetal risks and infant morbidity associated with maternal hyperglycemia. The greatest success in maintaining optimal glycemic stability throughout pregnancy comes from partnering with a multidisciplinary team and receiving targeted self-management education. Key components of care include antenatal testing and the effective use of self-management skills.

It is important to acknowledge that all pregnancies, including those complicated by diabetes, have the same goal, which is a healthy outcome for both mother and infant. This chapter begins with a review of the components of every pregnancy: adequate weight gain, healthy eating, and regular physical activity. An additional goal for pregnancies complicated by diabetes is to achieve glycemic stability without sacrificing weight gain, good nutrition, or physical activity.

Normal Pregnancy

Physiology of Pregnancy

The fetus depends on an adequate but not excessive supply of fuel from maternal sources. Glucose, which is transported across the placenta via facilitated diffusion, is the fuel source preferred by the fetus over amino acids and free fatty acids.[6] The first trimester is often characterized by lower maternal glucose levels than in nonpregnant women. Hormonal levels (estrogen, progesterone, human placental lactogen) progressively increase in the second and third trimesters, resulting in increased insulin resistance. Fetal growth accelerates in the third trimester as free fatty acids are mobilized for maternal energy needs. This allows for additional placental transfer of glucose to the developing fetus. The normal response to the increased insulin resistance in pregnancy is progressively increasing insulin secretion, which may be 100% above nonpregnant levels by the third trimester (see Figure 24.1).

Weight Gain

The 2009 guidelines from the Institute of Medicine (IOM) provide the basis for determining appropriate weight gain during pregnancy.[7] Weight gain categories are based on the woman's prepregnancy body mass index (BMI) established by the World Health Organization (see Table 24.1). A high BMI increases both maternal and fetal risks, including hypertension, preeclampsia, macrosomia, operative or difficult delivery, and gestational diabetes. It is interesting to note that over 50% of women in their childbearing years have a BMI of 25 or higher at conception.[8]

The amount of weight gained during pregnancy may affect pregnancy outcomes. Excessive gestational weight gain is associated with heavier infants and greater postpartum weight retention. A key recommendation for all health professionals is to identify women at risk for excessive gestational weight gain early in the pregnancy and intervene to help manage their weight gain.

However, the weight gain guidelines may change based on a 2019 meta-analysis on maternal obesity and childhood outcomes. This meta-analysis of over 196,000

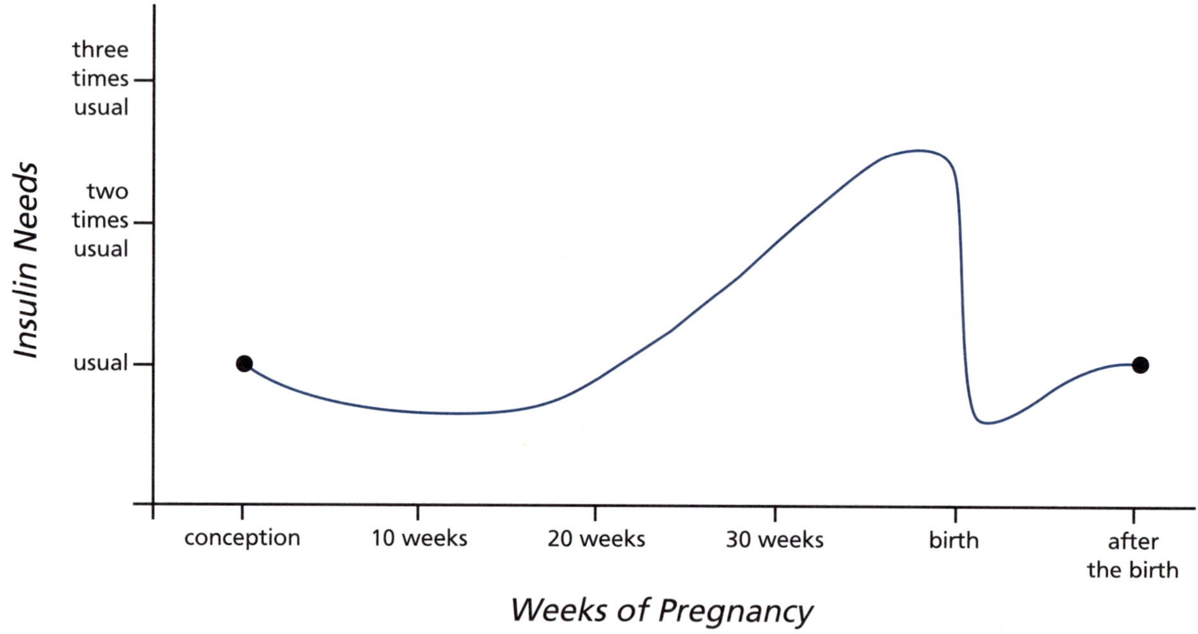

FIGURE 24.1 Normal Insulin Production in Pregnancy

Source: Reprinted with permission from *Pregnancy Planning and Care for Women With Diabetes* (Minneapolis, Minn: International Diabetes Center, 2012).

TABLE 24.1 Recommended Ranges of Total Weight Gain for Pregnant Women

Weight-for-Height Category	*Recommended Total Weight Gain (Singleton Gestation)*	*Weekly Weight Gain Rates in the Second and Third Trimesters (Singleton Gestation)*	*Recommended Total Weight Gain (Twin Gestation)*
Underweight (BMI* <18.6)	28–40 lb (12.7–18.2 kg)	1 lb (.5 kg)	
Normal weight (BMI 18.6–24.9)	25–35 lb (11.3–16 kg)	1 lb (.5 kg)	37–54 lb (16.8–24.5 kg)
Overweight (BMI 25.0–29.9)	15–25 lb (6.8–11.3 kg)	⅔ lb (.3 kg)	31–50 lb (14.1–22.7 kg)
Obese (BMI >30)	11–20 lb (4.5–9.0 kg)	½ lb (.25 kg)	25–42 lb (11.3–19.1 kg)

*BMI = weight/height^2

Source: National Academy of Sciences, *Weight Gain During Pregnancy: Reexamining the Guidelines* (Washington, DC: National Academy Press, 2009).

singleton pregnancies from Europe and North America addressed the relationships between gestational weight gain and clinical outcomes. This study showed lower risks for adverse outcomes, which included preeclampsia, gestational hypertension, gestational diabetes, cesarean delivery, preterm birth, small or large gestational age were associated with the following gestational weight gain ranges:

- BMI <18.5 kg/m^2 (underweight) – Weight gain 31 to <35 pounds (14.0 to <16.0 kg)
- BMI 18.5 to 24.9 kg/m^2 (normal weight) – Weight gain 22 to <40 pounds (10 to <18 kg)
- BMI 25.0 to 29.9 kg/m^2 (overweight) – Weight gain 4 to <35 pounds (2.0 to <16.0 kg)
- BMI 30.0 to 34.9 kg/m^2 (obesity class 1) – Weight gain 4 to <13 pounds (2.0 to <6.0 kg)
- BMI 35.0 to 39.9 kg/m^2 (obesity class 2) – Weight gain or loss 0 to <9 pounds (weight loss or gain of 0 to <4.0 kg)
- BMI ≥40.0 kg/m^2 (obesity class 3) – Weight gain 0 to <13 pounds (0 to <6.0 kg)

The IOM guidelines did not address weight gain among the various subclassifications of obesity nor did the guidelines evaluate the relationship between gestational weight gain and preeclampsia or GDM. This meta-analysis showed a stronger association with prepregnancy weight gain and adverse perinatal outcomes than gestational weight gain.[9]

Nutrition During Pregnancy

Most dietary recommendations for pregnant women without diabetes may be followed by women with diabetes. This includes appropriate weight gain and providing adequate nutrients for maternal and fetal health. Table 24.2 provides guidelines for the number of servings of fruit, vegetables, grains, dairy, meat, fats, and additional calories for a normal-weight woman who exercises less than 30 minutes a week.[10–12] Goals specific to diabetes will be addressed in subsequent sections.

Nutrition Requirements

Energy The dietary reference intakes (DRIs)[13,14] are used to determine the estimated energy requirements (EERs) in pregnancy, which are based on age, height, weight, and physical activity level. The EERs for pregnancy are as follows:

- *1st trimester:* Adult EER + 0
- *2nd trimester:* Adult EER + 160 kcal (8 kcal/wk × 20 wk) + 180 kcal
- *3rd trimester:* Adult EER + 272 kcal (8 kcal/wk × 34 wk) + 180 kcal

The 8 kcal per week represents the change in total energy expenditure due to pregnancy; the 180 kcal is the mean energy deposition during pregnancy. An example of estimated calorie needs for a 30-year-old woman with a BMI of 24.7 is provided in Table 24.3.

Protein The recommended dietary allowance (RDA) for protein in the nonpregnant woman is 0.8 g per kilogram per day, or 46 g per day. Protein requirements increase to 1.1 g per kilogram per day, or 25 g extra per day, for a singleton gestation and 50 g extra for twin pregnancies.[14]

Carbohydrate The DRI for carbohydrate in pregnant women aged 19 to 50 years is a minimum of 175 g per day.

TABLE 24.2 Sample Dietary Guidelines for Pregnancy*

	First Trimester	*Second Trimester*	*Third Trimester*	*Examples*
Total calories	1800	2200	2400	
Grains	6 servings	7 servings	8 servings	1 slice bread; ½ c potato, rice, pasta
Vegetables	2½ c	3 c	3 c	Carrots, broccoli, onion 2 c greens = 1 c vegetables
Fruits	1½ c	2 c	2 c	Whole fruit, juice
Milk	3 c	3 c	3 c	Milk, yogurt, cheese
Meat and beans	5 oz	6 oz	6½ oz	½ c beans = 1-oz serving of meat
Extras	290 calories	360 calories	410 calories	May come from additional food groups or from higher calorie, higher fat foods
Fats and oils	6 tsp	7 tsp	8 tsp	Oil, butter, nuts

*For a normal-weight woman who exercises less than 30 minutes per week

Source: MJ Franz, AB Evert, *American Diabetes Association Guide to Nutrition Therapy for Diabetes* (Washington, DC: American Diabetes Association, 2012).

TABLE 24.3 Example of EERs Before and During Pregnancy for a 30-Year-Old Woman With a BMI of 24.7 kg/m^2 (65 in [1.65 m] and 150 lb [68.0 kg])

Physical Activity Level	*Nonpregnant and First Trimester* *EER (kcal/d)*	*Second Trimester* *EER + 340 kcal**	*Third Trimester* *EER + 450 kcal**
Sedentary	1983	2300	2450
Low active	2203	2550	2650
Active	2479	2800	2950

*Calories rounded to the nearest 50

Source: MJ Franz, AB Evert, *American Diabetes Association Guide to Nutrition Therapy for Diabetes* (Washington, DC: American Diabetes Association, 2012).

This amount of carbohydrate provides an adequate source of glucose for fetal growth (approximately 33 g per day) and for the maternal brain.[14]

Vitamins and Minerals Adequate calcium, iron, folate, vitamin D, and magnesium intakes are especially important in pregnancy. Dietary reference intakes in pregnancy are listed in Table 24.4.

Safe Eating During Pregnancy

Nonnutritive Sweeteners

All nonnutritive sweeteners approved by the US Food and Drug Administration (FDA) are approved for use by the general public, which includes pregnant and lactating women.[15] However, the consensus of most registered dietitians (RDs) and diabetes care and education specialists is to limit the use to 3 servings or less during pregnancy and lactation.

Alcohol

Use of all alcoholic beverages during pregnancy is discouraged because of the risks of fetal alcohol spectrum disorders.[16]

Mercury-Contaminated Fish

The FDA has recommended that pregnant women and women of childbearing age avoid eating shark, swordfish, king mackerel, marlin, bigeye tuna, orange roughy, and tilefish (Gulf of Mexico) (https://www.fda.gov/food/consumers/advice-about-eating-fish). These fish often

TABLE 24.4 Dietary Reference Intakes for Pregnant and Lactating Women

Nutrient	*Pregnant Woman*	*Lactating Woman*
Protein (g)[1]	+25	+25
Vitamin A (mcg)		
14–18 years	750	1200
19–50 years	770	1300
Vitamin D (mcg)[2]	15	15
Vitamin K (mcg)		
14–18 years	75	75
19–50 years	90	90
Vitamin C (mg)		
14–18 years	80	115
19–50 years	85	120
Thiamin (mg)	1.4	1.4
Riboflavin (mg)	1.4	1.6
Niacin (mg NE)	18	17
Vitamin B_6 (mg)	1.9	2.0
Folate (mcg FE)	600	500
Vitamin B_{12} (mcg)	2.6	2.8
Calcium (mg)[2]		
14–18 years	1300	1300
19–50 years	1000	1000
Phosphorus (mg)		
14–18 years	1250	1250
19–50 years	700	700
Magnesium (mg)		
14–18 years	400	360
19–30 years	350	310
31–50 years	360	320
Iron (mg)		
14–18 years	27	10
19–50 years	27	9
Zinc (mg)		
14–18 years	12	13
19–50 years	11	12
Iodine (mcg)	220	290
Selenium (mcg)	60	70

Sources:

1. P Trumbo, S Schlicker, AA Yates, M Poos, "Dietary reference intakes for energy, carbohydrate, fiber, fat, fatty acids, cholesterol, protein and amino acids," J Am Diet Assoc. 102(2002):1621-30.
2. Institute of Medicine of the National Academies. Dietary Reference Intakes for Calcium and Vitamin D (Washington, DC: The National Academies Press, 2011).

contain high levels of methyl-mercury, a potent human neurotoxin, which readily crosses the placenta and has the potential to damage the fetal nervous system.[17] Women should consult their local health department for further fish advisories in their area.

Listeriosis

Food safety is of primary concern in pregnancy. The Centers for Disease Control and Prevention (CDC) estimates a fivefold increase in the risk of contracting listeriosis during pregnancy. Approximately one third of all listeriosis cases involve pregnant women. Listeriosis can be transmitted to the fetus via the placenta. The risks of listeriosis are preterm delivery, spontaneous abortion, and other complications. Pregnant women are advised to avoid the following:

- Deli meats, hot dogs, and luncheon meats, unless reheated until steaming hot
- Soft cheeses (such as feta, Brie, Camembert, blue-veined), queso blanco, and queso fresco (hard cheeses and pasteurized cheese are recommended)
- Refrigerated patés and meat spreads (canned and shelf-stable paté and meat spreads can be consumed)
- Refrigerated smoked seafood, unless cooked
- Raw or unpasteurized milk

Salmonella

Salmonella is another infection that can lead to complications during pregnancy. The complications include dehydration and bacteremia, which can lead to meningitis. Salmonella can be transmitted to the fetus, and babies born with salmonella infection may develop diarrhea or fever after birth. Pregnant women should avoid eating raw or undercooked eggs, poultry, and meat and unpasteurized milk or juice.

Physical Activity During Pregnancy

Physical activity guidelines for pregnancy and the postpartum period are as follows:[18,19]

- Healthy women who are not already highly active or performing vigorous-intensity activity should get at least 150 minutes of moderate-intensity aerobic activity per week during pregnancy and the postpartum period (see Table 24.5). However, there are certain obstetric or medical conditions that are contraindicated to physical activity in pregnancy (see Table 24.6).

TABLE 24.5 Examples of Safe Physical Activities During Pregnancy

• Walking	• Low-impact aerobics
• Swimming	• Jogging
• Water aerobics	• Strength training
• Stationary cycling	

TABLE 24.6 Absolute Contraindications for Physical Activity in Pregnancy

- Hemodynamically significant heart disease
- Restrictive lung disease
- Incompetent cervix/cervical cerclage
- Multiple gestation at risk of preterm labor
- Intrauterine growth retardation
- Persistent second- or third-trimester bleeding
- Placenta previa
- Preeclampsia or pregnancy-induced hypertension
- Premature labor or history of preterm labor
- Premature rupture of membranes
- Severe anemia

- Pregnant women who habitually engage in vigorous-intensity aerobic activity or are highly active can continue physical activity during pregnancy and the postpartum period, provided they remain healthy and discuss with their healthcare provider how and when activity should be adjusted over time.

Frequency and Duration of Physical Activity in Pregnancy

- *Goal of 30 minutes daily.* In the absence of medical or obstetric complications, pregnant women should participate in 30 minutes or more of moderate-intensity physical activity on most, if not all, days of the week.[16] Active women can continue similar activities during pregnancy.
- *Intervals as short as 10 minutes can be effective.* The physical activity can be short bouts of 10 minutes each, accumulated over the course of the day.
- *Sedentary lifestyle.* Pregnancy generally is not a time for a woman who was previously sedentary to initiate strenuous activity; however, walking is possible for most women, and a 15- to 20-minute walk can lower blood glucose by 20 to 40 mg/dL.

Breastfeeding

The EER for lactation is calculated from total energy expenditure, milk energy output, and energy mobilization from tissue stores.[14] In the first 6 months postpartum, lactating women experience an average weight loss of 0.8 kg per month, which is equivalent to 170 kcal per day. The milk energy output is approximately 500 kcal per day. As the infant is introduced to solid foods, usually at 6 months, the amount of milk produced is reduced and the milk energy output decreases to 400 kcal per day. The EER for lactation is as follows:

- *1st 6 months:* EER + 500 – 170 (milk energy output – weight loss)
- *2nd 6 months:* EER + 400 – 0 (milk energy output – weight loss)
- *RDA for protein:* 1.1 g per kilogram per day, or an additional 25 g per day (same as in pregnancy)[14]
- *RDA for carbohydrate:* 210 g per day[14]

Diabetes in Pregnancy

Preconception Care and Education

Evidence shows that intensive diabetes management can improve the perinatal outcome.[20] For women with preexisting diabetes, care should begin before conception, which is sometimes referred to as the "12-month pregnancy."

Case: Type 1 Diabetes—A Pregnancy With Preconception Care

PB, a 33-year-old woman with type 1 diabetes for 18 years, was referred by a diabetes treatment center to a maternal-fetal medicine specialist for obstetrical care. She was confirmed as 7 weeks pregnant during her first prenatal visit. This is her third pregnancy; her previous pregnancies ended in first-trimester spontaneous abortions 4 and 5 years ago (at 8 weeks and 10 weeks gestation, respectively). In planning for this pregnancy, PB was instructed by the diabetes center to delay conception until her blood glucose levels were at optimal levels (A1C <6.5%).

Case: Type 1 Diabetes—A Pregnancy With Preconception Care (continued)

Preconception Care and Education

PB delayed conception for 6 months using a low-dose progestin-only oral contraceptive agent until her A1C was 6.3%. The following protocol was established to achieve optimal diabetes stability before PB attempted conception:

- Discuss safe and realistic goals (her husband was included in the decision-making process).
- Assess any vascular complications; include a dilated retinal examination, thyroid function tests, kidney function testing to determine creatinine, creatinine clearance, and microalbumin, and an EKG. She had proliferative retinopathy and received laser photocoagulation therapy 7 years ago. Her last episode of diabetic ketoacidosis (DKA) occurred 3 years ago, and she began experiencing neuropathy in her feet at age 24.
- Refer for genetic counseling because of a family history of diabetes. PB's father has type 2 diabetes, and her 25-year-old brother was diagnosed with type 1 diabetes at age 9.
- Refer to an RD for adjustments to her food plan.
- Begin folic acid supplementation of 400 mcg per day.
- Assess her self-management skills, including insulin administration, glucose monitoring, and treatment of hypoglycemic episodes.
- Continue contraception until glucose goals are attained.

Care and Education During Pregnancy

Pathophysiology in Type 1 Diabetes

PB began her pregnancy with planning and implementing efforts to optimize her glycemic stability and improve the outcomes.

Diabetes Management During Pregnancy

At her first prenatal visit, PB brought her last laboratory tests, from 10 weeks ago, and blood glucose records. Her A1C was 6.3% and hemoglobin and hematocrit were 13.8 mg/dL and 40.6%, respectively. Her recent assessment of kidney function (24-hour urine for protein and creatinine) was within normal limits. Her BMI was 22.4. Her fasting blood glucose ranged from 75 to 115 mg/dL (4.2 to 6.4 mmol/L), premeal 58 to 132 mg/dL (3.2 to 7.4 mmol/L), and 1 hour postprandial 115 to 145 mg/dL (6.4 to 8.1 mmol/L). PB monitors her blood glucose 7 times a day (fasting, premeal, 1 hour postmeal, and bedtime), and her insulin regimen is 4 injections per day, with rapid-acting insulin before meals and a long-acting insulin analog (detemir) before bedtime.

Complications

Care and education are important to achieve and maintain optimal glycemic levels and improve perinatal outcome. PB had proliferative diabetic retinopathy and is at higher risk for progression of the condition during pregnancy. She has also experienced DKA in the past. Since conception was delayed until her glycemic levels were in optimal control, the risk for fetal complications was decreased.

Healthy Coping

Facing some stressful and fearful situations, PB needed support from the diabetes care team and her family. The diabetes center recommended continuous subcutaneous insulin infusion (CSII), which PB had avoided in the past but was now considering because of the pregnancy. She indicated her willingness to comply with all instructions to ensure that this pregnancy was carried to term, but also expressed cautious optimism because of her past obstetric history. She was referred to a social worker to discuss her concerns.

Healthy Eating

PB denied use of alcohol and drugs. With early morning nausea, occasional vomiting, and an aversion to cooking odors, her appetite has decreased in the past 2 weeks.

Care Plan

As a result of preparations made early in the pregnancy and even before conception, the following elements of care were planned as optimal management during pregnancy:

- Maternal and fetal surveillance and testing (eg, nuchal translucency, ultrasound, nonstress test, biophysical profile, maternal serum alpha fetal protein, and amniocentesis/chorionic villus sampling [PB opted not to have the either procedure])
- Referral to an ophthalmologist for a baseline eye exam to detect changes during pregnancy
- Referral to an RD for medical nutrition therapy (MNT)
- Referrals to other specialists, as necessary

Diabetes Education

The following were identified as topics for which PB required education and/or intervention:

- *Diabetic ketoacidosis prevention:* Teach PB how to prevent DKA.
- *Risks:* Discuss with PB and her husband the risks associated with type 1 diabetes and pregnancy.

(continued)

Case: Type 1 Diabetes—A Pregnancy With Preconception Care (continued)

- *Intensity of care:* Explain how prenatal care is more intensive than preconception care and includes frequent obstetrical visits and tests.
- *Hypoglycemia:* Assess the husband's knowledge of signs and symptoms of hypoglycemia and how to treat.
- *Assessment of social-emotional well-being:* Assess PB's response to feelings, since the 2 earlier pregnancies ended in miscarriage; if necessary, refer the couple to a social worker or behavioral health specialist to discuss their feelings regarding this pregnancy.

Medical Nutrition Therapy

PB was referred to an RD to evaluate her eating habits and was provided information on the following:

- Weight gain guidelines according to her prepregnancy BMI[5,21]
- Managing nausea and vomiting to avoid hypoglycemia
- Managing other gastrointestinal discomforts that may occur (eg, heartburn, constipation, ptyalism)
- Use of nonnutritive sweeteners during pregnancy
- Food safety issues
- Physical activity, if no contraindications
- Infant feeding plans
- Keeping food records

To avoid hypoglycemia, PB had to maintain consistency in her meal and snack times and portion sizes. Her insulin-to-carbohydrate ratios may be different during the pregnancy. For example, the insulin-to-carbohydrate ratio at breakfast may be greater than at other meals because of increased cortisol and growth hormone levels that appear to contribute to morning glucose intolerance. Monitoring of blood glucose levels, blood or urine ketones, appetite, and weight gain guided the RD in developing an appropriate individualized food plan and in making adjustments to this plan throughout the pregnancy.[22]

Insulin Therapy

Aspects of insulin therapy that needed to be addressed through diabetes education included glucose targets during pregnancy and the need to adjust her insulin regimen as the pregnancy progressed.

- *Glucose targets.* Optimal blood glucose stability is necessary to decrease the risk of complications in pregnancy. Treatment of hypoglycemia is necessary if blood glucose levels are below 60 mg/dL (3.3 mmol/L). Changes in blood glucose recommendations for pregnancy were discussed (lower than prepregnancy values). PB's last episode of DKA was 3 years ago. The signs, symptoms, and management of DKA were discussed. More frequent self-monitoring of her blood glucose levels is appropriate, especially if she experiences nocturnal hypoglycemia.
- *Changing insulin requirements.* PB was told that her insulin regimen would change throughout the pregnancy. Her requirements might decrease during the first trimester but increase in the second and even triple by the third trimester. The benefits of CSII were discussed.

PB decided to delay switching to the insulin pump until after delivery. She was engaged with her diabetes and pregnancy regimen. She did not miss any appointments with her healthcare provider, diabetes care and education specialist, or RD. Blood glucose records were consistently kept and verified by her glucose meter, as were food records, which were e-mailed to the dietitian. The results of both maternal and fetal surveillances were normal, and PB discovered during an ultrasound appointment that she was having a girl! PB and her husband attended childbirth education classes offered at the hospital where she would deliver.

Diabetes Care During Labor and Delivery

PB's blood glucose levels were frequently monitored, and insulin and glucose were administered as necessary. At 39 weeks gestation and after 6 hours of labor, she vaginally delivered baby Brianna, a 3,540-g girl.

Postpartum Care and Education

Lactation

PB decided very early in the pregnancy that she would breastfeed. Brianna spent a day in the neonatal intensive care unit to be assessed for any anomalies or complications. With no complications, she was reunited with her mother. Because PB knew her milk production might be delayed, she began pumping soon after delivery. She noticed a drop in her glucose level whenever Brianna nursed. PB received a visit from the lactation consultant during her hospital stay, and the diabetes nurse educator called her to discuss postpartum glycemic changes.

Assessment Phone Call

Two weeks after delivery, the diabetes nurse educator phoned PB again to assess how she was adjusting to motherhood. PB told her that breastfeeding was going well and Brianna was gaining weight. PB's insulin requirements had decreased, which necessitated more frequent glucose monitoring. To assess for postpartum depression, the diabetes care and

Case: Type 1 Diabetes—A Pregnancy With Preconception Care (continued)

education specialist asked PB how she felt emotionally; PB denied any emotional changes.

Office Visit

PB made an appointment with the diabetes care and education specialist to discuss changes to her regimen during the postpartum period. The diabetes care and education specialist stressed the need to maintain optimal glycemic levels for the duration of the breastfeeding period and while weaning. During the appointment, PB informed the diabetes care and education specialist that although she was happy being a new mother, she wanted to wait at least 2 years before attempting to conceive again. The diabetes care and education specialists reviewed contraceptives that were safe while breastfeeding and after weaning, and discussed postpartum depression. After her 6-week postpartum checkup, PB was scheduled to return to the diabetes center for care and to make an appointment with the RD to discuss weight loss and adjustments to her food plan.

Preconception care, as demonstrated with PB's case, is key to improving outcomes in pregnancies complicated by diabetes. Both the American Diabetes Association (ADA) and the American College of Obstetricians and Gynecologists (ACOG) recommend that diabetes care and education begin before conception.[1,5] Sufficient time must be allowed to evaluate the mother's health status and to normalize or maximize glycemic stability, thereby offering the best chance for the fetus.

Case: Type 2 Diabetes—A Pregnancy Requiring Hospitalization

LR is a 27-year-old Hispanic woman who, at 13 weeks' gestation, was referred to a high-risk obstetrical clinic for her first pregnancy. She had fainted at home and was taken to the emergency room, where the pregnancy was confirmed by ultrasound. She was admitted from the emergency room when her random blood glucose level was 210 mg/dL (11.7 mmol/L). At her initial prenatal visit, LR weighed 248 lb.

Preconception Care and Education

LR never received preconception counseling. She was diagnosed with type 2 diabetes 4 years ago and was prescribed metformin (Glucophage®, Bristol-Myers Squibb), 1000 mg twice a day, but stopped taking it a year ago. When asked why, she replied, "I sometimes forget to take my medication."

Care and Education During Pregnancy

Pathophysiology of Type 2 Diabetes

LR presented for her first visit with many challenges, which included an unstable home environment. She needed the help of a comprehensive diabetes care team.

Diabetes Management During Pregnancy

LR was unsure of her weight prior to this pregnancy, but weighed 248 lb at her initial prenatal visit; she is 62.5 inches tall. Her A1C was 11.0% and hematocrit was 38.7 mg/dL. She complained of recurrent urinary tract infections (UTIs) and is currently taking antibiotics.

Assessment

It is important to assess why LR discontinued the diabetes treatment plan, including her medications. Her family history includes diabetes in both maternal and paternal grandfathers. She has experienced some significant changes in her life, including an unplanned pregnancy and a recent separation; additional information is needed about her current living conditions. Referral to a social worker or mental health professional would be helpful in establishing baseline information on her willingness and ability to follow a care plan.

- What is her current relationship with her husband? Is there anyone who could assist her during the pregnancy?
- What is her financial situation? Does she have health insurance? If not, is she able to purchase diabetes supplies such as insulin and syringes, test strips, and lancets?
- Is she willing to follow an intensive insulin regimen and monitor her blood glucose levels multiple times daily?

Complications

LR has been experiencing frequent UTIs and might be vulnerable to other complications associated with obesity—such as chronic hypertension, obstructive sleep apnea, preeclampsia, higher rate of cesarean sections, and difficult delivery. Careful and comprehensive assessment for complications was required, and appropriate interventions were initiated. At each subsequent visit, LR was screened for UTI.

Insulin Therapy

LR was started on an insulin regimen of 4 injections daily: lispro before meals, detemir at night. She monitors her blood glucose levels 4 times daily (fasting and 1-hour postprandial). She was immediately started on insulin to normalize her glycemic levels. The initial insulin initiation was calculated at 1.5 units per kilogram of actual body weight. The insulin

(continued)

Case: Type 2 Diabetes—A Pregnancy Requiring Hospitalization (continued)

dose may increase to 2.0 units per kilogram because of third trimester insulin resistance. Insulin dose is typically higher In women with type 2 diabetes than in women with type 1 diabetes because they are typically more insulin resistant than women with type 1 diabetes in the third trimester.

Medical Nutrition Therapy

LR received MNT when first diagnosed with type 2 diabetes but followed the food plan for only about 6 months. She found that the food plan from her current admission was difficult to follow at home. The original food plan was modified by the RD to include LR's food preferences. LR was income-eligible for WIC and Food Stamps and a referral was made to these programs. By the third visit with the dietitian, LR was following the food plan. She had decided to formula-feed the baby.

Diabetes Education

LR needed information about the risks she and her baby may encounter, healthy and reasonable expectations regarding weight gain, mental preparation for the increase in antenatal testing, and support regarding her use of the food plan.

Risks

LR needed assistance in understanding that obese pregnant women with type 2 diabetes are at higher risk for adverse pregnancy outcomes than pregnant women without diabetes.

- *Weight.* She received information on weight gain guidelines and the importance of avoiding weight loss to decrease the risk for starvation ketosis and intrauterine growth retardation. She was informed that calorie restriction is not recommended during pregnancy.
- *Food plan.* She was given information on how women with type 2 diabetes may benefit from a lower calorie food plan of no fewer than 1800 calories a day. Effective implementation of MNT could help LR avoid ketosis and provide adequate nutrients.
- *Medical care.* Maternal and fetal monitoring would begin according to the gestational week. Because of the elevated A1C at conception, in addition to the usual laboratory testing in diabetes and pregnancy, LR would be offered anatomy scan (level 2 ultrasound) to assess fetal anatomy as well as an amniocentesis or chorionic villus sampling to detect chromosomal abnormalities. She learned that frequent monitoring was necessary to assess fetal well-being.
- *Glycemic stability.* She was informed about the value of good glycemic management in the short and long term, for her and her baby's health.

LR works as a part-time school bus aide and set up appointments with the diabetes care and education specialist between bus runs. She expressed gratitude for the assistance. She met with the social worker and was referred for financial assistance to help with insulin and monitoring supplies. The result of the nuchal transparency test (screening test to detect trisomy 21 (Down's syndrome) was negative. Having learned from the diabetes care and education specialist that maternal glycemic levels can affect the fetus, LR followed her medication and monitoring schedule.

Preconception Counseling for Women With Preexisting Diabetes

Preconception care is a set of preventive and management interventions that identify and modify risk factors that may affect pregnancy outcome.[23,24] The CDC recommends incorporating preconception care into the routine health care of all women of childbearing age. However, since more than half of all pregnancies in the United States are unplanned or unintended, most women do not receive preconception care, including those with preexisting diabetes, prediabetes, or previous GDM.[24] The ACOG recommends preconception counseling for women with preexisting diabetes as a beneficial and cost-effective service.[25] Preconception counseling that focuses on achieving euglycemia prior to and during the critical period of organogenesis may help prevent anomalies.

In a study that examined preconception counseling rates in managed care, 52% of the women recalled a discussion on glucose management with their health-care provider, and only 37% received advice on family planning.[26] Women with type 2 diabetes tend not to be referred for preconception care as often as their type 1 diabetes counterparts.[27] An Australian study showed that while 27.8% of women with type 1 diabetes received preconception counseling, only 12% of those with type 2 diabetes received the same services.[28]

Elevated maternal glucose levels during organogenesis are associated with higher rates of congenital anomalies and spontaneous abortions. The risk of complications decreases if the woman with diabetes enters pregnancy in optimal blood glucose stability. The lowest risk of congenital anomalies is associated with an A1C level that is less than 6.5% at conception.[29] An effective method of contraception should be used until the desired glycemic results are achieved.

According to the ACOG Practice Bulletin on pregestational diabetes mellitus. effective forms of reversible (non-permanent) contraception include intrauterine devices or implantable progestin, which do not appear to affect glycemic stability. Other options include low-dose combination oral contraceptives for women who are non-smokers and without vascular disease. Women with diabetes and vascular disease should be prescribed progestin-only pills.[2] ADA does not specify which type of contraception is recommended for women with preexisting diabetes. Their recommendation is the same as for women without diabetes as the risk of an unplanned pregnancy outweighs the risk of any contraception option.[29]

A pregnant woman with preexisting diabetes may or may not have received self-management instructions prior to conception. She may not be aware of the importance of optimal glycemic stability and how best to avoid the complications associated with hyperglycemia in pregnancy, such as congenital anomalies and macrosomia. Without preconception counseling, a woman may not be prepared to apply problem-solving and self-management skills to the critical situations that may arise quickly in early pregnancy or in emergency situations that may require hospitalization. Plans for diabetes education during pregnancy must thus factor in whether the woman had preconception care. Topics that may be covered, particularly in the first trimester, include:

- Keeping glycemic levels at optimal levels
- Mild to severe hypoglycemia as a result of increased insulin sensitivity
- Increased visits with the diabetes team at the beginning of pregnancy
- Continuation of successful self-management skills

Preconception care for the woman with preexisting diabetes is conducted with a multidisciplinary team. The initial preconception visit consists of a comprehensive medical and obstetrical history, physical examination, laboratory evaluation, and management plan. The woman should be referred for evaluations of her renal and retinal status, peripheral and autonomic neuropathy, hypoglycemic risk, peripheral vascular disease, and thyroid.[20] Certain medications, such as statins, angiotensin II receptor blockers, and angiotensin converting enzyme inhibitors, are contraindicated during pregnancy. Healthcare providers will generally change these medications to those less teratogenic to the fetus. Women with type 2 diabetes or prediabetes on oral glucose-lowering medications will most likely switch to insulin. According to the ADA's position statement on preconception care, the woman should be seen at 1- to 2-month intervals until her A1C results indicate stable glycemic levels and the risk and status of her diabetes complications have decreased.[30] When these 2 goals are achieved, contraception can be discontinued; however, preconception care should continue until pregnancy occurs.

The 2019 ADA Standards of Medical Care also recommend that women with preexisting diabetes be counseled on the risk of development and/or progression of diabetic retinopathy. Eye examinations should occur before pregnancy.[27]

Pathophysiology

In the first trimester, women with type 1 diabetes may actually experience a decrease in their insulin requirements as glycemic levels fall and insulin sensitivity increases.[22,31] However, if the glycemic levels are elevated around conception and organogenesis, the risk of congenital malformations and spontaneous abortions increases. As the pregnancy progresses, the absence of maternal pancreatic beta cell function increases the concentration of glucose, fatty acids, ketones, and amino acids transported across the placenta to the fetus. Exogenous insulin requirements may increase two- to threefold over pre-pregnant amounts to maintain euglycemia and reduce the risk of fetal complications. Pedersen hypothesized that maternal hyperglycemia is the primary reason for fetal hyperinsulinemia resulting from the overstimulation of fetal pancreatic beta cells.[32] Other factors that affect fetal growth include insulin growth factors, leptin, and tumor necrosis factor.[33]

Women with type 2 diabetes may also experience hypoglycemia in early pregnancy. Hyperglycemia in the first trimester will also increase the risk of poor perinatal outcome. As insulin resistance increases, beta cell function declines while glucose levels rise. In both types of diabetes, glycemic levels worsens because of the effects of elevated maternal and placental hormonal levels. Whether type 1 or type 2 diabetes, self-management education should prepare the woman for the expected increase in insulin requirements in the second and third trimesters when hormone levels increase, resulting in greater insulin resistance.

Complications

Maternal

Diabetes can affect the health of the mother and the fetus in T1DP and T2DP. Complications may have predated or develop during the pregnancy. Specific complications are described below.

Diabetic Retinopathy Hormones, such as growth hormone and insulin-like growth factor (IGF-1), along with the rise in estrogen, progesterone, and cortisol levels, may accelerate retinopathy.[34,35] Rosenn et al[36] found that pregnancy-induced hypertension or chronic hypertension was the most important risk factor associated with the progression of retinopathy in pregnancy. Rapid normalization of blood glucose can cause acute progression of retinopathy.[37] Pregnant women with diabetes and no background or mild retinopathy are less likely to have progression than those with advanced retinopathy. In most situations, background retinopathy that occurs during pregnancy regresses after delivery. If the woman has untreated proliferative retinopathy, pregnancy should be delayed until after laser photocoagulation.

Diabetic Nephropathy Hypertension, increased glomerular filtration rate, increased protein intake and excretion, and poor glycemic management are factors that contribute to the development of diabetic nephropathy. Diabetic nephropathy is associated with poor pregnancy outcome. Optimal maternal hypertensive and glycemic management may improve renal function and slow the progression of nephropathy during and after pregnancy. Angiotensin converting enzyme inhibitors are contraindicated during pregnancy because of potential fetal risks.

Diabetic Neuropathy Diabetic neuropathy can be divided into peripheral neuropathy (eg, numbness, tingling, or burning in the feet) and autonomic neuropathy (eg, gastroparesis). There are few studies on the effect of pregnancy on diabetic neuropathy. Gastroparesis is often associated with poor glycemic stability; women with severe gastroparesis should not become pregnant, because of the association of gastroparesis with maternal (pulmonary edema) and fetal complications (intrauterine fetal restriction and preterm labor). However, glycemic management may improve the symptoms of slow gastric emptying.

Hypertension Hypertension in pregnancy is classified into 4 categories based on guidelines by the ACOG Task Force in Hypertension in Pregnancy (see Table 24.7).[38] The incidence of hypertensive disorders in pregnancy, including preeclampsia, is higher in women with diabetes as a result of poor glycemic management.[39]

Diabetic Ketoacidosis Women with type 1 diabetes are at greater risk of developing diabetic ketoacidosis (DKA) than women with type 2 diabetes. According to the ADA's Standards of Medical Care in Diabetes, the risk of diabetic ketoacidosis occurs at blood glucose levels that are lower than those of the nonpregnant woman with diabetes.[29] Diabetic ketoacidosis increases the risk of fetal demise. Other factors associated with DKA include infections, hyperemesis, gastroparesis, corticosteroids, beta-sympathomimetic agents for tocolysis, and insulin pump failure.[40,41]

Polyhydramnios Polyhydramnios is defined as excessive amniotic fluid and is associated with an increased risk of preterm birth, placental abruption, and fetal anomalies. Diabetes (maternal hyperglycemia) is a risk factor for polyhydramnios.

Complications Associated With Obesity Obesity is a risk factor associated with a higher incidence of perinatal mortality and morbidity.[7,42] Complications associated with obesity in pregnancy include chronic hypertension, obstructive sleep apnea, preeclampsia, increased UTIs, and higher rates of cesarean and difficult deliveries in the mother.[42]

Fetal

Congenital Malformations Congenital anomalies occur during organogenesis (the first 8 weeks of gestation) and are more common in women with preexisting diabetes.[29] In a large Danish study that compared pregnancy outcomes in T1DP with a nondiabetes population, the perinatal complications in the former group

TABLE 24.7 Hypertensive Disorders in Pregnancy

Preeclampsia–eclampsia	Hypertension in association with thrombocytopenia, impaired liver function, the new development of renal insufficiency, pulmonary edema, or new-onset cerebral or visual disturbances
Chronic hypertension	Hypertension that predates pregnancy
Preeclampsia superimposed on chronic hypertension	Chronic hypertension in association with preeclampsia
Gestational hypertension	BP elevation after 20 weeks of gestation in the absence of proteinuria

Source: Hypertension in Pregnancy (Washington, DC: The American College of Obstetricians and Gynecologists, 2013).

were higher in women with increasing A1C levels and poor self-care.[43] Wren et al found a fivefold increase in the risk of cardiovascular malformations in infants born to women with preexisting diabetes compared with women without diabetes.[44] Birth defects associated with preexisting diabetes in pregnancy are listed in Table 24.14.

Fetal demise. Women with preexisting diabetes and without prenatal care or seek care late during the pregnancy are at higher risk of late-term fetal demise. Fetal demise at late term is also associated with higher HbA1C values.[2]

Protecting Pregnant Women From Influenza

Since pregnancy is considered an immunocompromised state, influenza is more likely to cause severe illness than in women who are not pregnant. The CDC's Advisory Committee on Immunization Practice and ACOG recommend that all adults receive an annual influenza vaccine. This includes pregnant women and the vaccine can be safely given in any trimester. No studies or data have reported any adverse effects of pregnant women receiving the flu vaccine except for one small retrospective case-control study. This small study suggested a possible association between a certain type of flu vaccine given early in the first trimester and spontaneous abortion in women who also received the same vaccine In the previous flu season. However, this study was noted to have major flaws nor has not been replicated.

The fetus is also protected from the flu virus and women who were vaccinated were less likely to be hospitalized; this included less hospital admissions for their infants.

Only persons who have a severe allergy to the flu vaccine should not be vaccinated. This does not include persons with a mild allergy to eggs indicated by hives. People with mild egg allergies are still encouraged to get the vaccine.

Flu season in the United States is typically from October to May; and the influenza vaccine should ideally be given around the end of October.

Sources: The Centers for Disease Control and Prevention Influenza, on the Internet at http://www.cdc.gov/flu/highrisk/qa_vacpregnant.htm

(Reference: American College of Obstetricians and Gynecologists. Committee Opinion. Number 732. "Influenza vaccination during pregnancy," Obstet Gynecol. 131(2018): e109-14)

Other Fetal Complications Other problems associated with unstable glucose levels in the infant include macrosomia, neonatal hypoglycemia, respiratory distress syndrome, neonatal hypocalcemia, polycythemia, and hyperbilirubinemia.

Macrosomia Macrosomia is defined as infant birth weight greater than 4,000 or 4,500 g.[45] Macrosomic infants have trunks and shoulders that are disproportionately larger than the head. A cesarean section is often indicated to prevent birth trauma if the infant birth weight exceeds 4,500 g.[46]

Neonatal Hypoglycemia Neonatal hypoglycemia in the newborn is dependent on the age of the infant and whether the infant is asymptomatic or symptomatic for hypoglycemia. An asymptomatic infant is fed within 1 hour after birth and the blood glucose level is checked after 30 minutes. If the initial blood glucose screen is less than 25 mg/dL (1.9 mmol/L), the infant is re-fed and checked in 1 hour. If the result after 1 hour is still less than 25 mg/dL (1.9 mmol/L), the infant will be given intravenous glucose. The target glucose screen is greater than 45 mg/dL (2.5 mmol/L), and in the preterm infant, less than 25 mg/dL (1.4 mmol/L). Risks associated with neonatal hypoglycemia include seizures, cerebral damage, and death.[47]

Respiratory Distress Syndrome Respiratory distress syndrome (RDS) is a condition commonly seen in premature infants in which the lungs are not fully developed. This is caused by a deficiency of surfactant that is necessary for inflating the lungs. Infants born with RDS have difficulty breathing and may require supplemental oxygen at birth.[32]

Neonatal Hypocalcemia Neonatal hypocalcemia is a total serum calcium concentration less than 8 mg/dL (2 mmol/L) in term infants or less than 7 mg/dL (1.75 mmol/L) in preterm infants.[32] Pregnant women with diabetes tend to have higher than normal ionized calcium levels. While it is not well understood, hypocalcemia in the infants of women with diabetes may be caused by lower parathyroid concentrations. Higher maternal ionized calcium concentration may suppress the fetal parathyroid glands.

Polycythemia Babies born with polycythemia have a hematocrit greater than 65%.[32] This increase in red blood cells could result in hypoxia caused by insufficient oxygen to fetal tissues.

Hyperbilirubinemia Hyperbilirubinemia is a common condition in newborns that is characterized by

TABLE 24.8 AADE7 Self-Care Behaviors® for Diabetes and Pregnancy*

Healthy coping	Refer to childbirth education Understand the necessity of a higher degree of intensive care, including more frequent healthcare visits Obtain support and referral, as necessary Offer support and referral if needed Guide development of a positive and cooperative response to lifestyle changes; emphasize benefits to the baby GDM—Acknowledge common emotional reactions to the diagnosis: fear, anger, guilt
Healthy eating	Consume adequate calories to avoid weight loss and ketone production Consume adequate nutrients for maternal stores and fetal growth and development; consume adequate intakes of fruit, vegetables, dairy, and protein Avoid alcohol and other substances that could be harmful to the fetus Avoid foods that can lead to foodborne illnesses Minimum carbohydrate intake of 175 g per day Manage total and per-meal carbohydrate based on food plan and medications Match carbohydrate with rapid-acting or bolus insulin using insulin-to-carbohydrate ratio Avoid high-carbohydrate, low-nutrient foods, such as sweetened soft drinks May need to reduce/restrict foods with a high glycemic index
Being active	Participate in daily physical activity, if no contraindications Carry extra carbohydrate for hypoglycemia prevention, if taking oral glucose-lowering agents or insulin
Monitoring	Monitor fasting, premeal, and postmeal blood glucose levels; frequency and targets determined by healthcare provider Test ketones as instructed by healthcare provider Keep food and blood glucose records as instructed by healthcare team Self-monitoring of blood glucose is used to make therapy adjustments Continuous glucose monitoring may be used to assess trends in blood glucose levels A1C is not used to determine the need for therapy adjustments
Taking medications	Understand that insulin requirements increase as pregnancy progresses Understand that certain oral glucose-lowering agents and other medications for cardiometabolic risk may be discontinued until after delivery GDM—Women with GDM may need glucose-lowering medication in addition to MNT
Reducing risks	Identify and treat hypoglycemia for women using glucose-lowering medications Understand risk of maternal hyperglycemia on fetal outcome Manage weight to decrease long-term health risks Understand the importance of fetal surveillance (eg, kick counts, serial ultrasounds) GDM—Describe risk of developing type 2 diabetes postpartum; encourage lifestyle changes that lead to diabetes prevention
Problem solving	Identify symptoms and treatment of hypoglycemia and hyperglycemia Identify criteria for when to contact the healthcare provider Schedule follow-up visits with healthcare providers and diabetes care and education specialists to review self-management skills

*These behaviors apply to all pregnant women with diabetes unless otherwise specified.

the yellowing of the skin and eyes. This is caused by an increase in the level of bilirubin after birth. A total serum bilirubin level above 5 mg/dL (0.28 mmol/L) in the neonate is considered abnormal.[32]

AADE7 Self-Care Behaviors® During Pregnancy: Preexisting Diabetes

The AADE7 Self-Care Behaviors® provide a framework to assess and evaluate outcomes throughout pregnancy in women with preexisting or gestational diabetes (see Table 24.8). The following section covers managing women with preexisting diabetes.

Healthy Eating

An individualized food plan is important to optimize blood glucose stability. Medical nutrition therapy for preexisting diabetes in pregnancy has 4 important goals:

- Assist in appropriate gestational weight gain
- Avoid maternal ketosis
- Provide adequate nutrients for maternal and fetal health
- Minimize blood glucose excursions

Energy Requirements

Adequate calories are necessary to provide for fetal growth and to avoid ketonemia from either ketoacidosis or accelerated starvation ketosis in all pregnant women.[21] Adjustments to the food plan may be necessary to compensate for erratic blood glucose levels caused by fluctuating hormonal levels.

Carbohydrate Guidelines for Preexisting Diabetes

The amount and distribution of calories and carbohydrates are individualized and based on the woman's food preferences, blood glucose records, and physical activity level. Mealtime insulin must match the amount of mealtime carbohydrate to keep glucose levels in the target range before and after eating. Many women use an insulin-to-carbohydrate ratio to determine mealtime insulin. Since insulin requirements increase substantially during pregnancy, the insulin-to-carbohydrate ratio will change frequently during the second half of the pregnancy.

Being Active

The ADA recommends at least 150 minutes of moderate-intensity aerobic physical activity every week for persons with diabetes.[29] Regular exercise has been shown to improve blood glucose levels, reduce cardiovascular risk factors, contribute to weight loss, and improve well-being. In pregnancy, physical activity and exercise promote physical fitness and may prevent excessive weight gain. Pregnant women with medical or obstetric complications, including diabetes, should be carefully evaluated by their obstetric care providers prior to their provider making recommendations on physical activity participation during pregnancy.[18,48] If there are no contraindications, pregnant women with diabetes are encouraged to participate in regular physical activity.

Diabetes, Pregnancy, and Physical Activity Self-Care Instructions

Diabetes education should include the following:

- Explain to the woman that, as with any physical activity for persons with diabetes, planning, adjustments, and education for safety are needed.
- Instruct the woman using insulin or oral glucose-lowering agents to always carry additional carbohydrate in case of hypoglycemia.
- Advise the woman to always carry a medical ID (such as a bracelet) which identifies her as having diabetes.
- Advise the woman to test her blood glucose before and after physical activity.
- Teach the woman to palpate her uterus during physical activity to detect contractions.
- Caution the woman against becoming dehydrated, overheated, tachycardic (heart rate >140 bpm), or dyspneic.
- Advise the woman of contraindications for physical activity in pregnancy, which include abnormally high or low blood glucose levels (see Table 24.9).

Monitoring

Although there is a lack of agreement regarding precise glucose thresholds and timings, maintaining normal blood glucose levels remains the ultimate goal in the management of diabetes and pregnancy. Table 24.10 summarizes the ranges of plasma glucose targets recommended by the ADA, the ACOG, and other experts. Diabetes management is monitored through measurements of glycemic levels, ketones, and A1C as discussed below.[20]

Blood Glucose

Self-monitoring of blood glucose (SMBG) is needed pre- and postprandially in T1DP to evaluate the effectiveness of rapid-acting or short-acting insulin. No studies have specifically compared preprandial with postprandial

TABLE 24.9 Physical Activity Guidelines for Pregnant Women With Preexisting Diabetes

- Discuss with healthcare provider to determine safety, type, and duration of the physical activity.
- Get screened for proliferative retinopathy, neuropathy, and cardiovascular disease.
- Monitor blood glucose levels before, during, and after physical activity.
- Add carbohydrate if the glucose level before physical activity is <100 mg/dL (5.6 mmol/L) and the woman is taking insulin.
- Avoid vigorous activity in the presence of ketones. However, physical activity does not need to be postponed if the woman feels well and urine and/or blood ketones are negative.
- Be aware of immediate and prolonged hypoglycemia after the physical activity.
- Carry a readily available form of glucose at all times to treat hypoglycemia, if necessary.
- Avoid injecting insulin into an extremity to be used during exercising.
- Inject insulin 1 hour prior to exercising.
- If blood glucose level is >250 mg/dL, check urine for ketones; if ketones are present, delay exercise until glucose levels are more stable and ketones are resolved.
- Avoid physical activity during peak insulin action times.
- Learn to palpate uterus to detect contractions.

Sources: Adapted from American Diabetes Association, "Lifestyle management: standards of medical care in diabetes—2019," *Diabetes Care* 42 (2019): S46-60; JL Kitzmiller, L Jovanovic, F Brown, D Coustan, DM Reader, eds, *Managing Preexisting Diabetes and Pregnancy* (Alexandria, Va: American Diabetes Association, 2008); GD Harris, RD White, "Diabetes management and exercise in pregnant patients with diabetes," *Clin Diabetes* 23, no. 4 (2005): 165-8; American College of Obstetricians and Gynecologists, Committee Opinion No. 650, "Physical activity and exercise during pregnancy and the postpartum period," *Obstet Gynecol* 126 (2015): 135-42; MW Carpenter, "The role of exercise in pregnant women with diabetes mellitus," *Clin Obstet Gynecol* 43 (2000): 56-64.

TABLE 24.10 Blood Glucose Goals in Normal and Preexisting Diabetes Pregnancy

	Daily Mean Glucose (mg/dL)	*Fasting, Premeal, Nighttime Glucose (mg/dL)*	*1 Hour Postprandial Glucose (mg/dL)*	*2 Hour Postprandial Glucose (mg/dL)*	*A1C (%)*
Normal pregnancy, mean ± SD					
Capillary glucose by meter	82.0 ± 5.8	69.3 ± 5.7	108.4 ± 6.0		5.0 ± 0.4
Continuous interstitial glucose	83.7 ± 18	76.6 ± 11.5	105.3 ± 12		
Preexisting diabetes					
Goals before and during early pregnancy	<125	60–119	100–149		<6.0–6.5
Goals during second and third trimesters	<110	60–99	<140	<120	<6.0

Sources: JL Kitzmiller, L Jovanovic, F Brown, D Coustan, DM Reader, eds, *Managing Preexisting Diabetes and Pregnancy* (Alexandria, Va: American Diabetes Association, 2008); American College of Obstetricians and Gynecologists, "Pregestational diabetes mellitus," ACOG Bulletin #201 2018, *Obstet Gynecol* 132 (2018): e228-48; American Diabetes Association, "Management of diabetes and pregnancy," *Diabetes Care* 39 Suppl 1 (2016): S94-8.

blood glucose monitoring in T2DP. Studies in women with T1DP and GDM have shown that postprandial testing is more closely associated with a lower incidence of maternal and fetal complications. Blood glucose records are verified by the use of memory meters to help identify glucose patterns. Because alternate site testing may not identify rapid changes in blood glucose concentrations characteristic of pregnant women, finger-stick testing is best in pregnancy.[20]

Continuous glucose monitoring, or CGM, is a system which monitors glucose from interstitial fluid. This system can provide real-time or retrospective information and assist the healthcare provider and the user in making informed decisions regarding diabetes management. In recent years, automated insulin delivery systems have been developed that increase and decrease insulin delivery based on CGM derived glucose levels to begin to approximate physiologic insulin delivery. One system, a hybrid closed-loop system uses an algorithm for delivering basal insulin and boluses for meals are inputted manually. There are few studies on the use of the closed-loop system in pregnancy. One study showed women who used the closed loop system overnight were more in the target range than women who used sensor-augmented pump therapy.[49]

Additional information on CGM and hybrid closed-loop system is found in chapter 18, Glucose Monitoring.

Ketone Testing

According to the ADA, women with type 1 diabetes and, to a lesser extent, women with type 2 diabetes are at risk for DKA.[29] As previously mentioned earlier in this chapter, DKA occurs at blood glucose levels that are lower than those of nonpregnant persons with diabetes. Ketone testing is necessary during illness, weight loss, or a reduction in calorie intake caused by nausea and/or vomiting. The presence of ketones may indicate impending DKA. The woman should be instructed to contact her healthcare provider immediately if moderate or large ketones are present in her urine. Although no studies have shown how ketosis may affect the fetus, 2 studies have suggested an association between elevated plasma ketone levels and poor glucose levels with lower IQ scores in offspring.[50,51] If the woman is positive for ketones because of an inadequate food intake, an RD will need to evaluate the food plan to determine the appropriate calorie level.

A1C

The goal of A1C in early gestation is <6% to 6.5% (42-48 mmol/L) without undue risk of hypoglycemia in the mother.[29] Measurements of A1C may be obtained monthly because of alteration in red blood cell kinetics during pregnancy. An A1C of <6% is recommended in the second and third trimesters, as it is associated with the lowest risk of large-for-gestational-age infants.

Time in Range

While the A1C has been used for many years as the standard for glucose management, its accuracy is affected by other factors, such as iron deficiency anemia, hemoglobinopathies and pregnancy. CGMs are now used in establishing standardized metrics to identify time in ranges for glycemic management. An international consensus panel has targets of glycemic levels in pregnancy. The time in range (TIR) in pregnancy is 63 to 140 mg/dL (3.5-7.8 mmol/L) with the percentage of readings of TIR: >70%, and time below range (TBR): <4% and time above range (TAR) <25%.[52]

Taking Medication

Euglycemia is the goal of a pregnancy complicated by diabetes. Combining medications with a food plan is necessary for the successful management of pregnancy and preexisting diabetes. This section describes medications used during pregnancy and precautions for use. Also see chapter 17, on pharmacologic therapies for glucose management.

Insulin and Insulin Analogs

The use of rapid-acting insulin analogs (lispro, aspart) in pregnancy has yielded results comparable to short-acting insulin.[53–56] In pregnancy, intensive insulin therapy requiring 3 or 4 injections is used to achieve the best glycemic level. One example of an insulin regimen in pregnancy is as follows:

- *Morning:* Intermediate- and rapid-acting analog or short-acting insulin and intermediate-acting insulin
- *Lunch:* Rapid-acting insulin analog
- *Dinner:* Rapid-acting analog or short-acting insulin
- *Bedtime:* Intermediate-acting insulin or long-acting insulin analog

Until June 2015, the FDA used the following lettering system to categorize all drugs used in pregnancy: A, B, C, D, and X. Category A drugs were any medications in adequate well-controlled studies in pregnant women that had shown no increased risk of abnormalities in any trimester of pregnancy. Category B was classified as animal studies that revealed no evidence of harm to the fetus; however, there were no adequate well-controlled studies done in pregnant women. Category C showed an adverse effect in animal studies, but no adequate well-controlled studies were done in pregnant women. Category D demonstrated a risk to the fetus in adequate well-controlled or observational studies in pregnant women; however, the benefits of therapy may outweigh the potential risk. All drugs in Category X were contraindicated during pregnancy because animal and human studies demonstrated positive evidence of fetal abnormalities or risks. In place of the FDA lettering system, medications used during pregnancy and lactation are now categorized into 3 groups: pregnancy, lactation, and males and females of reproductive potential.[57]

Insulin lispro, aspart detemir, and regular and NPH, along with oral glucose-lowering agents glyburide and metformin, were classified as Category B. Insulin glulisine, glargine, and degludec were classified as Category C.

Insulin Requirements (Daily Dose)

Insulin requirements in pregnancy are based on current weight, gestational age, blood glucose monitoring results, and caloric intake. The total daily dose per kilogram per day has a different range in each trimester (see Table 24.11).

Pump Therapy

Continuous subcutaneous insulin infusion therapy delivers insulin in a pattern similar to the normal physiologic secretion of insulin. Insulin pump therapy lowers the amount of circulating basal insulin, thereby decreasing the incidence of premeal hypoglycemia while efficiently managing the more dramatic rise in postprandial glucose common during pregnancy.[58] Other advantages of insulin pump therapy during pregnancy include more rapid and predictable insulin absorption, decreased severe hypoglycemia, enhanced lifestyle flexibility, and simplified morning sickness management.[59] Basal rates are often decreased in the first trimester because of increased insulin sensitivity. As insulin resistance begins to increase in the second trimester, the basal rate may eventually increase by 50% or more. The mealtime bolus will also increase as the carbohydrate-to-insulin ratio also increases as the pregnancy progresses.[60] Women continuing on insulin pump therapy after delivery postpartum were shown to have significantly lower A1C levels 1 year after delivery compared with women receiving multiple daily injections of insulin.[61]

TABLE 24.11 Insulin Requirements During Pregnancy

	Insulin (units/kg)
First trimester	0.7–0.8
Second trimester	0.8–1.0
Third trimester	0.9–1.2

Source: American College of Obstetricians and Gynecologists, "Pregestational diabetes mellitus," Practice bulletin no. 201, *Obstet Gynecol* 132 (2018): e228-48.

Pregnant women using insulin pumps must be highly motivated. Complications can arise, such as frequent and severe hyperglycemia, if there is an interruption in the delivery of insulin or an infection at the infusion site.[62]

Oral Glucose-Lowering Agents

Insulin is the preferred agent for managing blood glucose levels in women with T1DP or T2DP. Traditionally, women with T2DP were switched to insulin for glycemic management. However, studies in pregnant women with polycystic ovary syndrome have shown that metformin can be used without adverse outcomes. Recent studies using metformin in women with T2DP showed less maternal weight gain, pregnancy-induced hypertension, neonatal hypoglycemia, and neonatal intensive care than in the insulin group.[63,64]

Tocolytic Agents

Tocolytic agents such as ritodrine and terbutaline, used to treat premature labor, have been reported to cause deterioration of blood glucose levels and ketosis in pregnant women with diabetes.[20] These agents should not be the first line of therapy for women with diabetes; if they are used, blood glucose levels must be carefully monitored.

Problem Solving

Pregnant women with preexisting diabetes and no preconception care will need to learn self-management skills quickly to achieve and maintain euglycemia throughout the remainder of their pregnancies. Specifically, they must develop the flexibility to make adjustments to the care plan if they experience gastrointestinal discomforts during pregnancy. These adjustments include the following:

- Recognizing and treating hypoglycemic episodes
- Consistency in monitoring
- More frequent interactions with the healthcare team, including (1) discussing food plan adjustments with the RD, (2) follow-up diabetes education visits to assess self-management skills, and (3) when to contact the appropriate healthcare provider to discuss the care plan

Nausea and vomiting occur more often during the first and early second trimesters and most frequently in the morning ("morning sickness"); however, a woman may experience these symptoms at any time in pregnancy. Hypoglycemia may occur if the woman is experiencing nausea and vomiting and is unable to eat or is limited in the amount of food consumed. All pregnant women with diabetes should be instructed on sick-day rules and how to treat hypoglycemia, especially if on insulin or oral glucose-lowering medications. If vomiting occurs after taking a premeal rapid-acting or short-acting insulin dose, glucagon may be administered to help prevent hypoglycemia until the vomiting subsides. The woman should contact her healthcare provider if the vomiting becomes severe.[65]

Hyperemesis gravidarum is a severe and persistent form of nausea and vomiting characterized by weight loss, ketosis, dehydration, nutritional deficiencies, and electrolyte imbalance. Hospitalization for treatment, which could include rehydration, antiemetics, or enteral or parenteral nutrition, may be necessary to manage the vomiting.

Reducing Risks of Diabetes Complications

Women with preexisting diabetes have a higher incidence of poor perinatal outcomes than women with GDM. If the woman did not receive preconception care, hospitalization may be necessary to begin intensive diabetes management and education. Indications for hospitalization include the following:

- Hyperemesis
- Maternal hyperglycemia with ketones
- Non-engagement with previous instructions
- Obstetric complications, such as preeclampsia or preterm labor

Self-management skills reinforced or taught for the first time during pregnancy will have long-term benefits for the mother by establishing good habits that continue beyond the postpartum period. As glycemic levels remain within normal ranges, the woman's risk of developing long-term complications associated with diabetes is reduced.

Reducing risks also involves surveillance to assess the well-being of the fetus. The woman may be referred to other testing centers, such as genetics, for fetal assessment (see Table 24.12).

Healthy Coping

Women with preexisting diabetes may feel overwhelmed and not be prepared for the degree of intensive care associated with pregnancy. This includes the occasional uncomfortableness of a growing fetus, interaction with a new healthcare provider or team (obstetrician and/or perinatal center), and more frequent healthcare visits and testing. Diabetes education will help the woman to emotionally prepare for more intensive care.

- *Changes to insulin regimen.* Women with T1DP will have their insulin regimen changed several times during the pregnancy.
- *Injections.* Women with T2DP may be resistant to more frequent monitoring or switching from oral agents to insulin injections.

A referral for childbirth education classes is helpful for the expectant mother to learn about the physical and emotional changes of pregnancy. The usual topics of discussion in childbirth classes include labor and delivery, relaxation, breathing techniques, and medical interventions.

See chapter 4 for more information on addressing barriers to self-management. If a woman is not able to cope, a referral to a psychologist or social worker who understands diabetes is recommended.

TABLE 24.12 Maternal and Fetal Testing

- Cell-free fetal DNA test—this noninvasive prenatal test screens for Down syndrome (trisomy 21), trisomy 18, trisomy 13, or an abnormality in the sex chromosome. This test is performed after the 10th week of pregnancy.
- Ultrasonography—provides an image of the fetal anatomy, assess fetal growth, and estimates the delivery date.
- Nuchal translucency—an ultrasound that measures the fetal nuchal translucency thickness, which is the skin fold area behind the nape of the neck. This test is performed at 10 to 14 weeks gestation and is a risk predictor for chromosomal abnormalities and congenital cardiac defects.
- Maternal serum alpha fetal protein—a test performed early in the second trimester which may indicate neural tube defect or Down syndrome in the fetus.
- Amniocentesis or chorionic villus sampling—invasive tests in which amniotic fluid is extracted for fetal analysis.
- Nonstress testing—measures fetal heart rate acceleration in response to fetal activity.
- Biophysical profile—a noninvasive test that combines an ultrasound with nonstress testing to measure fetal movement, heart rate, breathing rate, muscle tone, and amniotic fluid.
- Fetal kick counts—the mother keeps track of fetal activity by counting the number of kicks or movements within a certain time period.

Diabetes Care During Labor and Delivery

When to deliver a woman with preexisting diabetes will depend on the condition of the mother and the fetus. An earlier delivery (before 39 weeks) may be indicated if the woman is in poor glycemic stability, has vascular disease or nephropathy, or a past fetal demise. If the woman is well managed and her antenatal testing results are normal, she may deliver at 39/07 to 39 6/7 weeks. A pregnancy that is beyond 39 6/7 weeks is not recommended in women with preexisting diabetes.[2]

The key to successful intrapartum management is to monitor blood glucose levels frequently and administer insulin and glucose as necessary. The following is an example of a regimen used to manage blood glucose levels during labor and delivery:

1. Administer the usual dose of intermediate-acting insulin at bedtime.
2. Withhold the morning dose of insulin and begin an intravenous infusion of normal saline.
3. Once active labor begins or the glucose level decreases to less than 70 mg/dL (3.9 mmol/L), change the infusion to dextrose to keep blood glucose levels below 110 mg/dL (6.1 mmol/L).[25] The rate of dextrose administered is 2.0 to 2.5 mg per kilogram per minute.
4. Measure maternal blood glucose values every hour.
5. Administer insulin by continuous intravenous infusion as necessary to maintain euglycemia and help prevent neonatal hypoglycemia.[22]

Postpartum Care

After the birth of her infant, the mother with diabetes will face new challenges. Her focus and attention will shift from self-care to caring for her baby. Postpartum care and education should begin prior to her hospital discharge. This time can be used to review the self-management skills learned during pregnancy and continued later at home.

After the woman has been at home with her infant for a couple of weeks, a follow-up phone call by a diabetes care and education specialist is appropriate. About 6 weeks after delivery, the woman should have a scheduled office visit with both the diabetes care and education specialist and the RD. Topics for education include the following:

- Glycemic management with decreasing insulin requirements
- More frequent SMBG
- Balancing infant care with self-care for the new mother
- Postpartum depression and stress
- Readjusting the insulin regimen or resuming oral glucose-lowering medications
- Readjusting the food plan, whether breastfeeding or not
- Weight loss or weight management
- Family planning and contraception

Lactation

Unless contraindicated, breastfeeding should be strongly encouraged in women with diabetes. Women with type 2 diabetes may be switched from insulin to oral glucose-lowering medication. Key education points on lactation and diabetes are the following:

- *Insulin:* Breastfeeding mothers may require less insulin because of the calories expended during nursing. The insulin dosage will vary and may need to be frequently readjusted. A small snack either before or during breastfeeding may help to avoid hypoglycemia and frequent dosage adjustments.
- *Oral glucose-lowering medications:* Glipizide, glyburide, metformin, and acarbose are considered compatible with breastfeeding.[20,66,67]
- *Monitoring:* Breastfeeding mothers may need more frequent SMBG because of hypoglycemic episodes.

Gestational Diabetes Mellitus

For many years, gestational diabetes mellitus (GDM) was defined as any degree of glucose intolerance with onset of or first recognition during pregnancy.[68] This definition facilitated a uniform strategy for detection and classification of GDM, but its limitations were recognized for many years. It has been suspected that women who develop GDM in the first trimester actually have undiagnosed diabetes. Since 2010, the ADA has recommended that women at high risk for diabetes be tested at the first prenatal visit for diabetes using standard criteria. If the woman tests positive, she should receive the diagnosis of overt, not gestational, diabetes. (See chapter 13 of this text.) Because of this change, the definition of GDM is now "diabetes diagnosed in the second or third trimester of pregnancy that is not clearly either type 1 or type 2 diabetes."[68]

At the first prenatal appointment, women at high risk for developing GDM or for undiagnosed type 2 diabetes should be identified and screened. If diagnosed with type 2 diabetes, they will need immediate treatment to normalize glucose levels, as discussed earlier in this chapter. All women, except those diagnosed with preexisting diabetes, should be screened for abnormal glucose tolerance between 24 and 28 weeks of pregnancy. Table 24.18 shows the risk categories, characteristics, and the timing of glucose testing to be considered at the first prenatal visit.

Recommendations on Screening and Diagnosis of GDM

The diagnosis and screening recommendations for GDM have changed several times since the original criteria were accepted at the First International Conference-Workshop on GDM in 1979. Beginning in 2001, the ADA and the ACOG recommended the 2-step method using the Carpentar-Coustan criteria for all women between 24 and 28 weeks gestation.

In January 2011, the ADA accepted the recommendations of the International Association of Diabetes and Pregnancy Study Group (IADPSG) to revise the diagnostic criteria for GDM, based on the results of the Hyperglycemia and Adverse Pregnancy Outcome (HAPO) study.[69] In September 2011, the ACOG did not accept the IADPSG recommendations.[70] In March 2013, the National Institutes of Health held the Consensus Conference on the Diagnosis of Gestational Diabetes. The consensus panel concluded there is insufficient evidence to adopt a 1-step approach, such as that proposed by the IADPSG, and recommended the continuation of the 2-step approach.[71] In 2014 the ADA rescinded its exclusive support for the IADPSG diagnostic criteria for GDM and stated that both methods are acceptable.

Currently in the United States, 2 methods are used to diagnose GDM: the 2-step approach using the 100-g oral glucose tolerance test (OGTT) following a positive result from the 50 gram Oral Glucose Challenge Test and the 1-step approach using the 75-g OGTT. The US Preventive Services Task Force (USPSTF) recommends screening for GDM in asymptomatic pregnant women after 24 weeks of gestation.[72]

2-Step Approach: Using 100-g OGTT

The first step is a 50-g glucose challenge test (GCT) given at any time of the day. The cutoff for the 1-hour test is not clear. ACOG and ADA recommend that healthcare providers select ≥130 or ≥135 or ≥140 mg/dL (7.2, 7.5, or 7.8 mmol/L) as a single consistent cutoff based on factors such as community prevalence rates.[73] If the result 1 hour later is greater than the cutoff, then the second step, a 100-g OGTT, is scheduled. The woman reports to the lab, having fasted for at least 8 hours and having consumed a normal carbohydrate load of at least 150 g for 3 days. Blood is drawn at fasting and at 1, 2, and 3 hours. The woman cannot smoke, is required to stay seated and resting, and may drink only water, if necessary. The diagnosis of GDM is made when 2 or more of the 4 values are equal to or greater than the criteria in Table 24.13.

1-Step Approach: Using 75-g OGTT

Following the same criteria for a 2-step OGTT, the woman reports to the lab, having fasted for at least 8 hours and having consumed a normal carbohydrate load of at least 150 g for 3 days. Blood is drawn at fasting and at 1 and 2 hours. The diagnosis of GDM is made when 1 or more of 3 values is equal to or greater than the criteria in Table 24.13.

TABLE 24.13 Current Methods to Diagnose GDM

	2-step method	*1-step method*
	Step 1: 50-g GCT If ≥ 130 or ≥135 or ≥140 mg/dL, then go to step 2 (100-g OGTT)	Step 1: 75-g OGTT
	Step 2: 100-g OGTT	
	2 abnormal values needed for diagnosis	*1 abnormal value needed for diagnosis*
Fasting	≥95 mg/dL (5.3 mmol/L)	≥92 mg/dL (5.1 mmol/L)
1 hour	≥180 mg/dL (10.0 mmol/L)	≥180 mg/dL (10.0 mmol/L)
2 hour	≥155 mg/dL (8.6 mmol/L)	≥153 mg/dL (8.5 mmol/L)
3 hour	≥140 mg/dL (7.8 mmol/L)	

Case—Part 1: A Pregnancy With GDM

MA has a number of risk factors for GDM:

- She is a member of a high-risk ethnic group.
- She is both older and overweight.
- She has a history of a large-for-gestational-age infant.
- Her mother and grandmother had type 2 diabetes.

At MA's first prenatal appointment, her obstetrician determined she was at high risk for GDM and might have undiagnosed diabetes. After her appointment, MA had an A1C drawn. The result was 5.4% indicating that she did not have diabetes or pre-diabetes. Between the 24th and 28th weeks of pregnancy, she will be screened for gestational diabetes. MA was concerned and wanted to manage her weight gain better during pregnancy.

At 26 weeks, MA took the first step, a 50 g glucose challenge test (GCT) and the result was 155 mg/dL (8.6 mmol/L), which was abnormal. She returned within a week for the 3-hour, 100-g OGTT. Her results are shown in the table.

MA was diagnosed with GDM because at least 2 of the 4 tests were equal to or greater than the diagnostic criteria.

Blood Glucose After 100 g of Glucose	*Criteria: 2 or More Results Equal to or Greater Than:*	*MA's Test Results*
Fasting	95 mg/dL (5.3 mmol/L)	93 mg/dL (5.2 mmol/L)
1 hour	180 mg/dL (10.0 mmol/L)	210 mg/dL (11.7 mmol/L)
2 hour	155 mg/dL (8.6 mmol/L)	176 mg/dL (9.8 mmol/L)
3 hour	140 mg/dL (7.8 mmol/L)	132 mg/dL (7.3 mmol/L)

The OGTT determines the diagnosis; however, it is interesting to ask whether the OGTT also predicts her course with GDM. There appears to be a continuous relationship between increasing maternal glycemia and morbidities of pregnancy, so the higher the number the greater the likelihood MA will need insulin therapy.

Case—Part 2: Clinical Outcomes and Initial Therapy

What clinical targets needed to be set for MA? Glucose management was primary as blood glucose levels within the normal range help prevent macrosomia and a large-for-gestational-age infant, as MA had in her last pregnancy.

- *Self-monitoring.* MA was taught SMBG and asked to test her fasting and after-meal glucose levels.
- *Weight gain.* MA needed to manage weight gain. Her BMI of 27 gave her a weight gain target for the pregnancy of 15 to 25 lb.
- *Records.* She needed to eat a healthy diet, so she was asked to record her food intake as well as blood glucose values; these records would be assessed at a follow-up visit in 1 or 2 weeks.

Because MA's fasting result on the OGTT was less than 95 mg/dL (5.3 mmol/L), initial therapy for GDM was MNT.

Case—Part 3: Self-Management Education Begins

MA's healthcare provider referred her to the diabetes education center. Her first appointment was within a week of diagnosis, at 29 weeks gestation.

The diabetes care and education specialist discovered that MA was very motivated to follow through with the protocol. Because her mother and grandmother had diabetes, she was familiar with blood glucose monitoring, as well as how to inject insulin. MA was surprised that her blood glucose targets were so much lower than the blood glucose values she saw her family members obtain. She was instructed to record

Case—Part 3: Self-Management Education Begins (continued)

her blood glucose test results 4 times per day on her food record form.

- *Healthy eating.* MA was very motivated to change her diet. She stopped drinking regular soda after she was diagnosed with GDM. She readily admitted that she probably eats too much and likes high-fat foods, but is willing to cut back on the fat and portions.
- *Being active.* MA was physically active at work. She was busy at home with her family but did not intentionally walk or exercise. MA considered whether a daily walk after dinner would be beneficial to her glucose management and desire to manage weight gain.
- *Behavior-change goals.* MA and her diabetes team set up 2 behavior-change goals at the first visit:
  1. Test blood glucose every morning before breakfast and 1 hour after the start of each meal
  2. Follow the food plan; count carbohydrates and record food intake

Case—Part 4: Focus on the Food Plan

To help MA understand and quickly begin using the food plan, the RD worked with her to create a sample 1-day intake that incorporates the changes suggested in this chapter. The RD assessed that MA would be capable of learning carbohydrate counting. The food plan gave a suggested starting range of carbohydrate choices based on the sample food plan they developed together. MA was instructed to record all of the food and beverages she consumed during the next week and return in 1 week. The chart below shows a typical day's intake for MA on the left and the new food plan and sample menu on the right. Also shown below is a table summarizing the RD's recommendations for modifying MA's food intake.

Typical Day	*Typical Day's Intake*	*New Food Plan*	*Sample Menu*
Breakfast, 9 AM	Cornflakes, whole milk, fruit, coffee	*Breakfast, 9 AM (2 carb choices)*	Slice of toast with peanut butter, 1 c 1% milk
		Snack, 11 AM (1–2 carb choices)	A piece of fruit
Lunch, 1 PM	Hamburger or sandwich, fries or chips, and 20-oz regular soda from a fast-food restaurant near work	*Lunch, 1 PM (4 carb choices)*	Sandwich, fruit, small container (6-oz) yogurt
		Snack, 4 PM (1–2 carb choices)	Carrots, ¼ c peanuts
Dinner, 8 PM	Traditional Mexican dinner of 4 tortillas made with rice, beans, chicken	*Dinner, 8 PM (4–5 carb choices)*	2 rice-and-bean tortillas, chicken strips, salad, 1 c low fat milk
		Bedtime snack, 11 PM (1–2 carb choices)	1 tortilla with cheese, ½ c juice

(continued)

Case—Part 4: Focus on the Food Plan (continued)

SUMMARY OF DIETITIAN'S RECOMMENDATIONS FOR MODIFYING MA'S FOOD INTAKE

Topic	*MA's Typical Intake*	*Recommendations*
Number of meals and snacks	3 meals, no snacks	Add small morning, afternoon and bedtime snacks
Intake of high-carbohydrate foods	Drinks regular soda Does not eat desserts (eg, cookies, ice cream, pastries, candy) regularly	Discontinue regular soda. May use diet soda, but she is encouraged to drink water. Good she does not have a sweet tooth
Total amount of carbohydrate at each meal and snack	Breakfast about 4 carbs Lunch about 8 carbs Dinner about 8 carbs	Reduce total carbs per meal; try 3–4 carbs per meal and test postmeal; add snacks
Estimate of calorie intake and weight-gain goal	Has gained 10 lb BMI category: overweight	Weight gain seems on track Gain 1/2 lb per week Weight gain goal 15–25 lb
Fat content of diet	Uses whole milk Prepares tortillas and beans with lard	Reduce fat content of milk to 2%, 1%, or skim Cook using monounsaturated oil; use less oil/fat
Anticipation of potential problems	Cornflakes at breakfast Fast foods	Avoid processed cereal at breakfast Avoid fast foods if postmeal reading is too high
Adequate nutrition in all food groups	Fruit: 1 serving per day Milk: on cereal only Protein: 2 servings per day Vegetables: at dinner	Increase fruit intake; add between meals or at lunch Increase milk to 3–4 servings per day; drink milk instead of soda Protein intake adequate Add another serving of vegetables with lunch or between meals

Case—Part 5: Therapy Evolves as Pregnancy Progresses

Medical Nutrition Therapy

At 30 weeks gestation, MA had her follow-up visit with the diabetes care and education specialists, 1 week after her initial visit. The diabetes care and education specialists assessed her progress and discussed the following points:[74]

- What her glucose levels were and how often she met her target levels
- How often she was able to follow her meal plan
- Whether she felt confident in her ability to count carbohydrates
- How often she found her hunger satisfied
- How happy she was with her weight gain

Most of MA's blood glucose readings were in target. The glucose readings that were too high were explained by errors in counting carbohydrates. She understood the errors and was willing to adjust her food intake. All elevated postmeal glucose

Case—Part 5: Therapy Evolves as Pregnancy Progresses (continued)

readings were after the dinner meal. MA and her diabetes care and education specialists agreed that adding a daily walk after dinner would help postmeal glucose levels. Her weight did not change. The RD's overall assessment was that the food plan would provide for MA's calorie needs and satisfy her appetite.

Exercise Prescription

The diabetes care team provided MA guidance on implementing a safe physical activity plan that could help her manage her blood glucose level after meals. MA agreed to start with a daily walk after dinner.

Behavior Change

Like other women with gestational diabetes, MA had to learn and implement diabetes self-management in a very short period of time.

Case—Part 6: Achieving Glucose Stability

At 33 Weeks

MA returned to her healthcare provider with food, blood glucose, and activity records. Her weight was 167, up 1 lb. She was comfortable with her food plan, and all blood glucose values were in target range.

At 36 Weeks

MA had her final visit for GDM management. She had done well and was happy with her blood glucose values. The diabetes care and education specialists discussed her risk for developing diabetes postpartum and explained the strategies for diabetes prevention. MA had made many changes in her eating and activity habits that she planned to continue after delivery. She saw GDM as an opportunity to make changes that improved the health of her whole family. Now she was looking forward to delivery.

Case Wrap-up

At 39½ weeks, MA delivered an 8 lb, 2 oz (3,685 g) baby boy. Baby M's blood glucose was tested at 1 hour, and it was 70 mg/dL (3.9 mmol/L). He started breastfeeding and could stay with his mother in her room. During her hospital stay, MA's fasting blood glucose level was tested the day after delivery. It was in the normal range. When she left the hospital, she was instructed to continue testing her blood glucose levels once a week—fasting and 2 hours after eating—and to return in 6 weeks for an evaluation of glucose stability.

At her 6-week postpartum visit, all blood glucose values were within the normal (nonpregnant) range: fasting <100 mg/dL (5.5 mmol/L) and 2 hour <140 mg/dL (7.8 mmol/L). To confirm that she did not have diabetes, her healthcare provider ordered a 75-g OGTT. MA's test results were in the normal range. She continued with her food plan, walked every evening with her husband, and remained pleased to have lost 6 lb; she was feeling great. Her healthcare provider discussed that she is at a high risk for developing type 2 diabetes and supported the excellent lifestyle changes she had already made. MA was instructed to return annually for a blood glucose test.

MA was told that if she becomes pregnant again, her risk for developing GDM again is 30% to 65%.[11] She was also made aware of factors that increase her risk: the amount of weight gained between pregnancies, hip-to-waist ratio, and diet composition.

Complications of GDM

Recent research has described a strong continuous association between maternal glucose concentrations and perinatal complications, even at glucose levels below the current diagnosis of GDM.[68] Gestational diabetes mellitus primarily develops in the second half of pregnancy and is not associated with the risk for congenital anomalies that occur with preexisting diabetes. (See Table 24.14.) Hyperglycemia in the second trimester is associated with an increased risk for macrosomia, cesarean section, difficult delivery, and neonatal hypoglycemia. Explanations of these complications are found earlier in the chapter.

AADE7® in GDM

This section highlights the unique guidelines and recommendations for gestational diabetes. The reader should refer to Table 24.8, which describes the goals for all pregnancies.

TABLE 24.14 Congenital Malformations in Infants Born to Women With Preexisting Diabetes

Cardiovascular	
Transposition of great vessels	Coarctation or interruption of the aortic arch
Ventricular septal defect	Hydroplastic left ventricle
Atrial septal defect	Truncus arteriosus
Tetralogy of Fallot	Ebstein anomaly
Single umbilical artery	Pulmonary stenosis
Hypertrophic cardiomyopathy	Tricuspid valve dysplasia
Aortic stenosis	Double-outlet right ventricle (DORV)
Central nervous and skeletal	
Sacral agenesis	Arnold-Chiari anomaly
Microcephaly	Anencephaly
Macrocephaly	Hydrocephaly
Holoprosencephaly	Neural tube defects
Absent corpus callosum	
Genitourinary	
Renal agenesis	Micropenis
Hydronephrosis	Hypospadias
Ureteral duplication	Cryptorchidism
Anal/rectal atresia	Ambigious genitalia
Hypoplastic vagina	
Gastrointestinal	
Duodenal atresia	Omphalo-enteric cyst
Anorectal atresia	Microcolon
Pyloric stenosis	
Musculoskeletal	
Cauddal dysgenesis	Limb reduction
Craniosynostosis	Club foot
Costovertebral anomalies	Polysyndactyly
Other	
Cleft palate	

Sources: MM Agha, RH Glazer, R Moineddin, G Booth, "Congenital abnormalities in newborns of women with pregestational diabetes: a time-trend analysis, 1994 to 2009," *Birth Defects Research (Part A)*. 106(2016):831-9.

S Liu, J Rouleau, JA Leon, et al, "Impact of pre-pregnancy diabetes mellitus on congenital anomalies, Canada, 2001-2012," *Health Promot Chronic Dis Prev Can*. 35(2015):79-84.

VM Allen, BA Armson, "Teratogenicity associated with pre-existing and gestational diabetes," *J Obstet Gynaecol Cab* 29, no. 11 (2007).

Healthy Eating for GDM

Carbohydrate Guidelines for Gestational Diabetes The Evidence-Based GDM Nutrition Practice Guidelines of the Academy of Nutrition and Dietetics suggest dividing carbohydrate intake into 3 small-to-moderate meals with 2 to 4 snacks. (Duarte-Gardea,[74] Academy of Nutrition and Dietetics Gestational Practice Guideline). This eating pattern accommodates the pregnant woman well because the amount of food tolerated at a time decreases as the pregnancy progresses. An initial food plan would suggest the following carbohydrate ranges for each meal and snack:

- *Breakfast:* 15 to 45 g
- *Lunch and dinner:* 45 to 75 g each
- *Snacks:* 15 to 45 g

The most difficult blood glucose level to manage is the postbreakfast value, due to higher hormonal levels in the morning. Consensus is to restrict carbohydrate at breakfast time to 15 to 45 g.[74] Breakfast cereals are often discouraged, as the total amount of carbohydrate is higher than 45 g and postmeal blood glucose levels are higher than with other food choices. The glycemic index may help explain why some foods produce higher postmeal glucose levels. Highly processed breakfast cereals, sweetened beverages, fast foods, and pizza are frequently found to raise postmeal levels higher than less processed, higher fiber foods with the same amount of total carbohydrate.

The Academy of Nutrition of Nutrition and Dietetics Evidence-Analysis Library reviewed and graded the literature regarding nutrition therapy for gestational diabetes and wrote practice guidelines to direct care of individuals with GDM. The guidelines are published in the Journal of Nutrition and Dietetics. In Table 24.15 below are summarized some of the key components of nutrition therapy.

Being Active for GDM

Just as physical activity improves glucose tolerance in type 2 diabetes, it also improves glucose levels in GDM. If there are no contraindications for physical activity (see Table 24.6), women with GDM should undertake 30 minutes per day of low-impact activity.

Monitoring for GDM

Glucose Monitoring Monitoring fasting and postmeal glycemic levels is recommended for women with GDM. Recommended glucose targets for both 1 hour and 2 hours postmeal are provided in Table 24.16; however, there is no definitive research to support 1-versus 2-hour testing. Research using continuous glucose monitoring indicated that the peak glucose is reached 80 minutes after eating.[80,81] In another study, a comparison of 2 breakfast meals with different glycemic indexes found that the peak postbreakfast time was earlier with the high-glycemic-index foods. The researchers also identified a large intersubject variability in the timing of the peak.[82] There is limited research regarding the frequency of testing. As previously stated, the goal is to achieve euglycemia, and whatever amount of testing is needed to achieve that goal is recommended.

Ketone Testing Routine ketone testing for women with GDM is not recommended by any of the national professional organizations.

A1C The A1C test is the standard for overall glucose management, but its role in GDM is not clear. However, the A1C may be used in women diagnosed with GDM in the first trimester.

Taking Medication for GDM

Euglycemia is the goal of a pregnancy complicated by diabetes. Most women with GDM (about 70%-85%) are able to use MNT alone for glucose management, which means that 15% to 30% of women will need additional pharmacologic therapy for glucose management.[29] This section describes medications used for managing GDM. Also see the section on taking medications for preexisting diabetes.

Insulin Therapy in GDM

Insulin therapy is still the preferred treatment when endogenous insulin production is inadequate. There is no one insulin regimen that has been shown to be the most effective in managing women with GDM. Rapid-acting insulin analogs and NPH insulin are the most commonly used types of insulin in a GDM pregnancy.[83] See the section Insulin and Insulin Analogs earlier in this chapter.

There is no protocol for starting insulin therapy in GDM; the ADA position statement recommends that SMBG guide the doses and timing of the insulin regimen.[1] Many women who need insulin during pregnancy require basal insulin coverage with NPH insulin twice daily, or 1 injection if using detemir. Insulin resistance continues to increase dramatically during the third trimester, which means insulin doses need to be adjusted

TABLE 24.15 Medical Nutrition Therapy Practice Guidelines for Gestational Diabetes

Calorie Prescription	– Individualize the calorie prescription based on a thorough nutrition assessment with guidance from relevant references (DRI and IOM) and encourage adequate calorie. – No definitive research suggests there is a specific optimal calorie intake for women with GDM or if calorie needs are different than women without GDM. – In a study of obese women only, gestational weight gain slowed after women with GDM reportedly consumed 30% below their caloric requirements without adverse effects.
Macronutrient Requirement	– Provide adequate amounts of macronutrients to support pregnancy, with guidance from Dietary Reference Intakes (DRI). – DRI for all pregnant women recommends a minimum of 175 g carbohydrate, a minimum of 71 g protein (or 1.1g/kg/d protein) and 28 g fiber.

Carbohydrate Prescription	– Individualize both the amount and type of carbohydrate based on nutrition assessment, treatment goals, blood glucose response, and the person's needs.
	– Limited evidence does not confirm an ideal amount of carb for women with GDM.[75]
	– Several studies showed positive effects on glycemic management and neonatal/fetal and maternal outcomes with varying amounts and types of carb.
	  – Low (<55) and medium (55–69) glycemic index diets with diets containing a range of 36.7% to >60% carb[76–77]
	  – DASH diets with greater than 65% carb[78]

Carbohydrate and Post-Breakfast Glycemia	– Individualize both the amount and type of carbohydrate based on nutrition assessment, treatment goals, blood glucose response, and the person's needs.
	– If the person experiences elevated post-prandial breakfast glucose, modify the amount or the type of carbohydrate to achieve glucose targets. Research supports:
	  – lower overall amount of carb
	  – lower glycemic index without lower amount of carb
	– No research supports restricting individual foods such as milk or fruit.

Source: Adapted from Academy of Nutrition and Dietetics Gestational Diabetes Evidence-Based Nutrition Practice Guidelines. JAND 2018.

TABLE 24.16 Target Plasma Glucose in Gestational Diabetes and Pregnancy (Preexisting and GDM)

Testing Time	*ADA*[1]	*ACOG*[2]
Fasting	≤95 mg/dL (5.3 mmol/L)	95 mg/dL (5.3 mmol/L)
1 hour after meals	≤140 mg/dL (7.8 mmol/L)	<140 mg/dL (7.8 mmol/L)
2 hours after meals	≤120 mg/dL (6.7 mmol/L)	<120 mg/dL (6.7 mmol/L)

Sources:

1. American Diabetes Association, "Standards of medical care in diabetes. Management of diabetes in pregnancy," *Diabetes Care.* 42 Suppl 1(2019):S165-72.
2. American College of Obstetricians and Gynecologists. Practice Bulletin. Number 201. Pregestational diabetes mellitus. Obstet Gynecol. 132(2018):e228-48.
3. American College of Obstetricians and Gynecologists. Practice Bulletin Number 190. Gestational diabetes mellitus. Obstet Gynecol. 131(2018):e49-64.

weekly until about 36 to 37 weeks of pregnancy. The dose of insulin at delivery is about 1.0 unit per kilogram.[84]

Noninsulin Therapies for GDM

Glyburide Historically, adding insulin was the only option for the woman with GDM. In 2000, the *New England Journal of Medicine* published an article that compared glyburide and insulin in women with gestational diabetes.[86] Langer et al demonstrated that the oral hypoglycemic agent glyburide is a clinically effective alternative to insulin. Sulfonylurea drugs were not used in pregnancy because of concern about teratogenicity and neonatal hypoglycemia. Initially it was reported that glyburide was not detected in cord serum of the infant; subsequent studies suggest that it is present in concentrations averaging approximately 70% of maternal levels.[87]

The use of glyburide by providers rose significantly, from 6% in 2000 to 64% in 2011.[89] It has become the most common treatment of GDM. However, a recent systematic review of the use of glyburide, metformin, and insulin has raised concerns.[90] Comparing these 3 medications in 15 studies with over 2,500 patients showed that glyburide is considered inferior to insulin and metformin due to higher risk of neonatal hypoglycemia and macrosomia.

Metformin The use of metformin for the management of GDM has been increasing over the past few years. It is known to cross the placenta; however, no adverse effects on the fetus have been demonstrated.[29] A systematic review which compared glyburide, metformin, and insulin for the management of GDM identified metformin and insulin as "slightly better than insulin"alone and reported that glyburide should not be used.[89] Metformin use is associated with a lower risk of hypoglycemia and less weight gain but slightly increases the risk of prematurity. The dose should begin at 500 mg per day and titrated as usual up to 2,000 mg per day.

Diabetes medications not recommended during pregnancy include thiazolidinediones, dipeptidyl peptidase-4 (DPP-4) inhibitors, GLP-1 agonists, and sodium-glucose co-transporter 2 (SGLT2) inhibitors.[29]

Healthy Coping for GDM

Although GDM is short-lived, major lifestyle changes during the middle of pregnancy can be stressful and emotional. A study in which interviews of pregnant women explored stress and anxiety after the diagnosis of GDM identified 3 themes:[91]

- *Stress related to GDM diagnosis and the perception of a high-risk pregnancy.* Concern that the pregnancy was not a "normal" pregnancy created fears and stress.
- *Stress over losing control of GDM during the process of dietary management.* Women felt frustrated when trying to follow the food plan, yet glucose levels remained out of target. Women using insulin therapy exhibited more stress.
- *Anxiety related to the fear of maternal and infant complications.* Fear of having a big baby and not wanting to have a cesarean section was a common concern, along with the fear that diabetes would remain after delivery.

Diabetes care and education specialists should be aware that the diagnosis of GDM is often perceived with increased stress, anxiety, and fears. Allow time in the visit to address concerns and answer questions, and provide adequate follow-up visits to support the individual who has been expected to make significant lifestyle changes very quickly.

Postpartum Follow-Up After GDM

Women with a history of GDM should be screened for diabetes 6 to 12 weeks after delivery using the 75-g OGTT for nonpregnant individuals.[68] If the results are normal, testing should be repeated at 3-year intervals. More frequent testing may be considered depending on the initial results and risk status (see Table 24.17).

Diabetes Prevention for Women With a History of GDM and Their Offspring

All women should be actively encouraged to breastfeed their infants during the first year of life. Breastfeeding has been associated with decreasing the woman's risk of becoming overweight later in life and developing metabolic syndrome and type 2 diabetes.[92]

Women with a history of GDM are at high risk for developing type 2 diabetes. The risk factors for the development of type 2 diabetes are the same as those for the development of gestational diabetes (see Table 24.18). It has often been stated that GDM unmasks the metabolic dysfunction that has already begun that leads to type 2 diabetes. A systematic review and meta-analysis of studies reported that women who had gestational diabetes have at least a seven-fold increased risk for the development of type 2 diabetes.[93]

The good news is that in people with risk factors for diabetes, many studies have shown that diabetes can be prevented or the onset delayed (see chapter 1 for study details). A large trial in the United States called the Diabetes Prevention Program (DPP) reported that the incidence of diabetes was reduced by 58% in the lifestyle study arm compared with placebo.[94] People in this group

TABLE 24.17 Criteria for the Diagnosis of Diabetes
At 6-12 weeks' postpartum, use only 2-hour OGTT using a 75-g glucose load*
1. FPG (fasting plasma glucose) ≥126 mg/dL (7.0 mmol/L) **OR**
2. ≥200mg/dL (11.1 mmol/L)
Other criteria to diagnosis diabetes may be used for yearly screening
3. A1C ≥6.5% **OR**
4. RPG (random plasma glucose) ≥200 mg/dL (11.1 mmol/L)

*In the absence of unequivocal hyperglycemia, criterion 1 should be confirmed by repeat testing.

Source: American Diabetes Association, "Standards of medical care in diabetes—2019," *Diabetes Care* 42 Suppl 1 (2019): S17.

TABLE 24.18 Risk Assessment at First Prenatal Visit

Risk Category	*Characteristics*	*Timing of Glucose Testing*
High risk	BMI ≥30 First-degree relative with diabetes Women who delivered a baby weighing >9 lb or were diagnosed with GDM A1C of 5.7% or impaired fasting glucose (IFG) on previous testing High-risk ethnic group Polycystic ovary syndrome (PCOS)	Test for type 2 diabetes using accepted diagnostic criteria at first prenatal visit (see chapter 15) If normal glucose levels at first prenatal visit, then glucose challenge test (GCT) between 24 and 28 weeks; if abnormal, diagnose with diabetes or prediabetes and begin glucose management
Normal risk	Does not fit other categories	See Table 24.13 for the 1-step and 2-step methods to test and diagnose for GDM
Low risk	<25 years of age No history of poor obstetrical outcome No first-degree family history of diabetes Normal weight or underweight Low-risk ethnic group	Not routinely screened Screened based on clinician assessment

participated in a lifestyle-modification program with the goals of reducing weight by 7% and being active at least 150 minutes per week.

Within the DPP trial were 350 women who had a history of GDM. In an analysis that compared these 350 women with the 1,416 women who had a pregnancy without GDM, the researchers found that women with a history of GDM were more likely to develop diabetes and that lifestyle intervention was less successful in preventing the onset of diabetes.[95] What messages should the diabetes care and education specialist give to women with a history of GDM?

- If the woman is considering becoming pregnant, emphasize the importance of having excellent glucose stability before conception. Earlier in this chapter, the importance of good glucose stability in women with preexisting diabetes who become pregnant was emphasized. Women with a history of GDM should follow the same guidelines to ensure their A1C is in a normal range before conception.
- Recurrence of GDM in a subsequent pregnancy is not expected, although it is common; one systematic review reported that recurrence rates ranged from 30% to 84%. The predictor of recurrence was ethnicity; non-Hispanic whites had the lowest recurrrence.[96] In another study, the risk for developing GDM increased with each subsequent GDM pregnancy.[97]
- Reinforce the importance of diabetes prevention as mentioned above. Women who have lost weight and increased their activity level do not necessarily have GDM in a second or third pregnancy and will reduce their risk of developing type 2 diabetes as they age.

As described earlier in this chapter, the Hyperglycemia Adverse Outcome Trail (HAPO) was designed to examine the association of increasing degrees of untreated maternal glycemia, less severe than overt diabetes, with adverse pregnancy outcomes and to unify the approach to the diagnosis of GDM. The primary outcome showed a strong continuous linear relationship with adverse outcomes and maternal glycemia. The secondary outcomes included long-term follow-up of offspring of women in this study. In two studies published in 2019 of over 4,000 racially and ethnically diverse offspring at 10 to14 years of age shows that untreated maternal hyperglycemia was associated with higher prevalence of IGT, highlighting the importance of seeking normal glycemia during pregnancy for the long-term effects on the offspring. Diabetes runs in families and families can work together to establish a healthy lifestyles to prevent the development of diabetes.[98]

Focus on Education: Preexisting Diabetes and Pregnancy

Key Points

Preconception counseling (also care) has become the key for good perinatal outcomes. An increasing number of women are developing type 2 diabetes during their childbearing years. Growing, too, is the number of women with type 1 diabetes desiring to have children.

Encourage the woman to see herself as a vital part of the multidisciplinary team. The woman's willingness to work together with the other members of the healthcare team before and during her pregnancy can result in an improved outcome.

Teaching Strategies

The diabetes care and education specialist has many opportunities to make important contributions during a woman's pregnancy and to assist her in planning for motherhood. From preconception to postpartum care, the mother and her infant will benefit from the diabetes care and education specialist's involvement.

Relieve the stress. Diabetes care and education specialists are pivotal in helping coordinate the woman's care to decrease the anxiety and stress of the mother-to-be. Women with preexisting diabetes may be concerned about preterm delivery or their infants having major malformations.

Set attainable goals during the pregnancy. Attending to the immediate issues of glycemic management, pregnancy care, and diabetes self-management, the care and education specialist assists the woman in establishing achievable goals for the pregnancy. As the pregnancy progresses, the care and education specialist and the woman (family also, if needed) will frequently review the goals and revise if necessary.

Develop the opportunity to improve the woman's long-term health. The care and education specialist assists the woman in establishing goals and habits that can last beyond pregnancy and childbearing—the woman gains knowledge that can be of value in subsequent pregnancies and lowers her risk of long-term complications.

Messages for Persons With Diabetes

Motivation is key to the success of a good outcome in pregnancy.

Expect more intense care and monitoring requirements. In a pregnancy complicated by diabetes, additional testing and monitoring may be necessary during the pregnancy. Glycemic management within the optimal range is necessary to decrease the risk of congenital malformations and spontaneous abortions. Periodic adjustments in insulin dosage and food intake may require more frequent SMBG.

Pay attention to food plans and weight gain. Weight gain goals will be established based on the IOM guidelines. Medical nutrition therapy will be based on current eating habits and the DRIs for pregnant women.

Expect changes in medication. Medication therapy may change frequently during pregnancy as hormones impact insulin needs. Medications may also change at delivery and in the postpartum phase.

Breastfeed to attain immunological benefits. Breastfeeding is encouraged because of the immunological benefits to the mother and infant. Lactation may be delayed because of early separation of the infant; however, pumping the breasts soon after delivery can establish a steady milk supply.

Focus on Education: GDM

Teaching Strategies

Enable timely initial visits. New referrals should be seen as soon as possible–within 1 week of referral.

Involve team in glucose goals. Achieve target glucose stability as quickly as possible, within the context of a healthy pregnancy; get to know team members in obstetrics-gynecology, endocrinology, and family medicine and involve them in agreeing on targets, curriculum handouts, and content.

Take action and offer support. Women with GDM need more support than the person with type 1 diabetes or type 2 diabetes, as there is so much to learn and implement in just a few weeks.

Offer hope for a healthy future. Present the information that implementing lifestyle changes now may lead to diabetes prevention as well as reduce an individual's chances of developing other chronic diseases, including cardiovascular disease.

Model the lifestyle. Consider how you and your team can best model positive approaches to lifestyle changes intended to lead to diabetes prevention and a reduction in obesity, cardiovascular disease, and cancer.

Messages for Persons With Diabetes

Use your diabetes team. Diabetes care and education specialists, clinicians, and specialty services are available to help you in any way to understand and manage GDM.

Manage GDM. Good management balances glucose stability with the goals of a healthy pregnancy.

Be comfortable with insulin. Do not be afraid of adding insulin, as it is a hormone your body makes, not a drug; during the pregnancy, you may need extra insulin, via injection, to keep blood glucose at target levels.

Guard your own health after delivery. Knowing you had GDM is a clear signal that you are at risk for developing diabetes. Take steps to prevent diabetes by improving your eating and exercise habits and maintaining an appropriate weight after your baby is born. These healthy habits will not only help you but help your whole family.

Health Literacy for Pregnancy With Preexisting Diabetes or GDM

Health literacy is defined as the degree to which individuals have the capacity to obtain, process, and understand basic health information and the services needed to make appropriate health decisions.[99] It includes the ability to interpret health information presented by healthcare providers and to make decisions based on an understanding of the information.[100] If the person with diabetes lack the necessary skills to understand what is said or written, it could result in a negative impact on their health. The American Medical Association considers poor health literacy as a stronger predictor of a person's health than age, income, employment status, education level, and race.[101]

Although health literacy is not necessarily based on reading ability, reading ability is of particular concern in persons with low literacy skills, especially women of childbearing age. If a woman has difficulty understanding the information or following directions, this may affect either her health or the health of her child. Women with diabetes may be even more vulnerable to poorer outcomes if they are unaware of the health consequences associated with diabetes and pregnancy. Low health literacy in pregnant women with preexisting diabetes may affect the birth outcome. In a study of 74 pregnant women with preexisting diabetes, those with low functional literacy were less likely to have received preconception care.[102]

The ACOG recommends the following general health literacy guidelines when working with women:

- Tailor speaking and listening skills to the individual women.
- Tailor the health information to the intended user.
- Develop written materials that keep the message simple.

Focus on Practice

When providing education and care for pregnant women with preexisting diabetes or gestational diabetes, be sure to establish a good relationship with the obstetrics department.

- Diabetes care and education specialists who work with pregnant women with diabetes are, in most cases, already working with individuals with type 1 diabetes or type 2 diabetes. They probably have good relationships with clinicians who work in primary care, internal medicine, and endocrinology.
- Work together to agree on the referral process, the method of documentation, and the message that communication is important for consistent care for the person with diabetes.

Include comprehensive preconception, prenatal, postpartum, and interconception self-management education as part of your program.

- Be prepared to discuss preconception care with women with type 1 diabetes or type 2 diabetes.
- Consider multicultural concerns for GDM, type 1 diabetes, or being pregnant with type 2 diabetes.
- Provide appropriate care during the postpartum period (ie, breastfeeding and nutritional and insulin management, taking medication); provide referrals for pediatricians, endocrinologists, and other providers involved in preconception, prenatal, postpartum, and interconception care.
- Work with service providers such as WIC (Women, Infants, and Children) or other social services to coordinate appropriate care.

References

1. American Diabetes Association. Standards of medical care in diabetes. Glycemic targets. Diabetes Care. 2019;39 Suppl 1:S61-70.
2. American College of Obstetricians and Gynecologists, "Pregestational diabetes mellitus," Practice bulletin no. 201, Obstet Gynecol. 2018;132:e228-48.
3. Engelgau MM, Herman WH, Smith PJ, et al. The epidemiology of diabetes and pregnancy in the US, 1988. Diabetes Care. 1995;18:1029-33.
4. American College of Obstetricians and Gynecologists. Committee Opinion Number 504. Screening and diagnosis of gestational diabetes mellitus. Obstet Gynecol. 2013;122:406-15.
5. Hartling L, Dryden DM, Guthrie A, et al. Screening and Diagnosing Gestational Diabetes Mellitus. Evidence Report/Technology Assessment No. 210. AHRQ Publication No. 12(13)-E021-EF. Rockville, Md: Agency for Healthcare Research and Quality; 2012.
6. Koos BJ, Moore PJ. Maternal physiology during pregnancy. In: DeCherney AH, Nathan L, eds. Current Obstetric and Gynecologic Diagnosis and Treatment. New York: Lange Medical Books/McGraw-Hill; 2003:154-62.
7. Institute of Medicine. Weight Gain During Pregnancy: Reexamining the Guidelines. Washington, DC: National Academy Press; 2009.
8. American College of Obstetricians and Gynecologists. Committee Opinion Number 548. Obesity in pregnancy. Obstet Gynecol. 2013;121:213-7 (reaffirmed 2018).
9. Voerman E, Santos S, Inskip H, et al. Association of gestational weight gain with adverse maternal and infant outcomes. The Life Cycle Project—Maternal Obesity and Childhood Outcomes Study Group. JAMA. 2019;321(17):1702-15.
10. Franz MJ, Evert AB. American Diabetes Association Guide to Nutrition Therapy for Diabetes. Washington, DC: American Diabetes Association; 2012.
11. American College of Obstetricians and Gynecologists. Your Pregnancy and Childbirth: Month by Month. 5th ed. Washington, DC: American College of Obstetricians and Gynecologists; 2010.
12. Widen E, Siega-Riz AM. Prenatal nutrition: a practical guide for assessment and counseling. J Midwifery Womens Health. 2010;55:540-9.
13. Institute of Medicine of the National Academies. Dietary Reference Intakes for Calcium and Vitamin D. Washington, DC: The National Academies Press; 2011.
14. Institute of Medicine of the National Academies. Dietary Reference Intakes: Energy, Carbohydrate, Fiber, Fat, Fatty Acids, Cholesterol, Protein, and Amino Acids. Washington, DC: The National Academies Press; 2002.
15. Academy of Nutrition and Dietetics. Position of the Academy of Nutrition and Dietetics: use of nutritive and nonnutritive sweeteners. J Acad Nutr Diet. 2012;112:739-58.
16. Williams JF, Smith VC; Committee on Substance Abuse. Fetal alcohol spectrum disorders. Pediatrics. 2015;136(5):e1395-406 (cited 2016 Jun 14). On the Internet: http://pediatrics.aappublications.org/content/pediatrics/136/5/e1395.full.pdf.

17. Food and Drug Administration. Fish: what pregnant women and parents should know. 2014 (cited 2016 Jun 20). On the Internet at: http://www.fda.gov/downloads/Food/FoodborneIllness Contaminants/Metals/UCM400358.pdf. Now: Food and Drug Administration. Advice about eating fish: for women who are or might become pregnant, breastfeeding mothers, and young children. 2019 July 30. http://fda.gov./food/consumers /advice-about-eating-fish.

18. American College of Obstetricians and Gynecologists. Committee Opinion Number 650. Physical activity and exercise during pregnancy and the postpartum period. Obstet Gynecol. 2015;126:e135-42 (cited 2016 May 15). On the Internet at: http://www.acog.org/-/media/Committee-Opinions/Committee -on-Obstetric-Practice/co650.pdf?dmc=1.

19. US Department of Health and Human Services. Physical Activity Guidelines Advisory Committee final report (cited 2013 May 31). On the Internet at: http://www.health.gov/PAGuidelines /Report/Default.aspx.

20. Kitzmiller JL, Jovanovic L, Brown F, Coustan D, Reader DM, eds. Managing Preexisting Diabetes and Pregnancy. Alexandria, Va: American Diabetes Association; 2008.

21. Abrams BF, Laros RK Jr. Prepregnancy weight, weight gain and birth weight. Am J Obstet Gynecol. 1986;154:503-9.

22. Landon MB, Gabbe SG. Diabetes mellitus. In: Barron WM, Lindheimer MD, Davison JM, eds. Medical Disorders in Pregnancy. St. Louis, Mo: Mosby; 2000:71-100.

23. Centers for Disease Control and Prevention. Recommendations to improve preconception health and health care—United States. MMWR Morb Mortal Wkly Rep. 2006;55(RR06):1-23.

24. Guttmacher Institute. Unintended pregnancy in the United States. Fact sheet. 2016 Mar (cited 2016 Oct 11). On the Internet at: https://www.guttmacher.org/sites/default/files/pdfs/pubs /FB-Unintended-Pregnancy-US.pdf.

25. American College of Obstetricians and Gynecologists. Pregestational diabetes mellitus. Practice bulletin No. 201. Obstet Gynecol. 2018;132:e228-48.

26. Kim C, Ferrara A, McEwen LN, Marrero DG, Gerzoff RB, Herman WH; TRIAD Study Group. Preconception care in managed care: the translating research into action for diabetes study. Am J Obstet Gynecol. 2005;192(1):227-32.

27. Dunne F. Type 2 diabetes and pregnancy. Sem Fetal Neonatal Med. 2005;10:333-9.

28. McElduff A, Ross GP, Lagström JA, et al. Pregestational diabetes and pregnancy: an Australian experience. Diabetes Care. 2005;28:1260-1.

29. American Diabetes Association. Standards of medical care in diabetes. Management of diabetes in pregnancy. Diabetes Care. 2019;42 Suppl 1:S165-72.

30. American Diabetes Association. Preconception care of women with diabetes. Diabetes Care. 2004;27 Suppl 1:S76-8.

31. Catalano PM, Buchanan TA. Metabolic changes during normal and diabetic pregnancies. In: Reece EA, Coustan DR, Gabbe SG, eds. Diabetes in Women: Adolescence, Pregnancy, and Menopause. Philadelphia: Lippincott Williams & Wilkins; 2004:129-45.

32. Pedersen J. The Pregnant Diabetic and Her Newborn. 2nd ed. Baltimore: Williams & Wilkins; 1977.

33. Eidelman AI, Samueloff A. The pathophysiology of the fetus of the diabetic mother. Semin Perinatol. 2002;26:232-6.

34. Jovanovic L. Diabetic retinopathy. In: Reece EA, Coustan DR, Gabbe SG, eds. Diabetes in Women: Adolescence, Pregnancy, and Menopause. 3rd ed. Philadelphia: Lippincott Williams & Wilkins; 2004:371-82.

35. Lauszus FF, Klebe JG, Bek T, et al. Increased serum IGF-I during pregnancy is associated with progression of diabetic retinopathy. Diabetes. 2003;52:852-6.

36. Rosenn B, Miodovnik M, Kranias G, et al. Progression of diabetic retinopathy in pregnancy: association with hypertension in pregnancy. Am J Obstet Gynecol. 1992;166:1214-8.

37. Brinchmann-Hansen O, Dahl-Jorgensen K, Hanssen KF, et al. Effects of intensified insulin treatment on various lesions of diabetic retinopathy. Am J Ophthalmol. 1985;100:644-53.

38. Report of the National High Blood Pressure Education Program Working Group on High Blood Pressure in Pregnancy. Am J Obstet Gynecol. 2000;183:S1-22.

39. Hinton AC, Sibai BM. Hypertensive disorders in pregnancy. In: Reece EA, Coustan DR, Gabbe SG, eds. Diabetes in Women: Adolescence, Pregnancy, and Menopause. 3rd ed. Philadelphia: Lippincott Williams & Wilkins; 2004:363-70.

40. de Veciana M. Diabetes ketoacidosis in pregnancy. Semin Perinatol. 2013;37:267-73.

41. Bahai BM, Viteri OA. Diabetic ketoacidosis in pregnancy. Obstet Gynecol. 2014;123:167-78.

42. Academy of Nutrition and Dietetics. Position of the Academy of Nutrition and Dietetics: obesity, reproduction, and pregnancy outcomes. J Acad Nutr Diet. 2016;116(4):677-91.

43. Jensen DM, Damm P, Moelsted-Pedersen L, et al. Outcomes in type 1 diabetic pregnancies. Diabetes Care. 2004;27:2819-23.

44. Wren C, Birrell G, Hawthorne G. Cardiovascular malformations in infants of diabetic mothers. Heart. 2003;89:1217-20.

45. American College of Obstetricians and Gynecologists. Fetal macrosomia. ACOG Practice Bulletin No. 22. Washington, DC: American College of Obstetricians and Gynecologists; 2000.

46. Coustan DR. Delivery: timing, mode, and management. In: Reece EA, Coustan DR, Gabbe SG, eds. Diabetes in Women: Adolescence, Pregnancy, and Menopause. 3rd ed. Philadelphia: Lippincott Williams & Wilkins; 2004:433-9.

47. American Academy of Pediatrics; Committee on Fetus and Newborn. Postnatal glucose homeostasis in late-preterm and term infants. Pediatrics. 2011;127:575-9.

48. US Department of Health and Human Services. Physical Activity Guidelines Advisory Committee final report (cited 2016 Oct 11). On the Internet at: https://health.gov/paguidelines/report/.

49. Stewart ZA, Wilinska ME, Hartnell S, et al. Closed-loop insulin delivery during pregnancy in women with type 1 diabetes. N Engl J Med. 2016;375:644-54.

50. Rizzo T, Metzger BE, Burns WJ, et al. Correlations between antepartum maternal metabolism and child intelligence. N Engl J Med. 1991;325:911-6.

51. Churchill JA, Berendes HW. Intelligence of children whose mothers had acetonuria during pregnancy. In: Perinatal Factors Affecting Human Development. Pan American Health Organization Scientific Publication. Washington, DC: Pan American Health Organization; 1969;185:300.

52. Battelino T, Danne T, Bergenstal RM, et al. Clinical targets for continuous glucose monitoring data interpretation: recommendations from the International Consensus on time in range. Diabetes Care. 2019; https://doi.org/10.2337/dci19-0028.

53. Lapolla A, Dalfrà MG, Fedele D. Insulin therapy in pregnancy complicated by diabetes: are insulin analogs a new tool? Diabetes Metab Res Rev. 2005;21:241-52.

54. Gamson K, Chia S, Jovanovic L. The safety and efficacy of insulin analogs in pregnancy. J Matern Fetal Neonatal Med. 2004;15:26-34.

55. Garg SK, Frias JP, Anil S, Gottlieb PA, MacKenzie T, Jackson WE. Insulin lispro therapy in pregnancies complicated by type 1 diabetes: glycemic control and maternal and fetal outcomes. Endocr Pract. 2003;9:187-93.

56. Cypryk K, Sobczak M, Pertyńska-Marczewska M, et al. Pregnancy complications and perinatal outcome in diabetic women treated with Humalog (insulin lispro) or regular human insulin during pregnancy. Med Sci Monit. 2004;10:129-32.

57. Federal Register. Content and format of labeling for human prescription drug and biological products; requirements for pregnancy and lactation labeling. 2014 (cited 2016 May 9). On the Internet at: https://federalregister.gov/a/2014-28241.

58. Rudolf MC, Coustan DR, Sherwin RS, et al. Efficacy of the insulin pump in the home treatment of pregnant diabetics. Diabetes. 1981;30:891-5.

59. Kitzmiller J, Younger D, Hare J, et al. Continuous subcutaneous insulin therapy during early pregnancy. Obstet Gynecol. 1985;66:606-11.

60. Mathiesen MJM, Secher AL, Ringholm L, et al. Change in basal rates and bolus calculator settings in insulin pumps during pregnancy in women with type 1 diabetes. J Matern Fetal Neonatal Med. 2014;27:724-8.

61. Gabbe SG. New concepts and applications in the use of the insulin pump during pregnancy. J Matern Fetal Med. 2000;9:42-5.

62. Radermecker RP, Scheen AJ. Continuous subcutaneous insulin infusion with short-acting insulin analogues or human regular insulin: efficacy, safety, quality of life, and cost-effectiveness. Diabetes Metab Res Rev. 2004;20:178-88.

63. Hickman MA, McBide R, Boggess KA, Strauss R. Metformin compared with insulin in the treatment of pregnant women with overt diabetes: a randomized controlled trial. Am J Perinatol. 2013;30:483-90.

64. Ainuddin JA, Karim N, Zaheer S, et al. Metformin treatment in type 2 diabetes in pregnancy: an active controlled, parallel-group, randomized, open label study in patients with type 2 diabetes in pregnancy. J Diabetes Res. 2015;2015:325851. On the Internet at: http://dx.doi.org/10.1155/2015/325851.

65. Coustan DR, ed. Medical Management of Pregnancy Complicated by Diabetes. 5th ed. Alexandria, Va: American Diabetes Association; 2013.

66. Feig DS, Briggs GG, Koren G. Oral antidiabetic agents in pregnancy and lactation: a paradigm shift? Ann Pharmacother. 2007;41:1147-80.

67. Glatstein MM, Djokanovic N, Garcia-Bournissen F, et al. Use of hypoglycemic drugs during lactation. Can Fam Physician. 2009;55:371-3.

68. American Diabetes Association. Standards of medical care in diabetes. Classification and diagnosis of diabetes mellitus. Diabetes Care. 2019;42 Suppl 1:S13-28.

69. HAPO Study Cooperative Research Group. Hyperglycemia and adverse pregnancy outcomes. N Engl J Med. 2008;358(19): 1991-2002.

70. American College of Obstetricians and Gynecologists. Committee Opinion Number 504. Screening and diagnosis of gestational diabetes mellitus. Obstet Gynecol. 2011;118:751-3.

71. VanDorsten JP, Dodson WC, Espeland MA, et al. National Institutes of Health Consensus Development Conference Statement: diagnosing gestational diabetes mellitus. NIH Consens State Sci Statements. 2013;29(1):1-30.

72. Moyer VA. Screening for gestational diabetes mellitus: U.S. Preventive Task Force recommendation statement. Ann Intern Med. 2014;60(6):414-20.

73. American Diabetes Association. American Diabetes Association standards of medical care in diabetes—2019. ACOG Pract Bull. 2018 Feb.

74. Academy of Nutrition and Dietetics. Evidence Analysis Library. Gestational diabetes (cited 2016 Jun 30). On the Internet: http://andeal.org.

75. Perichart-Perera O, Balas-Nakash M, Rodriguez-Cano A, et al. Low glycemic index carbohydrates versus all types of carbohydrates for treating diabetes in pregnancy: a randomized clinical trial to evaluate the effect of glycemic control. Int J Endocrinol. 2012;2012:296017.

76. Moreno-Castilla C, Hernandez M, Bergua M, et al. Low-carbohydrate diet for the treatment of gestational diabetes mellitus. Diabetes Care. 2013;36:2233-8.

77. Hernandez TL, Van Pelt RE, Anderson MA, et al. A higher-complex carbohydrate diet in gestational diabetes achieves glucose targets and lowers postprandial lipids: a randomized crossover study. Diabetes Care. 2014;37(5):1254-62.

78. Asemi Z, Samimi M, Tabassi Z, Esmaillzadeh A. The effect of DASH diet on pregnancy outcomes in gestational diabetes: a randomized control trial. Eur J Clin Nutr. 2014;68:490-5.

79. Viana LV, Gross JL, Azevedo MJ. Dietary interventions in patients with gestational diabetes mellitus: a systematic review and meta-analysis of randomized clinical trials on maternal and newborn outcomes. Diabetes Care. 2014;37:3345-55.

80. Ben-Haroush A, Yogev Y, Rosenn B, Hod M, Langer O. The postprandial glucose profile in the diabetic pregnancy. Am J Obstet Gynecol. 2004;191(2):576-81.

81. Yogev Y, Ben-Haroush A, Chen R, Rosenn B, Hod M, Langer O. Diurnal glycemic profile in obese and normal weight non-diabetic pregnant women. Am J Obstet Gynecol. 2004;191:949-53.

82. Louie JCY, Markovic TP, Ross GP, et al. Timing of peak blood glucose after breakfast meals of different glycemic index in women with gestational diabetes. Nutrients. 2013;5:1-9.

83. Metzger BE, Buchanan TA, Coustan DR. Summary and recommendations of the Fifth International Workshop-Conference on Gestational Diabetes Mellitus. Diabetes Care. 2007;30 Suppl 2:S251-60.

84. American Diabetes Association. Gestational diabetes mellitus (position statement). Diabetes Care. 2004;27 Suppl 1:S88-90.

85. de Veciana M, Major CA, Morgan MA, et al. Postprandial versus preprandial blood glucose monitoring in women with gestational diabetes mellitus requiring insulin therapy. N Engl J Med. 1995;333:1237-41.

86. Langer O, Conway D, Berkus M, Xenakis EM, Gonzales O. A comparison of glyburide and insulin in women with gestational diabetes mellitus. N Engl J Med. 2000;343:1134-8.

87. Society of Maternal-Fetal Medicine Publication Committee. SMFM Statement: Pharmacological treatment of gestational diabetes. May 2018.

88. Dhulkotia JS, Ola B, Fraser R, Farrell T. Oral hypoglycemic agents vs insulin in management of gestational diabetes: a systematic review and metaanalysis. Am J Obstet Gynecol. 2010;203:457.e1-9.

89. Thorkelson SJ, Anderson KR. Oral medication for diabetes in pregnancy: use in a rural population. Diabetes Spectr. 2016;29(2):98-101.

90. Balsells M, Garcia-Patterson A, Sola I, et al. Glibenclamide, metformin and insulin for the treatment of gestational diabetes: a systematic review and meta-analysis. BMJ. 2015;350:h102.

91. Hui AL, Sevenhuysen G, Harvey D, Salamon E. Stress and anxiety in women with gestational diabetes during dietary management. Diabetes Educ. 2014;40(5):668-77.

92. Gunderson EP, Hedderson MM, Chiang V, et al. Lactation intensity and postpartum maternal glucose tolerance and insulin resistance in women with recent GDM: the SWIFT cohort. Diabetes Care. 2012;35(1):50-6.

93. Bellemy L, Casas JP, Hingorani AD, Williams D. Type 2 diabetes after gestational diabetes: a systematic review and meta-analysis. Lancet. 2009;373:1773-9.

94. Diabetes Prevention Program Research Group. Reduction in the incidence of type 2 diabetes with lifestyle intervention or metformin. N Engl J Med. 2002;346(6):393-403.

95. Ratner RE, Costa AC, Metzger BE, et al. Prevention of diabetes in women with a history of gestational diabetes: effects of metformin and lifestyle interventions. J Clin Endocrinol Metab. 2008 Dec;93(12):4774-9.

96. Kim C, Berger DK, Chamany S. Recurrence of gestational diabetes mellitus. Diabetes Care. 2007;30(5):1314-19.

97. Getahun D, Fassett MJ, Jacobsen SJ. Gestational diabetes: risk of recurrence in subsequent pregnancies. Am J Obstet Gynecol. 2010 Nov;203(5):467.e1-6.

98. Brown FM, Isganaitis E, James-Todd T. Much to HAPO-FUS About: Increasing maternal glycemia in pregnancy is associated with worsening childhood glucose metabolism. Diabetes Care. 2019;42:393-5.

99. US Department of Health and Human Services. Health literacy (cited 2016 July 5). On the Internet: https://nnlm.gov/outreach/consumer/hlthlit.html.

100. American College of Obstetrics and Gynecology. ACOG Committee Opinion No. 391. Health literacy. Obstet Gynecol. 2007;110:1489-91.

101. American Medical Association Ad Hoc Committee on Health Literacy for the Council on Scientific Affairs. Health literacy: report of the Council on Scientific Affairs. JAMA. 1999;281:552-7.

102. Endres LK, Sharp LK, Haney E, Dooley SL. Health literacy and pregnancy preparedness in pregestational diabetes. Diabetes Care. 2004;27:331-4.

CHAPTER 25

Cardiovascular Complications of Diabetes

JoAnn Sperl-Hillen, MD

Key Concepts

- Diabetes is a major cause of cardiovascular (CV) events. Despite advances in detection and treatment, heart attacks and strokes continue to be the leading cause of complications, disability, and premature death for people with diabetes.
- Increased effort is needed to identify modifiable risk factors earlier in people with diabetes for intervention with education and preventive treatments.
- Important modifiable risk factors are obesity, hypertension, dyslipidemia, hyperglycemia, tobacco use, and underuse of antiplatelet therapy in individuals with heart disease.
- Calculation of CV risk using the American College of Cardiology (ACC)/American Heart Association (AHA) Pooled Cohort Equation can support individualized treatment recommendations and may be a useful tool for patient counseling, education, and shared decision making.
- A multidisciplinary strategy that includes lifestyle and multiple pharmacologic considerations, care coordination, and frequent follow-up is recommended to treat CV risk.
- One of several sodium-glucose cotransporter 2 inhibitors (SGLT2s) and glucagon-like peptide 1 receptor agonists (GLP1 agonists) with demonstrated CV benefit should be considered for people with type 2 diabetes and CV disease. The SGLT2s may be preferred for those with congestive heart failure.
- The prevalence of CV disease differs among sex, racial, and ethnic groups in the United States. Special attention may be warranted for high-risk subgroups.

Introduction

With the dramatic global increase in the number of people with type 2 diabetes mellitus (T2DM), CV complications are particularly significant due to the associated frequency, morbidity, mortality, and economic consequences.[1,2] The incidence of CV events in both the diabetic and the nondiabetic populations has diminished since the 1950s following a highly significant improvement in blood pressure (BP) and cholesterol management, although trends may be reversing more recently.[3] The incidence of diabetes and prediabetes has doubled,[4,5–7] and abnormal glucose carries important prognostic implications with decreased probability of event-free survival.[8,9] Even though diabetes is underreported on death certificates, it is still the seventh-leading reported cause of death in the United States.[10] People with diabetes are at least twice as likely as people without diabetes to have heart disease or strokes, and their risk of death is at least twice that of people of similar age without diabetes.[11] Sixty-five percent of deaths in people with diabetes are due to either coronary or cerebrovascular events.[12–14]

The increased annual cost to individual patients related to CVD is substantial compared to T2DM alone, contributing to an enormous global population impact.[15]

> People with diabetes have 2 to 3 times the risk of stroke, myocardial infarction (MI), and sudden death as those without diabetes.

This chapter begins by describing the importance of recognizing and treating CV risk factors early and aggressively. It discusses methods for quantifying CV risk and clinical considerations helpful in engaging patients in the process of treating modifiable risk. It includes a discussion of issues and challenges for patients related to common CV problems and ends with pearls for practice, a worthwhile to-do list for diabetes care and education specialists.

Manifestations of Cardiovascular Disease

Coronary Heart Disease

- Angina
- Myocardial infarction
- Congestive heart failure

Cerebrovascular Disease

- Cerebrovascular accident (stroke)
- Transient ischemic attack

Peripheral Artery Disease

- Lower extremity ischemia

The Relationship Between Diabetes and Cardiovascular Disease

Epidemiology of Diabetes and Cardiovascular Disease

A number of large epidemiologic studies have shown that chronic hyperglycemia, as evaluated by fasting blood glucose or A1C, is an independent risk factor for cardiovascular disease (CVD).[16] Cardiovascular risk increases by approximately 28% for each 1% increase in A1C[17,18] and a similar effect was found for peripheral artery disease (PAD).[19] Studies have also demonstrated that increased levels of A1C are correlated with increased carotid intima-media thickness (IMT), a measure of early atherosclerosis.[20] Pooled data from a meta-analysis suggest that a 1% increase in A1C is associated with a 1.2- to 1.3-fold increased risk of CVD, including coronary events, stroke, and PAD.[21] People with type 1 diabetes mellitus (T1DM) are at a tenfold increased risk for CV events overall,[21,22] and those who are between the ages of 20 and 39 are at a fivefold increased risk.[23] Because of these sobering statistics, it is highly recommended that CV risk factors—particularly dyslipidemia, smoking, and hypertension—be aggressively addressed in both T1DM and T2DM populations.[24,25,26]

Why Is the Risk of CV Events Higher in People With Diabetes?

Research has shown that a rupture of weakened areas within plaques of partially occluded blood vessels often leads to acute coronary and cerebral thrombosis.[27] Diabetes, insulin resistance, and glucose intolerance are also associated with a state of enhanced thrombosis by affecting platelets and production of clotting factors, increasing the development of thrombi that cause acute events. In acute coronary events, endothelial function is altered in ways that accelerate atherosclerotic change, including increased vasospasm, enhanced thrombosis, and increased local inflammatory responses.[28]

Factors contributing to cardiometabolic risk are described in Figure 25.1. Factors such as hyperlipoproteinemia, smoking, diabetes, and hypertension disturb endothelial function in a variety of ways. Further, the effects of these factors appear to be synergistic rather than just additive. Increasing evidence suggests that both hyperglycemia and insulin resistance affect vascular function, and when both are present, the effects are much greater than when either is present alone.[29] Chronic hyperglycemia and insulin resistance may produce vasoconstrictive substances and advanced glycation end products that disturb endothelial function and affect the vessel walls by causing increased stiffness and decreased compliance of the arterial wall.[30] Other risk factors for decreased arterial compliance include advanced age, hypertension, presence of components of the metabolic syndrome, microalbuminuria, central obesity, and low cardiopulmonary fitness.

Post-prandial hyperglycemia excursions may also play a role in the pathophysiology of microvascular and macrovascular complications of diabetes. Epidemiologic data support the association of postprandial hyperglycemia and increased CV risk.[31,32] A number of epidemiologic studies and glycemic intervention studies suggest that postprandial spikes in blood glucose and triglycerides (TGs) may each play a greater role in CVD than either average or fasting glucose.[32–36] Several interventional studies targeting postprandial hyperglycemia support the hypothesis that reducing postprandial glucose excursions may decrease CV risk in people with prediabetes and diabetes.[37–39]

Can Better Glycemic Management in People With T2DM Prevent CV Events?

Despite the strong observational association between diabetes and macrovascular disease, the evidence has been controversial about whether and to what extent improved glycemic management can reduce the risk of events, particularly in T2DM.[40] In the United Kingdom Prospective Diabetes Study (UKPDS) study, there was a 16% reduction in myocardial infarction (MIs) in the intensively treated group, but this effect missed statistical significance,[41] and the effect of glycemic stability was much less

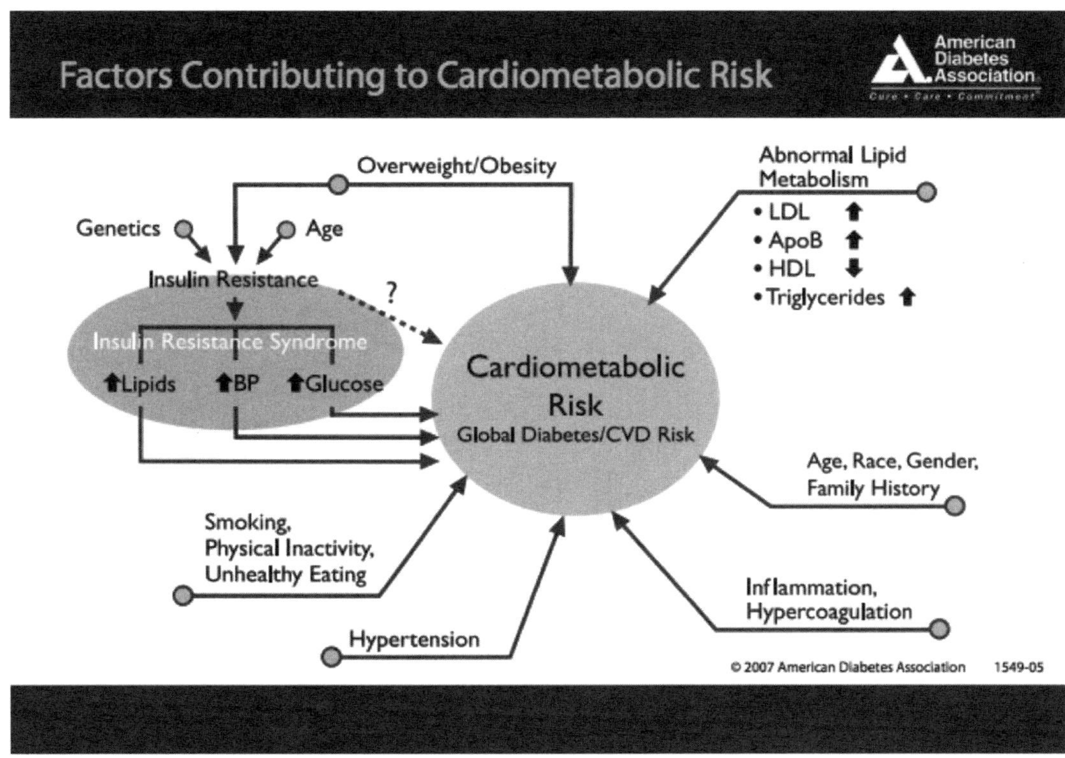

FIGURE 25.1 **Factors Contributing to Cardiometabolic Risk in Persons with Diabetes**

Source: Reproduced with permission from the American Diabetes Association, "Factors contributing to cardiometabolic risk" (cited 2014 Mar 14), on the Internet at http://professional.diabetes.org/UserFiles/File/Resources%20for%20Professionals/CMR_Chart.pdf.

than the effect of hypertension or hyperlipidemia stability. Interestingly, after the UKPDS study ended, the hemoglobin A1C difference between the intensive and control groups was lost within 1 to 2 years but there was a significant reduction in MI, diabetes-related death, and all-cause mortality after 10 years in the intensively treated group.[42]

Three large randomized trials failed to show a significant effect of more intensive glycemic management on their primary CV event outcomes. The Action to Control Cardiovascular Risk in Diabetes (ACCORD) study randomly assigned 10,251 people with established type 2 diabetes (mean duration 10 years) and at least 2 CVD risk factors to a strategy targeting A1C <6.0% versus 7.0% to 7.9%.[43] The intensive and control group patients achieved median A1C levels of 6.4% and 7.5%, respectively. The ACCORD study was stopped early due to increased all-cause mortality in the intensively treated group.[44] The study was insufficiently powered to determine the cause of increased mortality; however, despite a lower MI rate trend in the intensive group, a higher rate of fatal MI was observed.

The Action in Diabetes and Vascular Disease: Preterax and Diamicron Modified Release Controlled Evaluation (ADVANCE) trial randomly assigned 11,140 people with T2DM to either standard care goals (local guidelines) or to a target A1C ≤6.5%.[45] Enrolled subjects had an A1C of 7.2% at baseline and had had diabetes for, on average, 8 years. The intensive group achieved a median A1C of 6.3%, compared with the standard group A1C of 7.0%. Although microvascular disease (primarily nephropathy) was reduced in the intensively treated group, there was no difference in the rate of vascular events between the 2 groups.[43]

The Veterans Administration Diabetes Trial (VADT) randomly assigned 1,791 people with T2DM to standard or intensive therapy.[46] Enrolled subjects were 97% male and had had diabetes for 11.5 years and a baseline median A1C of 9.4%. The median A1C achieved in the intensive group was 6.9%, compared with 8.5% in the standard therapy group.[43] There were no significant differences in major CV event or any component of the outcome. There were no observed differences in microvascular complications (except for progression of albuminuria), and rates of hypoglycemia were significantly higher in the intensive therapy group. Results of a 10-year long-term follow-up study of VADT subjects revealed less CV events in the more intensively treated group but no improvement in survival.[47]

These well-designed interventions failed to show that more intensively treated glycemic management significantly reduced the rates of cardiovascular events. However, the inconsistency in results between these trials and UKPDS may have been related to the characteristics of the patients who received interventions in these trials. For example, patients in the UKPDS study were younger and had a more recent diabetes diagnosis than those in later interventional trials such as ACCORD, in which subjects had had diabetes longer and had a greater degree of preexisting suboptimal glycemic levels and insulin use at study entry. Another prominent theory is that cardiovascular events are associated with hypoglycemia,[48] and hypoglycemia rates differed significantly in these trials. The implication that early intervention is beneficial, whereas later intervention may be less effective, is supported by further analyses of the VADT, which suggest that duration of diabetes interacts with effects of intensive management; subjects with a shorter duration of diabetes appear to benefit more from intensive management, whereas those with longer duration appear to either receive no benefit or even have adverse effects. Newly diagnosed persons with diabetes who are pharmacologically treated for hyperglycemia have reduced risk of CV events compared with those who are untreated.[49] A lesser degree of preexisting CVD, as measured by coronary calcium scores, may also predict greater benefit from intensive glycemic management.[43]

Studies suggest that glycemic stability may have greater CV benefits in people with diabetes if started early in the disease process.

The Effects of Specific Glucose Lowering Drugs on CV Outcomes

Rosiglitazone (Avandia, GlaxoSmithKline) was implicated in a meta-analysis as a drug that increased CV risk in some studies.[50] This analysis precipitated a Food and Drug Administration (FDA) box warning for the heart-related risks in 2007 which was reversed in 2013 after further study and review.[51] However, due to the lingering questions related to CV safety of T2DM drugs, the FDA has since required larger and more comprehensive CV safety outcome studies.[52] The results of these studies thus far show that the effect of diabetes treatment on CV outcomes varies by medication and medication class as described below:

1. *Metformin:* Most experts conclude from the UKPDS study that metformin is cardioprotective, but the data are insufficient to draw strong conclusions.[53] Given widespread acknowledgment that metformin as the best first line treatment for T2DM, it is unlikely that additional CV studies are forthcoming.[54]
2. *SGLT2 inhibitors* (canagliflozin, empagliflozin) reduce cardiovascular risk in people with T2DM and high risk for CVD and reduce rates of hospitalization for heart failure.[55–57] Empagliflozin significantly reduced all-cause mortality in those with T2DM and established CVD.[57] The benefits of SGLT2 inhibitors must be weighed against high costs and reported risks including bone fractures (canagliflozin), diabetic ketoacidosis (rare), genitourinary infections, volume depletion hypotension, increased LDL cholesterol, and Fournier's gangrene.[58]
3. *GLP1 receptor agonists* (liraglutide, semaglutide) have favorable cardiovascular and chronic kidney disease (CKD) end points and composite indices of CKD in high risk subjects.[59,60]
4. *DPP-4 inhibitors* – sitagliptin showed cardiovascular benefit in those with acute coronary syndrome, but saxagliptin and alogliptin were not of proven cardiovascular benefit and may increase hospital admissions for heart failure.[61,62]

The differences in CV outcomes in these studies may be related to intrinsic properties of the medications, study design, or differences in patient characteristics of the study populations. Of note is that even though the mean A1C reduction was only 0.4% in the studies of empagliflozin and liraglutide, an impressive reduction in mortality was observed.[63]

Considerations for T1DM

The major predictor of CVD in people with T1DM appears to be duration of the disease.[64] Several lines of evidence support the long-term effects of glycemic stability on macrovascular risk. Pancreas transplantation normalizes glucose and has been shown to reduce increased carotid IMT to normal within 2 years of successful transplantation.[65] In a study of kidney transplant patients, the group that received a subsequent islet transplant had improved cardiac function and stabilization of carotid IMT compared with the kidney-alone group.[66]

Long-term follow-up of the Diabetes Control and Complications Trial (DCCT) cohort has provided interesting data about the impact of intensive management on the development of macrovascular disease in T1DM. After the DCCT ended in 1992, most participants were enrolled in a long-term follow-up study, the Epidemiology of Diabetes Interventions and Complications (EDIC) study. Glycemic stability, as determined by A1C, between the 2 groups remained minimally different for 4 years; however, by the fifth year after the DCCT ended, there was no difference between the 2 groups. Carotid IMT was measured from 1994 to 1996 and again 4 years later. Progression of carotid IMT was associated with a number of conventional risk factors, including age, systolic blood pressure, smoking, the ratio of low-density lipoprotein cholesterol (LDL-C) to high-density lipoprotein cholesterol (HDL-C), and albuminuria. Most important, progression of carotid IMT 6 years after the DCCT ended was closely associated with allocation to the intensive therapy group during the 6.5 years of the DCCT.[67] Subsequent data from the same group found that early intensive management of glycemia reduced all CV events by 42%, and nonfatal MI, cerebrovascular accident, and CV death by 57%. These effects were mediated by glycemic management during the DCCT. Thus, the combined DCCT/EDIC studies proved that early intensive management of T1DM decreases the risk of both microvascular and macrovascular complications.[68]

Assessing CV Risk

Using a CV Risk Calculator

An assessment of cardiometabolic risk gives the diabetes care and education specialist and the patient a picture of the patient's health and potential risk of CV events. Patients with known coronary heart disease (CHD), regardless of age, are generally considered to have a 10-year CV risk of 20% or higher. In addition, most men with diabetes aged 50 years and older and most women aged 60 years and older with at least 1 additional major CV risk factor (eg, hypertension, smoking, dyslipidemia, albuminuria, family history of CVD) have a 10-year CV risk of 10% or greater. However, outside of these generalizations, studies show that clinicians are often inaccurate in their predictions of CV risk without the support of risk model calculations.[69]

Many methods of estimating 10-year CV risk, such as the Framingham and Reynolds risk scores, have been recommended over the years.[73] The ACC/AHA Guideline on the Treatment of Blood Cholesterol to Reduce Atherosclerotic CV Risk in Adults recommends using the Pooled Cohort Equation.[73,74] The Pooled Cohort Equation for 10-year risk of atherosclerotic CV disease (ASCVD) has advantages over Framingham CHD risk estimations because it was developed using pooled cohorts that included participants from several large randomized and geographically dispersed cohort studies sponsored by the National Heart, Lung, and Blood Institute (NHLBI).[75] Data needed to calculate the ACC/AHA 10-year CV risk include the following:

- Age
- Sex
- Systolic blood pressure
- Total cholesterol
- HDL cholesterol
- Hypertension treatment (yes/no)
- Diabetes status (yes/no)
- Race (non-Hispanic white or non-Hispanic African American)

One notable gap in the Pooled Cohort Equation is the lack of ethnic-specific risk algorithms for Hispanic-American and Asian-American populations. When compared with non-Hispanic whites, the estimated 10-year risk for ASCVD is generally lower in these populations and higher in American-Indian populations. Until better algorithms are developed for these populations, providers may consider using the equations for non-Hispanic whites for these patients. However, it is important to remember that the risks may be overestimated for Hispanic Americans and Asian Americans.[75]

Young individuals, even with significant CV risk factors, generally do not have high 10-year CV risk. However, extensive epidemiological, pathological, and basic science data indicate that the development of atherosclerosis, the precursor of ASCVD, occurs over decades and is related to long-term and cumulative exposure to causal, modifiable risk factors. Thus, a life-course perspective on risk assessment and prevention should be considered for younger individuals aged 20 to 59 years without known ASCVD. The ACC/AHA recommends that using a 30-year or lifetime ASCVD risk assessment can help with counseling on lifestyle and healthy behavior[75,76] (Table 25.1).

The use of CV risk predictions can guide education and engagement efforts and influence patient behavior.[70] Although more research is needed in this area, two systematic reviews support the conclusion that risk assessment plus counseling is associated with favorable

TABLE 25.1 Examples of ASCVD Risk Calculations Using the ACC/AHA Pooled Cohort Equation

	Black Male Age 70	*White Female Age 50*	*White Female Age 48*
Total cholesterol (TC)	230 mg/dL	180 mg/dL	180 mg/dL
HDL-C	35 mg/dL	50 mg/dL	55 mg/dL
Systolic blood pressure (SBP)	159 mm Hg	135 mm Hg	130 mm Hg
Hypertension treatment?	Yes	Yes	No
Diabetes?	Yes	Yes	Yes
Smoker?	Yes	Yes	No
Calculated 10-year ASCVD risk	70%	10%	2%
10-year ASCVD risk with optimal risk factors*	9%	1%	1%
Lifetime ASCVD risk	Not useful in older patients	50% (would be 8% with optimal risk factors)*	39% (would be 8% with optimal risk factors)*
Recommendations to consider	Stop smoking, initiate high-intensity statin therapy, intensify blood pressure therapy, encourage lifestyle modifications	Stop smoking, initiate high-intensity statin therapy, encourage lifestyle modifications	Initiate moderate-intensity statin therapy, encourage lifestyle modifications

Abbreviations: ASCVD, atherosclerotic cardiovascular disease; HDL-C, high-density lipoprotein cholesterol.

*Optimal risk factors include TC 170 mg/dL, HDL-C 50 mg/dL, SBP 110 mm Hg, not taking medications for hypertension, no diabetes.

changes in patient knowledge and intention to change and with provider prescribing behavior and risk factor management.[71,72] Although there is not much evidence to support the best way to approach a patient discussion about cardiovascular risk, one study showed that patients had higher risk perception and willingness for therapy when shown lifetime risk estimates compared to 10-year estimates.[77]

The ACC/AHA guideline suggests estimation of 10-year and lifetime risk for ASCVD using a Web-based calculator available at http://my.americanheart.org/cvriskcalculator or http://www.cardiosource.org/science-and-quality/practice-guidelines-and-quality-standards/2013-prevention-guideline-tools.aspx. The calculator can also be downloaded to a mobile device as an app from several sources, including iTunes. The calculator is easy to use and requires minimal input of patient data. The calculation can give the clinician a picture of a patient's total risk for CV events in the next 10 years and can be used for educational and counseling purposes to influence patient behavior.

Instruction Opportunity—Explaining CV Risk Calculator Results to Patients[77,78]

The 10-year ACC/AHA Pooled Risk Equation predicts hard ASCVD events (MI, CHD death, stroke, and fatal stroke). To give the patient some context for his or her risk, it can be useful to inform him or her what the risk would be for a patient of the same age, gender, and race if the other CV risk factors were optimal.

- To describe 10-year ASCVD risk (valid for patients over age 40), results can be explained to the patient as, "You have an X% chance of having a heart attack or stroke in the next 10 years. A patient of your age, race, and gender who has optimal risk factors has a Y% chance of having a heart attack or stroke in the next 10 years."
- For describing CV risk in younger patients (aged 21-39 years), it is more useful to use a 30-year risk calculator. Results can be explained to the patient as, "You have an X% chance of having a heart attack or stroke in the next 30 years. A person of the same age, gender, and race with optimal CV risk factors has a Y% chance of having a heart attack or stroke in the next 30 years."

Case Example—Using a CV Risk Calculator and Explaining Results to a Patient

MS, a 50-year-old white woman, is seeing you today for diabetes education. She has T2DM and a body mass index (BMI) of 32. She has a history of hypertension that has been well managed with lisinopril. She does not take any lipid medications. She is a smoker with no other known significant health issues. Her blood pressure is 135/84 mm Hg. Her most recent labs were as follows: A1C 6.6%, total cholesterol 180 mg/dL, HDL-C 50 mg/dL, TGs 140 mg/dL, and LDL-C 102 mg/dL. You want to help MS understand her future risk of heart attack and stroke. You use the online risk calculator to determine her 10-year CV risk is 19% and lifetime risk is 50%. The calculator informs you with optimal risk factor management the 10-year risk would be 1% and lifetime risk 8%. You initiate the following conversation with MS:

MS, your risk of having a stroke or heart attack in the next 10 years is 19%. This means that if you were in a group of 100 persons with the same danger, we would expect about 19 people to have a heart attack or stroke in the next 10 years. If 100 people of the same age and gender were to have optimal management of cholesterol, blood pressure, and smoking, we would expect 1 person to have a heart attack or stroke in the next 10 years.

Your risk of having a heart attack or stroke in your lifetime is 50%. This means that in a group of 100 persons with the same danger as you, we would expect 50 of them to have a heart attack or stroke in their lifetime. With optimal management of cardiovascular risk, we would expect 8 people to have a heart attack or stroke in their lifetime.

CVD Risk-Reduction Strategy

Understanding and prioritizing modifiable CV risk factors can facilitate earlier intervention with education and treatment. Because many patients have multiple risk factors, it is important to recognize and emphasize the relative priorities of the patient's individualized risk factors when communicating about CV risk reduction. The priority for clinical attention should always be on the modifiable risk factors.

Nonmodifiable Risk Factors

In the prevention and management of CV events, the emphasis is on CV risk reduction in patients with the potential to reverse (modify) their risk with lifestyle and pharmacologic interventions. Age, sex, family history/genetics, and race/ethnicity are examples of nonreversible risk factors. However, nonmodifiable risk factors can still influence clinical decision making in these ways:

- *Family history/genetics.* Genetics plays a role in the development of complications of CVD, but currently, clinically useful gene markers are not available. Family history of premature heart disease (often defined as CHD before age 55 for men or 65 for women in a first-degree relative) is associated with increased risk of future CHD, independent of other established risk factors. Men with a family history of premature heart disease have about a 50% higher lifetime risk of both CHD and CVD mortality than men without a family history.[79] However, adding data related to family history to the risk equation models does not improve the classification of clinically relevant risk for individuals.[75,80] Therefore, family history of premature CHD is useful information and can influence clinical judgment, but the information is not necessary for CV risk calculation.
- *Age.* There is a relationship between both age and duration of diabetes and CV risk. The older the individual and the longer he or she has had diabetes, the higher the risk for CV problems. The general health of the patient and long-term prognosis may influence CV risk factor management. Aggressive treatment to prevent long-term complications is not warranted for very elderly patients and others with limited life expectancy.
- *Sex.* Before menopause, there is a sex-protective factor for females without diabetes (but not with diabetes) for CVD events.[81] Some clinicians tend to take women's CV complaints less seriously than men's.[81] The CV risks of women with diabetes should be taken as seriously as those of men.
- *Race/ethnicity.* African Americans with diabetes have a higher incidence of macrovascular disease than whites with diabetes,[82] and Mexican Americans with diabetes have an increased risk of peripheral vascular disease.[64] Peripheral artery disease is also prevalent in African Americans and Hispanics with diabetes.

Take a Multifactorial Treatment Approach

Taking a multifactorial treatment approach to managing modifiable risk factors in people with T2DM improves patient outcomes. The STENO-2 study instituted intensive behavioral and pharmacologic therapy to target hyperglycemia, hypertension, dyslipidemia, and microalbuminuria for 80 people with established T2DM and microalbuminuria. Most patients were also treated with aspirin. Although few patients reached target goals for all interventions, those in the more aggressively treated intervention group had significant reductions in CVD, retinopathy, nephropathy, and autonomic neuropathy and a 20% decrease in all-cause mortality after 13 years of follow-up.[83]

The National Quality Forum, a nonprofit organization that reviews, endorses, and recommends standardized health performance measures to improve patient outcomes, has endorsed a multifactorial measure for optimal diabetes care.[84,85] Table 25.2 describes evidence-based guideline recommendations for the modifiable CV risk factors.

TABLE 25.2 National Guidelines for Treating CV Risk Factors for Adults With Diabetes

Clinical Domain	*Subgroup*	*Achievable Goal*	*Source*	*Individual Considerations*
Lipids[1]	Age >21 with ASCVD	High-intensity statin	2019 ACC/AHA	Excludes patients with NYHA Class II-IV congestive heart failure and renal disease on dialysis. Use moderate-intensity statin for patients at higher risk for adverse effects who would otherwise be candidates for high-intensity statin.
	Age >21 with LDL ≥190 mg/dL	High-intensity statin	2019 ACC/AHA	
	Age 40–75 with LDL ≥70 without multiple risk factors	Moderate intensity statin	2019 ACC/AHA	
	Age 40–75 with multiple risk factors	high-intensity statin	2019 ACC/AHA	
	Age <40, age >75	Individualize	2019 ACC/AHA	Consider statins in patients with significant CV risk
Blood pressure[2]	Adults age 18 and older	<140/90 mm Hg	2019 ADA	Consider a lower SBP target of <130 mm Hg for certain individuals such as younger patients and those with albuminuria if it can be reached without undue treatment burden
A1C	Adults	<8%	2019 ADA	Lower A1C goal recommended if achievable without difficulty
Aspirin for secondary prevention	Adults	Low-dose aspirin use	2019 ADA and 2016 USPSTF	Assess and consider GI bleeding risks
Aspirin for primary prevention	Adults under 40 over age 70 and over Or people of any age who are at increased risk for bleeding	aspirin not recommended	2019 ADA[2] 2019 ACCAHA[3]	Under 50, benefit is too low Age 70 and over, risks are too high

(continued)

TABLE 25.2 National Guidelines for Treating CV Risk Factors for Adults With Diabetes (continued)

Clinical Domain	*Subgroup*	*Achievable Goal*	*Source*	*Individual Considerations*
	Adults age 40–70 at higher risk for ASCVD	Might be considered if not at increased bleeding risk	2019 ACC/AHA[3]	
Tobacco	All who use tobacco products	Cessation	2019 ACC/AHA[3]	

Abbreviations: ACC/AHA, American College of Cardiology and the American Heart Association; ADA, American Diabetes Association; USPSTF, United States Preventive Services Task Force; JNC8, Eighth Joint National Committee; LDL, low-density lipoprotein; ASCVD, atherosclerotic cardiovascular disease; NYHA, New York Heart Association; CV, cardiovascular; CHD, coronary heart disease; CKD, chronic kidney disease; ACEI, angiotensin-converting enzyme inhibitor; ARB, angiotensin receptor blocker.

*K Bibbins-Domingo, "Aspirin Use for the Primary Prevention of Cardiovascular Disease and Colorectal Cancer: U.S. Preventive Services Task Force Recommendation Statement," *Ann Intern Med* 164, no. 12 (2016): 836-45.

[1] SM Grundy, NJ Stone, "2018 American Heart Association/American College of Cardiology Multisociety guideline on the management of blood cholesterol: primary prevention," JAMA Cardiol. 4(5)(2019):488–9. doi:https://doi.org/10.1001/jamacardio.2019.0777.

[2] ADA standards of care. Cardiovascular Disease and Risk Management Diabetes Care. 2019;42(Suppl 1): S110.

[3] Arnett DK, Blumenthal RS, Albert MA, et al. 2019 ACC/AHA Guideline on the Primary Prevention of Cardiovascular Disease. Journal of the American College of Cardiology. September 2019;74(10). DOI: 10.1016/j.jacc.2019.03.009

Instruction Opportunity—Communicating the "Multifactorial" Approach to Patients

The "D5" terminology is a way of communicating to patients the importance of a multifactorial approach to CV risk reduction.[86] D5 communicates goals for glycemia, blood pressure, lipids, tobacco, and aspirin use. It uses a simple message to make it easier for people with diabetes to set and achieve goals to better manage the disease: "When you achieve D5 success, you reduce your risk of complications such as heart attack, stroke, and problems with your kidneys, eyes, and nervous system." While target levels for the components should be individualized, attention to all D5 goals is appropriate and beneficial for almost all people with diabetes.

The D5 message is a simple way to help patients understand the importance of a multifactorial treatment approach to reducing their risk of heart attack and stroke. Figure 25.2 is an example of patient information on the Internet to help communicate the D5 message: "The D5 represents 5 goals you need to achieve to reduce your risk for complications."

For patients with multiple risk factors outside target/goal range, help them set priorities for treating their risk factors. There are different ways to set priorities, but exploring the following can be helpful:

- *Distance from clinical goal.* Treating the risk factors furthest from goal usually has a greater impact on reducing cardiovascular risk than treating risk factors already close to goal.
- *Fewest risk of side effects.* Although starting a new medication class can be more clinically, a relatively simple adjustment of existing medication can be easier for patients than prescribing a new medication, especially if there are concerns about potential interactions and side effects.
- *Patient preference.* Engagement can be improved by learning if the person with diabetes strongly prefers or fears a particular treatment.
- *Current therapy.* For patients not at goal on near-maximum pharmacologic treatment, additional assessment for possible barriers to engagement and psychosocial issues should be pursued before further intensifying treatment.

FIVE GOALS. ONE REASON: LIVING WELL.

If you have diabetes, it is important to take steps to manage your conditions. The D5 represents 5 goals you need to achieve to reduce your risk for complications.

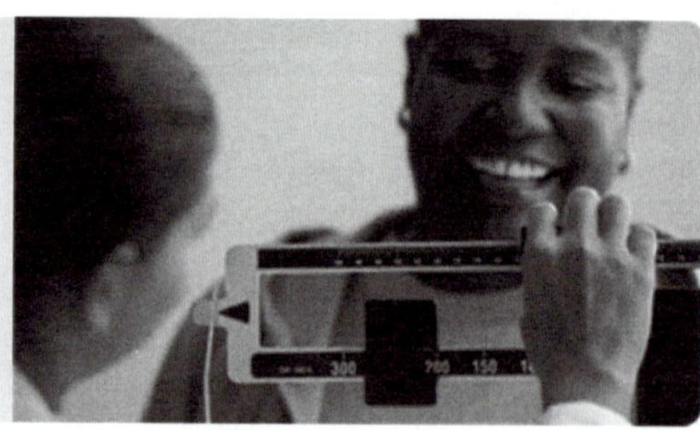

You achieve the D5 when you meet all five goals:

1. Your blood pressure is less than 140/90 mmHG
2. Your bad cholesterol, LDL, is less than 100 mg/dl
3. Your blood sugar, A1c, is less than 8%
4. You are tobacco-free
5. You take an aspirin as appropriate

The D5 was created to make it easier for people with diabetes to work together and set and achieve goals to better manage the disease. When you achieve D5 success, you reduce your risk for complications such as heart attack, stroke and problems with your kidneys, eyes and nervous system.

Diabetes (dye-uh-BEE-teez) occurs when there is too much glucose (sugar) in the blood and not enough in the cells of your body. This can interfere with your body's ability to convert food into energy needed for daily life.

EXPLORE THE D5 GOALS ▶

FIGURE 25.2 **Setting Goals to Achieve the "D5."**

Source: Re Minnesota Community Measurement (MNCM), http://mncm.org/reports-and-websites/the-d5/.

Lifestyle Management (Diet, Physical Activity, and Weight Loss)

Diet

Rates of obesity in the US population have increased as a result of less-healthy eating patterns and decreased physical activity. Thus, the benefits of a therapeutic lifestyle change go well beyond reducing CVD in people with diabetes. As a result, the American Diabetes Association (ADA), the AHA, and the American Cancer Society are working together to effect lifestyle changes to reduce rates of diabetes, heart disease, and cancer.[87] The effects of a healthy diet include improvement in weight, blood pressure,[88] and dyslipidemia and reduced CV event rates.[89–91]

The diet with the strongest evidence to improve CV outcomes is the Mediterranean diet, which is characterized by high intake of olive oil, fruit, nuts, vegetables, and cereals; moderate intake of fish and poultry; low intake of dairy products, red meat, processed meat, and sweets; and wine in moderation at meals.[91] In the randomized PREDIMED study of persons at high CV risk but without known CVD, a Mediterranean diet supplemented with extra-virgin olive oil or nuts significantly reduced the incidence of major CV events (relative risk reduction of 30%).[91]

The DASH dietary pattern also has strong evidence to support improvement in CV risk factors. The diet is high in vegetables, fruits, low-fat dairy products, whole grains, poultry, fish, and nuts and low in sweets, sugar-sweetened beverages, and red meats. The DASH dietary pattern is low in saturated fat, total fat, and cholesterol. It is rich in potassium, magnesium, calcium, protein, and fiber. Studies demonstrated that the DASH diet, compared with typical American diets of the 1990s, can lower blood pressure by about 5 to 6 mm Hg and LDL-C by 11 mg/dL without changes in body weight.[76]

Weight Loss

Among overweight and obese adults, analysis of observational data shows that the greater the BMI, the higher the risk of CVD, T2DM, and all-cause mortality in both sexes. The current BMI cut points for overweight (BMI $\geq$25.0 kg/m^2) and obesity (BMI $\geq$30.0 kg/m^2) compared with normal weight (BMI 18.5 to <25.0 kg/m^2) are associated with elevated risk of fatal CHD. Lifestyle changes that produce even modest, sustained weight loss of 3% to 5% produce clinically meaningful health benefits. Greater weight loss reduces blood pressure, improves LDL-C and HDL-C, and reduces the need for medications to manage blood pressure, glucose, and lipids, as well as further reduces TGs and blood glucose. Overweight and obese individuals who would benefit from weight loss should be invited to participate in a comprehensive lifestyle program consisting of a lower calorie diet and increased physical activity through the use of behavioral strategies.[92]

Overweight and obese individuals who would benefit from weight loss should be invited to participate in a comprehensive lifestyle program consisting of a lower calorie diet and increased physical activity through the use of behavioral strategies.[92]

The Look AHEAD study was designed to examine whether weight loss in overweight persons with T2DM would decrease CV morbidity and mortality. A total of 5,145 individuals in 16 study centers were randomly assigned either to intensive lifestyle intervention promoting weight loss and physical activity or to a control group with basic education. More patients in the intervention group experienced weight loss (not a large difference), reduced A1C, and improved fitness and CV risk factors (except LDL) than did patients in the control group. Nevertheless, the study was stopped early after 10 years due to futility (no difference in CV outcome).[93] While this was disappointing to some, many experts believed that the weight loss achieved in the intensive group was too small to see the hypothesized effect. The positive news from this study is that, despite the modest between-group differences, the intervention did result in many other desirable outcomes, such as improvements in kidney disease, eye disease, depression, and quality of life; fewer hospitalizations; enhanced mobility; and reduced medication use.

Bariatric Surgery[94,95]

Glycemic stability is one of the major benefits of bariatric surgery. In a multicenter longitudinal study (LABS) in over 2,300 participants, 60% to 70% of patients with diabetes at baseline (nearly 30% of those undergoing Roux-en-Y gastric bypass) achieved remission up to 7 years after Roux-en-Y gastric bypass, and less than 1.5% developed new-onset diabetes.[96] Improved glycemic management generally translates into fewer diabetes-related vascular complications. In two retrospective studies in patients with type 2 diabetes, compared with medical treatment, bariatric surgery was associated with lower incidences of coronary artery disease (1.6 vs. 2.8 percent), neuropathy (7 vs. 21 percent), nephropathy (5 vs. 10 percent), and retinopathy (7 vs. 11 percent) at five years.[94,97] (See "Outcomes of bariatric surgery", section on 'Diabetes mellitus'.)

In obese adults, bariatric surgery (also called metabolic surgery) generally results in a more favorable impact on obesity-related comorbid conditions than usual care, conventional medical treatment, lifestyle intervention, or medically supervised weight loss. Randomized trials have shown a benefit of metabolic surgery compared to medical therapy in the short term (1-3 years) on numerous patient outcomes including need for glucose-lowering medications, quality of life, and improvement in CV risk factors in patients with type 2 diabetes.[98–102] Among obese persons with diabetes at baseline who achieve a 20% to 35% weight loss 2 to 3 years after bariatric surgery, fasting glucose and insulin are reduced, and diabetes remission is more likely. In longitudinal studies, 60% to 70% of patients with diabetes at baseline achieve remission up to 7 years after Roux-en-Y bypass.[94] However, longer-term follow-up (10 years) shows that diabetes and hypertension may recur over time in individuals who see improvement in the short term.[78] Evidence is emerging from nonrandomized studies that bariatric surgery may be associated with reduced rates of CV events, microvascular complications, and deaths in obese adults.[95,103] In observational studies, the benefits of metabolic surgery were higher in patients with diabetes as well as those who were younger and those with BMI greater than 50 kg/m^2.[104]

Bariatric surgery should be a consideration for adults with diabetes with BMI ≥40 kg/m^2 (≥37.5 kg/m^2 for Asian-Americans). Surgery may also be an option for adults with BMI 35.0 to 39.9 kg/m^2 (32.5-37.4 kg/m^2 for Asian-Americans) if hyperglycemia is inadequately managed with optimal lifestyle and medical management.[105] It is advisable to refer patients for metabolic surgical consultations to high-volume experienced centers. Despite encouraging data, safety risks associated with bariatric surgery include surgical complications, vitamin deficiencies, gallstones, and anemia; the risks need to be balanced with potential benefits.

Adults with diabetes and a BMI ≥35 who are motivated to lose weight and have not achieved satisfactory management of hyperglycemia with lifestyle and medical management may be candidates for bariatric surgery. People with diabetes may experience a greater magnitude of weight loss than people without diabetes.[104] Consider offering a referral to an experienced bariatric surgeon for consultation and evaluation.[92]

Physical Activity

A number of prospective epidemiologic studies have shown the benefits of physical activity on reducing CV events.[106] More recent data indicate the same effect is present in people with diabetes. A prospective study of more than 1,700 persons with T2DM found that moderate-to-high levels of exercise decreased total and CV mortality. Although smoking and higher levels of blood pressure, BMI, and cholesterol were associated with a higher risk of death from CVD, the effect of exercise was independent of these risk factors.[107] Among men and women, 40 minutes of moderate-to-vigorous aerobic physical activity 3 or 4 times per week decreases systolic and diastolic blood pressure, on average, by 2 to 5 mm Hg and 1 to 4 mm Hg, respectively.[76] When sedentary adults aged 55 to 75 years initiate a program of regular supervised physical training, they can experience a significant reduction in metabolic markers of CV risk and a lower rate of abnormal exercise stress test results and angina pectoris.[76,108]

Smoking Cessation

Nearly 20% of deaths from CVD can be directly linked to cigarette smoking. Stopping smoking can reduce the risk of coronary death by 50% within 1 year.[109] A number of randomized clinical trials have shown that brief counseling for smoking cessation is efficacious and cost-effective. For the patient motivated to quit, the combination of pharmacologic therapy such as nicotine replacement and counseling is more effective than either treatment alone.[110]

Three commonly used medications to support smoking cessation are:

- Nicotine replacement therapy, which helps by replacing the nicotine from cigarettes. Each type (eg, gum, lozenge, patch, nasal spray, inhaler) comes with different instructions.
- Bupropion, a non-nicotine pill that acts on neurotransmitters, "chemical messengers" that carry messages to cells in the brain. This medication should be taken for 1 to 2 weeks before stopping smoking. Possible side effects include abdominal pain, constipation, decreased appetite, dizziness, dry mouth, sweating, nausea or vomiting, trembling or shaking, and trouble sleeping.
- Varenicline produces nicotine effects to ease withdrawal symptoms and lessens the satisfaction of smoking by blocking the effects of nicotine. This medication should be started 1 week before quitting smoking. Possible side effects include nausea, insomnia, headache, abdominal pain, constipation, and flatulence. Some people have had changes in behavior, including hostility, agitation, depression, and suicidal thoughts, while on or after stopping varenicline.[111]

Side effects of these medications can lessen or disappear as the body adjusts to treatment. All of these medications should be taken under the direction of a doctor. Strategies addressing the motivational, behavioral, and social aspects of smoking cessation are also very important and should be used in combination with smoking cessation medications. Many state and national phone and online resources are available for free to help patients stop smoking (eg, http://smokefree.gov).

Lipid Management

Statins

Thirty years have passed since publication of the MRFIT study, which attempted to prove that lowering total cholesterol through diet would reduce CV events.[112] Since then, a plethora of articles have investigated the role of statins for lipid lowering, including the landmark Scandinavian Simvastatin Survival Study (4S) and CARDS Study.[113] Although the studies were not limited to only people with diabetes, most included a large diabetes subgroup. Studies have shown benefits from statin therapy for secondary prevention in people with established coronary disease[114,115] and for primary prevention in people with diabetes with no evidence of preexisting CVD.[115] A meta-analysis of 6 primary prevention studies and 8 secondary prevention studies showed relative risk reductions of 22% and 24%, respectively, through use of statins in people with T2DM.[116] In another meta-analysis of statin therapy for primary prevention with more than 18,000 patients followed for a mean of 4.3 years, all-cause mortality decreased 9% and vascular mortality decreased 13% for each mmol/L (38 mg/dL) reduction in LDL.[117–121] The benefits of statin therapy are also observed in people with diabetes at lower LDL levels and moderate CVD risk.[115,122] Although statin use increases the risk of developing diabetes, the CV event rate reduction outweighs the risk of incident diabetes.[123,124]

In the absence of severe hypertriglyceridemia (TGs >1000 mg/dL), the first priority of lipid therapy is statin use. The 2019 ADA Standards of Medical Care[105] recommend statin use for most individuals with T1DM or T2DM:

- All ages with ASCVD or 10-year ASCVD risk >20% (high intensity)
- Patients age 40 to 75 and over without ASCVD disease (moderate intensity)

Statin therapy can be considered for individuals with diabetes who are younger than 40 or older than 75, based on consideration of additional risk factors influencing ASCVD risk, benefits and adverse effects, drug-drug interaction potential, and patient preferences. Coronary artery calcium scores (CACs) may help to make decisions about statin use in younger patients or if patients are indecisive about statin use.

The ACC/AHA recommends considering high-intensity therapy rather than moderate intensity for people with diabetes who have risk enhancers such as more than 10 years of type 2 diabetes or 20 years of type 1 diabetes, microalbuminuria, chronic kidney disease, retinopathy, neuropathy, or ABI <0.9.[125]

Examples of high-intensity statin therapy are daily doses of atorvastatin, 40 to 80 mg, or rosuvastatin, 20 to 40 mg. Examples of moderate-intensity therapy are daily doses of atorvastatin, 10 to 20 mg; rosuvastatin, 5 to 10 mg; and simvastatin, 20 to 40 mg.[73] The FDA does not recommend initiation of high-dose simvastatin (80 mg) due to increased risk of myopathy and rhabdomyolysis. In addition, increasing doses of simvastatin beyond 40 mg per day could be harmful. Statins are contraindicated in pregnancy, and extreme caution should be used if considering statin therapy in women of childbearing age.

Statin therapy is less evidence-based in those on hemodialysis, those with New York Heart Association (NYHA) class II-IV heart failure (Table 25.2), and those who are older than age 75 unless clinical ASCVD is present. In 4 randomized controlled trials reviewed, there was insufficient information on which to base recommendations in patients with these comorbidities; therefore, individualized assessment is needed to evaluate reduction benefit, adverse effects, drug-drug interactions, and other cautions.[73]

Statin Safety

Patients predisposed to adverse effects of statins (eg, those with impaired renal or hepatic function, other serious coexisting conditions, a history of statin intolerance, concomitant use of drugs affecting statin metabolism, or unexplained elevation of alanine aminotransferase [ALT] levels that are 3 times the upper limit of normal; and those who are age >75) should use moderate-intensity statin therapy when high-intensity therapy would otherwise be recommended.[126] Baseline ALT before statin initiation should be checked and monitored at follow-up if symptoms suggest hepatotoxicity (eg, unusual fatigue or weakness, loss of appetite, abdominal pain, dark-colored urine, jaundice). It is also reasonable to measure baseline creatinine kinase (CK) before statin initiation in individuals at risk for adverse muscle events based on personal or family history of statin intolerance or muscle disease, and in individuals receiving concomitant drug therapy that increases myopathy risk.

Statin Intolerance

It is estimated that statin intolerance occurs in about 10% to 15% of patients (but is probably over-diagnosed by many practitioners).[127,128] Common side effects (muscle tenderness, stiffness, cramping, weakness, or generalized fatigue) can be experienced by patients in anticipation that statins may be harmful.[129] True statin side effects usually occur within 3 to 6 months of statin initiation or intensification, are usually bilateral and symmetrical, and may worsen with exercise.[130,131] A reasonable approach to addressing statin intolerance is to remove the statin for 2 to 4 weeks (symptoms or biomarker abnormalities should resolve if due to the statin) and then rechallenge with a low dose of a different statin.[132] Most experts agree that statin intolerance criteria should include the inability to tolerate at least 2 different statins at doses required to reduce a person's CV risk sufficiently from their baseline.[126]

Dietary Modification

Lifestyle modification (eg, heart-healthy diet, regular exercise, avoidance of tobacco, maintenance of a healthy weight) is also a critical component of the management of hyperlipoproteinemia.[73,76] Dietary modification, as discussed earlier in detail, can include the following recommendations:

- Consume a diet that consists largely of vegetables, fruits, and whole grains; includes low-fat dairy products, poultry, fish, legumes, nontropical vegetable oils, and nuts; and limits intake of sweets, sugar-sweetened beverages, and red meats.
- Reduce intake of saturated fat to 5% to 6% of total calories and minimize *trans* fat from partially hydrogenated vegetable oils.

LDL-C Monitoring

Screening for lipid abnormalities using a fasting lipid profile is recommended in most adults with diabetes at the time of diagnosis and at least every 5 years or more frequently if indicated. Lipid testing is recommended prior to statin initiation to determine the recommended intensity of statin therapy and periodically thereafter to monitor response to therapy and inform engagement with the therapy. However, because the guidelines no longer emphasize target LDL levels for most individuals, the need for annual assessment of cholesterol levels in patients with diabetes on stable therapy is eliminated.[126]

It is reasonable to do follow-up lipid testing after statin initiation to consider a dose reduction if LDL values are consistently lower than 40 mg/dL or to consider whether high-intensity statin treatment is sufficient in very high risk individuals. The aim of high-intensity therapy is to lower the LDL by 50% or more.[125]

Lipid levels are best measured after an overnight fast, because postprandial TG elevations may interfere with evaluation of the lipid profile. Calculation of LDL-C is often inaccurate with elevated TGs, and most laboratories do not report the LDL-C if the TG level is greater than 400 mg/dL. In this case, the direct LDL-C assay may be useful.

Triglyceride Treatments

Hypertriglyceridemia should be addressed with dietary and lifestyle changes. Severe hypertriglyceridemia (≥1,000 mg/dL) warrants immediate pharmacologic therapy with a fibrate, niacin, or fish oil to reduce the risk of acute pancreatitis. In the absence of severe hypertriglyceridemia, the pharmacologic intervention with fibrates or niacin, in addition to statin therapy, is not recommended to achieve HDL and TG goals. Combinations of statins with other pharmacotherapy such as fibrates and niacin were studied in large clinical trials (ACCORD and Aim High, respectively) and did not reduce CV event rates more than statin therapy alone.[134–136] Moreover, in ACCORD, *reversible* worsening of renal function occurred more often with fenofibrate.[103]

However, niacin, fenofibrate, ezetimibe, and bile acid sequestrants can all lower LDL cholesterol, and these drugs may be considered in patients intolerant of statin therapy. Gemfibrozil therapy reduced CVD events by 24% in men with diabetes and previous CVD, low HDL, and modestly elevated triglycerides.[136] Fenofibrate resulted in fewer nonfatal MIs and coronary revascularizations but no signficant difference in total coronary mortality.[133] Niacin therapy can increase blood glucose at doses required to improve lipids, and intensification of glycemic therapy may be needed.

Ezetimibe and proprotein convertase subtilisin-kexin 9 (PCSK9) Inhibitors

For some patients with diabetes and established coronary heart disease who have persistently elevated LDL (LDL >70 mg/dl) or less than 50% LDL lowering despite engagement with high intensity statin therapy, addition of ezetimibe or PCSK9 inhibitors should be considered. Ezetimibe is the preferred first option based on lower cost.[105,137–139]

PCSK9 inhibitors are monoclonal antibodies that inactivate PCSK9, resulting in increased lifespan of LDL receptors in hepatocytes and consequent clearing of more LDL cholesterol from the bloodstream. The drugs require parenteral administration, are very expensive (alirocumab was launched at a list price of $14,600 per patient per year), and will result in higher net costs to healthcare systems if future use of these drugs becomes more widespread.[140]

The ADA and ACC/AHA guidelines emphasize the importance of statin therapy in people with diabetes. Most people with diabetes should receive at least moderate-intensity statin therapy. For patients who do not tolerate the intended intensity statin, maximally tolerated statin doses should be used.[105]

Hypertension Management

Numerous studies have shown that blood pressure reduction in people with diabetes and hypertension can reduce overall CV mortality and, in particular, the incidence of stroke. This effect is shown with even modest reductions in blood pressure; for example, in the UKPDS, the intensive group reached a mean blood pressure of 144/82 mm Hg, compared with the control group's 154/87 mm Hg. Diabetes-related death was reduced by 32% and stroke by 44%.[141] There was a nonsignificant 21% reduction in MI with blood pressure control. Most studies have shown the same pattern: a dramatic reduction in stroke and total CV mortality and a less dramatic effect on MI.[142]

Blood Pressure Measurement Technique

Blood pressure should be checked at every routine visit, and at least yearly, for all people with diabetes. Blood pressure should be checked accurately with appropriate cuff size and the patient in a seated position, feet on the floor with arm supported at heart level, after 5 minutes of rest without talking. Automated office blood pressures (AOBP) measurement recording the average of 2 to 3 blood pressure readings conducted in this way using a fully automated oscillometric sphygomanometer result in a mean systolic BP approximately 14.5 mm Hg lower than routine office BP measurement. Use of automated blood pressure cuffs can also eliminate the interpretation bias and digit preference observed in manual auscultatory measurements.[143,144]

Patients with elevated blood pressure should have blood pressure confirmed on a separate day. The diabetes care and education specialist should stress that patients with an elevated blood pressure reading should return for a repeat blood pressure in a timely fashion. There are no strict guidelines for the time frame for a repeat blood pressure, but a reasonable time frame is within 2 to 4 weeks if the situation is not urgent, and within days if blood pressure is ≥180/110 mm Hg. Too often in many care systems, patients with elevated blood pressure are lost to follow-up for long periods.

Home and ambulatory blood pressure monitoring may help with diagnosis and management of hypertension—especially when there is a discrepancy between office and home readings (eg, "white coat hypertension"). Ambulatory blood pressure measurements correlate with CVD risk better than office measurements. Asleep systolic blood pressure mean and sleep-time relative to systolic blood pressure decline are the most significant predictors of CVD events.[145] Recommended ambulatory blood pressure thresholds for men, without compelling clinical indications for more aggressive treatment, are 135/85 mm Hg for awake and 120/70 mm Hg for asleep systolic blood pressure/diastolic blood pressure means. Recommended thresholds for higher-risk persons with diabetes, CKD, or CHD are often 15/10 mm Hg lower.

Blood Pressure Goals

There is strong and non-controversial evidence to support blood pressure treatment goals of less than 140/90 for people with diabetes.[105] In 2017, the American College of Cardiology/American heart Association (ACC/AHA) announced new categories for blood pressure that defined a normal blood pressure as <120/80 mm Hg and Stage 1 hypertension as an SBP of 130 to 139 mm Hg or a dBP 80 to 89 mm Hg, with a recommended threshold for pharmacologic treatment of ≥ 130/80 mm Hg and a BP goal of <130/80 mm Hg.[146] This lower treatment goal was mostly based on the results of the SPRINT trial, which showed a significantly lower rate of CV events and death in patients aged >50 years with high CV risk but without diabetes assigned to a goal of blood pressure <120 mm Hg compared with <140 mm Hg. The Hypertension Optimal Treatment (HOT) Study, a randomized trial published in 1998 which targeted lower diastolic blood pressures for people with diabetes, demonstrated additional CV benefits down to a diastolic blood pressure target of 80 mm Hg.[147]

However, these lower BP goals recommended by ACC/AHA have been controversial.[148,149] The ACCORD trial, which examined whether a systolic blood pressure of <120 mm Hg would provide greater benefit than a systolic blood pressure of 130 to 139 mm Hg in persons with T2DM, found that neither the primary outcome (overall CV event rates) nor microvascular complications were significantly reduced in the more intensively treated group.[150] Although strokes were reduced to a small degree, serious adverse events (eg, syncope, hyperkalemia) occurred at a higher rate in the intensively treated group.[151] Another large trial, ADVANCE, showed reduced mortality rates in the more intensively treated group, but the achieved mean systolic blood pressure was 135 mm Hg.[152]

Amidst the controversy over the ACC/AHA guideline, the ADA Standards continue to recommend a blood pressure of <140 mm Hg for most people with diabetes, with the option of a lower target of <130 mm Hg for certain individuals such as younger patients and those with albuminuria if it can be reached without undue treatment burden.[105]

Treatment of Hypertension

Evaluation of people with hypertension and diabetes begins by addressing lifestyle factors that may contribute to hypertension and CV risk. This is clearly in the purview of the diabetes care and education specialist. Lifestyle modification is a mainstay of treatment for *all* individuals with prehypertension and hypertension. Suggested lifestyle changes may include the following:

- Weight reduction
- Adoption of the DASH eating plan
- Dietary sodium reduction
- Increased physical activity
- Moderation of alcohol consumption
- Avoidance of nonsteroidal anti-inflammatory drugs (NSAIDs)

Numerous clinical trials have explored the benefits of specific antihypertensive pharmacotherapy on CV outcomes. The largest of these was ALLHAT, which compared chlorthalidone (a thiazide diuretic), amlodipine (a dihydropyridine calcium-channel blocker [CCB]), lisinopril (an angiotensin-converting enzyme [ACE] inhibitor), and doxazosin (alpha blocker).[153] The doxazosin arm of the study was discontinued due to increased incidence of heart failure, and the remaining 3 arms of the study showed decreased rates of fatal and nonfatal MI. Chlorthalidone was superior to amlodipine and lisinopril in preventing new-onset heart failure, although the benefit may have been due to greater blood pressure lowering observed in the chlorthalidone group.

Angiotensin-converting enzyme inhibitors and angiotensin-receptor blockers (ARBs) may have several advantages in people with diabetes, including relatively low toxicity and additional renal protection. However, many experts have concluded from the data that the achieved blood pressure, rather than the specific drug class used, is the primary determinant of benefit. Recommendations for choice of initial medications thiazide diuretics, calcium channel blockers, ACE inhibitors, and ARBs.[146] For the general black population, including those with diabetes, initial antihypertensive treatment should include a thiazide diuretic or CCB. In the general population with CKD, regardless of diabetes status, an ACE inhibitor or ARB therapy is recommended for initial or add-on therapy to improve kidney outcomes. The main objective of blood pressure management is to attain and maintain the recommended blood pressure goal by reinforcing medication and lifestyle changes and intensifying pharmacologic therapy, if indicated. Angiotensin-converting enzyme inhibitors and ARBs should not be used together. If blood pressure remains uncontrolled on first line therapies, evaluate the person with diabetes for issues related to regimen engagement, secondary causes such as obstructive sleep apnea, interfering substances such as NSAIDs, and consider addition of a mineralocorticoid receptor agonist such as spironolactone or eplerenone. Referral[154] to a hypertension specialist may be indicated for patients whose blood pressure goal cannot be attained using the above strategy with 3 or more drugs.[155] Full details of medical nutrition therapy, lifestyle modification, and specific pharmacologic treatment (including dosing, contraindications, and side effects) of hypertension are included in chapters 16 and 20.

Instruction Opportunity—Supporting Patients in Achieving Blood Pressure Goals

Most people with T2DM need at least 2 or 3 medications to achieve blood pressure goals (a mean of 2.3 drugs was required in ACCORD patients with a systolic blood pressure goal of 130-139 mm Hg, and 3.4 drugs for patients with a goal of <120 mm Hg).[156] Setting this expectation early in the educational process may help. The level of blood pressure achieved is generally considered more important than the choice of drugs used to achieve the goal.

Assess persons with diabetes routinely for potential barriers to regimen engagement, such as medication taking, cost of medications, and side effects. Many persons with diabetes with adequate knowledge of their medications still lack motivation to take their medications as directed. To adequately address lack of engagement, the World Health Organization recommends a model that addresses information, motivation, and behavioral skills (IMB model).[157] Help patients keep track of their medication schedule and engage with their medication plan with tables of medications, their purpose, and when to take them. Explain that, even if hypertension is asymptomatic, it is very important to continue treatment to prevent heart attacks and strokes.

Pharmacists, nurses, and dietitians, if available in the patient's care system, can facilitate pharmacologic management using medication protocols (if within their practice scope and licensure). For patients with established hypertension, home blood pressure telemonitoring with phone-based case management can result in lower mean blood pressure and a higher percentage of patients achieving recommended blood pressure targets.[158,159]

Appropriate Use of Aspirin

One of the earliest studies of antiplatelet agents, the Early Treatment Diabetic Retinopathy Study,[160] was designed primarily to determine the effect of aspirin therapy on retinopathy. The study found that aspirin had no significant effect on retinopathy but that it decreased the rate of MI by 28%.[161] As a result, for quite some time, aspirin was recommended for most patients with diabetes for primary cardiovascular prevention. However, more recently, randomized controlled trials of aspirin use in patients with and without diabetes have either not shown benefit or have shown some benefit but with increased risk of bleeding. A summary of these studies is as follows:

- ASCEND: 15,480 patients with diabetes and no known CVD randomized to aspirin 100 mg or placebo. After a mean of 7.4 years, the primary CV outcome was reduced by 12%, but major bleeding was significantly increased.[162]
- ARRIVE: 12,546 patients randomized to aspirin versus placebo. No benefit to the primary CV endpoint. GI bleeding was significantly increased.[163]
- ASPREE: 19,114 patients including 11% with diabetes, no benefit on the primary CV end point. GI bleeding was significantly increased.[164]

Based on these studies, the ACC/AHA recommends that aspirin not be administered on a routine basis for primary prevention of ASCVD among adults age 70 or over or among adults of any age who are at increased risk of bleeding. Low dose aspirin (75-100 mg) might be considered for primary prevention of ASCVD among select adults age 40-70 who are higher ASCVD risk but not at increased risk for bleeding.

For secondary CV prevention in patients with a history of known CHD, ischemic stroke, transient ischemic attack, and/or PAD, the benefits of aspirin generally outweigh the risks (for patients untreated with other anticoagulants or other antiplatelet drugs and with no history of gastrointestinal ulcer or bleeding). Aspirin is also sometimes recommended for primary prevention of stroke in patients with a history of atrial fibrillation if anticoagulants cannot be used.

Other considerations in the balance of benefits and harms of aspirin therapy include a strong family history of CHD, a positive test for urinary albumin, and a family history of colon cancer (aspirin may be protective in this situation). Other patient factors can increase the risk of gastrointestinal bleeding and should be considered when balancing the benefits and harms of aspirin therapy. Nonsteroidal anti-inflammatory drugs combined with aspirin roughly quadruples the risk for serious gastrointestinal bleeding compared with aspirin alone. The rate of serious bleeding is 2 to 3 times higher in patients with a history of gastrointestinal ulcer. Enteric-coated or buffered preparations do not clearly reduce aspirin's gastrointestinal effects.

Aspirin is not usually recommended for patients taking other anticoagulants or antiplatelet agents. Dual antiplatelet therapy with clopidogrel and aspirin may increase risks, but combination therapy is associated with a reduction in the risk of CV events compared with aspirin alone in patients with symptoms of acute coronary syndrome.[165] Antiplatelet therapy is also indicated to reduce the risk of MI, stroke, or vascular death in individuals with PAD. Aspirin in daily doses of 75 to 325 mg is usually recommended for PAD, but clopidogrel (75 mg per day) is an effective alternative. The combination of aspirin and clopidogrel can be considered in patients with symptomatic PAD, including intermittent claudication, limb ischemia, or history of amputation.[165,166] The FDA has approved clopidogrel for the reduction of ischemic events in patients with PAD.

The optimum dose of aspirin for preventing CVD events is not known. The ADA states that 75 to 162 mg/day is optimal.[105]

Aspirin Use for Primary Prevention of CV Events

The decision to use aspirin is best individualized using a shared decision-making approach with a fully informed patient. For primary ASCVD prevention, aspirin is not recommended for any adult with increased risk of bleeding or for adults over age 70. Aspirin can be considered for adults age 40-70 with high ASCVD risk but not at increased risk of bleeding.

Instruction Opportunity—Using Aspirin Appropriately

Aspirin has been heavily marketed for prevention of CV events. Because aspirin is available over the counter, many patients take it without the knowledge or recommendation of their provider. It is important that the patient's providers are aware of aspirin use and that it is documented in the medication list. Patients must understand that aspirin is not without risk and that their risk of gastrointestinal hemorrhage must be balanced with the possible benefits of CV and CRC risk reduction. The decision to use aspirin is best individualized using a shared decision-making approach with a fully informed patient. Patients who take aspirin should be advised to avoid NSAIDs and to seek prompt medical attention for signs or symptoms of gastrointestinal bleeding (eg, dark stools, vomiting blood, bright red blood from the rectum, syncope, lightheadedness).

ACE Inhibitors or ARBs for Patients With Increased Urinary Albumin Excretion

Increased urinary albumin excretion indicates endothelial dysfunction and can help predict CV events. Persons with diabetes and microalbuminuria have 2 to 8 times the risk of CV events than persons with diabetes without microalbuminuria.[167] Both the presence of increased urinary albumin and its progression predict increased coronary mortality in T2DM.[168] Angiotensin-converting enzyme inhibitors or ARBs are recommended for patients with urinary albumin to prevent progression of renal disease[155] and may also significantly reduce the risk of CV events in patients beyond their blood pressure–lowering effect.[169]

Nontraditional and Emerging New CV Risk Factors

Traditional risk factors such as diabetes, hypertension, smoking, and dyslipidemia are generally understood to explain only about 50% to 60% of the variability in CV risk. Thus, the past decade has seen a concerted effort to identify other risk factors to help predict CV events in individuals for more accurate risk assessment. Some nontraditional biomarkers associated with CV risk are high-sensitivity C-reactive protein (hs-CRP), lipoproteins, apolipoproteins A-I and B, CKD testing such as glomerular filtration rate and microalbuminuria, fibrinogen, white blood cell count, cystatin C, homocysteine (Hcy), B-type natriuretic peptide, CAC scores, ankle-brachial index (ABI), and carotid IMT.[170] The ACC/AHA guideline indicates that assessments of family history of premature CVD and measurement of hs-CRP, CAC scores, and ABI show promise for clinical use based on limited data.[75] However, the ACC/AHA guideline workgroup concluded that evidence is insufficient that these markers can improve the CV risk prediction over the recommended Pooled Cohort Equation. Likewise, the addition of family history of CHD or BMI did not improve discrimination of the model.[75] However, if a risk-based treatment decision is uncertain after quantitative ASCVD risk assessment, assessment of 1 or more of family history, hs-CRP, CAC score, or ABI may help inform treatment decision-making.[126] The USPSTF concluded that "current evidence is insufficient to assess the balance of benefits and harms of using the nontraditional risk factors studied to screen asymptomatic men and women with no history of CHD to prevent CHD events."[171(p474)]

Nontraditional Therapies to Lower CV Risk

Supplements with vitamins and antioxidants such as A, C, and E and multivitamins with folic acid have been touted as CV risk-reduction strategies, but evidence does not support their use. In the NORVIT study, vitamin B_6 and folate increased the risk of MI by 21%. The SEARCH study revealed that the addition of vitamin E to simvastatin, an HMG-CoA reductase inhibitor, also increased the risk of CV events.[172] An analysis of data from the HOPE and HOPE-TOO studies found that vitamin E supplementation in people with diabetes or CVD did not reduce the rate of major CV events and may have increased the risk of heart failure.[173] Beta carotene supplementation could also be dangerous and should be discouraged.[174] The USPSTF recommends that patients who take vitamins be encouraged to take the dosages recommended in the dietary reference intakes of the Institute of Medicine.[175] Inappropriate use of antioxidants and vitamins not only blunts the protective effects of other therapies but often creates the misperception that "natural" therapies are always better than drugs, diverting the patient from proven therapies.

CV Risk Management Issues Specific to Children and Adolescents

An observed linear increase in T1DM and T2DM in childhood is expected to significantly increase the prevalence of diabetes in youth over the next 40 years (2010 to 2050). The prevalence of T1DM is projected to triple and T2DM to quadruple, with the greatest increase in youth in minority racial/ethnic groups.[176] The prevalence of having at least 2 CVD risk factors is about 21% (roughly 92% of youth with T2DM and 14% of youth with T1DM).[177] The implications of this increase are staggering. A continuation of this increase in the number of young people with T2DM will lead to a massive increase in microvascular and macrovascular disease over the next 3 decades.[178] Strategies for weight, lipid, and blood pressure management in youth with diabetes are needed to prevent or delay the development of CVD as these youth mature.

> Strategies for weight, lipid, and blood pressure management in youth with diabetes are critical to prevent or delay the development of CVD as these youth mature.

Blood Pressure Management in Children and Adolescents

Normal blood pressures for age, sex, and height and appropriate methods for determination are available at http://www.nhlbi.nih.gov/health/prof/heart/hbp/hbp_ped.pdf. The 2018 ADA Standards of Medical Care in Diabetes discuss screening for and management of hypertension for children and adolescents with diabetes and make this recommendation.[179] Blood pressure should be measured at all routine visits, and elevated blood pressure should be confirmed on 3 separate days. The target is a blood pressure below the 90th percentile for age, sex, and height.

Treatment including dietary intervention, exercise, and weight management should be initiated in youth with high-normal blood pressure consistently above the 90th percentile. If blood pressure targets are not reached within 3 to 6 months of lifestyle intervention, pharmacologic treatment should be considered. Hypertension in childhood is defined as an average systolic or diastolic blood pressure ≥95th percentile for age, sex, and height percentile confirmed on at least 3 separate days. Pharmacologic treatment for hypertension should be considered as soon as the diagnosis is confirmed. See chapter 20 for details on pharmacologic interventions for hypertension in youth.

Lipid Management for Children and Adolescents

Universal lipid screening is recommended for children between the ages of 9 and 11 and again in early adulthood between the ages of 17 and 21. For children with a significant family history of CVD, the National Heart, Lung, and Blood Institute recommends obtaining a fasting lipid panel beginning at 2 years of age. The 2018 ADA Standards of Medical Care in Diabetes recommend obtaining a fasting lipid profile in children 10 years of age and older soon after the diagnosis (after glucose stability has been established).[179] If lipids are abnormal, annual monitoring is reasonable. If LDL cholesterol values are within the accepted risk level (<100 mg/dL [2.6 mmol/L]), a lipid profile repeated every 5 years is reasonable.

Pharmacotherapy for children younger than 10 is generally not recommended and should be used only under the direction of a pediatric lipid specialist. Pharmacotherapy is advocated for children 10 and older with diabetes if LDL is refractory to nonpharmacotherapy and CV risk factors are present. Pharmacotherapy can be recommended for people with diabetes and LDL ≥160 mg/dL or ≥130 mg/dL if other CV factors (hypertension, smoking, BMI >95th percentile, HDL <40 mg/dL) or high-risk conditions (eg, CKD, heart transplant, Kawasaki disease with coronary aneurysm, chronic inflammatory diseases, HIV, nephritic syndrome) are present. Neither long-term safety nor CV outcome efficacy has been established for statins in children, and they are not approved for children younger than 10. Statins are Category X in pregnancy and should be used cautiously in postpubertal girls.[124]

Coronary Artery Disease

How Does Coronary Artery Disease Present?

Coronary artery disease (CAD) most often presents with either angina pectoris or MI. Chest pain is a common symptom that may or may not be angina or MI. Persons with diabetes are at very high risk for CAD and should be educated about the warning signs (Table 25.3).

Autonomic neuropathy, which is common in people with long-standing diabetes, often includes cardiac denervation, which may result in the atypical chest pain of coronary ischemia. Rather than angina pectoris or substernal pain, the patient may experience only weakness, diaphoresis, dyspnea, or nausea with the onset of ischemia or infarction.

Patients who show evidence of autonomic neuropathy should be educated about atypical cardiac symptoms.

Should Patients Be Screened for CAD?

Diagnostic tests are used when there is a clinical indication of disease. The question remains whether additional

TABLE 25.3 Warning Signs of CAD

	Angina	*MI*
Etiology	Coronary ischemia; partial occlusion of coronary artery (may be caused by 70%–80% narrowing of 1 or more coronary vessels); usually gradual onset	Sudden total occlusion of coronary artery, often caused by 40%–50% occlusion; vulnerable soft plaque with thin fibrous caps that rupture and release necrotic, lipid-filled material into the artery that can initiate a thrombus and occlude an artery
Quality	Squeezing, tightness, pressure or heavy weight on the chest; more discomfort than pain	Intense, severe squeezing or crushing pain
Location	Diffuse over chest, radiating to neck, lower jaw, or left arm	Midsternal pain radiating to arms, neck, and jaw; epigastric pain
Timing	Rarely lasts more than 5 minutes; remits when precipitating activity is stopped (may be triggered by exercise, sexual intercourse, cold weather, cocaine use)	30–60 minutes
Associated symptoms	Dyspnea, diaphoresis, cold and clammy skin, fatigue, syncope	Diaphoresis, nausea, vomiting, weakness, dyspnea, sense of impending doom, paleness
Notes	Elderly and those with diabetic autonomic neuropathy may have no pain	Autonomic neuropathy may cause loss of pain sensation; may present with onset of diabetic ketoacidosis in people with T1DM; in patients suspected of having MI, advise chewing a full-strength aspirin and call 911

cardiac testing to screen for CAD in asymptomatic patients improves patient outcomes. Several important questions need to be asked when considering screening for CAD in people with diabetes:

- Who should be screened?
- Why should they be screened?
- How should they be screened?

Some studies suggest that everyone with T2DM should be considered to have CAD.[180] However, screening the more than 23 million people in the United States with T2DM would be very expensive. So how do clinicians decide who should be screened?

Studies have not demonstrated improved CV outcomes when asymptomatic people with diabetes underwent cardiac stress testing or screening with adenosine SPECT myocardial perfusion scanning.[181,182] The lack of effect may reflect the general improvement in CV outcomes as a result of more aggressive management of dyslipidemia and hypertension. Intensive medical therapy for CV risk factors is indicated for high-risk patients, regardless of results of screening tests, and seems to provide outcomes equal to those of invasive revascularization.[183,184] Therefore, current evidence does not show cost-effectiveness or benefits to routine cardiac screening of people with diabetes without cardiac symptoms and with a normal EKG.

CAC for cardiovascular risk assessment may be useful in selected asymptomatic adults at intermediate CV risk (10-year risk 10% to 20%) if the results might change clinical management by reclassifying the person into a higher CV risk group. However, these newer noninvasive coronary artery screenings can lead to potentially unnecessary invasive testing and result in cardiac procedures such as angiography and bypass, such that the benefits of noninvasive testing should be balanced with these costs and risks.[105]

The ADA practice guidelines suggest that patients with typical or atypical cardiac symptoms or abnormal resting EKGs are candidates for more cardiac testing. Most often, the initial screening is exercise EKG without or with echocardiography. The EKG leads are placed in the standard locations for a 12-lead EKG. The individual then begins to walk on a level treadmill at a slow pace. The speed and incline of the treadmill are gradually increased until symptoms or EKG abnormalities occur. In the stress echocardiogram, the myocardium is imaged by sonography during exercise. Areas of abnormal motion indicate ischemia. Pharmacologic stress echocardiography or nuclear imaging should be considered for patients who are unable to exercise.

Instruction Opportunity—Preparing Patients for an Exercise Stress Test

Patients usually fast before exercise stress testing. Significant hyperglycemia or hypoglycemia may interfere with the ability to exercise at an appropriate level. Although the stress test is usually limited to 12 to 15 minutes, it may be enough to precipitate hypoglycemia during or shortly after the exercise in people taking long-acting insulin or sulfonylureas.

Potential hypoglycemia reactions induced by stress testing should be discussed with the patient. This type of hypoglycemia is usually short-lived and can be treated with oral anticoagulants. It can often be avoided by withholding sulfonylureas and short-acting insulins until the first meal after the test.

Treatment of Acute MI

Treatment of acute MI in people with diabetes is similar to that in people without diabetes. Treatment may include thrombolytic agents, coronary angioplasty, stents, and revascularization. Outcomes may be worse for people with diabetes. Despite advances in cardiac care over the past 4 decades, the presence of diabetes still doubles the risk of death after MI.[185] Once the patient is stable, the cardiologist may perform testing to evaluate short-term risk and therapies (eg, exercise stress testing, echocardiogram, coronary angiogram). In some cases, further revascularization may be performed.

Hyperglycemia in a person with MI increases the risk of death and congestive heart failure (CHF) whether or not the person had a diagnosis of diabetes before admission.[186] There is increasing evidence that MI may be the initial presentation of diabetes.[187] The Diabetes Mellitus, Insulin Glucose Infusion in Acute Myocardial Infarction (DIGAMI) trial studied the effect of aggressive diabetes management in the immediate post-MI period with an intravenous insulin-glucose drip and 3 months of a 4-shot regimen. Patients randomly assigned to the intensive protocol had significantly reduced mortality. The risk reduction was greatest in those classified as low risk who were not previously treated with insulin.[188] However, the follow-up DIGAMI 2 study did not confirm the findings of DIGAMI; there was no significant difference in mortality between the intensively and non-intensively treated groups.[189] Thus, current recommendations for the treatment of diabetes in people with acute MI do not differ from those of other hospitalized patients. Insulin is the drug of choice: intravenous insulin for patients in critical care units and subcutaneous insulin for other patients. Long-term diabetes management for these patients does not differ from that of high-risk patients previously described.

Risk-factor management and education begin in the hospital. Diabetes management should be stressed and the patient prepared for post-discharge lifestyle changes and risk-factor reduction. A statin, an ACE inhibitor, a beta-blocker, and an antiplatelet agent are often instituted as soon as possible if there are no contraindications.

Instruction Opportunity—Educating Patients After an MI

Persons with an MI undergo a major psychological trauma. They are often discharged from the hospital within days after an uncomplicated MI, usually with a myriad of unanswered and unasked questions. The following are important education topics:

- *Follow-up care.* Schedule appointments with the physician, diabetes care and education specialist, mental health counselor, and cardiac rehabilitation team, as needed.
- *Medications.* Most people with an MI go home with many new medications, including a statin, an ACE inhibitor, a beta-blocker, aspirin, and perhaps another antiplatelet agent in addition to their diabetes medication, which may well be new or intensified at this time (see Treatment of Acute MI section above).
- *Exercise.* Some people with a recent MI may be afraid to exercise, and some, in the throes of denial, may overdo it. Cardiac rehabilitation programs enable the individual to work with a trained clinical team to carefully increase exercise in a supervised setting. A cardiac rehabilitation center can be an excellent venue for your diabetes self-management education program as well.
- *Therapeutic lifestyle change.* This includes smoking cessation and medical nutrition therapy.
- *Psychosocial issues.* Up to one third of people with MI have significant depressive symptoms afterward, and major depression occurs in nearly one fifth.[190] Depression, which is common in people with diabetes, is associated with a twofold to threefold increase in risk of death in the first 6 months after MI.[191] Another study of highly stressed individuals after MI found that home nursing visits were associated with a significant reduction in subsequent fatal and nonfatal cardiac events.[192]
- *Sexual activity.* Many patients are concerned about safely resuming sexual activity. Sexual dysfunction may be common, and its treatment should be discussed with the patient.

How Should Patients Be Prepared for Elective Cardiac Catheterization and Angioplasty?

Issues to discuss with the patient and the physician include the following:

- *Timing and food consumption.* Whenever possible, elective cardiac catheterization for people taking insulin should be scheduled in the morning. In most cases, the patient fasts after midnight for an early-morning procedure. If the procedure is later in the day, a light meal may be allowed up to 2 to 4 hours before.
- *Diabetes medications.* Advise the patient about whether to decrease or withhold certain diabetes medications.
  - —In general, there is no reason to change evening or bedtime insulin or oral agents if morning self-monitored glucose is acceptable.
  - —Persons on insulin pumps should continue their normal basal insulin infusion.
  - —Sulfonylureas, secretagogues, and acarbose should be held on the morning of the procedure and resumed when the person resumes normal eating.
  - —Metformin is held the morning of the procedure and resumed when creatinine has been rechecked and it is certain that the angiogram dye has caused no adverse renal effects.
- *Hyperglycemia and hypoglycemia.* Planning should include addressing hyperglycemia and hypoglycemia before and during the procedure.
- *Hydration.* Patients should be instructed to increase fluid intake to enhance excretion of the angiogram dye.
- *Steroid pretreatment.* In patients with a history or risk of allergy to the angiogram dye, steroids such as prednisone may be given the day before and the day of the procedure. Most patients note a significant increase in their glucose for 2 to 3 days after beginning an oral steroid. Patients should be adequately prepared for this effect so they can appropriately adjust their medication.

Cerebrovascular Disease

Atherosclerosis affecting the central nervous system presents in 3 characteristic ways:

- Transient ischemic attack
- Cerebrovascular accident
  —*Ischemic:* Thrombotic, embolic, or systemic hypotension
  —*Hemorrhagic:* Intracranial or subarachnoid
- Vascular dementia

What Causes a Cerebrovascular Accident?

About 80% of strokes are ischemic, and the rest are hemorrhagic. By definition, a cerebrovascular accident (CVA) is tissue death resulting from disruption from either hemorrhage or ischemic infarction. Ischemic CVA may be caused by atherosclerotic disease in intracranial or extracranial arteries. The process may be intrinsic to the affected artery, as in atherosclerotic thrombi, or the result of embolus from either the heart or extracranial arteries. The clinical presentation depends on the area of the brain served by the affected arteries.

Ischemic strokes are more likely to occur at a younger age in African Americans, when hypertension is present, and when there is a history of MI.[82] Most thrombotic and embolic strokes occur in persons older than 40, but this may be less predictive in the future because today's youth with T2DM will reach their 40s with a history of almost 30 years of diabetes.

Is a Stroke Preventable?

Hypertension, including isolated systolic hypertension, is the most important risk factor for stroke. Diabetes and smoking also contribute to stroke risk. Smoking increases the prevalence of extracranial occlusive arterial disease and more than doubles the risk of stroke. Diabetes is also associated with a doubling of stroke risk, affecting both small and large arteries. Statin therapy has been shown to decrease the risk of fatal and nonfatal stroke.[193]

Effective antihypertensive therapy, statin therapy, and smoking cessation have been shown to decrease stroke risk.[141,194]

What Is a Transient Ischemic Attack?

Transient ischemic attack (TIA), sometimes called "mini stroke" by lay people, is classically defined as the sudden onset of a neurologic deficit that lasts less than 24 hours and is not associated with a permanent residual defect. Transient ischemic attack is presumably caused by a transient decrease in blood supply, causing focal ischemia in the area of the brain that produces the symptoms.

The syndromes caused by TIA depend on the pathogenesis and location. Transient ischemic attacks may be caused by decreased flow in a large artery, either intracranial or extracranial. Less often, an embolus from a larger artery or the heart results in a TIA. Transient ischemic attack may result from lesions in either the anterior (carotid) or posterior (vertebral) circulation. The symptoms of ischemia differ significantly because these vascular beds supply areas of the brain with markedly different functions.

Initial evaluation of a person with a suspected TIA starts with a carefully taken history. In most cases, the episode has passed by the time the person is seen by a clinician. It is important to differentiate an ischemic event from a metabolic event such as hypoglycemia. Although seizure disorders, syncope, and migraine auras may mimic TIA symptoms, it is important to first rule out TIA. Urgent medical attention and evaluation of patients with TIA symptoms, even if they have disappeared, are important. Risk of CVA in the months after a TIA is very high. From 11% to 20% of patients with a TIA have a CVA in the next 90 days; half of the strokes occurred in the first 2 days.[195,196]

Transient ischemic attacks occur suddenly, with symptoms that may have passed by the time the patient is seen. They require urgent evaluation and referral due to the high risk of stroke.

Instruction Opportunity—Recognizing Signs of a TIA or Stroke

The AHA promotes the acronym FAST as an easy way to help patients remember the warning signs and symptoms of stroke.[197] According to the AHA's Web site, FAST is described as the following:

- Face drooping—Does one side of the face droop or is it numb? Ask the person to smile. Is the smile uneven?
- Arm weakness—Is one arm weak or numb? Ask the person to raise both arms. Does one arm drift downward?
- Speech difficulty—Is speech slurred? Is the person unable to speak or hard to understand? Ask the person to repeat a simple sentence, like "The sky is blue." Is the sentence repeated correctly?
- Time to call 9-1-1—If someone shows any of these symptoms, even if the symptoms go away, call 9-1-1 and get the person to the hospital immediately. Check the time so you'll know when the first symptoms appeared.

TABLE 25.4 Early-Warning Symptoms of Stroke

The Stroke Association has publicized these early-warning symptoms of stroke and recommends that the person or witness call 911 if they occur:

- Sudden numbness or weakness of the face, arm, or leg, especially on one side of the body
- Sudden confusion, trouble speaking or understanding
- Sudden trouble seeing in 1 or both eyes
- Sudden trouble walking, dizziness, or loss of balance or coordination
- Sudden, severe headache with no known cause

Source: Stroke Association, "Stroke Symptoms" (last reviewed 2019 Dec 22, cited 2019 Dec 22), on the Internet at: https://www.stroke.org/en/about-stroke/stroke-symptoms

Symptoms of cerebrovascular disease may mimic those of hypoglycemia. See the early-warning symptoms of stroke in Table 25.4. Current therapeutic approaches to thrombotic CVA (the most common form in diabetes) call for early institution of thrombolytic agents. Transient ischemic attacks may be an early warning of an impending CVA. Thus, early identification is essential. Educating people with diabetes about the difference between a hypoglycemic episode and a TIA or an early CVA is clearly important. Many of these symptoms are similar to the symptoms of hypoglycemia; there is no perfect way to distinguish them other than to test glucose during an episode.

Peripheral Artery Disease

Peripheral artery disease is the third most important manifestation of atherosclerosis after coronary and cerebral disease. An estimated 12 million people in the United States have PAD, although it is difficult to estimate its prevalence, because more than half of those with PAD are asymptomatic or have atypical symptoms. About one third have classic symptoms of intermittent claudication, and about one sixth have more severe ischemia. Data from the Framingham study suggest that roughly 20% of people with PAD have diabetes; these data are likely to be an underestimate, given the frequency of asymptomatic PAD.[198] A survey of people with diabetes older than 50 found the prevalence of PAD by ABI determination to be almost 30%.[90] People with long-standing diabetes and PAD may have atypical symptoms due to neuropathy and may not present for medical care until a neurogenic or ischemic ulcer or gangrene develops.

The increased risk of PAD in diabetes is likely to be caused by the same etiologic factors as those of other vascular beds, including hypertension, dyslipidemia, tobacco, and endothelial dysfunction. Thus, the clinical diagnosis of PAD should raise concern about other vascular beds, including the coronary arteries, renal arteries, and cerebral vessels. Patients with PAD are at increased risk for CV events, including stroke, renovascular hypertension, MI, and sudden death.

One in three people with diabetes older than 50 likely has PAD.[199]

How Does PAD Present in People With Diabetes?

The pattern of PAD in those whose primary risk factor is diabetes is different from the pattern in those with other risk factors, such as smoking and hypertension. In the presence of diabetes, PAD occurs more often in the distal arteries—those below the knee (femoral-popliteal and tibial). Other risk factors, such as hypertension and smoking, are associated with a more proximal (aortic, iliac, and proximal femoral) arterial distribution.

The effects of PAD are determined by its progression, presence of symptoms, and associated CV risk. Although most patients with PAD remain stable, more than one fourth have progression of symptoms over 5 years, with amputation occurring in about 4%. One fifth have a CV event within 5 years. Severe ischemia carries a greater risk; 30% have an amputation, and fatality rates approach 20% in 6 months.[200] Although these data are from the general population and there have been no long-term follow-up studies of people with diabetes, event rates are likely to be even higher in people with diabetes.

How Is PAD Detected and Diagnosed?

Screening for and diagnosing PAD is important for 2 reasons. First, the presence of PAD indicates that the person is at increased risk for other events, including stroke and MI. Second, PAD contributes to disability, particularly in those with diabetes. Much of the difference between people with PAD with diabetes and those with PAD without diabetes can be explained by peripheral neuropathy.[201] Adverse effects of PAD include diminished walking ability, with slower walking and shorter walking distances. This leads to deconditioning, which contributes to diminished quality of life and progressive disability.

People with diabetes and PAD are more prone to sudden events, including arterial thrombosis, neuroischemic ulceration, and infection. These events lead to critical limb ischemia and increased risk of amputation. By diagnosing PAD in its early stages, preventive measures can be instituted to diminish its progression or elective revascularization in a threatened limb can be arranged before amputation is necessary.

Evaluation for PAD begins with a carefully taken history and physical assessment. The classic symptom of PAD is *intermittent claudication*. The patient complains of pain, cramping, or aching in the calves, thighs, or buttocks. This pain recurs with walking and is relieved by rest. This pattern differs from that of diabetic peripheral neuropathy, in which pain is usually exacerbated by rest and relieved by walking. The pain of spinal stenosis also increases with walking and may be confused with claudication. As PAD progresses, it may cause ischemic pain at rest, tissue loss, or gangrene. The combination of PAD and peripheral neuropathy places the person with diabetes at greater risk for lower-limb amputation.

The diabetes care and education specialist should ask the patient about symptoms of claudication, pain at rest, and limitations to walking. A carefully taken exercise history often uncovers symptoms of claudication; patients often do not volunteer this information, so it is important to seek it. The pattern of the pain will help differentiate PAD from neuropathy. Peripheral artery disease may cause a wide variety of symptoms, ranging from no symptoms to severe leg pain at rest. It is also important to identify patients with risk factors, such as smoking and hypertension, in addition to their diabetes. Because the person with PAD is at increased risk for other vascular events, eliciting a history of chest pain or atypical angina symptoms is important. Unfortunately, a stroke history is usually self-evident, but a history of TIAs may indicate atherosclerosis in the cerebral circulation.

The physical assessment for diabetic foot problems is part of every diabetes visit. "Shoes and socks off" should be the rule. The ischemic foot may be pale or have *dependent rubor*, a deep red color when the foot is hanging down but pallor on elevation. There is hair loss on the distal foot and toes; cool, dry, atrophic skin; and dystrophic toenails. The dorsalis pedis and posterior tibial pulses should be palpated; if they are absent, the popliteal pulse should be palpated as well. It is important to note that palpating pulses is a skill that takes practice and has a high rate of false-negative and false-positive results.

Ankle-Brachial Index

The ABI is a ratio of the systolic pressure at the ankle (posterior tibial or dorsalis pedis pulses) and the brachial artery. The ABI has been found to be a reasonably accurate, reproducible measure for the screening and detection of PAD and its severity. The ABI is determined by placing the blood pressure cuff just above the ankle and inflating it to above systolic pressure. A simple handheld Doppler device is used to detect the systolic pulse in the dorsalis pedis and posterior tibial arteries as the cuff is slowly deflated. The same procedure is used in both feet and 1 arm. To obtain a ratio, the systolic pressure in each of the 4 lower limb arteries is divided by the brachial systolic pressure. The higher value in each limb is the ABI for that limb (Table 25.5). The ADA recommends that an ABI be considered part of initial screening, because many patients with PAD are asymptomatic.

TABLE 25.5 ABI Diagnostic Criteria
Normal: 1.00–1.40
Borderline: .91–.99
Abnormal: ≤.90
Elevated pressures (>1.40) may indicate poorly compressible arteries and the presence of arterial calcification. If so, the ABI may not represent the true degree of obstruction.

Source: TW Rooke, AT Hirsch, S Misra, et al, "2011 ACCF/AHA Focused Update of the Guideline for the Management of Patients With Peripheral Artery Disease (updating the 2005 guideline): a report of the American College of Cardiology Foundation/American Heart Association Task Force on Practice Guidelines," *J Am Coll Cardiol* 58, no. 19 (2011): 2020–45.

An abnormal ABI is indicative of, but not diagnostic of, PAD and necessitates a referral to a vascular laboratory for more formal testing. In addition, patients with poorly compressible arteries should be considered for formal vascular testing if there is a high degree of suspicion for PAD. Patients with PAD are generally treated with aggressive support for smoking cessation, daily use of antiplatelet agents, and endovascular and open surgical revascularization for critical limb ischemia. Patients with claudication, absent pedal pulses, or abnormal ABI should be referred to a vascular specialist for further evaluation.

Congestive Heart Failure

Congestive heart failure is a major contributor to morbidity and mortality in the United States, affecting an estimated 5 million people. Common treatments of CHF include sodium restriction, diuretics, ACE inhibitors, and beta-blockers. Thiazolidinedione treatment should be avoided in patients with symptomatic CHF. Metformin use should be individualized for patients with pharmacologically treated heart failure; it may be used in patients with stable CHF with normal renal function but should be discontinued in unstable or hospitalized patients.[202] Current evidence does not support use of statins in patients with NYHA Class II-IV CHF (Table 25.6).[73]

TABLE 25.6 NYHA Functional Classification of Heart Failure

NYHA Class	*Symptoms*
I	Cardiac disease without symptoms and/or limitation in ordinary physical activity (eg, shortness of breath when walking or climbing stairs)
II	Mild symptoms (mild shortness of breath and/or angina) and slight limitation during ordinary activity
III	Marked limitation in activity due to symptoms, even during mild activity (eg, walking short distances [20–100 meters])
	Comfortable only at rest
IV	Severe limitations. Symptoms experienced even while at rest. Most patients are bedbound.

Focus on Education

Teaching Strategies

Stress that management of CV risk factors is as important as glycemic management for people with diabetes.

Help patients understand their personal ASCVD risk. Calculate ASCVD risk and explain what the numbers mean in terms that patients can understand.

Use a multifactorial risk-reduction approach. Cardiovascular risk reduction requires addressing all of the patient's modifiable risk factors. Cardiovascular risk can be lowered the most by achieving the "D5 goals": managing hypertension, achieving lipid goals, smoking cessation, blood glucose management, and use of antiplatelet therapy, when appropriate.

Individualize the approach with the person with diabetes and use shared decision making to help him or her prioritize treatment strategies based on the risk factors furthest from goal, complexity of the treatment recommendations, and current therapy.

Consider the cardiovascular benefits of different glucose-lowering therapies when selecting treatment options for patients with high cardiovascular risk.

Review and individualize instructions. Educational needs are highly individualized. When preparing for education and care planning, spend time preparing and individualizing the treatment options. Have appropriate descriptive materials, take-home handouts, and media for viewing in the clinical setting and reviewing at home.

Information, individualization, shared decision making, skill building, and follow-up are the keys to care.

Messages for Persons With Diabetes

People with diabetes are at higher risk for heart attacks and strokes.

Prevention of heart attacks and strokes requires multiple treatments, such as statin use, blood pressure management, tobacco cessation, blood glucose management, and aspirin use, if appropriate. Achieving these targets significantly reduces your risk of complications such as heart attack and stroke, as well as problems with your kidneys, eyes, and nervous system.

Support is available for smoking cessation. If you have diabetes, smoking is like adding fuel to a fire. Work with your healthcare team to find the support you need to quit smoking.

Heart-healthy eating, physical activity, and stress management benefit all aspects of well-being. Healthy lifestyle behaviors will benefit not just CV health but your overall quality of life.

The AHA recommends statin therapy for most people with diabetes.

Know your numbers. Monitor how changes in your lifestyle and medication affect your blood pressure and A1C.

Health Literacy

The American Heart Association acknowledges that limited health literacy is highly prevalent in the United States and a barrier to their national goals to reduce the rates of heart disease. Numerous studies have found that CV care outcomes can be improved with targeted patient education and improved clinician communication skills that consider patients' health literacy. One study found that only half of clinicians took appropriate action to properly communicate with and educate low-literacy patients—even when the clinicians knew about their patients' literacy level.[203] Everyone, regardless of age, income, or education level, is at risk for low health literacy. Help patients make decisions by describing the nature of the decision, assessing their understanding, eliciting their preferences, and discussing the alternatives, risks and benefits, and related uncertainties.

Social and cultural variances among patients create barriers in understanding health care. Some perceptions can influence the patients' view of and engagement with the treatment regimen. Many patients choose treatment options that seem logical based on their interpretation of the conditions; however, patients often misinterpret the conditions. Ask patients what the information means to them or what they will do differently based on what they have learned. Also, normalizing that it is common to feel overwhelmed about this information allows you to ask, "What is most confusing for you about this information?"

Evaluate health numeracy, the ability to reason and apply simple numerical concepts. Innumeracy can cause patients to make poor health-related decisions because of inaccurate perceptions of the information. Basic numeracy involves counting pills or using a calendar to schedule an appropriate date for an appointment. Analytical numeracy enables patients to understand if blood pressure, cholesterol, and blood glucose levels are within normal range and to determine whether screening tests are necessary. Statistical health numeracy enables patients to weigh the risks and benefits of treatment options. Recognizing poor health numeracy can help the clinician convey the information more appropriately.

Numbers can be a powerful motivator for change in cases of "silent" diseases like hypertension and diabetes. However, patients need to know the meaning of the numbers and track any changes. They need to understand the norm and how their test results deviate from it.

Positive psychological well-being, such as optimism, has also been associated with cardiovascular health and improved outcomes. Mindfulness-based programs and positive psychological interventions could potentially promote well-being, although more research on the efficacy of these interventions is needed.[204,205]

Diabetes care and education specialists can maximize learning among persons with diabetes with low health literacy by doing the following:[206]

- Assess health literacy skills of persons with diabetes
- Use simple language instead of medical terminology
- Show or draw pictures
- Limit information given at each interaction, and repeat instructions
- Use a "teach back" or "show me" approach to confirm understanding
- Be respectful, caring, sensitive, and interested
- Consider mindfulness-based programs to promote a positive sense of well-being
- Consider the result: It is not what you know but what the person with diabetes knows.

Focus on Practice

If not readily available, create care processes for doing efficient assessment of CV risk factors and 10-year ASCVD risk.

Develop team-based CV care and education protocols for your institution. Collaborate with all departments, including nutrition, pharmacy, nursing, primary care providers, and specialists.

If within the scope of your practice, develop consensus and approval for simple protocol-driven adjustment of statin and blood pressure therapies.

Create systems with reminders, case management, and quality-improvement mechanisms.

Use continuous quality improvement methods, with measurement performance for optimal diabetes care, feedback, and benchmarking.

Select CVD as a quality focus because it is relevant to all health plan populations. Establish appropriate baseline measurements and performance goals. Identify barriers to quality CV care and prevention.

Identify appropriate target population for intervention. Compare CV performance data with goals. Pay attention to healthcare disparities due to race, ethnicity, or sex.

Consider the financial benefits of total CV risk management, which through the prevention of serious complications can reduce the economic burden of diabetes to health plans, employers, persons with diabetes and society.

References

1. American Diabetes Association. Economic costs of diabetes in the U.S. in 2007. Diabetes Care. 2008;31(3):1-20.
2. International Diabetes Federation. IDF Diabetes Atlas. 6th ed. Brussels, Belgium: International Diabetes Federation; 2013.
3. Preis SR, Hwang SJ, Coady S, et al. Trends in all-cause and cardiovascular disease mortality among women and men with and without diabetes mellitus in the Framingham Heart Study, 1950 to 2005. Circulation. 2009;119(13):1728-35.
4. Wilhelmsen L, Welin L, Svardsudd K, et al. Secular changes in cardiovascular risk factors and attack rate of myocardial infarction among men aged 50 in Gothenburg, Sweden. Accurate prediction using risk models. J Intern Med. 2008 Jun;263(6):636-43.
5. Norhammar A, Tenerz A, Nilsson G, et al. Glucose metabolism in patients with acute myocardial infarction and no previous diagnosis of diabetes mellitus: a prospective study. Lancet. 2002 Jun;359(9324):2140-4.
6. Bartnik M, Malmberg K, Norhammar A, Tenerz A, Ohrvik J, Rydén L. Newly detected abnormal glucose tolerance: an important predictor of long-term outcome after myocardial infarction. Eur Heart J. 2004 Nov;25(22):1990-7.
7. Hu DY, Pan CY, Yu JM; China Heart Survey Group. The relationship between coronary artery disease and abnormal glucose regulation in China: the China Heart Survey. Eur Heart J. 2006 Nov;27(21):2573-9. Epub 2006 Sep 19.
8. Lenzen M, Ryden L, Ohrvik J, et al. Diabetes known or newly detected, but not impaired glucose regulation, has a negative influence on 1-year outcome in patients with coronary artery disease: a report from the Euro Heart Survey on diabetes and the heart. Eur Heart J. 2006 Dec;27(24):2969-74.
9. Ritsinger V, Tanoglidi E, Malmberg K, et al. Sustained prognostic implications of newly detected glucose abnormalities in patients with acute myocardial infarction: long-term follow-up of the Glucose Tolerance in Patients with Acute Myocardial Infarction cohort. Diab Vasc Dis Res. 2015 Jan;12(1):23-32.
10. Center for Disease Control and Prevention. National diabetes statistics report, 2017. Atlanta, GA: Centers for Disease Control and Prevention, U.S. Dept of Health and Human Services; 2017.
11. National Centers for Disease Control and Prevention. National diabetes statistics report 2014. www.cdc.gov/data/statistics/statistics-report.html.
12. Gorina Y, Lentzner H. Multiple causes of death in old age. Aging Trends. 2008 Feb;(9):1-9.
13. Centers for Disease Control and Prevention. National diabetes fact sheet, 2011 (cited 2014 Mar 3). On the Internet at: http://www.cdc.gov/diabetes/pubs/pdf/ndfs_2011.pdf.
14. National Diabetes Information Clearinghouse. Diabetes, heart disease, and stroke. 2013 Aug (cited 2014 Mar 3). On the Internet at: http://diabetes.niddk.nih.gov/dm/pubs/stroke/.
15. Einarson TR, Acs A, Ludwig C, Panton UH. Economic burden of cardiovascular disease in type 2 diabetes: a systematic review. Value Health. 2018;21(7): 881-90.
16. Coutinho M, Gerstein HC, Wang Y, Yusuf S. The relationship between glucose and incident cardiovascular events: a metaregression analysis of published data from 20 studies of 95,783 individuals followed for 12.4 years. Diabetes Care. 1999;22(2):233-40.
17. Turner RC, Millns H, Neil HA, et al. Risk factors for coronary artery disease in non-insulin dependent diabetes mellitus: United Kingdom Prospective Diabetes Study (UKPDS: 23). BMJ. 1998 Mar 14;316(7134):823-8.
18. Khaw KT, Wareham N, Luben R, et al. Glycated haemoglobin, diabetes, and mortality in men in Norfolk cohort of European Prospective Investigation of Cancer and Nutrition (EPIC-Norfolk). BMJ. 2001 Jan 6;322(7277):15-8.
19. Muntner P, Wildman RP, Reynolds K, Desalvo KB, Chen J, Fonseca V. Relationship between HbA1c level and peripheral arterial disease. Diabetes Care. 2005 Aug;28(8):1981-7.
20. Selvin E, Coresh J, Golden SH, Boland LL, Brancati FL, Steffes MW. Glycemic control, atherosclerosis, and risk factors for cardiovascular disease in individuals with diabetes: the atherosclerosis risk in communities study. Diabetes Care. 2005 Aug;28(8):1965-73.
21. Selvin E, Marinopoulos S, Berkenblit G, et al. Meta-analysis: glycosylated hemoglobin and cardiovascular disease in diabetes mellitus. Ann Intern Med. 2004 Sep 21;141(6):421-31.
22. Krolewski AS, Kosinski EJ, Warram JH, et al. Magnitude and determinants of coronary artery disease in juvenile-onset, insulin-dependent diabetes mellitus. Am J Cardiol. 1987 Apr 1;59(8):750-5.
23. Dorman JS, Tajima N, LaPorte RE, et al. The Pittsburgh Insulin-Dependent Diabetes Mellitus (IDDM) Morbidity and Mortality Study: case-control analyses of risk factors for mortality. Diabetes Care. 1985 Sep-Oct;8 Suppl 1:54-60.
24. Miller J, Silverstein J. Risk factors for cardiovascular disease in children with diabetes. Practical Diabetology. 2004;23(2):13-8.
25. American Diabetes Association. Management of dyslipidemia in children and adolescents with diabetes. Diabetes Care. 2003 Jul;26(7):2194-7.
26. Orchard TJ, Forrest KY, Kuller LH, Becker DJ. Lipid and blood pressure treatment goals for type 1 diabetes: 10-year incidence data from the Pittsburgh Epidemiology of Diabetes Complications Study. Diabetes Care. 2001 Jun;24(6):1053-9.
27. Libby P, Ridker PM, Maseri A. Inflammation and atherosclerosis. Circulation. 2002 Mar 5;105(9):1135-43.
28. Davignon J, Ganz P. Role of endothelial dysfunction in atherosclerosis. Circulation. 2004 Jun 15;109(23 Suppl 1):III27-32.
29. Golden SH, Folsom AR, Coresh J, Sharrett AR, Szklo M, Brancati F. Risk factor groupings related to insulin resistance and their synergistic effects on subclinical atherosclerosis: the atherosclerosis risk in communities study. Diabetes. 2002 Oct;51(10):3069-76.

30. Stehouwer C. The many faces of vascular dysfunction in diabetes. Paper presented at: 20th Camillo Golgi Lecture; delivered at European Association for the Study of Diabetes; 2005; Athens, Greece.

31. Bonora E, Muggeo M. Postprandial blood glucose as a risk factor for cardiovascular disease in type II diabetes: the epidemiological evidence. Diabetologia. 2001 Dec;44(12):2107-14.

32. Ceriello A. Postprandial hyperglycemia and diabetes complications: is it time to treat? Diabetes. 2005 Jan;54(1):1-7.

33. DECODE Study Group, European Diabetes Epidemiology Group. Glucose tolerance and cardiovascular mortality: comparison of fasting and 2-hour diagnostic criteria. Arch Intern Med. 2001 Feb 12;161(3):397-405.

34. Rodriguez BL, Lau N, Burchfiel CM, et al. Glucose intolerance and 23-year risk of coronary heart disease and total mortality: the Honolulu Heart Program. Diabetes Care. 1999 Aug;22(8):1262-5.

35. Bonora E. Postprandial peaks as a risk factor for cardiovascular disease: epidemiological perspectives. Int J Clin Pract Suppl. 2002 Jul;129:5-11.

36. Ceriello A, Taboga C, Tonutti L, et al. Evidence for an independent and cumulative effect of postprandial hypertriglyceridemia and hyperglycemia on endothelial dysfunction and oxidative stress generation: effects of short- and long-term simvastatin treatment. Circulation. 2002 Sep 3;106(10):1211-8.

37. Chiasson JL, Josse RG, Gomis R, Hanefeld M, Karasik A, Laakso M. Acarbose treatment and the risk of cardiovascular disease and hypertension in patients with impaired glucose tolerance: the STOP-NIDDM trial. JAMA. 2003 Jul 23;290(4):486-94.

38. Hanefeld M, Cagatay M, Petrowitsch T, Neuser D, Petzinna D, Rupp M. Acarbose reduces the risk for myocardial infarction in type 2 diabetic patients: meta-analysis of seven long-term studies. Eur Heart J. 2004 Jan;25(1):10-6.

39. Esposito K, Giugliano D, Nappo F, Marfella R. Regression of carotid atherosclerosis by control of postprandial hyperglycemia in type 2 diabetes mellitus. Circulation. 2004 Jul 13;110(2):214-9.

40. Huang ES, Meigs JB, Singer DE. The effect of interventions to prevent cardiovascular disease in patients with type 2 diabetes mellitus. Am J Med. 2001 Dec 1;111(8):633-42.

41. Intensive blood-glucose control with sulphonylureas or insulin compared with conventional treatment and risk of complications in patients with type 2 diabetes (UKPDS 33). UK Prospective Diabetes Study (UKPDS) Group. Lancet. 1998 Sep 12;352(9131):837-53.

42. Holman RR, Paul SK, Bethel MA, Matthews DR, Neil HA. Ten-year follow-up of intensive glucose control in type 2 diabetes. N Engl J Med. 2008 Oct 9;359(15):1577-89.

43. Skyler JS, Bergenstal R, Bonow RO, et al. Intensive glycemic control and the prevention of cardiovascular events: implications of the ACCORD, ADVANCE, and VA diabetes trials: a position statement of the American Diabetes Association and a scientific statement of the American College of Cardiology Foundation and the American Heart Association. Diabetes Care. 2009 Jan;32(1):187-92.

44. Gerstein HC, Miller ME, Byington RP, et al. Effects of intensive glucose lowering in type 2 diabetes. N Engl J Med. 2008 Jun 12; 358(24):2545-59.

45. Patel A, MacMahon S, Chalmers J, et al. Intensive blood glucose control and vascular outcomes in patients with type 2 diabetes. N Engl J Med. 2008 Jun 12;358(24):2560-72.

46. Duckworth W, Abraira C, Moritz T, et al. Glucose control and vascular complications in veterans with type 2 diabetes. N Engl J Med. 2009 Jan 8;360(2):129-39.

47. Hayward RA, Reaven PD, Wiitala WL, et al. Follow-up of glycemic control and cardiovascular outcomes in type 2 diabetes. N Engl J Med. 2015 Jun 4;372(23):2197-206.

48. Johnston SS, Conner C, Aagren M, Smith DM, Bouchard J, Brett J. Evidence linking hypoglycemic events to an increased risk of acute cardiovascular events in patients with type 2 diabetes. Diabetes Care. 2011 May;34(5):1164-70.

49. Anselmino M, Wallander M, Norhammar A, Mellbin L, Ryden L. Implications of abnormal glucose metabolism in patients with coronary artery disease. Diab Vasc Dis Res. 2008 Nov;5(4):285-90.

50. Nissen SE, Wolski K. Effect of rosiglitazone on the risk of myocardial infarction and death from cardiovascular causes. N Engl J Med. 2007 Jun 14;356(24):2457-71.

51. Komajda M, Curtis P, Hanefeld M, et al. Effect of the addition of rosiglitazone to metformin or sulfonylureas versus metformin/sulfonylurea combination therapy on ambulatory blood pressure in people with type 2 diabetes: a randomized controlled trial (the RECORD study). Cardiovasc Diabetol. 2008;7:10.

52. Hirshberg B, Raz I. Impact of the U.S. Food and Drug Administration cardiovascular assessment requirements on the development of novel antidiabetes drugs. Diabetes Care. 2011 May;34 Suppl 2:S101-6.

53. Holman RR, Paul SK, Bethel MA, Matthews DR, Neil HA. 10-year follow-up of intensive glucose control in type 2 diabetes. N Engl J Med. 2008 Oct 9;359(15):1577-89. doi: 10.1056/NEJMoa0806470. Epub 2008 Sep 10.

54. Griffin SJ, Leaver JK, Irving GJ. Impact of metformin on cardiovascular disease: a meta-analysis of randomised trials among people with type 2 diabetes. Diabetologia. 2017;60(9):1620–29. doi:10.1007/s00125-017-4337-9.

55. Zinman B, Wanner C, Lachin JM, et al. Empagliflozin, cardiovascular outcomes, and mortality in type 2 diabetes. N Engl J Med. 2015;373:2117-28. DOI: 10.1056/NEJMoa1504720.

56. Neal B, Perkovic V, Mahaffey KW, et al. CANVAS Program Collaborative Group. Canagliflozin and cardiovascular and renal

events in type 2 diabetes. N Engl J Med. 2017;377:644–57. doi: 10.1056/NEJMoa1611925.

57. Zelniker TA, Wiviott SD, Raz I, et al. SGLT2 inhibitors for primary and secondary prevention of cardiovascular and renal outcomes in type 2 diabetes: a systematic review and meta-analysis of cardiovascular outcome trials. Lancet. 2019 Jan 5; 393(10166):31-9. doi: 10.1016/S0140-6736(18)32590-X. Epub 2018 Nov 10.

58. American Diabetes Association. Pharmacologic approaches to glycemic treatment: Standards of Medical Care in Diabetes, American Diabetes Association. Diabetes Care. 2019 Jan; 42(Suppl 1): S93.

59. Marso SP, Daniels GH, Brown-Frandsen K, et al. Liraglutide and cardiovascular outcomes in type 2 diabetes. N Engl J Med. 2016 Jul 28;375(4):311-22. doi: 10.1056/NEJMoa1603827. Epub 2016 Jun 13.

60. Marso SP, Bain SC, Consoli A, et al. Semaglutide and cardiovascular outcomes in patients with type 2 diabetes. N Engl J Med. 2016 Nov 10;375(19):1834-44. Epub 2016 Sep 15.

61. Scirica BM, Bhatt DL, Braunwald E, et al; the SAVOR-TIMI 53 Steering Committee and Investigators. Saxagliptin and cardiovascular outcomes in patients with type 2 diabetes mellitus. N Engl J Med. 2013;369:1317-26. Abstract.

62. White WB, Cannon CP, Heller SR, et al; the EXAMINE Investigators. Alogliptin after acute coronary syndrome in patients with type 2 diabetes. N Engl J Med. 2013;369:1327-35. Abstract.

63. Wanner C. Empagliflozin and progression of kidney disease in type 2 diabetes. N Engl J Med. 2016 Jul 28;375(4):323-34.

64. Stern M. Diabetes in Hispanic Americans. In: National Diabetes Data Group, eds. Diabetes in America. 2nd ed. Bethesda, Md: National Institute of Diabetes and Digestive and Kidney Diseases; 1995:631-60.

65. Larsen JL, Colling CW, Ratanasuwan T, et al. Pancreas transplantation improves vascular disease in patients with type 1 diabetes. Diabetes Care. 2004 Jul;27(7):1706-11.

66. Fiorina P, Gremizzi C, Maffi P, et al. Islet transplantation is associated with an improvement of cardiovascular function in type 1 diabetic kidney transplant patients. Diabetes Care. 2005 Jun;28(6):1358-65.

67. Nathan DM, Lachin J, Cleary P, et al. Intensive diabetes therapy and carotid intima-media thickness in type 1 diabetes mellitus. N Engl J Med. 2003 Jun 5;348(23):2294-303.

68. Nathan DM, Cleary PA, Backlund JY, et al. Intensive diabetes treatment and cardiovascular disease in patients with type 1 diabetes. N Engl J Med. 2005 Dec 22;353(25):2643-53.

69. Pignone M, Phillips CJ, Elasy TA, Fernandez A. Physicians' ability to predict the risk of coronary heart disease. BMC Health Serv Res. 2003;3:13.

70. Moons KG, Kengne AP, Woodward M, et al. Risk prediction models: I. Development, internal validation, and assessing the incremental value of a new (bio)marker. Heart. 2012 May;98(9):683-90.

71. Sheridan SL, Crespo E. Does the routine use of global coronary heart disease risk scores translate into clinical benefits or harms? A systematic review of the literature. BMC Health Serv Res. 2008;8:60.

72. Sheridan SL, Viera AJ, Krantz MJ, et al. The effect of giving global coronary risk information to adults: a systematic review. Arch Intern Med. 2010 Feb 8;170(3):230-9.

73. Stone NJ, Robinson J, Lichtenstein AH, et al. 2013 ACC/AHA Guideline on the Treatment of Blood Cholesterol to Reduce Atherosclerotic Cardiovascular Risk in Adults: a Report of the American College of Cardiology/American Heart Association Task Force on Practice Guidelines. Circulation. Epub 2013 Nov 12.

74. Grundy SM, Stone NJ. 2018 American Heart Association/ American College of Cardiology Multisociety guideline on the management of blood cholesterol: primary prevention. JAMA Cardiol. 2019;4(5):488–489. doi:https://doi.org/10.1001/jamacardio.2019.0777.

75. Goff DC Jr, Lloyd-Jones DM, Bennett G, et al. 2013 ACC/ AHA Guideline on the Assessment of Cardiovascular Risk: a Report of the American College of Cardiology/American Heart Association Task Force on Practice Guidelines. J Am Coll Cardiol. Epub 2013 Nov 7.

76. Eckel RH, Jakicic JM, Ard JD, et al. 2013 AHA/ACC Guideline on Lifestyle Management to Reduce Cardiovascular Risk: a Report of the American College of Cardiology/American Heart Association Task Force on Practice Guidelines. Circulation. Epub 2013 Nov 12.

77. Navar AM, Wang TY, Mi X, et al. Influence of cardiovascular risk communication tools and presentation formats on patient perceptions and preferences. JAMA Cardiol. 2018.

78. Magnani JW, Mujahid MS, Aronow HD, et al. Health literacy and cardiovascular disease: fundamental relevance to primary and secondary prevention: a scientific statement from the American Heart Association. Circulation. 2018;138(2): e48-e74.

79. Bachmann JM, Willis BL, Ayers CR, Khera A, Berry JD. Association between family history and coronary heart disease death across long-term follow-up in men: the Cooper Center Longitudinal Study. Circulation. 2012 Jun 26;125(25):3092-8.

80. Sivapalaratnam S, Boekholdt SM, Trip MD, et al. Family history of premature coronary heart disease and risk prediction in the EPIC-Norfolk prospective population study. Heart. 2010 Dec;96(24):1985-9.

81. Kuhn FE, Rackley CE. Coronary artery disease in women: risk factors, evaluation, treatment, and prevention. Arch Intern Med. 1993 Dec 13;153(23):2626-36.

82. Tull E, Roseman J. Diabetes in African Americans. In: National Diabetes Data Group, eds. Diabetes in America. 2nd ed. Bethesda, Md: National Institute of Diabetes and Digestive and Kidney Diseases; 1995:613-30.

83. Gaede P, Vedel P, Larsen N, Jensen GV, Parving HH, Pedersen O. Multifactorial intervention and cardiovascular disease in patients with type 2 diabetes. N Engl J Med. 2003 Jan 30;348(5):383-93.

84. National Quality Forum (cited 2014 Mar 3). On the Internet at: http://www.qualityforum.org.

85. NQF technical report 2015. http://www.qualityforum.org.

86. MN HealthScores. The D5 for diabetes. 2013. On the Internet at: http://mncm.org/reports-and-websites/the-d5/.

87. Eyre H, Kahn R, Robertson RM, et al. Preventing cancer, cardiovascular disease, and diabetes: a common agenda for the American Cancer Society, the American Diabetes Association, and the American Heart Association. Stroke. 2004 Aug;35(8):1999-2010.

88. Chobanian AV, Bakris GL, Black HR, et al. The Seventh Report of the Joint National Committee on Prevention, Detection, Evaluation, and Treatment of High Blood Pressure: the JNC 7 report. JAMA. 2003 May 21;289(19):2560-72.

89. Expert Panel on Detection, Evaluation, and Treatment of High Blood Cholesterol in Adults. Executive Summary of the Third Report of the National Cholesterol Education Program (NCEP) Expert Panel on Detection, Evaluation, and Treatment of High Blood Cholesterol in Adults (Adult Treatment Panel III). JAMA. 2001 May 16;285(19):2486-97.

90. Pi-Sunyer X, Blackburn G, Brancati FL, et al. Reduction in weight and cardiovascular disease risk factors in individuals with type 2 diabetes: one-year results of the look AHEAD trial. Diabetes Care. 2007 Jun;30(6):1374-83.

91. Estruch R, Ros E, Salas-Salvado J, et al. Primary prevention of cardiovascular disease with a Mediterranean diet. N Engl J Med. 2013 Apr 4;368(14):1279-90.

92. Jensen MD, Ryan DH, Apovian CM, et al. 2013 AHA/ACC /TOS Guideline for the Management of Overweight and Obesity in Adults: a Report of the American College of Cardiology/American Heart Association Task Force on Practice Guidelines and the Obesity Society. Circulation. 2013 Nov 12.

93. Wing RR, Bolin P, Brancati FL, et al. Cardiovascular effects of intensive lifestyle intervention in type 2 diabetes. N Engl J Med. 2013 Jul 11;369(2):145-54.

94. Fisher DP, Johnson E, Haneuse S, et al. Association between bariatric surgery and macrovascular disease outcomes in patients with type 2 diabetes and severe obesity. JAMA. 2018;320(15):1570.

95. O'Brien R, Johnson E, Haneuse S, et al. Microvascular outcomes in patients with diabetes after bariatric surgery versus usual care: a matched cohort study. Ann Intern Med. 2018;169(5):300. Epub 2018 Aug 7.

96 Courcoulas AP, King WC, Belle SH, et al. Seven-Year Weight Trajectories and Health Outcomes i he Longitudunal Assessment of Baritric Surgery (LABSO Study. JAMA Surg. 2018;153(5):427-434.

97 Aminian A, Zajichek A, Arterburn DE, et al. Association of Metabolic Surgery With Major Adverse Cardiovascular Outcomes in Patients With Type 2 Diabetes and Obesity AMA. 2019;322(13):1271-1282. doi:10.1001/jama.2019 .14231.

98. Schauer PR, Kashyap SR, Wolski K, et al. Bariatric surgery versus intensive medical therapy in obese patients with diabetes. N Engl J Med. 2012 Apr 26;366(17):1567-76. doi: 10.1056/NEJMoa1200225. Epub 2012 Mar 26.

99. Schauer PR, Bhatt DL1, Kirwan JP1,et al. Bariatric Surgery versus Intensive Medical Therapy for Diabetes—5-Year Outcomes. N Engl J Med. 2017 Feb 16;376(7):641-51. doi: 10.1056 /NEJMoa1600869.

100. Kashyap SR, Bhatt DL, Wolski K, et al. Metabolic effects of bariatric surgery in patients With moderate obesity and type 2 diabetes: Analysis of a randomized control trial comparing surgery with intensive medical treatment. Diabetes Care. Vol 36, August 2013:2175-82.

101. IIkramuddin S, Korner J, Lee WJ, et al. Roux-en-Y gastric bypass vs intensive medical management for the control of type 2 diabetes, hypertension, and hyperlipidemia: the Diabetes Surgery Study randomized clinical trial. JAMA. 2013 Jun 5; 309(21):2240-9. doi: 10.1001/jama.2013.5835.

102. Halperin, F, Ding, SA, Simonson, DC, et al. Roux-en-Y gastric bypass surgery or lifestyle with intensive medical management in patients with type 2 diabetes feasibility and 1-year results of a randomized clinical trial. JAMA Surg. 2014;149(7):716-26. doi:10.1001/jamasurg.2014.514.

103. Sjostrom L, Peltonen M, Jacobson P, et al. Bariatric surgery and long-term cardiovascular events. JAMA. 2012 Jan 4; 307(1):56-65.

104. Arterburn D, Wellman R, Emiliano A, et al. Comparative effectiveness and safety of bariatric procedures for weight loss: a pcornet cohort study. Ann Intern Med. 30 Oct 2018;169:741–50. doi: 10.7326/M17-2786. [Epub ahead of print].

105. American Diabetes Association. Standards of care in diabetes. Cardiovascular Disease and Risk Management. Standards of Medical Care 2020. American Diabetes Association. Diabetes Care. 2019;42(Suppl 1): S110.

106. Sigal RJ, Kenny GP, Wasserman DH, Castaneda-Sceppa C. Physical activity/exercise and type 2 diabetes. Diabetes Care. 2004 Oct;27(10):2518-39.

107. Hu G, Jousilahti P, Barengo NC, Qiao Q, Lakka TA, Tuomilehto J. Physical activity, cardiovascular risk factors, and mortality among Finnish adults with diabetes. Diabetes Care. 2005 Apr;28(4):799-805.

108. Petrella RJ, Lattanzio CN, Demeray A, Varallo V, Blore R. Can adoption of regular exercise later in life prevent metabolic risk for cardiovascular disease? Diabetes Care. 2005 Mar;28(3):694-701.

109. Samet JM. The 1990 Report of the Surgeon General: The Health Benefits of Smoking Cessation. Am Rev Respir Dis. 1990 Nov;142(5):993-4.

110. U.S. Preventive Services Task Force. Counseling and interventions to prevent tobacco use and tobacco-caused disease in adults and pregnant women: U.S. Preventive Services Task Force reaffirmation recommendation statement. Ann Intern Med. 2009 Apr 21;150(8):551-5.

111. Chantix [package insert]. New York: Pfizer (last revised 2012 Dec, cited 2014 Mar 14). On the Internet at: http://labeling.pfizer.com/showlabeling.aspx?id=557.

112. The multiple risk factor intervention trial (MRFIT): a national study of primary prevention of coronary heart disease. JAMA. 1976 Feb 23;235(8):825-7.

113. Randomised trial of cholesterol lowering in 4444 patients with coronary heart disease: the Scandinavian Simvastatin Survival Study (4S). Lancet. 1994 Nov 19;344(8934):1383-9.

114. Pyorala K, Pedersen TR, Kjekshus J, Faergeman O, Olsson AG, Thorgeirsson G. Cholesterol lowering with simvastatin improves prognosis of diabetic patients with coronary heart disease: a subgroup analysis of the Scandinavian Simvastatin Survival Study (4S). Diabetes Care. 1997 Apr;20(4): 614-20.

115. Colhoun HM, Betteridge DJ, Durrington PN, et al. Primary prevention of cardiovascular disease with atorvastatin in type 2 diabetes in the Collaborative Atorvastatin Diabetes Study (CARDS): multicentre randomised placebo-controlled trial. Lancet. 2004 Aug 21;364(9435):685-96.

116. Vijan S, Hayward RA. Pharmacologic lipid-lowering therapy in type 2 diabetes mellitus: background paper for the American College of Physicians. Ann Intern Med. 2004 Apr 20;140(8):650-8.

117. Shepherd J, Barter P, Carmena R, et al. Effect of lowering LDL cholesterol substantially below currently recommended levels in patients with coronary heart disease and diabetes: the Treating to New Targets (TNT) study. Diabetes Care. 2006 Jun;29(6):1220-6.

118. Collins R, Armitage J, Parish S, Sleigh P, Peto R. MRC/BHF Heart Protection Study of cholesterol-lowering with simvastatin in 5963 people with diabetes: a randomised placebo-controlled trial. Lancet. 2003 Jun 14;361(9374):2005-16.

119. Sever PS, Poulter NR, Dahlof B, et al. Reduction in cardiovascular events with atorvastatin in 2,532 patients with type 2 diabetes: Anglo-Scandinavian Cardiac Outcomes Trial—lipid-lowering arm (ASCOT-LLA). Diabetes Care. 2005 May;28(5):1151-7.

120. Taylor F, Ward K, Moore TH, et al. Statins for the primary prevention of cardiovascular disease. Cochrane Database Syst Rev. 2011(1):CD004816.

121. Baigent C, Blackwell L, Emberson J, et al. Efficacy and safety of more intensive lowering of LDL cholesterol: a meta-analysis of data from 170,000 participants in 26 randomised trials. Lancet. 2010 Nov 13;376(9753):1670-81.

122. Kearney PM, Blackwell L, Collins R, et al. Efficacy of cholesterol-lowering therapy in 18,686 people with diabetes in 14 randomised trials of statins: a meta-analysis. Lancet. 2008 Jan 12;371(9607):117-25.

123. Sattar N, Preiss D, Murray HM, et al. Statins and risk of incident diabetes: a collaborative meta-analysis of randomised statin trials. Lancet. 2010 Feb 27;375(9716):735-42.

124. American Diabetes Association. Standards of medical care in diabetes—2014. Diabetes Care. 2014;37 Suppl 1:S14-80.

125. Arnett DK, Blumenthal RS, Albert MA, et al.2019 ACC/AHA guideline on the primary prevention of cardiovascular disease: a report of the American College of Cardiology/American Heart Association Task Force on Clinical Practice Guidelines. J Am Coll Cardiol. 2019. [Epub ahead of print].

126. Keaney JF Jr, Curfman GD, Jarcho JA. A pragmatic view of the new cholesterol treatment guidelines. N Engl J Med. 2014 Jan 16;370(3):275-8.

127. Joy TR, Hegele RA. Narrative review: statin-related myopathy. Ann Intern Med. 2009 Jun 16;150(12):858-68.

128. Banach M, Rizzo M, Toth PP, et al. Statin intolerance—an attempt at a unified definition. Position paper from an International Lipid Expert Panel. Arch Med Sci. 2015 Mar 16;11(1):1-23.

129. Finegold JA, Manisty CH, Goldacre B, Barron AJ, Francis DP. What proportion of symptomatic side effects in patients taking statins are genuinely caused by the drug? Systematic review of randomized placebo-controlled trials to aid individual patient choice. Eur J Prev Cardiol. 2014 Apr;21(4):464-74.

130. Jacobson TA. The safety of aggressive statin therapy: how much can low-density lipoprotein cholesterol be lowered? Mayo Clin Proc. 2006 Sep;81(9):1225-31.

131. Rosenson RS, Baker SK, Jacobson TA, Kopecky SL, Parker BA; the National Lipid Association's Muscle Safety Expert Panel. An assessment by the Statin Muscle Safety Task Force: 2014 update. J Clin Lipidol. 2014 May-Jun; 8(3 Suppl):S58-71.

132. Parker BA, Capizzi JA. Effect of statins on skeletal muscle function. Circulation. 2013 Jan 1;127(1):96-103.

133. Keech A, Simes RJ, Barter P, et al. Effects of long-term fenofibrate therapy on cardiovascular events in 9795 people with type 2 diabetes mellitus (the FIELD study): randomised controlled trial. Lancet. 2005 Nov 26;366(9500):1849-61.

134. Ginsberg HN, Elam MB, Lovato LC, et al. Effects of combination lipid therapy in type 2 diabetes mellitus. N Engl J Med. 2010 Apr 29;362(17):1563-74.

135. Boden WE, Probstfield JL, Anderson T, et al. Niacin in patients with low HDL cholesterol levels receiving intensive statin therapy. N Engl J Med. 2011 Dec 15;365(24):2255-67.

136. Rubins HB, Robins SJ, Collins D, et al. Gemfibrozil for the secondary prevention of coronary heart disease in men with low levels of high-density lipoprotein cholesterol: Veterans Affairs High-Density Lipoprotein Cholesterol Intervention Trial Study Group. N Engl J Med. 1999 Aug 5;341(6):410-8.

137. Giugliano RP, Cannon CP, Blazing MA, et al. Benefit of adding ezetimibe to statin therapy on cardiovascular outcomes and safety in patients with versus without diabetes mellitus: results from IMPROVE-IT (improved reduction of outcomes: vytorin efficacy international trial). Circulation. 2018 Apr 10;137(15):1571-82. PMID: 29263150.

138. Sabatine MS, Giugliano RP, Keech AC, et al; FOURIER Steering Committee and Investigators. evolocumab and clinical outcomes in patients with cardiovascular disease. N Engl J Med. 2017 May 4;376(18):1713-22. PMID: 28304224.

139. Squizzato A, Suter MB, Nerone M, et al. PCSK9 inhibitors for treating dyslipidemia in patients at different cardiovascular risk: a systematic review and a meta-analysis. Intern Emerg Med. 2017 Oct;12(7):1043-53. PMID: 28695455.

140. Writing Committee; Lloyd-Jones DM, Morris PB, Ballantyne CM, et al. 2016 ACC Expert Consensus Decision Pathway on the role of non-statin therapies for LDL-cholesterol lowering in the management of atherosclerotic cardiovascular disease risk: a report of the American College of Cardiology Task Force on Clinical Expert Consensus Documents. J Am Coll Cardiol. 2016 Jul 5;68(1):92-125.

141. Tight blood pressure control and risk of macrovascular and microvascular complications in type 2 diabetes: UKPDS 38. UK Prospective Diabetes Study Group. BMJ. 1998 Sep 12; 317(7160):703-13.

142. Sowers J. Treatment of hypertension in patients with diabetes. Arch Intern Med. 2004;164:1850-7.

143. Beevers G, Lip GY, O'Brien E. ABC of hypertension: blood pressure measurement. Part II—conventional sphygmomanometry: technique of auscultatory blood pressure measurement. BMJ. 2001 Apr 28;322(7293):1043-7.

144. Keary L, Atkins N, Molloy E, Mee F, O'Brien E. Terminal digit preference and heaping in blood pressure measurement. J Hum Hypertens. 1998;12:787-8.

145. Hermida RC, Smolensky MH, Ayala DE, Portaluppi F. 2013 ambulatory blood pressure monitoring recommendations for the diagnosis of adult hypertension, assessment of cardiovascular and other hypertension-associated risk, and attainment of therapeutic goals. Chronobiol Int. 2013 Apr;30(3): 355-410.

146. Whelton PK, Carey RM, Aronow WS, et al. ACC/AHA/AAPA/ABC/ACPM/AGS/APhA/ASH/ASPC/NMA/PCNA Guideline for the prevention, detection, evaluation, and management of high blood pressure in adults: a report of the American College of Cardiology/American Heart Association Task Force on Clinical Practice Guidelines. Hypertension. 2018 Jun;71(6):e13-e115. doi: 10.1161/HYP.0000000000000065 . Epub 2017 Nov 13.

147. Hansson L, Zanchetti A, Carruthers SG, et al. Effects of intensive blood-pressure lowering and low-dose aspirin in patients with hypertension: principal results of the Hypertension Optimal Treatment (HOT) randomised trial. HOT Study Group. Lancet. 1998 Jun 13;351(9118):1755-62.

148. AAFP. Guidelines developed by external organizations not endorsed by the AAFP. 2017. https://www.aafp.org/patient-care/clinical-recommendations/non-endorsed.html.

149. de Boer IH, Bakris G, Cannon CP. Blood pressure targets for people with diabetes and hypertension: comparing the ADA and the ACC/AHA recommendations. March 15, 2018. doi:10.1001/JAMA. 2018;319(13):0642.

150. Cooper-DeHoff RM, Gong Y, Handberg EM, et al. Tight blood pressure control and cardiovascular outcomes among hypertensive patients with diabetes and coronary artery disease. JAMA. 2010 Jul 7;304(1):61-8.

151. Cushman WC, Evans GW, Byington RP, et al. Effects of intensive blood-pressure control in type 2 diabetes mellitus. N Engl J Med. 2010 Apr 29;362(17):1575-85.

152. Patel A, MacMahon S, Chalmers J, et al. Effects of a fixed combination of perindopril and indapamide on macrovascular and microvascular outcomes in patients with type 2 diabetes mellitus (the ADVANCE trial): a randomised controlled trial. Lancet. 2007 Sep 8;370(9590):829-40.

153. ALLHAT Officers and Coordinators for the ALLHAT Collaborative Research Group. Major outcomes in high-risk hypertensive patients randomized to angiotensin-converting enzyme inhibitor or calcium channel blocker vs diuretic: the Antihypertensive and Lipid-Lowering Treatment to Prevent Heart Attack Trial (ALLHAT). JAMA. 2002 Dec 18; 288(23):2981-97.

154. Williams B, MacDonald TM, Morant S, et al. British Hypertension Society's PATHWAY Studies Group. Spironolactone versus placebo, bisoprolol, and doxazosin to determine the optimal treatment for drug-resistant hypertension (PATHWAY-2): a randomised, double-blind, crossover trial. Lancet. 2015 Nov 21;386(10008):2059-68. Epub 2015 Sep 20. PMID: 26414968.

155. James PA, Oparil S, Carter BL, et al. 2014 evidence-based guideline for the management of high blood pressure in adults: report from the panel members appointed to the Eighth Joint National Committee (JNC 8). JAMA. 2014 Feb 5;311(5):507-20.

156. Cushman WC, Evans GW, Byington RP, et al. Effects of intensive blood-pressure control in type 2 diabetes mellitus. N Engl J Med. 2010 Apr 29;362(17):1575-85.

157. World Health Organization. Adherence to long-term therapies: evidence for action. 2003. On the Internet at: http://www.who.int/chp/knowledge/publications/adherence_report/en/.

158. Margolis KL, Asche SE, Bergdall AR, et al. Effect of home blood pressure telemonitoring and pharmacist management on blood pressure control: a cluster randomized clinical trial. JAMA. 2013 Jul 3;310(1):46-56.

159. Margolis KL, Asche SE, Bergdall AR, et al. A successful multifaceted trial to improve hypertension control in primary care: Why did it Work? J Gen Intern Med. 2015 Nov; 30(11): 1665–72.

160. Early Treatment Diabetic Retinopathy Study Research Group. Effects of aspirin treatment on diabetic retinopathy.

ETDRS report number 8. Ophthalmology. 1991 May; 98(5 Suppl):757-65.

161. ETDRS Investigators. Aspirin effects on mortality and morbidity in patients with diabetes mellitus. Early Treatment Diabetic Retinopathy Study report 14. JAMA. 1992 Sep 9; 268(10):1292-300.

162. ASCEND Study Collaborative Group. Effects of aspirin for primary prevention in persons with diabetes mellitus. N Engl J Med. 2018 Oct 18;379(16):1529-1539. doi: 10.1056/NEJMoa1804988. Epub 2018 Aug 26.

163. Gaziano JM, Brotons C, Coppolecchia R, et al. Use of aspirin to reduce risk of initial vascular events in patients at moderate risk of cardiovascular disease (ARRIVE): a randomised, double-blind, placebo-controlled trial. Lancet. 2018 Sep 22; 392(10152):1036-46. doi: 10.1016/S0140-6736(18)31924-X. Epub 2018 Aug 26.

164. McNeil JJ, Wolfe R, Woods RL. Effect of aspirin on cardiovascular events and bleeding in the healthy elderly. N Engl J Med. 2018 Oct 18;379(16):1509-18. doi: 10.1056/NEJMoa1805819. Epub 2018 Sep 16.

165. Walker CW, Dawley CA, Fletcher SF. Aspirin combined with clopidogrel (Plavix) decreases cardiovascular events in patients with acute coronary syndrome. Am Fam Physician. 2007 Dec 1;76(11):1643-5.

166. Rooke TW, Hirsch AT, Misra S, et al. 2011 ACCF/AHA Focused Update of the Guideline for the Management of Patients With Peripheral Artery Disease (updating the 2005 guideline): a report of the American College of Cardiology Foundation/American Heart Association Task Force on Practice Guidelines. J Am Coll Cardiol. 2011 Nov 1; 58(19):2020-45.

167. Park HY, Schumock GT, Pickard AS, Akhras K. A structured review of the relationship between microalbuminuria and cardiovascular events in patients with diabetes mellitus and hypertension. Pharmacotherapy. 2003 Dec;23(12):1611-6.

168. Spoelstra-de Man AM, Brouwer CB, Stehouwer CD, Smulders YM. Rapid progression of albumin excretion is an independent predictor of cardiovascular mortality in patients with type 2 diabetes and microalbuminuria. Diabetes Care. 2001 Dec;24(12):2097-101.

169. Yusuf S, Sleight P, Pogue J, Bosch J, Davies R, Dagenais G. Effects of an angiotensin-converting-enzyme inhibitor, ramipril, on cardiovascular events in high-risk patients. The Heart Outcomes Prevention Evaluation Study Investigators. N Engl J Med. 2000 Jan 20;342(3):145-53.

170. Myers GL, Christenson RH, Cushman M, et al. National Academy of Clinical Biochemistry Laboratory Medicine Practice guidelines: emerging biomarkers for primary prevention of cardiovascular disease. Clin Chem. 2009 Feb;55(2):378-84.

171. US Preventive Services Task Force. Using nontraditional risk factors in coronary heart disease risk assessment: US Preventive Services Task Force recommendation statement. Ann Intern Med. 2009 Oct 6;151(7):474-82.

172. Brown BG, Cheung MC, Lee AC, Zhao XQ, Chait A. Antioxidant vitamins and lipid therapy: end of a long romance? Arterioscler Thromb Vasc Biol. 2002 Oct 1; 22(10):1535-46.

173. Lonn E, Bosch J, Yusuf S, et al. Effects of long-term vitamin E supplementation on cardiovascular events and cancer: a randomized controlled trial. JAMA. 2005 Mar 16;293(11): 1338-47.

174. Omenn GS, Goodman GE, Thornquist MD, et al. Risk factors for lung cancer and for intervention effects in CARET, the Beta-Carotene and Retinol Efficacy Trial. J Natl Cancer Inst. 1996 Nov 6;88(21):1550-9.

175. US Preventive Services Task Force. Routine vitamin supplementation to prevent cancer and cardiovascular disease: recommendations and rationale. Ann Intern Med. 2003 Jul 1;139(1):51-5.

176. Imperatore G, Boyle JP, Thompson TJ, et al. Projections of type 1 and type 2 diabetes burden in the U.S. population aged <20 years through 2050: dynamic modeling of incidence, mortality, and population growth. Diabetes Care. 2012 Dec;35(12):2515-20.

177. Rodriguez BL, Fujimoto WY, Mayer-Davis EJ, et al. Prevalence of cardiovascular disease risk factors in U.S. children and adolescents with diabetes: the SEARCH for diabetes in youth study. Diabetes Care. 2006 Aug;29(8):1891-6.

178. Dean H, Flett B. Natural history of type 2 diabetes diagnosed in childhood: long term follow-up in young adult years. Diabetes. 2002;51 Suppl 2:A24.

179. American Diabetes Association. Children and adolescents: standards of medical care in diabetes-2018. Diabetes Care. 2018 Jan;41(Suppl 1):S126-S136. doi: 10.2337/dc18-S012.

180. Haffner SM, Lehto S, Ronnemaa T, Pyorala K, Laakso M. Mortality from coronary heart disease in subjects with type 2 diabetes and in nondiabetic subjects with and without prior myocardial infarction. N Engl J Med. 1998 Jul 23; 339(4):229-34.

181. Young LH, Wackers FJ, Chyun DA, et al. Cardiac outcomes after screening for asymptomatic coronary artery disease in patients with type 2 diabetes: the DIAD study: a randomized controlled trial. JAMA. 2009 Apr 15;301(15):1547-55.

182. Wackers FJ, Young LH. Lessons learned from the detection of ischemia in asymptomatic diabetics (DIAD) study. J Nucl Cardiol. 2009 Nov-Dec;16(6):855-9.

183. Frye RL, August P, Brooks MM, et al. A randomized trial of therapies for type 2 diabetes and coronary artery disease. N Engl J Med. 2009 Jun 11;360(24):2503-15.

184. Boden WE, O'Rourke RA, Teo KK, et al. Optimal medical therapy with or without PCI for stable coronary disease. N Engl J Med. 2007 Apr 12;356(15):1503-16.

185. Braunwald E. Shattuck lecture—cardiovascular medicine at the turn of the millennium: triumphs, concerns, and opportunities. N Engl J Med. 1997 Nov 6;337(19):1360-9.

186. Wahab NN, Cowden EA, Pearce NJ, Gardner MJ, Merry H, Cox JL. Is blood glucose an independent predictor of mortality in acute myocardial infarction in the thrombolytic era? J Am Coll Cardiol. 2002 Nov 20;40(10):1748-54.

187. Norhammar A, Tenerz A, Nilsson G, et al. Glucose metabolism in patients with acute myocardial infarction and no previous diagnosis of diabetes mellitus: a prospective study. Lancet. 2002 Jun 22;359(9324):2140-4.

188. Malmberg K. Prospective randomised study of intensive insulin treatment on long term survival after acute myocardial infarction in patients with diabetes mellitus. DIGAMI (Diabetes Mellitus, Insulin Glucose Infusion in Acute Myocardial Infarction) Study Group. BMJ. 1997 May 24;314(7093): 1512-5.

189. Mellbin LG, Malmberg K, Norhammar A, Wedel H, Ryden L. The impact of glucose lowering treatment on long-term prognosis in patients with type 2 diabetes and myocardial infarction: a report from the DIGAMI 2 trial. Eur Heart J. 2008 Jan;29(2):166-76.

190. Ziegelstein RC. Depression in patients recovering from a myocardial infarction. JAMA. 2001 Oct 3;286(13):1621-7.

191. Carinci F, Nicolucci A, Ciampi A, et al. Role of interactions between psychological and clinical factors in determining 6-month mortality among patients with acute myocardial infarction. Application of recursive partitioning techniques to the GISSI-2 database. Gruppo Italiano per lo Studio della Sopravvivenza nell' Infarto Miocardico. Eur Heart J. 1997 May;18(5):835-45.

192. Frasure-Smith N. In-hospital symptoms of psychological stress as predictors of long-term outcome after acute myocardial infarction in men. Am J Cardiol. 1991 Jan 15;67(2):121-7.

193. Taylor F, Huffman MD, Macedo AF, et al. Statins for the primary prevention of cardiovascular disease. Cochrane Database Syst Rev. 2013;1:CD004816.

194. Kawachi I, Colditz GA, Stampfer MJ, et al. Smoking cessation and decreased risk of stroke in women. JAMA. 1993 Jan 13;269(2):232-6.

195. Johnston SC, Gress DR, Browner WS, Sidney S. Short-term prognosis after emergency department diagnosis of TIA. JAMA. 2000 Dec 13;284(22):2901-6.

196. Streifler JY, Eliasziw M, Benavente OR, et al. The risk of stroke in patients with first-ever retinal vs hemispheric transient ischemic attacks and high-grade carotid stenosis. North American Symptomatic Carotid Endarterectomy Trial. Arch Neurol. 1995 Mar;52(3):246-9.

197. American Heart Association/American Stroke Association. Spot a stroke. Stroke warning signs and symptoms (cited 2014 Mar 12). On the Internet at: http://www.strokeassociation.org/STROKEORG/WarningSigns/Stroke-Warning-Signs-and-Symptoms_UCM_308528_SubHomePage.jsp.

198. Murabito JM, D'Agostino RB, Silbershatz H, Wilson WF. Intermittent claudication: a risk profile from the Framingham Heart Study. Circulation. 1997;96:44-9.

199. US Department of Health and Human Services, National Institutes of Health, National Heart, Lung, and Blood Institute. Facts about peripheral arterial disease (P.A.D.). 2006 Aug (cited 2014 Mar 14). On the Internet at: https://www.nhlbi.nih.gov/health/public/heart/pad/docs/pad_extfctsht_general_508.pdf.

200. Golomb BA, Dang TT, Criqui MH. Peripheral arterial disease: morbidity and mortality implications. Circulation. 2006 Aug 15;114(7):688-99.

201. Dolan NC, Liu K, Criqui MH, et al. Peripheral artery disease, diabetes, and reduced lower extremity functioning. Diabetes Care. 2002 Jan;25(1):113-20.

202. American Diabetes Association. Standards of medical care in diabetes—2013. Diabetes Care. 2013 Jan;36 Suppl 1:S11-66.

203. Powell CK, Kripalani S. Brief report: resident recognition of low literacy as a risk factor in hospital readmission. J Gen Intern Med. 2005 Nov;20(11):1042-4.

204. Kubzansky LD, Huffman JC, Boehm JK, et al. Positive psychological well-being and cardiovascular disease: JACC health promotion series. J Am Coll Cardiol. 2018;72(12): 1382-96.

205. Labarthe DR, Kubzansky LD, Boehm, JK, et al. Positive cardiovascular health. J Am Coll Cardiol. 2016;68(8):860.

206. American Diabetes Association. Improving care and promoting health in populations: standards of medical care in diabetes—2018. Diabetes Care. 2018; 41(Suppl 1):S7-12. https://doi.org/10.2337/dc18-S001.

CHAPTER 26

Eye Disease Related to Diabetes

Szilárd Kiss, MD

Key Concepts

- The population of persons with diabetes is susceptible to a considerable number of eye conditions that can lead to blindness. These generally occur more frequently and at a younger age in people with diabetes than in the general population.
- Early diagnosis and treatment can prevent or delay vision loss from eye disorders.
- Early treatment of diabetic retinopathy can prevent severe vision loss.
- Diabetic retinopathy, the leading cause of blindness among individuals aged 20 to 74 years in the United States,[1] is often present before the person notices any visual changes.
- Tight management of blood glucose levels, blood pressure, blood lipids, and smoking cessation help prevent severe vision loss due to diabetic retinopathy.
- Diabetes care and education specialists need to encourage persons with diabetes to have annual retinal evaluations, whether or not they are experiencing any visual symptoms.

Introduction

Diabetes is the leading cause of blindness among adults aged 20 to 74 years in the United States. The literature suggests that 8,000 to 23,000 new cases of legal blindness associated with diabetes present annually.[2–6] Various ocular conditions are 25 times more common among people with diabetes than in the general population.[4] Of people with diabetes who are on work disability, 15% to 20% have some visual impairment.[7]

As people advance in age, they are more at risk for certain eye conditions, such as glaucoma and cataracts. People with diabetes have an even greater risk for these conditions, which often present earlier in age in these individuals than in the general population. Poorly managed diabetes creates a more serious condition called diabetic retinopathy, which affects the retina.

The retina is the light-sensing tissue lining the inner surface of the eye. The cornea and the lens create an image of the visual world on the retina, which serves a function analogous to film in a traditional camera or to a charge-coupled device and complementary metal oxide semiconductor image sensor in a digital camera. Light striking the retina initiates a cascade of chemical and electrical events that ultimately trigger nerve impulses that are then sent to various visual centers of the brain via the optic nerve. Disorders of the retina typically affect either central or peripheral vision. Figure 26.1 identifies parts of the eye that are discussed in this chapter.

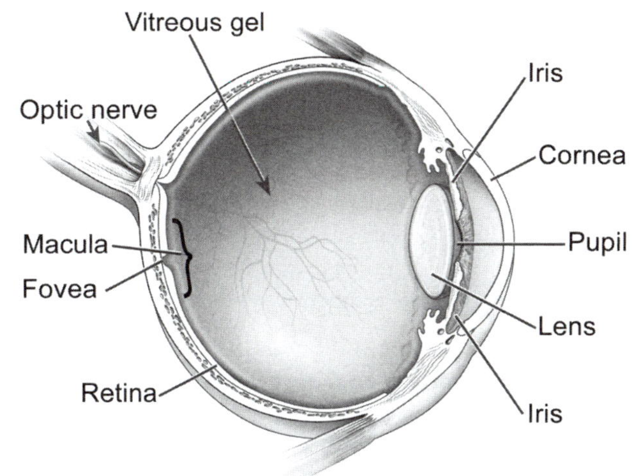

FIGURE 26.1 Normal Eye

Source: National Eye Institute, National Institutes of Health, Reference #NEA08.

Diabetic retinopathy is the most severe form of diabetic eye disease. Diabetic retinopathy results from leaky blood vessels and the growth of abnormal blood vessels in the retina. Within 1 year of developing diabetic retinopathy, 5% to 10% of patients will progress to a more advanced stage.[3]

The number of Americans aged 40 years and older with retinopathy is estimated to triple by 2050, to 16.0 million for all diabetic retinopathy and 3.4 million for vision-threatening diabetic retinopathy.[8]

This chapter focuses on eye diseases associated with diabetes mellitus. For each ocular condition, the epidemiology, risk factors, clinical findings, stages of the disease, and appropriate treatments are outlined.

- *Common eye diseases.* Common eye diseases are discussed first, including cataracts, glaucoma, and other ocular manifestations that occur more frequently in people with diabetes.
- *Diabetic retinopathy.* Information on diabetic retinopathy is presented next. Major clinical studies and current treatment strategies for diabetic retinopathy are outlined. The text emphasizes how appropriate and timely therapy can prevent severe visual loss in up to 90% of cases.[9]

Cataracts

Cataracts are one of the leading causes of reversible blindness in the world today, and at least 300,000 to 400,000 new cases of visually disabling cataracts occur annually in the United States. The rate of cataracts for individuals with diabetes is significantly higher than that of the general population, with faster progression to vision loss.[8] With early detection, close monitoring, and timely surgical intervention, visual impairment due to cataracts is reversible. Cataracts are a vision-impairing disease characterized by a gradual, progressive thickening and opacification of the lens. The lens is the eye structure in charge of focusing images on the retina. The lens's transparent intraocular tissue helps bring rays of light to focus on the retina.

The most common patient complaint is of a progressive gradual decrease in visual acuity at distance and at near, but patients may also complain of a decrease in contrast sensitivity in brightly lit environments, disabling glare during the day, and/or glare from the headlights of oncoming cars at night. The progression of cataracts frequently results in a mild-to-moderate degree of myopic shift or increase in nearsightedness. Consequently, presbyopic patients may report an improvement in their near

Case: Reluctance in Self-Care Leads to Vision Loss

MG is a 50-year-old male who was diagnosed with type 2 diabetes 10 years ago. His blood glucose levels have ranged from 100 to 355 mg/dL (5.6 to 19.7 mmol/L) in the past 3 months. He has insisted, however, that he is doing fine because he does not "feel" that his diabetes is causing any problems. He is using oral medications to manage his diabetes and lives a sedentary lifestyle; he was referred to the ophthalmologist by his family physician to rule out diabetic retinopathy. Findings from the initial examination were as follows:

- Best-corrected visual acuity was 20/40 in the right eye and 20/20 in the left eye. Since MG had never checked his vision 1 eye at a time before, he had never noticed the difference in visual acuity between both eyes.
- Intraocular pressure (IOP) was 19 mm Hg on the right eye and 22 mm Hg on the left eye.
- Slitlamp biomicroscopy revealed a 2+ posterior subcapsular cataract in the right eye and mild cataract changes in the left eye.
- The fundus examination revealed a 0.5 cup-to-disc (C/D) ratio of the optic nerves.
- A few retinal microaneurysms were also noted without macular edema or neovascularization at this point.

Diagnosis

Because of the fundus examination finding and the IOP measurement, MG was considered a glaucoma suspect. He was diagnosed as follows:

- Mild nonproliferative diabetic retinopathy in both eyes
- Posterior subcapsular cataract in the right eye
- Glaucoma suspect

The findings and the importance of ocular follow-up were explained to MG. The ophthalmologist discussed the presence of cataract changes and explained that since these changes did not interfere with MG's daily activities, they did not warrant surgery at this time. MG was advised to schedule a follow-up visit within 8 to 12 months. He was also referred to a glaucoma specialist for evaluation of possible glaucoma.

vision and less need for reading glasses—an experience commonly called "second sight." Patients must be told that this change is temporary and that as the cataracts develop further, they will eventually lose this temporary benefit. In some cases, patients with cataracts may present with monocular diplopia that is not corrected with use of spectacles or prisms. These cases can usually be solved with cataract surgery.

The Eye Diseases Prevalence Research Group (EDPRG) estimates that in the year 2000, 20.5 million people over age 40 in the United States had a cataract in either eye.[10] The group predicts this number will increase to 30.1 million by the year 2020. The number of cases of cataracts among African Americans and whites 40 years and older with diabetes is expected to increase 235% by 2050.[8] This increase is significantly more pronounced for minorities, especially those who are older. For example, the number of cataract cases in African-American women 75 years and older who have diabetes is projected to increase by 637% between 2005 and 2050.[8]

How Do Cataracts Form?

When the blood glucose level is high, the aqueous glucose levels are also elevated. The glucose diffuses through the lens capsule and increases its concentration within the crystalline lens. This results in a glycosylation of lens proteins. Some of the glucose is converted by the intracellular enzyme aldose reductase into sorbitol. This causes alterations in lens permeability and results in cataract formation.[11]

Cortical Cataract

A special type of cataract, known as a cortical cataract, is seen in many individuals with diabetes. It has a "snowflake" appearance with bilateral, widespread subcapsular changes. Often, it has an abrupt onset and an acute course. These cataracts are seen most often in the younger person whose diabetes is not well managed. These lens changes mature rapidly and result in total opacification over a period of a few weeks with very significant visual loss. This "true diabetic cataract" is becoming rarer as better programs to manage diabetes have been available.

Common Senile Cataract

Common senile cataracts (nuclear sclerotic cataracts and posterior subcapsular cataracts) occur more frequently and at younger ages, and progress more rapidly in persons afflicted with diabetes than in the general population.[12]

What Treatment Options Are Available?

The only treatment option for cataracts is surgical cataract extraction and placement of an intraocular lens implant. Cataract surgery is a very safe and relatively quick procedure in which the patient can have total visual recovery within days if there is no other pathology affecting the vision. With current cataract extraction techniques, this procedure can be done as soon as the person notices any change in visual acuity. Since there is no real visual acuity cutoff at which the surgery is performed, the patient must be told that the timing of the procedure is flexible and not medically urgent, and must also be informed of all possible risks of surgery.

Complications

Diabetes is not a contraindication for cataract surgery. However, cataract surgery can stimulate additional problems for persons with diabetes, especially if the cataract surgery results in a capsulotomy (rupture in the bag that holds the lens). In this case, the angiogenic factors produced by the retina that can cause proliferative diabetic retinopathy flow from the posterior segment forward to reach the iris. This, in turn, may stimulate neovascular glaucoma, a recognized complication of cataract surgery in individuals with diabetes.[11] Proper stabilization of any diabetic retinopathy prior to cataract extraction can significantly reduce the risk of the development of these complications. In addition, in some cases, lens extraction may be needed to improve retinal surveillance.[13]

The appropriate management of individuals with diabetes who are undergoing cataract surgery is an evolving task. Cataract surgery with more modern techniques, such as phacoemulsification, may not cause the progression of diabetic retinopathy, as had been suggested by earlier studies using older cataract extraction techniques.[14] More important, it remains unclear whether the progression of diabetic retinopathy in some patients following cataract surgery is a result of the surgery itself or a reflection of the natural progression of the disease.

Recent small case series suggest that adjunctive use of anti-inflammatory (either steroids or nonsteroidal anti-inflammatory drugs) or anti-vascular endothelial growth factor (anti-VEGF) agents at the time of cataract surgery may improve visual recovery from surgery, decrease the incidence of postsurgical macular edema, and perhaps even decrease the progression of diabetic retinopathy.[15,16] These data may be most applicable to persons who have poorly managed diabetes and who require cataract surgery prior to full treatment of their diabetic retinopathy.

However, larger prospective clinical trials are still needed to confirm these results and to recommend these medications for all persons with diabetes undergoing cataract surgery.

Glaucoma

Glaucoma is the second-leading cause of blindness in the United States after cataracts, with more than 1.6 million people having significant visual impairment.[17] Glaucoma is the leading cause of blindness in African Americans.[18] There are several categories of glaucoma, which are based on chronology or etiology. Those most commonly associated with diabetes are the following:

- Primary open-angle glaucoma
- Neovascular glaucoma

Primary Open-Angle Glaucoma

Primary open-angle glaucoma (POAG) is described as a multifactorial optic neuropathy (optic nerve disease) characterized by a chronic and progressive loss of optic nerve fibers (clinically, this can be evaluated according to the optic nerve C/D ratio, which usually ranges from 0.1 to 0.4). Such loss develops in the presence of an open anterior chamber angle (the eyes' main drainage system), characteristic visual-field abnormalities, and IOP that is too high for the continued health of the eye (normal IOP ranges from 8 to 22 mm Hg). Because of the silent nature of the disease, patients usually do not present with any visual complaints until late in the course. At this time, patients present with complaints of a constriction in the visual field (decrease in peripheral vision) or a decrease in visual acuity. Although there is still controversy, some epidemiologic studies show that POAG is found more often in individuals with type 2 diabetes than in age-matched individuals without diabetes.[19–21]

Treatment of POAG is limited to the reduction of IOP. This is mainly performed through topical medications (eyedrops) and occasionally via laser or incisional surgery. The US Preventive Services Task Force (USPSTF) concluded in the March 2005 recommendation statement Screening for Glaucoma that there is good evidence that screening can detect increased IOP and early POAG in adults.[22] The USPSTF also found good evidence that early treatment of adults with increased IOP detected by screening reduces the number of persons who develop small visual-field defects and allows for early treatment to prevent progression. However, the task force did not find sufficient evidence to determine the extent to which screening, with earlier detection and treatment, would reduce impairment in vision-related function or quality of life. Harms associated with treatment of increased IOP and early POAG include local eye irritation and an increased risk for cataracts. Further research is needed to clarify the balance between the benefit from early treatment and the given known harm of early screening for glaucoma.

Initial evaluation of a patient suspected of having POAG includes measurement of IOP and central corneal thickness, examination of the angle structures via gonioscopy, evaluation and documentation of optic nerve head and retinal nerve fiber layer, and testing of the visual field by automated static threshold perimetry. Medical therapy (eg, eyedrops) is presently the most common initial intervention for treating POAG. Laser trabeculoplasty and filtering surgery are other treatment options and are typically second or third line. These 3 interventions lower IOP and decrease the progression of the visual field cut. Since glaucoma cannot be cured, patients with POAG require lifetime monitoring and therapy. The monitoring for POAG consists of IOP measurement, visual field testing, and optic nerve head and retinal nerve fiber layer evaluation, typically carried out several times a year. For patients diagnosed with glaucoma, engagement with the treatment plan as well as regular follow-up examinations by an ophthalmologist or optometrist is essential to maintaining vision.

Among Americans with diabetes, the number of persons with POAG is expected to substantially increase by 2050 for all demographic groups, but particularly for Hispanics in all age groups and African Americans 50 years and older.[8] There is a projected twelvefold increase from 2005 to 2050 in the number of Hispanics with diabetes 65 years and older with glaucoma.

Glaucoma and Diabetes

In addition to POAG, a great visual threat to persons having both glaucoma and diabetes is development of neovascular glaucoma.

Neovascular Glaucoma

Neovascular glaucoma (NVG) is a secondary glaucoma. Retinal ischemia is the most common and important mechanism in NVG. Significantly higher vascular endothelial growth factor (VEGF)[23] levels occur in the ocular fluids of individuals with proliferative diabetic retinopathy than in persons with nonproliferative diabetic retinopathy. Even higher levels of VEGF are found in the ocular fluids of patients with NVG. Patients presenting with NVG may experience ocular pain or redness, multicolored halos, or headache, and some patients may be asymptomatic.

The management of NVG is related to the stage of the disease and the level of diabetic retinopathy. The lasering of the peripheral retina, called panretinal photocoagulation (PRP), remains an important treatment of both NVG and proliferative diabetic retinopathy. Panretinal photocoagulation is a type of laser surgery delivered in a scatter pattern throughout the peripheral fundus; its intent is to cause a regression of abnormal blood vessels (neovascularization). Panretinal photocoagulation reduces the areas of retinal ischemia, and thus production of VEGF and other angiogenic factors is also reduced. In cases where PRP treatment does not lower the pressure, filtration surgery or the implantation of a drainage device may be necessary to control the pressure and salvage the optic nerve.[24]

Given the prominent role of VEGF in the pathogenesis of NVG, several case series have indicated that the adjunctive use of anti-VEGF drugs, such as ranibizumab or bevacizumab, may be useful for the treatment of NVG either at the time of PRP treatment or even at the time of glaucoma surgery.[25,26] Although the outcomes in these small case series are extremely promising, larger randomized trials are required prior to recommending these medications for all patients with NVG.

Central Retinal Vein Occlusion

Central retinal vein occlusion (CRVO) is a retinal vascular disorder commonly seen in persons with a history of high blood pressure and/or diabetes mellitus.[27] The exact pathogenesis of the occlusion of the central retinal vein is not known. Various local and systemic factors play a role in the pathological closure of the central retinal vein. Clinically, CRVO presents with variable sudden visual loss. The fundus eye exam may show retinal hemorrhages, dilated tortuous retinal veins, cotton-wool spots (soft exudates that represent infarcts of the nerve fiber layer of the retina), macular edema (swelling or thickening in the central part of the retina), and swelling of the optic nerve. Central retinal vein occlusion can be divided into 2 clinical types:

- Nonischemic CRVO
- Ischemic CRVO

Nonischemic CRVO is the milder form of the disease. It may present with good vision, a few retinal hemorrhages and cotton-wool spots, no relative afferent pupillary defect (abnormality in the pupils' reaction to light), and good blood perfusion to the retina. Nonischemic CRVO may resolve fully with good visual prognosis, or it may progress to the ischemic type.

Ischemic CRVO is the severe form of the disease. Usually, ischemic CRVO presents with severe visual loss, extensive retinal hemorrhages and cotton-wool spots, presence of relative afferent pupillary defect, and/or poor blood perfusion to the retina. In addition, the disease may result in NVG and a painful blind eye.

No known effective medical treatment is available for either prevention or treatment of CRVO. If an underlying systemic medical condition is found, treatment may be indicated, but this rarely reverses the vein occlusion.[28] Treatment may, however, help prevent the opposite eye from developing a vascular occlusion. Various medical modalities for the treatment of CRVO have been advocated by multiple authors with varying success in preventing complications and preserving vision. Laser photocoagulation is the treatment of choice in the management of various complications associated with retinal vascular diseases (diabetic retinopathy, branch retinal vein occlusion). That is why PRP has been used in the treatment of neovascular complications of CRVO such as NVG for numerous years. Guidelines on treatment modalities and follow-up care of patients with CRVO were provided by the Central Vein Occlusion Study (CVOS),[29] a multicenter prospective study sponsored by the National Eye Institute.

Intraocular Steroids

The role of intravitreal glucocorticoids is promising. Ozurdex (0.7 mg dexamethasone intravitreal implant) was the first drug approved by the Food and Drug Administration (FDA) that was indicated specifically for the treatment of macular edema secondary to central and branch retinal vein occlusions.[30] Patients receiving this intravitreal implant, which provides a sustained release of dexamethasone over a 6-month period, were not only more likely to gain vision following CRVO but also more likely to gain more vision.[31–33]

Antiangiogenic Therapy With Anti-VEGF Agents

Anti-vascular endothelial growth factor agents were more recently approved for the treatment of macular edema secondary to CRVO and branch retinal vein occlusion (BRVO). Anti-VEGF agents injected directly into the eye are now considered the standard treatment for edema in both BRVO and CRVO. These agents work by limiting macular edema and improving vision by reducing vascular permeability. In 2 large phase III trials in patients with macular edema following BRVO or CRVO, monthly injections of ranibizumab (Lucentis®, Genentech/Roche) 0.5 mg into the eye were associated with significantly greater improvement in vision compared with sham injections.[34,35] With continued monitoring and frequent injections, the benefits of ranibizumab were sustained for 12 months and beyond.[36]

In September 2012, aflibercept (Eylea®, Regneron; VEGF trap-eye) was also approved by the FDA for treatment of macular edema associated with CRVO. In the phase III pivotal trials, nearly 60% of patients receiving intravitreal injections of aflibercept 2 mg monthly achieved at least a 15-letter improvement in visual acuity from baseline over 6 months compared with less than 20% in the control group. Additionally, patients receiving aflibercept achieved, on average, a 20-letter improvement in vision compared with placebo.[37,38] These gains in vision were sustained with close monitoring and continued injections over 12 months.[39]

Neuropathies

Prolonged diabetes is a risk factor in the development of a number of neuropathies. The mechanism responsible for the observed neurological defects is believed to be an injury that damages the small vessels nourishing the nerves. Defects of this nature that affect the eye include the following:

- Ischemic optic neuropathy
- Ocular palsies
- Diabetic corneal neuropathy

Ischemic Optic Neuropathy

Ischemic optic neuropathy refers to irreversible optic nerve damage due to loss of blood flow to the nerve. Patients present with complaints of loss of central field and/or a characteristic altitudinal visual field defect. This ocular complication occurs more frequently in persons with diabetes than in the general population and can lead to permanent visual loss.

Ocular Palsies

Ocular palsies result from ischemia to the third, fourth, and sixth cranial nerves. Impairment of extraocular muscle function leads to strabismus (crossing of the eyes) or diplopia (double vision). In most cases this condition is temporary, and normal function usually returns within a few months—however, it is very important that any patient reporting new onset of double vision be immediately referred back to his or her primary eye doctor for evaluation.

Diabetic Corneal Neuropathy

Diabetic corneal neuropathy can lead to severe dry eye and corneal ulcers. (The cornea is the transparent front part of the eye that covers the iris, pupil, and anterior chamber and provides most of the eyes' optical power.) In addition to these corneal epithelial problems, the corneal endothelium has an increased incidence of dysfunction in individuals with diabetes.[40,41] Usually, these patients complain of tearing, occasional ocular pain, and blurry vision. This condition needs to be treated with topical lubricants to decrease the occurrence of further complications.

Other Visual Impairments

Blurring of Vision

Blurring of vision due to instability of blood glucose may be related to osmotic changes in the lens of the eye. This problem commonly occurs at the onset of diabetes and during periods of fluctuating blood glucose levels. Most often, the patient may just need to be reassured that this condition is transient, and should be instructed to delay testing for new refractive lenses until the blood glucose has been stabilized for 6 to 8 weeks. However, all persons with diabetes with a blurring of vision should get a dilated fundus exam in order to evaluate for potentially vision-threatening causes of the blurriness.

Temporary Visual Changes

Temporary visual changes such as dimming of vision, bright flashing lights, or double vision may be experienced during periods of hypoglycemia (low blood glucose levels).[2,42,43]

Diabetic Retinopathy

Diabetic retinopathy is the leading cause of legal blindness among working-aged people in the United States. It is the most common and most important eye disease affecting people with diabetes. Symptoms often do not appear until the late stages of this condition. Delay in treatment decreases effectiveness of therapy. Progression of diabetic retinopathy can be rapid once it is identified. Early recognition is imperative to prevent vision loss.

Diabetic retinopathy[3,5,42,44] occurs when the microvasculature that nourishes the retina is damaged. This damage is caused by elevated blood glucose levels as well as high blood pressure. The damage permits leakage of blood components through the vessel walls. The retina is a layer of nerve tissue at the back of the eye that is responsible for converting light into the electrical signals interpreted by our brains. It is analogous to the film in a camera. These images are relayed along the optic nerve to the brain. Any disturbance to the retina can cause visual symptoms, most often decreased visual acuity. Unlike the changes in the lens that may lead to a cataract, which can be removed and replaced with an artificial intraocular lens, once the retina is severely damaged, permanent visual disturbance results. At this time, the retina cannot be replaced by an artificial retina.

There are many theories regarding the pathogenic mechanisms that lead to the development of diabetic eye disorders. The most popular of these theories relate to abnormalities of (1) protein glycosylation, (2) aldose reductase activity, and (3) glycosylated hemoglobin. All of these mechanisms can result in a relative tissue hypoxia, which may be the final common pathway.[11]

The first clinical findings of diabetic retinopathy are abnormalities of the retinal blood vessels. For instance, the first identifiable lesion is a microaneurysm located within 30° of the center of the macula.[45] (The macula is the small central area of the retina surrounding the fovea; it is the area of acute central vision used for reading and discriminating fine detail and color. A microaneurysm is a minute bubble in the wall of a small blood vessel.) After these first abnormalities are detected, more will tend to occur.

Preventing Blindness

Diabetic retinopathy, the most common and most important eye disease affecting persons with diabetes, is the nation's leading cause of legal blindness.

Intervention impedes the leading cause of blindness in persons with diabetes. Without appropriate intervention, diabetic retinopathy can progress from a mild asymptomatic form to a severe, rapidly progressing and blinding condition.

Retinopathy is staged from its mildest form, using the term *nonproliferative* (mild, moderate, and severe), to its most advanced form, called *proliferative retinopathy*.[46] Table 26.1 summarizes the stages. Retinopathy is often detectable within 5 years of the onset of diabetes.[2,3] Since type 2 diabetes may go undetected for well over 5 years after its onset, 21% of persons with type 2 diabetes already have retinopathy at the time of initial diagnosis.

Ninety percent of people who are diagnosed with either type 1 diabetes or type 2 diabetes and are less than 30 years of age will develop nonproliferative retinopathy within 20 years after the initial diagnosis, and 50% will progress to sight-threatening proliferative retinopathy.[47]

The number of people with diabetic retinopathy and sight-threatening diabetic retinopathy is expected to triple by 2050 to over 16 million people.[8] There's even a larger growth projected for Hispanics and African Americans, especially among those 65 years and older.

TABLE 26.1 Diabetic Retinopathy—International Clinical Disease Severity Scale

No apparent retinopathy	No abnormalities
Mild nonproliferative diabetic retinopathy	Microaneurysms only
Moderate nonproliferative diabetic retinopathy	More than just microaneurysms but less than severe nonproliferative diabetic retinopathy
Severe nonproliferative diabetic retinopathy	Any of the following: More than 20 intraretinal hemorrhages in each of 4 quadrants Definite venous beading in 2 or more quadrants Prominent intraretinal microvascular abnormalities in 1 or more quadrants And no signs of proliferative diabetic retinopathy
Proliferative diabetic retinopathy	One or both of the following: Neovascularization Vitreous or preretinal hemorrhage

Source: CP Wilkinson, FL Ferris III, RE Klein, et al; Global Diabetic Retinopathy Project Group, "Proposed international clinical diabetic retinopathy and diabetic macular edema disease severity scales (review)," *Ophthalmology* 110, no. 9 (2003), 1677-82.

Case—Part 2: Poor Follow-up Prevents Timely Intervention

Three years passed. MG had missed all of his follow-up appointments with the ophthalmologist after the initial exam, but he saw the glaucoma specialist once. The glaucoma specialist had started him on eyedrops to control the eye pressure, but MG stopped using them 2 years ago. He returned to the retina service approximately 3 years after his initial examination. By this time, he noticed his vision had decreased, and he had started seeing several "cobwebs," especially in the right eye.

- On examination, he had a visual acuity of 20/200 in the right eye and 20/40 in the left.
- IOP was 22 and 21 mm Hg, respectively, in the right and left eyes.
- A 2+ posterior subcapsular cataract was noted (unchanged since last visit) on the right eye and mild cataract on the left eye.
- On the fundus exam, the C/D ratio was unchanged from the last visit.
- The retinal evaluation revealed that MG had progressed to a more severe stage of diabetic retinopathy with neovascularization at the disc. Multiple intraretinal hemorrhages, microaneurysms, and cotton-wool spots along with hard exudates were noted within the macular area. There were several areas of retinal thickening (edema) on both eyes.
- Fluorescein angiography, macular optical coherence tomography, and visual field tests were performed. They showed a large amount of dye leakage from both eyes, macular thickening, and visual field defects in both eyes.

Diagnosis

- Proliferative diabetic retinopathy
- Clinically significant macular edema
- Subcapsular cataract in right eye
- Primary open-angle glaucoma

Treatment

- MG was given laser treatment (PRP and focal laser) in both eyes according to standards of care and scheduled for follow-up in 6 to 8 weeks.
- He was also referred to the glaucoma specialist to restart glaucoma treatment.

Follow-up

Six weeks later, MG's visual acuity was 20/80 in the right eye and 20/30 in the left eye, and significant improvement was noted in the retinal exam. There was regression of the neovascularization and improvement of the macular edema. He saw the glaucoma specialist, who restarted him with glaucoma eyedrops. His IOP was reduced to 14 mm Hg on both eyes. For 2 years, MG continued his eye examinations as indicated and remained stable.

The progression of eye disease might have been prevented in this case or at least delayed through continued close treatment and ongoing observation of the patient's eye disease. Application of effective teaching strategies might have helped this man realize the implications of his self-care choices and motivate him to engage in successful comprehensive self-management.

Risk Factors

The development and progression of retinopathy correlate strongly with the degree of glycemic stability and the duration of diabetes.[5,6,42]

The severity of hyperglycemia is the key alterable risk factor associated with the development and progression of diabetic retinopathy.[48–50] Hyperglycemia and blood pressure are modifiable risk factors. Blood pressure stability and blood lipid stability are important.

Glucose Management

The relationship of hyperglycemia severity to the development and progression of diabetic retinopathy was demonstrated in the Diabetes Control and Complications Trial (DCCT) for type 1 diabetes and in the UK Prospective Diabetes Study (UKPDS) for type 2 diabetes.[49,51] The data resulting from these studies emphasized the importance of achieving tight blood glucose stability in all persons with diabetes in an attempt to decrease the severity of its complications. Once retinopathy is present, duration of diabetes appears to be less of a factor than hyperglycemia; therefore, it must be stressed to the person with diabetes and healthcare providers that maintaining target blood glucose levels will greatly determine progression to the later, more advanced stages of diabetic retinopathy.[50] (See chapter 23, Acute Hyperglycemia.)

Blood Pressure

Another important alterable factor is high blood pressure. Epidemiologic studies and clinical trials have repeatedly implicated hypertension as an important modifiable risk factor for the development of diabetic retinopathy.[52] Each 10-mm Hg increase in systolic blood pressure has been associated with an approximately 10% increased risk of early retinopathy and a 15% increased risk of proliferative diabetic retinopathy or diabetic macular edema (DME). In the UKPDS, persons with type 2 diabetes and hypertension who had tight blood pressure management had a 37% reduction in the risk of microvascular disease, a 34% reduction in the rate of progression of retinopathy, and a 47% reduction in the deterioration of visual acuity.[53,54]

Hyperlipidemia

Although there have been several studies on the relationship between lipid abnormalities and the development of diabetic retinopathy, this association, in contrast to other risk factors like hyperglycemia and hypertension, has been somewhat inconsistent.[55] In the Wisconsin Epidemiologic Study of Diabetic Retinopathy (WESDR), total serum cholesterol was not a significant factor in the severity of retinopathy but was significantly associated with the presence (odds ratio 1.65) and severity of hard exudates in subjects with young-onset diabetes.[56] The Australian Diabetes, Obesity and Lifestyle Study reported that cholesterol was not associated with diabetic retinopathy,[57] while the Singapore Malay Eye Study reported that higher body mass index and higher total and LDL cholesterol levels were associated with a lower prevalence of diabetic retinopathy (odds ratio 0.75).[58] In the DCCT study, researchers showed that severity of retinopathy was associated with increasing triglycerides and inversely associated with HDL cholesterol.[59] In the Fenofibrate Intervention and Event Lowering in Diabetes (FIELD) trial, treatment with fenofibrate, a lipid-lowering medication taken by mouth, reduced the need for laser treatment in patients with vision-threatening diabetic retinopathy by approximately 30%.[60] Results from the ACCORD-Eye study were similar to those of the FIELD study. Here, too, treatment with fenofibrate was associated with a 40% decrease in retinopathy progression.[60] In both studies, patients with preexisting diabetic retinopathy derived greater benefit from oral fenofibrate therapy.

Other Risk Factors

Smoking has also been linked to the development and progression of vision-threatening diabetic retinopathy.[61] There is less agreement concerning the importance of other factors such as age, clotting factors, renal disease, and use of specific types of high blood pressure medication.[50,62–64]

Evidence Base

Several large clinical studies have provided excellent information on the natural history and effective treatment strategies that can prevent severe vision loss. These studies include 5 major clinical trials: the DCCT,[49,65,66] the Diabetic Retinopathy Study (DRS),[67,68] the Early Treatment Diabetic Retinopathy Study (ETDRS),[69,70] the Diabetic Retinopathy Vitrectomy Study (DRVS),[71,72] and the UKPDS.[51,53,73]

Natural History

In its earliest stages, diabetic retinopathy, termed *nonproliferative diabetic retinopathy* (NPDR), is characterized by retinal vascular abnormalities. These include microaneurysms (which are seen as sacular outpouchings along weakened vascular walls), intraretinal hemorrhages that may appear as dots or a flame shape, and cotton-wool spots. Increased retinal vascular leakage (permeability) can occur in this or later stages of retinopathy and may result in retinal thickening (edema) and fluid deposits (hard exudates). *Clinically significant macular edema* (CSME) is a term used frequently for retinal thickening and/or hard exudates that either involve the center of the macula or threaten to infiltrate it.

As retinopathy progresses, there is a gradual closure of the retinal vessels, which results in decreased perfusion and ischemia. Signs of increased ischemia include vascular abnormalities (eg, beading, loops), intraretinal microvascular abnormalities that appear as dilated capillaries that arise around ischemic areas where there is capillary closure, and increased retinal hemorrhages and exudation.

The more advanced and vision-threatening stage, proliferative diabetic retinopathy (PDR), is characterized by the growth of new blood vessels along the surface of the retina (neovascularization). These vessels may extend to the vitreous cavity using the posterior vitreous surface as a scaffold. (The vitreous is the transparent, colorless, gelatinous mass that fills the rear two thirds of the eyeball, between the lens and the retina.) The blood vessels are fragile and rupture easily. For this reason, neovascularization in the optic disc (NVD) or neovascularization elsewhere (NVE) is prone to bleeding, which ultimately results in a vitreous hemorrhage. (The optic disc is the ocular end of the optic nerve; it denotes the exit of retinal nerve fibers from the eye and entrance of blood vessels to the eye.) This and other fibrous proliferation may result in epiretinal membrane formation, vitreoretinal traction bands, retinal tears, and ultimately retinal detachments.[74] See Tables 26.1 and 26.2 for specific classifications of diabetic retinopathy stages and findings, including macular edema.

TABLE 26.2 Diabetic Macular Edema—International Clinical Disease Severity Scale	
Diabetic macular edema apparently absent	No apparent retinal thickening or hard exudates in posterior pole
Diabetic macular edema apparently present	Some retinal thickening or hard exudates in posterior pole
Mild diabetic macular edema	Some retinal thickening or hard exudates in posterior pole, but distant from the center of the macula
Moderate diabetic macular edema	Retinal thickening or hard exudates approaching the center of the macula but not involving the center
Severe diabetic macular edema	Retinal thickening or hard exudates involving the center of the macula

Source: CP Wilkinson, FL Ferris III, RE Klein, et al; Global Diabetic Retinopathy Project Group, "Proposed international clinical diabetic retinopathy and diabetic macular edema disease severity scales (review)," *Ophthalmology* 110, no. 9 (2003), 1677-82.

Diabetic Macular Edema

The macula is the specialized portion of the retina responsible for central vision. Macular edema is leakage of fluid and exudate from the vessels into the macula. This is a serious consequence that affects the primary area of focus.[3,5] Macular edema may accompany NPDR or PDR. Table 26.2 outlines the progression and severity of macular edema.

Clinically significant macular edema, as defined by the ETDRS, exists with any of the following findings:

- Retinal thickening within 500 μm of the center of the fovea (the central pit in the macula that produces the sharpest vision)
- Hard exudates within 500 μm of the center of the fovea with adjacent retinal thickening
- At least 1 disc area (1.5 × 1.5 mm) of retinal thickening, any part of which is within 1 disc diameter (~1.5 mm) of the center of the fovea[75]

Focal edema is associated with hard exudate rings that result from leakage of the microaneurysms. Diffuse edema results from the breakdown of the blood-retinal barrier with leakage from microaneurysms, retinal capillaries, and arterioles. Clinically significant macular edema results when retinal thickening and exudates are sufficient enough to threaten or impair the central vision. Visual loss may vary from mild blurring to a visual acuity of 20/200 or less (legal blindness). (The higher the bottom number, the more vision is decreased. Normal visual acuity is 20/20.) The risk for development of CSME is 10% to 15% for all persons having diabetes for 15 to 20 or more years.

Clinically significant macular edema is determined through a dilated pupil, by slitlamp biomicroscopy, and/or by stereoscopic fundus photography. Fluorescein angiography is a study used to evaluate the retinal vessels, and it helps guide treatment and monitor progression and therapeutic results. Macular edema that is not clinically significant may be observed. Clinically significant macular edema was traditionally treated with laser surgery by using focal argon photocoagulation to seal the leaking blood vessels. Focal photocoagulation is a laser technique directed to abnormal blood vessels with specific areas of focal leakage to reduce chronic fluid leakage in patients with macular edema.

Over the last five years, in patients with symptomatic visual loss associated with DME, the treatment paradigm for DME has shifted away from focal/grid laser photocoagulation toward intravitreal pharmacotherapeutics, principally anti-VEGF medications, as first-line therapy.[76] Six prospective clinical trials examining the effect of intravitreal ranibizumab in the treatment of DME (READ-2, RESOLVE, RESTORE, RISE, RIDE, and DRCR.net protocol I) have all demonstrated improved visual outcomes with anti-VEGF therapy compared with laser treatment alone.[76] In the RISE and RIDE studies, for example, over 40% of patients receiving monthly ranibizumab injections for 2 years gained 15 letters of vision improvement compared with 15% of patients who were treated with laser alone. With continued close monitoring and repeated injections, this gain was sustained for the entire 3-year duration of the study. Ranibizumab 0.3 mg is approved by the FDA for the treatment of DME and may be used in combination with focal/grid laser photocoagulation. Similar to ranibizumab, aflibercept intravitreal therapy is also FDA approved for the treatment of diabetic macular edema.[77] In 2 prospective, randomized, phase 3 clinical trials, VISTA(DME) and VIVID(DME), patients with DME received either intravitreal aflibercept injection (IAI) 2 mg every 4 weeks (2q4), IAI 2 mg every 8 weeks after 5 initial monthly doses (2q8), or macular laser photocoagulation.[78] At week 52, IAI demonstrated significant superiority in visual function and OCT anatomic endpoints over laser. This superiority of aflibercept injections over laser photocoagulation was sustained out to week 100. Interestingly, in the clinical trials in which patients received anti-VEGF therapy for the treatment of diabetic macular edema, a significant portion of patients also experienced an improvement in the severity of diabetic retinopathy. For example, even out to week 100, well over 30% of patients in VIVID and VISTA who received IAI experienced a ≥2 step improvement in the DRSS score compared with approximately 10% of patients who received laser.[77] A similar result was noted in trials with ranibizumab.

Pharmacotherapy with longer acting intravitreal corticosteroids also remains a treatment option for many patients, especially in refractory cases of DME. The 0.7 mg dexamethasone biodegradable intravitreal implant (Ozurdex, DEX implant) slowly releases corticosteroid over many months and is FDA approved for the treatment of DME. The DEX implant demonstrated superior efficacy compared with sham injections in patients with DME in two 3-year randomized prospective clinical trials.[79] Unlike anti-VEGF therapies that require monthly or bimonthly injections, the DEX implant has the potential for efficacy out to 6 months following a single intravitreal injection. Similar to the DEX implant, the fluocinolone acetonide intravitreal implant (FA, Iluvien®) is an injectable, non-erodible corticosteroid implant that is FDA approved for the treatment of DME.[80] The FA implant releases corticosteroid for up to 3 years following a single intravitreal injection. Both the DEX and FA implants have the potential to not only significantly decrease the treatment burden associated with monthly intravitreal anti-VEGF injections but also address more broad mechanisms underlying DME, including the proinflammatory pathway. Importantly, elevated intraocular pressure (including glaucoma requiring incisional surgery) and cataract formation remain significant side effects of both the DEX and FA implants.

With the options of focal/grid laser photocoagulation, intravitreal anti-VEGF therapy, and long-acting corticosteroid implants all currently available for the successful treatment of DME, individualized therapeutic discussions are extremely important in order to determine the most appropriate treatment plan based on each person's safety and efficacy profile as well as treatment burden (eg, number of required intravitreal injections).

Proliferative Diabetic Retinopathy

Proliferative diabetic retinopathy (PDR) occurs when abnormal blood vessels appear in the retina as a result of diabetic damage. This represents a severe form of diabetic retinopathy that has the potential to lead to severe blindness from bleeding (vitreous hemorrhage) and/or retinal detachment. Until recently, the traditional treatment of PDR involved application of hundreds to thousands of laser spots to the peripheral retina (PRP) in order to prevent vision loss. Panretinal photocoagulation, however, can damage the retina, causing peripheral vision loss and worsening of DME. Therefore, similar to what has occurred with the treatment of DME, the shift has begun away from PRP toward pharmacotherapy with injection of anti-VEGF medications as first-line and adjunctive therapy in patients with PDR. The recently published Diabetic Retinopathy Clinical Research Network Protocol S compared PRP with intravitreal injections of ranibizumab for PDR. Patients were randomly assigned to receive PRP treatment or a series of intravitreal ranibizumab injections. The study found that vision outcomes and surgery rates were not inferior in the injection group compared with the PRP group.[81] Secondary outcomes, such as visual field evaluations and the occurrence of DME, indicate improved functional results with ranibizumab, supporting injections as a possible alternative treatment of PDR. Longer term follow-up with anti-VEGF therapy is needed before it too replaces PRP as the treatment of choice.

Eye Examination

The initial diabetic eye examination should include the following components at a minimum:

- Best corrected visual acuity
- Intraocular pressure
- Ocular motility
- Gonioscopy (a test to visualize the anterior chamber angle and help classify glaucoma), when indicated
- Slitlamp biomicroscopy (examining the lens and other structures at the front of the eye)
- Dilated funduscopy including stereoscopic examination of the posterior pole
- Examination of the peripheral retina and vitreous

Other studies such as diagnostic imaging are performed when indicated.

Frequency of Examination

Recommended frequencies of diabetic eye exams, for both type 1 diabetes and type 2 diabetes, are listed in the following sidebar. See chapter 24 for information on progression of retinopathy as a maternal complication in pregnancy; see also the first case study's discussion of preconception care in that chapter.

Recommended Frequency of Eye Examination for Persons With Diabetes

- *Type 1 diabetes:* Individuals with type 1 diabetes should have a routine diabetic eye exam at puberty, if diabetes is diagnosed by then, and within 3 to 5 years of receiving a diagnosis of diabetes. Thereafter, individuals should have an annual exam and an exam when pregnant.
- *Type 2 diabetes:* All persons with type 2 diabetes should be referred for an ophthalmic evaluation at the time of diagnosis.[82] Individuals should schedule a routine diabetic eye exam yearly thereafter as well as when pregnant.

Type 1 Diabetes

Type 1 diabetes usually has an abrupt onset; therefore, one can usually determine how long a person has had diabetes. Diabetic retinopathy usually becomes apparent as early as 6 to 7 years after onset of the disease, but since the development of vision-threatening retinopathy is rare in children prior to puberty,[83,84] ophthalmic examination is recommended to begin 3 to 5 years after the diagnosis of type 1 diabetes and every year thereafter.[74,85] The eye care provider may need to evaluate the patient more often if progression of retinopathy warrants it.

Type 2 Diabetes

At the time an individual is diagnosed with type 2 diabetes, the disease has usually been present for an undetermined period of time. For this reason, up to 3% of those diagnosed with diabetes at age 30 years and older have CSME at the time of the initial diagnosis.[76] Almost 30% of patients will have some manifestation of diabetic retinopathy at diagnosis. Thus, it is imperative that a patient diagnosed with type 2 diabetes get a full eye evaluation shortly after the diagnosis.

The onset and diagnosis of type 1 diabetes typically occur at an earlier age than that of type 2 diabetes. Most people with an initial diagnosis of type 1 diabetes will not show any ocular manifestations at the time of diagnosis. However, a great majority of those individuals will develop diabetic retinopathy at some point during their lifetime.[61] This is in contrast to people with type 2 diabetes, who are typically diagnosed at an older age and may have changes in the eyes due to diabetes at the time of initial diagnosis. Consequently, both persons with type 1 diabetes and those with type 2 diabetes require careful ophthalmic surveillance and management throughout their lifetime to ensure that treatable causes of vision loss are addressed appropriately.

TABLE 26.3 Suggested Schedule for Ophthalmologic Examination

Stage of Retinopathy	*Frequency of Examination*
No retinopathy	Annually
Mild nonproliferative retinopathy	Annually
Moderate nonproliferative retinopathy	Within 6–12 months
Clinically significant macular edema or proliferative retinopathy	Every 3–4 months
Proliferative retinopathy with high-risk characteristics	Individualized to patient needs

Source: M Bernbaum, T Stich, "Eye Disease and Adaptive Diabetes Education for Visually Impaired Persons," in MJ Franz, ed, *A Core Curriculum for Diabetes Educators: Diabetes and Complications,* 5th ed (Chicago: American Association of Diabetes Educators, 2003), 131.

Table 26.3 summarizes the recommended frequency of ophthalmologic examinations based on the stage of retinopathy.

Care Process

The primary purpose of evaluating and managing diabetic retinopathy is to prevent, retard, or reverse loss of vision. Doing so maintains and/or improves vision-related quality of life (see sidebar for self-management and self-care strategies). Once diabetic retinopathy is established, treatment is provided according to its severity scale or retinopathy stage (see Tables 26.1 and 26.2).

Early treatment reduces visual loss by 50% after 3 years.[86] Within 1 year of diagnosis of eye disease, 5% to 10% of patients will progress to a more advanced stage.[3] These guidelines are thus imperative:

- Normal-to-mild nonproliferative retinopathy requires observation and should be reexamined annually.[85]
- Moderate nonproliferative retinopathy without macular edema should be reexamined within 6 to 12 months, as disease progression is common.[63]
- Mild-to-moderate nonproliferative retinopathy with CSME should be treated with focal argon photocoagulation to seal leaking blood vessels.

Vision improves in only a minority of patients; for the majority, the goal of laser photocoagulation treatment is to stabilize visual acuity.

Patients with CSME and excellent visual function should be considered for treatment before visual loss occurs. When treatment is deferred because the center of the macula is not involved or imminently threatened, the patient should be observed at least every 3 to 4 months for progression.[74] Severe NPDR and (non-high-risk) PDR have similar clinical courses. Consequently, subsequent recommendations and treatment are similar, as shown in the ETDRS.

Importance of Self-Management Education and Self-Care

Treatment of retinopathy begins with preventive measures such as optimizing blood glucose, lipids, and blood pressure. Smoking cessation may also be of value. Routine annual screening and follow-up by an ophthalmologist or optometrist are essential to ensure that any intervention is appropriately timed.[3,5,42,44,75,86,87]

Patient education about the following topics is an important part of the care process:[74]

- Maintaining near-normal glucose levels
- Maintaining near-normal blood pressure
- Lowering serum lipid levels

Laser Surgery

In eyes with severe diabetic retinopathy, the risk of progression to proliferative disease is 50% to 75% within 1 year. The ETDRS also studied the value of laser surgery for these patients. Panretinal photocoagulation should be considered and should not be delayed if the eye has reached the high-risk proliferative stage (if neovascularization of the optic disc is extensive or vitreous/preretinal hemorrhage has occurred recently). Careful follow-up at 3 to 4 months is important. The goal of laser therapy is to reduce the risk of visual loss. The ETDRS protocol provides detailed guidelines for treatment.[88,89] The patient should be seen for a follow-up visit every 1 to 4 weeks until completion of PRP and then every 2 to 4 months thereafter.

When PRP is to be carried out in eyes with macular edema, it is preferable to perform focal photocoagulation before PRP. There is evidence that PRP may exacerbate macular edema and may cause moderate visual loss compared with untreated eyes.[69] Panretinal laser photocoagulation should not be delayed if the diabetic retinopathy is in the high-risk stage. In these cases, panretinal and focal photocoagulation may be performed concomitantly.[74]

Similar to the treatment of DME, pharmacotherapy with intravitreal anti-VEGF treatment will likely have a future role in the therapy for and prevention of proliferative diabetic retinopathy.[90] However, while these studies are still ongoing, the standard therapy remains PRP.

Vitreous Surgery

In cases of high-risk PDR, photocoagulation may not be delivered due to cataracts or severe vitreous or preretinal hemorrhage. In other cases, active PDR may persist despite extensive PRP. In these cases, it may be necessary to perform vitreous surgery. Vitreous surgery is frequently indicated in patients with tractional retinal detachment and in nonclearing vitreous hemorrhage precluding PRP. Patients with vitreous hemorrhage and rubeosis iridis (neovascularization of the iris) should also be considered for prompt vitrectomy and intraoperative photocoagulation, as demonstrated in the DRVS.[71,72]

Other Treatments Being Investigated

Different drugs are currently being studied for the management of diabetic retinopathy. Some of these drugs include the administration of short- and long-acting corticosteroids for DME. Other drugs with antiangiogenic activity (inhibitors of the vascular endothelial growth factor) are also being studied. Review of the available literature by the American Academy of Ophthalmology indicates that anti-VEGF pharmacotherapy, via repeated intravitreal injection into the eye, either alone or in combination with focal laser photocoagulation, is a safe and effective treatment of DME over several years' time.[76] Further evidence is required to support the long-term safety and comparative efficacy of anti-VEGF agents.

Ancillary Tests

If used appropriately, a number of tests ancillary to the clinical examination may enhance patient care. These include the following:

- *Color fundus photography.* This is a more reproducible technique than a clinical examination for detecting diabetic retinopathy in clinical research studies. However, clinical examination is superior for detecting retinal thickening and identifying fine-caliber neovascularization (NVD or NVE).
- *Fluorescein angiography.* This is a clinically valuable test for selected patients with diabetic retinopathy and can be used as a guide for treating DME.[75] It is also helpful as a means for evaluating areas of retinal ischemia or the cause of unexplained decreased visual acuity.
- *Ultrasonography (echography).* This is a valuable test for diabetic eyes with opaque media. The test should be considered when media opacities preclude exclusion of retinal detachment or retinal masses by indirect ophthalmoscopy.

- *Optical coherence tomography.* Provides high-resolution (5 µm) imaging of vitreoretinal interface, retina, and subretinal space. Optical coherence tomography can be useful for quantifying retinal thickness and macular edema and identifying vitreomacular traction.[91]

Counseling and Referral

The ophthalmologist or optometrist has the responsibility to not only manage eye disease but also ensure that people with diabetes are referred for appropriate management of their systemic condition.[42]

An important aspect of treatment is meeting the patient's needs in adapting to loss of vision.[71,92–95] To help alleviate anxiety and depression, an offer of psychosocial counseling should be made before there is actual deterioration of vision. Chapters 10 (Problem Solving) and 4 (Healthy Coping) can be of value in assessing and addressing anxiety and depression and in learning how to work with a patient to recognize and manage these issues.

Low-vision evaluation is indicated as soon as vision loss impacts normal daily activities. Referral to rehabilitation services as early as possible will allow the person to acquire adaptive skills and maintain participation and independence in work and recreational activities. Patients need information and instruction in adaptive diabetes self-care as soon as vision is compromised, preferably before adaptive equipment is required.

The extent of vision impairment and the individual's ability to adapt to the vision loss must be evaluated before undertaking adaptive education. The adaptive education and training needs of persons with preexisting eye disease due to other causes may differ from those of persons experiencing a new onset of diabetic retinopathy. The diabetes care and education specialist can play a key role in referring patients with visual impairment to the proper rehabilitative and psychosocial services.

Focus on Education

Teaching Strategies

Provide hope and support, and prevent vision loss. Most diabetic eye diseases can be managed without significant visual loss if they are diagnosed and managed in a timely manner. Visual impairment and blindness do not have to be part of diabetes. The primary purpose of managing retinopathy is to prevent, retard, or reverse loss of vision. In addition, consistent, frequent monitoring of blood pressure, blood glucose, and lipids is needed.

Prepare adequately for those with visual impairment. Teaching methods need to include large print, magnifiers, and the option of recording the instructor's information or directions or obtaining prerecorded instructions. Provide hands-on time and extra time for return demonstration when teaching people with varied levels of visual capacity.

Appropriately assess and reassess patients' needs and capacity for self-care management. Persons with visual impairment and diabetes face daily challenges that are multifactorial. Their visual limitations significantly impact their daily tasks. Review daily routines and strategize accordingly for modifying the needed activities.

Focus on one task at a time. Reevaluate implementation of the task, adjust accordingly, and then add another task. This way, you will minimize confusion or the feeling of being overwhelmed with all that has to be done. Also, each successfully accomplished task will increase the confidence in making the new task a reality!

Help with adapting to loss of vision. Anxiety and depression can negatively influence patients' confidence in their ability to manage their diabetes. Reassess their willingness and readiness to self-manage on an ongoing basis, as their attitude and confidence will change with the acceptance and overall perspective of the condition.

Strategize for timely referrals. Rehabilitative and psychosocial services are available, and referral needs to be made promptly to prepare patients for vision loss as well as help them adapt to vision already lost. Assisting patients with the task instead of telling them to do it on their own will ensure its implementation.

Messages for Persons With Diabetes

Maintain good diabetes management. Keeping blood glucose, blood pressure, and lipids under or at target levels, along with smoking cessation, helps preserve vision.

Use your support network. A support network is instrumental to successful diabetes care with or without visual impairment. Invite family or significant others to attend education sessions for support and to assist in "helping" roles. Ensure, however, that "helpers" do not take over, for example, when vision is compromised.

Ask about vision changes. Blurriness may be temporary due to elevated blood glucose. Wait until blood glucose resolves before considering eye glasses or changes in lenses.

Discuss eye care. Be knowledgeable about screening to protect vision and other reasons to consult an eye care specialist. Understand what the recommendations are for diabetic eye examinations, for both initial visits and follow-up. Identify the frequency of eye care visits that will best protect vision for the individual.

Protect vision through eye examinations. Knowing the current status of eye disease and what symptoms to watch for is important. Schedule a retinal evaluation by an ophthalmologist or optometrist to assess eye condition. This examination is not just a fitting for glasses; it is a dilated eye exam. Use the appointment to ask questions like these: What condition are my eyes in? What can I do to keep my vision? Is it okay to exercise? and What do I need to change?

Seek out specialists when help is needed. To help alleviate anxiety and depression and begin the process of adapting to loss of vision, psychosocial counseling is appropriate to include *before* deterioration of vision occurs.

Health Literacy and Numeracy

There is no "typical" vision-impaired patient. Use different approaches for low-vision patients and blind patients. You can use print with special equipment and materials for low vision. The extent of visual disability within patients who are blind can depend on their eyes' physical sensory impairment, the duration of the onset of vision impairment, and the way in which that impairment occurred. Vision may also fluctuate or may be influenced by factors such as inappropriate lighting, light glare, or fatigue. The best way to know which education approach to use is to ask the patient, "What works best for you?" Individualize strategies based on the patient's preferences and skill of communication (Braille, speed listening).

Communicate effectively with your patients.

- Identify yourself and your role.
- Call a patient by name if you want his or her attention.
- Use descriptive words such as *straight*, *forward*, and *left* in relation to the patient's body orientation. Avoid nondescriptive terms such as *over there*, *here*, and *this*.
- Describe in detail pertinent visual occurrences of the learning activities.
- Offer to read written information.
- Do not speak loudly to people with visual impairments.
- Use a projector to show step-by-step instructions.
- Appropriately label objects used for identification.
- Use an actual object for demonstrations.
- Use a tape recorder.
- Make all handouts available in an appropriate form such as regular print, large print, or Braille, depending on the patient's preferences.
- Enlist the aid of a special education professional, if needed, for teaching the task of taking insulin or monitoring glucose.

Put a meaning to the task. Motivation to self-manage diabetes among visually impaired patients varies. Explore their health belief system and confidence in their ability to apply the information learned. Use a confidence scale to assess whether they are able, willing, and ready to do a specific task. For example, ask, "What do you think can be done for you to use a meter to test your blood glucose?"

Minimize the use of "unrealistic optimism"—for example, "Bad things are unlikely to happen when . . ." versus "Good things are likely to happen when . . ."—as patients' perception of their ability to handle things can be very unpredictable. Also, their responses can be defensive, and they can be skeptical of information that is inconsistent with their attitudes or preferences. The best approach is not to make any assumptions about health literacy or patients' ability to do things.

Focus on Practice

Clinician style. Be empathetic, accepting, supportive of self-efficacy, and collaborative.

Skills. Utilize active listening, open-ended questions, and summarizing.

Tools. Use appropriate teaching and behavioral change approaches.

Collaboration. Utilize the expertise of other professionals to help patients realize their full potential in achieving their clinical care goal and enjoying their life.

Ongoing support. People need to be reminded more often than they need to be instructed. Create a series of functional messages and directions that can be used to maintain a healthy routine and tasks.

Program Planning

Anticipate a need for alternatives to traditional patient handouts. As blood glucose levels change, patients may experience short-term blurred vision or reoccurring blurriness, as well as more permanent vision changes. When preparing your teaching materials, accommodate this change by using one or more of the following alternative methods for conveying information:

- Enlarged-print handouts
- Transferring materials from black on white to white on black
- Audio recording
- Schedule a time outside the scheduled visit/classroom if needed to clarify information and to reinforce and encourage participants

References

1. Fong DS, Aiello LP, Ferris FL III, Klein R. Diabetic retinopathy. Diabetes Care. 2004;27(10):2540-53.
2. Klein R, Klein BEK. Vision disorders in diabetes. In: National Diabetes Data Group, eds. Diabetes in America. 2nd ed. Bethesda, Md: National Institutes of Health; 1995:293-337.
3. Ferris FL III, Davis MD, Aiello LM. Treatment of diabetic retinopathy (review). New Engl J Med. 1999;341:667-78.
4. Javitt JC, Aiello LP. Cost effectiveness of detecting and treating diabetic retinopathy. Ann Intern Med. 1996;124:164-9.
5. Aiello LP, Gardner TW, King GL, et al. Diabetic retinopathy (technical review). Diabetes Care. 1998;21(1):143-56.
6. Aiello LP, Cavallerano J, Bursell SE. Diabetic eye disease. Endocrinol Metab Clin North Am. 1996;25:271-91.
7. Harris MI. Summary. In: National Diabetes Data Group, eds. Diabetes in America. 2nd ed. Bethesda, Md: National Institutes of Health; 1995:1-13.
8. Saaddine JB, Honeycutt AA, Venkat Narayan KM, Zhang X, Klein R, Boyle JP. Projection of diabetic retinopathy and other major eye diseases among people with diabetes mellitus: United States, 2005-2050. Arch Ophthalmol. 2008;126(12):1740-7.
9. Ferris FL III. How effective are treatments for diabetic retinopathy? JAMA. 1993;269:1290-1.
10. Congdon N, Vingerling JR, Klein BE, et al; Eye Diseases Prevalence Research Group. Prevalence of cataract and pseudophakia/aphakia among adults in the United States. Arch Ophthalmol. 2004;122(4):487-94.
11. Feman SS. Diabetes and the eye. In: Duane's Clinical Ophthalmology on CD-ROM. Philadelphia: Lippincott Williams & Wilkins; 2004.
12. Ederer F, Hiller R, Taylor HR. Senile lens change in diabetes in two population studies. Am J Ophthalmol. 1981;91:381-95.
13. Flanagan DW. Current management of established diabetic eye disease. Eye. 1993;7:302-8.
14. Shah AS, Chen SH. Cataract surgery and diabetes. Curr Opin Ophthalmol. 2010;21(1):4-9.
15. Cheema RA, Al-Mubarak MM, Amin YM, Cheema MA. Role of combined cataract surgery and intravitreal bevacizumab injection in preventing progression of diabetic retinopathy: prospective randomized study. J Cataract Refract Surg. 2009 Jan;35(1):18-25.
16. Kim SY, Yang J, Lee YC, Park YH. Effect of a single intraoperative sub-Tenon injection of triamcinolone acetonide on the progression of diabetic retinopathy and visual outcomes after cataract surgery. J Cataract Refract Surg. 2008;34(5):823-6.
17. Leske MC. The epidemiology of open-angle glaucoma: a review. Am J Epidemiol. 1983;118:166-91.
18. Sommer A, Tielsch JM, Katz J, et al. Racial differences in the cause-specific prevalence of blindness in east Baltimore. N Engl J Med. 1991;325(20):1412-7.
19. Becker B. Diabetes mellitus and primary open-angled glaucoma. Am J Ophthalmol. 1971;71:1-16.
20. Klein BE, Klein R, Jensen SC. Open-angle glaucoma in older onset diabetes: the Beaver Dam Eye Study. Ophthalmology. 1994;101:1173-7.
21. Dielemans I, de Jong PTVM, Stolk R, et al. Primary open-angle glaucoma, intraocular pressure, and diabetes mellitus in the general elderly population: the Rotterdam Study. Ophthalmology. 1996;103:1271-5.
22. US Preventive Services Task Force. Screening for glaucoma (recommendation statement). Ann Fam Med. 2005;3:171-2.
23. Aiello LP, Avery RL, Arrig PG. Vascular endothelium growth factor in ocular fluid of patients with diabetic retinopathy and other retinal disorders. N Engl J Med. 1994;331:1480-7.
24. Molteno ACB, VanRooyen MNB, Bartholomew RS. Implants for draining neovascular glaucoma. Br J Ophthalmol. 1977;61:120-5.

25. Ciftci S, Bayezit Sakalar Y, Unlu K, Keklikci U, Caca I, Dogan E. Intravitreal bevacizumab combined with panretinal photocoagulation in the treatment of open angle neovascular glaucoma. Eur J Ophthalmol. 2009;19:1029-34. Epub 2009 Jun 25.

26. Chen CH, Lai IC, Wu PC, et al. Adjunctive intravitreal bevacizumab-combined trabeculectomy versus trabeculectomy alone in the treatment of neovascular glaucoma. J Ocul Pharmacol Ther. 2010;26(1):111-8.

27. The Eye Disease Case-Control Study Group. Risk factors for central retinal vein occlusion. Arch Ophthalmol. 1996;114:545-54.

28. Schwab PJ, Okun E, Fahey FJ. Reversal of retinopathy in Waldenstrom's macroglobulinemia by plasmapheresis: a report of two cases. Arch Ophthalmol. 1960;64:515-21.

29. Central Vein Occlusion Study Group. A randomized clinical trial of early panretinal photocoagulation for ischemic central vein occlusion: the Central Vein Occlusion Study Group N report. Ophthalmology. 1995;102(10):1434-44.

30. Kuno N, Fujii S. Biodegradable intraocular therapies for retinal disorders: progress to date. Drugs Aging. 2010 Feb 1; 27(2):117-34.

31. Schwartz SG, Flynn HW Jr. Pharmacotherapies for diabetic retinopathy: present and future. Exp Diabetes Res. 2007; 2007:52487.

32. Grover D, Li TJ, Chong CC. Intravitreal steroids for macular edema in diabetes. Cochrane Database Syst Rev. 2008 Jan 23; 1:CD005656.

33. Allergan. Safety and efficacy of a new treatment in vitrectomized subjects with diabetic macular edema [study in recruiting stage] (cited 2010 Oct 18). On the Internet at: http://www.clinicaltrials.gov.

34. Brown DM, Campochiaro PA, Singh RP, et al. Ranibizumab for macular edema following central retinal vein occlusion: six-month primary end point results of a phase III study. Ophthalmology. 2010;117(6):1124-33.

35. Campochiaro PA. Ranibizumab for macular edema following branch retinal vein occlusion: six-month primary end point results of a phase III study. Ophthalmology. 2010; 117(6):1102-12.

36. Campochiaro PA. Sustained benefits from ranibizumab for macular edema following central retinal vein occlusion: twelve-month outcomes of a phase III study. Ophthalmology. 2011;118(10):2041-9.

37. Boyer D, Heier J, Brown DM, et al. Vascular endothelial growth factor Trap-Eye for macular edema secondary to central retinal vein occlusion: six-month results of the phase 3 COPERNICUS study. Ophthalmology. 2012;119(5):1024-32.

38. Holz FG, Roider J, Ogura Y, et al. VEGF Trap-Eye for macular oedema secondary to central retinal vein occlusion: 6-month results of the phase III GALILEO study. Br J Ophthalmol. 2013;97(3):278-84.

39. Brown DM, Heier JS, Clark WL, et al. Intravitreal aflibercept injection for macular edema secondary to central retinal vein occlusion: 1-year results from the phase 3 COPERNICUS study. Am J Ophthalmol. 2013;155(3):429-37.

40. Schultz RO, Peters MA, Sobocinski K. Diabetic corneal neuropathy. Trans Am Ophthalmol Soc. 1983;81:107-24.

41. Busted N, Olsen T, Schmitz O. Clinical observations on the corneal thickness and the corneal endothelium in diabetes mellitus. Br J Ophthalmol. 1982;65:687-90.

42. Frank KJ, Dieckert JP. Diabetic eye disease: a primary care perspective. South Med J. 1996;89:463-70.

43. Cox DJ, Kiernan BD, Schroeder DB, Cowley M. Psychosocial sequelae of visual loss in diabetes. Diabetes Educ. 1998;24:481-4.

44. Sanders R, Wilson M. Diabetes-related eye disorders. J Natl Med Assoc. 1993;85:104-8.

45. Feman SS. The natural history of the first clinically visible features of diabetic retinopathy. Trans Am Ophthalmol Soc. 1994;92:745-73.

46. Wilkinson CP, Ferris FL III, Klein RE, et al. Proposed international clinical diabetic retinopathy and diabetic macular edema disease severity scales. Ophthalmology. 2003;110:1677-82.

47. Deshpande AD, Harris-Hayes M, Schootman M. Epidemiology of diabetes and diabetes-related complications. Phys Ther. 2008 Nov;88(11):1254-64.

48. Klein R, Klein BE, Moss SE, et al. Glycosylated hemoglobin predicts the incidence and progression of diabetic retinopathy. JAMA. 1988;260:2864-71.

49. The Diabetes Control and Complications Trial (DCCT) Research Group. The effect of intensive treatment of diabetes on the development and progression of long-term complications in insulin-dependent diabetes mellitus. N Engl J Med. 1993;329:977-86.

50. Davis MD, Fisher MR, Gangnon RE, et al. Risk factors for high-risk proliferative diabetic retinopathy and severe visual loss: Early Treatment Diabetic Retinopathy Study Report #18. Invest Ophthalmol Vis Sci. 1998;39:233-52.

51. UK Prospective Diabetes Study (UKPDS) Group. Intensive blood-glucose control with sulphonylureas or insulin compared with conventional treatment and risk of complications in patients with type 2 diabetes (UKPDS 33). Lancet. 1998;352:837-53.

52. Mohamed Q, Gillies MC, Wong TY. Management of diabetic retinopathy: a systematic review. JAMA. 2007;298:902-16.

53. UK Prospective Diabetes Study Group. Tight blood pressure control and risk of macrovascular and microvascular complications in type 2 diabetes (UKPDS 38). BMJ. 1998;317:703-13.

54. Snow V, Weiss KB, Mottur-Pilson C. The evidence base for tight blood pressure control in the management of type 2 diabetes mellitus. Ann Intern Med. 2003;138:587-92.

55. Lim LS, Wong TY. Lipids and diabetic retinopathy. Expert Opin Biol Ther. 2012;12(1):93-105.

56. Klein BE, Moss SE, Klein R, Surawicz TS. The Wisconsin Epidemiologic Study of Diabetic Retinopathy: XIII. Relationship of serum cholesterol to retinopathy and hard exudate. Ophthalmology. 1991;98:1261-5.

57. Tapp RJ, Shaw JE, Harper CA. The prevalence of and factors associated with diabetic retinopathy in the Australian population. Diabetes Care. 2003;26:1731-7.

58. Wong TY, Cheung N, Tay WT. Prevalence and risk factors for diabetic retinopathy: the Singapore Malay Eye Study. Ophthalmology. 2008;115:1869-75.

59. Lyons TJ, Jenkins AJ, Zheng D, et al. Diabetic retinopathy and serum lipoprotein subclasses in the DCCT/EDIC cohort. Invest Ophthalmol Vis Sci. 2004;45(3):910-8.

60. Keech AC, Mitchell P, Summanen PA, et al. Effect of fenofibrate on the need for laser treatment for diabetic retinopathy (FIELD study): a randomised controlled trial. Lancet. 2007 Nov 17;370(9600):1687-97.

61. Klein R, Lee KE, Gangnon RE, Klein BEK. The 25-year incidence of visual impairment in type 1 diabetes mellitus: the Wisconsin Epidemiologic Study of Diabetic Retinopathy. Ophthalmology. 2010;117(1):63-70.

62. Klein R, Klein BE, Moss SE, et al. The Wisconsin Epidemiologic Study of Diabetic Retinopathy: IX. Four-year incidence and progression of diabetic retinopathy when age at diagnosis is less than 30 years. Arch Ophthalmol. 1989;107(2):237-43.

63. Klein R, Klein BE, Moss SE, et al. The Wisconsin Epidemiologic Study of Diabetic Retinopathy: X. Four-year incidence and progression of diabetic retinopathy when age at diagnosis is 30 years or more. Arch Ophthalmol. 1989;107(2):244-9.

64. Klein R, Sharrett AR, Klein BE, et al. The association of atherosclerosis, vascular risk factors, and retinopathy in adults with diabetes: the atherosclerosis risk in communities study. Ophthalmology. 2002;109:1225-34.

65. The Diabetes Control and Complications Trial (DCCT). The relationship of glycemic exposures (HbA1c) to the risk of development and progression of retinopathy. Diabetes. 1995;44:968-83.

66. The Diabetes Control and Complications Trial (DCCT) Research Group. The effect of intensive diabetes treatment on the progression of diabetic retinopathy in insulin dependent diabetes mellitus. Arch Ophthalmol. 1995;113:36-51.

67. The Diabetic Retinopathy Study (DRS) Research Group. Report no. 14. Indications for photocoagulation treatment of diabetic retinopathy. Int Ophthalmol Clin. 1987;27:239-53.

68. The Diabetic Retinopathy Study (DRS) Research Group. DRS report no. 3. Four risk factors for severe visual loss in diabetic retinopathy. Arch Ophthalmol. 1979;97:654-5.

69. Early Treatment Diabetic Retinopathy Study Research Group. ETDRS report no. 9. Early photocoagulation for diabetic retinopathy. Ophthalmology. 1991;98:766-85.

70. Early Treatment Diabetic Retinopathy Study Research Group. ETDRS report no. 19. Focal photocoagulation treatment of diabetic macular edema: relationship of treatment effect to fluorescein angiographic and other retinal characteristics at baseline. Arch Ophthalmol. 1995;113:1144-55.

71. The Diabetic Retinopathy Vitrectomy Study Research Group. Diabetic Retinopathy Vitrectomy Study report no. 2. Early vitrectomy for severe vitreous hemorrhage in diabetic retinopathy: two-year results of a randomized trial. Arch Ophthalmol. 1985;103:1644-52.

72. The Diabetic Retinopathy Vitrectomy Study Research Group. Diabetic Retinopathy Vitrectomy Study report no. 5. Early vitrectomy for severe vitreous hemorrhage in diabetic retinopathy: four-year results of a randomized trial. Arch Ophthalmol. 1990;108:958-64.

73. UK Prospective Diabetes Study (UKPDS) Group (UKPDS 34). Effect of intensive blood-glucose control with metformin on complications in overweight patients with type 2 diabetes. Lancet. 1998;352:854-65.

74. American Academy of Ophthalmology Quality of Care Committee Retina Panel. Preferred Practice Pattern for Diabetic Retinopathy. San Francisco: American Academy of Ophthalmology; 2003.

75. Early Treatment Diabetic Retinopathy Study Research Group. ETDRS report no. 1. Photocoagulation for diabetic macular edema. Arch Ophthalmol. 1985;103:1796-806.

76. Ho AC, Scott IU, Kim SJ, et al. Anti-vascular endothelial growth factor pharmacotherapy for diabetic macular edema: a report by the American Academy of Ophthalmology. Ophthalmology. 2012;119(10):2179-88.

77. Brown DM, Schmidt-Erfurth U, Do DV, et al. Intravitreal aflibercept for diabetic macular edema: 100-week results from the VISTA and VIVID studies. Ophthalmology. 2015 Oct;122(10):2044-52. doi:10.1016/j.ophtha.2015.06.017. Epub 2015 Jul 18.

78. Korobelnik JF, Do DV, Schmidt-Erfurth U, et al. Intravitreal aflibercept for diabetic macular edema. Ophthalmology. 2014 Nov;121(11):2247-54. doi:10.1016/j.ophtha.2014.05.006. Epub 2014 Jul 8.

79. Boyer DS, Yoon YH, Belfort R Jr, et al. Three-year, randomized, sham-controlled trial of dexamethasone intravitreal implant in patients with diabetic macular edema. Ophthalmology. 2014 Oct;121(10):1904-14. doi:10.1016/j.ophtha.2014.04.024. Epub 2014 Jun 4.

80. Campochiaro PA, Brown DM, Pearson A, et al. Long-term benefit of sustained-delivery fluocinolone acetonide vitreous inserts for diabetic macular edema. Ophthalmology. 2011 Apr;118(4):626-35.e2. doi:10.1016/j.ophtha.2010.12.028.

81. Writing Committee for the Diabetic Retinopathy Clinical Research Network. Panretinal photocoagulation vs intravitreous ranibizumab for proliferative diabetic retinopathy: a randomized clinical trial. JAMA. 2015 Nov 24;314(20):2137-46. doi:10.1001/jama.2015.15217.

82. Klein R, Klein BE, Moss SE, et al. The Wisconsin Epidemiologic Study of Diabetic Retinopathy: III. Prevalence and risk of diabetic retinopathy when age of diagnosis is 30 or more years. Arch Ophthalmol. 1984;102:527-32.

83. Klein R, Klein BE, Moss SE, et al. Retinopathy in young-onset diabetic patients. Diabetes Care. 1985;8:311-5.

84. Krolewski AS, Warram JH, Rand LI, et al. Risk of proliferative diabetic retinopathy in juvenile onset type I diabetes: a 40-year follow-up study. Diabetes Care. 1986;9:443-52.

85. Klein R, Klein BE, Moss SE, et al. The Wisconsin Epidemiologic Study of Diabetic Retinopathy: II. Prevalence and risk of diabetic retinopathy when age at diagnosis is less than 30 years. Arch Ophthalmol. 1984;102:520-6.

86. The Diabetic Retinopathy Study Research Group. Preliminary report on effects of photocoagulation therapy. Am J Ophthalmol. 1976;81:383-96.

87. Ferris F. Early photocoagulation in patients with either type I or type II diabetes. Trans Am Ophthalmol Soc. 1996;94:505-37.

88. Early Treatment Diabetic Retinopathy Study Research Group. ETDRS report no. 2. Treatment techniques and clinical guidelines for photocoagulation of diabetic macular edema. Ophthalmology. 1987;94:761-74.

89. Early Treatment Diabetic Retinopathy Study Research Group. ETDRS report no. 3. Techniques for scatter and local photocoagulation treatment of diabetic retinopathy. Int Ophthalmol Clin. 1987;27:254-64.

90. Tremolada G, Del Turco C, Lattanzio R, et al. The role of angiogenesis in the development of proliferative diabetic retinopathy: impact of intravitreal anti-VEGF treatment. Exp Diabetes Res. 2012;2012:728325.

91. Strom C, Sander B, Larsen N, et al. Diabetic macular edema assessed with optical coherence tomography and stereo fundus photography. Invest Ophthalmol Vis Sci. 2002;43:241-5.

92. Bernbaum M, Albert SG. Referring patients with diabetes and vision loss for rehabilitation—who is responsible? Diabetes Care. 1996;19:175-7.

93. Bernbaum M, Albert SG, Duckro PN. Psychosocial profiles in patients with visual impairment due to diabetic retinopathy. Diabetes Care. 1988;11:551-7.

94. Jacobson AM. Current concepts: the psychological care of patients with insulin-dependent diabetes mellitus. N Engl J Med. 1996;334:1249-53.

95. Wulsin LR, Jacobson AM, Rand LI. Psychosocial adjustment to advanced proliferative diabetic retinopathy. Diabetes Care. 1993;16:1061-6.

CHAPTER 27

Diabetic Kidney Disease

Elizabeth Van Dril, PharmD, BCPS, BCACP

Key Concepts

- Early detection and diagnosis of chronic kidney disease is essential for preventing and/or delaying further disease progression.
- Cardiovascular disease is the most common cause of death in persons with chronic kidney disease.
- For persons with type 2 diabetes and chronic kidney disease a sodium-glucose cotransporter 2 inhibitor should be considered for the treatment of hyperglycemia to reduce the risk of kidney disease progression and/or cardiovascular events.
- Initial antihypertensive treatment for persons with diabetes and chronic kidney disease (stage 3 or greater or stage 1 or 2 with severely increased albuminuria) should consist of an angiotensin-converting enzyme inhibitor or angiotensin receptor blocker.

Introduction

The spectrum of changes in the kidney that occur among individuals diagnosed with diabetes that cannot be attributed to other causes has been called *diabetic nephropathy*, or preferably, *diabetic kidney disease* (DKD).[1] The spectrum of DKD ranges from those with mild disease in the form of microalbuminuria to more overt disease that is characterized by persistent albuminuria, hypertension, and a progressive decline in kidney function, which may lead to renal replacement therapies (RRTs; ie, hemodialysis, peritoneal dialysis, or transplantation) and/or premature mortality from cardiovascular disease (CVD). Appropriate and timely intervention may delay or prevent microalbuminuria from progressing to kidney failure.[1,2]

Chronic kidney disease (CKD) is a growing public health problem in the United States, with its current prevalence estimated at 15% of the population.[3] Recent statistics from the United States Renal Data System (USRDS) indicate that diabetes is the most common comorbid risk factor for CKD; however, the prevalence of CKD among individuals with diabetes has decreased from 44 to 36 percent over the past 20 years. This is likely due to the innovative therapeutic approaches that have improved the management of diabetes and its complications, and therefore increased the life expectancy of these individuals.

Rates of obesity in the United States continue to rise, affecting 39.8% of adults and 18.5% of youth in 2015–2016.[4] The growing obesity epidemic has contributed to the increase in prevalence of diabetes with current trends in the U.S. estimating that the prevalence will increase from 1 in every 10 adults to 1 in every 3 adults by the year 2050.[5,6] As persons with diabetes receive earlier diagnoses, they have the potential for longer durations of suboptimal glycemic management. If not well managed over time, the incidence of complications, such as CKD, will increase and influence the number of individuals eligible for conservative renal management and/or RRTs.

Historically, persons with DKD initiating dialysis had the highest rate of mortality among the 3 leading causes of kidney failure (ie, diabetes, hypertension, and glomerulonephritis).[7] More recent data demonstrate an overall decline in mortality among ESRD patients, and this increased lifespan may be a primary reason for continued growth of this patient population.[3] Regardless of the risk factors implicated in its development, the primary cause of death among persons with CKD is CVD. The presence of diabetes and CVD as comorbidities in CKD further increases the risk for death. In 2016, persons with CKD alone had an adjusted mortality rate of 47 deaths per 1,000 patient-years, while the mortality rate for those with CKD with both diabetes and CVD was almost tripled at 138 deaths per 1,000 patient-years.[3] Among dialysis patients, cardiovascular causes (ie, arrhythmias, cardiac arrest, congestive heart failure, acute myocardial infarction, atherosclerotic heart disease) accounted for 48% of all deaths in this population. Thus, a comprehensive treatment approach for

CKD should integrate the proactive management of diabetes as well as primary and secondary prevention strategies for CVD.

Kidney Function in Health and Disease

The kidney is an intricate vital organ that maintains homeostasis within the body through regulation of fluid volume, sodium and potassium levels, acid-base ratios, and calcium-phosphorus balance.[8] The kidney is one of the main detoxifying organs of the body; it excretes waste products such as excess water, electrolytes, metabolites, drugs, and other potentially harmful toxins. Lastly, it supplies endocrine functions necessary to maintain bone health, blood pressure, normal metabolism, and red blood cell production.

To fully appreciate the kidney's diverse functions, it is important to first review its complex structure. The urinary system is composed of the kidneys, ureters, bladder, and urethra.[9] The outer core of each kidney is encapsulated by a fibrous, rigid sheath that forms the renal cortex, and directly underneath this cortex is the medulla. Individual nephrons, the functional units of the kidney, and their collecting tubules transverse these 2 segments. Each kidney has over 1 million nephrons. Within each nephron are several components:[9]

- *Glomerulus and Bowman's capsule.* A network of capillaries, known as a tuft, make up the branches of small arteries in the glomerulus. Through this tuft of afferent and efferent arterioles, blood flows into and out of the kidney. The exchange of waste products occurs at the Bowman's capsule. Each day, approximately 180 L of filtrate pass through the kidneys at the glomerulus; however, almost 99% of this filtrate is reabsorbed through the remainder of the urinary system, resulting in the production of only 1–2 L of urine per day.
- *Proximal convoluted tubule.* This section of the nephron, which is directly connected to the Bowman's capsule, is the main location where glucose, sodium, bicarbonate, potassium, chloride, calcium, phosphate, and other solutes are reabsorbed after being filtered at the glomerulus. Sodium-potassium ATPase pumps as well as osmotic reabsorption with the aforementioned solutes make the proximal convoluted tubule the primary site for water reabsorption.
- *Loop of Henle.* This is the site where urine is concentrated or diluted. The process is largely dictated by the fluid requirements of the body.
- *Distal convoluted tubule.* This short tubule contains the macula densa at the area adjacent to the ascending limb of the loop of Henle. The specialized cells of the macula densa sense fluctuations in the filtrate's sodium and chloride concentrations and emit signals to adjust afferent arteriole blood flow, and therefore glomerular hydrostatic pressure, to regulate the glomerular filtration rate. This process is termed tubuloglomerular feedback. The distal convoluted tubule is also the site responsible for regulating pH, sodium, potassium, and calcium levels.
- *Collecting duct.* Secretion of potassium is a major function of the collecting duct and is primarily regulated by the hormone, aldosterone. As urine is produced in the nephrons, it flows from the collecting duct to the main cavity of the renal pelvis, then on to the ureter into the bladder, and then it is expelled through the urethra.

Renal Physiology

Through glomerular filtration, reabsorption, and tubular secretion, the kidneys are able to regulate the chemical composition of the blood and eliminate metabolic waste.[8] Homeostatic regulation of the urine osmolality is controlled by the distal convoluted tubules and collecting ducts.[9] Reabsorption and transport of water greatly varies with cellular permeability and is largely affected by secretion of antidiuretic hormone (ADH) from the pituitary gland.[10] As plasma osmolality increases in a dehydrated condition, ADH secretion increases so that water is conserved by the kidneys; the opposite is true in a hypervolemic state.

The kidneys are also one of the sites responsible for maintaining calcium and phosphorus levels.[11] Parathyroid hormone (PTH), secreted by the parathyroid glands, plays an integral role in maintaining these levels. The hormone maintains this balance by enhancing calcium and phosphorus absorption from the gastrointestinal tract, resorption from the bone, and reabsorption at the proximal tubule of the kidney. During episodes of increased calcium intake, there is a transitory rise in circulating levels of calcium with a subsequent decrease in PTH secretion. This results in less calcium being reabsorbed at the kidneys and increases the amount excreted. The inverse occurs during periods of low dietary calcium intake. Parathyroid hormone synthesis and release also respond to variations in circulating levels of serum phosphorus, irrespective of serum calcium or vitamin D levels. Additionally, the final step in the activation of vitamin D occurs within the kidneys. Vitamin D is essential for assisting with calcium absorption from the intestinal lumen and maintains calcium-phosphorus homeostasis and overall bone health with the help of calcitonin and PTH.

It is evident that multiple functions of the kidneys are regulated by a number of hormones; however, the kidneys themselves are responsible for the production of certain hormones that are vital to the endocrine system as well.[10] For instance, renin and erythropoietin are produced and released by the kidneys to stimulate effects in the cardiovascular and hematopoietic systems, respectively. Renin, an enzyme, is vital to regulating blood pressure and is secreted by the kidneys in response to a decrease in blood volume. Renin acts to convert angiotensinogen to angiotensin I, which is further converted to angiotensin II by angiotensin-converting enzyme. Angiotensin II serves as a powerful vasoconstrictor and triggers the release of aldosterone, which enhances sodium and water retention. Erythropoietin, a hormone secreted by the kidneys, acts by stimulating the bone marrow to produce red blood cells, and its deficiency in advanced stages of CKD is implicated in the development of anemias. As evident from the discussion of their many functions and role in maintaining homeostasis in multiple systems, the kidneys are one of the most vital organs in the body and why multiple complications arise when their function declines.

Disorders of Renal Function

Kidney impairment may be either sudden, causing acute kidney injury, or progressive in nature, as in CKD.

Chronic Kidney Disease

The National Kidney Foundation–Kidney Disease Outcomes Quality Initiative (NKF-KDOQI) develops evidence-based practice guidelines for the management and treatment of all stages and related complications of kidney disease. It published its first set of guidelines for the evaluation, classification, and stratification of CKD in 2002, which helped to standardize the language associated with kidney disease because synonymous terms were easily confused.[12] Commonly used terms such as *pre-dialysis*, *pre-ESRD*, and *chronic renal insufficiency* were replaced with a formal staging system. In 2012, KDIGO (Kidney Disease: Improving Global Outcomes) published an updated guideline to provide recommendations for the evaluation and management of CKD based on evidence published since 2002.[2] This guideline update clarified the definition of CKD and revised recommendations for its classification based cause, glomerular filtration rate (GFR) and albuminuria category.

Diagnosis of Chronic Kidney Disease

Chronic kidney disease is defined by structural or functional abnormalities of the kidney, as outlined by either of the criteria below, for >3 months:[2]

- GFR <60 mL/min/1.73 m^2 (Stages 3a–5)
- Persistent albuminuria
  - —Urine albumin-to-creatinine ratio (UACR) ≥30 mg/g creatinine or ≥3 mg/mmol creatinine
  - —Albumin excretion rate (AER) ≥30 mg/24 hours
- Other manifestations of kidney damage
  - —Urine sediment abnormalities
  - —Electrolyte and other abnormalities due to tubular disorders
  - —Abnormalities detected by histology or imaging
  - —History of kidney transplantation

Stages of CKD

The updated standardized CKD classification and staging system using GFR and degree of albuminuria was outlined by KDIGO in 2012.[2] This information is summarized in Table 27.1. Glomerular filtration rate is estimated from serum creatinine using a number of validated formulas; however, KDIGO specifically recommends the Chronic Kidney Disease Epidemiology Collaboration (CKD-EPI) equation over other equations.

Acute Kidney Injury

Persons with acute kidney injury (AKI) typically present with a rapid elevation in serum creatinine and blood urea nitrogen (BUN), with a corresponding rapid decline in estimated glomerular filtration rate (eGFR) over a relatively short time period. Diabetes itself increases the risk for AKI compared to persons without diabetes, and the presence of preexisting CKD, exposure to nephrotoxic agents, and the use of medications that affect pre-renal and intrarenal hemodynamics are also known risk factors for acute injury.[13] These medications include antihypertensive medications that are often used in the management of persons with CKD (eg, diuretics and renin-angiotensin-aldosterone system [RAAS] inhibitors), and can reduce glomerular filtration by decreasing intravascular volume and/or altering renal blood flow.

TABLE 27.1 Staging of CKD and Prognosis by GFR and Albuminuria Category

GFR Categories (Description and Range)					Persistent Albuminuria Categories (Description and Range)		
					A1	*A2*	*A3*
					Normal to mildly increased	*Moderately increased*	*Severely increased*
	CKD Stage		*Quantitative Description*	*eGFR (mL/min/1.73 m²)*	*<30 mg/g <3 mg/mmol*	*30–300 mg/g 3–30 mg/mmol*	*>300 mg/g >30 mg/mmol*
			At increased risk, CKD risk factors	≥60			
	1	G1	Normal or high eGFR	≥90	Low risk*	Moderately increased risk	High risk
	2	G2	Mildly decreased eGFR	60–89	Low risk*	Moderately increased risk	High risk
	3	G3a	Mildly to moderately decreased eGFR	45–59	Moderately increased risk	High risk	Very high risk
		G3b	Moderately to severely decreased eGFR	30–44	High risk	Very high risk	Very high risk
	4	G4	Severely decreased eGFR	15–29	Very high risk	Very high risk	Very high risk
	5	G5	Kidney failure, ESRD	<15	Very high risk	Very high risk	Very high risk

*Low risk if no other markers of kidney disease

Abbreviations: CKD, chronic kidney disease; eGFR, estimated glomerular filtration rate; ESRD, end-stage renal disease

Adapted from: Kidney Disease: Improving Global Outcomes (KDIGO) CKD Work Group, "KDIGO 2012 clinical practice guideline for the evaluation and management of chronic kidney disease," *Kidney Int Suppl.* 3(2013):1–150.

Regardless of its cause, identification and management in a timely manner are paramount to reducing the morbidity and mortality associated with AKI, as each episode increases the risk for CKD progression.[14]

Diabetic Kidney Disease

Long-standing and/or suboptimal management of diabetes can result in a type of CKD known as diabetic kidney disease. Its clinical diagnosis is made based on the presence of albuminuria and/or reduced eGFR (<60mL/min/1.73 m^2) in the absence of other primary causes of CKD.[15] Not all kidney disease that is found in persons with diabetes represents DKD. The presentation of DKD usually occurs with diabetes of long-standing duration, retinopathy, albuminuria without hematuria, and progressive decline in eGFR. In some cases of type 2 diabetes, DKD can occur without the presence of retinopathy and may be present at diagnosis because diabetes may be present for many years before the diagnosis is made.

Pathophysiology

Hyperglycemia plays a role in the pathogenesis of DKD. Alteration in tubuloglomerular feedback occurs, resulting in dilation of the afferent arterioles, increased renal blood flow, and hyperfiltration at the glomerulus.[16] Accelerated formation of non-enzymatic advanced glycation end-products (AGEs) in tissues is directly correlated with hyperglycemia, and an increase in circulating AGEs parallels the severity of renal dysfunction.[17] Glycosylation of proteins in the capillary basement membrane may stimulate mesangial expansion, a common structural abnormality in DKD. Glycation of albumin can also contribute to its loss across the glomerular basement membrane.

Other hormonal imbalances, aside from insulin insufficiency or resistance, have been implicated in the pathogenesis of DKD. Growth hormone and glucagon, both of which are elevated in the presence of hyperglycemia, have been shown to cause glomerular hyperfiltration.[17]

Neurohormonal activation results in changes in circulating levels of angiotensin II, catecholamines, and prostaglandins.[16] Increased concentrations and altered responsiveness to these vasoactive hormones promote glomerular hypertension, characterized by increased pressure and flow across the glomerular membrane, and therefore results in hyperfiltration. Hyperfiltration, a consequence of glomerular hypertension coupled with vasodilation of afferent arterioles, increases glomerular protein filtration, leading to proteinuria and glomerulosclerosis with consequent destruction of nephrons.

Risk Factors

Risk factors for DKD may be classified as modifiable and nonmodifiable, and are summarized in Table 27.2. Modifiable risk factors implicated in the onset of DKD also contribute to its rate of progression in individuals with a diagnosis; therefore, these risk factors should continue to be evaluated and managed through advanced stages of kidney disease. Table 27.3 further elaborates guideline recommendations for the focus of kidney-related care as individuals progress through various stages of renal impairment.

Nonmodifiable Risk Factors Age, gender, ethnicity, family history of CKD, and duration of diabetes are considered nonmodifiable risk factors for DKD.[18] Advanced age is the most common risk factor for DKD given renal

TABLE 27.2 Risk Factors for Onset and Progression of Diabetic Kidney Disease

Modifiable risk factors	*Nonmodifiable risk factors*
Hyperglycemia Elevated blood pressure Dyslipidemia Obesity and metabolic syndrome Smoking Exposure to nephrotoxic agents	Advanced age (>60 years-old) Ethnicity Genetic factors Family history of diabetic kidney disease, type 2 diabetes, hypertension, and insulin resistance Longer duration of diabetes

Sources: National Kidney Foundation, "KDOQI clinical practice guideline for diabetes and CKD: 2012 update," *Am J Kidney Dis.* 60(2012):850–86.; American Diabetes Association, "Standards of medical care in diabetes—2019," *Diabetes Care.* 42(2019) Suppl 1:S1–193.; V Harjutsalo, PH Groop, "Epidemiology and risk factors for diabetic kidney disease," *Adv Chronic Kidney Dis.* 21(2014):260–6.

TABLE 27.3 Focus of Kidney-related Care by CKD Stage

CKD Stage†				*Focus of kidney-related care*			
Stage		*eGFR (mL/min/1.73 m²)*	*Evidence of kidney damage*	*Diagnose cause of kidney injury*	*Evaluate and treat risk factors for CKD progression*	*Evaluate and treat CKD complications*	*Prepare for renal replacement therapy*
No clinical evidence of CKD		≥60	–				
1	G1	≥90	+	✔	✔		
2	G2	60–89	+	✔	✔		
3	G3a	45–59	+/–	✔	✔	✔	
	G3b	30–44					
4	G4	15–29	+/–		✔	✔	✔
5	G5	<15	+/–			✔	✔

† CKD Stages 1 and 2 are defined by evidence of kidney damage (+), while stages 3 to 5 are defined by reduced eGFR with or without evidence of kidney damage (+/–).

*Markers of kidney damage include albuminuria (urine albumin-to-creatinine ratio >30 mg/g Cr), urine sediment abnormalities, electrolyte, and other abnormalities due to tubular disorders, histological, pathological or structural abnormalities, or history of kidney transplantation.

Adapted from: American Diabetes Association, "Standards of medical care in diabetes—2019," *Diabetes Care.* 42(2019) Suppl 1:S1–193.

function naturally declines with increasing age. It is estimated that renal function decreases approximately 1 mL/minute/year for patients in the general population over the age of 40 years.[19] The prevalence of CKD was highest in patients 60 years of age and older at 32.2% in 2013–2016, which demonstrated a decrease compared to a prevalence of 33.1% in this population for the 2009–2012 period.[3] Conversely, the rate of CKD has been rising in younger populations, with its prevalence increasing from 5.5 to 6.3% in populations aged 20–39 years and from 8.3% to 10.4% in those aged 40–59 years over this same time period.

The most recent population data from the USRDS shows that 16.7% of females and 12.9% of males in the United States have established CKD, suggesting that females have a slightly higher risk of kidney disease in the general population.[3] Men were historically thought to be more susceptible to DKD compared to women in the presence of both type 1 and type 2 diabetes; however, recent evidence suggests that the risk for the development and progression of nondiabetic nephropathy is lower for females but that this protection disappears in the presence of diabetes.[20,21]

There are well-documented race/ethnic differences in the rate of DKD and subsequent cases of ESRD. The prevalence of DKD Is approximately two- to threefold higher in African Americans, Hispanics, and Asians compared to Caucasians.[22] The risk for DKD is up to 18-fold higher in Native Americans compared to Caucasians. In an analysis examining the rates of nonproteinuric versus proteinuric DKD by ethnicity, minorities were at higher risk for proteinuric DKD, and therefore increased risk for faster progression to ESRD, compared to non-Hispanic whites.

Evidence also supports a strong genetic predisposition for DKD. Familial clustering of kidney disease has been observed in persons with type 1 and type 2 diabetes.[23–25] This may in part be due to the genes associated with modifiable risk factors. For example, a parental history of type 2 diabetes, hypertension, cardiovascular disease, and insulin resistance are all considered individual risk factors for the development of kidney disease in persons with diabetes, suggesting that these disorders are linked to DKD by a complex interrelated genetic predisposition.[25]

The risk of developing DKD increases with the duration of diabetes. The incidence of DKD historically peaked 15 to 20 years after a diagnosis of type 1 diabetes.[26,27] Given that type 2 diabetes may be present but undetected for some time prior to an official diagnosis, the true duration of disease before the development of DKD is unknown. However, for those without DKD present at their diagnosis of type 2 diabetes, early implementation of intensive lifestyle interventions may delay the onset of disease complications, including DKD.[28] Therefore, age at onset and resulting duration of type 2 diabetes may not be a fully nonmodifiable risk factor.

Modifiable Risk Factors The presence of hyperglycemia, elevated blood pressure, dyslipidemia, obesity, and smoking are well-documented modifiable risk factors for the onset and progression of DKD.[1,15,18] Optimization of antihyperglycemic therapy to achieve near normoglycemia has been shown to prevent the onset and delay the progression of DKD in several landmark trials.[29–33] In the Diabetes Control and Complications Trial (DCCT) evaluating persons with type 1 diabetes, intensive glycemic management lowered the risk for microalbuminuria by 34%, and in individuals with microalbuminuria at baseline, the risk for further disease progression was reduced by 56%.[29] The U.K. Prospective Diabetes Study (UKPDS) demonstrated that individuals with type 2 diabetes had a 25% relative risk reduction in microvascular complications, which included fatal and nonfatal renal failure, when intensive antihyperglycemic therapy was initiated.[30] Additionally, for every 1% drop in A1C, there was a 37% reduction in risk for complications.[34]

Hypertension is another major risk factor for the development of DKD.[2,15,35] Elevations in blood pressure have shown to correlate with increases in albuminuria, and a number of studies have substantiated the inverse relationship between blood pressure and GFR; that is, as blood pressure rises, the GFR drops.[18,36] Persons with DKD often present with dyslipidemia, typically characterized by abnormally high plasma levels of low-density lipoprotein (LDL), very low-density lipoprotein (VLDL), intermediate-density lipoprotein, and triglycerides, and abnormally low levels of high-density lipoprotein (HDL) cholesterol.[37] Metabolic syndrome, characterized by abdominal obesity in the presence of the aforementioned modifiable risk factors (ie, hyperglycemia, hypertension, and dyslipidemia) independently increases the risk for DKD by approximately 3.75-fold after adjustment for traditional risk factors.[38] Additionally, smoking is a known risk factor for the development of microvascular and macrovascular complications of diabetes and results in poor outcomes in dialysis and transplantation.[2,15]

Concurrent Complications From Diabetes The presence of existing retinopathy and neuropathy in persons with diabetes may indicate an increased risk for also developing DKD, yet there is evidence to suggest that this is not always the case.[15] In a study of persons with both type 1 and type 2 diabetes, retinopathy was present in the majority of persons with type 1 diabetes and macroalbuminuria independent of the presence of hypertension.[39] In contrast, up to 47.5% of persons with type 2 diabetes did not have signs of retinopathy despite the presence of hypertension and overt proteinuria. Thus, while it is rare for persons with type 1 diabetes to develop CKD without retinopathy, it is considered to have only moderate sensitivity and specificity for the presence of DKD in persons with type 2 diabetes.[40]

Progression of Disease

Rates of decline in GFR are highly variable in individuals with DKD. Age and the presence of risk factors, such as hypertension, dyslipidemia, or poor glycemic management, may dictate the rate of disease progression. In the absence of medical intervention, 80% of persons with type 1 diabetes will progress to albuminuria (>300 mg per day) in 10 to 15 years.[41] Progression rates cited in the literature vary widely; however, generally trend according to type of diabetes:

- *Type 1 diabetes.* In individuals with type 1 diabetes with albuminuria, approximately 50% will develop ESRD within 10 years, and 75% within 20 years.
- *Type 2 diabetes.* In the absence of clinical interventions, only 20% to 40% of individuals with type 2 diabetes with microalbuminuria will progress to albuminuria. Of those who develop albuminuria, 20% are expected to progress to ESRD within 20 years.

Persons diagnosed with CKD experience a permanent decrease in GFR that occurs over a period of months to years. Eventually, progression through the stages of CKD leads to the fifth and final stage, which requires RRT in the form of dialysis or transplantation to sustain life. Although RRTs are discussed, the focus of this chapter is on strategies to delay or prevent progression of disease.

Screening and Detection

Recommended Frequency of Screening for DKD

- *Type 1 diabetes:* 5 years after diagnosis; annually thereafter
- *Type 2 diabetes:* At diagnosis and annually thereafter; also during pregnancy

As discussed previously, DKD is a clinical diagnosis made based on presence of albuminuria and/or eGFR <60 ml/min/1.73 m^2 attributed to diabetes.[15] Measurement of urinary albumin and estimation of glomerular filtration rate are therefore the primary screening tests used to detect CKD. After an official diagnosis, these tests are also used to monitor disease progression, detect superimposed kidney diseases (eg, AKI), estimate risk for complications, facilitate appropriate medication dosing, and determine when patients require specialized nephrology care.

Frequency of Screening

In type 2 diabetes, hyperglycemia may have been present but undetected for an extended period prior to an official diagnosis. This may result in varying degrees of complications, including renal impairment, upon identification of disease. Thus, screening for DKD should be performed at the time of diagnosis of type 2 diabetes and annually thereafter.[15] Given the clinical course of disease onset in persons with type 1 diabetes, DKD is unlikely to be present at diagnosis; however, these patients have a progressive risk of overt nephropathy and kidney failure as the duration of diabetes increases. As a result, annual screening starting 5 years after diagnosis of type 1 diabetes facilitates appropriate early detection.

Albuminuria

Measurement of the urinary albumin-to-creatinine ratio (UACR) in a random spot urine collection is the recommended screening method for albuminuria.[15] While a timed or 24-hour urine collection was historically the "gold standard" for quantification of albuminuria, missed or improperly timed samples and the burden of the collection process make it neither a cost-effective nor an efficient method to assess for albuminuria. Additionally, because variations in hydration status and resulting urine concentration can affect urinary albumin, spot measurements of albumin alone without simultaneous measurement of creatinine are not recommended due to the risk for false-positive and false-negative results.

A normal UACR is defined as <30 mg/g creatinine, while abnormal urinary albumin excretion is classified as moderately increased if 30 to 300 mg/g creatinine (A2 albuminuria, formerly termed "microalbuminuria") and severely increased if >300 mg/g creatinine (A3 albuminuria, formerly termed "macroalbuminuria").[2] Two of three spot UACRs, preferably from first-void urine samples, collected within a 3- to 6-month period, must be abnormal to be able to diagnose albuminuria.[2,15] Confirmation of an abnormal measurement is required due to natural variability in urinary albumin excretion. For example, UACR can increase independently of renal function in the presence of infection, fever, recent strenuous exercise, menstruation, extensive hyperglycemia, and heart failure.[15]

Estimating Glomerular Filtration Rate

Glomerular filtration rate is the best overall index of kidney function, as it measures the cumulative filtration rates of the functioning nephrons within the kidney.[42] A normal GFR in a healthy, young adult is typically 120 to 130 mL/min/1.73 m^2, but will vary depending on age, sex, and body size and declines naturally with age. While GFR cannot be measured directly, kidney function can be estimated from endogenous filtration markers, such as serum creatinine levels (SCr), and other variables, such as gender, age, weight, and race, using validated formulas. These formulas include the Cockcroft-Gault formula, Modification of Diet in Renal Disease (MDRD) Study equation, and the Chronic Kidney Disease Epidemiology Collaboration (CKD-EPI) equation.

Cockcroft-Gault Formula

The Cockcroft-Gault formula was originally developed in 1973 and is used to estimate creatinine clearance (CrCl) rather than GFR, as it does not adjust for body surface area.[42] The equation was derived from a study of 249 males with CrCl ranging from 30 to 130 mL/min, making the formula less reliable in more diverse patient populations and individuals with lower kidney function. An additional limitation to its use in estimating kidney function is the discrepancy that arises with use of ideal body weight, actual body weight, or adjusted body weight in the equation for individualized dosing, depending on the clinical scenario. The Cockcroft-Gault formula also assumes that SCr is at steady state for its calculation of CrCl and is therefore less reliable in instances of rapidly changing kidney function.

In 2010, the National Kidney Foundation (NKF) led the initiative to standardize creatinine assays in clinical laboratories.[42] While other formulas used to estimate GFR were either originally designed or re-expressed to account for these standardized assays, the Cockcroft-Gault formula has not been re-expressed for use with these standardized assays resulting in GFR estimates that are higher and less accurate than estimates derived from non-standardized assays.[43] Due to these documented inaccuracies, the Cockcroft-Gault formula is no longer preferred for clinical use.[42,43]

Modification of Diet in Renal Disease Study Equation

In 1999, the MDRD Study equation was derived using data from 1,628 CKD patients whose GFR ranged from 5 to 90 mL/min/1.73 m^2.[42] The 4-variable equation uses age, sex, race, and SCr to estimate GFR, and is widely used to stage CKD. It does not require body weight because the results are normalized to a body surface area of 1.73 m^2, which is the generally accepted mean for adults.

The MDRD Study equation provides a more accurate estimation of GFR than those from the Cockcroft-Gault formula or direct measurements from 24-hour urine collections.[42,44] Its utility is questionable in patients with mild-to-moderate renal insufficiency, as the equation consistently underestimates GFR in individuals with normal renal function (GFR >60 mL/min/1.73 m^2), thereby overestimating the prevalence of CKD Stages 1 and 2 in the general population. The MDRD Study equation has demonstrated reasonable accuracy in nonhospitalized patients and those with severe renal impairment, and is generally regarded as more accurate than the Cockcroft-Gault formula in older and obese patients.[45,46] Due to the complexity of the calculation, MDRD Study equation calculators are available through mobile applications, integrated into medical software, and available online. For example, the NKF Web site has calculators for multiple formulas to estimate GFR, including the MDRD Study equation, and can be located at https://www.kidney.org/professionals/KDOQI/gfr_calculator.

Chronic Kidney Disease Epidemiology Collaboration Equation

Similar to the MDRD Study equation, the CKD-EPI equation uses age, sex, race, and SCr to estimate GFR.[47] The equation was developed in 2009 from a cohort of 8,254 Caucasian and African American individuals with and without diabetes and solid organ transplants aged 18 to 97 years, whose GFR ranged from 2 to 198 mL/min/1.73 m^2. It was then validated in a separate cohort of 3,896 people with a similarly diverse age (18-93 years-old) and GFR range (2-200 mL/min/1.73 m^2).

Compared to the MDRD Study equation, the CKD-EPI equation is substantially more accurate at higher levels of GFR (>60 mL/min/1.73 m^2) and has demonstrated similar accuracy in individuals with lower levels of GFR (<60 mL/min/1.73 m^2) and those with CKD.[42] As a result, the NKF and the 2012 KDIGO guidelines now recommend that clinical laboratories use the CKD-EPI equation to report eGFR, and it appears to be emerging as the preferred method for staging CKD.[42,48,49] While its utility in drug dosing is emerging, it is generally recommended that clinicians use the estimation method that provides the most accurate assessment of GFR.[49] Thus, most medications in the treatment of type 2 diabetes have transitioned to eGFR-based renal dosing recommendations using the CKD-EPI equation and have updated their published prescribing information accordingly. Online calculators are also available for the CKD-EPI equation, and an example can be found on the NKF Web site.

Implications of Screening

Early Identification Is Essential

Early identification and improved awareness of DKD facilitates appropriate management that may have the following desired effects:

- Prevent or delay the progression to ESRD
- Improve clinical outcomes of related complications of DKD

Despite disseminating these screening recommendations in the form of major evidence-based guidelines for diabetes care, the most recent data from USRDS indicates that CKD screening rates can be improved. Claims data indicated that testing for albuminuria was conducted for only 41.8% of Medicare persons with a diagnosis of diabetes in 2016.[3] This may contribute to the continued poor awareness of CKD in patients with early stages of their disease. For example, only 15% of patients with both hypertension and diabetes who were classified by laboratory measures as having CKD were aware of their kidney disease.[3] Awareness improved among individuals with stage 4 CKD, with 57% of patients with severe renal impairment reporting that they had the condition. This is likely secondary to improving referral mechanisms to specialized nephrology care in advanced stages of CKD. In 2018, the USRDS reported that 25% of patients with any CKD claim in 2015 were seen by a nephrologist over the subsequent year, while in 2016, 41.1% of patients with stage 3 CKD and approximately two thirds with

Case Study: New Onset DKD in Prolonged Hyperglycemia

MG is a 64-year-old widowed African-American woman who was diagnosed with type 2 diabetes approximately 10 years ago. She was referred to the primary care clinic for intensive diabetes education and self-management training after being lost to follow-up for the past 2 years. Her blood pressure this visit is 148/92 mmHg (up from 138/86 mmHg last visit) with a heart rate of 99 bpm. Her is height 5 ft 3 in, and weight is 190 lb (BMI 33.65 kg/m^2). MG does not smoke tobacco and she drinks approximately 1–2 glasses of wine per week.

From the most recent laboratory results, it is evident MG is currently at Stage 3 CKD, with an eGFR of 46 mL/min/1.73 m^2. MG's spot urine albumin-to-creatinine ratio should be repeated over the next 3 to 6 months to confirm the patient has moderately increased albuminuria (A2 albuminuria; 30–300 mg/g creatinine); however, this would not change recommendations for management at this time.

The diagnosis of DKD is substantiated by the elevation in the fasting blood glucose level and A1C, which have likely been unchanged over the past 1 to 2 years given the loss to follow-up. MG is slightly anemic (hemoglobin <11.0 g/dL). MG is also at considerable cardiovascular risk, not only because of the presence of albuminuria, but also because she presented with uncontrolled hypertension, dyslipidemia, and obesity. Regarding her medications, MG is currently taking metformin 1,000 mg twice daily and glipizide 5 mg twice daily prior to meals for her type 2 diabetes, and ibuprofen 200 mg 2 to 4 tablets daily for knee pain.

Laboratory parameter	*Result*	*Reference Range*
Glucose, fasting (mg/dL)	175	<140
Creatinine (mg/dL)	1.4	0.6–1.2
eGFR (mL/min/1.73 m^2)	46	90–120
A1C (%)	8.5	<5.6
TC (mg/dL)	236	<200
LDL-C (mg/dL)	130	<100
HDL-C (mg/dL)	45	>40
TG (mg/dL)	345	<150
UACR (mg/g creatinine)	195	<30
Calcium (mg/dL)	8.9	8.4–9.5
Phosphorus (mg/dL)	4.0	2.7–4.6
Hemoglobin (g/dL)	10.1	>11.0
PTH (pg/mL)	65	35–70

stage 4 CKD or higher visited a nephrologist.[3] These data highlight the importance of early and regular screening for DKD and appropriate timing of referrals to specialized nephrology care to enhance patients' awareness of their condition and facilitate timely management of kidney disease, its complications, and comorbidities that are contributing to its progression.

Prevention and Delaying the Progression of CKD

Early Implementation of Interventions Are Key

The onset and rate of progression of DKD, as well as the increase in cardiovascular risk that results, may be mitigated by several interventions, including the following:[1,2,15]

- Optimizing glycemic management
- Optimizing blood pressure management
- Reducing risk of CVD
- Engaging in recommended levels of physical activity
- Attaining and maintaining a healthy body weight
- Achieving and maintaining smoking cessation, if applicable
- Eliminating or minimizing the use of nephrotoxic agents

These interventions are most effective when implemented early.

Multiple risk factors implicated in the onset and progression of DKD overlap with risk factors associated with increased cardiovascular risk. Therefore, targeting modifiable risk factors may reduce the risk of CVD in individuals with CKD and prevent the progression to ESRD.[2] For persons with diabetes and CKD stages 1 to 4, the focus of kidney-related care is identification and treatment of risk factors for CKD progression.[15] This includes evidence-based treatment of hyperglycemia and hypertension, measures to reduce cardiovascular risk, lifestyle modifications, and avoidance of nephrotoxic agents.[2,15]

Optimizing Glycemic Management

Optimizing glycemic management is the mainstay of therapy for preventing or delaying further disease progression. The American Diabetes Association (ADA) recommends measurement of the glycated hemoglobin A1C (A1C) as an effective tool to guide the management of persons with diabetes; however, nephrologists have reservations about its use, as the A1C may not consistently correlate with average blood glucose levels in patients with kidney disease.[15] Persons with advanced stages of DKD may have anemia of chronic disease with lower than normal hemoglobin levels. Erythrocyte survival times become shorter as eGFR falls, resulting in lower than expected A1C values when compared to individuals' glucose levels.[50] Although there have been several studies demonstrating a wide variability in the relationship between glucose and A1C levels at various stages of CKD, including hemodialysis, the clinical significance of this variability is considered to be negligible.[50–54] Thus, for persons with diabetes and CKD, A1C is still considered the best clinical indicator of long-term glycemic stability, particularly if interpreted with consideration of self-monitoring blood glucose measurements.[1]

Increased attention has been given to weighing the benefits of achieving recommended A1C goals against the risk of hypoglycemia in persons with diabetes. While there is extensive evidence that intensive treatment for glycemic management has nephroprotective effects, these studies have demonstrated an increased incidence of hypoglycemia in persons with type 1 and type 2 diabetes.[29–33] Additionally, in the Action to Control Cardiovascular Risk in Diabetes (ACCORD) trial, intensive glycemic management resulted in a significant increase in mortality and hypoglycemia in persons with type 2 diabetes and CKD at baseline.[55,56] As a result, KDOQI updated its recommendations to avoid intensifying treatment in persons with diabetes and CKD due to the risk associated with hypoglycemia.[1] The ADA Standards of Medical Care align with this recommendation, with an A1C goal of less than 7% for the general population, and go further to recommend less intensive goals in patients with CKD and substantial comorbidity.[15] Specifically, in older adults with end-stage illnesses, such as ESRD, an A1C goal of less than 8.5% may be appropriate to minimize the risk of hypoglycemia.

When evaluating the risk-benefit profile during the selection of glycemic treatment goals, it is important to be mindful of the patient's life expectancy, comorbid conditions, risk for hypoglycemia, and the financial burden of treatment. Recommended goals for A1C and corresponding fasting and bedtime glucose levels for various stages of CKD and complexities of comorbid conditions in older adults are summarized in Table 27.4; however, these recommendations may also be applied to younger patients with extensive comorbidities at high risk of hypoglycemia. To attain A1C goals and prevent the progression of DKD without undesired hypoglycemia and weight gain,

TABLE 27.4 Considerations for Glycemic Treatment Goals in Older Adults With Diabetes

Patient characteristics/ health status	*Rationale*	*Reasonable A1C goal*	*Fasting or preprandial glucose*	*Bedtime glucose*
Healthy (few coexisting chronic illnesses, intact cognitive and functional status)	Longer remaining life expectancy	<7.5% (58 mmol/mol)	90–130 mg/dL (5.0–7.2 mmol/L)	90–150 mg/dL (5.0–8.3 mmol/L)
Complex/intermediate (≥3 coexisting chronic illnesses* or ≥2 instrumental ADL impairments or mild-to-moderate cognitive impairment)	Intermediate remaining life expectancy, high treatment burden, hypoglycemia vulnerability, fall risk	<8.0% (64 mmol/mol)	90–150 mg/dL (5.0–8.3 mmol/L)	100–180 mg/dL (5.6–10.0 mmol/L)
Very complex/poor health (long-term care or end-stage chronic illnesses** or moderate-to-severe cognitive impairment or ≥2 ADL dependencies)	Limited remaining life expectancy makes benefit uncertain	<8.5% (69 mmol/mol)	100–180 mg/dL (5.6–10.0 mmol/L)	110–200 mg/dL (6.1–11.1 mmol/L)

* Coexisting chronic illnesses are conditions serious enough to require medications or lifestyle management and may include arthritis, cancer, heart failure, depression, emphysema, falls, hypertension, incontinence, stage 3 or worse CKD, myocardial infarction, and stroke.

**The presence of a single end-stage chronic illness, such as stages 3 to 4 heart failure or oxygen-dependent lung disease, CKD requiring dialysis, or uncontrolled metastatic cancer, may cause significant symptoms or impairment of functional status and significantly reduce life expectancy.

Adapted from: American Diabetes Association, "Standards of medical care in diabetes—2020," *Diabetes Care.* 43(2020) Suppl 1:S1–212.

implementation of dietary modifications, recommended levels of physical activity, optimal non-insulin antihyperglycemic medications, as well as insulin therapy, as necessary, are recommended.[15]

Non-Insulin Antihyperglycemic Medications

When reviewing non-insulin antihyperglycemic options for persons with type 2 diabetes, a patient's preferences and chronic comorbidities should be considered in the selection of therapies. First and foremost is the safety of medications in the setting of declining renal function, the second consideration being the potential for reducing cardiovascular and renal clinical outcomes with the use of certain therapies. The publication of the Food and Drug Administration (FDA)-mandated outcomes trials to assess the cardiovascular safety of all new antihyperglycemic therapies has had a significant impact on the recommendations for the treatment of type 2 diabetes in the setting of chronic kidney disease.[15]

Metformin continues to be recognized as the first-line therapy option for persons with type 2 diabetes. It is now approved for use in CKD stages 1 to 3.[57] Recommendations for metformin dosing and monitoring as DKD progresses are summarized in Table 27.5. Initial cardiovascular outcomes trials evaluating select sodium-glucose cotransporter-2 (SGLT2) inhibitors (ie, empagliflozin, canagliflozin, dapagliflozin) and glucagon-like peptide-1 (GLP-1) receptor agonists (ie, liraglutide, semaglutide, dulaglutide) in persons with type 2 diabetes and either established CVD or at high risk for CVD, have demonstrated a reduction in progression of DKD as various secondary endpoints.[58–63] Additionally, multiple SGLT2 inhibitors and GLP-1 receptor agonists have also demonstrated a significant reduction in cardiovascular death alone or cardiovascular risk via reduction in the primary composite endpoint of cardiovascular death, nonfatal myocardial infarction, and nonfatal stroke.[58–61,63]

The Canagliflozin and Renal Events in Diabetes with Established Nephropathy Clinical Evaluation (CREDENCE) trial evaluated persons with type 2 diabetes and chronic DKD (UACR >300 mg/g, and eGFR 30 to <90 mL/min/1.73 m^2) on guideline-recommended, maximum tolerated RAAS inhibitors, with relatively optimized glycemic and blood pressure levels.[64] Investigators found that canagliflozin significantly decreased the primary composite endpoint of ESRD, doubling of SCr, or death from renal or cardiovascular causes by 30% compared to placebo. Additionally, the renal-specific composite outcome (ie, ESRD, doubling of SCR or renal death), was reduced by 34% with the use of canagliflozin. Prior to the publication of this data, there were no SGLT2 inhibitors approved for use when eGFR<45 mL/min/1.73 m^2 due to loss of antihyperglycemic efficacy; however, it is important to note that the renal and cardiovascular benefits seen in the CREDENCE trial were maintained in patients with Stage 3b CKD.

Trials of other SGLT2 inhibitors in patients with CKD at baseline are ongoing to confirm this benefit; however, the ADA has updated their recommendations based on these landmark trials.[65,66] For persons with type 2 diabetes and DKD with an eGFR ≥30 mL/min/1.73 m^2 and specifically those with severely increased albuminuria (>300 mg/g creatinine), a SGLT2 inhibitor is recommended to decrease the risk of CKD progression, cardiovascular events, or both independent of baseline A1C or individualized A1C goal.[15] While the evidence for preventing the progression of CKD is less robust with GLP-1 receptor agonists, they may also be considered in patients with CKD to reduce the risk of cardiovascular events and/or the progression of albuminuria.

Other non-insulin therapies have not demonstrated reductions in cardiovascular or renal outcomes; however, they may still be considered appropriate treatment options for type 2 diabetes in the setting of CKD. Dipeptidyl peptidase-4 (DPP-4) inhibitors are a reasonable option given their neutral effect on body weight, limited adverse effect profile, and modest A1C-lowering.[15] Caution should be exhibited with the use of saxagliptin and alogliptin given the increased risk for heart failure hospitalization associated with these agents in the SAVOR-TIMI trial and post-hoc analysis of the EXAMINE trial, respectively.[67,68] If patients are expected to have endogenous insulin production remaining, glipizide or glimepiride may be considered and are preferred to other agents in the pharmacologic class due to their short duration of action and limited ability to accumulate in renal impairment.[15] Glyburide should not be used with an eGFR <60 mL/min/1.73 m^2 and should be avoided in older persons with type 2 diabetes without CKD at baseline due to the natural decline in renal function that is expected with increasing age.[1,15,69] Thiazolidinediones are generally not recommended in CKD due to potential for fluid retention.[15] Specifically, the use of rosiglitazone has demonstrated increased risk for acute myocardial infarction and heart failure hospitalizations and heart failure-related death, and risks for these adverse outcomes may be accentuated in a CKD population with an elevated baseline risk for CVD.[70,71]

Limited evidence is available for the treatment of persons with type 2 diabetes and CKD using amylin, alpha-glucosidase inhibitors, bile acid sequestrants, and dopamine agonists, and therefore, their use should be reserved for when other non-insulin medications are not tolerated or indicated and patients are not amenable to the initiation of insulin therapy. Table 27.5 provides recommendations for renal dose adjustments for non-insulin therapies and may provide guidance as to when to consider these agents in the treatment of persons with type 2 diabetes and CKD.

Insulin

Insulin therapy is the most effective agent to lower A1C, although its use is not without risks in the setting of kidney disease. Increased insulin resistance, reduced gluconeogenesis, and impaired insulin degradation are present in persons with diabetes with CKD.[1] Reduced kidney gluconeogenesis may limit the ability of a person with diabetes with declining blood glucose levels to defend against hypoglycemia. Renal degradation of insulin accounts for approximately one third of the body's ability to catabolize insulin. As kidney function declines, exogenous insulin acts longer and in an unpredictable manner, characterized by recurrent or severe hypoglycemia in some individuals. Additionally, anorexia that may present in advanced stages of CKD prior to starting dialysis will result in dietary changes that may reduce glucose consumption and further impact a person with diabetes' insulin requirements. Thus, the challenge in predicting insulin requirements in various stages of CKD results in the need for frequent evaluation to be able to properly individualize therapy especially as disease progresses.

Optimizing Blood Pressure Management

Appropriate management of hypertension slows the decline of GFR in persons with DKD.[1,2,15] The risk of persons with type 1 or type 2 diabetes with hypertension and established CKD progressing to ESRD is reduced when these individuals are treated with an angiotensin-converting enzyme (ACE) inhibitors or angiotensin receptor blockers (ARBs).[72–74] While both CKD and hypertension are independent risk factors for CVD, their coexistence further increases the risk for CVD and cerebrovascular events, especially in the presence of proteinuria.[75] Thus, optimizing the management of hypertension is paramount to delaying the progression of kidney disease as well as reducing overall cardiovascular risk.

To slow the progression of CKD, a blood pressure goal of <130/80 mmHg is recommended for adults with hypertension and CKD by the American College of Cardiology (ACC)/American Heart Association (AHA) multisociety clinical practice guidelines for the management of high blood pressure.[76] The ADA generally recommends

TABLE 27.5 Dose Adjustment for Insulin and Non-Insulin Medications for Diabetes in CKD

Medication class and agents	*Recommended dose adjustment*
Biguanides	
Metformin	eGFR ≥45 mL/min/1.73 m²: No dose adjustment necessary eGFR 30–44 mL/min/1.73 m²: Reduce dose to 1000 mg/day if already receiving therapy and do not initiate if renal function is persistently in this range eGFR <30 mL/min/1.73 m²: Contraindicated
Sodium-glucose cotransporter-2 (SGLT2) Inhibitors	
Dapagliflozin	eGFR ≥45 mL/min/1.73 m²: No dose adjustment necessary eGFR 30–44 mL/min/1.73 m²: Not recommended eGFR <30 mL/min/1.73 m²: Contraindicated
Canagliflozin	eGFR ≥60 mL/min/1.73 m²: Initiate at 100 mg daily; may increase to 300 mg eGFR 45–59 mL/min/1.73 m²: Dose is limited to 100 mg daily; do not increase eGFR 30–44 mL/min/1.73 m² with albuminuria (>300 mg/day): Dose is limited to 100 mg daily; do not increase eGFR <30 mL/min/1.73 m² or dialysis: Do not initiate For those already initiated on therapy whose eGFR declines to <30 mL/min/1.73 m² with albuminuria (>300 mg/day), therapy can be continued at 100 mg daily until transplant or dialysis, then discontinue
Empagliflozin	eGFR ≥45 mL/min/1.73 m²: No dose adjustment necessary eGFR <45 mL/min/1.73 m²: Do not initiate and continued use is not recommended if renal function is persistently in this range
Ertugliflozin	eGFR ≥60 mL/min/1.73 m²: No dose adjustment necessary eGFR 30–59 mL/min/1.73 m²: Do not initiate and continued use is not recommended if renal function is persistently in this range eGFR <30 mL/min/1.73 m²: Contraindicated
Glucagon-like peptide (GLP)-1 receptor agonists	
Exenatide	CrCl <30 mL/min: Not recommended
Exenatide, extended release	eGFR <45 mL/min/1.73 m²: Not recommended
Liraglutide	No dose adjustment is recommended in patients with renal impairment. There is limited data in patients with ESRD.
Dulaglutide	No dose adjustment is recommended in patients with renal impairment including ESRD. There is limited data in patients with ESRD.
Lixisenatide	eGFR ≥30 mL/min/1.73 m²: No dose adjustment is necessary eGFR 15–29 mL/min/1.73 m²: No dose adjustment provided by manufacturer labeling; however, exposure increased in these patients eGFR <15 mL/min/1.73 m²: Not recommended
Semaglutide	No dose adjustment is recommended in patients with renal impairment
Dipeptidyl peptidase 4 (DPP-4) inhibitors	
Sitagliptin	eGFR ≥45 mL/min/1.73 m²: 100 mg daily eGFR 30–44 mL/min/1.73 m²: 50 mg daily eGFR <30 mL/min/1.73 m²: 25 mg daily ESRD, hemodialysis or peritoneal dialysis: 25 mg daily, administered without regard to timing of dialysis

(continued)

TABLE 27.5 Dose Adjustment for Insulin and Non-Insulin Medications for Diabetes in CKD (continued)	
Medication class and agents	*Recommended dose adjustment*
Saxagliptin	eGFR ≥45 mL/min/1.73 m^2: 5 mg daily eGFR <45 mL/min/1.73 m^2: 2.5 mg daily ESRD, hemodialysis: 2.5 mg daily, administered post-dialysis ESRD, peritoneal dialysis: Not studied
Linagliptin	No dose adjustment necessary
Alogliptin	CrCl ≥60 mL/min: 25 mg daily CrCl 30–59 mL/min: 12.5 mg daily CrCl <30 mL/min: 6.25 mg daily ESRD, hemodialysis: 6.25 mg daily, administered without regard to timing of dialysis ESRD, peritoneal dialysis: Not studied
First-generation sulfonylureas	
Tolazamide	Avoid use in CKD
Tolbutamide	Avoid use in CKD
Second-generation sulfonylureas	
Glipizide	eGFR <50 mL/min/1.73 m^2: Initiate conservatively at 2.5 mg daily ESRD: Initiate conservatively at 2.5 mg daily
Glipizide, extended release	Initiate conservatively at 2.5 mg daily
Glimepiride	Initiate conservatively at 1 mg daily
Glyburide	Avoid use in CKD
Meglitinides	
Repaglinide	CrCl 20–40 mL/min: Initiate conservatively at 0.5 mg with meals CrCl <20 mL/min: Not studied
Nateglinide	eGFR <30 mL/min/1.73 m^2: Initiate conservatively at 60 mg with meals
Thiazolidinediones	
Pioglitazone	No dose adjustment necessary Generally not recommended in CKD due to potential for fluid retention
Rosiglitazone	No dose adjustment necessary Generally not recommended in CKD due to potential for fluid retention
Alpha-glucosidase inhibitors	
Acarbose	CrCl <25 mL/min or SCr >2 mg/dL: Not recommended
Miglitol	CrCl <25 mL/min or SCr >2 mg/dL: Not recommended
Amylin analog	
Pramlintide	eGFR ≥15 mL/min/1.73 m^2: No dose adjustment is necessary ESRD: Not studied
Dopamine receptor agonist	
Bromocriptine mesylate	Not studied in patients with renal impairment

(continued)

TABLE 27.5 Dose Adjustment for Insulin and Non-Insulin Medications for Diabetes in CKD (continued)

Medication class and agents	*Recommended dose adjustments*
Basal insulins	
Degludec	No dose adjustments are provided in the manufacturer labeling; insulin requirements may be reduced due to changes in insulin clearance or metabolism.
Glargine	
Detemir	
Neutral Protamine Hagedorn (NPH)	
Bolus insulins	
Aspart	No dose adjustments are provided in the manufacturer labeling; insulin requirements may be reduced due to changes in insulin clearance or metabolism.
Lispro	
Glulisine	
Regular	

Sources: American Diabetes Association. Standards of medical care in diabetes—2019. *Diabetes Care.* 42(2019) Suppl 1:S1–193.; K Lipska, C Bailey, S Inzucchi, "Use of metformin in the setting of mild-to-moderate renal insufficiency," *Diabetes Care.* 34(2011):1431–7; Farxiga [package insert]. Princeton, NJ: Bristol-Myers Squibb Company; 2020.; Invokana [package insert]. Titusville, NJ: Janssen Pharmaceuticals, Inc.; 2020.; Jardiance [package insert]. Ridgefield, CT: Boehringer Ingelheim Pharmaceuticals, Inc.; 2014.; Steglatro [package insert]. Whitehouse Station, NJ: Merck & Co., Inc.; 2017.; Byetta [package insert]. Wilmington, DE: AstraZeneca Pharmaceuticals; 2018.; Bydureon BCise [package insert]. Wilmington, DE: AstraZeneca Pharmaceuticals; 2019.; Victoza [package insert]. Plainsboro, NJ: Novo Nordisk Inc.; 2018.; Trulicity [package insert]. Indianapolis, IN: Eli Lilly and Company; 2018.; Adlyxin [package insert]. Bridgewater, NJ: Sanofi-Aventis US LLC; 2016.; Ozempic [package insert]. Plainsboro, NJ: Novo Nordisk, Inc.; 2017.; Januvia [package insert]. Whitehouse Station, NJ: Merck and Co Inc.; 2019.; Onglyza ([package insert]. Wilmington, DE: AstraZeneca Pharmaceuticals; 2018.; Tradjenta [package insert]. Ridgefield, CT: Boehringer Ingelheim Pharmaceuticals; 2017.; Nesina [package insert]. Deerfield, IL: Takeda Pharmaceuticals America Inc.; 2016.; National Kidney Foundation, "KDOQI clinical practice guideline for diabetes and CKD: 2012 update," *Am J Kidney Dis.* 60(2012):850–86; JC Arjona Ferreira, M Marre, N Barzilai, et al, "Efficacy and safety of sitagliptin versus glipizide in patients with type 2 diabetes and moderate-to-severe chronic renal insufficiency," *Diabetes Care.* 36(2013):1067–73; RY Gianchandani, S Neupane, JJ Iyengar, M Heung, "Pathophysiology and management of hypoglycemia in end-stage renal disease patients: a review," *Endocr Pract.* 23(2017):353–62; Glucotrol XL [package insert]. New York, NY: Pfizer, Inc.; 2018.; Amaryl [package insert]. Bridgewater, NJ: Sanofi-Aventis US LLC; 2013.; Prandin [package insert]. Plainsboro, NJ: Novo Nordisk, Inc.; 2017.; Starlix [package insert]. East Hanover, NJ: Novartis Pharmaceuticals Corporation; 2018.; Actos [package insert]. Deerfield, IL: Takeda Pharmaceuticals America Inc.; 2011.; Avandia [package insert]. Research Triangle Park, NC: GlaxoSmithKline; 2019.; Precose [package insert]. Wayne, NJ: Bayer HealthCare Pharmaceuticals Inc.; 2011.; Glyset [package insert]. Germany: Bayer HealthCare Pharmaceuticals Inc.; 2016.; Symlin [package insert]. Wilmington, DE: AstraZeneca Pharmaceuticals; 2014.; Cycloset [package insert]. Tiverton, RI: VeroScience, LLC; 2017.

a blood pressure target of <140/90 mmHg in individuals with diabetes; however, they also suggest that a lower target (<130/80 mmHg) may be suitable in persons with diabetes and CKD given their increased risk for CKD progression and CVD mortality.[15]

Antihypertensive Therapy

Initiation of an ACE inhibitor or ARB is recommended as the first-line therapy for the treatment of high blood pressure in individuals with DKD (stage 3 or greater or stage 1 or 2 with severely increased albuminuria [>300mg/g creatinine]).[15,76] Treatment of individuals with hypertension and moderately increased albuminuria (30-300 mg/g creatinine) with an ACE inhibitor or ARB has shown reduced progression to advanced albuminuria and decreased rates of cardiovascular events, but no benefit in terms of reduced progression to ESRD.[77,78] Thus, the use of an ACE inhibitor or ARB as the first agent to treat high blood pressure in persons with diabetes and moderately increased albuminuria (30-300 mg/g creatinine) is reasonable.[15] Serum creatinine and potassium levels should be monitored within 1 to 2 weeks of starting treatment with an ACE inhibitor or ARB and periodically thereafter to assess for acute increases in creatinine or hyperkalemia, respectively.

Multiple guidelines recommend against the use of an ACE inhibitor with an ARB, as several studies have found that their concomitant use provided no cardiovascular or renal benefit and increased the risk of adverse events, particularly hyperkalemia and AKI.[15,76] The combination of a direct renin inhibitor and ARB (or ACE inhibitor) is also contraindicated in the management of patients with CKD and high blood pressure due to the unacceptably high rates of hyperkalemia and hypotension seen in clinical trials.[76]

If further blood pressure lowering is required after initiation and titration of an ACE inhibitor or ARB to its maximum tolerated dose, an alternative first-line agent for the management of hypertension, such as a dihydropyridine calcium channel blocker or thiazide or thiazide-like diuretic, may be considered.[15,76] Clinicians should be mindful that some thiazide diuretics (ie, hydrochlorothiazide) lose their blood pressure–lowering effect in advanced CKD (CrCl <30 mL/min), which may necessitate transitioning to other thiazide-like diuretics or alternative antihypertensive classes.

The addition of a dihydropyridine calcium channel blocker to an ACE inhibitor or ARB in patients with hypertension and DKD may be the preferred combination regimen based on the results from the Avoiding Cardiovascular Events through Combination Therapy in Patients Living with Systolic Hypertension (ACCOMPLISH) trial.[79] The ACCOMPLISH trial evaluated treatment with the ACE inhibitor, benazepril, and either the dihydropyridine calcium channel blocker, amlodipine, or thiazide diuretic, hydrochlorothiazide, in patients with hypertension at high cardiovascular risk, including those with type 2 diabetes and CKD. Combination treatment with benazepril-amlodipine demonstrated a reduction in the primary composite endpoint of death from cardiovascular causes, nonfatal myocardial infarction, nonfatal stroke, hospitalization for angina, resuscitation after sudden cardiac arrest, and coronary revascularization compared to benazepril-hydrochlorothiazide. Therefore, the selection of add-on antihypertensive therapy in patients with DKD and high blood pressure should take into consideration a variety of patient-specific factors, including current kidney function, serum electrolyte levels, and an assessment of cardiovascular risk.

Restriction of dietary sodium to <1,500 to 2,300 mg/day is recommended to reduce blood pressure and associated cardiovascular risk.[15,76] Implementation of the Dietary Approaches to Stop Hypertension (DASH) eating plan, which is rich in fruits, vegetables, whole grains, and low-fat dairy products, and limits saturated and total fat, may facilitate weight loss and is recommended for patients with high blood pressure.[76] The DASH diet alone is associated with a 11 mmHg decrease in systolic blood pressure in individuals with hypertension and therefore is an important lifestyle modification to limit the adverse effects of high blood pressure in patients with DKD.

Further Cardiovascular Risk Reduction

As previously discussed, the primary cause of death in patients with CKD is CVD, and the presence of diabetes as a comorbid condition further increases the risk of cardiovascular death.[3] Both reduced eGFR (<60mL/min/1.73 m^2) and albuminuria (>30 mg/g creatinine) are recognized as independent risk factors for CVD, and this risk is multiplied when both factors are present.[80] The relationship between these factors may be related to genetic predisposition, endothelial dysfunction, associated hypertension, insulin resistance, atherogenic dyslipidemias, hyperglycemia, and anemia.[1]

Current recommendations are to initiate moderate-intensity statin therapy for primary prevention of CVD in adults aged 40 to 75 years with diabetes and low-density lipoprotein cholesterol (LDL-C) ≥70 mg/dL, regardless of the patient's estimated 10-year risk of atherosclerotic cardiovascular disease (ASCVD).[15,80] Further intensification of statin therapy should be considered in adults with diabetes and multiple risk factors for CVD (eg, CKD) or patients aged 50–75 years, as well as those with established CVD.[80] The recommendations from the ADA align with those from the combined ACC/AHA guidelines for blood cholesterol, advocating for high-intensity statin therapy in patients with an estimated 10-year ASCVD risk ≥20% or those with multiple CVD risk factors, and patients with established CVD.[15] Increasing rates of earlier-onset type 2 diabetes, and the subsequent prolonged lifetime exposure to hyperglycemia and atherogenic risk factors (ie, insulin resistance, hypertension, dyslipidemia) has substantially increased the risk of cardiovascular morbidity and mortality of young adults.[81] As a result, the ACC/AHA guidelines for the management of blood cholesterol now recommend statin therapy in patients with prolonged duration of diabetes (≥10 years of type 2, ≥20 years of type 1) or in the presence of albuminuria (≥30 mg/g creatinine), eGFR <60 mL/min/1.73 m^2, retinopathy, neuropathy, or ankle-brachial index <0.9.[80]

Both diabetes and CKD serve as individual risk factors for CVD and are therefore compelling indications for statin therapy in adults with LDL-C ≥70 mg/dL; however, initiation of statin therapy in patients with advanced CKD requiring dialysis is not recommended.[80] This is due to the proposed lower rate of deaths due to atherosclerotic causes in dialysis patients and the lack of benefit of statin initiation seen in randomized controlled trials. Patients with advanced CKD requiring dialysis that were initiated on a statin prior to starting dialysis may continue to derive cardiovascular benefit once on dialysis, and therefore, it may be reasonable to continue statin therapy.

Engaging in Physical Activity

Regular physical activity has been shown to improve glycemic management, decrease cardiovascular risk, maintain healthy weight, and improve overall well-being.[2,15] After appropriate screening to ensure there is no underlying cardiovascular disease, adults with diabetes with or without kidney disease are recommended to engage in at least 150 minutes per week of moderate- to vigorous-intensity aerobic exercise distributed over at least 3 days, with no more than 2 consecutive days without physical activity.[15] Participating in resistance training (eg, exercise with free weights or weight machines) for 2 to 3 sessions per week on nonconsecutive days is also recommended. All adults with diabetes, specifically those with type 2 diabetes, should be encouraged to decrease the proportion of daily sedentary behavior. Counseling patients to briefly stand and walk or perform other light physical activities helps to avoid extended sedentary periods and may improve glycemic levels. No specific exercise recommendations or restrictions exist for patients with DKD.

Healthy Weight Management

Studies of calorie restriction for weight management in individuals with type 2 diabetes have reduced A1C by 0.3% to 2.0%, decreased medication dose requirements, and improved quality of life.[15] Maintaining weight loss over a period of 5 years has shown to sustain these improvements in glycemic management. Patients with CKD are recommended to maintain a normal body weight, or a body mass index of 20 to 25 kg/m^2.[2] The ADA reports that at least a 5% reduction in body weight is needed in obese persons with type 2 diabetes to see improved glucose, lipid, and blood pressure levels, and if safe and feasible, more intensive weight loss goals (ie, 15%) may be appropriate to optimize these clinical benefits.[15] An overall healthy eating plan with some degree of calorie restriction in conjunction with weight loss medications and/or metabolic surgery should be considered in select individuals with type 2 diabetes to reduce body weight, A1C, and risk for CVD. A structured weight loss plan should include guidance on medical nutrition therapy from a registered dietitian or registered dietitian nutritionist with experience in diabetes and weight management, as well as knowledge of dietary restrictions that are individualized for those with varying degrees of renal impairment.

Smoking Cessation

Smoking is associated with both micro- and macrovascular complications in persons with diabetes; therefore, cessation is recommended to reduce the risk for CVD and CKD progression.[2,15] All patients should be advised to avoid cigarettes and other tobacco products, as well as e-cigarettes.[15] Smoking cessation therapy should be offered to all patients that continue to use tobacco products as a standard component of diabetes care. Pharmacologic therapy when added to counseling in a motivated patient significantly increases the likelihood of a successful quit attempt, and treatment selection must be based on patient preference and safety in the setting of declining kidney function.[15,82] For example, varenicline requires dose adjustment in severe renal impairment (CrCl <30 mL/min) and ESRD.[82] Bupropion should be used with caution in CKD due to the potential for accumulation of the parent drug and its metabolite; however, there have been no clinical manifestations of this accumulation, and dose adjustments are available for advanced stages of CKD. It is also recommended that nicotine replacement therapy, including the gum, lozenge, and patch, be used with caution in severe renal impairment; however, no specific dose adjustments are available.

Avoidance of Nephrotoxic Agents

The presence of medications that are known nephrotoxins may worsen renal impairment; therefore, such substances should be avoided in patients at risk for and with known CKD.[2] Nephrotoxic medications that may be encountered in the treatment of diabetes or comorbidities include nonsteroidal anti-inflammatory drugs (NSAIDs), including cyclooxygenase-2 (COX 2) inhibitors, lithium, calcineurin inhibitors, select antimicrobial agents (eg, aminoglycosides, amphotericin B), and radiocontrast dye. Additionally, the use of NSAIDs is also contraindicated in patients on a combination of both diuretics and ACE inhibitors or ARBs due to risk of AKI and worsening renal function.[83]

Other Care Considerations

Dietary Modifications

Dietary recommendations for patients with DKD are similar to those for persons with diabetes without reduced kidney function. That is, no single eating pattern has been shown to be effective for all individuals with diabetes.[15] Specifically, there is no ideal distribution of carbohydrates, protein, and fat consumption for these patients, but rather, macronutrient distribution should be based on an individual's metabolic goals and current eating pattern and preferences. In general, emphasis should be placed on increasing non-starchy vegetable intake, limiting added sugars and refined carbohydrates, and choosing whole over highly processed foods whenever possible.[84] Mediterranean-style and plant-based diets are examples of healthy eating patterns for patients with DKD; however, low- or very low-carbohydrate dietary plans are not recommended in patients with renal impairment.

Historically, dietary recommendations for patients with advanced CKD focused on protein restriction to reduce albuminuria and limit disease progression.[2] Recent evidence demonstrates that reducing the amount of daily protein intake to <0.8g/kg/day may result in improvements in albuminuria, but has no clinically significant effect on the rate of eGFR decline.[84] Additionally, studies have shown that a low-protein diet may promote malnutrition in individuals with DKD.[85–88] The updated ADA consensus report on nutrition therapy for adults with prediabetes and diabetes no longer recommends restricting dietary protein in individuals with non-dialysis dependent DKD to less than the average protein intake.[84] Therefore, the recommended protein intake for patients with DKD should be 1 to 1.5 g/kg/day or 15% to 20% of total calorie intake, but should not exceed 1.3 g/kg/day, as excessively high levels of protein intake are associated with increased albuminuria, more rapid eGFR decline, and CVD mortality.[15,84]

Other considerations for those with impaired renal function include individualizing dietary intake based on the degree of renal failure and laboratory values. In general, limiting sodium, potassium, and phosphorus in the diet are important for fluid, electrolyte, and mineral balance.[8,11] The goal is to prevent complications associated with renal impairment including worsening hypertension and/or volume overload, hyperkalemia, and associated cardiac arrythmias, as well as hyperphosphatemia. Hyperphosphatemia causes urticaria and may trigger increased parathyroid hormone production, which can result in bone density changes including renal osteodystrophy.[11]

Nephrology Referral

Referral to a physician with specialized training in the care of kidney disease should be considered when there is uncertainty in the etiology of CKD, complications of declining renal function arise (ie, anemia, resistant hypertension, metabolic bone disease, electrolyte disturbances), severe albuminuria (>300 mg/g creatinine) persists, or in patients with CKD stage 4 or greater.[2,15] Studies have demonstrated reductions in healthcare cost, improved quality of care, and slowed progression to dialysis when patients that develop stage 4 CKD consult with a nephrologist.[89] Additionally, individuals with a 10% to 20% or greater risk of kidney failure within 1 year should be referred to initiate planning for RRT.[2] Several validated risk prediction tools are available to calculate the likelihood of progression to kidney failure and assist in this clinical decision making.

The provision of kidney-related care should not be limited to specialists' visits. Other physicians and members of the multidisciplinary care team should regularly educate patients on the importance of treating hyperglycemia and hypertension to preserve kidney function, the progressive nature of CKD, and the potential need for RRT.

Case Study: New Onset DKD in Prolonged Hyperglycemia

Use of a 24-hour food recall and diet history revealed that MG was following a high-protein diet 6 months ago and initially lost 10 lb, but was not able to follow the low-carbohydrate plan. MG had regained over 15 lb. She generally skipped breakfast, ate a salad for lunch at her desk, drank diet sodas throughout the day, and sometimes ordered food in or stopped at a local fast-food restaurant for dinner. MG rarely cooked since the death of her husband last year. MG remarked that she often ate a lot at night when she was feeling the most "out of sorts."

Patient-specific treatment goals to prevent or delay the progression of DKD are listed below and further applied to the AADE7 Self-Care Behaviors®

- Optimizing glycemic management
- Optimizing blood pressure management
- Implementing measures to reduce cardiovascular risk
- Engaging in regular physical activity
- Attaining and maintaining a healthy weight with a safe and effective eating plan
- Minimizing the use of nephrotoxic agents

Healthy Eating

- Recommendations for the implementation of dietary patterns for MG should be focused on glycemic management, blood pressure reduction, and weight loss.
- Following a Mediterranean diet and implementing recommendations from the DASH eating plan may benefit glycemic and blood pressure management, respectively, as well as reduce overall cardiovascular risk.
- Education on how to review macronutrient content of foods should be reviewed, along with how to balance meal planning throughout the day to limit fluctuations in blood glucose.

(continued)

Case Study: New Onset DKD in Prolonged Hyperglycemia (continued)

- Encouraging MG to limit her consumption of fast-food and takeout should reduce sodium and saturated fat intake to further improve her blood pressure, lipid panel, and overall cardiovascular risk.
- A low-carbohydrate, high-protein diet should not be recommended for MG, as high levels of protein intake (>1.3 g/kg/day) are associated with increased albuminuria, more rapid decline in eGFR, and death from CVD. Rather, MG should be counseled to maintain a normal protein intake of 1 to 1.5 g/kg/day to maintain a well-rounded diet and reduce the risk of malnutrition that may occur with more stringent protein restrictions.

Healthy Coping and Problem Solving

- MG's feelings about the loss of her husband and the frequency of her nighttime dietary indiscretions needed to be considered when determining whether a referral to a mental health professional might be warranted. The presence of diabetes, CKD, and her other comorbidities is a high psychological burden. Consulting with a mental health specialist may increase the likelihood of MG successfully implementing treatment recommendations to improve the management of her chronic disease states.
- MG should be advised to identify and engage in familial and friends/peer support systems and partake in available networking opportunities.
- Being active in her treatment plan, learning how to complete routine self-monitoring blood glucose, and being empowered to take on the responsibility of following dietary, physical activity, and pharmacotherapy recommendations will be key to MG's success managing her chronic conditions.

Being Active

- Appropriate physical activity should be recommended for MG to facilitate weight loss, lower blood pressure, improve glycemic management, and reduce the risk for CKD progression and CVD.
- MG should engage in at least 150 minutes per week of moderate- to vigorous-intensity aerobic exercise distributed over at least 3 days. She should be instructed to go no more than 2 consecutive days without exercise.
- Recommend that MG participate in resistance training using free weights or weight machines for 2 to 3 sessions every week.
- When confined to activities that require long periods of sitting, encourage MG to break up sedentary periods by briefly standing or taking a quick walk every 30 minutes.

Taking Medication and Reducing Risks

- *Glycemic management.* MG is not meeting her glycemic goals for her type 2 diabetes; therefore, modification of her therapy is recommended.
  - —With MG's most recent eGFR being ≥45 mL/min/1.73 m², metformin can be continued at its current dose of 2,000 mg/day, which is also its clinically maximum effective dose. The dose of metformin would need to be adjusted if eGFR falls to 30 to 44 mL/min/1.73 m², and discontinued if persistently <30 mL/min/1.73 m². She should be educated to discontinue (hold) metformin in times of acute illness, if unable to maintain adequate fluid status (eg, vomiting, diarrhea, or dehydration), or with an acute decline in renal function as reduced clearance increases the risk of lactic acidosis. Metformin use should be re-evaluated by monitoring eGFR every 3 to 6 months with progression of CKD.
  - —Given MG's newly diagnosed CKD, guideline recommendations for add-on therapy after metformin now advocate for a SGLT2 inhibitor to reduce the risk of kidney disease progression and/or cardiovascular events. Starting a SGLT2 inhibitor will also modestly reduce her blood pressure, which is also not at goal, and facilitate weight loss. Completing repeat monitoring of SCr and eGFR 1 to 2 weeks after initiation of a SGLT2 inhibitor may be warranted to ensure that the transient decrease in eGFR returns to baseline, similar to the concept of monitoring therapy with the initiation of ACE inhibitors or ARBs.
  - —After optimizing glycemic management with a SGLT2 inhibitor, it may be prudent to reassess MG's glipizide therapy. Given sulfonylureas increase the risk for hypoglycemia and contribute to weight gain, continued use of glipizide may not best align with MG's overall care goals.
  - —Consider the use of a GLP-1 receptor agonist with demonstrated cardiovascular and renal benefit (ie, liraglutide, semaglutide, or dulaglutide) if further antihyperglycemic therapy is needed after discontinuation of glipizide. Treatment with 1 of the aforementioned GLP-1 receptor agonists would further reduce MG's risk for CKD progression,

(continued)

Case Study: New Onset DKD in Prolonged Hyperglycemia (continued)

reduce CVD morbidity and mortality, and facilitate further weight loss.

- *Blood pressure management.* A diagnosis of hypertension was confirmed with two elevated blood pressure readings during two separate clinic visits. MG likely has worsening blood pressure control secondary to declining kidney function. Initiation of an ACE inhibitor or ARB should be recommended to provide blood pressure-lowering, reduce the progression to advanced albuminuria, and decrease rates of cardiovascular events. Again, repeat monitoring of SCr and eGFR, as well as serum potassium is warranted 1 to 2 weeks after initiation of RAAS inhibitor therapy to verify that the transient decline in kidney function returns to baseline, and to ensure that the patient has not developed hyperkalemia. Both RAAS inhibiting agents and SGLT2 inhibitors cause a transient decrease in eGFR through the dilation of efferent arterioles and constriction of afferent arterioles, respectively. Thus, some clinicians may recommend separating their initiation by 1 to 2 weeks or at least until repeat laboratory measurements confirm that MG tolerated the initiation of 1 agent before adding another.
- *Reducing CVD risk.* MG is indicated for at least moderate-intensity statin therapy based on her age (40-75 years-old), diagnosis of diabetes, and LDL-C ≥70 mg/dL. This recommendation is independent of her estimated 10-year ASCVD risk. The presence of multiple general ASCVD risk factors (ie, uncontrolled hypertension, obesity, eGFR <60 mL/min/1.73 m^2, albuminuria, type 2 diabetes duration ≥10 years) and her age (50-75 years-old) advocate for high-intensity statin therapy for MG to prevent an initial cardiovascular event. Recommending atorvastatin 40 mg daily or rosuvastatin 20 to 40 mg daily would be appropriate for MG, with a goal of achieving a LDL-C reduction of ≥50% from baseline.
- *Avoiding nephrotoxic agents.* The regular use of NSAIDs and other nephrotoxic agents in patients with CKD is not recommended. NSAIDs are known to worsen kidney function, and their concomitant use with ACE inhibitors and diuretics is contraindicated due to the increased risk of AKI. While MG is not currently receiving diuretic therapy per se, initiation of a SGLT2 inhibitor may have a diuretic-like effect and reduce plasma volume; therefore, MG should be warned of the risk of continuing self-treatment with ibuprofen, especially if initiated on a SGLT2 inhibitor for her diabetes and an ACE inhibitor or ARB for her hypertension, as recommended above. Pending MG has no contraindications to acetaminophen, it may be recommended as an alternative for as needed relief of knee pain. If acetaminophen does not provide adequate pain relief, recommending MG follow-up with her primary care physician for further evaluation and management would be most appropriate.

Monitoring

Lastly, MG was told about the importance of keeping regular follow-up appointments with her primary care team to manage her chronic conditions. Regular laboratory monitoring of kidney function will permit monitoring of disease progression, enable continuous reassessment of the safety and efficacy of medications and permit timely dose adjustments when necessary, and will help to determine when referral to a nephrologist is necessary if her CKD continues to progress. The nephrology care team would collaboratively monitor for disease progression and manage the complications of CKD, and, if appropriate, prepare MG for further treatment options for kidney failure.

Management of End-Stage Renal Disease

The term ESRD represents the final stage of kidney disease, where the accumulation of toxins, electrolytes, and fluids that are normally excreted by the kidneys leads to death unless removed by RRT.[16] Once kidney failure results (CKD stage 5), options for RRT are available as either maintenance dialysis or transplantation:

- *Hemodialysis:* In-center or at home
- *Peritoneal dialysis:* Continuous ambulatory, continuous cyclic, or intermittent
- *Transplantation:* Kidney or kidney-pancreas

Individuals diagnosed with kidney failure and their family members or caregivers need to be involved in the planning and treatment decisions for ESRD. This part of the chapter reviews therapeutic options for RRT and the effects of such modalities on glycemic management. Since the individual diagnosed with kidney failure will likely be closely followed by a specialized healthcare team associated with a dialysis treatment facility (ie, nephrologist, clinical pharmacist, nurse, dietitian, social worker), it is important for the patient and family to feel comfortable discussing issues relating to RRT with the nephrology care team.

Hemodialysis

Hemodialysis (HD) is a process of filtering the blood to remove extra fluid and nitrogenous wastes, and maintain appropriate electrolyte levels and acid-base balance. The blood of the person being treated is circulated and cleansed outside the body.[90] With effective dialysis treatments, uremia can be treated and the life expectancy of the individual can be prolonged. The process is described below, with related factors for consideration noted after the description.

The filter used for HD is a semipermeable membrane.[90] The membrane, a thin material with holes, permits passage of small solutes but retains larger particles. During dialysis, the patient's blood passes on one side of the membrane while the dialysate (prepared dialysis solution) passes on the other side of the membrane. The dialysate removes fluid and solutes (waste products) from the blood by diffusive clearance. Blood is withdrawn through a needle inserted into a specially prepared blood vessel, usually a synthetic graft or an arteriovenous fistula using the patient's own blood vessels located in the forearm, upper arm, or thigh. Prior to maturation of the arteriovenous fistula or arteriovenous graft, a long-term hemodialysis catheter (ie, permcath) may be utilized temporarily as the dialysis access. The needle is attached by plastic tubing to a HD machine. A pump keeps blood moving through the dialyzer as waste and fluid are filtered out across the semipermeable membrane into the dialysate. The cleansed blood returns to the patient through another needle in the same or an adjacent blood vessel. Hemodialysis can be performed in an ambulatory setting or in the patient's home.

Treatment Considerations Treatments are usually 3 to 4 hours long, and performed on average 3 times per week. Because fluid and waste products are not being appropriately removed 24 hours per day, individuals treated with HD should follow individualized meal plans and recommendations for fluid restriction as directed by their nephrology care team. Hemodialysis can be performed in an ambulatory setting or in the patient's home. Conventional home HD requires both the patient and the family members or caregivers to be trained on the use of the machine and insertion of the needles. The treatment times are similar to those in ambulatory care settings. Nocturnal home HD is a newer option for patients who have to go to school or work or have other commitments during the day. Each session lasts 6 to 8 hours and is performed every other night, or more often as prescribed by a nephrologist. In the case of nocturnal home HD, fluids and waste materials are removed more slowly and often. Another option is short daily dialysis, which is performed for 2 hours every day. Limiting fluid and waste accumulation between HD sessions often reduces the clinical effect of between-treatment complications, which may include electrolyte derangements and increased plasma volume resulting in worsening hypertension, left ventricular hypertrophy, and heart failure.

Glycemic Management Patients with advanced kidney disease demonstrate increased insulin resistance, reduced gluconeogenesis, and decreased rates of insulin catabolism.[1,91] Thus, insulin requirements may fluctuate depending on the net balance between tissue sensitivity and insulin metabolism. While insulin is the preferred antihyperglycemic therapy for patients on HD, these factors make it difficult to predict insulin requirements and necessitate more frequent follow-up for dose adjustments to individualize therapy, especially during the initiation stage.[91] Other factors that can alter glucose levels for individuals receiving HD include the glucose concentration in the dialysate, fluctuations in appetite on dialysis versus nondialysis days, decreased activity on dialysis days, and emotional stress. Additionally, glucose is a small molecule that easily passes into the dialysate, while insulin formulations are large proteins that are not filtered; therefore, insulin requirements may decrease with the initiation of HD and more frequent glucose monitoring may be required during this time. Inquiring about individual glycemic patterns, dietary habits, and activity levels on dialysis compared to nondialysis days will help elucidate the fluctuations in blood glucose levels. Byproducts of hyperglycemia in HD include polydipsia, which may negatively impact fluid restriction recommendations, and cellular shifts in potassium that can elevate serum levels and place individuals at risk for complications of hyperkalemia, especially if electrolyte abnormalities exist at baseline.

Peritoneal Dialysis

Peritoneal dialysis (PD) takes place inside the body, employing the body's own capillary and serosal membranes.[90] Blood is filtered through the peritoneal membrane that lines the abdominal cavity. Surgery is required to place a catheter through an opening in the wall of the abdominal cavity where it is then tunneled underneath the skin before exiting to the outside to help prevent infection. This opening allows the dialysate to be instilled into the peritoneal cavity, and waste products then pass from the bloodstream into the dialysate. Once diffusion occurs and the dialysate is saturated with waste products, it is drained and replaced with new dialysate. Currently, 3 types of PD are used:

- *Continuous ambulatory peritoneal dialysis (CAPD).* This is a manual method of performing PD in which the dialysate is exchanged manually by the patient 3 to 5 times throughout the day. The patient infuses fluid into the abdomen and gravity naturally allows it to move through the body. The entire process, including the connection of a new bag of dialysate, emptying and filling for each exchange typically takes the patient 30 to 40 minutes. A nighttime dwell may be instilled at bedtime for solute removal while the patient sleeps. The dialysate passes from a plastic bag through the catheter and stays in the patient's abdomen with the catheter sealed and is drained upon awakening. Patient that are "low transporters," meaning that it takes longer for waste products and fluid to cross the peritoneal membrane, are ideal candidates for CAPD.
- *Continuous cyclic peritoneal dialysis (CCPD).* This is similar to CAPD except a machine that is connected to the catheter automatically fills and drains the dialysate from the patient's abdomen. Like CAPD, CCPD is performed every day; however, unlike CAPD, CCPD is usually performed only at night in a series of automated exchanges that occur while the patient sleeps; usually over an 8- to 12-hour period with or without a mid-day exchange.
- *Intermittent peritoneal dialysis (IPD).* This form of dialysis uses the same type of machine as CCPD to fill and drain the dialysate from the patient's abdomen; however, intermittent peritoneal dialysis treatments take longer than CCPD. This type of dialysis is most often performed in an institutional setting.

Treatment Considerations Peritoneal dialysis is often a preferred treatment modality because of its ability to limit fluctuations in serum chemistries and fluid status. Peritoneal dialysis allows for the removal of uremic toxins on a daily basis, and generally does not require as stringent dietary or fluid restrictions as HD.[92,93]

Typically dextrose or a nonabsorbable carbohydrate, such as icodextrin, is included to increase the hypertonicity of the dialysate since PD relies on hypertonicity to drive solute removal, rather than concentration gradients as in HD.[90] Despite increased absorption of glucose from dextrose-containing solutions, intraperitoneal administration of insulin by adding it to the dialysate has been proposed to assist with glycemic management.[94] Such administration allows for continuous delivery of insulin into the portal circulation. When insulin is instilled into the abdominal cavity with the dialysate, there may be some loss of insulin activity due to delayed absorption secondary to dilution, or through its adsorption to the dialysate bag; therefore, supplemental subcutaneous insulin may still be required. Intraperitoneal insulin can also be an additional source of bacterial contamination in the dialysate during CAPD, resulting in peritonitis and increased total insulin requirements. These limitations coupled with the increasing costs of insulin therapy, may limit the utility of intraperitoneal administration of insulin.

An additional consideration with the use of PD is the presence of gastroparesis. Gastroparesis is a neuropathic complication often associated with long-standing hyperglycemia.[95] Patients with gastroparesis at baseline may experience considerable nausea and/or vomiting with the initiation of PD. This is due to the increased intra-abdominal pressure that arises with extra fluid volume in the abdominal space and can further result in malnutrition. In addition, delays in gastric emptying caused by gastroparesis and mismatched insulin pharmacokinetics despite optimal administration timing may result in erratic glucose levels characterized by postprandial hyper- and/or hypoglycemia. If optimal management does not occur with CAPD, patients may benefit from IPD or alternatively decreasing the volume exchanged during the day and increasing the volume of the nighttime dwell to limit the effects of gastroparesis throughout the day.

Glycemic Management Factors that can affect blood glucose levels for individuals on PD include the following:

- Concentration of the dialysate
- Method(s) of insulin delivery (eg, intraperitoneal, subcutaneous, or both)
- Infection (peritonitis)
- Gastroparesis

To understand the effect of these factors on the variability of blood glucose levels, the practitioner should assess the following:

- Glucose concentration of the dialysate (eg, 1.5%, 2.5%, or 4.25%)
  —Glucose contained in dialysate increases need for antihyperglycemic therapy
- Type and amount of insulin, as well as the route of insulin delivery
- Any clinical signs of infection

In PD patients who need better ultrafiltration due to hypervolemia or in persons with diabetes, an icodextran solution (7.5%) may be substituted for traditional dextrose-containing dialysate.[90] Since icodextran is a glucose polymer and produces maltose upon metabolism, there is a potentially deleterious effect when glucometers requiring glucose dehydrogenase pyrroloquinolinequinone (GDH-PQQ) cofactor-based test strips are used.[96] The GDH-PQQ cofactor-based test strips use a methodology that cannot distinguish between glucose and non-glucose sugars, including maltose, xylose, and galactose.[97] As a result, these non-glucose sugars may be read by such test strips as a falsely elevated serum glucose level, thereby masking a hypoglycemic episode or causing inappropriately aggressive insulin management. The consequences may lead to serious injury or death. Table 27.6 contains a list of GDH-PQQ cofactor-based test strips that were included in this FDA safety alert.

TABLE 27.6 GDH-PQQ Test Strips With Associated Meters

Roche Diagnostics

- Accu-Chek Comfort Curve test strips for use with the following meters:

Accu-Chek Complete, Advantage, Voicemate

- Accu-Chek Aviva test strips for use with the following meters:

Accu-Chek Aviva meters

- Accu-Chek Compact test strips for use with the following meters:

Accu-Chek Compact meters and Compact Plus meters

- Accu-Chek Go test strips for use with Accu-Chek Go meter
- Accu-Chek Active test strips for use with Accu-Chek Active meters

Abbott Diabetes Care

- FreeStyle test strips for use with FreeStyle, FreeStyle Flash, and FreeStyle Freedom meters
- FreeStyle Lite test strips for use with FreeStyle Lite meters

Home Diagnostic

- TRUE test strips for use with TRUE result meters and TRUE 2 go meters

Smiths Medical

- Abbott Diabetes Care FreeStyle test strips for use with CoZmonitor blood glucose module

Insulet

- Abbott Diabetes Care FreeStyle test strips for use with OmniPod Insulin Management System

Source: US Food and Drug Administration. Advice for patients: serious errors with certain blood glucose monitoring test strips. MedWatch-FDA Safety Information and Adverse Event Reporting Program (cited 2019 June 29). On the Internet at: http://www.fda.gov/MedicalDevices/Safety/AlertsandNotices/PatientAlerts/ucm177189.htm#attachment [archived].

Kidney Transplantation

Kidney transplantation can be performed using a kidney from a living related donor, a living unrelated donor, or a suitable cadaveric donor.[98] Once transplantation has occurred, immunosuppressive medications are required throughout the recipient's life to prevent the body from rejecting the transplanted organ. Individuals with diabetes often have altered insulin requirements following transplantation as a result of the newly functioning kidney once again catabolizing insulin, immunosuppression with corticosteroid therapy that has hyperglycemic effects, and the fact that individuals may experience a notable increase in appetite, which necessitates increased antihyperglycemic therapy to maintain glycemic targets.[99]

Glycemic Management Following transplantation, blood glucose levels may be altered by the following factors:[99]

- Degree of functionality (ie, insulin degradation capacity) of the transplanted kidney
- Therapy for prevention of transplant rejection
  - —Immunosuppressant agents, specifically, corticosteroids, cyclosporine, and tacrolimus, may contribute to posttransplant diabetes
- Increased appetite and ability to consume a more liberal diet with subsequent carbohydrate consumption
- Presence of infection
  - —Transplant recipients are more susceptible to infection due to immunosuppression therapy

Simultaneous Transplant: Kidney and Pancreas

Persons with type 1 diabetes may be considered for a simultaneous kidney-pancreas transplantation.[99] A kidney-pancreas transplantation restores both glucose metabolism and kidney function. Criteria for patient selection vary by transplant center.

Post-transplantation Diabetes Mellitus (PTDM)

Post-transplantation Diabetes Mellitus (PTDM), formerly called New Onset Diabetes After Transplant (NODAT), occurs when the diagnosis of diabetes is made following a solid organ transplant, including renal transplant. Certain medications and other factors related to the transplantation process are associated with an increased risk for developing PTDM. Corticosteroid therapy is known to contribute to PTDM; however, there is evidence that calcineurin inhibitors and rapamycin inhibitors may increase this risk as well.[100] Kidney allografts from deceased donors express higher levels of cytokine pro-inflammatory markers compared to living donor transplants, which also poses an increased risk for PTDM. Additionally, infections with hepatitis C virus and cytomegalovirus have both been associated with increased rates of PTDM.

Those at high risk for PTDM should be screened for post-transplantation glucose abnormalities, with the oral glucose tolerance test (OGTT) considered the gold standard for diagnosing PTDM.[101] Post-prandial glucose readings and A1C levels may also be considered as expanded screening tools. Transient hyperglycemia is present in 90% of kidney allograft recipients during the first few weeks after transplant; therefore, a formal diagnosis of PTDM should only be made when patients have stable allograft function, are on maintenance immunosuppression therapy, and in the absence of acute infections. A consensus panel on the management of PTDM recommended that insulin be used for the treatment of transient hyperglycemia in the early post-transplant period (days 1-8), insulin with oral agents be considered for post-transplant days 8 to 45, and to begin screening for PTDM starting at day 46 post-transplantation, with subsequent treatment if necessary.

Treatment of PTDM includes traditional diabetes management strategies including lifestyle modifications, oral medications and/or insulin therapy as needed.[101] Historically, the use of newer antihyperglycemic therapies in the treatment of PTDM was limited as there was a lack of safety and efficacy data in this population, and their effects on immunosuppressive therapy was unknown. Retrospective and small, randomized controlled studies of DPP-4 inhibitors have since demonstrated their safety and efficacy in the treatment of PTDM.[102–105] Additionally, a single-center, double-blind, randomized, controlled trial resulted in improved glycemic management without excess adverse events when empagliflozin was used to treat individuals with PTDM after kidney transplant compared to placebo.[106] Small studies of GLP-1 receptor agonists have examined the safety and efficacy of these agents, with a focus being the effect of their ability to delay gastric emptying on levels of immunosuppressive therapy. Infusion with a GLP-1 agonist demonstrated short-term improvements in glucose-induced insulin secretion and glucagon suppression in patients with PTDM.[107] There are studies of GLP-1 receptor agonists for the treatment of DM in patients with renal and other solid organ transplants, and evidence that liraglutide does not alter tacrolimus trough levels in patients with kidney transplant; however, prospective clinical trials examining the role of GLP-1 receptor agonists specifically in the treatment of PTDM are lacking.[108–110] While the evidence is promising for newer agents, especially those that help to reduce cardiovascular risk in the post-transplant population, further studies are needed to determine the optimal antihyperglycemic therapy with regard to clinical safety and efficacy outcomes for patients with PTDM.

Summary

Despite medical advances in DKD, the morbidity and mortality of individuals with diabetes on RRT are higher than among those who do not have diabetes. Regular screening, early detection, and treatment with appropriate referrals are essential in the management of kidney disease to preserve residual renal function. Intensive glycemic and hypertensive management focused on minimizing proteinuria have been shown to be effective in slowing disease progression; however, evidence to recommend restrictions in dietary protein is lacking. Malnutrition may result from such restrictive diets and may have a significant impact on survival and treatment outcomes. The interrelated nature of diabetes, CKD, and CVD requires a comprehensive treatment approach that integrates the proactive management of diabetes as well as primary and secondary prevention strategies for CVD.

Focus on Education

Teaching Strategies

Explain the importance of screening for kidney disease and monitoring its progression after its diagnosis. In type 1 diabetes, screening with a spot urine albumin-to-creatine ratio should occur annually starting 5 years after diagnosis. In type 2 diabetes, screening should occur annually starting at diagnosis.

Emphasize the importance of cardiovascular risk reduction. Medical management minimizes further loss of kidney function and reduces the risk of complications, the most common being the risk of cardiovascular disease. This will likely involve pharmacologic interventions to manage hyperglycemia, hypertension, and dyslipidemia. Certain therapies used to lower blood sugar in diabetes have demonstrated benefit in lowering the risk for cardiovascular events and preventing the progression of kidney disease.

Messages for Persons With Diabetes

Incorporate recommended lifestyle modifications. Making lifestyle changes to lower and maintain weight, as well as optimizing blood glucose and blood pressure levels will help to prevent further progression and minimize complications of kidney disease. Increasing levels of physical activity by small amounts (eg, 5-10 minutes/week) each week and modifying eating patterns to assist with blood glucose and blood pressure-lowering by adjusting 1 meal or snack at a time will help achieve these broader goals. Communicate with your clinicians if the diet and exercise recommendations are not realistic to implement.

Utilize a healthcare professional and personal support network. It takes time and effort to implement the self-care behaviors required to successfully manage diabetic kidney disease. Having a well-rounded healthcare team will ensure that your therapeutic plan is being reevaluated on an ongoing basis, as the best recommendations for the management of kidney disease are updated regularly based on new research. Additionally, a support system at home can reduce the likelihood of reverting back to unhealthy lifestyle habits and their involvement in discussions about care options, particularly in advanced kidney disease, will help to provide clarity in the decision-making process.

Focus on Practice

Treatment strategies should be tailored based on kidney function, age, and other patient-specific factors. Shifting the focus from preventative care for diabetic kidney disease, to delaying its progression, and finally to dialysis care requires different clinical interventions and management considerations.

Create a system to remain up-to-date in the management of diabetic kidney disease. Comprehensive evaluation of the patient and their care goals should be an ongoing process, with consideration of both established and emerging evidence with new antihyperglycemic therapies to optimize the care of patients' diabetes, chronic kidney disease, and cardiovascular risk.

References

1. National Kidney Foundation. KDOQI clinical practice guideline for diabetes and CKD: 2012 update. Am J Kidney Dis. 2012;60:850-86.
2. Kidney Disease: Improving Global Outcomes (KDIGO) CKD Work Group. KDIGO 2012 clinical practice guideline for the evaluation and management of chronic kidney disease. Kidney Int Suppl. 2013;3:1-150.
3. United States Renal Data System. 2018 USRDS annual data report: epidemiology of kidney disease in the United States. Bethesda, MD: National Institutes of Health, National Institute of Diabetes and Digestive and Kidney Diseases; 2018.
4. Hales CM, Carroll MD, Fryar CD, Ogden CL. Prevalence of obesity among adults and youth: United States, 2015–2016. NCHS data brief, no 288. Hyattsville, MD: National Center for Health Statistics; 2017.
5. Centers for Disease Control and Prevention. National diabetes statistics report: estimates of diabetes and its burden in the United States, 2017. Atlanta, GA: United States Department of Health and Human Services; 2017.
6. Boyle JP, Thompson TJ, Gregg EW, Barker LE, Williamson DF. Projection of the year 2050 burden of diabetes in the US adult population: dynamic modeling of incidence, mortality, and prediabetes prevalence. Popul Health Metr. 2010; 8:29.
7. United States Renal Data System. 2015 USRDS annual data report: Epidemiology of kidney disease in the United States. Bethesda, MD: National Institutes of Health, National Institute of Diabetes and Digestive and Kidney Diseases; 2015.
8. Renal physiology: Introduction. In: Barrett KE, Barman SM, Brooks HL, Yuan JJ, eds. Ganong's Review of Medical Physiology, 26e. New York, NY: McGraw-Hill; 2019.
9. Renal function & micturition. In: Barrett KE, Barman SM, Brooks HL, Yuan JJ, eds. Ganong's Review of Medical Physiology, 26e. New York, NY: McGraw-Hill; 2019.
10. Regulation of Extracellular Fluid Composition & Volume. In: Barrett KE, Barman SM, Brooks HL, Yuan JJ, eds. Ganong's Review of Medical Physiology, 26e. New York, NY: McGraw-Hill; 2019.

11. Hormonal control of calcium & phosphate metabolism & the physiology of bone. In: Barrett KE, Barman SM, Brooks HL, Yuan JJ, eds. Ganong's Review of Medical Physiology, 26e. New York, NY: McGraw-Hill; 2019.

12. National Kidney Foundation. K/DOQI clinical practice guidelines for chronic kidney disease: evaluation, classification, and stratification. Am J Kidney Dis. 2002;39 Suppl 1:S1-266.

13. James MT, Grams ME, Woodward M, et al.; CKD Prognosis Consortium. A meta-analysis of the association of estimated GFR, albuminuria, diabetes mellitus, and hypertension with acute kidney injury. Am J Kidney Dis. 2015;66:602-61.

14. Thakar CV, Christianson A, Himmelfarb J, Leonard AC. Acute kidney injury episodes and chronic kidney disease risk in diabetes mellitus. Clin J Am Soc Nephrol. 2011;6: 2567-72.

15. American Diabetes Association. Standards of medical care in diabetes—2020. Diabetes Care. 2020;43 Suppl 1:S1-212.

16. Bargman JM, Skorecki KL. Chronic kidney disease. In: Jameson J, Fauci AS, Kasper DL, et al, eds. Harrison's Principles of Internal Medicine, 20e. New York, NY: McGraw-Hill; 2018.

17. Harvey KS. Nutrition and pharmacologic approaches. In: Byham-Gray LD, Burrowes JD, Chertow GS, eds. Nutrition in Kidney Disease. Totowa, NJ: Humana Press, Springer Publications Inc.; 2008.

18. Harjutsalo V, Groop PH. Epidemiology and risk factors for diabetic kidney disease. Adv Chronic Kidney Dis. 2014;21: 260-6.

19. MacGregor MS. How common is early chronic kidney disease? A background paper prepared for the UK Consensus Conference on early chronic kidney disease. Nephrol Dial Transplant. 2007;22 Suppl 9:ix8-18.

20. Maric C. Sex, diabetes and the kidney. Am J Physiol Renal Physiol. 2009;296:F680-8.

21. Pavkov ME, Mason CC, Bennett PH, et al. Change in the distribution of albuminuria according to estimated glomerular filtration rate in Pima Indians with type 2 diabetes. Diabetes Care. 2002;25:859-64.

22. Bhalla V, Zhao B, Azar KM, et al. Racial/ethnic differences in the prevalence of proteinuric and nonproteinuric diabetic kidney disease. Diabetes Care. 2013;36:1215-21.

23. Seaquist E, Goetz FC, Rich S, Barbosa J. Familial clustering of diabetic kidney disease: evidence for genetic susceptibility to diabetic nephropathy. N Engl J Med. 1989;320:1161-5.

24. Rich S. Genetics of diabetes and its complications. J Am Soc Nephrol. 2006;17:353-60.

25. Harjutsalo V, Katoh S, Sarti C, Tajima N, Tuomilehto J. Population-based assessment of familial clustering of diabetic nephropathy in type 1 diabetes. Diabetes. 2004;53:2449-54.

26. Andersen AR, Christiansen JS, Andersen JK, Kreiner S, Deckert T. Diabetic nephropathy in type 1 (insulin-dependent) diabetes: an epidemiological study. Diabetologia. 1983;25:496-501.

27. Krolewski AS, Warram JH, Christlieb AR, Busick EJ, Kahn CR. The changing natural history of nephropathy in type I diabetes. Am J Med. 1985;78:785-94.

28. Tuomilehto J, Lindstrom J, Eriksson JG, et al. Prevention of type 2 diabetes mellitus by changes in lifestyle among subjects with impaired glucose tolerance. N Engl J Med. 2001;344:1343-50.

29. Diabetes Control and Complications Trial Group. The effect of intensive treatment of diabetes on the development and progression of long-term complications in insulin-dependent diabetes mellitus. N Engl J Med. 1993;329:977-86.

30. UK Prospective Diabetes Study (UKPDS) Group. Intensive blood-glucose control with sulphonylureas or insulin compared with conventional treatment and risk of complications in patients with type 2 diabetes (UKPDS 33). Lancet. 1998;352:837-53.

31. UK Prospective Diabetes Study (UKPDS) Group. Effect of intensive blood glucose control with metformin on complications in overweight patients with type 2 diabetes (UKPDS 34). Lancet. 1998;352:854-65.

32. Patel A, MacMahon S, Chalmers J, et al.; ADVANCE Collaborative Group. Intensive blood glucose control and vascular outcomes in patients with type 2 diabetes. N Engl J Med. 2008;358:2560-72.

33. Ismail-Beigi F, Craven T, Banerji MA, et al.; ACCORD Trial Group. Effect of intensive treatment of hyperglycaemia on microvascular outcomes in type 2 diabetes: an analysis of the ACCORD randomised trial. Lancet. 2010;376:419-30.

34. Stratton IM, Adler AI, Neil HA, et al. Association of glycaemia with macrovascular and microvascular complications of type 2 diabetes (UKPDS 35): prospective observational study. BMJ. 2000;321:405-12.

35. Leehey DJ, Zhang JH, Emanuele NV, et al.; VA NEPHRON-D Study Group. BP and renal outcomes in diabetic kidney disease: the Veterans Affairs Nephropathy in Diabetes Trial. Clin J Am Soc Nephrol. 2015;10:2159-69.

36. Stanton R. Clinical challenges in diagnosis and management of diabetic kidney disease. Am J Kidney Dis. 2014;63 Suppl 2:S3-21.

37. Jenkins AJ, Lyons TJ, Zheng D, et al. Lipoproteins in the DCCT/ EDIC cohort: associations with diabetic nephropathy. Kidney Int. 2003;64:817-28.

38. Thorn LM, Forsblom C, Fagerudd J, et al. Metabolic syndrome in type 1 diabetes: association with diabetic nephropathy and glycemic control (the FinnDiane study). Diabetes Care. 2005;28:2019-24.

39. Wolf G, Müller N, Mandecka A, Müller UA. Association of diabetic retinopathy and renal function in patients with types 1 and 2 diabetes mellitus. Clin Nephrol. 2007;68:81-6.

40. He F, Xia X, Wu XF, Yu XQ, Huang FX. Diabetic retinopathy in predicting diabetic nephropathy in patients with type 2 diabetes and renal disease: a meta-analysis. Diabetologia. 2013;56:457-66.

41. American Diabetes Association. Nephropathy in diabetes. Diabetes Care. 2004;27 Suppl 1:S79-83.

42. National Kidney Foundation. Frequently asked questions about GFR estimates (cited 2019 June 22). On the Internet at: https://www.kidney.org/sites/default/files/12-10-4004_FAQ-ABE.pdf.

43. Stevens LA, Manzi J, Levey AS, et al. Impact of creatinine calibration on performance of GFR estimating equations in a pooled individual patient database. Am J Kidney Dis. 2007;50:21-35.

44. Levey AS, Coresh J, Greene T, et al. Using standardized serum creatinine values in the Modification of Diet in Renal Disease Study equation for estimating glomerular filtration rate. Ann Intern Med. 2006;145:247-54.

45. Coresh J, Stevens LA. Kidney function estimating equations: where do we stand? Curr Opin Nephrol Hypertens. 2006;15:276-84.

46. Stevens LA, Coresch J, Feldman HI, et al. Evaluation of the modification of diet in renal disease study equation in a large diverse population. J Am Soc Nephrol. 2007;18:2749-57.

47. Levey AS, Stevens LA, Schmid CH, et al. A new equation to estimate glomerular filtration rate. Ann Intern Med. 2009;150:604-12.

48. Becker BN, Vassalotti JA. A software upgrade: CKD testing in 2010. Am J Kidney Dis. 2010;55:8-10.

49. Matzke GR, Aronoff GR, Atkinson AJ Jr, et al. Drug dosing consideration in patients with acute and chronic kidney disease-a clinical update from Kidney Disease: Improving Global Outcomes (KDIGO). Kidney Int. 2011;80:1122-37.

50. Freedman BI, Shihabi ZK, Andries L, et al. Relationship between assays of glycemia in diabetic subjects with advanced chronic kidney disease. Am J Nephrol. 2010;31:375-9.

51. Morgan L, Marenah CB, Jeffcoate WJ, Morgan AG. Glycated proteins as indices of glycaemic control in diabetic patients with chronic renal failure. Diabet Med. 1996;13:514-9.

52. Joy MS, Cefalu WT, Hogan SL, Nachman PH. Long-term glycemic control measurements in diabetic patients receiving hemodialysis. Am J Kidney Dis. 2002;39:297-307.

53. Riveline JP, Teynie J, Belmouaz S, et al. Glycaemic control in type 2 diabetic patients on chronic haemodialysis: use of a continuous glucose monitoring system. Nephrol Dial Transplant. 2009;24:2866-71.

54. Ng JM, Cooke M, Bhandari S, Atkin SL, Kilpatrick ES. The effect of iron and erythropoietin treatment on the A1C of patients with diabetes and chronic kidney disease. Diabetes Care. 2010;33:2310-3.

55. Miller ME, Bonds DE, Gerstein HC, et al.; ACCORD Investigators. The effects of baseline characteristics, glycaemia treatment approach, and glycated haemoglobin concentration on the risk of severe hypoglycaemia: post hoc epidemiological analysis of the ACCORD study. BMJ. 2010;340:b5444.

56. Papademetriou V, Lovato L, Doumas M, et al.; ACCORD Study Group. Chronic kidney disease and intensive glycemic control increase cardiovascular risk in patients with type 2 diabetes. Kidney Int. 2015;87:649-59.

57. Lipska K, Bailey C, Inzucchi S. Use of metformin in the setting of mild-to-moderate renal insufficiency. Diabetes Care. 2011;34:1431-7.

58. Zinman B, Wanner C, Lachin J, et al. Empagliflozin, cardiovascular outcomes, and mortality in type 2 diabetes. N Engl J Med. 2015;373:2117-28.

59. Marso S, Daniels G, Brown-Frandsen K, et al. Liraglutide and cardiovascular outcomes in type 2 diabetes. N Engl J Med. 2016;375:311-22.

60. Marso S, Bain S, Consoli A, et al. Semaglutide and cardiovascular outcomes in patients with type 2 diabetes. N Engl J Med. 2016;375:1834-44.

61. Neal B, Perkovic V, Mahaffey KW, et al. Canagliflozin and cardiovascular and renal events in type 2 diabetes. N Engl J Med. 2017;377:644-57.

62. Wiviott SD, Raz I, Bonaca MP, et al. Dapagliflozin and cardiovascular outcomes in type 2 diabetes. N Engl J Med. 2019;380:347-57.

63. Gerstein HC, Colhoun HM, Dagenais GR, et al. Dulaglutide and cardiovascular outcomes in type 2 diabetes (REWIND): a double-blind, randomised placebo-controlled trial. Lancet. 2019;394:121-30.

64. Perkovic V, Jardine MJ, Neal B, et al. Canagliflozin and renal outcomes in type 2 diabetes and nephropathy. N Engl J Med. 2019;380:2295-306.

65. Boehringer Ingelheim. The study of heart and kidney protection with empagliflozin (EMPA-KIDNEY). NLM identifier: NCT03594110 (cited 2019 June 7). On the Internet at: https://clinicaltrials.gov/ct2/show/NCT03594110.

66. AstraZeneca. A study to evaluate the effect of dapagliflozin on renal outcomes and cardiovascular mortality in patients with chronic kidney disease (Dapa-CKD). NLM identifier: NCT03036150 (cited 2019 June 7). On the Internet at: https://clinicaltrials.gov/ct2/show/NCT03036150.

67. Scirica B, Bhatt D, Braunwald E, et al. Saxagliptin and cardiovascular outcomes in patients with type 2 diabetes mellitus. N Engl J Med. 2013;369:1317-26.

68. Zannad F, Cannon CP, Cushman WC, et al. Heart failure and mortality outcomes in patients with type 2 diabetes taking alogliptin versus placebo in EXAMINE: a multicentre, randomized, double-blind trial. Lancet. 2015;385:2067-76.

69. 2019 American Geriatrics Society Beers Criteria® Update Expert Panel. American Geriatrics Society 2019 updated AGS Beers Criteria® for potentially inappropriate medication use in older adults. J Am Geriatr Soc. 2019;67:674-94.

70. Nissen S, Wolski K. Effect of rosiglitazone on the risk of myocardial infarction and death from cardiovascular causes. N Engl J Med. 2007;356:2457-71.

71. Home PD, Pocock SJ, Beck-Nielsen H, et al. Rosiglitazone evaluated for cardiovascular outcomes in oral agent combination therapy for type 2 diabetes (RECORD): a multicentre, randomised, open-label trial. Lancet. 2009;373:2125-35.

72. Lewis EJ, Hunsicker LG, Bain RP, Rohde RD; Collaborative Study Group. The effect of angiotensin-converting-enzyme inhibition on diabetic nephropathy. N Engl J Med. 1993;329:1456-62.

73. Brenner BM, Cooper ME, de Zeeuw D, et al.; RENAAL Study Investigators. Effects of losartan on renal and cardiovascular outcomes in patients with type 2 diabetes and nephropathy. N Engl J Med. 2001;345:861-9.

74. Lewis EJ, Hunsicker LG, Clarke WR, et al.; Collaborative Study Group. Renoprotective effect of the angiotensin-receptor antagonist irbesartan in patients with nephropathy due to type 2 diabetes. N Engl J Med. 2001;345:851-60.

75. Matsushita K, van der Velde M, Astor BC, et al. Association of estimated glomerular filtration rate and albuminuria with all-cause and cardiovascular mortality in general population cohorts: a collaborative meta-analysis. Chronic Kidney Disease Prognosis Consortium. Lancet. 2010;375:2073-81.

76. Whelton PK, Carey RM, Aronow WS, et al. 2017 ACC/AHA/AAPA/ABC/ACPM/AGS/APhA/ASH/ASPC/NMA/PCNA guideline for the prevention, detection, evaluation, and management of high blood pressure in adults: a report of the American College of Cardiology/American Heart Association Task Force on Clinical Practice Guidelines. Hypertension. 2018;71:1269-324.

77. Heart Outcomes Prevention Evaluation Study Investigators. Effects of ramipril on cardiovascular and microvascular outcomes in people with diabetes mellitus: results of the HOPE study and MICRO-HOPE substudy. Lancet. 2000;355:253-9.

78. Parving HH, Lehnert H, Brochner-Mortensen J, et al.; Irbesartan in Patients with Type 2 Diabetes and Microalbuminuria Study Group. The effect of irbesartan on the development of diabetic nephropathy in patients with type 2 diabetes. N Engl J Med. 2001;345:870-8.

79. Jamerson K, Weber MA, Bakris GL, et al. Benazepril plus amlodipine or hydrochlorothiazide for hypertension in high-risk patients. N Engl J Med. 2008;359:2417-28.

80. Grundy SM, Stone NJ, Bailey AL, et al. 2018 AHA/ACC/AACVPR/AAPA/ABC/ACPM/ADA/AGS/APhA/ASPC/NLA/PCNA guideline on the management of blood cholesterol: a report of the American College of Cardiology/American Heart Association Task Force on Clinical Practice Guidelines. Circulation. 2019;139:e1082-143.

81. American Diabetes Association. TODAY2 Study: Youth-onset type 2 diabetes more severe than adult-onset disease (cited 2019 June 29). On the Internet at: https://www.adameetingnews.org/live-updates/session-coverage/today2-study-youth-onset-type-2-diabetes-more-severe-than-adult-onset-disease.

82. Formanek P, Salisbury-Afshar E, Afshar M. Helping patients with ESRD and earlier stages of CKD to quit smoking. Am J Kidney Dis. 2018;72:255-66.

83. Lapi F, Azoulay L, Yin H, Nessim SJ, Suissa S. Concurrent use of diuretics, angiotensin converting enzyme inhibitors, and angiotensin receptor blockers with non-steroidal anti-inflammatory drugs and risk of acute kidney injury: nested case-control study. BMJ. 2013;346:e8525.

84. Evert AB, Dennison M, Gardner CD, et al. Nutrition therapy for adults with diabetes or prediabetes: a consensus report. Diabetes Care. 2019;42:731-54.

85. Meloni C, Tatangelo P, Cipriani S, et al. Adequate protein dietary restriction in diabetic and nondiabetic patients with chronic renal failure. J Ren Nutr. 2004;14:208-13.

86. Dussol B, Iovanna C, Raccah D, et al. A randomized trial of low-protein diet in type 1 and in type 2 diabetes mellitus patients with incipient and overt nephropathy. J Ren Nutr. 2005;15:398-406.

87. Robertson L, Waugh N, Robertson A. Protein restriction for diabetic renal disease. Cochrane Database Syst Rev. 2007;4:CD002181.

88. Pan Y, Guo LL, Jin HM. Low-protein diet for diabetic nephropathy: a meta-analysis of randomized controlled trials. Am J Clin Nutr. 2008;88:660-6.

89. Smart NA, Dieberg G, Ladhani M, Titus T. Early referral to specialist nephrology services for preventing the progression to end-stage kidney disease. Cochrane Database Syst Rev. 2014;6:CD007333.

90. Liu KD, Chertow GM. Dialysis in the treatment of renal failure. In: Jameson J, Fauci AS, Kasper DL, et al, eds. Harrison's Principles of Internal Medicine, 20e. New York, NY: McGraw-Hill; 2018.

91. K/DOQI Workgroup. K/DOQI clinical practice guidelines for cardiovascular disease in dialysis patients. Am J Kidney Dis. 2005;45 Suppl 3:S1-153.

92. Pagenkemper JJ. Nutrition management of diabetes in chronic kidney disease. In: Byham-Gray LD, Wiesen K, eds. A Clinical Guide to Nutrition Care in Kidney Disease. Chicago, IL: American Dietetic Association; 2004.

93. Pagenkemper JJ. Diabetes mellitus. In: Byham-Gray LD, Burrowes JD, Chertow GS, eds. Nutrition in Kidney Disease. Totowa, NJ: Humana Press, Springer Publications Inc.; 2008.

94. Quellhorst E. Insulin therapy during peritoneal dialysis: pros and cons of various forms of administration. J Am Soc Nephrol. 2002;13 Suppl 1:S92-6.

95. Etemad B. Gastrointestinal complications of renal failure. Gastroenterol Clin North Am. 1998;27:875-92.

96. Williams M, Garg R. Glycemic management in ESRD and earlier stages of CKD. Am J Kidney Dis. 2014;63 Suppl 2:S22-38.

97. US Food and Drug Administration. FDA public health notification: potentially fatal errors with GDH-PQQ glucose monitoring technology. MedWatch-FDA Safety Information and Adverse Event Reporting Program (cited 2019 June 29). On the Internet at: http://www.fda.gov/Safety/MedWatch/SafetyInformation/SafetyAlertsforHumanMedicalProducts/ucm177295.htm [archived].

98. Azzi J, Milford EL, Sayegh MH, Chandraker A. Transplantation in the treatment of renal failure. In: Jameson J, Fauci AS, Kasper DL, et al, eds. Harrison's Principles of Internal Medicine, 20e. New York, NY: McGraw-Hill; 2018.

99. Kent PS. Transplantation. In: Byham-Gray LD, Burrowes JD, Chertow GS, eds. Nutrition in Kidney Disease. Totowa, NJ: Humana Press, Springer Publications Inc.; 2008.

100. Shivaswamy V, Boerner B, Larsen J. Post-transplant diabetes mellitus: causes, treatment, and impact on outcomes. Endocr Rev. 2016;37:37-61.

101. Sharif A, Hecking M, de Vries AP, et al. Proceedings from an international consensus meeting on posttransplantation diabetes mellitus: recommendations and future directions. Am J Transplant. 2014;14:1992-2000.

102. Boerner BP, Miles CD, Shivaswamy V. Efficacy and safety of sitagliptin for the treatment of new-onset diabetes after renal transplantation. Int J Endocrinol. 2014;2014:617-38.

103. Lane JT, Odegaard DE, Haire CE, et al. Sitagliptin therapy in kidney transplant recipients with new-onset diabetes after transplantation. Transplantation. 2011;92:e56-57.

104. Werzowa J, Hecking M, Haidinger M, et al. Vildagliptin and pioglitazone in patients with impaired glucose tolerance after kidney transplantation: a randomized, placebo controlled clinical trial. Transplantation. 2013;95:456-62.

105. Halden TAS, Asberg A, Vik K, Hartmann A, Jenssen T. Short-term efficacy and safety of sitagliptin treatment in long-term stable renal recipients with new-onset diabetes after transplantation. Nephrol Dial Transplant. 2014;29:926-33.

106. Halden TAS, Kvitne KE, Midtvedt K, et al. Efficacy and safety of empagliflozin in renal transplant recipients with posttransplant diabetes mellitus. Diabetes Care. 2019;42:1067-74.

107. Halden TA, Egeland EJ, Asberg A, et al. GLP-1 restores altered insulin and glucagon secretion in posttransplantation diabetes. Diabetes Care. 2016;39:617-24.

108. Liou JH, Liu YM, Chen CH. Management of diabetes mellitus with glucagonlike peptide-1 agonist liraglutide in renal transplant recipients: a retrospective study. Transplant Proc. 2018;50:2502-5.

109. Singh P, Pesavento TE, Washburn K, Walsh D, Meng S. Largest single-centre experience of dulaglutide for management of diabetes mellitus in solid organ transplant recipients. Diabetes Obes Metab. 2018;21:1061-65.

110. Pinelli NR, Patel A, Salinitri FD. Coadministration of liraglutide with tacrolimus in kidney transplant recipients: a case series. Diabetes Care. 2013;36:e171-2.

C H A P T E R 2 8

Diabetic Neuropathies

Eric L. Johnson, MD
Aaron I. Vinik, MD, PhD, FCP, MACP
Etta J. Vinik, MA (Ed)

Key Concepts

- Management of diabetic neuropathy is complex, and the key to success is to separate out the underlying pathological processes in each particular clinical presentation. The specific syndrome guides the treatment.
- Diabetic neuropathy, which includes somatic and autonomic neuropathies, is associated with considerable morbidity and mortality and has a significant impact on quality of life.
- The pathogenesis of neuropathy is still poorly understood. Recent studies on new agents that target the pathophysiological mechanisms have led to a better understanding of the pathogenesis of diabetic neuropathy as well as the pain mechanisms for the different types of pain syndromes.
- Small-fiber neuropathy may lead to foot ulceration and subsequent gangrene and amputation.
- Large-fiber neuropathy produces numbness and ataxia, impairs quality of life, and may lead to falls and fractures.
- Somatic and autonomic neuropathies are among the most common long-term complications of diabetes as well as the common precursor of prediabetes.
- Focal mononeuropathies involving single nerves occur and, for the most part, resolve spontaneously.
- Entrapments occur in one third of persons with diabetes and are treated medically or surgically.
- Diabetic neuropathies are not always recognized or diagnosed by healthcare providers
- A careful history and detailed physical examination, together with objective testing, are essential for the diagnosis.
- A number of simple tests done in the clinic are useful for detecting diabetic neuropathy and predicting complications, such as foot ulcers and gangrene.
- Standard and validated quantitative measures of disease progression are now available and allow better interpretation of responses to different treatments and study results.
- The newer symptomatic treatment modalities, based on etiologic factors, have potential for making a significant impact on morbidity and mortality.
- Preventive strategies and education for person with diabetes are key in reducing complication rates and mortality.

Introduction

Diabetic neuropathy (DN) is not a single entity; rather, it is a number of different syndromes, each with a range of clinical and subclinical manifestations. Effective management is based on recognizing the particular manifestation and underlying pathogenesis of the particular form of DN in each person with diabetes and using this information to initiate therapy at a level that ideally avoids undesirable side effects.

Translation of the science of neuropathy into clinical care is a major challenge for diabetes care providers. It requires knowledge on the one hand and careful attention to person with diabetes histories, symptoms, and signs on the other. The emergence of the study of neuropathy is a science in its own right, enhanced by technological and biological advances. However, the scientific and person with diabetes communities still await major research breakthroughs in understanding the complete pathophysiology and etiology of neuropathy.

Different syndromes can now be distinguished by different affected nerve fibers. The artful healthcare provider, through mindful interaction with the person with diabetes, appropriate testing, and a carefully honed skill set, is able to delineate the different but often intertwined neuropathic entities and administer individualized treatment.

State of the Disease

Diabetic neuropathy is the most common form of neuropathy in developed countries and is responsible for at least half of all nontraumatic amputations.[1] These disorders are among the most frequent complications of diabetes mellitus and a significant cause of morbidity and mortality. The major morbidity is foot ulceration, which can lead to gangrene and, ultimately, to limb loss. The true prevalence is not known, and reports vary from 10% to 90%, depending on the criteria and methods used to define neuropathy.[2–8] Estimates of diabetes-related amputation vary greatly from 78 to 704 per 100,000 person years, with a relative risk of diabetic versus nondiabetic varied from 7.4 to 41.3.[7] The lifetime risk of foot ulcers until recently was generally believed to be 15% to 25%, recent data suggest that the figure may be as high as 34%.[9] The national annual direct cost of foot ulcers in the United States has been estimated at approximately $9 billion to $13 billion.[10] Diabetic neuropathy is clearly a huge global economic burden; on an individual level, it also has a tremendous impact on the quality of life (QOL) of a person with diabetes.[1,11,12] The trend was noted to potentially be reversing in January 2012, when the Centers for Disease Control and Prevention (CDC) issued a press release on the results of a study showing a dramatic decline in diabetes-related foot ulcers in the United States by 65%. Importantly, the study also showed that this decline was restricted to those demographic areas where persons with diabetes had access to diabetes care that included education on foot care.[13] Other studies have confirmed a decrease in some populations.[7,14] Areas that are more problematic include underserved populations in rural and inner-city areas.[7]

It may not be completely accurate to characterize a decrease in relative risk of limb loss across heterogenous populations.[7]

Overall, diabetic neuropathy has a tremendous impact on the QOL of persons with diabetes, predominantly by causing parasthesias, pain, weakness, ataxia, and incoordination predisposing to diabetic foot ulcers, limb loss, falls, and fractures.[10] Chronic, persistent pain accounts for 40% of person with diabetes visits in a primary care setting, and about 20% of the presenting persons with diabetes attest to enduring pain for more than 6 months.[11] Persistent neuropathic pain significantly interferes with QOL, impairing sleep and recreation; it also significantly impacts emotional well-being and is associated with, if not the cause of, depression, anxiety, loss of sleep, and lack of engagement with treatment.[12]

Meanwhile, healthcare professionals are being confronted by new challenges related to results of studies showing that the autonomic neuropathy in its cardiovascular form is associated with at least a threefold increased risk for mortality.[2,14,15,16] More recently, autonomic imbalance between the sympathetic and the parasympathetic nervous systems has been implicated as a predictor of cardiovascular risk.[14,16]

Resting heart rate and measures of effort-related cardiac autonomic dysfunction have been acknowledged as predictors of cardiovascular events in asymptomatic persons with type 2 diabetes.[17] Diagnosis of autonomic neuropathy (AN) is also associated with poorer QOLl with a mortality rate of approximate 25% to 50% within 5 to 10 years.[5,6,16,18]

A Problem Diabetes Education Can Address

Diabetes care and education specialists have a major opportunity to assist in preventing the painful, devastating, and costly complications of DN.

- Although DN is highly prevalent in the diabetes population, healthcare providers may not recognize it.[19]
- When DN is recognized, providers may regard it as a single disease (rather than a heterogeneous group of disorders)

This chapter offers suggestions for dealing with these problems. Diabetes care and education specialists have the following opportunities to assist persons with diabetes affected by these common, painful, and potentially devastating diabetes complications:

- Acquire more information about neuropathy
- Recognize the different components of the disease
- Elicit useful information from persons with diabetes by asking the right questions
- Use the information to guide interventions

The diabetes care and education specialist can play a significant role by teaching the importance of controlled blood glucose blood pressure, lipids, with lifestyle modifications and meticulous foot care. These remain essential measures to reduce the risk of macrovascular and microvascular disease.

This chapter includes information on DN and new information on AN and its effect on QOL, and explains the cardiovascular component as a predictor of mortality. It emphasizes the importance of addressing persistent neuropathic pain as a difficult-to-manage clinical problem. Additionally, it exhorts the diabetes care and education specialist to counsel persons with diabetes on the risks of falling and strategies to prevent falls.

This chapter also provides information about new research on different treatment modalities that not only relieve neuropathic symptoms but also provide hope for changing the course of the disease.

Overview of DNs

This chapter describes different aspects of DN, explains the various nomenclatures, presents a clear and comprehensible classification of this complex disease state, and describes treatment options for specific neuropathic disorders.

As mentioned, DNs are a heterogeneous group of disorders that include abnormalities ranging from subclinical to clinical manifestations. Diabetes-related neuropathies have been classified on the basis of their clinical manifestations as well as anatomical findings[20] (see Table 28.1). Most of the pathology of DN occurs in the peripheral (surrounding) nervous system, although there may be some central nerve involvement. The peripheral nerve system is composed of the ANS (sympathetic and parasympathetic) and the sensorimotor nervous system. Autonomic nerves control *involuntary* functions (eg, breathing, heartbeat), while sensory nerves send information from the skin and internal organs about sensory perception (eg, hot and cold sensation), and motor nerves send commands from the brain to the body (eg, "Remove your hand from the hot stove"), thus controlling voluntary functions.[10]

Implications for Diabetes Education and Care

Because of the prevalence of neuropathy, and because it is an insidious and often silent disease, diabetes care and education specialists are advised to bring even the slightest suspicion of sensory and autonomic neuropathy to the provider's attention for nerve function testing. Table 28.2 lists the evidence-graded recommendations for screening.

Recommendations: American Diabetes Association

- All persons with diabetes should be assessed for diabetic peripheral neuropathy starting at diagnosis of type 2 diabetes and 5 years after the diagnosis of type 1 diabetes and at least annually thereafter. B
- Assessment for distal symmetric polyneuropathy should include a careful history and assessment of either temperature or pinprick sensation (small-fiber function) and vibration sensation using a 128-Hz tuning fork (for large-fiber function). All persons with diabetes should have annual 10-g monofilament testing to identify feet at risk for ulceration and amputation. B
- Symptoms and signs of autonomic neuropathy should be assessed in persons with diabetes with microvascular complications. E

Source: American Diabetes Association Diabetes Care 2019 Jan; 42(Supplement 1): S124-38.

TABLE 28.1 Clinical DNs: Classification

Rapidly Reversible Neuropathy	• Sexual dysfunction related to autonomic neuropathy
• Hyperglycemic neuropathy	• Bladder dysfunction related to autonomic neuropathy
Generalized Symmetrical Polyneuropathy	• Sudomotor dysfunction related to autonomic neuropathy
• Acute sensory neuropathy	• Pupillomotor and visceral (metabolic) response related to autonomic neuropathy
• Chronic sensorimotor neuropathy (distal diabetic polyneuropathy)	**Focal and Multifocal Neuropathies**
Small-fiber neuropathy	• Focal-limb
Large-fiber neuropathy	• Cranial neuropathy
Autonomic Neuropathy	• Proximal-motor neuropathy (amyotrophy)
• Cardiac autonomic neuropathy	• Truncal radiculoneuropathy
• Gastrointestinal disorders related to autonomic neuropathy	• Coexisting chronic inflammatory demyelinating neuropathy

Sources: Adapted from AJ Boulton, AI Vinik, JC Arezzo, et al, "Diabetic neuropathies: a statement by the American Diabetes Association," *Diabetes Care* 28, no. 4 (2005): 956-62; PK Thomas, JD Ward, PJ Watkins, "Diabetic neuropathy," in H Keen, J Jarrett, eds, *Complications of Diabetes* (London: Edward Arnold Publishing Company, 1982): 109-36.

TABLE 28.2 ADA Evidence-Grading System for Clinical Practice Recommendations

Level of Evidence	*Description*
A	Clear evidence from well-conducted, generalizable, and randomized controlled trials that are adequately powered, including the following: • Evidence from a well-conducted multicenter trial • Evidence from a meta-analysis that incorporated quality ratings in the analysis Compelling nonexperimental evidence (ie, the "all or none" rule developed by the Center for Evidence-Based Medicine at Oxford) Supportive evidence from well-conducted, randomized controlled trials that are adequately powered, including the following: • Evidence from a well-conducted trial at 1 or more institutions • Evidence from a meta-analysis that incorporated quality ratings in the analysis
B	Supportive evidence from well-conducted cohort studies, including the following: • Evidence from a well-conducted cohort study or registry • Evidence from a well-conducted meta-analysis of cohort studies Supportive evidence from a well-conducted case-control study
C	Supportive evidence from poorly controlled or uncontrolled studies, including the following: • Evidence from randomized clinical trials with 1 or more major or 3 or more minor methodological flaws that could invalidate the results • Evidence from observational studies with high potential for bias (such as case series with comparison to historical controls) • Evidence from case series or case reports Conflicting evidence with the weight of evidence supporting the recommendation
E	Expert consensus or clinical experience

Source: Standards of Medical Care in Diabetes—2020 American Diabetes Association Diabetes Care 2020 Jan; 43 (Supplement 1):S52

Diagnosis/Clinical Assessment Tools

Scoring Systems

Symptoms of neuropathy can vary markedly from 1 person with diabetes to another, making the correct assessment of these disorders difficult at times. For this reason, standardized, validated symptom questionnaires with similar scoring systems have been developed for measuring the severity of symptoms and the degree of reproducible neuropathic deficits. These include the Michigan Neuropathy Screening Instrument,[21] the Neuropathy Symptom Score for neuropathic symptoms, and the Neuropathy Disability Score or the Nerve Impairment Score (NIS) for neuropathic deficits.[22] The Neurologic Symptom Score[23,24] has 38 items that capture symptoms of muscle weakness, sensory disturbances, and autonomic dysfunction and are useful for follow-up with a person with diabetes and for assessing a person with diabetes responses to treatment.

The neurological history and examination are central to care of a person with diabetes and should always be performed initially and then at all subsequent visits.

Screening Recommendations

Combinations of more than 1 test have more than 87% sensitivity in detecting chronic sensorimotor neuropathy.[25,26] Longitudinal studies have shown that these simple tests are good predictors of foot-ulcer risk.[27] Numerous composite scores to evaluate clinical signs of DN, such as the NIS, are useful in documenting and monitoring neuropathic deficits.[28]

Objective Devices for the Diagnosis of Neuropathy

The neurological examination should focus on the lower extremities and should always include an accurate foot inspection for deformities, ulcers, fungal infection, muscle wasting, hair distribution or loss, and the presence or absence of pulses. Sensory modalities should be assessed using simple handheld devices such as the following:

- Touch—cotton wool or soft brush
- Vibration—128-Hz tuning fork
- Pressure—1-g and 10-g SWM
- Pinprick—Wartenberg wheel or a pin
- Temperature—testing with cold or warm objects or NeuroQuick (Schweers)[29]

Finally, the Achilles reflexes should be tested[25,30] (Table 28.3). Figure 28.1 describes how to use a monofilament.

Diagnosis of early distal symmetric polyneuropathy (DSP) is challenging. Nerve conduction studies (NCS) are often normal. Skin biopsy for intraepidermal nerve fiber density has better sensitivity but is invasive.

Quantitative Sensory Testing

Quantitative sensory testing (QST) is of value in detecting subclinical neuropathy, assessing progression, and predicting risk for foot ulceration.[28,31] These standardized measures of vibration and thermal thresholds also play an important role in multicenter clinical trials as primary efficacy end points, as do QOL measures.[10]

Moreover, assessment of thermal thresholds is a key element in the diagnostic pathway of small-fiber polyneuropathy.[32,33] A consensus subcommittee of the American Academy of Neurology stated that QST received a Class II rating as a diagnostic test, with a type B strength of recommendation.[34]

Skin Biopsy and Intraepidermal Nerve Fiber Density

Skin biopsy has become a widely used tool to investigate small-caliber sensory nerves, including somatic unmyelinated intraepidermal nerve fibers (IENFs), dermal myelinated nerve fibers, and autonomic nerve fibers in peripheral neuropathies and other conditions.[35–37] The importance of the skin biopsy as a diagnostic tool for DSP is increasingly being recognized.[38–40] This technique

TABLE 28.3 Examination—Bedside Sensory Tests

Sensory Modality	*Nerve Fiber*	*Instrument*	*Associated Sensory Receptors*
Vibration	Aβ (large)	128-Hz tuning fork	Ruffini corpuscle mechanoreceptors
Pain (pinprick)	C (small)	Neuro-tips	Nociceptors for pain and warmth
Pressure	Aβ, Aα (large)	1-g and 10-g monofilament	Pacinian corpuscle
Light touch	Aβ, Aα (large)	Wisp of cotton	Meissner's corpuscle
Cold	Aδ (small)	Cold tuning fork	Cold thermoreceptors

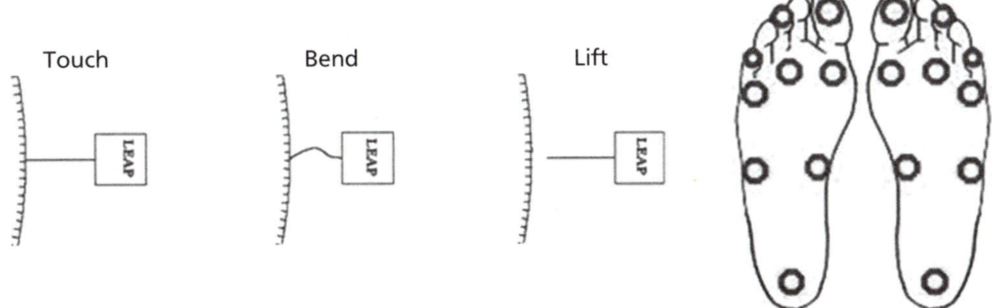

1. **Touch:** Use a smooth motion to touch the filament to the skin on the foot. Touch the filament along the side of and NOT directly on an ulcer, callus, or scar. Touch the filament to the skin for 1-2 seconds.
2. **Bend:** Push hard enough to make the filament bend as shown above.
3. **Lift:** Touch the filament to both of the feet in the sites circled on the drawing above. Place a (+) in the circle if the individual can feel the filament at that site and a (–) if the individual cannot feel the filament at that site.

FIGURE 28.1 Monofilament Testing

Source: US Department of Health and Human Services, Health Resources and Services, "Lower Extremity Amputation Prevention (LEAP)" (cited 2019 Dec 23), on the Internet at: http://www.hrsa.gov/hansensdisease/leap/.

quantitates small epidermal nerve fibers through antibody staining of the pan-axonal marker protein gene product 9.5 (PGP 9.5). Though minimally invasive (3-mm diameter punch biopsy), it enables a direct study of small fibers, which cannot be evaluated by nerve conduction velocity studies. It has led to the recognition of small-nerve-fiber syndrome as part of prediabetes and diabetes (Figure 28.2). When persons with diabetes present with "burning foot or hand syndrome," evaluation for prediabetes and diabetes is necessary. Therapeutic lifestyle changes[41] can result in nerve fiber regeneration, reversal of the neuropathy, and alleviation of symptoms. Different techniques for tissue processing and nerve fiber evaluation exist. For diagnostic purposes in peripheral neuropathies, the recent guidelines from the Joint Task Force of the European Federation of Neurological Societies and the Peripheral Nerve Society should be applied.[42] Quantification of IENF density appears to be more sensitive than sensory nerve conduction study or sural nerve biopsy in diagnosing small-fiber neuropathy.

Corneal Confocal Microscopy

Corneal confocal microscopy is a noninvasive technique used to detect small-nerve-fiber loss in the cornea, as it correlates with both increasing neuropathic severity and reduced IENF density in persons with diabetes.[43,44] A novel technique of real-time mapping permits an area of 3.2 mm² to be mapped with a total of 64 theoretically nonoverlapping single 400 µm² images.[45]

Contact Heat-Evoked Potentials

Contact heat-evoked potentials (CHEPs) have been studied in healthy controls, in persons newly diagnosed with diabetes, in persons with established diabetes, and in persons with prediabetes. It appears that CHEPs are capable of detecting small-fiber neuropathy in the absence of other indices, and that CHEPs correlate with quantitative sensory perception and objective tests of small-fiber function such as the cooling detection threshold and cold pain.[46,47]

Sudomotor Function

Changes in peripheral ANS function are an early manifestation of distal small-fiber neuropathy.[7] Sudomotor dysfunction is one of the earliest detectable neurophysiologic abnormalities in distal small-fiber neuropathies. Sweat glands are innervated by small, unmyelinated sympathetic C-nerve fibers that are responsible for the sweat response. Skin biopsies have confirmed that epidermal C-nerve fibers are reduced in persons with diabetes.[48] Thus, sudomotor function represents an attractive tool to evaluate the peripheral and autonomic nervous systems in people with diabetes mellitus.[49] The various techniques of sudomotor function testing, each with its strengths and weaknesses, are very sensitive and specific in the detection of distal small-fiber neuropathy. Most of these techniques, however, have remained underutilized in clinical practice due to lack of availability, results variability, and technical demands of the tests—most of them being tedious, cumbersome, and time-consuming. SUDOSCAN™ (Impeto Medical) is a device designed to precisely evaluate sweat gland function based on sweat chloride concentrations through reverse iontophoresis and chronoamperometry.[50–52] This is a simple noninvasive test that is easy to perform. Persons with diabetes place their hands and feet on the

IENF Loss in Small-Fiber Neuropathy

Control

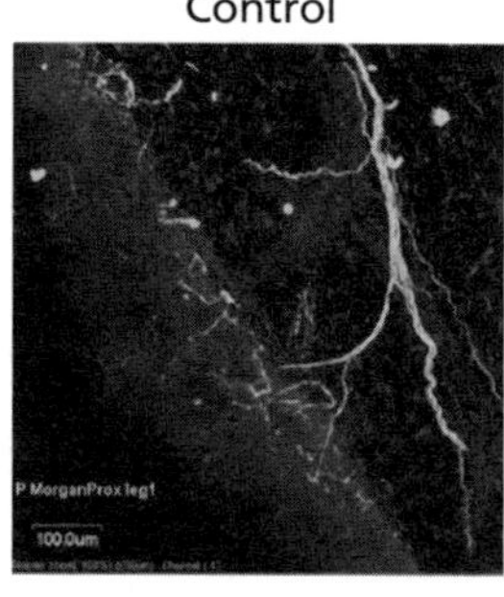

Metabolic syndrome

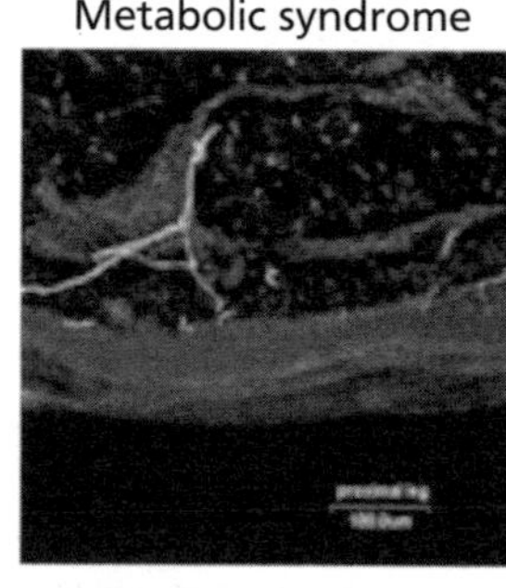

Diabetes

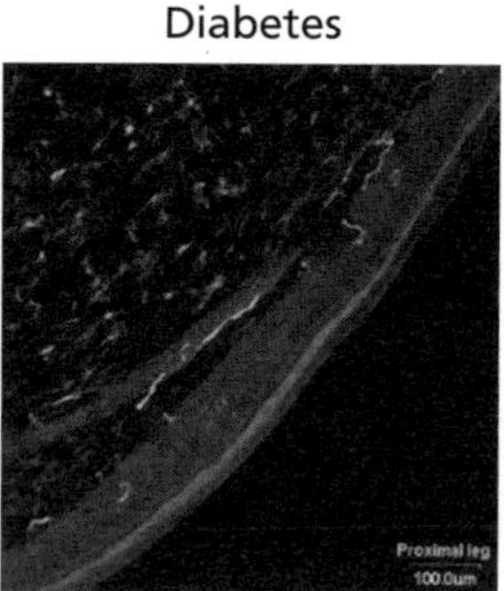

FIGURE 28.2 **Loss of Cutaneous Nerve Fibers That Stain Positive for the Neuronal Antigen PGP 9.5 in Metabolic Syndrome Diabetes**

Sources: AI Vinik, J Ullal, HK Parson, CM Casellini, "Diabetic neuropathies: clinical manifestations and current treatment options," *Nat Clin Pract Endocrinol Metab* 2 (2006): 269-81; GL Pittenger, M Ray, NI Burcus, P McNulty, B Basta, AI Vinik, "Intraepidermal nerve fibers are indicators of small-fiber neuropathy in both diabetic and nondiabetic patients," *Diabetes Care* 27 (2004): 1974-9; G Pittenger, A Mehrabyan, K Simmons, et al, "Small fiber neuropathy is associated with the metabolic syndrome," *Metab Syndr Relat Disord.* 3 (2005): 113-21.

electrodes and stand still for 2 to 3 minutes. Neither special subject preparation nor specially trained medical personnel are needed. The reproducibility of this sweat function measurement has been successfully validated in different studies, and inter-device reproducibility has been confirmed through measurements with 2 different devices.[52,53,54,55,56]

Nerve Conduction Velocity

The use of electrophysiologic measures (measures of nerve conduction velocity [NCV]) in both clinical practice and multicenter clinical trials is recommended.[7,57] Refer also to the review article recommending measurement of nerve conduction amplitudes in the clinic as well as in clinical trials.[58]

In persons with type 2 diabetes, NCV abnormalities in the lower limbs increased from 8% at baseline to 42% after 10 years of disease.[59] A slow progression of NCV abnormalities in persons with type 1 diabetes was observed in the Diabetes Control and Complications Trial (DCCT).[60] In fact, NCV plays a key role in ruling out other causes of neuropathy and is essential for the identification of focal and multifocal neuropathies.[33,61] It is important to recognize that persons with diabetes with painful, predominantly small-fiber neuropathy may have normal NCV study results.

QOL Measures

The effect of neuropathy per se on the QOL of the person with diabetes is widely recognized. A number of instruments have been developed and validated to assess QOL in DN. The Norfolk QOL-DN questionnaire is a validated tool that addresses specific symptoms and the impact of large, small, and autonomic nerve-fiber functions; the tool has been used in clinical trials and is available in 38 validated language versions.[7] The NeuroQol[62] measures persons' with diabetes perceptions of the impact of neuropathy and foot ulcers.

The diagnosis of distal polyneuropathy is mainly clinical, aided by specific diagnostic tests according to the type and severity of the neuropathy; however, nondiabetic causes of neuropathy must always be excluded, depending on the clinical findings.

Many people in the United States and abroad are unaware that they have neuropathy. In a study in Romania, 25,000 persons with diabetes were screened for neuropathy using the Norfolk QOL-DN questionnaire. Although they self-reported that they did not have neuropathy, 6,615 were found to have neuropathy according to the criteria in the screening tool.

This large number of people with undisclosed neuropathy underscores the need to have good diagnostic techniques and an awareness for persons with diabetes and health professionals to recognize symptoms and signs of neuropathy.[63]

The spectrum of clinical neuropathic syndromes described in persons with diabetes includes dysfunction of almost every segment of the somatic peripheral and autonomic nervous systems[64]—thus the adage "Knowing neuropathy means to know the whole of medicine." Distinguishing each syndrome by its pathophysiologic, therapeutic, and prognostic features is feasible. This theme will be reiterated throughout the chapter.

Conditions Mimicking DN[8]

A number of conditions can be mistaken for painful DN:

- Intermittent claudication—the pain is exacerbated by walking
- Morton's neuroma—the pain and tenderness are localized to the intermetatarsal space and may be elicited by applying pressure with the thumb in the appropriate intermetatarsal space
- Osteoarthritis—the pain is confined to the joints, made worse with joint movement or exercise, and associated with morning stiffness that improves with ambulation
- Radiculopathy—the pain originates in the shoulder, arm, thorax, or back and radiates into the legs and feet
- Charcot neuroarthropathy—the pain is localized to the site of the collapse of the bones of the foot, and the foot is hot rather than cold
- Plantar fasciitis—shooting or burning pain in the heel with each step and exquisite tenderness in the sole of the foot
- Tarsal tunnel syndrome—pain and numbness radiate from beneath the medial malleolus to the sole and are localized to the inner side of the foot

In contrast, DSP pain is bilateral, symmetrical (covering the whole foot and particularly the dorsum), and worse at night, interfering with sleep.

Implications for Diabetes Education and Care

Diabetes care and education specialists should take note of the conditions that mimic DN.

Recognize that the most important differential diagnoses from the general medicine perspective include neuropathies caused by alcohol abuse, uremia, hypothyroidism, vitamin B_{12} deficiency, peripheral arterial disease, cancer, inflammatory and infectious diseases, elevated mercury levels, celiac disease, and neurotoxic drugs.[65]

Classification and Diagnostic Assessment of Distal Symmetric Diabetic Polyneuropathies

Chronic Sensorimotor Neuropathy

Chronic sensorimotor neuropathy (also referred to as distal diabetic polyneuropathy or distal symmetric polyneuropathy) is the most common form of diffuse neuropathy in diabetes. Chronic sensorimotor neuropathy primarily involves the sensory nerves. Sensory symptoms are more prominent than motor symptoms and usually involve the lower limbs. Symptoms include pain, paresthesia, hyperesthesia, deep aching, and burning and sharp stabbing sensations similar to but less severe than those described in ASN. In addition, persons with diabetes may experience negative symptoms such as numbness in the feet and legs that in time leads to painless foot ulcers and subsequent amputations if the neuropathy is not promptly recognized and treated. Unsteadiness is also frequently seen due to abnormal proprioception and muscle sensory function.[66,67] Alternatively, some persons with diabetes may be completely asymptomatic and signs may be discovered only by a detailed neurological examination.

Sensory deficits occur in the distal portions of the limbs, spreading over time from the toes to the legs and then from the fingers to the arms in a "stocking-glove" pattern, involving small-nerve fibers, large-nerve fibers, or both. Distal symmetric polyneuropathy is frequently accompanied by AN. All persons with diabetes with DSP are at increased risk of neuropathic complications such as foot ulceration and Charcot neuroarthropathy (see Figure 28.3).

Because of the lack of agreement on the definition and diagnostic assessment of neuropathy, several consensus conferences were convened to overcome the current problems, the most recent of which has redefined the minimal criteria for the diagnosis of typical distal symmetric diabetic polyneuropathies (DSPN), as summarized below.[7]

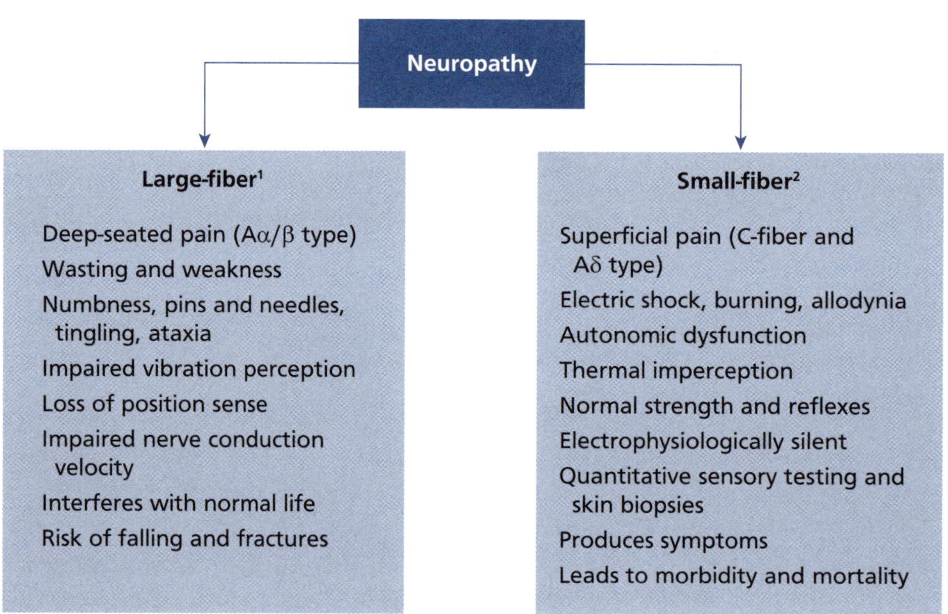

FIGURE 28.3 **Clinical Presentation of Small- and Large-Fiber Neuropathies**

[1]Aα fibers are large myelinated fibers that are in charge of motor functions and muscle control. Aα/β fibers are also large myelinated fibers, with sensory functions such as perception to touch, vibration, and position.

[2]Aδ fibers are small myelinated fibers responsible for pain stimuli and cold perception. Small C-fibers can be myelinated or unmyelinated and have both sensory (warm perception and pain) and autonomic functions (blood pressure and heart rate regulation, sweating, gastrointestinal tract and genitourinary tract).

Source: Modified from original diagram by A Vinik, C Casellini, A Nakave, C Patel, "Diabetic neuropathies," edited by R Rushakoff (cited 18 Oct 2016). On the Internet at: http://diabetesmanager.pbworks.com/w/page/17680180/Diabetic%20Neuropathies.

Toronto Classification of DSPN[7]

1. *Possible DSPN:* The presence of symptoms or signs of DSPN may include the following: symptoms—decreased sensation, positive neuropathic sensory symptoms (eg, "asleep numbness," prickling or stabbing pain, burning or aching pain) predominantly in the toes, feet, or legs; signs—symmetric decrease of distal sensation or unequivocally decreased or absent ankle reflexes.
2. *Probable DSPN:* The presence of a combination of symptoms and signs of neuropathy including any 2 or more of the following: neuropathic symptoms, decreased distal sensation, or unequivocally decreased or absent ankle reflexes.
3. *Confirmed DSPN:* The presence of an abnormality of nerve conduction and either a symptom (or symptoms) or a sign (or signs) of neuropathy confirm DSPN. If nerve conduction is normal, a validated measure of small-fiber neuropathy (with class 1 evidence) may be used. To assess for the severity of DSPN, several approaches are recommended: the graded approach outlined above and in Table 28.2; various continuous measures of sum scores of neurologic signs, symptoms, or nerve test scores; scores of function of activities of daily living; or scores of predetermined tasks or of disability.
4. *Subclinical DSPN:* The presence of no signs or symptoms of neuropathy is confirmed with abnormal nerve conduction or a validated measure of small-fiber neuropathy (with class 1 evidence). Definition 1, 2, or 3 can be used for clinical practice, and definition 3 or 4 can be used for research studies.
5. *Small-fiber neuropathy:* Small-fiber neuropathy should be graded as follows: (1) possible: the presence of length-dependent symptoms and/or clinical signs of small-fiber damage; (2) probable: the presence of length-dependent symptoms, clinical signs of small-fiber damage, and normal sural nerve conduction; and (3) definite: the presence of length-dependent symptoms, clinical signs of small-fiber damage, normal sural nerve conduction, and altered IENF density at the ankle and/or abnormal thermal thresholds at the foot.[30]

The diagnosis of DSPN should rest on the findings of the clinical and neurological examinations, that is, the presence of neuropathic symptoms (positive and negative, sensory and motor) and signs (sensory deficit, allodynia and hyperalgesia, motor weakness, absence of reflexes).[68,69] Symptoms alone have poor diagnostic accuracy in predicting the presence of polyneuropathy. Signs are better predictors than symptoms. Multiple signs are better predictors than a single sign. Relatively simple examinations are as accurate as complex scoring systems. Thus, both symptoms and signs should be assessed.

The basic neurological assessment comprises the general medical and neurological history, inspection of the feet, and neurological examination of sensation using simple semiquantitative bedside instruments such as the 10-g Semmes Weinstein Monofilament (SWM) or Neuropen® (Owen Mumford)[70] (to assess touch/pressure); NeuroQuick (Schweers)[71] or Tip Therm® (tip therm GmbH)[72] (to assess temperature); calibrated Rydel-Seiffer tuning fork (to assess vibration); pinprick (to assess pain); and deep tendon reflexes (to assess the knee and ankle). In addition, assessment of joint position and motor power may be indicated. The normal range for the tuning fork on the dorsal distal joint of the great toe is ≥5/8 scale units in persons 21 to 40 years old, ≥4.5/8 in those 41 to 60 years old, ≥4/8 in individuals 61 to 71 years old, and ≥3.5/8 in those 72 to 82 years old.[73]

The following findings should alert healthcare providers to consider causes for DSPN other than diabetes and referral for a detailed neurological workup: (1) pronounced asymmetry of the neurological deficits; (2) predominant motor deficits, mononeuropathy, or cranial nerve involvement; (3) rapid development or progression of the neuropathic impairments; (4) progression of the neuropathy despite optimal glycemic control; (5) symptoms from the upper limbs; (6) family history of nondiabetic neuropathy; and (7) diagnosis of DSPN cannot be ascertained by clinical examination.[74]

Implications for Diabetes Education and Care

A comprehensive clinical examination is key to the diagnosis of chronic sensorimotor neuropathy. Examine feet in detail to detect ulcers, calluses, and deformities, and inspect footwear at every visit. Check shoes for stones, buttons, or other loose items that are potentially harmful to insensate feet. All persons with chronic sensorimotor neuropathy are at increased risk of foot ulceration and Charcot neuroarthropathy.

Subtypes of DSPN

Rapidly Reversible Hyperglycemic Neuropathy

Reversible abnormalities of nerve function with distal sensory symptoms may occur in persons with recently diagnosed or poorly controlled diabetes. These are unlikely to be caused by structural abnormalities, as recovery soon follows restoration of euglycemia.[32]

Rapidly reversible hyperglycemic neuropathy usually presents with distal sensory symptoms, and whether these abnormalities result in an increased risk of developing chronic neuropathies in the future remains unknown.[21,75]

Implications for Diabetes Education and Care

In people recently diagnosed with diabetes or those with poorly controlled diabetes, the opportunity exists to reverse neuropathy. A concerted effort to encourage the individual to achieve this goal by tight blood glucose control is essential. The individual must be advised and understand that the pain may get worse with initiation of glycemic control before it gets better. During the early phase of glycemic control, when the blood vessels are constricted, blood is shunted away from the damaged area, exacerbating the pain. Later, the body adapts by dilating the blood vessels and increasing the blood flow.

Acute Sensory Neuropathy

Acute sensory neuropathy (ASN) is a variant of chronic sensorimotor neuropathy that is characterized by severe pain, wasting, weight loss, depression, and in males, erectile dysfunction.[76] Persons with diabetes report, especially in the feet, unremitting burning, deep pain, and hyperesthesia. Other symptoms include sharp, stabbing, or electric shock–like sensations in the lower limbs that appear more frequently during the night. Signs are usually absent with a relatively normal clinical examination, except for allodynia (interpretation of all stimuli as painful, even light touch). Occasionally, ankle reflexes are absent or reduced.[77] Acute sensory neuropathy is usually associated with poor glycemic control but may also appear after rapid improvement of glycemia. It has been hypothesized that changes in blood glucose flux produce alterations in epineurial blood flow, leading to ischemia.[78] Other authors propose an immune-mediated mechanism.[79]

Implications for Diabetes Education and Care

The key to management of ASN is achieving blood glucose stability.[31] Most persons with diabetes also require medication for neuropathic pain.[80] The natural history of this disease is resolution of symptoms within 1 year.[81]

Small-Nerve-Fiber Neuropathy

Small-nerve-fiber neuropathy often presents with pain, but without objective signs or electrophysiologic evidence of nerve damage. Table 28.4 lists clinical manifestations of small-fiber neuropathies.

TABLE 28.4 Small-Fiber Neuropathies: Clinical Manifestations
Small, thinly myelinated Aδ and unmyelinated C fibers are affected
Symptoms are prominent; pain is the C-fiber type: burning, superficial, and associated with allodynia (interpretation of all stimuli—ie, touch—as painful)
Late in the condition, progression to numbness and hypoalgesia (lack of sensation)
Abnormal cold and warm thermal sensation
Defective autonomic function with decreased sweating; dry skin; impaired vasomotion; the vascular responses to vasoconstrictive and vasodilative stimuli, whose net effect acts on blood flow; and the presentation of a cold foot
Reflexes and motor strength are remarkably intact
Nerve conduction velocity studies show no deficit
Loss of cutaneous nerve fibers is shown on skin biopsies using PGP 9.5 staining
Diagnosed clinically by reduced sensitivity to 1-g SWM and pricking sensation using the Wartenberg wheel or similar instrument[1]
Risk is foot ulceration, subsequent gangrene, and amputation
Abnormalities in thresholds for warm thermal perception, neurovascular function, pain, quantitative sudorimetry, and quantitative autonomic function tests[2,3]

Sources:

1. AJ Boulton, RA Malik, JC Arezzo, JM Sosenko, "Diabetic somatic neuropathies," *Diabetes Care*. 27(2004):1458-86.
2. AI Vinik, ML Nevoret, CM Casellini, "The new age of sudomotor function testing: a sensitive and specific biomarker for diagnosis, estimation of severity, monitoring progression, and regression in response to intervention," *Front Endocrinol* (Lausanne). 6(2015):94.
3. CM Casellini, HK Parson, MS Richardson, ML Nevoret, AI Vinik, "SUDOSCAN, a noninvasive tool for detecting diabetic small fiber neuropathy and autonomic dysfunction," *Diabetes Technol Ther*. 18(6)(2016):391-8. Epub 2016 Apr 8.

Ulceration, Gangrene, and Amputation Are Risks With Small-Fiber Neuropathy

With small-fiber neuropathy, the greatest risk is for foot ulceration and subsequent gangrene and amputation.

As previously mentioned, small, unmyelinated nerve fibers are affected early in diabetes and are not reflected in NCV studies. Other methods that do not depend on conduction, such as QST or skin biopsy with quantification of IENFs, are necessary to identify these cases.[79,82] However, NCV plays a key role in ruling out other causes of neuropathy and is essential for the identification of focal neuropathies and entrapments as well as multifocal neuropathies.[32,61] Also, as mentioned, the importance of the skin biopsy as a diagnostic tool for chronic sensorimotor neuropathy is increasingly being recognized.[38–40]

Pain Mechanism in Small-Fiber Neuropathy

The mechanism for pain in small-fiber neuropathy is not well understood.[83] Hyperglycemia may be a factor in lowering the pain threshold. However, too rapid or overzealous lowering of A1C greater than 1% per month may result in severe pain called *neuritis*.[84] A striking amelioration of symptoms with the intravenous administration of insulin *can* be achieved.[85] The disappearance of pain may not necessarily reflect nerve recovery but rather nerve death. When persons with diabetes volunteer the loss of pain, progression of the neuropathy must be excluded by careful examination and specific small-fiber testing.[86]

Large-Nerve-Fiber Neuropathies

Large-nerve-fiber neuropathies may involve sensory and/or motor nerves. These tend to be the neuropathies of *signs*, with a lesser degree of *symptoms*. Large fibers mediate motor function, vibration perception, position sense, and cold thermal perception. Unlike the small-nerve fibers, these myelinated, rapidly conducting fibers begin in the toes and have their first synapse in the medulla oblongata. (Myelin is a fatlike substance that forms a sheath around certain nerve fibers.) These fibers tend to be affected first because of their length and the tendency in diabetes for nerves to "die back." Because they are myelinated, they are the fibers represented in the electrophysiologic nerve conduction studies, and subclinical abnormalities in nerve function are readily detected.

The symptoms may be minimal: sensation of walking on cotton, floors feeling strange, or the inability to turn the pages of a book or to discriminate among coins. Large-nerve-fiber neuropathy produces numbness, ataxia, and incoordination, impairing daily living activities and causing falls and fractures.[39] See Table 28.5 for clinical manifestations of large-fiber neuropathies.

Combinations of Large- and Small-Fiber Damage

Most persons with diabetes with chronic sensorimotor neuropathy have a "mixed" variety of neuropathy, with both large-nerve-fiber and small-nerve-fiber damage. Early in the course of the neuropathic process, multifocal sensory loss might also be found. In some individuals, severe distal muscle weakness can accompany the sensory loss, resulting in an inability to stand on the toes or heels. Some grading systems use this as a definition of severity.

Definition of Neuropathic Pain

A definition of peripheral neuropathic pain in diabetes, adapted from a definition proposed by the International Association for the Study of Pain,[87] is "pain arising as a direct consequence of abnormalities in the peripheral somatosensory system in people with diabetes."[7]

TABLE 28.5 Large-Fiber Neuropathies: Clinical Manifestations
Large myelinated Aα/β fibers are affected and may involve sensory and/or motor nerves
Impaired vibration perception and position sense are often the first objective evidence
Abnormal tendon reflexes
Pain is described as deep-seated gnawing, dull, a "toothache" in the bones of the feet, or crushing or cramplike pain (called type A-d nerve fibers)
Sensation of walking on cotton, floors feeling strange, inability to turn pages of a book or to discriminate among coins
Sensory ataxia (waddling like a duck)
Wasting of small muscles of feet with hammertoes
Weakness of hands and feet
Shortening of the Achilles tendon with pes equines (horses' foot)
Increased blood flow (hot foot)
Higher risk of falls, fractures, and development of Charcot neuroarthropathy
Most persons with diabetes have a mixture of large- and small-nerve-fiber involvement

A grading system for the degree of certainty of the diagnosis of neuropathic pain has been proposed. It is based on 4 simple criteria, namely,

1. whether the pain has a distinct neuroanatomical distribution,
2. whether the history of the person with diabetes suggests the presence or absence of a lesion or disease of the peripheral or central somatosensory system,
3. whether either of these findings is supported by at least 1 confirmatory test, and
4. whether there is an abnormality of nerve conduction.[87]

Degree of certainty is defined according to the number of criteria met: 1 to 4 (definite neuropathic pain), 1 and 2 plus 3 or 4 (probable neuropathic pain), or only 1 and 2 (possible neuropathic pain). There is no consensus on their diagnostic validity, since neuropathic pain is a composite of pain and other sensory symptoms associated with nerve injury. For example, sensory deficits, abnormal spontaneous or induced sensations such as paresthesias (eg, tingling), spontaneous attacks of electric shock–like sensations, and allodynia preclude a simple definition (see below).

The Diagnosis of Neuropathic Pain

The diagnosis of neuropathic pain—as opposed to pain from causes other than neuropathy—is made by taking a careful history. Persons with diabetes should be queried during the office visit as to whether they are experiencing tingling, burning, or pain at rest in their feet. A positive response warrants further investigation and screening for painful diabetic peripheral neuropathy (PDPN). Somatosensory, motor, or autonomic bedside evaluation can be done and is complemented by use of one of the pain screening tools (DN4, Pain DETECT, etc).[88] The physician should ensure that all features of pain, such as distribution, quality, severity, timing, associated symptoms, and exacerbating and relieving factors (if any), are recorded. In particular, the presence of numbness, burning, tingling, lightning pain, stabbing, and prickling should be recorded, as is done in the Norfolk QOL tool,[89] the Neuropathy Total Symptom Score-6 (NTSS-6) questionnaire,[90] and the Pain DETECT.[88] Pain intensity and quality should be assessed using pain intensity scales (Visual Analogue Scale or a numerical rating scale)[91] and pain questionnaires (Brief Pain Inventory [BPI] and the Neuropathic Pain Symptom Inventory [NPSI]). A number of tools and questionnaires have been developed to quantify the impact of pain on sleep, on mood, and on QOL, mainly to be used in clinical trials. In clinical practice, the BPI Interference, the Profile of Moods, or the hospital scale for anxiety and depression can provide a simple measure of the impact of pain on QOL. Persons with diabetes can self-report their responses to treatment by using a diary to record the course of painful symptoms and their impact on daily life.[89,92] These questionnaires, pain inventories, and self-reporting diaries are most useful for outcome measures in clinical trials on drugs used for pain relief. Validated scoring systems for symptoms and signs are available in the form of questionnaires or checklists, such as the Neuropathy Symptom Score and the Michigan Neuropathy Screening Instrument Questionnaire for symptoms, and the Michigan Neuropathy Screening Instrument and the Neuropathy Disability Score for signs.[21,93]

Distinction Between Nociceptive and Non-nociceptive Pain

Because of its complexity, the presentation of pain poses a diagnostic dilemma for the clinician who needs to distinguish between neuropathic non-nociceptive pain arising as a direct consequence of a lesion or disease of the somatosensory system and nociceptive pain that is due to trauma, inflammation, or injury. It is imperative to try to establish the nature of any predisposing factor, including the pathogenesis of the pain, if one is to be successful in its management. First line medications may be useful (see below). Persons with diabetes can also be encouraged to find solutions, using targeted pain-centered strategies such as biofeedback or diversion. The inciting injury may be focal or diffuse and may involve single or, more likely, multiple mechanisms such as metabolic disturbances encompassing hyperglycemia, dyslipidemia, glucose fluctuations, or intensification of therapy with insulin. On the other hand, the injury might embrace autoimmune mechanisms, neurovascular insufficiency, deficient neurotrophism, oxidative and nitrosative stress, and inflammation.[80,94] Because pain syndromes in diabetes may be focal or diffuse, proximal or distal, acute or chronic, each has its own pathogenesis, and the treatment must be tailored to the underlying disorder if the outcome is to be successful. The presence of diabetes must be established, if this has not already been done.

A number of self-administered questionnaires have been developed, validated, translated, and subjected to cross-cultural adaptation to both diagnose and distinguish neuropathic as opposed to non-neuropathic pain: Leeds Assessment of Neuropathic Symptoms and Signs (LANSS) Pain Scale, Douleur Neuropathique en 4 Questions (DN4), Neuropathic Pain Questionnaire (NPS), Pain DETECT, and ID-Pain.[89,94–100] Assessment questionnaires such as the Short-Form McGill Pain Questionnaire, the BPI, and the NPSI assess pain quality and intensity.[94,101,102]

According to Initiative on Methods, Measurement and Pain Assessment in Clinical Trials, the following pain characteristics should be evaluated to assess the efficacy and effectiveness of chronic pain treatment:[103]

1. pain intensity measured on a 0 to 10 numerical rating scale;
2. physical functioning, assessed by the Multidimensional Pain Inventory and Brief Pain Inventory (BPI) Interferences scale;
3. emotional functioning, assessed by the Beck Depression Inventory and Profile of Mood States; and
4. patient rating of overall improvement, assessed by the Patient Global Impression of Change.

Laboratory Tests to Evaluate Neuropathic Pain

Since neuropathic pain is subjective, no tests can objectively quantify this pain in humans. Tests of pain in animal studies are really measures of reaction time to heat or other stimuli, which is one of the reasons for failure of translation of animal studies to humans. Thus, laboratory tests do not reflect spontaneous pain but rather the function of the nociceptive system and, ultimately, with QST, the evoked positive sensory phenomena associated with neuropathic pain (ie, hyperalgesia and allodynia). This means that the results of laboratory tests become useful only in the context of a comprehensive clinical examination. Other tests were discussed earlier in the chapter.

Evaluation of pain intensity is essential for monitoring the response to therapy. There are a number of symptom-based screening tools, such as the NTSS-6, BPI, QOL-DN, SF-36 Health Survey (a short-form, 36-question health survey), Visual Analog Scale for Pain Intensity, NeuroQol, and Norfolk Neuropathy Symptoms Score. With the Visual Analog Scale, the person with diabetes marks the intensity of his or her pain on a scale from 0 to 10, allowing an assessment of the response to intervention. Simultaneously, the person with diabetes should complete a QOL tool, such as the Norfolk QOL-DN, which needs to include comorbidities such as anxiety, depression, and sleep interference.

Pharmacologic Therapeutic Modalities for Diabetic Neuropathic Pain

Treatment Based on Pathogenic Concepts of Pain

Painful symptoms in DSPN may constitute a considerable management problem. The efficacy of a single therapeutic agent is not the rule, and simple analgesics are usually inadequate to control the pain. There is agreement that persons with diabetes should be offered the available therapies in a stepwise fashion.[104–107] Effective pain treatment considers a favorable balance between pain relief and side effects without implying a maximum effect. The following general considerations in the pharmacotherapy of neuropathic pain require attention:

- The appropriate and effective drug has to be tried and identified in each person with diabetes by carefully titrating the dose based on efficacy and side effects.
- Lack of efficacy should be judged only after 2 to 4 weeks of treatment using an adequate dose.
- Because the evidence from clinical trials suggests only a maximum response of ≈50% for any monotherapy, analgesic combinations may be useful.
- Potential drug interactions have to be considered given the frequent use of polypharmacy in persons with diabetes.

Treatment With Evidence Grade Indicated

- Optimize glucose control to prevent or delay the development of neuropathy in persons with diabetes with type 1 diabetes **A** and to slow the progression of neuropathy in persons with diabetes with type 2 diabetes. **B**
- Assess and treat persons with diabetes to reduce pain related to diabetic peripheral neuropathy **B** and symptoms of autonomic neuropathy and to improve quality of life. **E**
- Pregabalin, duloxetine, or gabapentin are recommended as initial pharmacologic treatments for neuropathic pain in diabetes. **A**

Source: American Diabetes Association Diabetes Care 2020 Jan; 43(Supplement 1):S151.

A recent meta-analysis in which duloxetine was indirectly compared with pregabalin and gabapentin for the treatment of PDPN concluded that these 3 drugs have comparable efficacy and tolerability.[108] Some studies have analyzed healthcare costs in persons with PDPN treated with pregabalin, duloxetine, or other usually used drugs. In general, all studies showed similar results, with a good cost-effective profile for both drugs.[109–111]

Other medications including tapentadol have indications for diabetic neuropathic pain. Tapentadol has opiod type effects and should be used cautiously. Tricyclic antidepressants, venlafaxine, carbamazepine, and topical capsaicin (or patch) are not approved for the treatment of painful DPN, but may be effective and considered for the treatment of painful DPN. Any opioids for management of chronic neuropathic pain carry the risk of addiction and should be avoided.[112]

Guard Against Amputation

Recent statistics show that diabetes/foot-care education has proved effective in preventing amputations. Unfortunately, this type of education is not universally accessible and persons with diabetes still need to be reminded to take care of their feet.

Implications for Diabetes Education and Care

Reinforce information and instruction on foot care so persons with diabetes routinely inspect and attend to problems affecting their feet. Address the goal of management and prevention of foot complications with education and self-management skills. Encourage preventive strategies to emphasize the following:

- Proper care of nails, calluses, and injuries
- Proper-fitting footwear
- Daily inspection of feet and shoes
- Follow-up care as recommended
- In special populations, such as the visually impaired, the diabetes care and education specialist should encourage persons with diabetes to have a family member check their feet once a day if possible, or at least once a week with prompt medical treatment of abnormalities
- A referral to a podiatrist for care of nails and to check for calluses and ulcers
- Cushioned shoes that fit well and thick, padded socks
- Proper cleaning and drying of feet
- Avoid going barefoot
- Avoid temperature extremes

Severe weakness is rare and, if present, should raise the question of a possible nondiabetic neuropathy, such as Guillain-Barré syndrome, chronic inflammatory demyelinating polyneuropathy, or monoclonal gammopathies.[14,32,34] Another important point is that chronic sensorimotor neuropathy is frequently accompanied by DAN, which is easily determined by the methods discussed below.

Risk of Falling

There is a heightened awareness of the risk of falling in an older population of people with type 2 diabetes, most of whom show evidence of at least mild to moderate neuropathy as defined by the 1989 San Antonio criteria (2 or more of the following: abnormal signs and symptoms, nerve conduction testing, autonomic function testing, and QST). It would certainly be remiss to exclude this important issue from a chapter on neuropathy.

The normal aging process is associated with an increased risk of falling, fall-related injury, and subsequent loss of functional ability. For older individuals, the chance of falling and injury generally increases if they also develop age-related diseases like type 2 diabetes, often exhibiting greater impairments in balance and altered gait dynamics compared with healthy individuals of a similar age.[110–115] It has been suggested that the risk of falling for older individuals with diabetes is increased because they need to compensate for age as well as disease-related factors that can impact their balance and stability. Age-related physiological changes that potentially affect balance include loss of lower limb muscle strength and power, changes in muscle function, and slower reaction times.[116,117] The person with diabetes also has to compensate for disease processes like DN, with its confounding factors such as proximal muscle weakness and loss of proprioception, as well as the effects of hypoglycemia, which contribute to a loss of stability and balance. Additionally, the person with diabetes may be receiving treatment for hypertension, hyperlipidemia, cardiac disease, and depression.

These are additional risk factors for unsteadiness, loss of balance, and falls, and so are the medications used to treat them.[118] Reduced physical activity with aging is a common factor related to the decline in postural stability and is also linked to an increased risk of falls.[112,118,119] It is also well known that the normal process of aging is often associated with a slower speed of cognitive processing (as measured by increased reaction time,[120,121] slower postural reactions,[118,122] and decreased strength and muscle function[123]; all are essential factors for optimal balance control).[119] Unfortunately, many older individuals tend to exhibit slower reaction times.[119,120] This slowness in movement responses translates to balance tasks where older individuals at increased risk of falling also respond more slowly to changes in posture. The benefits of strength and endurance training on gait, balance, and fall risk have been well established for older, healthy individuals,[123,124] but this approach has now been shown to apply to older individuals with type 2 diabetes.[125]

A recent study[119] found that a low-intensity exercise intervention in older individuals with diabetes resulted in a reduction in the risk of falls, with concurrent improvement in a number of physiological and postural assessments. The researchers showed that effective interventions can be easily implemented in this high-risk population to prevent or lower the risk of falls. By following a basic exercise program, a high-risk group demonstrated improved balance, increased lower limb strength, improvements in proprioceptive function, faster reaction times, and, consequently, decreased risk of falling. The results of this study lend strong support for the practice of prescribing supervised exercise, gait, and balance training to older individuals with type 2 diabetes to alleviate some of the risk factors associated with falls.

Implications for Diabetes Education and Care

In general, an exercise program geared toward improving strength, gait, and balance can result in improvements in a range of risk factors for falls, impacting positively on sensory, motor, and cognitive processes. The ability to respond quickly and appropriately to any external perturbation is an essential component for correcting oneself to avoid a possible fall.[122,126]

As with persons with diabetes entering any exercise program, the following guidelines and understanding the to caveats are imperative:

- Check feet for ulcers, cuts, sores, or blisters; previous amputations of toes; or partial foot and toe amputations.
- Test sensation in the feet using a monofilament or tuning fork.
- Check that shoes selected for exercise fit well, provide support, and are cushioned.
- Test blood pressure and pulse from a lying to a standing position. If blood pressure falls (orthostasis), the person with diabetes may have autonomic dysfunction. Refer to a physical therapist for training using compensatory exercise.
- Test for abnormal cardiovascular response to exercise (refer to section on autonomic neuropathy in this chapter for more information).
- Test whether person with diabetes is able to stand on 1 leg for 3 seconds (if not, caution experienced trainer to modify exercise appropriately).
- Test whether person with diabetes is able to get up from a chair with no supporting arms. If not, reinforce the need to deal with this deficit, suggest gentle building of gluteus muscles in addition to supervised gait, and balance training.
- Encourage helpful interventions such as a cane or walker to person with diabetes with balance and gait problems.
- Encourage the use of nonslip bath and shower mats. Recommend that all unattached floor rugs, which may be hazardous for tripping and falling, be removed from the home.
- Encourage the use of safety grab bars in areas such as the bath or shower.
- Check visual and auditory acuity. Deficits in these functions are risk factors for many types of possible accidents.

Case: Neuropathic Pain

CM, a 48-year-old woman with an 18-year history of type 2 diabetes, returned to see her primary care provider after a 2-year absence. Her complaint was numbness and pain in both feet. She has a medical history of obesity, hypertension, dyslipidemia, and nonproliferative retinopathy.

Physical Signs

Blood pressure (BP) 152/88 mm Hg, heart rate 80 beats per minute, body mass index (BMI) 38.9

Microaneurysms on ophthalmoscopic examination

2/6 Systolic ejection murmur

Normal thyroid, carotids, heart, abdomen, lungs

Dorsalis pedis pulses 1+ symmetrically

Calluses over fifth metatarsal heads and lateral edge of great toes, bilaterally

Ankle jerks absent

Vibratory sense absent

Touch pressure absent (5.07 Semmes-Weinstein monofilament [SWM])

Medications

Metformin 1000 mg bid

Glipizide 10 mg/d

Basal Insulin (glargine, detemir, degludec, 32 units/hs)

Lisinopril 20 mg

Aspirin 81 mg/d

Atorvastatin 40 mg/d

Multivitamin 1 tablet daily

(continued)

Case: Neuropathic Pain (continued)

Questions to Consider

What is the significance of the physical findings (especially the calluses and the absence of ankle jerks, vibratory sense, and touch pressure)?

How common is the problem of nerve impairment?

Is this a typical presentation?

What investigations should be conducted?

Diagnosis and Initial Treatment

CM's healthcare provider ordered the following tests and obtained the results noted:

Electrolytes: normal

Thyroid function test (TSH): 2.0 (normal <4.0 u/mL)

B_{12}: 250 (normal 450 pg/mL)

A1C: 9.5% (healthy range 4.1%-6.5%), her individualized target is <7%

Albumin/creatinine ratio: 98 g/mg (normal <30)

eGFR: 48 (Normal ≥ 60)

Serum creatinine 1.4 (normal 0.5–1.3)

Liver function tests show minor elevations

Triglycerides: 298 mg/dL (normal <150)

Cholesterol: 187 mg/dL (normal <200)

HDL cholesterol 31 (target >50)

LDL cholesterol 98 (target <100)

CM had previously mentioned numbness and pain. What other questions are appropriate to ask about the discomfort in her feet?

When CM described her pain, she mentioned 3 kinds:

Constant, diffused, sharp, burning

Knifelike lightning episodes that occur occasionally at night

Dull, gnawing "bone" pain, similar to a toothache

Is there any significance to these descriptions? What do they reveal? Into which of the following categories does her pain fit:

Distal symmetric polyneuropathy?

Acute or chronic (greater or less than 6 months)?

Small- or large-fiber?

What initial approach to the management of her neuropathic discomfort would you recommend?

She may benefit from insulin titration or addition of rapid acting insulin with meals or a GLP-1 agonist. As well, a DPP-IV Inhibitor (not with GLP-1) or SGLT-2 Inhibitor may be appropriate additions. Be aware that SGLT-2 Inhibitors carry a warning for possible increase in distal amputation risk. If any of these are done, her polypharmacy may be reduced with stoppage of glipizide.

At the time, topical over the counter capsaicin 0.025% 4 times per day was suggested. Capsaicin 8% patch for treating painful diabetic peripheral neuropathy also available for use.[127]

Finding Acceptable Pain Relief

One Month Later

CM returned for follow-up. Her basal insulin had been titrated upward, and her overall glycemic levels appeared improved; however, she required further pain relief. In addition to improved glycemic levels, what agents would you have suggested?

Three Months Later

CM returned for continued follow-up. Her A1C had declined to 7.4% (4.1%-6.5%) with the addition of a GLP-1 agonist.

Subsequent Follow-Up

CM had some relief of her DPN discomfort from over the counter capsaicin and A1C improvement. One year later, she again complained of burning, superficial (just below the skin) discomfort. In this Instance, we could consider pregabalin, gabapentin, or duloxetine. These may also be first line choices according the American Diabetes Association's Standards of Care.[112] Tricyclic antidepressants, venlafaxine, carbamazepine, and topical capsaicin, although not approved for the treatment of painful DPN, may be effective and considered for the treatment of painful DPN.[112] The use of extended-release Tapentadol is not recommended as first- or second-line therapy.[128] Any opioids for management of chronic neuropathic pain carry the risk of addiction and should be avoided.[112]

Emphasize Foot Care

Loss of lower body sweating can cause dry, brittle skin that cracks easily, predisposing one to ulcer formation that can lead to limb loss. Alert **persons with diabetes** to pay special attention to foot care, as many individuals do not recognize or treat problems.

Autonomic Neuropathy

Autonomic neuropathy (AN) is often referred to in the diabetic population as diabetic autonomic neuropathy (DAN). Refer to the guidelines from the American Association of Clinical Endocrinologists[57] and the American Diabetes Association.[1,112]

Autonomic neuropathy significantly impacts survival and QOL:

- Although serious and common, AN (or DAN) is among the least recognized and poorly understood complications of diabetes.[129]
- The reported prevalence of AN varies widely (7.7%-90.0%), depending on the study population and methods used for diagnosis.[130,131]
- Autonomic dysfunction has recently been shown to be a predictor of cardiovascular dysfunction.[17,18,54,60]

The ANS supplies all organs in the body and consists of an afferent system and an efferent system, involving both the parasympathetic and the sympathetic nervous systems. Autonomic neuropathy may involve any system in the body. Involvement of the ANS can occur as early as the first year after diagnosis, and major manifestations are cardiovascular, gastrointestinal, and genitourinary system dysfunction.[63,132]

Disturbances in the ANS may be *functional* (eg, gastroparesis with hyperglycemia and ketoacidosis) or *organic*, wherein nerve fibers are actually lost. This creates great difficulty in diagnosing and treating as well as establishing true prevalence rates. Many conditions affect the ANS (AN is not unique to diabetes); thus, the diagnosis of DAN rests with excluding other causes. Subclinical involvement may be widespread, whereas clinical symptoms and signs may be focused within a single organ.

Symptoms

The following are some common symptoms of AN:

- Reduced exercise tolerance
- Syncope
- Orthostatic tachycardia
- Orthostatic bradycardia
- Orthostatic hypotension
- Edema
- Paradoxical supine or nocturnal hypertension
- Intolerance to heat (due to defective thermoregulation)
- Gastrointestinal and genitourinary dysfunction

Table 28.6 lists the most common clinical features, diagnostic methods, and treatment options for AN.

Cardiac Autonomic Neuropathy

Cardiovascular dysfunction is associated with abnormalities in heart rate control and vascular dynamics. Parasympathetic nerves slow the heart rate, and sympathetic nerves increase the speed and force of heart contractions and stimulate the vascular tree to increase the blood pressure. The Consensus Panel on Diabetic Neuropathy, after extensive review of the literature, recently concluded that the prevalence of confirmed CAN in unselected people with type 1 diabetes or type 2 diabetes is approximately 20%, but it can be as high as 65% with increasing age and diabetes duration.[133] Clinical correlates or risk markers for CAN are age, diabetes duration, glycemic levels, microvascular complications (peripheral polyneuropathy, retinopathy, and nephropathy),[15] hypertension, and dyslipidemia. Established risk factors for CAN are glycemic stability in type 1 diabetes, and a combination of hypertension, dyslipidemia, obesity, and glycemic stability in type 2 diabetes.[133]

Additional factors that have emerged as identifying susceptibility to cardiovascular events with intensification of glycemic management include duration of diabetes 12 to 15 years, impaired renal function, coronary artery calcification, a previous cardiovascular event, being African American, being female, a history of neuropathy or numb feet, and loss in HRV.[4,134,135]

The Cardiovascular Autonomic Neuropathy Subcommittee of the Toronto Consensus Panel on Diabetic Neuropathy recommends CAN screening to all asymptomatic persons with type 2 diabetes at diagnosis and all persons with type 1 diabetes after 5 years of disease—in particular, those at greater risk for CAN because of a history of poor glycemic stability (hemoglobin A1C >7%), the presence of 1 major cardiovascular risk factor (hypertension, dyslipidemia, or smoking), or the presence of macro- or microangiopathic complications (level of evidence B).[136]

The subcommittee also suggested that CAN screening might be required in asymptomatic persons with

TABLE 28.6 AN: Clinical Features, Diagnosis, and Treatment

Symptoms	*Tests*	*Treatments*
Cardiac		
Resting tachycardia, exercise intolerance	HRV, MUGA thallium scan, MIBG scan	Graded supervised exercise, ACE inhibitors, β-blockers
Postural hypotension, dizziness, weakness, fatigue, syncope	HRV, supine and standing BP, catecholamines	Mechanical measures, clonidine, midodrine, octreotide, erythropoietin
Gastrointestinal		
Gastroparesis, erratic glucose control	Gastric emptying study, barium study	Frequent small meals, prokinetic agents (metoclopramide, domperidone, erythromycin)
Abdominal pain, early satiety, nausea, vomiting, bloating, belching	Endoscopy, manometry, electrogastrogram	Antibiotics, antiemetics, bulking agents, tricyclic antidepressants, pyloric botox, gastric pacing
Constipation	Endoscopy	High-fiber diet and bulking agents, osmotic laxatives, lubricating agents Lubiprostone and linaclotide are recommended*
Diarrhea (often nocturnal, alternating with constipation)	None	Soluble dietary fiber, gluten and lactose restriction, anticholinergic agents, cholestyramine, antibiotics, somatostatin, pancreatic enzyme supplements, tincture opium
Sexual Dysfunction		
Erectile dysfunction	H&P, HRV, penile-brachial pressure index, nocturnal penile tumescence	5′- phosphodiesterase inhibitors; PG E1 injections, devices, or prostheses; sex therapy; psychological counseling
Vaginal dryness	None	Vaginal lubricants
Bladder Dysfunction		
Frequency, urgency, nocturia, urinary retention, incontinence	Cystometrogram, postvoiding sonography	Bethanechol, intermittent catheterization
Sudomotor Dysfunction		
Anhidrosis, heat intolerance, dry skin, hyperhidrosis	Quantitative sudomotor axon reflex, sweat test, skin blood flow	Emollients and skin lubricants, scopolamine, glycopyrrolate, botulinum toxin, vasodilators
Pupillomotor and Visceral Dysfunction		
Visual blurring, impaired adaptation to ambient light, Argyll-Robertson pupil	Pupillometry, HRV	Care with driving at night
Impaired visceral sensation: silent myocardial infarction, hypoglycemia unawareness		Recognition of unusual presentation of myocardial infarction, control of risk factors, control of plasma glucose levels

Abbreviations: ACE, angiotensin-converting enzyme; BP, blood pressure; H&P, history and physical examination; HRV, heart rate variability; MI, myocardial infarction; MIBG, metaiodobenzylguanidine; MUGA, multigated angiography; PG, prostaglandin

*Lubiprostone, is a bicyclic fatty acid derived from prostaglandin E1 that acts by specifically activating chloride channels in the apical aspect of gastrointestinal epithelial cells, producing a chloride-rich solution. These solutions soften the stool, increase gut motility, and promote spontaneous bowel movements (SBMs). Symptoms of constipation such as pain and bloating are usually improved within 1 week, and SBM may occur within 1 day. Unlike many laxative products, lubiprostone does not produce tolerance, dependency, or altered serum electrolyte concentration. There is no rebound effect; it does not penetrate beyond the GI tract; it is rapidly metabolized without involvement of the cytochrome P450. The actions occur in the stomach and duodenum (RJ Hamilton, ed, Tarascon Pocket Pharmacopoeia [Burlington, Ma: Jones & Bartlett Learning, 2013]). Linaclotide, activates neurons that stimulate the relief of bicarbonate and chloride into the intestines, resulting in an increase in intestinal fluid and gastric transit. It is approved by the FDA for chronic idiopathic constipation as well as irritable bowel syndrome, a common disorder that affects the large intestine (colon), commonly presenting with cramping, abdominal pain, and constipation alternating with diarrhea. Persons with diabetes need to be treated 30 minutes before the first meal of the day with 145 or 290 mcg once daily. It has no major interactions but can cause diarrhea, abdominal pain, and bloating—some of the symptoms it has been designed to treat!

Source: Copyright © 2005 American Diabetes Association. Adapted with permission from AJ Boulton, A Vinik, J Arezzo, et al, "Diabetic neuropathies (position statement)," *Diabetes Care* 28, no. 4 (2005): 956-62.

diabetes for preoperative risk assessment before major surgical procedures (level of evidence C).[133]

Morbidity and Mortality in CAN

Cardiac autonomic neuropathy is a significant cause of morbidity and mortality and is associated with a high risk of cardiac arrhythmias and sudden death, possibly related to silent myocardial ischemia. Cardiovascular disease remains the main cause of excess mortality among persons with type 1 diabetes or type 2 diabetes. Reduced HRV as a marker of autonomic dysfunction has been shown to have dire consequences in terms of morbidity. The first sign of cardiac impairment is usually resting tachycardia. The 3 major associated syndromes are the following:[137]

- Cardiac denervation syndrome
- Abnormal cardiovascular response to exercise
- Orthostatic (postural) hypotension

Cardiac Denervation Syndrome

Cardiac denervation is defined as a fixed heart rate that does not change in response to stress, exercise, breathing patterns, or sleep. This syndrome results from both parasympathetic and sympathetic system impairment. Initially, parasympathetic tone decreases, which causes a relative increase in sympathetic tone and an increase in heart rate. Progressive impairment of sympathetic tone then causes a gradual slowing of the heart. Over time, both parasympathetic and sympathetic tone become impaired.[26] Initially, a fixed heart rate of 100 to 120 beats per minute is common. In the later stages, the fixed heart rate will be in the range of 80 to 100 beats per minute. The heart rate is unresponsive to stress, exercise, or tilting.[114,115] In the later stages, the person may suffer myocardial ischemia or myocardial infarction (MI) without experiencing pain. The resulting delay or failure to seek treatment contributes to increasing mortality rates. These persons are also at risk for cardiac arrhythmias and sudden death.[26]

Diagnostic Tests Methods of CAN assessment in clinical practice include assessment of symptoms and signs, cardiovascular autonomic reflex tests based on heart rate and blood pressure, and ambulatory blood pressure monitoring.[133]

Cardiovascular autonomic reflex tests assess cardiovascular autonomic function through time-domain heart rate response to deep breathing, Valsalva maneuver, and postural change and by measuring the end-organ response, that is, heart rate and blood pressure changes. Although indirect autonomic measures, they are considered the gold standard in autonomic testing. Heart rate variations during deep breathing, Valsalva maneuver, and lying-to-standing (heart rate tests) are indices mainly of parasympathetic function, whereas the orthostatic hypotension, the blood pressure response to a Valsalva maneuver, and sustained isometric muscular strain provide indices of sympathetic function. Autonomic balance can be measured using time and frequency domain analyses of autonomic function including the standard deviation of normal RR intervals and the root mean squared of the standard deviation of the normal RR intervals. These tests are noninvasive, safe, clinically relevant (they correlate with tests of peripheral nervous system function), easy to carry out, sensitive, specific, reproducible, and standardized, and therefore they are considered consolidated gold-standard measures of autonomic function.

There is now strong evidence of inflammation with activation of inflammatory cytokines in persons with diabetes. These changes correlate with abnormalities in sympathetic-vagal balance. Several investigations have shown the neuroregulatory role for the ANS being a key instrument in the inflammatory process.

Person with diabetes suffer from severe orthostasis, postural hypotension, exercise intolerance, enhanced intraoperative instability, and an increased incidence of silent MI and ischemia. Several agents have become available for the correction of functional defects in the ANS. Restoration of autonomic balance is possible and has been shown with therapeutic lifestyle changes, increased physical activity, diabetes treatment, beta-adrenergic blockers, and potent antioxidants such as alpha-lipoic acid. There are prospects for pathogenesis-oriented intervention.

Caveats for Exercise With Autonomic Neuropathy
Autonomic dysfunction impairs exercise tolerance, reduces response in heart rate and blood pressure, and blunts increases in cardiac output in response to exercise. Persons with diabetes who are likely to have CAN should be tested for cardiac stress before undertaking an exercise program. Persons with CAN need to rely on their perceived exertion, not heart rate, to avoid hazardous levels of intensity of exercise.[138,139] Presently, there is inadequate evidence to recommend routine screening of asymptomatic persons with diabetes with an exercise EKG test. Emerging data support the futility of stress imaging testing in identifying persons with diabetes with preclinical coronary artery disease, particularly those individuals with high-risk features and comorbidities, such as longstanding disease, CAN, multiple chronic renal failures, resting ECG abnormalities, and peripheral artery disease. Rather, a simple bedside evaluation of heart rate variability (HRV) in response to a Valsalva maneuver has the

greatest sensitivity of predicting a major adverse cardiovascular event.[140]

Implications for Diabetes Education and Care Teach persons with diabetes with cardiac denervation syndrome to avoid heavy exercise, aerobic exercise, and straining themselves. Stress testing is a requirement before initiating any type of exercise program. In addition, these persons with diabetes should be carefully evaluated prior to initiation of intensive insulin therapy because of the risk of hypoglycemia with possible hypoglycemic unawareness, which can result in cardiac arrhythmias.[26]

Abnormal Cardiovascular Response to Exercise

Some people with DAN may lose their normal increased cardiac output and vascular tone response to exercise and become hypotensive with aerobic activity.[26] If an individual becomes faint or dizzy while exercising, the individual's blood pressure should be checked immediately. If needed, provide therapy or seek an intervention by a healthcare provider.

Postural Hypotension

Blood pressure is normally maintained upon standing by a sympathetic reflex that increases the heart rate and by peripheral vascular resistance in association with an increase in norepinephrine levels. Orthostatic hypotension is defined as a drop in systolic blood pressure of more than 30 mm Hg or a diastolic drop of more than 10 mm Hg within 2 minutes of changing from a supine position to a standing position. This syndrome occurs late in diabetes and signals advanced autonomic impairment.

Orthostatic hypotension, which results from blood pooling in the feet, can occur without symptoms but is often accompanied by dizziness, light-headedness, weakness, visual impairment, or syncope.[26] This places the person with diabetes at risk for injury from falls. All persons with diabetes must have their blood pressure and pulse rates assessed in the lying, sitting, and standing positions. Symptomatic persons with diabetes should have this test at each office visit. Greater accuracy in the assessment can be achieved by having the person with diabetes rest in a supine position and then stand quietly while the blood pressure is measured at 1-minute intervals for 3 to 5 minutes.[26]

Treatment of symptoms involves raising the head of the bed 30° at night, increasing venous pressure with supportive elastic whole-body stockings (or stockings that go to at least the waist and are applied while the person is supine), and wearing an antigravity suit. Other therapies include correcting hypovolemia, midodrine, octreotide, and erythropoietin (refer to Table 28.6). Florinef is not recommended, because it usually causes hypertension and fluid retention before alleviating orthostasis.

Implications for Diabetes Education and Care Persons with diabetes should receive education on the proper application and use of elastic body stockings, which need to be waist high (knee- and thigh-high stockings that cut into the leg are hazardous, as they may restrict the blood supply). Persons with diabetes should also receive instruction on rising slowly from a recumbent position. Graded, supervised exercise to improve strength and balance is recommended, as well as nutritional counseling on salt intake. Liberalize salt intake to >6 g per day. Silent MI, respiratory failure, amputations, and sudden death ("dead in bed") are hazards for persons with diabetes with CAN.[141,142] Therefore, it is imperative to make this diagnosis early so that appropriate intervention can be instituted.[143]

Treatment of the Underlying Cause of CAN

Treatment of the underlying cause of AN can include management of the following:

- Hyperglycemia
- Lipids to include statins, PCSK-9 Inhibitors, ezetimibe
- Blood pressure, to include beta blockers or calcium channel blockers for rhythm control
- Use of antioxidants[131,144]
- Angiotensin-converting enzyme (ACE) inhibitors [145,146]
- Angiotensin receptor blockers

These treatments are designed to minimize the effects of hyperglycemia, dyslipidemia, hypertension, oxidative and nitrosative stress, and compromised nerve function.

Gastrointestinal Disorders Related to AN

If the nerves are affected by AN, gastric emptying of both liquids and solids may be delayed. Vagal nerve dysfunction is usually responsible for motility.

Upper Gastrointestinal Dysfunction

Most upper gastrointestinal dysfunction involves the esophagus, stomach, and upper small intestine. Symptoms of gastroparesis (delayed gastric emptying) can include heartburn, reflux, anorexia, early satiety, nausea, abdominal bloating, erratic blood glucose levels due to delayed absorption of food, and vomiting undigested food eaten several hours or days earlier.[147,148] Signs associated with gastroparesis include weight loss and a succussion splash (a splashing sound made during body movement) over the upper left quadrant of the abdomen, although delayed gastric emptying can also occur without symptoms.[147,148]

Diagnosis A barium series of the upper gastrointestinal tract is useful to rule out obstruction. A solid-phase gastric emptying phase study is the most specific way to diagnose delayed gastric emptying.[123,124] The recommended blood glucose level for the test is <240 mg/dL (13.32 mmol/L). A blood glucose level >240 mg/dL impairs gastric emptying. Gastroscopy may be needed to exclude a bezoar.

It is important to recognize the effect of new classes of drugs on gastric emptying, such as the "incretin effect." Broadly speaking, they can be divided into agents that enhance insulin secretion and agents that are insulin sensitizers. In the latter class are the glucagon-like peptide-1 (GLP-1) receptor agonists and the glucose-dependent insulin secretagogues. The GLP-1 drugs modulate numerous functions in humans. Native incretins are secreted upon ingestion of food, promote satiety, and reduce appetite. They stimulate insulin only in the presence of an increased blood glucose level and suppress the postprandial secretion of glucagon. More importantly, they slow the rate of gastric emptying, thereby lowering the postprandial rise in glucose levels. The GLP-1 receptor agonists exenatide, dulaglutide, semaglutide,and liraglutide are synthetic analogs of the naturally occurring hormone in humans, are capable of slowing gastric emptying. All are capable of causing weight loss, but caution must be exercised in persons with diabetes with gastroparesis in whom side effects can be exacerbated. Nausea is a common side effect of these medications.[149–151]

Implications for Diabetes Education and Care Normalizing blood glucose levels may improve gastric emptying. The presence of gastroparesis complicates balancing insulin doses with food absorption. Frequent monitoring of pre- and postprandial blood glucose levels is required to detect hypoglycemia and hyperglycemia and determine the insulin dose. Rapid-acting insulin should be used cautiously for some persons with diabetes with gastroparesis, although some find it useful if taken after the meal.

Treatment includes the following:

- Referral to a dietitian for a low-fat, low-fiber diet
- Use of multiple small and mostly liquid meals eaten throughout the day
- Referral to a gastroenterologist
- Medications to decrease inhibition of gastric motility, such as metoclopramide or erythromycin may be useful. Metoclopramide is limited by the possibilities of parkinsonism or extrapyramidal effects. Erythromycin may cause diarrhea or lose its effect over time. Domperidone is available outside of the United States.[112]
- In the most severe stages, gastric pacemaker may be necessary.[112]

Lower Intestinal Tract Dysfunction

Lower intestinal tract dysfunction is the result of damage to the efferent autonomic nerves and leads to hypotonia and poor contraction of the smooth muscles to the gut, which results in constipation.

Constipation is fairly common and has been reported in up to 60% of all persons with diabetes. Treatment involves increasing fiber in the diet while avoiding excess fiber* in persons with diabetes with gastroparesis. Diabetes care and education specialists should encourage judicious use of laxatives, adequate hydration, increased activity, stool softeners, bulk laxatives such as psyllium, Polyethylene Glycol 3350 powder, and medications such as metoclopramide or neostigmine to increase intestinal motility.[147,152]

Diarrhea can also occur as a result of both decreased small intestinal motility and hypermotility without bacterial overgrowth.[147,148] Although constipation is more common, diarrhea is usually more troublesome to persons with diabetes. Diarrhea may be nocturnal, intermittent with constipation, and associated with fecal incontinence; it may occur without cramping or pain. Treatment involves the use of antibiotics (eg, tetracycline or metronidazole) to decrease the bacterial overgrowth. It is better to drive the bowel (eg, with metoclopramide or erythromycin) than to inhibit motility. Nonetheless, medications that may be useful for slowing intestinal motility are loperamide, codeine, and diphenoxylate hydrochloride and atropine sulfate. However, care should be exercised as withdrawal may aggravate the situation. Fiber and psyllium may increase stool bulk and consistency but may present problems with aggravating gastroparesis. In addition, some persons with diabetes may benefit from biofeedback, relaxation, and bowel training.

---

*Normal dietary fiber guidelines are as follows:

Females: 21 to 26 g per day
Males: 30 to 38 g per day
Progressively decrease the number of grams for males and females over the age of 50

The average American consumes only 14 g of fiber per day. The regular fiber intake of persons with diabetes should be calculated and adjusted accordingly.

Early treatment of diarrhea may help prevent the development of incontinence.[147,148]

Implications for Diabetes Education and Care Include a discussion of how these symptoms are related to diabetes. Stress the need to inform providers of symptoms to allow for early detection and treatment. Explain with care diagnostic tests, test results, and therapies.

Sexual Dysfunction Related to AN

Sexual dysfunction is common among people with diabetes. As many as 75% of men and 35% of women experience sexual problems due to DN.[153] Male sexual dysfunction involves erectile dysfunction and retrograde ejaculation. Retrograde ejaculation is unusual and may respond to use of an antihistamine, desipramine, or phenylephrine.[154]

Male Sexual Dysfunction

Erectile dysfunction (ED) occurs in men with diabetes at an earlier age than in the general population. The incidence of ED in men with diabetes aged 20 to 29 years is 9% and increases to 95% by 70 years of age. Erectile dysfunction may be the presenting symptom of diabetes. More than 50% notice the onset of ED within 10 years of the diagnosis, but it may precede the other complications of diabetes. The etiology of ED in diabetes is multifactorial. Neuropathy, vascular disease, diabetes management, nutrition, endocrine disorders, and psychogenic factors as well as drugs used in the treatment of diabetes and its complications play a role.[153,154] Diagnosis of the cause of ED is made by a logical stepwise progression.[154,155]

Diagnostic Assessments Assessments should include a careful medical and sexual history; physical and psychological evaluations; blood test for diabetes and levels of testosterone, prolactin, and thyroid hormones; a test for nocturnal erections; and tests to assess penile, pelvic, and spinal nerve function, penile blood supply, and blood pressure. A simple test of autonomic function using HRV will exclude a neurologic cause of ED. A flowchart can assist in defining the problem.[153,154]

The healthcare provider must ask questions to help distinguish the various forms of organic ED from those that are psychogenic in origin. The physical examination must include an evaluation of the ANS, vascular supply, and hypothalamic-pituitary-gonadal axis.

Autonomic neuropathy causing ED is almost always accompanied by loss of ankle jerks and absence or reduction of vibration sense over the large toes. More direct evidence of impairment of penile autonomic function can be obtained by demonstrating normal perianal sensation, assessing the tone of the anal sphincter during a rectal exam, and ascertaining the presence of an anal wink. These measurements are easily and quickly done at the bedside and reflect the integrity of sacral parasympathetic divisions.

A test for nocturnal penile tumescence (NPT) distinguishes psychogenic from organic dysfunction. Normal NPT defines psychogenic ED, and a negative response to vasodilators implies vascular insufficiency. However, the NPT test is not so simple. It is much like having a sphygmomanometer cuff inflate over the penis many times during the night while the person with diabetes is trying to sleep.

Treatment of ED A number of treatment modalities are available, and each treatment has positive and negative effects. Therefore, persons with diabetes must be made aware of both aspects before making a therapeutic decision. Before considering any form of treatment, every effort should be made to have the person withdraw from alcohol and eliminate smoking. If possible, the person with diabetes should be removed from drugs that are known to cause ED, and metabolic control should be optimized.

Research has revealed that the ability to have and maintain an erection depends on nitric oxide and cyclic guano monophosphate (cGMP). Agents such as sildenafil, vardenafil, and tadalafil exert their effect by increasing nitric oxide and cGMP levels that may be low in men with diabetes. These may be prescribed in a presumptive trial before the need of additional testing. Before any of these agents are prescribed, ischemic heart disease must be excluded. These medications are absolutely contraindicated in persons being treated with nitroglycerine or other nitrate-containing drugs. Severe hypotension and fatal cardiac events can occur.[156]

Direct injection of prostacylin into the corpus cavernosum will induce satisfactory erections in a significant number of men. Also, surgical implantation of a penile prosthesis may be appropriate. The less expensive type of prosthesis is a semirigid, permanently erect type that may be embarrassing and uncomfortable for some men. The inflatable type is 3 times more expensive and subject to mechanical failure, but it avoids the embarrassment caused by other devices.

Implications for Diabetes Education and Care The advent of therapies such as sildenafil, vardenafil, and tadalafil has created a new era of openness regarding sexual issues. Current recommendations include continuous low-dose therapy rather than as-needed dosing. However, many persons with diabetes may still be reticent about their sexual function. The diabetes diabetes care and education specialist should be aware that a problem may exist and alert the physician. When appropriate, including both sexual partners in selecting therapy is extremely important. Review all therapeutic options as well as their costs and benefits. Although these drugs facilitate erections, stimulation is also necessary. This should be explained to both partners.

Female Sexual Dysfunction

Women with diabetes mellitus may experience decreased sexual desire, difficulties in arousal, and pain during sexual intercourse. They also have decreased vaginal lubrication even if stimulated.[157] However, female sexual dysfunction, decreased vaginal lubrication, vaginal flushing, and delayed or absent orgasmic response need further assessment.

Sexual difficulties in women with diabetes that are not related to AN include loss of libido (possibly related to depression as a result of diabetes and its complications), hormonal fluctuations/menopause, and frequent occurrence of yeast and other vaginal infections. More recently it has been shown that the sodium-glucose co-transporter 2 (SGLT2) inhibitors increase urinary glucose secretion; therefore, they should be avoided in women who are susceptible to fungal infections and in men with previous episodes of balanitis. Warnings have been inserted in or on the packaging of SGLT2 inhibitor products regarding genitourinary infections and Fournier's gangrene, an ischemic condition of the genitals which can occur in men and women.

Implications for Diabetes Education and Care Diabetes care and education specialists need to address sexual concerns because these issues may be difficult for persons with diabetes to discuss. Discuss sexual function, the potential for diabetes-related problems, and the need to bring problems to the attention of providers. Offer to include persons' with diabetes partners in the discussion and point out the importance of their inclusion in treatment decisions. Management includes application of estrogen or lubricating vaginal creams and referral to a gynecologist. Offer the person with diabetes and her partner referral for counseling with a sex therapist.

Bladder Dysfunction Related to AN

In AN, the motor function of the bladder is unimpaired, but afferent fiber damage results in diminished bladder sensation. Symptoms of a neurogenic bladder are usually insidious and progressive. In the early stages, the sensation of the need to void may be blunted. This infrequent urination may be misinterpreted as decreased polyuria due to improved blood glucose levels. In later stages, difficulty in emptying the bladder, dribbling, and overflow incontinence may occur.[26] The urinary bladder can be enlarged to more than 3 times its normal size. Persons with diabetes are seen with bladders filled to their umbilicus, yet they feel no discomfort. Loss of bladder sensation occurs with diminished voiding frequency, and the person is no longer able to void completely. An untreated neurogenic bladder often leads to urinary tract infections as a result of urinary stasis. These frequent infections may accelerate deterioration of renal function. More than 2 urinary tract infections per year among men and 3 among women indicate the need for further evaluation of bladder function.

Diagnosis

Bladder insensitivity is diagnosed by a cystometrogram. A post-voiding residual of greater than 150 cc confirms bladder dysfunction or cystopathy, which may put the person with diabetes at risk for urinary infections.

Treatment of Cystopathy

A person with diabetes with cystopathy should be instructed to palpate his or her bladder. If unable to initiate micturition with a full bladder, the person with diabetes should be instructed to use Crede's maneuver (massage or put pressure on the lower portion of the abdomen just above the pubic bone) to start the flow of urine. The principal aim of the treatment should be to improve bladder emptying and reduce the risk of urinary tract infection. Parasympathomimetics such as bethanechol are sometimes helpful, although frequently they do not help to completely empty the bladder. Extended sphincter relaxation can be achieved with an α_1-blocker such as doxazosin or tamsulosin. Self-catheterization can be particularly useful, with the risk of infection generally being low with proper technique.

Implications for Diabetes Education and Care

Stress the need for frequent, complete urination; the signs and symptoms of urinary tract infections; and the importance of early treatment of infections. Teach persons with diabetes to palpate for bladder fullness.

Sudomotor Dysfunction (Sweating Disturbances) Related to AN

Excessive perspiration (hyperhidrosis) of the upper body, often related to eating (gustatory sweating), and deficiency of sweat (anhidrosis) of the lower body are characteristic features of AN. Gustatory sweating accompanies the ingestion of certain foods, particularly spicy foods and cheeses. The administration of glycopyrrolate (antimuscarinic compound) has been suggested for persons with diabetes who experience gustatory sweating.[78] Symptomatic relief can be obtained by avoiding the specific food irritant.

Implications for Diabetes Education and Care

Persons with diabetes rarely think to report abnormal sweating. However, this symptom is a red flag for the potential for heat stroke and foot ulcers. A careful history and examination of the feet for dryness and fissures are important to conduct at each visit.[26] Education for persons with diabetes should include inspection for fissures and lubrication for dry feet; avoidance of hot, spicy, or other offending foods; and prevention of hyperthermia and heat stroke.

Research studies have shown defective blood flow in the small capillary circulation.[158–160] The clinical counterpart is dry, cold skin; loss of sweating; and development of fissures and cracks that are portals of entry for organisms leading to infectious ulcers and gangrene. This is an example of the value of research translating into clinical care. Awareness of the consequences of defective blood flow and education toward behaviors for preventing fissures and cracks can protect against the ravages of foot ulcers and gangrene.

Pupillomotor and Visceral (Metabolic) Response Related to AN

Abnormal Pupillary Response

The iris is innervated by both parasympathetic and sympathetic nerve fibers. Sympathetic nerve fibers cause the pupils to dilate and are generally more severely affected. Abnormal pupillary responses are related to duration of diabetes.[27] Slow dilation of pupils in response to darkness may be observed during clinical examination. Persons with diabetes may report slow adaptation when entering a dark room.

Implications for Diabetes Education and Care Stress using caution during night driving, the importance of turning on lights when entering a dark room, and using nightlights in darkened hallways and bathrooms to help prevent injuries.

Hypoglycemia Unawareness

Blood glucose concentration is normally maintained during starvation or increased insulin action by an asymptomatic parasympathetic response with bradycardia and mild hypotension, followed by a sympathetic response with glucagon and epinephrine secretion for short-term glucose counterregulation and growth hormone and cortisol in long-term regulation. The release of catecholamine alerts the person to take the required measures to prevent coma due to low blood glucose. The absence of warning signs of impending neuroglycopenia is known as *hypoglycemic unawareness*. Failure of glucose counterregulation can be confirmed by the absence of glucagon and epinephrine responses to hypoglycemia that is induced by a standard, controlled dose of insulin.[161]

In persons with type 1 diabetes mellitus, the glucagon response is impaired with diabetes duration of 1 to 5 years, and after 14 to 31 years of diabetes, the glucagon response is almost undetectable. The glucagon response is not present in those with AN. However, a syndrome of hypoglycemic autonomic failure occurs with intensification of diabetes management and repeated episodes of hypoglycemia. The exact mechanism is not understood, but it does represent a real barrier to physiologic glycemic stability. In the absence of severe autonomic dysfunction, hypoglycemic unawareness associated with hypoglycemia is at least partly reversible. It is important to reduce the previous target and goals and to set new levels.[162]

Persons with diabetes with hypoglycemia unawareness and unresponsiveness pose a significant management problem for the healthcare team. Although AN may improve with intensive therapy and normalization of blood glucose, there is a risk to the person with diabetes, who may become hypoglycemic (without being aware of it) and be unable to mount a counterregulatory response. Following are some recommendations:

- Intensive basal bolus or pump with a continuous glucose monitor In general, modify individual goals for glucose and A1C levels in these persons with diabetes to avoid the possibility of hypoglycemia.[163]

Further complicating management for some persons with diabetes is the development of a functional autonomic insufficiency associated with intensive insulin treatment, which resembles AN in all relevant aspects. In these instances, relaxing therapy, as for the person with diabetes with bona fide AN, is prudent. If hypoglycemia occurs in these persons with diabetes at a certain glucose level, it will take a lower glucose level to trigger the same symptoms in the next 24 to 48 hours. Avoidance of hypoglycemia for a few days will result in recovery of the adrenergic response.

Implications for Diabetes Education and Care Include prevention of hypoglycemia, appropriate treatment, the value of frequent home blood glucose monitoring, using

Case: Complexities of AN

RK is a 36-year-old white nonobese man (height 5 ft 7 in, weight 142 lb) with a 15-year history of type 1 diabetes. His diabetes has been poorly managed for many years on a regimen of a single dose of 35 units of 70/30 insulin per day without regular blood glucose monitoring. He has had repeated admissions to hospitals for diabetic ketoacidosis and has resisted attempts at intensification of treatment or improved monitoring.

Over the past few weeks, RK developed intractable burning pain in his feet, a sensation he described as a "dog gnawing at the bones" and like having a "toothache in the feet." He found it unbearable to have his feet come into contact with the bedclothes, and putting on his shoes and socks in the morning was close to impossible. The pain was worse at night, and he was getting little sleep.

Symptoms

- Constantly tired, weak, apathetic, lethargic, and incapable of carrying out his normal daily activities
- Had become significantly depressed by the pain and was not eating well
- Felt bloated and full after eating only little bits of food, and occasionally vomited and could taste food on his breath that he had eaten maybe a day or 2 before
- Irregular bowels, varied from marked constipation to explosive diarrhea, with episodes sometimes so sudden and forceful he would soil himself
- Erectile dysfunction

Physical Signs

- A lean individual who displayed signs of weakness
- Resting blood pressure: 80/64 mm Hg; heart rate: 96 beats per minute
- On standing, blood pressure fell to 50/40 mm Hg; heart rate did not change
- Proliferative retinopathy
- No known cardiovascular disease

Question to Consider

- What kind of neuropathy does RK have?

Diagnosis

RK had clear evidence of mixed sensory motor polyneuropathy with AN. Which tests should be ordered?

The following tests were ordered, with results as noted:

- Gastric emptying study: Gastroparesis: documented with a gastric emptying time of 55 minutes for solid foods (normal <17 minutes)
- Lipids: Cholesterol: 132 mg/dL (normal 110–200 mg/dL); triglycerides: 101 mg/dL (normal 40–149 mg/dL); HDL 40, LDL 110
- A1C: 11.5% target <7%
- Urine protein: 500 mg (normal <250 mg for 24 hours); creatinine: 1.7 mg/dL (normal 0.5–1.2 mg/dL); BUN: 40 mg/dL (normal 6–22 mg/dL); eGFR: 70
- Supine norepinephrine: 196 pg/mL, rising to 369 pg/mL after standing 15 minutes
- Resting cardiac ejection fraction: 61% (normal >60%), no increase with maximal exercise
- Resting heart rate: 100 beats per minute (normal 60–80 beats per minute)
- Beat-to-beat HRV: 12 beats per minute between deep inspiration; expiration E:I ratio: 1.01 (normal >1.3)
- Valsalva ratio: 1.06 (normal >1.10)
- Orthostatic pulse: Heart rate response to standing (the 30:15 ratio): 1.0 (normal >1.0)
- Orthostatic systolic pressure drop: 36 mm Hg (normal <30 mm Hg); RK became quite dizzy

Treatment

What would you suggest to help manage RK's hyperglycemia?

Intensive education and implementation of basal/bolus multiple daily injection insulin with a continuous glucose monitor (hypoglycemia unawareness history) or a pump and continuous glucose monitor should be implemented. If psychological issues are diagnosed, he should receive behavioral health intervention. What about his painful neuropathy?

- Medications to consider for painful neuropathy are gabapentin, pregabalin, or duloxetine.
- How would you address the autonomic neuropathy? Focused on symptoms. See Table 28.6.
- What can be done for the orthostasis? See treatments in Table 28.6.
- Is there anything that would improve gastric emptying? Frequent small meals, maybe prokinetic agents (metoclopramide, domperidone, erythromycin).
- This chapter's section on AN helps readers answer questions raised in this case.

caution while driving, and wearing appropriate diabetes identification. Teach family members the signs and treatment of hypoglycemia, including glucagon administration. Blood glucose awareness training may improve functional capacity.[134,164] Continuous glucose monitoring is very helpful, as alarms can be set to notify the person with diabetes when his or her glucose level drops below the target level.

Focal and Multifocal Neuropathies

The various focal neuropathies are acute and unpredictable. They are not specific to diabetes and are not related to the duration of diabetes. There are no strategies for prevention or early detection. Focal neuropathies are generally classified into the following types:

- Mononeuropathies
- Entrapment syndromes

The primary symptom of focal neuropathies is acute local pain.

Focal Limb Neuropathies

Focal limb neuropathies are usually due to entrapments. Entrapment syndromes start slowly and progress and persist unless intervention is prescribed. Carpal tunnel syndrome (compression or entrapment of the median nerve of the wrist) occurs 3 times as frequently in people with diabetes compared with healthy populations[61,165] and is found in up to one third of people with diabetes.[61] The diagnosis can be made by a careful history and physical and confirmed by electrophysiological studies.

Treatment consists of resting, aided by placement of a wrist splint in a neutral position to avoid repetitive trauma. Anti-inflammatory medications and steroid injections are sometimes useful. Surgery should be considered if weakness appears and medical treatment fails.[32,166]

Mononeuropathies

Mononeuropathies occur primarily in older people; the onset is acute and associated with pain, and their course is self-limiting, resolving within 6 to 8 weeks. They are due to vascular obstruction.[167] Mononeuropathies, characterized by their acute onset, should be distinguished from entrapment syndromes (see Table 28.7).

TABLE 28.7 Mononeuropathies Versus Entrapment Syndrome

Feature	*Mononeuropathy*	*Entrapment Syndrome*
Onset	Sudden	Gradual
Pattern	Single nerve, but may be multiple	Single nerve exposed to trauma
Nerves involved	Cranial nerves III, VI, VII; ulnar; median; peroneal	Median, ulnar, peroneal, medial and lateral plantar
Natural history	Resolves spontaneously	Progressive
Treatment	Symptomatic	Rest, splints, local steroids, diuretics, surgery

Source: Adapted with permission from Elsevier from A Vinik, A Mehrabyan, "Diabetic neuropathies," *Med Clin North Am* 88, no. 4 (2004): 954.

Cranial Neuropathies

Cranial neuropathies in persons with diabetes are less common and occur more often in older individuals with a long duration of diabetes.[168] The third cranial nerve is most often affected. The onset is generally abrupt with headache, eye pain, or dysesthesias of the upper lid preceding palsy. The person with diabetes is unable to move the eye. After a few weeks the pain subsides and ocular function improves, with full recovery in 3 to 5 months. Diplopia can be caused by opthalmoplegias of cranial nerves 4 and 6 as well. These also often resolve on their own.[169]

Implications for Diabetes Education and Care Assure the person with diabetes that this is a temporary situation that will soon resolve. Suggest the use of an eye patch for the affected eye. The physician should rule out ruptured communicating artery aneurysm or stroke.

Proximal-Motor Neuropathy (Amyotrophy)

Proximal-motor neuropathy typically occurs in older people (50-60 years of age) with type 2 diabetes and presents with severe pain and unilateral or bilateral muscle weakness and atrophy in proximal thighs. Pathogenesis is still unclear, although immune-mediated epineurial microvasculitis is the culprit in some cases. Immunosuppressive therapy is recommended using high-dose steroids or intravenous immunoglobulin.[170]

Implications for Diabetes Education and Care Treatment of proximal neuropathies can be very rewarding, as 91% are due to the coexistence of chronic inflammatory demyelinating polyneuropathy and respond to intravenous immunoglobulin therapy. For those who fail to respond, immunosuppressive agents such as etanercept (Enbrel®, Amgen) or azathioprine (Imuran®, Prometheus Laboratories Inc) may be effective.[171,172]

Chronic Inflammatory Demyelinating Polyneuropathy

When an unusually severe, predominantly motor and progressive polyneuropathy develops in persons with diabetes, chronic inflammatory demyelinating polyneuropathy should be considered. Progressive motor deficit and progressive sensory neuropathy in spite of optimal glycemic stability, together with typical NCV findings and an unusually high cerebrospinal-fluid protein level, suggest the possibility of an underlying demyelinating neuropathy. This neuropathy occurs 11 times more frequently in people with diabetes than in those without diabetes.[171,173–175]

Implications for Diabetes Education and Care The diagnosis is often overlooked, but it is very important to recognize the condition because it is treatable. Immunomodulatory therapy with intravenous immunoglobulin or immunotherapy can produce a relatively rapid and substantial improvement.[175]

Diabetic Truncal Radiculoneuropathy

Diabetic truncal radiculoneuropathy affects middle-aged to elderly persons, especially males. (Radiculopathy is the disease condition of the nerve roots in spinal nerves.) Pain is the most important symptom, occurring in a girdle-like distribution over the lower thoracic or abdominal wall, unilaterally or bilaterally distributed. Pain and/or loss of sensation is usually worse at night. Motor weakness is rare. Resolution generally occurs within 4 to 6 months.

Implications for Diabetes Education and Care Non-narcotics or simple analgesics may help control the pain, which generally subsides in 6 to 24 months. The distribution of pain and sensory disturbance is clinically diagnosed by an experienced clinician.

Treatment of DN Based on Pathogenetic Mechanisms

See Serhiyenko and Serhiyenko[2] for a complete discussion of therapies.

Glycemic and Metabolic Management

Studies have shown a relationship between hyperglycemia and the development and severity of DN. The DCCT research group reported that clinical and electrophysiological evidence of neuropathy was reduced by 50% in persons with type 1 diabetes treated intensively with insulin.[176] In the UK Prospective Diabetes Study, management of blood glucose was associated with improvement in vibration perception.[177,178]

Vascular Risk Factors and DN

The Steno trial, using multifactorial intervention, reported a reduction in the development of AN in people with type 2 diabetes.[146] The EURODIAB, a prospective study that included 3,250 persons with diabetes across Europe, showed that the incidence of neuropathy is also associated with potentially modifiable cardiovascular risk factors, including a raised triglyceride level, BMI, smoking, and hypertension.[179]

Treatment and Prevention

Treatment and prevention of neuropathy should include measures to reduce both microvascular and macrovascular risk factors (hyperglycemia, blood pressure, and lipid management) and lifestyle modifications (exercise and weight reduction, smoking cessation, a diet rich in omega-3 fatty acids, and avoidance of excess alcohol consumption).[146]

Oxidative Stress

A number of studies have shown that hyperglycemia causes oxidative stress in tissues, including peripheral nerves that are susceptible to complications of diabetes. Studies show that hyperglycemia induces an increased presence of markers of oxidative stress, such as superoxide and peroxynitrite ions, which are now measurable in tissues and in body fluids. Persons with diabetic peripheral neuropathy have a reduced internal antioxidant defense mechanism against free radicals.[180]

Treatment

Therapies known to reduce oxidative stress are recommended.[181] Those under investigation include aldose reductase inhibitors (ARIs), γ-linolenic acid, and alpha-lipoic acid.

- *Aldose reductase inhibitors* reduce the flux of glucose through the polyol pathway, inhibiting tissue accumulation of sorbitol and fructose. (Sorbitol is a crystalline alcohol that is the intermediate product in the metabolism of glucose in the nerve and other tissues.) Newer ARIs are currently being explored,[182] but it is becoming clear that these agents may be insufficient per se, and combinations of treatments may be needed.[166]
- *γ-Linolenic acid* can cause significant improvement in clinical and electrophysiological tests for neuropathy.[183]
- *Alpha-lipoic acid*, or thioctic acid, has been used for its antioxidant properties and for its thiol-replenishing redox-modulating properties. It may have favorable influence on microcirculation

and reversal of some symptoms of neuropathy.[184] Ongoing studies will examine its long-term effects on electrophysiology and clinical assessments.[185]

Some of the research studies mentioned above could provide models for the translation of the results of clinical trials involving neuropathy into preventive medicine and optimal clinical care. However, the art of a skilled healthcare provider will still be required to interact fully with the person with diabetes and maximize the outcomes of translational research.

Controversies in Neuropathy Management

Mechanical Measures

Transcutaneous Electrical Nerve Stimulation

Transcutaneous electrical nerve stimulation (TENS, or electrotherapy) may be helpful and is one of the more benign therapies for painful neuropathy.[186,187] Caveat: It is important to move the electrodes around to identify sensitive areas and obtain maximal relief.

Static Magnetic Field Therapy

Static magnetic field therapy has been reported to be of benefit, but blinding in these studies was difficult.[188] It is very easy to determine when there is a magnet in a shoe of the person with diabetes. For this reason, it is difficult to do a blinded study.

Frequency-Modulated Electromagnetic Neural Stimulation

Frequency-modulated electromagnetic neural stimulation (FREMS) has been shown to induce a significant reduction in daytime and nighttime pain. In addition, a significant increase in tactile threshold was detected using SWM, lowering of the vibration detection threshold, and improved motor nerve conduction velocity using a biosthesiometer. There was an extra benefit shown in measures of QOL using the SF-36 Health Survey, in terms of general health, physical, and social functioning.[189] This finding suggests that FREMS may be an active, safe method to improve symptoms of neuropathy with the possibility of enhancing neurological function.

Infrared Light

Infrared light had benefits in a study of 27 persons with diabetes whose extremities were treated for 2 weeks with sham or active infrared. There was reportedly a reduction in the number of insensate sites in persons with diabetes with mild neuropathy, but not in those with greater sensory loss. Improved balance was also reported but was not quantified objectively. Clearly, these observations need to be extended for longer periods, and more objective measures need to be applied to evaluate responsiveness to treatment.[190]

Implanted Spinal Cord Stimulation

An implanted spinal cord stimulator was used in a series of persons with diabetes with severe painful neuropathy who were unresponsive to conventional therapy.[191] However, this should be recommended only in very resistant cases, as it is invasive, expensive, and unproven in controlled studies.

Vibration

Vibration on the sole of the foot below the individual's threshold for 30 to 60 seconds has been shown to enhance sensitivity, neurotransmission, and vibration detection threshold.[192] Although monofilament application to the sole of the foot after vibration resulted in enhanced detection, this enhancement did not apply to the big toe. The ability to amplify signals from the neuropathic foot may have relevance for protecting feet from injury and possibly even enhancing postural stability. These studies need to be expanded to a longer term to determine the durability of their effects.

Surgical Treatment of Neuropathy

Tarsal Tunnel Release

The role of tarsal tunnel release in the management of the person with diabetes who has a painful foot syndrome remains controversial.[61] The major problem is the application of tarsal tunnel release in persons with diabetes with diabetic peripheral neuropathy *in general* and not *specifically* for those persons with diabetes with tarsal tunnel entrapment syndrome (TTS). Tarsal tunnel entrapment syndrome is not difficult to diagnose clinically when DSPN is not severe and NCV is moderately abnormal. Mild symmetric peroneal and tibial NCV abnormality with intact ankle jerks and sensation of the dorsal aspect of the foot with the above-mentioned clinical signs are the most important diagnostic features of TTS. When the neuropathy is severe, diagnosis may be impossible. A positive Tinel sign, tapping just below the medial malleolus, may be helpful but may also simply reflect nerve damage in peripheral neuropathy, a negative sign suggesting that nerve damage predicts a poor outcome of surgery. Caveat: If persons with diabetes are carefully selected, release of the tibial nerve through the tarsal tunnel in the person with diabetes may improve plantar sensibility and help prevent plantar ulceration and ultimate lower extremity amputation. Several studies lend credence to this notion, though some are subject to design flaws.[193,194]

Summary

The following are key issues in DN:

- Diabetic neuropathies are among the most common long-term complications of diabetes, although they are not always fully recognized by healthcare providers.
- Management of the disease is complex.
- A thorough history and detailed physical examination, together with the aid of simple tests (performed in the clinic), are essential for the diagnosis.
- More advanced testing may be needed for some persons with diabetes.
- In each particular clinical situation, the best treatment option should be determined on the basis of the underlying pathological process, the clinical presentation, and cost in relation to effectiveness.
- There has been increasing understanding of the pathogenesis of DN over the past decades, and new therapies are currently being studied that hold promise for the treatment of this disease.

This chapter addressed the challenges facing diabetes care and education specialists and suggested opportunities for dealing with DN. The message is powerful: DN is not a single entity but rather a number of different syndromes, each with a range of clinical and subclinical manifestations. Effective management is based on recognizing the particular manifestation and underlying pathogenesis of the particular form of DN in each person with diabetes and using this information to initiate therapy at a level that improves QOL for the person with diabetes.

Focus on Education

Teaching Strategies

Assess daily neuropathy-related pain management. Diabetic neuropathy includes somatic and autonomic neuropathies, is associated with considerable morbidity and mortality, and has a significant impact on QOL. Ask persons with diabetes the following questions:

- How does your pain impact your daily routine?
- What is your pain management strategy?
- How do you navigate the healthcare system to utilize all of the resources and support available to you?

Focus on prevention. Help persons with diabetes see how desirable glucose levels can minimize the possibility of neuropathies.

Reverse neuropathies.

- Inform the person with diabetes about potential treatment options. Offer assurance that treatment of many of the neuropathies can lead to eliminating or minimizing pain and discomfort. Some conditions are due to coexistence of other problems and respond to therapy.
- Diabetic neuropathy is not a single disease (but rather a heterogeneous group of disorders), and it might require multiple treatment approaches.

Diagnose neuropathies. Often neuropathies are overlooked or "tolerated" as a natural progression of a disease. The key is screening, early detection, and treatment. Emphasis needs to be placed on routine annual and semiannual exams. Detection can be difficult; thus, clinicians are to inspect feet and skin at every visit to detect changes or symptoms.

Control neuropathies. Neuropathies can be controlled by treatment. Associated pain can be treated with nonnarcotics or simple analgesics.

Messages for Persons With Diabetes

The key is screening, early detection, and treatment.

- Keep track of your scheduled screening and its follow-up plan.
- Create a daily routine to examine/screen and care for your feet or other neuropathy-impacted system.
- Follow the prescribed medication or therapy recommended.
- Keep track of your pain management—what triggers pain, what it takes to relieve it, and how long it takes to manage the symptoms—and communicate with your healthcare providers about it.

Manage the ABCs (A1C, blood pressure, and cholesterol) to maintain optimal targets. Blood glucose, blood pressure, lipids, and lifestyle modifications are essential measures to reduce the risk of macrovascular disease, which contributes to DN.

Manage your pain. Read about the condition and its treatment, openly describe and talk about pain associated with neuropathies, and use medications (prescription and over-the-counter) appropriately. Relieving pain improves QOL and allows for clearer problem solving.

Attend all checkups. Schedule appointments in advance and note them on the calendar. Make this a priority. Identification and early treatment increase good response and reduction in symptoms. Insist that the healthcare provider look at your skin and feet at every visit and talk about the pain and problems to look for with neuropathies.

Follow medication and treatment regimens. Pay attention to timing of medicines. Use only the supplements advised by the healthcare team. Routinely review medicines with a pharmacist and the healthcare team; this is advisable to offer the best combination of treatments.

Diabetic neuropathies do not have to limit you from enjoying good QOL. Whether you are experiencing pain or working on minimizing or eliminating it, multiple treatment approaches are available to help you in your efforts. Different healthcare professionals can help in different ways. Ask your doctor to direct you to someone qualified to help with your needs.

Diabetic neuropathies can have an impact on your work, your relationships, and your ability to manage your diabetes. Talk to the diabetes care team about getting support with coping and overcoming challenges that will come with all the changes to your life.

Health Literacy

Persons with diabetes might be embarrassed to talk about some of the symptoms associated with DN. Request their permission to ask them a few questions about it or tell them why you need to examine them. Explain why you do what you are doing.

Demonstrate the treatment strategies when possible or use visuals to outline treatment steps. Allow people to verbalize or demonstrate back to you what they will do (let them teach you).

Create reminders for daily care. Establish a routine that allows for the treatment to be part of the usual daily tasks and monitor progress.

Help persons with diabetes explore the following:

- How treatment cost, treatment regimen, and other factors affect their engagement
- The costs and consequences of not engaging with the treatment regimen
- Therapy-related problems
- Development of solutions
- Selection of therapies
- Follow-up to assess outcomes

Consider that age, race, gender, income, education, intelligence, actual seriousness of the disease, and the efficacy of the treatment may be associated with engagement with the treatment regimen.

Encourage persons with diabetes to seek social support. Social support allows person with diabetes to be accountable for their care. Also, peer-to-peer support helps persons with diabetes explore options and validate their feelings and attitudes, and facilitates general discussions about care.

Focus on Practice

Establish a network of appropriate referral services for DNs. Effective management is based on recognizing the particular manifestation and underlying pathogenesis of the particular form of DN. Treatment modalities are individualized at all care levels to ultimately improve QOL for the person with diabetes.

Integrate DN management into the diabetes self-management education. There has been increasing understanding of the pathogenesis of DN over the past decades, and new therapies are currently being studied that hold promise for the treatment of this disease.

Examine access to care for people with DN. There is a significantly higher direct medical cost for individuals diagnosed with a diabetic complication of neuropathy.

References

1. Boulton AJM, Armstrong DG, Kirsner RS, Attinger CE, Lavery LA, Lipsky BA, Mills JL Sr., Steinberg JS. Diagnosis and Management of Diabetic Foot Complications. Arlington (VA): American Diabetes Association; 2018 Oct.
2. Serhiyenko VA, Serhiyenko AA. Cardiac autonomic neuropathy: Risk factors, diagnosis and treatment World J Diabetes. 2018 Jan 15;9(1):1-24. doi: 10.4239/wjd.v9.i1.1. Review.
3. Vinik AI, Maser RE, Ziegler D. Neuropathy: the crystal ball for cardiovascular disease. Diabetes Care. 2010;33:1688-90.
4. Vinik AI, Maser RE, Ziegler D. Autonomic imbalance: prophet of doom or scope for hope? Diabet Med. 2011;28:643-51.
5. Levitt NS, Stansberry KB, Wychanck S, Vinik AI. Natural progression of autonomic neuropathy and autonomic function tests in a cohort of IDDM. Diabetes Care. 1996;19:751-4.
6. Rathmann W, Ziegler D, Jahnke M, Haastert B, Gries FA. Mortality in diabetic patients with cardiovascular autonomic neuropathy. Diabet Med. 1993;10:820-4.
7. Narres, M., Kvitkina, T., Claessen, H., Droste, S., Schuster, B., Morbach, S., ... Icks, A. (2017). Incidence of lower extremity amputations in the diabetic compared with the non-diabetic population: A systematic review. PloS one, 12(8), e0182081. doi:10.1371/journal.pone.0182081.
8. Vinik AI, Nevoret ML, Casellini C, Parson H. Diabetic neuropathy. Endocrinol Metab Clin North Am. 2013 Dec;42(4):747-87. doi:10.1016/j.ecl.2013.06.001.
9. Armstrong DG, Boulton AJM, Bus SA. Diabetic foot ulcers and their recurrence. N Engl J Med. 2017;376:2367–75.
10. Rice JB, Desai U, Cummings AK, et al. Burden of DFUs for medicare and private insurers. Diabetes Care. 2014;37:651–8.
11. Mantyselka P, Ahonen R, Kumpusalo E, Takala J. Variability in prescribing for musculoskeletal pain in Finnish primary health care. Pharm World Sci. 2001;23:232-6.
12. Jensen MP, Chodroff MJ, Dworkin RH. The impact of neuropathic pain on health-related quality of life: review and implications. Neurology. 2007;68:1178-82.
13. WebMD. CDC: Big drop in diabetes amputations. 2012 Jan 24. On the Internet at: http://www.webmd.com/diabetes/news/20120124/cdc-big-drop-diabetes-amputations.
14. Li Y, Rios Burrows N, Gregg EW, Albright A, Geiss LS. Declining rates of hospitalizations for nontraumatic lower limb-extremity amputation in the diabetic population aged 40 years or older: US, 1988-2008. Diabetes Care. 2012;35:273-7.
15. Dyck PJ, Kratz KM, Karnes JL, et al. The prevalence by staged severity of various types of diabetic neuropathy, retinopathy, and nephropathy in a population-based cohort: the Rochester Diabetic Neuropathy Study. Neurology. 1993;43:817-24.
16. Verrotti A, Prezioso G, Scattoni R, Chiarelli F. Autonomic neuropathy in diabetes mellitus Front Endocrinol (Lausanne). 2014 Dec 1;5:205. doi: 10.3389/fendo.2014.00205. eCollection 2014. Review.
17. Zafrir B, Azencot M, Dobrecky-Mery I, Lewis BS, Flugelman MY, Halon DA. Resting heart rate and measures of effort-related cardiac autonomic dysfunction predict cardiovascular events in asymptomatic type 2 diabetes. Eur J Prev Cardiol. 2016;23(12):1298-306.
18. Wulsin LR, Horn PS, Perry JL, Massaro J, D'Agostino R. Autonomic imbalance as a predictor of metabolic risks, cardiovascular disease, diabetes, and mortality autonomic imbalance predicts CVD, DM, mortality. J Clin Endocrinol Metab. 2015:jc20144123.
19. Herman WH, Kennedy L. Underdiagnosis of peripheral neuropathy in type 2 diabetes. Diabetes Care. 2005;28(6):1480-1.
20. Thomas PK, Ward JD, Watkins PJ. Diabetic neuropathy. In: Keen H, Jarrett J, eds. Complications of Diabetes. London, England: Edward Arnold Publishing Company; 1982:109-36.
21. Feldman EL, Stevens MJ, Thomas PK, Brown MB, Canal N, Greene DA. A practical two-step quantitative clinical and electrophysiological assessment for the diagnosis and staging of diabetic neuropathy. Diabetes Care. 1994;17:1281-9.
22. Young MJ, Boulton AJM, MacLeod AF, Williams DRR, Sonksen PH. A multicenter study of the prevalence of diabetic peripheral neuropathy in the United Kingdom hospital clinic population. Diabetologia. 1993;36:150-4.
23. Dyck PJ. Severity and staging of diabetic polyneuropathy. In: Textbook of Diabetic Neuropathy. Stuttgart, Germany: Thieme; 2003:170-5.
24. Dyck PJ. Detection, characterization and staging of polyneuropathy: assessed in diabetes. Muscle Nerve. 1988;11:21-32.
25. Pop-Busui R, Boulton AJ, Feldman EL, Bril V, Freeman R, Malik RA, Sosenko JM, Ziegler D. Diabetic Neuropathy: A Position Statement by the American Diabetes Association. Diabetes Care. 2017 Jan;40(1):136-154. doi: 10.2337/dc16-2042.
26. Vinik AI, Suwanwalaikorn S, Stansberry KB, Holland MT, McNitt PM, Colen LE. Quantitative measurement of cutaneous perception in diabetic neuropathy. Muscle Nerve. 1995;18:574-84.
27. Abbott CA, Carrington AL, Ashe H, et al. The North-West Diabetes Foot Care Study: incidence of, and risk factors for, new diabetic foot ulceration in a community-based patient cohort. Diabetes Med. 2002;19(5):377-84.
28. Dyck PJ, Davies JL, Litchy WJ, O'Brien PC. Longitudinal assessment of diabetic polyneuropathy using a composite score in the Rochester Diabetic Neuropathy Study cohort. Neurology. 1997;49(1):229-39.
29. Haanpaa ML, Backonja MM, Bennett MI, et al. Assessment of neuropathic pain in primary care. Am J Med. 2009;122 Suppl 10:S13-21.

30. Boulton AJ, Gries FA, Jervell JA. Guidelines for the diagnosis and outpatient management of diabetic peripheral neuropathy. Diabet Med. 1998;15:508-14.

31. Yarnitsky D, Sprecher E. Thermal testing: normative data and repeatability for various test algorithms. J Neurol Sci. 1994;125:39-45.

32. Boulton AJ, Malik RA, Arezzo JC, Sosenko JM. Diabetic somatic neuropathies. Diabetes Care. 2004;27:1458-86.

33. Cruccu G, Sommer C, Anand P, et al. EFNS guidelines on neuropathic pain assessment: revised 2009. Eur J Neurol. 2010;17:1010-8.

34. Shy ME, Frohman EM, So Y, Arezzo JC, Cornblath DC, Giuliani MJ; the subcommittee of the American Academy of Neurology. Quantitative sensory testing: report of the Therapeutic and Technology Assessment Subcommittee of the American Academy of Neurology. Neurology. 2003;602:898-906.

35. Pittenger G, Mehrabyan A, Simmons K, et al. Small fiber neuropathy is associated with the metabolic syndrome. Metab Syndr Relat Disord. 2005;3:113-21.

36. Lauria G, Hsieh S, Johansson O, et al. European Federation of Neurological Societies/Peripheral Nerve Society Guideline on the use of skin biopsy in the diagnosis of small fiber neuropathy. Report of a joint task force of the European Federation of Neurological Societies and the Peripheral Nerve Society. Eur J Neurol. 2010;17:903-12.

37. Lauria G, Bakkers M, Schmitz C, et al. Intraepidermal nerve fiber density at the distal leg: a worldwide normative reference study. J Peripher Nerv Syst. 2010;15:202-7.

38. Pittenger GL, Ray M, Burcus NI, McNulty P, Basta B, Vinik AI. Intraepidermal nerve fibers are indicators of small-fiber neuropathy in both diabetic and nondiabetic patients. Diabetes Care. 2004;27:1974-9.

39. Kennedy WR, Wendelschafer-Crabb G, Johnson T. Quantitation of epidermal nerves in diabetic neuropathy. Neurology. 1996;47:1042-8.

40. Polydefkis M, Hauer P, Griffin JW, McArthur JC. Skin biopsy as a tool to assess distal small fiber innervation in diabetic neuropathy. Diabetes Technol Ther. 2001;3(1):23-8.

41. Smith AG, Russell J, Feldman EL, et al. Lifestyle intervention for pre-diabetic neuropathy. Diabetes Care. 2006;29: 1294-9.

42. Joint Task Force of the EFNS and the PNS. European Federation of Neurological Societies/Peripheral Nerve Society Guideline on the use of skin biopsy in the diagnosis of small fiber neuropathy. Report of a joint task force of the European Federation of Neurological Societies and the Peripheral Nerve Society. J Periph Nerv Syst. 2010;15:79-92.

43. Quattrini C, Tavakoli M, Jeziorska M, et al. Surrogate markers of small fiber damage in human diabetic neuropathy. Diabetes. 2007;56:2148-54.

44. Tavakoli M, Quattrini C, Abbott C, et al. Corneal confocal microscopy: a novel noninvasive test to diagnose and stratify the severity of human diabetic neuropathy. Diabetes Care. 2010;33:1792-7.

45. Zhivov A, Blum M, Guthoff R, Stachs O. Real-time mapping of the subepithelial nerve plexus by in vivo confocal laser scanning microscopy. Br J Ophthalmol. 2010;94:1133-5.

46. Parson HK, Nguyen VT, Boyd AL, Vinik A. CHEPs detects neuropathic changes earlier than traditional clinical measures. Diabetes. 2009;58 Suppl 1 abstract:A220.

47. Parson HK, Nguyen VT, Orciga MA, Boyd AL, Casellini CM, Vinik AI. Contact heat-evoked potential stimulation for the evaluation of small nerve fiber function. Diabetes Technol Ther. 2013;15:150-7.

48. McArthur JC, Stocks EA, Hauer P, Cornblath DR, Griffin JW. Epidermal nerve fiber density: normative reference range and diagnostic efficiency. Arch Neurol. 1998;55:1513-20.

49. Illigens BM, Gibbons CH. Sweat testing to evaluate autonomic function. Clin Auton Res. 2009;19:79-87.

50. Mayaudon H, Miloche PO, Bauduceau B. A new simple method for assessing sudomotor function: relevance in type 2 diabetes. Diabetes Metab. 2010;36:450-4.

51. Gin H, Baudoin R, Raffaitin CH, Rigalleau V, Gonzalez C. Non-invasive and quantitative assessment of sudomotor function for peripheral diabetic neuropathy evaluation. Diabetes Metab. 2011;37:527-32.

52. Hubert D, Brunswick P, Calvet JH, Dusser D, Fajac I. Abnormal electrochemical skin conductance in cystic fibrosis. J Cyst Fibros. 2011;10:15-20.

53. Calvet JH, Dupin J, Winiecki H, Schwarz PEH. Assessment of small fiber neuropathy through a quick, simple and noninvasive method in a German diabetes outpatient clinic. Exp Clin Endocrinol Diabetes. 2012;120:1-4.

54. Mao F, Liu S, Qiao X, et al. SUDOSCAN, an effective tool for screening chronic kidney disease in patients with type 2 diabetes. Exp Ther Med. 2017;14(2): 1343-50. doi:10.3892/etm.2017.4689.

55. Casellini CM, Parson HK, Richardson MS, Nevoret ML, Vinik AI. SUDOSCAN, a noninvasive tool for detecting diabetic small fiber neuropathy and autonomic dysfunction. Diabetes Technol Ther. 2013;15:948-53.

56. Smith AG, Lessard M, Reyna S, Doudova M, Singleton JR. The diagnostic utility of SUDOSCAN for distal symmetric peripheral neuropathy. J Diabetes Complications. 2014;28:511-6.

57. Handelsman Y, Bloomgarden ZT, Grunberger G, et al. American Association of Clinical Endocrinologists and American College of Endocrinology—clinical practice guidelines for developing a diabetes mellitus comprehensive care plan—2015. Endocr Pract. 2015;21:1-87.

58. Vinik A, Nevoret M-L, Casellini C, Parson H. Diabetic neuropathy. Endocrinol Metab Clin North Am. 2013;42(4):747-87.

59. DCCT Research Group. The effect of intensive diabetes therapy on the development and progression of neuropathy. Ann Intern Med. 1995;122:561-8.

60. Partanen J, Niskanen L, Lehtinen J, Mervaala E, Siitonen O, Uusitupa M. Natural history of peripheral neuropathy in patients with non-insulin-dependent diabetes mellitus. N Engl J Med. 1995;333:89-94.

61. Vinik A, Mehrabyan A, Colen L, Boulton A. Focal entrapment neuropathies in diabetes. Diabetes Care. 2004;27(7): 1783-8.

62. Vileikyte L, Peyrot M, Bundy C, et al. The development and validation of a neuropathy- and foot ulcer-specific quality of life instrument. Diabetes Care. 2003;26(9):2549-55.

63. Veresiu AI, Bondor CI, Florea B, Vinik EJ, Vinik AI, Gavan NA. Detection of undisclosed neuropathy and assessment of its impact on quality of life: a survey in 25,000 Romanian patients with diabetes. J Diabetes Complications. 2015;29:644-9.

64. Vinik AI, Holland MT, LeBeau JM, Liuzzi FJ, Stansberry KB, Colen LB. Diabetic neuropathies. Diabetes Care. 1992;15:1926-75.

65. Young RJ, Ewing DJ, Clarke BF. Chronic and remitting painful diabetic polyneuropathy. Correlations with clinical features and subsequent changes in neurophysiology. Diabetes Care. 1988;11:34-40.

66. Cavanagh PR, Simoneau GG, Ulbrecht JS. Ulceration, unsteadiness, and uncertainty: the biomechanical consequences of diabetes mellitus. J Biomech. 1993;26 Suppl 1:23-40.

67. Katoulis EC, Ebdon-Parry M, Lanshammar H, Vileikyte L, Kulkarni J, Boulton AJ. Gait abnormalities in diabetic neuropathy. Diabetes Care. 1997;20:1904-7.

68. England JD, Gronseth GS, Franklin G, et al. Distal symmetric polyneuropathy: a definition for clinical research: report of the American Academy of Neurology, the American Association of Electrodiagnostic Medicine, and the American Academy of Physical Medicine and Rehabilitation. Neurology. 2005;64:199-207.

69. Vinik AI, Bril V, Litchy WJ, Price KL, Bastyr EJ III. Sural sensory action potential identifies diabetic peripheral neuropathy responders to therapy. Muscle Nerve. 2005 Nov;32(5):619-25.

70. Paisley AN, Abbott CA, van Schie CHM, Boulton AJM. A comparison of the Neuropen against standard quantitative sensory threshold measures for assessing peripheral nerve function. Diabet Med. 2002;19:400-5.

71. Ziegler D, Siekierka-Kleiser E, Meyer B, Schweers M. Validation of a novel screening device (NeuroQuick) for quantitative assessment of small nerve fiber dysfunction as an early feature of diabetic polyneuropathy. Diabetes Care. 2005;28:1169-74.

72. Viswanathan V, Snehalatha C, Seena R, Ramachandran A. Early recognition of diabetic neuropathy: evaluation of a simple outpatient procedure using thermal perception. Postgrad Med J. 2002;78:541-2.

73. Martina IS, van Koningsveld R, Schmitz PI, van der Meche FG, van Doorn PA. Measuring vibration threshold with a graduated tuning fork in normal aging and in patients with polyneuropathy. European Inflammatory Neuropathy Cause and Treatment (INCAT) group. J Neurol Neurosurg Psychiatry. 1998;65:743-7.

74. Ziegler D, Hidvegi T, Gurieva I, et al. Efficacy and safety of lacosamide in painful diabetic neuropathy. Diabetes Care. 2010;33:839-41.

75. Boulton AJ, Malik RA. Diabetic neuropathy. Med Clin North Am. 1998;82:909-29.

76. Thomas PK. Classification, differential diagnosis, and staging of diabetic peripheral neuropathy. Diabetes. 1997;46 Suppl 2:S54-7.

77. Oyibo SO, Prasad YD, Jackson NJ, Jude EB, Boulton AJ. The relationship between blood glucose excursions and painful diabetic peripheral neuropathy: a pilot study. Diabet Med. 2002;19(10):870-3.

78. Tesfaye S, Malik R, Harris N, et al. Arterio-venous shunting and proliferating new vessels in acute painful neuropathy of rapid glycaemic control (insulin neuritis). Diabetologia. 1996;39:329-35.

79. Sinnreich M, Taylor BV, Dyck PJ. Diabetic neuropathies. Classification, clinical features, and pathophysiological basis. Neurologist. 2005;11:63-79.

80. Vinik A. The approach to the management of the patient with neuropathic pain. In: Wartofsky L, ed. A Clinical Approach to Endocrine and Metabolic Diseases. Vol. 2. Chevy Chase, Md: The Endocrine Society; 2012:177-94.

81. Archer AG, Watkins PJ, Thomas PK, Sharma AK, Payan J. The natural history of acute painful neuropathy in diabetes mellitus. J Neurl Neurosurg Psychiatry. 1983;46:491-9.

82. Pittenger G, Simmons K, Anandacoomaraswamy D, Rice A, Barlow P, Vinik A. Topiramate improves intraepidermal nerve fiber morphology and quantitative neuropathy measures in diabetic neuropathy patients. J Peripher Nerv Syst. 2005; 10 Suppl 1.

83. Vinik A, Pittenger G, Barlow P, Mehrabyan A. Diabetic neuropathies: an overview of clinical aspects, pathogenesis, and treatment. In: LeRoith D, Taylor S, Olefsky J, eds. Diabetes Mellitus. 3rd ed. Philadelphia: Lippincott Williams and Wilkins; 2004:1331-63.

84. Gibbons CH, Freeman R. Treatment-induced neuropathy of diabetes: an acute, iatrogenic complication of diabetes. Brain. 2015 Jan;138(Pt 1):43-52.

85. Vinik A, Mehrabyan A. Understanding diabetic neuropathies. Emerg Med. 2004;36(5):39-44.

86. Vinik AI, Smith AG, Singleton JR, et al. Normative values for electrochemical skin conductances and impact of ethnicity on quantitative assessment of sudomotor function. Diabetes Technol Ther. 2016;18:391-8.

87. Treede RD, Jensen TS, Campbell JN, et al. Neuropathic pain: redefinition and a grading system for clinical and research purposes. Neurology. 2008;70:1630-5.

88. Bennett MI, Attal N, Backonja MM, et al. Using screening tools to identify neuropathic pain. Pain. 2007;127:199-203.

89. Vinik EJ, Hayes RP, Oglesby A, et al. The development and validation of the Norfolk QOL-DN, a new measure of patients'

perception of the effects of diabetes and diabetic neuropathy. Diabetes Technol Ther. 2005;7(3):497-508.

90. Bastyr E, Zhang D, Bril V; the MBBQ Study Group. Neuropathy Total Symptom Score-6 Questionnaire (NTSS-6) is valid instrument for assessing the positive symptoms of diabetic peripheral neuropathy (DPN). Diabetes. 2002; 51:A199.

91. Scholz J, Mannion RJ, Hord DE, et al. A novel tool for the assessment of pain: validation in low back pain. PLoS Med. 2009;6:e1000047.

92. Spallone V. La neuropatia diabetica dolorosa: approccio alla diagnosi e alla terapia di un problema emergente. Me Dia. 2009;9:1-14.

93. Young RJ. Structural functional interactions in the natural history of diabetic polyneuropathy: a key to the understanding of neuropathic pain? Diabet Med. 1993;10 Suppl 2:89 S-90.

94. Vinik A, Ullal J, Parson HK, Casellini CM. Diabetic neuropathies: clinical manifestations and current treatment options. Nat Clin Pract Endocrinol Metab. 2006;2:269-81.

95. Bouhassira D, Attal N, Fermanian J, et al. Development and validation of the Neuropathic Pain Symptom Inventory. Pain. 2004;108:248-57.

96. Bennett MI, Smith BH, Torrance N, Potter J. The S-LANSS score for identifying pain of predominantly neuropathic origin: validation for use in clinical and postal research. J Pain. 2005;6:149-58.

97. Krause S, Backonja M. Development of a neuropathic pain questionnaire. Clin J Pain. 2003;19(5):306-14.

98. Bouhassira D, Attal N, Alchaar H, et al. Comparison of pain syndromes associated with nervous or somatic lesions and development of a new neuropathic pain diagnostic questionnaire (DN4). Pain. 2005;114:29-36.

99. Freyhagen R, Baron R, Gockel U. Pain detect: a new screening questionnaire to detect neuropathic components in patients with back pain. Curr Med Res Opin. 2006;22:1911-20.

100. Portenoy R. Development and testing of a neuropathic pain screening questionnaire: ID Pain. Curr Med Res Opin. 2006;22:1555-65.

101. Dworkin RH, Turk DC, Revicki DA, et al. Development and initial validation of an expanded and revised version of the short-form McGill Pain Questionnaire (SF-MPQ-2). Pain. 2009;144:35-42.

102. Daut RL, Cleeland CS, Flanery RC. Development of the Wisconsin Brief Pain Questionnaire to assess pain in cancer and other diseases. Pain. 1983;17:197-210.

103. Dworkin RH, Turk DC, Wyrwich KW, et al. Interpreting the clinical importance of treatment outcomes in chronic pain clinical trials: IMMPACT recommendations. J Pain. 2008;9:105-21.

104. Finnerup NB, Otto M, McQuay HJ, Jensen TS, Sindrup SH. Algorithm for neuropathic pain treatment: an evidence based proposal. Pain. 2005;118:289-305.

105. Finnerup NB, Sindrup SH, Jensen TS. The evidence for pharmacological treatment of neuropathic pain. Pain. 2010;150:573-81.

106. Dworkin RH, O'Connor AB, Backonja M, et al. Pharmacologic management of neuropathic pain: evidence-based recommendations. Pain. 2007;132:237-51.

107. Dworkin RH, O'Connor AB, Audette J, et al. Recommendations for the pharmacological management of neuropathic pain: an overview and literature update. Mayo Clin Proc. 2010;85:S3-14.

108. Quilici S, Chancellor J, Lothgren M, et al. Meta-analysis of duloxetine vs. pregabalin and gabapentin in the treatment of diabetic peripheral neuropathic pain. BMC Neurol. 2009;9:6-19.

109. Burke J, Sanchez R, Joshi A, Cappelleri J, Kulakodlu M, Halpern R. Health care costs in patients with painful diabetic peripheral neuropathy prescribed pregabalin or duloxetine. Pain Pract. 2012;12:209-18.

110. De Salas-Cansado M, Perez C, Saldana MT, et al. An economic evaluation of pregabalin versus usual care in the management of community-treated patients with refractory painful diabetic peripheral neuropathy in primary care settings. Prim Care Diabetes. 2012;6:303-12.

111. Bellows BK, Dahal A, Jiao T, Biskupiak J. A cost-utility analysis of pregabalin versus duloxetine for the treatment of painful diabetic neuropathy. J Pain Palliat Care Pharmacother. 2012;26:153-64.

112. American Diabetes Association. Microvascular complications and foot care: standards of medical care in diabetes—2019. Diabetes Care 2020;43(Suppl. 1):S135–S151

113. Lord S, Sherrington C, Menz H, Close J. Falls in Older People: Risk Factors and Strategies for Prevention. 2nd ed. Cambridge, UK: Cambridge University Press; 2007.

114. Maurer MS, Burcham J, Cheng H. Diabetes mellitus is associated with an increased risk of falls in elderly residents of a long-term care facility. J Gerontol A Biol Sci Med Sci. 2005;60(9):1157-62.

115. Schwartz AV, Hillier TA, Sellmeyer DE, et al. Older women with diabetes have a higher risk of falls: a prospective study. Diabetes Care. 2002;25(10):1749-54.

116. Clark RD, Lord SR, Webster IW. Clinical parameters associated with falls in an elderly population. Gerontology. 1993;39(2):117-23.

117. Close JC, Lord SL, Menz HB, Sherrington C. What is the role of falls? Best Pract Res Clin Rheumatol. 2005;19(6): 913-35.

118. Tinetti ME, Kumar C. The patient who falls: "It's always a trade-off." JAMA. 2010;303(3):258-66.

119. Morrison S, Colberg SR, Mariano M, Parson HK, Vinik AI. Balance training reduces falls risk in older individuals with type 2 diabetes. Diabetes Care. 2010;33(4):748-50.

120. Dhesi JK, Bearne LM, Moniz C, et al. Neuromuscular and psychomotor function in elderly subjects who fall and

the relationship with vitamin D status. J Bone Miner Res. 2002;17(5):891-7.

121. Welford AT. Between bodily changes and performance: some possible reasons for slowing with age. Exp Aging Res. 1984;10(2):73-88.

122. Tucker MG, Kavanagh JJ, Morrison S, Barrett RS. Voluntary sway and rapid orthogonal transitions of voluntary sway in young adults, and low and high fall-risk older adults. Clin Biomech. (Bristol, Avon). 2009;24(8):597-605.

123. Fukagawa NK, Wolfson L, Judget J, Whipple R, King M. Strength is a major factor in balance, gait, and the occurrence of falls. J Gerontol A Biol Sci Med Sci. 1995;50 A:64-7.

124. Buckner DM, Cress ME, de Lateur BJ, et al. The effect of strength and endurance training on gait, balance, fall risk, and health services use in community-living older adults. J Gerontol. 1997;52 A(4):M218-24.

125. Won-Park S, Goodpaster B, Strotmeyer E, et al. Decreased muscle strength and quality in older adults with type 2 diabetes: the health, aging and body composition study. Diabetes. 2006;55(6):1813-8.

126. Lord S, Fitzpatrick R. Choice stepping reaction time: a composite measure of falls' risk in older people. J Gerontol A Biol Sci Med Sci. 2001;56(10):M627-32.

127. Vinik AI, Perrot S, Vinik EJ, et al. Capsasicin 8% patch repeat treatment plus standard of care (SOC) versus SOC alone in painful diabetic peripheral neuropathy: a randomised, 52-week, open-label, safety study. BMC Neurol. 2016;16:251:1-14. Open Access

128. Vinik AI, Shapiro DY, Rauschkolb C, et al. A randomized withdrawal, placebo-controlled study evaluating the efficacy and tolerability of tapentadol extended release in patients with chronic painful diabetic peripheral neuropathy. Diabetes Care. 2014;37:2302-9.

129. Boulton A, Vinik A, Arrezzo J, et al. Position statement: diabetic neuropathies. Diabetes Care. 2005;28(4):956-62.

130. Ziegler D, Dannehl K, Muhlen H, Spuler M, Gries FA. Prevalence of cardiovascular autonomic dysfunction assessed by spectral analysis, vector analysis, and standard tests of heart rate variation and blood pressure responses at various stages of diabetic neuropathy. Diabetes Med. 1992;9(9):806-14.

131. Vinik AI, Maser RE, Mitchell BD, Freeman R. Diabetic autonomic neuropathy. Diabetes Care. 2003;26(5):1553-79.

132. Zola BE, Vinik AI. Effects of autonomic neuropathy associated with diabetes mellitus on cardiovascular function. Coron Artery Dis. 1992;3:33-41.

133. Spallone V, Ziegler D, Freeman R, et al. Cardiovascular autonomic neuropathy in diabetes: clinical impact, assessment, diagnosis, and management. Diabetes Metab Res Rev. 2011;27:639-53.

134. Pop-Busui R, Evans G, Gerstein H, et al; the ACCORD Study Group. Effects of cardiac autonomic dysfunction on mortality risk in the Action to Control Cardiovascular Risk in Diabetes (ACCORD) trial. Diabetes Care. 2010;33:1578-84.

135. Calles-Escandon J, Lovato L, Simons-Morton D, et al. Effect of intensive compared with standard glycemia treatment strategies on mortality by baseline subgroup characteristics. Diabetes Care. 2010;33:721-7.

136. Tesfaye S, Vileikyte L, Rayman G, et al; Toronto Expert Panel on Diabetic Neuropathy. Painful diabetic peripheral neuropathy: consensus recommendations on diagnosis, assessment and management. Diabetes Metab Res Rev. 2011 Oct;27(7):629-38.

137. Tracey KJ. Reflex control of immunity. Nat Rev Immunol. 2009;9:418-28.

138. Vinik AI, Ziegler D. Diabetic cardiovascular autonomic neuropathy. Circulation. 2007;115(3):387-97.

139. Maser RE, Mitchell BD, Vinik AI, Freeman R. The association between cardiovascular autonomic neuropathy and mortality in individuals with diabetes: a meta-analysis. Diabetes Care. 2003;26(6):1895-901.

140. Vinik A, Maser RE. Letter to editor: screening for asymptomatic coronary artery disease in patients with type 2 diabetes. JAMA. 2009;302(7):735-6.

141. Ziegler D. Diabetic cardiovascular autonomic neuropathy: prognosis, diagnosis and treatment. Diabetes Metab Rev. 1994;10(4):339-83.

142. Valensi P. Diabetic autonomic neuropathy: what are the risks? Diabetes Metab. 1998;24:66-72.

143. Mancia G, Paleari F, Parati G. Early diagnosis of diabetic autonomic neuropathy: present and future approaches. Diabetologia. 1997;40:482-4.

144. Ziegler D, Gries FA. Alpha-lipoic acid in the treatment of diabetic peripheral and cardiac autonomic neuropathy. Diabetes. 1997;46 Suppl 2:S62-6.

145. Athyros VG, Didangelos TP, Karamitsos DT, Papageorgiou AA, Boudoulas H, Kontopoulos AG. Long-term effect of converting enzyme inhibition on circadian sympathetic and parasympathetic modulation in patients with diabetic autonomic neuropathy. Acta Cardiol. 1998;53(4):201-9.

146. Gaede P, Vedel P, Larsen N, Jensen GV, Parving HH, Pedersen O. Multifactorial intervention and cardiovascular disease in patients with type 2 diabetes. N Engl J Med. 2003;348(5):383-93.

147. Vinik A, Mehrabyan A. Gastrointestinal disturbances. In: Lebovitz H, ed. Therapy for Diabetes Mellitus and Related Disorders. 4th ed. Alexandria, Va: American Diabetes Association; 2004:424-39.

148. Jones KL, Russo A, Stevens JE, Wishart JM, Berry MK, Horowitz M. Predictors of delayed gastric emptying in diabetes. Diabetes Care. 2001;24(7):1264-9.

149. Drucker DJ, Nauck MA. The incretin system: glucagon-like peptide-1 receptor agonists and dipeptidyl peptidase-4 inhibitors in type 2 diabetes. Lancet. 2006;368:1696-1705.

150. Drucker DJ, Sherman SI, Gorelick FS, Bergenstal RM, Sherwin RS, Buse JB. Incretin-based therapies for the treatment of type 2 diabetes: evaluation of the risks and benefits. Diabetes Care. 2010;33:428-33.

151. Nauck MA, Vilsboll T, Gallwitz B, Garber A, Madsbad S. Incretin-based therapies: viewpoints on the way to consensus. Diabetes Care. 2009;32 Suppl 2:S223-31.

152. Horowitz SH, Ginsberg-Fellner F. Ischemia and sensory nerve conduction in diabetes mellitus. Neurology. 1979;29: 695-704.

153. Vinik AI, Richardson D. Erectile dysfunction in diabetes. Diabetes Reviews. 1998;6:16-33.

154. Richardson D, Vinik A. Etiology and treatment of erectile failure in diabetes mellitus. Curr Diab Rep. 2002;2(6):501-9.

155. Vinik A, Richardson D. Erectile dysfunction. In: Sinclair A, Finucane P, eds. Diabetes in Old Age. 2nd ed. Chichester, UK: John Wiley & Sons; 2001:89-102.

156. Vinik A, Mehrabyan A. Diagnosis and management of diabetic autonomic neuropathy. Compr Ther. 2003;29(2/3):130-45.

157. Enzlin P, Mathieu C, Vanderschueren D, Demyttenaere K. Diabetes mellitus and female sexuality: a review of 25 years' research. Diabet Med. 1998;15(10):809-15.

158. Stansberry KB, Hill MA, Shapiro SA, McNitt PM, Bhatt BA, Vinik AI. Impairment of peripheral blood flow responses in diabetes resembles an enhanced aging effect. Diabetes Care. 1997;20:1711-6.

159. Stansberry KB, Peppard HR, Babyak LM, Popp G, McNitt PM, Vinik AI. Primary nociceptive afferents mediate the blood flow dysfunction in non-glabrous (hairy) skin of type 2 diabetes: a new model for the pathogenesis of microvascular dysfunction. Diabetes Care. 1999;22:1549-54.

160. Haak ES, Usadel KH, Kohleisen M, Yilmaz A, Kusterer K, Haak T. The effect of alpha-lipoic on the neurovascular reflex arc in patients with diabetic neuropathy assessed by capillary microscopy. Microvasc Res. 1999;58:28-34.

161. Meyer C, Hering BJ, Grossmann R, et al. Improved glucose counterregulation and autonomic symptoms after intraportal islet transplants alone in patients with long-standing type I diabetes mellitus. Transplantation. 1998;66(2):233-40.

162. Cryer PE, Davis SN, Shamoon H. Hypoglycemia in diabetes. Diabetes Care. 2003;26:1902-12.

163. Vinik A. Diagnosis and management of diabetic neuropathy. Clin Geriatr Med. 1999;15(2):293-319.

164. Cox DJ, Gonder-Frederick L, Julian DM, Clarke W. Long-term follow-up evaluation of blood glucose awareness training. Diabetes Care. 1994;17(1):1-5.

165. Perkins B, Olaleye D, Bril V. Carpal tunnel syndrome in patients with diabetic polyneuropathy. Diabetes Care. 2002;25:565-9.

166. Vinik A, Mehrabyan A. Diabetic neuropathies. Med Clin North Am. 2004;88(4):947-99.

167. Vinik A, Mehrabyan A. Diabetic monoradiculopathy/amyoradiculopathy. In: Lebovitz H, ed. Therapy for Diabetes Mellitus and Related Disorders. 4th ed. Alexandria, Va: American Diabetes Association; 2004:416-23.

168. Watanabe K, Hagura R, Akanuma Y, et al. Characteristics of cranial nerve palsies in diabetic patients. Diabetes Res Clin Pract. 1990;10(1):19-27.

169. Greco D, Gambina F, Maggio F. Ophthalmoplegia in diabetes mellitus: a retrospective study. Acta Diabetologica. 2009;46:23.

170. James P, Dyck B, Windenbank A. Diabetic and nondiabetic lumbosacral radiculoplexus neuropathy: new insights into pathophysiology. Muscle Nerve. 2002;25:477-91.

171. Vinik AI, Anandacoomaraswamy D, Ullal J. Antibodies to neuronal structures: innocent bystanders or neurotoxins? Diabetes Care. 2005;28(8):2067-72.

172. Bourcier ME, Vinik AI. A 41-year-old man with polyarthritis and severe autonomic neuropathy. Ther Clin Risk Manag. 2008;4:837-42.

173. Sharma K, Cross J, Farronay O, Ayyar D, Sheber R, Bradley W. Demyelinating neuropathy in diabetes mellitus. Arch Neurol. 2002;59:758-65.

174. Krendel DA, Zacharias A, Younger DS. Autoimmune diabetic neuropathy. Neurol Clin. 1997;15(4):959-71.

175. Ayyar DR, Sharma KR. Chronic inflammatory demyelinating polyradiculoneuropathy in diabetes mellitus. Curr Diab Rep. 2004;4(6):409-12.

176. DCCT Research Group. The effect of intensive treatment of diabetes on the development and progression of long-term complications in insulin dependent diabetes mellitus. N Engl J Med. 1993;329:977-86.

177. UK Prospective Diabetes Study (UKPDS) Group. Effect of intensive blood-glucose control with metformin on complications in overweight patients with type 2 diabetes (UKPDS 34). Lancet. 1998;352:854-65.

178. UK Prospective Diabetes Study Group. Tight blood pressure control and risk of macrovascular and microvascular complications in type 2 diabetes: UKPDS 38. BMJ. 1998;317:703-13.

179. Tesfaye S, Chaturvedi N, Eaton SE, et al. Vascular risk factors and diabetic neuropathy. N Engl J Med. 2005;352(4):341-50.

180. Ziegler D, Sohr CG, Nourooz-Zadeh J. Oxidative stress and antioxidant defense in relation to the severity of diabetic polyneuropathy and cardiovascular autonomic neuropathy. Diabetes Care. 2004;27(9):2178-83.

181. Vincent AM, Russell JW, Low P, Feldman EL. Oxidative stress in the pathogenesis of diabetic neuropathy. Endocr Rev. 2004;25(4):612-28.

182. Bril V, Buchanan RA. Aldose reductase inhibition by AS-3201 in sural nerve from patients with diabetic sensorimotor polyneuropathy. Diabetes Care. 2004;27(10):2369-75.

183. Keen H, Payan J, Allawi J, et al. Treatment of diabetic neuropathy with linolenic acid. Diabetes Care. 1993;16:8-15.

184. Ziegler D, Nowak H, Kempler P, Vargha P, Low PA. Treatment of symptomatic diabetic polyneuropathy with the antioxidant alpha-lipoic acid: a meta-analysis. Diabetes Med. 2004;21(2):114-21.

185. Ziegler D, Low PA, Freeman R, Tritschler H, Vinik AI. Predictors of improvement and progression of diabetic polyneuropathy following treatment with alpha-lipoic acid for 4 years in the NATHAN 1 trial. J Diabetes Complications. 2016;30:350-6.

186. Somers DL, Somers MF. Treatment of neuropathic pain in a patient with diabetic neuropathy using transcutaneous electrical nerve stimulation applied to the skin of the lumbar region. Phys Ther. 1999;79:767-75.

187. Hamza MA, White PF, Craig WF, et al. Percutaneous electrical nerve stimulation: a novel analgesic therapy for diabetic neuropathic pain. Diabetes Care. 2000;23(3):365-70.

188. Weintraub MI, Wolfe GI, Barohn RA, et al. Static magnetic field therapy for symptomatic diabetic neuropathy: a randomized, double-blind, placebo-controlled trial. Arch Phys Med Rehabil. 2003;84(5):736-46.

189. Bosi E, Conti M, Vermigli C, et al. Effectiveness of frequency-modulated electromagnetic neural stimulation in the treatment of painful diabetic neuropathy. Diabetologia. 2005;48(5):817-23.

190. Leonard DR, Farooqi MH, Myers S. Restoration of sensation, reduced pain, and improved balance in subjects with diabetic peripheral neuropathy: a double-blind, randomized, placebo-controlled study with monochromatic near-infrared treatment. Diabetes Care. 2004;27(1):168-72.

191. Tesfaye S, Watt J, Benbow SJ, Pang KA, Miles J, MacFarlane IA. Electrical spinal-cord stimulation for painful diabetic peripheral neuropathy. Lancet. 1996;348:1698-701.

192. Khaodhiar L, Niemi JB, Earnest R, Lima C, Harry JD, Veves A. Enhancing sensation in diabetic neuropathic foot with mechanical noise. Diabetes Care. 2003;26(12):3280-3.

193. Wieman TJ, Patel VG. Treatment of hyperesthetic neuropathic pain in diabetics: decompression of the tarsal tunnel. Ann Surg. 1995;221:660-5.

194. Dellon A. Treatment of symptomatic diabetic neuropathy by surgical decompression of multiple peripheral nerves. Plast Reconstr Surg. 1992;89(4):689-97.

INDEX

Note: Tables and figures are indicated by italicized page numbers.

A

A1C assay, role in diagnosis, 386
A1C goals, 486
  for children with type 1 diabetes, *301*
  therapy intensification and, 577–578, *578*
A1C levels
  assessment on hospital admission, 363, *363*
  cardiovascular risk and, 784
  continuous glucose monitoring and, 555
  dental care and, 297
  for diabetes and pregnancy, 763
  diabetes self-management education and support and lower, 6
  diagnosis of type 1 diabetes and, 405, *405*
  diagnosis of type 2 diabetes and, *433*
  frequency of monitoring, 568
  for gestational diabetes mellitus, 773
  medical nutrition therapy and decreases in, 158
  monitoring metabolic management using, 567–568
  in prediabetes, 387
  renal disease and, 846
  standard of care for, *286*
  targets, 288, 568
  targets for type 1 diabetes, *404*
  targets for type 2 diabetes, 434
  tracking via app, 302
  treating cardiovascular risk factors and, *790*
AADE Scope of Practice, Standards of Practice, and Standards of Professional Performance for Diabetes Educators, 328
AADE7 Self-Care Behaviors®, 5, 7, 10
  barriers to diabetes self-management behaviors and, *312*
  continuum of outcomes related to diabetes education and, 171
  for coping skills training and cognitive therapy, 151
  for diabetes and pregnancy, *760,* 761–765
  documentation and, 77
  effectiveness of diabetes education and, 345
  framework for person-centered diabetes education and care and, 396
  for gestational diabetes mellitus, 771–775
  Goal Sheet, 91
  guiding goal setting, 47–49
  for healthy coping, 131
  for healthy eating, 157, *158*
  monitoring and, 263, 533
  outcomes for, 80, *81–86*
  peer support and, 142
  for physical activity, 183
  planning and, 55, 57
  prevention of diabetic ketoacidosis and, *732–733*
  prevention of hyperosmolar hyperglycemic state and, 739, *739–740*
  problem solving and, 307
  reviewing blood glucose results and, 591
  risk reduction and, 285
  self-efficacy and, 117
  transition to outpatient care and, 367, *367–368*
  type 2 diabetes and, 444
Abdomen, diabetic ketoacidosis and acute, 727–728
Academy of Nutrition and Dietetics (AND), 7, 22, 32, 98, 163, 452, 773
Acanthosis nigricans, 441
Acarbose (Precose®), 246, 435, *491–492, 500,* 500–501, *850*
Accelerometers, 225
Acceptable daily intake (ADI), 458
Acceptance, coping with chronic disease and, *143*
Access issues, identification of, 343
Accountable care organization (ACO), 5, 13
Accreditation, myths *vs.* facts about program, 340, *340*
Acebutolol (Sectral®), 635
Acidosis, diabetic ketoacidosis and, *726,* 727
Acidosis/anion gap, in diabetic ketoacidosis, 730
Action planning, 53
Action stage for exercise behavior change, 226, 228
Active learning, 72
Active listening, 44, 114
Activities of daily living, assessment of, 40–41
Activity Pyramid, 188, *189*
ACTOplus met® (pioglitazone/metformin), *523*
Acupressure, 716
Acupuncture, 711, 716
Acute care hospital, transitioning to, 372
Acute hyperglycemia
  case study, 722, 728–729, 734, 741
  defined, 721
  diabetic ketoacidosis, 721–734, *726*
  education, prevention, and treatment, 740–742
  euglycemic ketoacidosis, 721
  hyperosmolar hyperglycemic nonketonic syndrome, 735–740, *737, 739*
  hyperosmolar hyperglycemic state, 721
  inpatient concerns, 734–735, *735*
  preventing in institutional care setting, 741
  self-care behaviors in prevention of, 732, *732–733, 740*
  sick day management, *725,* 733–734
Acute kidney injury (AKI), 839–940
Acute sensory neuropathy (ASN), 876
Adjunctive naturopathic care (ANC), 710
Administration aids, 258
Adolescents
  blood pressure management in, 800
  blood pressure targets for, 289
  cardiovascular risk management issues specific to, 800–801
  coping skills for, 258
  developmental characteristics of each stage in, *419*
  developmental issues and effect on diabetes in, *415*
  diabetic dyslipidemia in, 616
  eating habits of, 419
  education for those with diabetes, 162, 163, 406
  healthy coping and, 142, 148–149
  hypertension in, 289–290, 629
  insulin injection therapy for, 408–410
  lipid management for, 291, 801
  managing diabetes in, 301, 354
  medication administration in, 257
  nutrition therapy in, 469
  physical activity and, 220
  providing diabetes self-management education to, 63
  psychosocial issues and, 419–421
  reproductive health issues and, 419–420
  risky behavior and, 419
  standards of care for lipids in, 291
  transitional care to young adulthood, 354–363
  type 2 diabetes in, 257–258, 432, 441–444
Adult learning theory, 72
Adults. *See also* Elderly adults; Older adults
  blood pressure targets for, 289
  education for those with type 1 diabetes, 406
  healthy coping and, 142, 149

hypertension treatment for, 289
principles of learning and, 63–64
standards of care for lipids in, 290–291
type 1 diabetes in, 425
Advanced Carbohydrate Counting, 174
Advanced glycation end-products (AGEs), 840
Advanced Practice Nurse (APN), 595
Advisory group for diabetes self-management education and support program, 335, 341–342
Advocacy
for diabetes policy, 21–23
for removing barriers to diabetes self-management, 76–77
Aerobic exercise, 192–195
carbohydrate increases for, *208*
combined with resistance training, 198
effect on diabetes management, 200–201
for older adults, *218,* 218–219
Affordable Care Act (ACA), 4, 566
Diabetes Care and Education Specialists and, 15–21
diabetes-related provisions, 16
goals of, 15
Aflibercept (Eylea®), 821
Afrezza®, *517,* 517–518
African Americans
angiotensin-converting enzyme inhibitors and, 632, 633
cataracts and, 819
complementary health approaches and, 651
diabetes self-management education groups for, 113–114
diabetic kidney disease and, 842
health risks of, 37
healthy coping and, 150
ischemic strokes in, 804
prevalence of diabetes and, 381
risk of cardiovascular disease in, 789
use of prayer, 712
Age
diabetes-related skills and, *353*
as factor influencing problem solving, 318
incidence of type 2 diabetes and, 432
risk for poor medication-taking behavior, 242
risk of cardiovascular disease and, 789
Agency for Healthcare Research and Quality (AHRQ), recommendations for discharge planning, 369, *369*
Agenda-setting, motivational interviewing and using, 118
Aging, diabetes and, 2, 440
Alaska Natives
Affordable Care Act protections for, 18
healthy coping and, 150
Native American medicine and, 709
Albiglutide, 435, 505
Albumin excretion, abnormalities of, 269, *269*
Albuminuria, 843–884
Alcohol-free nonprescription medications, 253
Alcoholism, 136
Alcohol use
adolescents and, 419
coping and, 150–151
diabetes and, 136
dyslipidemia/cardiovascular disease risk and, 466
glycemia and, 460–461
insulin pump therapy and, 596
moderate, 176
during pregnancy, 750
weight management and, 467–468
Aldactazide®, 630
Aldose reductase inhibitors, 893
Aldosterone, 839
Algoliptin, 508, *508, 850*
Algorithm, referring providers and, 339
Alirocumab (Praluent®), 621, 625, 796
Aliskiren (Tekturna®), 634
Allicin, 682
Alliinase, 682
Allithiamines, 678
Aloe, 654–655, *668*
Alogliptin (Nesina®), 247, 259, 365, 435, *492,* 508, *508,* 786, 848
Alpha-glucosidase inhibitors, 246
antihyperglycemic management and, 486
for chronic kidney disease, 848, *850*
for type 2 diabetes, 435
for type 2 diabetes management, *491, 500,* 500–501
weight management and, 464
Alpha-linolenic acid (ALA), 680
Alpha-lipoic acid (ALA), 677–678, *684,* 893–894
Alpha 1-receptor blockers, 639–640
Alternative medicine, 647, *648,* 703, 704
AltMedDex, 689
Alzheimer's disease, healthy coping and, 149
Ambulatory Glucose Profile (AGP), *564,* 564–565
American Academy of Family Physicians, 354
American Academy of Ophthalmology, 829
American Academy of Pediatrics, 289, 354, 357, 363
American Association of Clinical Endocrinologists (AACE), 405, 533
on continuous glucose monitoring, 552–553, 556
glycemic algorithm, 578, *580*
guidelines to improve quality of care, 576
target blood glucose goals, 434, 542–543, *543*
on use of insulin pumps during hospitalization, 599
American Association of Diabetes Educators (AADE)
guiding principles of diabetes self-management education and support and, 32
on language, 121
on ongoing diabetes self-management education and support, 98
American Cancer Society, 792
American College of Cardiologists, 465
American College of Cardiology/American Heart Association (ACC/AHA), 615, 787, 788
American College of Endocrinology (ACE)
blood glucose targets, 577, *578*
on continuous glucose monitoring, 552–553
American College of Obstetricians and Gynecologists, 217
American College of Physicians, 354, 361, 734
American College of Sports Medicine (ACSM), 190, 192, 194
American Diabetes Association (ADA), 5, 7, 22
on assessment for polyneuropathy, 869
blood glucose targets, 577, *578*
on blood pressure management for chronic kidney disease, 848, 851
Clinical Practice Recommendations, 70
on continuous glucose monitoring, 552, 556, 558
on daily aspirin use, 267
definition of hypertension, 289
on diabetes care in school settings, 418
diabetes risk survey, 381
educational materials, 251
Education Recognition Program, 340
evidence-grading system for clinical practice recommendations, *870*
on glycemic management in renal disease, 846
goals of medical nutrition therapy, 159
Going to College with Diabetes: A Self-Advocacy Guide for Students, 361
on graded exercise stress test, 187
guidelines to improve quality of care, 576
guiding principles of diabetes self-management education and support and, 32
on lifestyle changes to reduce rates of diabetes, heart disease, and cancer, 792
Nutrition Therapy Consensus Report, 456
Nutrition Therapy for Adults With Diabetes or Prediabetes, 452, 453–454
on ongoing diabetes self-management education and support, 98
on peer support, 414

physical activity recommendations, 413
prescription assistance resources, 245
on psychological and social assessments and diabetes management, 273
resources to aid in implementing standards of care, 296
on selecting CSII, 590
target blood glucose goals, 434, 542–543, *543*
on use of insulin pumps during hospitalization, 599
American Diabetes Association (ADA) Standards of Medical Care in Diabetes, 258, 452
on blood glucose targets, 735
on blood pressure goals, 797
on hypertension, 629
on lipid management in children, 801
on managing dyslipidemia, 616
American Diabetes Association Transitions Work Group, transition recommendations/guidelines, *359*
American ginseng *(Panax quinquefolius L.),* 661, *673*
American Heart Association (AHA), 194, 266, 289, 465, 792
American Heart Association/American College of Cardiology (AHA/ACC) Multi-Society High Blood Pressure Guidelines, 628–629
American Holistic Nurses Association, 707
American Indians
Affordable Care Act protections for, 18
Native American medicine and, 709
prevalence of diabetes and, 381
American Pharmacists Association Foundation, 120
Americans with Disabilities Act (ADA), 74
Amilotide (Midamor®), 630, 631
Amiodarone, 636
Amitriptiline (Elavil®), 641
Amlodipine (Norvasc®), *620,* 637, 638, 797, 852
Amputation
diabetes-related, 868
exercise modifications and, 215
foot-care education and preventing, 880
small-fiber neuropathy and risk of, 877
Amylin, 384, 848, *850*
Amylin analog, 5, 246
for glucose management, 509–510, *510*
for type 2 diabetes management, *493*
Anger, coping with chronic disease and, *143*
Angina, *801,* 801
Angiotensin-1 (AT-1), 627
Angiotensin-converting enzyme (ACE), 533, 627
glycemic algorithm, *580*
Angiotensin-converting enzyme inhibitors (ACEI), 269, 632–633
calcium channel blockers and, 637
for cardiac autonomic neuropathy, 886
for chronic kidney disease, 848
for congestive heart failure, 806
for hypertension, 290, 629, *630,* 798, 851–852
milk thistle and, 664
for patients with increased urinary albumin excretion, 799
Angiotensin II (AT-II), 627, 839, 843
Angiotensin II receptor blocker, 269
Angiotensin receptor blockers (ARBs), 633–634
for cardiac autonomic neuropathy, 886
for chronic kidney disease, 848
for hypertension, 290, 629, *630,* 798, 851–852
for patients with increased urinary albumin excretion, 799
1,5-Anhydroglucitrol blood test (GlycoMark™), 566
Ankle-brachial index (ABI), 271–272, 806
Anorexia nervosa, 136, *137,* 163
Antidiuretic hormone (ADH), 838
Anti GAD 65 antibody, 594
Antihyperglycemic management, 486–489
medications for, *490–493,* 490–504, *494, 496, 497, 498, 500, 501, 502, 503*
weight management and, 464
Antihypertensive agents, classes of, 629–641, *630*
Antiplatelet therapy, 267, *278,* 291, 799
Anti-vascular endothelial growth factor (anti-VEGF) agents, 819, 826–827, 829
Anxiety, 134–135
among children and adolescents, 148
gender and, 149
gestational diabetes mellitus and, 775
in school-aged children with type 1 diabetes, 417
Anxiety management, 146
Appraisal of Diabetes Scale, 144
Appreciate Inquiry, 551
Appreciative coaching, 39–40
Apps
diabetes management and, 66
for physical activity tracking, 225–226
self-management of diabetes using, 302
tracking diabetes goals via, 53
Areas to improve in diabetes education (AIDE), 341, *342*
Arguments, motivational interviewing and avoiding, 115–116
Aromatherapy, 711
Artificial pancreas (APS) technology, 14
Art therapy, 711
Asian Americans
angiotensin-converting enzyme inhibitors and, 633
complementary health approaches and, 651
diabetic kidney disease and, 842
healthy coping and, 150
Asian ginseng *(Panax ginseng),* 661, *673*
ASL (American Sign Language), 74
Aspart, *517, 851*
Aspart detemir, 764
Aspirin therapy, 254, *525*
appropriate use of, 798–799
instructing on use of, 799
for prevention of cardiovascular disease, 267, *790–791*
standards of card, 291
Assessment
activities of daily living and, 40–41
annual, for type 1 diabetes, 424
of atherosclerotic cardiovascular disease risk, 614–615
beginning, 35–39
of blood glucose monitoring, 363
of cardiovascular risk, 614–615, 787–789
caregivers and, 40
closing, 44–46
cognitive, 272–273
of cognitive impairment, 132
conducting, 35
of coping, 140–141
critical thinking in, 41
cultural considerations in, 36–37, *37,* 41
data for, *36*
of diabetes distress, 132–133
DSME/S step, 32–46, *35*
DSMS algorithm of care and, *33*
of education needs and readiness to change, 41–42, *42*
effective, characteristics of, 35, 39–41, *45*
family and, 40
formalized problem-solving, 315
goal setting and, 49–50
at hospital admission, 363–364, *364*
of hypoglycemia risk, 202
of initial monitoring, 265–266
lifestyle issues and, 39
of neuropathy, 293
of nutrition, 168–169
of practice setting, 40
pre-activity, 185–186
setting tone for, 38
skills for, 43
special populations and, 40
for starting diabetes self-management education and support program, 328–331

strategies for, 43–46
of stress, 146–147
tips for quick, 38–39
Assessment, for coping
chronic disorders, *143,* 143–144
developmental age and stage, 141–142
family system roles and responsibilities, 142–143
financial resources and insurance, 143
psychosocial factors of social support, 142
Association for the Advancement of Medical Instrumentation, 267
Association of Diabetes Care and Education Specialists (ADCES), 4, 5, 7, 9, 19, 22, 183, 361. *See also* American Association of Diabetes Educators (AADE)
Competencies for Diabetes Care and Education Specialists, 329
Diabetes Education Accreditation Program (DEAP), 340
educational materials, 251
guidelines for practice, 10
guiding principles of diabetes self-management education and support and, 32
nutrition therapy and, 452
on peer support, 414
person-centered diabetes education and care and, 396
Project Vision, 8
resources to aid in implementing standards of care, 296
on selecting CSII, 590
technology and, 66
on use of insulin pumps during hospitalization, 599
Atenolol (Tenormin®), 635
Atherosclerosis, 804
Atherosclerotic cardiovascular disease (ASCVD), 787, 788, *788*
aspirin therapy to prevent, 799
beta-blockers and, 635
death due to, 613
Atherosclerotic cardiovascular disease (ASCVD), 615, 616
Athlete's foot treatment, 255–256
The Athlete's Guide to Diabetes, 210
Atlas of Diabetes, 2
Atorvastin (Lipitor®), 618, *620*
Attention-deficit/hyperactivity disorder (ADHD), 132, 149
Audiovisual materials, *60,* 71–72
Australian Paediatric Endocrine Group and the Australia Diabetes Society, transition recommendations/guidelines, *360*
Autism, healthy coping and, 149
Autoimmune disorders associated with type 1 diabetes, 422–423, 425
Autoimmunity, type 1 diabetes and, 390–391
Automated office blood pressure (AOBP) measurement, 796
Autonomic nerves, 869
Autonomic nervous system (ANS), 626, 883
Autonomic neuropathy (AN), *869,* 883, *884*
bladder dysfunction and, *884,* 889
cardiac, 883–886, *884*
caveats for exercise with, 885–886
clinical features, diagnosis, and treatment, *884*
exercise modifications for, 213–214, *214*
gastrointestinal disorders and, *884,* 886–888
monitoring for, 271, *278*
pupillary and visceral response and, *884,* 890–892
sexual dysfunction and, 888–889
sudomotor dysfunction and, *884,* 889–890
symptoms, 883
treating underlying causes, 886
Autonomy, Transtheoretical Model and, 108, *108*
Autonomy motivation, 108, *108*
Autonomy support, 108, *108*
Avandamet® (rosiglitazone/metformin), *523*
Avandaryl® (rosiglitazone/glimepiride), *523*
Avoidance coping style, 144, 145–146
Ayurvedic medicine system, 709
Azathioprine, 892
Azilsartan (Edarbi®), 630, 633

B

Background insulin, 515
Balance exercise, 198, 202, 219
Bargaining stage, coping with chronic disease, *143*
Bariatric surgery, 464, 793
Barriers
identifying and addressing diabetes self-management, 74–75, *75*
identifying and assessing potential problems and, 309–311
influencing self-management, 300–301
to medication-taking, 242–243, *243*
to physical activity, 184, 222–224, *223–224*
to self-monitoring blood glucose levels, 536–542, *538*
types of, 309–310
Basal-bolus regimen of insulin injection therapy, 248, 409, 443
Basal calculations for pediatric population, *603*
Basal energy expenditure (BEE), 582
Basal insulin, 515
for chronic kidney disease, *851*
exercise-related hypoglycemia risk and, 203
second-generation, 587
titrating newer, *586*
for type 2 diabetes, 579–580, 585–586
Basal ratio, fine-tuning, 597–598
Baseline evaluation, 263–264
Beck-Depression-Inventory, 144
Bedside sensory tests, *871*
Bedtime, blood glucose monitoring at, 414
Behavior, observing, 50
Behavioral health, focus on, 8
Behavioral objectives
characteristics of, 51–53
differentiating from learning objectives, *51*
establishing collaboratively, 51
guide for writing, *52*
Behavioral Risk Factor Surveillance System, 37, 343
Behavior change
applying, 111–113
diabetes education and, 98
empowerment-based protocol for, 110–114, *112, 113*
for exercise, 226–228
health belief model, *101,* 101–102
lifestyle interventions and prevention of type 2 diabetes, 161
motivational interviewing and person empowerment, 120–121
motivational interviewing approach to, 114–121, *116*
patient empowerment and theories for, 110
person empowerment and behavior-change theories, 109–110
role in promoting healthy eating, 170–172, *172*
self-determination theory, 107–109, *108*
social cognitive theory, 102–104, *103*
theoretical approaches to, 100–109
theory and approach combination for, 109
theory of reasoned action and theory of planned behavior, 104–105, *105*
transtheoretical model, 105–107, *106*
Behavior-change rules, 229
Behavior-change strategies, physical activity and, 184
Being active, evaluating, *81*
Benazepril (Lotensin®), 632, 852
Benchmarking progress over time, 343
Benfotiamine, 678–679, *684*
Benzphetamine, *483*
Berberine, 655–656, *668–669*

Beta-blockers, 635–637
for congestive heart failure, 806
exercise-related blood glucose levels and, 204
Betaxolol (Kerlone®), 635
Bethanechol, 889
Biguanides, 246
for type 2 diabetes, 435, *491, 497,* 497–498
Bilberry, 679, *685*
Bile acid resins, 623–624
Bile acid sequestrants, 247, 796
for chronic kidney disease, 848
for type 2 diabetes, 435, *493, 503,* 503–504
Billable hours, 339
Binge eating disorder (BED), 136, *137,* 164
Biofeedback, 712, 716
Biopsychosocial model of adaptation to illness, 131
Biotin, 658
Bismuth subsalicylate (Pepto-Bismol®), 254
Bisoprolol (Zebeta®), 635
Bitter melon, 656–657, *669–670*
Bladder dysfunction, related to autonomic neuropathy, 889
Blended learning, *61*
Blindness
diabetes as cause of, 817
diabetic retinopathy and, 823
exercise modifications for, 212–213
Blood glucose. *See also* Pattern management
assessment on hospital admission, 363, *363*
effect of physical activity on, 200
factors that may raise or lower, *550*
hyperosmolar hyperglycemic state and, 736
methodology for interpreting, 581–586
role of hormones in exercise blood glucose levels, 200
self-management strategies for physical activity and, 206–207
Blood glucose meters, 407–408
Blood glucose monitoring, 4, 5, 533
1,5-anhydroglucitrol blood test, 566
continuous glucose monitoring, 552–566, *556, 557, 558, 560–561, 563, 564*
for diabetes and pregnancy, 761–763, *762*
fructosamine measurement, 566
identifying barriers to self-monitoring blood glucose, 536–542, *538*
ketone tests, 567
noninvasive, 566
prevention of hyperosmolar hyperglycemic state and, *739*
problem-solving tool for, *552*
self-monitoring, 533–534, *535*
type 1 diabetes and, 407–409
urine testing, 566–567
using the blood glucose data, *542,* 542–552, *543, 544, 546–547, 548, 549, 550, 552, 553, 554*
using the meter, 534–536, *536, 537*
Blood glucose targets, 542–547, *543,* 734–735, *735*
for exercise, 204–205
frequency of monitoring, 542–547, *544*
for type 1 diabetes, *404*
for type 2 diabetes, 434
Blood pressure
botanical and nonbotanical products used to lower, 654–676, *668–676*
classification of, 627, *628*
diabetic retinopathy and, 824–825
measuring, 266, *266*
reducing risks for high, 289
self-monitoring of, 298–299
standard of care for, *286*
treating cardiovascular risk factors and, *790*
Blood pressure cuff sizes, *266*
Blood pressure management
in children and adolescents, 800
for chronic kidney disease, 848–852
Blood pressure measurement technique, 796–797
Blood pressure monitoring, *266,* 266–267, *277*
Blood pressure targets, 434, 797, 798
Bloom's taxonomy
collaborative goal setting and, 51, *52*
competencies for practice and, 10–11
Blurred vision, 822
Board-Certified Advanced Diabetes Management® (BC-ADM®), 5, 9, 336
Body mass index (BMI)
physical activity and, 184
prevalence of diabetes and increased, 380
Bolus insulin, 515
adjustments for physical activity, 210, *210*
calculations for pediatric population, *603*
for chronic kidney disease, *851*
exercise-related hypoglycemia risk and, 203
Bolus ratio, fine-tuning, 597–598
Bone mineral density (BMD) test, 274–275
Bovine serum albumin (BSA), 390
Bowman's capsule, 838
BPI Interference, 878
Breastfeeding, 752, 766
Brief Pain Inventory (BPI), 878, 879
British Hypertension Society, 267
Bromocriptine (Cycloset®), 247, 435
Bromocriptine mesylate, *492, 501,* 501–502, *850*
Budget, for diabetes self-management education and support program, 333–334, *334*
Budget planning worksheet, 333, *334*
Bulimia nervosa, 136, *137,* 164
Bumetanide (Bumex®), 631
Bupropion, 794, 853
Burning foot or hand syndrome, 872
Business plan, for diabetes self-management education and support program, 331–333, *332–333*
Buy-in, for goals, 48
Buzzy® devices, 352

C

Calcium channel blockers, 629, 636, 637–638
Calcium levels, maintaining, 838
Calorie consumption, in children with type 1 diabetes, 412–413
Camps, 411, 417
Canagliflozin (Invokana®), 247, 435, *492, 502,* 502–503, 786, 847, *849*
Cancer risk, diabetes and, 396, *397*
Candesartan (Atacand®), 633
Candidiasis, 276–277
Capsulotomy, 819
Captopril (Capoten®), 632
Carbohydrate counting, 173–174, 454
children and, 413
Carbohydrate-counting skills, 591, 592
Carbohydrate guidelines, 761, 773
Carbohydrates
dietary reference intake for pregnant women, 749–750, *751*
glycemia and, 455–459
increases for aerobic activity in grams, *208*
intensified insulin therapy and budgeting, 591
sports drink with, 206
Carbohydrate snacks, 207
Cardiac autonomic neuropathy (CAN), 193, 883–886
abnormal response to exercise, 886
cardiac denervation syndrome, 885–886
clinical features, *884*
exercise modifications for, 213–214
morbidity and mortality in, 885
postural hypotension and, 886
treatment of underlying cause of, 886
Cardiac catheterization and angioplasty, preparing patients for elective, 803
Cardiac denervation syndrome, 885–886
Cardiac output (CO), hypertension and, 626
Cardiometabolic health, benefits of physical activity on, 183
Cardiometabolic risk factors, 784, *785*
Cardiovascular complications of diabetes, 783

Cardiovascular disease (CVD)
- atherosclerotic, 787, 788, *788,* 799
- diabetes relationship to, 784–787
- epidemiology in diabetes of, 784
- exercise modifications for, 212
- hyperosmolar hyperglycemic state and, 738
- kidney disease and, 215, 852
- lifestyle management for, 792–796
- manifestations of, 784
- modifiable risk factors, 789–791
- nonmodifiable risk factors, 789
- pathogenesis of in diabetes, 395–396
- reducing risks for, 288–291
- risk-reduction strategy for, 789–791, *790–791*
- type 1 diabetes and, 784, 786–787
- type 2 diabetes and risk of, 434

Cardiovascular events (CV events)
- aspirin for primary prevention of, 799
- diabetes and risk of, 784
- glycemic control and prevention of, 784–786
- type 1 diabetes and risk of, 784

Cardiovascular risk assessment, 614–615, 787–789
Caregivers, assessment and, 40
Care plan, for pregnant women with preexisting diabetes, 753
Carpal tunnel syndrome, 892
Carpentar-Coustan criteria, 767
Carvedilol (Coreg®), 636
Case studies, *61*
Catalyst to Better Diabetes Care Act of 2009, 15–16, 21
Cataracts, 817, 818–820
Catecholamine response, 205
Catecholamines, 383, 843
Celiac disease
- diabetes and, 164
- screening of children for, 264, 266
- type 1 diabetes and, 423

Center for Food Safety and Applied Nutrition Web site, 650
Centers for Disease Control and Prevention (CDC), 296
- accreditation standards from, 13
- Diabetes Prevention Program certification (DPP), 340
- Diabetes Report Card, 16, 18, 21
- DPP PreventT2 curriculum, 119
- on listeriosis during pregnancy, 751
- National Diabetes Education Program, 119
- National Diabetes Prevention Program, 17
- registry of diabetes prevention programs, 19
- on social determinants of health, 35

Centers for Medicare & Medicaid Services (CMS), 18, 55, 338–339, 344, 535, 735
Centers of Excellence for Depression, 21
Central-acting alpha-adrenergic agonists, 640–641
Cerebral edema, diabetic ketoacidosis and, 731
Cerebrovascular accident, 804
Cerebrovascular disease, 804–805
Certification
- of diabetes care and education specialists, 7, 9
- of diabetes educators, 6–7
- for staff of diabetes self-management education and support program, 336

Certification Board for Diabetes Care and Education (CBDCE), 7, 9
Certified Diabetes Care and Education Specialist® (CDCES), 9, 336
Certified Diabetes Care and Education Specialists (CDCES) credential, 120
Change talk, 114, 118–119
Charcot neuroarthropathy, 873
Chart/file audit, *89*
Checklists, *89*
- monitoring, *264, 277–278*

Checks, blood, 541
Children
- access to diabetes resources, 13
- blood pressure management in, 289–290, 800
- blood pressure targets, 289
- cardiovascular risk management issues specific to, 800–801
- coping skills for, 258
- developmental issues and effect on diabetes in, *415*
- developmental tasks, 351–354, *353*
- diabetes diagnosis in, 386
- diabetic dyslipidemia in, 616
- foot exams and, 294
- goal setting and, 49
- healthy coping and, 142, 148–149
- hypertension in, 629
- hypertension treatment for, 289–290
- insulin for normal glucose metabolism, 733
- insulin injection therapy for, 408–410
- lipid management for, 291, 801
- management of diabetes in, 301, *301*
- medication administration in, 256–258
- nutrition education for, 162–163
- nutrition therapy in, 469
- physical activity and, 220
- problem solving and, 318
- readiness to learn and, 63
- real-time continuous glucose monitoring for, 558
- rehydration in, 729
- role in diabetes management, 417–418
- self-monitoring of blood glucose and, 541
- teaching points for transitions, *357–358*
- type 2 diabetes in, 3, 5, 257–258, 432, 441–444
- use of complementary health approaches in, 706–707, 708
- use of insulin pump therapy in, 602–603, *603*

Children's Health Insurance Program (CHIP), 17–18, 20
Chiropractic medicine, 713
Chlorthalidone, 630, 642, 797
Choice of action, diabetes management and, 311
Cholesterol, 613
- dyslipidemia and, 465–466
- monitoring, 267

Cholestyramine (Questran®), *525,* 623
Choose Your Foods: Food Lists for Diabetes, 173, 174, 454, 456
Choose Your Foods: Plan Your Meals, 173
Chromium, 657–658, *670,* 688
Chromium deficiency, 657
Chromium supplementation, 460
Chronic Care Model, 5, 113
Chronic complications
- disparities in, 300–301
- reducing risks for, 288–294

Chronic disease
- Affordable Care Act and, 17, 18–19
- coping with, 131, *143,* 143–144
- normalization and, 46

Chronic hyperglycemia, 721
Chronic inflammatory demyelinating polyneuropathy, 893
Chronic kidney disease (CKD), 269, 292, 837–838, 839
- avoidance of nephrotoxic agents, 853
- cardiovascular risk reduction and, 852
- chronic kidney disease epidemiology collaboration equation, 844
- diagnosis of, 839
- dietary manipulation for, 844, 854
- hypertension medications and, 851–852
- insulin and, 848, *849–851*
- nephrology referral, 854
- oral medications, 847–848, *849–851*
- pharmacologic interventions, 847–848, *849–851*
- physical activity and, 852–853
- prevention and delay of, 846–856
- screening and detection, 845–846
- smoking cessation and, 853
- stages of, 839, *840*
- stage 1–4 treatment, *843*
- stage 5 treatment, 856–860
- weight management, 853

Chronic sensorimotor neuropathy, 874–875
Cimetidine, 255
Cinnamon *(Cinnamomum cassia),* 658–659, *670–671*
Clarification, asking for, 44
Clinical considerations for diabetes medications, 245–252
Clinical inertia, 300, 576
Clinically significant macular edema (CSME), 825
Clinical Practice Consensus Guidelines 2018: Nutritional Management in Children and Adolescents With Diabetes, 457
Clonidine patch (Catapres-TTS®), 640
Clonidine tablets (Catapres®), 640
Clopidogrel, 799
Closed-ended questions, 43
Closed loop delivery, insulin pumps and, 589
Clozapine (Clozaril®), 253
Coaching, appreciative, 39–40
Cochrane Review, 682, 689
Cockcroft-Gault formula, 844
Coenzyme Q10 (CoQ10), 679–680, *685–686*
Cognitive-affective self, 140, *141*
Cognitive assessment, 272–273
Cognitive behavioral therapy (CBT), 148, 164
Cognitive function, pattern management and, 577
Cognitive impairment, as factor influencing problem solving, 318
Cognitive overload, 71
Cognitive restructuring (CR), stress management and, 147
Cognitive science, supporting diabetes self-management education, 72–73
Colesevelam (Welchol®), 247, 435, *493, 503,* 503–504, 623
Colestipol (Colestid®), 623
Collaboration
  on educational goals, 47
  encouraging problem solving through, 312, 314
Collaboratively establishing goals, 51–53
Collecting duct, 838
College Diabetes Network, 361
Color fundus photography, 829
Combination oral medications, 244, *244*
  for type 2 diabetes, 522, *523–524*
Combination therapies for dyslipidemia, 625–626
Common senile cataracts, 819
Communication
  diabetes management and, 311
  for diabetes self-management education and support program management, 337–338
  medication-taking behavior and, 243–244
Communication principles of motivational interviewing, 115–117
Community approaches to diabetes self-management education, 76
Community health workers, 5, 323
Community living assistance services and supports, 20
Community needs, diabetes self-management education and support program and assessing, 330
Comorbid conditions, standard of care for, *286*
Competence, Transtheoretical Model and, 108
Competencies for Diabetes Care and Education Specialists, 35, 46, 54, 66–67, 91, 329
Competencies for practice, for Diabetes Care and Education Specialists, 10–11
Complementary and alternative medicine (CAM), 647, 703. *See also* Complementary health approaches
  alternative *vs.* complementary, 647
  concerns about, 652–653
  cost increases, 653
  ethnic groups and, 652
  "other ingredient" concerns, 652–653
  product variability, 652
  side effects and drug interactions, 652
  standardization lacking, 652
  supplements, 653–654
Complementary health approaches. *See also* Dietary supplements
  additional costs, 706
  alternative and integrative *vs.,* 703, 704
  aromatherapy (essential oils), 711
  art therapy, 711
  Ayurvedic medicine, 703
  bio-field therapies, 714–715
  case study, 705, 716
  for children, 706–707
  chiropractic medicine, 713
  concerns about, 704–706
  conventional medicine delays, 706
  defined, *648*
  education about, 707
  electromagnetic-based therapies, 715
  energy therapies, 714–715
  guided imagery, 711
  homeopathy, 703, 709
  hypnosis, 711
  impacts of, 705
  laughter, 712
  massage, 713
  meditation during pump therapy, 705
  mind and body–based methods, 703, 731–714
  mind-body interventions, 711–712
  mindfulness, 711–712
  modality variability, 705
  Native American medicine, 709–710
  naturopathy, 703
  patient support, 707–708
  pet therapy, 712
  prayer and meditation, 712
  Qigong, 713
  reflexology, 713
  relaxation, 712
  research on, 708, 715–716
  scientific study lacking on, 706
  Tai Chi, 713–714
  therapeutic touch/healing touch, 714–715
  Traditional Chinese medicine, 703, 711
  whole-body medical systems, 709–711
  yoga, 704, 714
Complementary *vs.* alternative *vs.* integrative medicine, 703, 704
Compliance approach to education, 67–68, *68*
Complications
  autoimmune-related, 422–423
  cardiovascular, 783
  of cataracts, 819–820
  chronic, 288–294, 300–301
  dermatological, 256
  diabetic ketoacidosis and preventing, 731
  fetal, 758–759
  of gestational diabetes mellitus, 771, *772*
  maternal, 757–758
  microvascular, 268
  monitoring, 265
  oral, 256
  pathogenesis in diabetes of, 395
  pregnancy, 757–761
  of type 2 diabetes, 434
Comprehensive Management of the Neuropathic Foot, 294
Computer-based teaching strategy, *60*
Conditioning, 189
Confidence rulers, 229
Conflict between person with diabetes and diabetes care education specialist, *315*
Congenital malformations
  fetal, 758–759
  in infants born to women with preexisting diabetes, 771, *772*
Congestive heart failure (CHF), 802, 806–807
Connected pens, 587
Consensus Statement on Glucose Monitoring, 533
Constipation, related to autonomic neuropathy, 887
Constraints, on diabetes management, 311
Consumer Lab (CL), 649
Contact heat-evoked potentials (CHEPs), 872

Contemplation stage for exercise behavior change, 226, 227
Continuous ambulatory peritoneal dialysis (CAPD), 858
Continuous glucose monitoring (CGM), 288, 298, 552–566
  A1C and, 555
  accuracy of, 554
  barriers to use, 560–561, *560–561*
  for diabetes and pregnancy, 762–763
  as gold standard, 575
  in hospitalized patients, 366
  how it works, 553–554
  insulin pump systems and integrated, 556–557
  interpretation skills for, 561–566, *563, 564*
  metrics for, *563*
  operational skills for, 558–561
  pattern management and, 576–577
  personal, 555–556, *556, 557, 558*
  positive glucose questioning, *554*
  professional, *556,* 557–558
  real-time *vs.* intermittently scanned, 556
  recommendation of, 581
  risk reduction and, 301–302
  safety and contraindications for, 559–560, *561*
  selecting device, 558, *558*
  self-monitoring of blood glucose *vs.,* 554 555
  sensor insertion and calibration, 559
  special populations and, 558–561
  type 1 diabetes and, 407, 408
  type 2 diabetes and, 434
Continuous peritoneal dialysis (CCPD), 858
Continuous quality improvement (CQI), 337, 341, 345
  case examples, *345–347*
Continuous subcutaneous insulin infusion (CSII), 411–412
  use of devices in hospital, 365–366
Control IQ, 589
Conventional medicine, complementary approaches and delays in use of, 706
Conversation maps, *61*
Cooking, 175
Cool-down, 189
Coping. *See* Healthy coping
Coping skills, 59
  for children and adolescents with diabetes, 258
Cormorbidities
  modifying exercise for, 211–221
  monitoring for, 265
Cornea, 817, *817*
Corneal confocal microscopy, 872
Coronary artery calcium scores (CACs), 795
Coronary artery disease (CAD), 801–803
  preparing patients for elective cardiac catheterization and angioplasty, 803
  presentation of, 801
  screening for, 801–802
  treatment of acute MI, 802–803
  warning signs of, *801*
Coronary heart disease (CHD), 614, 615
Coronary vascular (CV) outcomes, effects of glucose lowering drugs on, 786
Coronary vascular disease (CVD)
  nutrition therapy and, 465–466
  physical activity and, 183
Coronary vascular disease (CVD) risk, 466, 799–800
Correctional institution, transition to, 372–373
Correction boluses, 586, 592
Cortical cataract, 819
Corticosteroids, 827, 829
Cortisol, *201,* 383
Cost
  of continuous glucose monitoring, 559, *560*
  insulin omitted due to, 724
  of medications, 244–245, 441
  use of complementary health approaches and, 652, 706
Cough and cold products, 253
Council for Responsible Nutrition, 651
Counseling psychology, 110
Count Your Carbs: Getting Started, 174
Cousins, Norman, 712
COVID-19, 1–2
C-peptide levels, type 2 diabetes and, 441
Cranial neuropathies, 892
C-reactive protein, 800
Create Your Plate, 173
Critical thinking, assessment and, 41
Cultural barriers to access to diabetes self-management education and support, 13
Cultural competency, self-assessment of, 36–37, *37*
Cultural considerations in assessment, 41
Cultural identity, 140
Cultural issues
  as factor influencing problem solving, 318
  in goal setting, 49
  healthy eating and, 169
  physical activity and, 220–221
Curcumin, 667
Curriculum
  adding new content, 59, *59*
  for diabetes self-management education and support program, 335, *335*
  prioritizing and scaffolding content, 56
CYP3A4, *620*
CYP2C9, *620*
Cytochrome P-450 isoenzymes, interactions between common drugs and, *620*

D

Dabl Educational Trust Web site, 267
Daily activity, integrating before planned exercise, 221–222
Daily review, 43
Danatech, 316, 566
Dapagliflozin (Farxiga®), 247, 435, *492, 502,* 502–503, *849*
DARN (Desire, Ability, Reasons, Need), 48
DASH (Dietary Approaches to Stop Hypertension) eating pattern, 166, *167,* 454, 465, 467, 792, 852
Data
  collection tools, *89*
  making use of evaluation, 90
Data log, blood glucose, 408
Data management for continuous glucose monitoring or self-monitoring of blood glucose, 565–566
Dawn phenomenon, 596
Day care, insulin injection therapy at, 411
Decision making, empowerment approach and shared, 68
Decision tree, 317, *318, 319,* 323
Degludec, 512–513, 514, *517,* 585, 588, 764, *851*
Degludec/liraglutide (Xultophy®), 251, 252, 513
Dehydration
  diabetic ketoacidosis and, *726,* 727, 728, *728,* 729–730
  hyperosmolar hyperglycemic state and, 735
  physical activity and, 213
Delphi technique, 11
Dementia, healthy coping and, 149
Demographic barriers, to access to diabetes self-management education and support, 13
Demonstration, *60*
Denial stage, of coping with chronic disease, *143*
Dental care, 256, *287,* 297
Dependent rubor, 806
Depression, 133
  among children and adolescents, 148
  coping with chronic disease and, *143*
  monitoring, 272–273
  in school-aged children with type 1 diabetes, 417
  screening for, *135,* 273
Dermatologic products, topical, 255–256
Describing phenomena, 99
Detemir, 203, 443, 512–513, 514, *517,* 587, 588, *851*
Developmental age and stage, healthy coping and, 141–142
Developmental characteristics of adolescence, *419*

Developmental issues and effect on diabetes in children and adolescents, *415*
Deviation review, 43
Dexamethasone, 827
DEX implant (Ozurdex), 827
Diabetes. *See also* Metabolic disorder; Metabolic disorder, pathophysiology of; Type 1 diabetes (T1DM); Type 2 diabetes (T2DM)
  botanical and nonbotanical products used to treat complications, 677–688, *684–688*
  classification, 387–389
  criteria for diagnosis of, *775*
  diagnosed and uundiagnosed among U.S. adults, *380, 381*
  financial impact of, 3–4
  forms of, 2
  goals of medical nutrition therapy for, 159
  prevalence of, 2
Diabetes Advanced Network Access (DANA), 66, 408
Diabetes camps, 417
Diabetes Care and Education Specialist (DCES), 9–10
  Affordable Care Act and, 15–21
  being agile educator, 75–76, *76*
  clinical problem solving by, 313
  competencies for practice, 10–11
  continuous glucose monitoring and, 565
  defined, 9
  facilitated problem solving by, 313–314
  former and proposed domains for, *11*
  interpreting blood glucose results, 581–582
  new technologies and, 14–15
  productivity metrics for, *344*
  role in coping, 140
  role in diabetes self-management education and technology, 66
  role in promoting healthy eating, 157, 158
  role in risk reduction for diabetes-related complications, 396–397
  self-management of blood glucose and, 551–552, *553*
  standards for, 10
Diabetes Care Program of Nova Scotia, transition recommendations/guidelines, *360*
Diabetes caucus, 22
Diabetes devices, 361–362
Diabetes distress, 98, 132–133, 300
  questions to assess, 146–147
Diabetes Distress Scale, 135, 144, 146, 273
Diabetes Eating Problem Survey, 164
Diabetes education. *See* Diabetes self-management education (DSME)
Diabetes Education Accreditation Program (DEAP), 340
Diabetes education and care. *See also* Diabetes self-management education and support (DSMES)
  applying problem solving in, 313–315
  bilingual modules, 62
  diabetic neuropathy and, 868–869, 873–874
  distal symmetric diabetic polyneuropathies and, 875
  fall risk and, 881
  history of, 4–5
  neuropathic pain and, 880
  as profession, 6–7, *7*
  as specialty, 7
  strategies for older adults, 440–441
Diabetes educators, defined, 9
Diabetes Forecast magazine, 250, 257
Diabetes in Older Adults: A Consensus Report by the ADA/American Geriatric Society, 486
Diabetes Mellitus Types 1 and 2 Systematic Review and Guideline, 452, 456, 457, 458, 465
Diabetes nutrition education, outline for well-designed encounter, 169
Diabetes paraprofessional, 12
Diabetes Patient Advocacy Coalition (DPAC), 22
Diabetes Prevention Act of 2009, 22
Diabetes Prevention Program. *See* National Diabetes Prevention Program (NDPP)
Diabetes Quality Improvement Project, 344
Diabetes remission, 463
Diabetes Report Card, 16, 18, 21
Diabetes risk surveys, 381
Diabetes self-management, using problem solving in, 308–313
Diabetes self-management education (DSME), 31–91
  assessment, 32–46, *33, 34, 35, 36, 37, 42, 44*
  defined, 7
  evaluation/monitoring, 77–90, *78, 79, 81–86, 87, 89*
  5-step process of, 32
  goal-setting, 47–54, *51, 52*
  implementation, 66–77, *68, 75, 76*
  monitoring, 87–89
  objectives, 31
  planning, 54–66, *56, 57, 58, 59, 60–61, 62, 64–65*
  process, 87–89, 90–91
  providing support following, 76–77
  standards for, 32
  technology and, 66
Diabetes self-management education and support (DSMES), 6, 7–8
  acquisition of skills and knowledge and, 285
  algorithm, 32
  barriers and facilitators to access, 12–13
  curriculum, 54–55, *56*
  defined, 8, 31
  diabetic retinopathy and, 829
  goal of, 7
  inadequate reimbursement for, 13
  mission of, 98
  ongoing, 98
  others engaged in, 12
  problem solving and, 307–308
  providing at four critical times, 98
  providing on ongoing basis, 98
  standard of care for, *287*
Diabetes self-management education and support (DSMES) program management, 327–349
  adopt, adapt, or create a curriculum, 335, *335*
  areas to improve, *342*
  assess program operations and impact, 338–339
  budget, 333–334, *334*
  business plan, 331–333, *332–333*
  communication and, 337–338
  evaluation, monitoring, and documentation, 340–341
  front-end operations, 338
  goal setting, 331–333
  implementation, 336–340
  managing staff, 336–337
  marketing, 339–340
  meeting the standards, 340, *340*
  national standards for diabetes self-management education and support, 328, *329*
  ongoing quality improvement, 341, *345–347*
  organizational structure, 341–347
  planning, 333–336
  productivity metrics, *344*
  program manager, 327–328
  staff, 335–337
  starting, 328–36
Diabetes self-management education (DSME) team, implementation and, 66
Diabetes self-management education specialist (DSMES), self-assessment by, 35–39
Diabetes self-management education/training (DSME/T), role in promoting healthy eating, 168–170
Diabetes self-management support (DSMS), 330–331
  behavior change and ongoing, 344–345
  role in promoting healthy eating, 168–170

Diabetes self-management support (DSMS) programs, 98
Diabetes self-management training (DSMT), 31
Diabetes self-management training (DSMT) programs, healthy eating and, 158
Diabetes-specific problem-solving skill training, 315–316
Diabetes Technology Society, Blood Glucose Monitoring System (BGMS) Surveillance Program, 536
Diabetic autonomic neuropathy (DAN), 880, 883. *See also* Autonomic neuropathy (AN)
  clinical manifestations and symptoms of, *272*
  monitoring for, 271
Diabetic corneal neuropathy, 822
Diabetic dyslipidemia
  in children and adolescents, 616
  common patterns in, 613–615
  pharmacotherapy for, 617–626, *618, 620*
  treatment goals, 615–616, *616, 618*
Diabetic ketoacidosis (DKA), 495, 721
  adequate insulin to restore and maintain normal glucose metabolism, 733
  assessing, 725–728
  cognitive impairment and, 132
  diabulimia and, 138
  hyperglycemia and, *726*, 727
  inadequate insulin and, 723–724
  ingested glucose and, 722
  insulin pump therapy and, 598–600
  ketones and, 723
  markers, *726*, 727
  monitoring, 722–723
  pathology, 721–723
  precipitating factors, 726, 728–729
  precipitating situations, 723–724
  pregnancy and, 758
  preventing complications, 731
  prevention of, 724–725
  self-care behaviors to prevent, *732–733*
  SGLT2 inhibitors and risk of, 265
  signs, symptoms, and laboratory indicators, 725–728, *729*
  treatment, *728*, 728–734
  type 1 diabetes and, 404, 422
Diabetic kidney disease (DKD), 837–838. *See also* Chronic kidney disease (CKD)
  blood pressure management and, 848, 851
  case study, 845, 854–856
  dietary modifications for, 853–854
  exercise modifications for, 215–216
  nutrition therapy and, 468
  pathophysiology of, 840–841
  progression of, 843
  reducing risk for, 292–293
  risk factors, *841*, 841–842
  screening and detection, 843
Diabetic macular edema, 826–827
Diabetic nephropathy (DN), 268–269
  pregnancy and, 758
Diabetic neuropathy (DN), 293, 867
  ADA evidence-grading systems, *870*
  bedside sensory tests, *871*
  classification, *869*, 874–875
  conditions mimicking, 873
  definitions, 869
  diagnosis and clinical assessment tools, 870–874, *871*
  education and, 868–869, 873–874
  fall risks and, 880–881
  overview, 869
  pharmacologic therapies for pain from, 879–880
  pregnancy and, 758
  scoring systems, 870
  screening recommendations, 870
  state of disease, 868
  treatment, 893–895
  vascular risk factors, 893
Diabetic peripheral neuropathy (DPN), 269–271
Diabetic retinopathy, 817, 818, 822–827
  ancillary tests, 829–830
  blood pressure, 824–825
  care process, 828–830
  counseling and referral, 830
  glucose management, 824
  hyperlipidemia and, 825
  laser surgery for, 829
  natural history, 825
  pregnancy and, 757, 758
  preventing blindness from, 823
  proliferative, 825, 827
  reducing risk for, 292
  risk factors, 824–825
  self-management education and care and, 829
  smoking and, 825
  staging of, 823, *823*
  vitreous surgery for, 829
Diabetic truncal radiculoneuropathy, 893
Diabulimia, 138, 164
Diagnosis
  confirmation of diabetes, *386*, 387
  criteria for diabetes, 385–387
  nutrition, 169
  testing options for, *386*
  of type 1 diabetes, 404–407
  of type 2 diabetes, 433
Diarrhea, related to autonomic neuropathy, 887
Diet
  for lipid management, 795
  modification for chronic kidney disease, 853–854
  modification for renal disease, 844
  reducing coronary vascular disease in diabetes and, 792
Dietary behavior, usefulness of Transtheoretical Model for changes in, 107
Dietary Guidelines 2015–2020, 173
Dietary Guidelines for Americans (DGAC), 165, 465
Dietary reference intakes (DRIs), 455, 749, *751*
Dietary Supplement and Non-Prescription Drug Consumer Protection Act, 649
Dietary Supplement Health and Education Act (DHSEA) of 1994, 648–649
Dietary supplements, 255
  case study, 648, 688
  claims of manufacturers evaluated, 649–651
  complementary health approaches, 647–648, *648*
  concerns about use, 652–653
  defined, *648*
  to lower blood glucose, 654–676, *668–676*
  review of, 653–654
  safety categories, *654*
  self-care implications, 689–690
  special populations, 689–690
  testing of, 649
  to treat diabetes complications, 677–688, *684–688*
  users, 651–652
Dietary Supplement Verification Program (DSVP), 649
Diethylpropion (Tenuate®), *480*, 482–483, *483*
Diffuse edema, 826
Digital support for physical activity, 225
Digoxin, 636
Diltiazem (Cardizem®, Tiazac®), *620*, 636, 637, 638
Dipeptidyl peptidase (DPP), 100
Dipeptidyl peptidase-4 (DPP-4), 384, 393
Dipeptidyl peptidase (DPP) PreventT2 curriculum, 119
Dipeptidyl peptidase-4 inhibitors (DPP-4i), 5, 247
  antihyperglycemic management and, 486
  for chronic kidney disease, 848, *849–850*
  effect on cardiovascular outcomes, 786
  for glucose management, 507–509, *508*
  for type 2 diabetes, 435, *492–493*
  use in hospital, 365
  weight management and, 464

Diphenhydramine, 636
Direct instruction, 308–309
Direct knowledge, problem solving *vs.*, 308–309
Direct questions, 43
Direct renin inhibitors (DRIs), *630,* 634–635
Disabilities, diabetes self-management education for, 73–74
Discharge counseling, 368–370
Discharge planning, *367–368,* 367–371, *369, 370*
Discrepancy, motivational interviewing and developing, 116–117
Discussion, *60*
Disordered eating behavior, healthy eating and, 163–164. *See also* Eating disorders
Distal convoluted tubule, 838
Distal symmetric diabetic polyneuropathies (DSPN), 874–875
  subtypes, 875–877
  Toronto classification of, 875
Diuretics
  adverse effects, 631
  for congestive heart failure, 806
  dosing, 631
  drug interactions, 631
  for hypertension, *630,* 630–632
  instructions, 632
  loop, 630, 631
  mechanisms of action, 631
  monitoring, 632
  potassium-sparing, 630–631
  pregnancy, precautions, and contraindications, 631
  thiazide-like, 630, 631
DMEPOS (Durable Medical Equipment, Prosthetics, Orthotics, and Supplies) Competitive Bidding Program, 535
Docosahexaenoic acid (DHA), 680, 681
Documentation
  of diabetes self-management education and support program, 340–341
  of the diabetes self-management education process, 77, *78,* 91
Document literacy, 61
Docusate, 254
Domperidone, 887
Donut hole, 245
Dopamine agonists, 435, 848, *850*
Dopamine receptor agonists, 247
  for type 2 diabetes, *492, 501,* 501–502
Doxazosin (Cardura®), 639, 797, 889
Dreyfus Model, competencies for practice and, 10–11
Driver safety, 421, *421*
Drug-disease interactions, 522, *524–527,* 527
Drug-drug interactions, 522, *524–527,* 527
Drug-food interactions, 522
Drug interactions, 242, 252–253, 522, *524–527,* 527
Drug use, diabetes and, 136
"D5" terminology and CV risk reduction, 791, *792*
Dual-energy X-ray absorptiometry (DEXA or DXA) test, 275
Duetact® (pioglitazone/glimepiride), *523*
Dulaglutide (Trulicity®), 247, 435, *493, 506,* 507, *849*
Duloxetine, 879
Dyslipidemia
  alcohol and, 466
  nutrition therapy and, 465–466
  physical activity and, 466
  treatment goals, 615–616, *616, 618*

E

Early starvation state, 382
Eating. *See* Healthy eating
Eating Disordered Inventory 3, 164
Eating disorders, 136–138, *137*
  among children and adolescents, 148
  gender and incidence of, 149
  healthy eating and, 163–164
  ketoacidosis and, 723
  Screen for Early Eating Disorder Signs, 138, *139–140*
  screening questions, *138*
Eating Healthy With Diabetes: Easy Reading Guide, 173
Eating out, 175
Eating patterns, 165–167, *166–167*
Eating plans for people with diabetes, 452
Edarbyclor®, 630
Education
  about hyperosmolar hyperglycemic state, 738–739
  on complementary health approaches, 707
  as factor influencing problem solving, 318
  for people newly diagnosed with type 1 diabetes, 406–407
  to prevent diabetic ketoacidosis, 731, 734
  to prevent hyperglycemia, 740–741
Education for All Handicapped Act of 1975, 418
Education needs, assessment and prioritizing, 41–42, *42*
Education plan
  components, 57–63
  sample, *58*
  template, *57*
Education Recognition Program (ERP), 340
Educator accountability, 77, 79
e-educator, 66
Effectiveness categories, *653*
eHealth, 14, 104
Eicosapentaenoic acid (EPA), 680, 681
Elderly adults
  access to diabetes resources in long-term care settings, 13
  healthy coping and, 149
  real-time continuous glucose monitoring for, 558
  rehydration in, 737
  self-monitoring of blood glucose and, 541
Electrocardiogram (ECG) stress testing, 186
Electrolyte deficits, hyperosmolar hyperglycemic state and correction of, 738
Electrolyte imbalances
  correction of, 730–731
  diabetic ketoacidosis and, *726,* 727
Electrolytes, physical activity and, 209
Electromagnetic-based therapies, 715
Electronic health record (EHR), 13, 302, 370
Emotional symptoms of stress, 146
Emotion-focused coping, 145
Empagliflozin (Jardiance®), 247, 435, *492, 502,* 502–503, 786, *849*
Empathic responding, 114
Empathy, expressing, 115
Empowerment
  defined, 110
  of person with diabetes as problem solver, 315–316
  transition from adolescence to young adulthood and, 356
Empowerment approach to education, 67–68, *68*
Empowerment-based behavior-change protocol example, 109, 110–114
  applying, 111–113
  evidence base, 111–112
  steps and example questions, *113*
Enalapril (Vasotec®), 632
Endocannabinoid system, 385
Endocrine-disrupting chemicals (EDCs), type 2 diabetes and, 392
Endocrine Society, 301, 357
End-stage renal disease (ESRD), 269, 292–293, 842, 856–860
  hemodialysis, 856, 857
  kidney transplantation, 856, 859–860
  peritoneal dialysis, 856, 857–859
Energy expenditure, aerobic activity and, 192–193
Energy requirements during pregnancy, 749, *750,* 761
Energy restriction, 463
Energy systems during physical activity, 198–200, *199*
Entacapone (Comtan®), 641
Entrapment syndrome, *892,* 894
Environment, 311–313, 356

Environmental barriers, 310
ePARmed-X+ (Physical Activity Readiness Medical Examination), 186
Epidemic, defined, 1
Epidemiology of diabetes, 380
Epinephrine, metabolic effects of physical activity and, 200, *201*
Eplerenone (Inspra®), 630, 631
Eprosartan (Teveten®), 633
Erectile dysfunction (ED), related to autonomic neuropathy, 888–889
Ertugliflozin (Steglatro®), 247, *492, 502,* 502–503, *849*
Erythromycin, 887
Erythropoietin, 839, 886
Esomeprazole (Nexium®), 254
Essential oils, 711
Estimated energy requirements (EERs), 749, 752
Etanercept, 892
Ethnicity
  complementary health approaches and, 651
  health disparities linked to, 37
  healthy coping and, 150
  healthy eating and, 169
  lack of specific risk algorithms and, 787
  prevalence of diabetes and, 380–383
  rate of diabetic kidney disease and, 842
  recurrence of gestational diabetes mellitus, 776
  risk of cardiovascular disease, 789
Etzwiler, Donnell, 4
Euglycemia, as goal of pregnancy complicated by diabetes, 763
Euglycemic ketoacidosis, 721
European Association of the Study of Diabetes (EASD), guidelines to improve quality of care, 576
Evaluation and monitoring, 77–79
  AADE7 Self-Care Behaviors and, 80, *81–86*
  of diabetes self-management education and support program, 340–341
  of documentation, 77, *78,* 91
  DSME/S step, *35*
  of educator accountability, 77, 79
  of formative evaluation, 79, *79*
  of individual evaluation, 79–80
  of outcomes to evaluate, *78,* 80–89, *81–86, 87*
  of summative evaluation, 79, *79*
  tools for, 89, *89*
  using data from, 90
Evolocumab (Repatha®), 621, 625
Exchange Lists for Meal Planning, 454, 456
Exenatide (Byetta®, Bydureon®, Amylin®), 203, 247, 435, *493, 505,* 505–507, *849*
Exenatide LAR, *493, 505*
Exercise. *See also* Aerobic exercise; Physical activity; Resistance exercise
  with autonomic neuropathy, 885–886
  balance, 198
  defined, 185
  flexibility, 197–198
  general prescription for, 189–198
  modifying for comorbid health issues, 211–221
Exercise and Diabetes, 190
Exercise EKG, 802
Exercise physiologist (EP), 190
Exercise stress test, 802
Exercise training session format, 188–189
Exertion, rating of perceived, 193–194, *194*
Exogenous cannabinoids, 385
Expanded Health Belief Model (EHBM), 101
Expanding Access to DSMT Act, 22
Expectations
  for diabetes self-management education and support program, 328–329
  regarding transitional care, 356
Expert Committee on the Diagnosis and Classification of Diabetes Mellitus, 386
Explaining the phenomena, 99
Exubera®, 517
Eye, normal, *817*
Eye disease related to diabetes. *See also* Diabetic retinopathy
  blurred vision, 822
  cataracts, 817, 818–820
  central retinal vein occlusion, 821–822
  diabetic macular edema, *826,* 826–827
  glaucoma, 817, 820–821
  neuropathies, 822
  proliferative diabetic retinopathy, 827
Eye examination, *287,* 827–828
Ezetimibe/simvastatin (Vytorin®), 621
Ezetimibe (Zetia®), 615, 616, 621, 625, 626, 796

F

Facilitators, of physical activity, 224
Fall risk, 204, 258, 271, *275,* 470, 880–881
Family
  assessment and, 40
  goal setting and, 49
  healthy coping and, 142–143, 414
  support and education for children with type 1 diabetes, 406–407
Family history, risk of cardiovascular disease and, 789
FAST (face drooping, arm weakness, speech difficulty, time to call 9-1-1), 804
Fasting glucose test, type 2 diabetes and, *433*
Fasting plasma glucose (FPG), 386
Fasting postabsorptive state, 381–382
Fat
  dyslipidemia and dietary, 465–466
  glycemia and, 459
Fear of change, as factor influencing problem solving, 319
Fed state, 381
Feedback, closing assessment and, 44
Felodipine (Plendil®), *620,* 638
Female sexual dysfunction, related to autonomic neuropathy, 889
Fenofibrate (Tricor®, Antara®, Fenoglide®, Lipofen®, Lofibra®, Triglide®), 622, 623, 796
Fenugreek, 659–660, *671*
Fetal complications, 758–759
Fetal demise, women with preexisting diabetes and, 759
Fetal testing, *765*
Fiber, 458, 466
Fibric acid derivatives (fibrates), 622–623, 626
Financial barriers, to manage diabetes, 310–311
Financial impact of diabetes, 3–4
Financial resources, coping and, 143
Fingerstick blood glucose monitoring, 407
Fish oil (omega-3 fatty acids), 680–681, *686*
Fitness, defined, 185
FITT-VP, prescriptive exercise and, 190
5As (Assess, Advise, Agree, Assist, Arrange) in nutrition education, 171
Fixed combination insulin, *512,* 513, *517*
Flaxseed, 660–661, *671–672*
Flexibility, defined, 197
Flexibility exercise, 197–198
  effect on diabetes management, 202
  for older adults, 219
Flexner, Abraham, 6
Fluid replacement, 729–730
Fluids, physical activity and, 209
Fluocinolone acetonide intravitreal implant (Iluvien®), 827
Fluorescein angiography, 829
Fluoxetine, 690
Flu vaccination, 424
Fluvastatin (Lescol®), 618, *620*
Focal edema, 826
Focal limb neuropathies, 892–893
Focal photocoagulation, 826, 827, 829
Follow-up
  diabetes self-management education, 65
  for type 1 diabetes, 423–424
Food and Drug Administration (FDA), 14, 443
  approval of nonnutritive sweeteners, 458
  Center for Device and Radiological Health (CDRH), 14
  on dietary supplements, 689, 690
  dietary supplements and, 649–650

food labeling rule, 175
on glucose meter accuracy, 536
gluten-free labeling rule, 164
homeopathy and, 709
Medical Device Safety Communication email alerts, 15
Safety Information and Adverse Event Reporting Program, 14
warning about rosiglitazone, 786
Food labeling rule, 175
Food label reading, 174–175
Food plan for gestational diabetes mellitus, 769–770
Foot care, 294
standards of care for, 294–295
Foot exam, 270, 294
self-examination, 299
standard of care for, *287*
vibratory sensation exam, 270–271
visual foot inspection, *270*
Foot ulcers, 293, 868, 871
Formative evaluation, 79, *79*
Formulary, 373
Fosinopril (Monopril®), 632
Foster care, transition to, 363
Fostering Medical Innovation: Software Precertification Pilot Program, 14
Framework Analysis (FA) method, 14
Framingham Risk Score (FRS), 615
Free fatty acids (FFAs), 383, 391, 393
Frequency
of aerobic activity, 192–193, 195
of physical activity sessions, 190
of resistance exercise, 196
Frequency-modulated electromagnetic neural stimulation (FREMS), 894
Fructosamine measurement, 566
Fuel homeostasis, 381–383, *382*
Fuel metabolism, normal, 383–385
Furosemide (Lasix®), 631

G

Gabapentin, 879
Games, *60*
Gangrene, small-fiber neuropathy and risk of, 877
Garlic, 681–682, *686–687*
Gastric motility, insulin pump therapy and, 601
Gastrointestinal disorders
nonprescription medications for, 254–255
related to autonomic neuropathy, 886–888
Gastrointestinal tract, diabetes and, 164–165
Gastroparesis, 165
exercise modifications for, 214, *214*
insulin pump therapy and, 601
peritoneal dialysis and, 858
Gemfibrozil (Lopid®), 622, 623, 796
Gender, diabetes and, 2
Gender identity, healthy coping and, 149–150
Generalized symmetrical polyneuropathy, *869*
Generational differences in learning, 64–65, *64–65*
Generic medications, 245
Genetics
of cardiovascular disease, 789
diabetic kidney disease and, 842
of MODY, 395
of type 1 diabetes, 389–390
of type 2 diabetes, 392–393
Genitourinary conditions, nonprescription medications for, 255
Geographic barriers, to access to diabetes self-management education and support, 12
Geographic location, type 1 diabetes and, 403
Gestational diabetes mellitus (GDM), 2, 149–150, 389, 747, 766–777
AADE7 Self-Care Behaviors for, *760,* 771–775
case study, 768–771
complications of, 771, *772*
defined, 747
diabetes prevention for women with and their offspring, 775–777, *776*
exercise modifications for, 217–218
general exercise prescription for, 191
healthy coping for, 775
healthy eating for, 162, 773, *774*
incidence of, 747
insulin therapy for, 515–516, 773–774
monitoring for, 773, *774*
noninsulin therapies for, 774–775
physical activity and, 773
postpartum follow-up after, 775, *775*
recurrence of, 776
screening and diagnosis of, *767,* 767–771
taking medications for, 773–775
Gestational hypertension, *758*
Ghrelin, role in fuel metabolism, 385
Ginger, 661, *672,* 688
Gingivitis, 256
Ginseng, 661–662, *673,* 688
Glargine, 443, 512–513, 514, *517,* 585, 587, 588, 600, 764, *851*
Glargine/lixisenatide (Soliqua®), 251, 513
Glaucoma, 213, 817, 820–821
Gliflozin, 721
Glimepiride (Amaryl®), 248, 259, *490, 494,* 848, *850*
Glipizide (Glucotrol®), 248, 259, 435, *490, 494,* 848, *850*
Glomerular filtration rate, estimating, 844
Glomerulus, 838
Glooko, 565
Glucagon, 383, 384, 723
administration in school, 418
recommended doses, 422, *422,* 522, *522*
Glucagon-like peptide-1 (GLP-1), 384, *384,* 393, 504
Glucagon-like peptide-1 receptor agonists (GLP-1 RA), 247, 365
antihyperglycemic management and, 486
for chronic kidney disease, 847, *849*
effect on cardiovascular outcomes, 786
fixed ratio combination of basal insulin and, 251–252, 513
for glucose management, *505–506,* 505–507
for obesity management, *482,* 485, *485*
for post-transplantation diabetes mellitus, 860
for type 2 diabetes, 435, *493,* 579
use in older adults, 259
weight management and, 464
Glucometers, 373
Gluconeogenesis, 383
Glucophage® XR, 246
Glucose, as fuel source, 383
Glucose dehydrogenase pyrroloquinolinequinone (GDH-PQQ) test strips, 859, *859*
Glucose-dependent insulinotropic peptide (GIP), 384, 504
Glucose-dependent insulin-releasing polypeptide's role in fuel metabolism, 384
Glucose homeostasis, 383
Glucose level targets
above, 420
in gestational diabetes mellitus, *774*
type 1 diabetes and, 411
Glucose management, diabetic retinopathy and, 824
Glucose management indicator (GMI), 563–564
Glucose meters
adequate blood sample for, 539–540
care of, 539
coding, 539
control solution, 539
documenting results, 540–541
ensuring accuracy, 536, *536, 537*
guidelines for teaching individuals to operate, *537*
insurance coverage, 535–536
meeting individual needs for skills, 541–542
operational skills, 534–536
selecting, 534–535
use of strips, 536–539
using alternative sites appropriately, 540

Glucose monitoring, 207
for gestational diabetes mellitus, 773
pattern management and, 576–577
Glucose pattern management (GPM), 547–551
framework for, *549*
interpreting retrospective continuous glucose- monitoring results using, 562–564
postprandial glucose, 548–551
steps in, 547–548
timing of blood glucose checks, *550*
Glucose tolerance test, 405, *405*
Glucosidase inhibitors, use in children and adolescents, 444
Glucovance® (glyburide/metformin), *523*
Glulisine, *517, 851*
Glumetza®, 246
Glutamic acid decarboxylase (GAD), 391
Gluten-free labeling rule, 164
Glyburide (Diabeta®), 248, 435, *490, 494, 526,* 580, 764, 774–775, 848, *850*
Glycemia
alcohol and, 460–461
carbohydrates and, 455–459
personalized nutrition and, 461
physical activity and, 460
protein and fat and, 459
vitamin and mineral supplementation and, 459–460
Glycemic algorithm, 578, *580*
Glycemic control
algorithms for, *487, 488*
recommendations for, *578*
Glycemic criteria, for diabetes diagnosis, 379
Glycemic index (GI), 167–168, 457–458
Glycemic load (GL), 167–168, 457
Glycemic management
case study, 855–856
chronic kidney disease and, 846–848, *847*
diabetic neuropathy and, 893
hemodialysis and, 857
kidney transplantation and, 859
peritoneal dialysis and, 858–859
preventing CV events in people with type 2 diabetes, 784–786
stress and, 146
Glycemic stability, pregnancy and, 747–748
Glycemic targets, 287–288, 371
for children under 5 years of age, 421
individualization of, *579*
for type 1 diabetes, 404, *404*
Glycemic thresholds, 385–386, *386*
Glycogen, 723
metabolic effects of physical activity and, 200, *201*
Glycogenolysis, 383
Glycogen synthase deficiency, 388
Glynase®, 248
Glyxambi (empagliflozin/linagliptin), *524*
Goal setting
AADE7 Self-Care Behaviors™ for guiding, 47–49
collaborating on education, 47
collaborative, *51,* 51–53
considerations in, 47
criteria for, 46
for diabetes self-management education and support program, 331–333
directions for, 46–47
DSME/S step, *35,* 46–54
healthy living and, 133–134
outcome evaluation and, 80
patient skill assessment for, 49–50
for physical activity, 224
self-monitoring and, 50
SMART for, 51–53
strategies for, 49
theory for, 47
tools for, 53
Good manufacturing practices (GMPs), 649, 650
Got Transition web site, 357
Graded exercise stress test, *186,* 187, 212
"Graduate School," diabetes self-management education, 76
Group education, 69–71
Group settings for problem solving, 316–317, 323
Growth hormone, *201,* 383
Growth in children with type 1 diabetes, 412–413
Guided imagery, 711
Gut microbiome, role in fuel metabolism, 385
Gymnema, 662–663, *673*

H

Habit formation, for exercise, 192
Hahnemann, Samuel, 709
Handbook of Nonprescription Drugs, 650
Handouts
checklist for evaluating, *62*
interactive, 72
Harris Benedict equation, 582
Harvard School of Public Health, 381
Hawthorne effect, 709, 712
Healing Beyond Borders, 707
Health, 35
Health Belief Model (HBM), 101–102, 109, 120
constructs and applications, *101*
evidence base for, 102
Health beliefs, healthy eating and, 169
Healthcare Effectiveness Data and Information Set, 344
Healthcare inequities, barriers to diabetes self-management education and support and, 12
Health care policy, 21–23
Healthcare professionals, monitoring checklist for, *264*
Healthcare providers, 423–424
Healthcare systems in the United States, 13
Healthcare team, members of, *310*
Health claims, dietary supplements and, 649
Health disparities, linked to ethnicity and socioeconomic factors, 37
Health fairs, 76
Health home, 17
Health Information National Trends Survey (HINTS), 8
Health insurance exchanges, 17
Health-IT Usability Evaluation Model (Health-ITUEM), 14
Health literacy, 61–62, 438
assessing, *42*
defined, 344
pattern management and, 577
poor medication-taking behavior and, 243
Healthy coping, 138–146
adaptation to chronic disorder and, *143,* 143–144
assessment of, 140–141
avoidance coping, 145–146
defined, 131
developmental age and stage and, 141–142
for diabetes and pregnancy, *760,* 765
diabetes care and education specialist's role in, 140
dietary supplements and, 689
emotion-focused coping, 145
evaluating, *81*
family system and related roles and responsibilities, 142–143
financial resources and insurance coverage, 143
for gestational diabetes mellitus, 775
illness adjustment, 138–140, *141*
information-seeking coping, 145
maladaptive, 150–151
measuring, 144
mental health concerns, 131–138, *134, 135, 137, 138, 139–140*
outcomes, 151
preventing diabetic ketoacidosis and, *732*
preventing hyperosmolar hyperglycemic state and, *739*
problem-focused coping, 144–145
psychosocial factors of social support, 142
relapse prevention strategies, 148
special populations, 148–150
stress management, 146–148

styles of, 144–146
type 1 diabetes and, 414–421
type 2 diabetes and, 445
Healthy eating, 157–181, *312*
adolescents and, 419
behavior change role in, 170–172, *172*
case study, 160, 176
cross-cultural counseling, 169
for diabetes and pregnancy, *760,* 761
diabetes care and education specialist's role, 157
diabetes educators' core competencies, 158, 159
diabetes self-management education and DSMS, 168–170
dietary supplements and, 689
for eating disorders, 163–164
education, 172
effective approaches, 165–167, *166–167*
evaluating, *81*
for gestational diabetes mellitus, 162, 773
glycemic index and glycemic load, 167–168
intensified insulin therapy and, 591
key concepts, 157
meal-planning resources, *173,* 173–174
meal-planning skills, 175–176
medical nutrition therapy and, 158–168
Nutrition Care Process and Model and, 168–170
nutrition diagnosis, 169
nutrition intervention, 169–170
Nutrition Practice Guidelines, 170
outcomes, 161
patterns of, 165–167, *166–167*
in pregnancy, 161–162
preventing diabetic ketoacidosis and, *732*
prevention of hyperosmolar hyperglycemic state and, *739*
promoting, 158–168
self-management of, 172–173
social cognitive theory and, 103–104
theory into practice, 172–176
type 1 diabetes and, 161, 162–163, 412
type 2 diabetes and, 161, 163, 444
Healthy eating pattern, 453–454
Healthy Food Choices, 173
Healthy People 2020, 8, 37, 297, 327
Hearing Handicap Inventory for the Elderly Screening (HHIE-S), *295,* 295–296
Hearing impaired, working with, 74
Hearing impairment, 295–296
Heart rate reserve (HRR), 193
Helping the Student with Diabetes Succeed: A Guide for School Personnel, 418
Hemodialysis (HD), 856, 857
Hemorrhagic stroke, 804
Hepatic glucose, excess, 724
Hepatitis B vaccinations, 276, 296
High-density lipoproteins (HDL-C), 613
elevated TGs and, 614
monitoring, 267
reverse cholesterol transport, 614
targets, 290
Hispanics
complementary health approaches and, 651
diabetic kidney disease and, 842
health risks of, 37
healthy coping and, 150
prevalence of diabetes and, 380, 381
HMG-CoA reductase inhibitors (statins), 618–620
adverse effects, 619
dosing, 618–619
drug interactions, 619, *620*
instructions, 620
mechanism of action, 618
monitoring, 619
pregnancy, precautions, and contraindications, 619
Home, transition from rehabilitation facility to, 374
Home blood pressure monitoring, 266–267
Homeopathy, 709
Honey, 663–664, *673–674*
Honeymoon period, decreased insulin needs during, 409–410
Hormonal disorders, 388
Hormonal effects of physical activity, 198–200, *201*
Hormone Health Network, 357
Hormones, role in fuel metabolism, 383–385
Hospital, transition into, 363–367
A1C assessment on admission, 363, *363*
medication use in, 364–367
Hospitalization, use of insulin pumps during a, 599–600
Humulin®, *517*
Hydration
encouraging, 739–740
during physical activity, 209
Hydrochloroquine, 636
Hydrochlorothiazide (HCTZ), 630, 631, 633, 642, 852
Hyperbilirubinemia, 759, 761
Hyperchloremic acidosis, correcting, 730
Hyperemesis gravidarum, 765
Hyperglycemia. *See also* Acute hyperglycemia
age and management of, *353*
case study, 845
chronic, 721
cognitive impairment and, 132
defined, 721
detecting, 309
diabetic kidney disease and, 840
education to prevent, 740–741
in gestational diabetes mellitus, 771
hyperosmolar hyperglycemic state and severe, 736
insulin pump therapy and, *598,* 598–600
interpretation and management of, 205–206
in person with myocardial infarction, 802
preventing, 309, 741
preventing in an institutional care setting, 741
treatment of, 741–742
type 2 diabetes and, 431
Hyperlipidemia
diabetic retinopathy and, 825
red yeast rice for, 682, 683
Hyperosmolar hyperglycemic nonketotic syndrome, 735–736
Hyperosmolar hyperglycemic state (HHS), 721, 735–736
assessing, 736–737
dehydration and, 735, 736
high-risk individuals, 740
pathophysiology of, 735–736
precipitating situations, 736
self-care behaviors to prevent, *739,* 739–740
treatment of, *737,* 737–739
Hypertension, 620–621, 626–627
AHA/ACC Multi-Society High Blood Pressure Guidelines, 628–629
alcohol and, 467–468
blood pressure goals, 797
blood pressure measurement technique, 796–797
case study, 617, 638–639, 639
in children and adolescents, 629
classification of, *289,* 627, *628*
DASH eating plan and, 467
defined, 289
diabetic retinopathy and, 824–825
diagnosis of, 627–629
exercise modifications for, 212
goals for, 628–629
management of, 796–798
monitoring, *266,* 266–267
nutrition therapy and, 467–468
orthostatic, 267, 641
pharmacotherapy for, 629–642, *630*
physical activity and, 467
pregnancy and, 758, *758*
reducing risks for, 289
as risk factor for diabetic kidney disease, 842
sodium and, 467
treatment of, 289–290, *628,* 629, 630, 797–798
treatment-resistant, 641–642
weight loss and, 467

Hyperthyroidism, 273–274, 422
Hypertriglyceridemia, 796
Hypnosis, 711, 716
Hypoglycemia, 520–522
  age and management of, *353*
  assessment of risk, 202
  causes of, 520–521
  cognitive impairment and, 132
  defined, 421, 520
  detecting, 309
  exercise hypoglycemia management, 202–205
  as fear for parents of infants and toddlers with diabetes, 416
  fear of, 249, 251, 416
  insulin omitted to avoid, 723–724
  insulin pump therapy and, 593–594
  medication impact on, 202–204, *203*
  mild, 421
  moderate, 421
  older adults with type 2 diabetes and risk of, 440
  during pregnancy, 764–765
  pregnancy and type 1 diabetes and, 162
  preventing, 309, 413–414, 521
  pump therapy and, 588
  risk of in children with type 1 diabetes, 301
  severe, 421–422
  snacks and prevention of, 207–208
  strategies to prevent exercise-related, 203
  therapy adjustments to prevent hypoglycemia associated with physical activity, *211*
  treatment of, 521–522
  type 1 diabetes and, 421–422
  type 2 diabetes and, 522
Hypoglycemia suspend, sensor augmented pump therapy and, 589
Hypoglycemia unawareness, 271, 890
Hypokalemia, 731
Hypothermia, diabetic ketoacidosis and, 728
Hypothesis testing, 43, 50
Hypothetical situations, 43
Hypothyroidism, 274, 422
Hypotonia, diabetic ketoacidosis and, 728
Hyzaar®, 630

I

Ibuprofen, 253
Icodextrin, 858
Icosapent ethyl (Vascepa®), 623, 626
Ideal self, 140, *141*
IDF Road Map Programme, 22
Illness adjustment, 138, 140
Imipramine (Janimime®, Tofranil®), 641
Immediate outcomes, 80, *81–82,* 171
Immunizations, 296–297
  monitoring, 275–276
  recommended, 296–297
  standard of care for, *287*
Impaired fasting glucose (IFG), 383
Implanted spinal cord stimulation, 894
Implementation, 66–77
  being an agile educator, 75–76, *76*
  cognitive science and, 72–73
  diabetes self-management education team, 66
  disabilities and, 73–74
  DSME/S step, *35*
  identifying and addressing barriers, 74–75, *75*
  individual *vs.* group, 69–70
  learning theory and, 72
  managing education session challenges, 70
  outpatient education, 70–71
  problem-based learning, 68–69
  providing support following diabetes self-management education, 76–77
  standards of practice, 66–67
  strategies for, 67–68, *68*
  teaching environment, 73
  teaching materials and audiovisual materials, 71–72
  thoughtful use of technology and, 73
Implementation, of diabetes self-management education and support program, 336–340
Importance rulers, 229
Improvement stage, of exercise progression, *191,* 192
Incidence, defined, 3
Incretin-based therapies, 504–509, *505–506, 508, 510*
Incretin effect, 384, 887
Incretin (intestinal) hormones, 384, 393
Incretin mimetics, 5
Indapamide, 631
Independence at Home Medical Practice Demonstration Program, 18
Individual education, 69–70
Individual evaluation, 79–80
Individualized menus, 173
Individual options in problem solving, 316
Infants with type 1 diabetes
  coping and, 142
  education about, 406
  insulin injection therapy for, 409
  psychosocial issues, 416
Influencing, 99
Influenza, protecting pregnancy women from, 759
Influenza vaccine, 296
Information gathering skills, *45*
Information-seeking, healthy coping and, 144
Information-seeking coping, 145
Information technology needs, of diabetes self-management education and support program, 336
Infrared light, 894
Infusion set, 588–589
Inhalation devices, for insulin, 516–518
Initial stage, of exercise progression, *191,* 191–192
Injection aids, 250
Innovative medical therapies, access to, 20
Inpatient assessments, 40
Inpatient education, 70
Inpatient hyperglycemia concerns, 734–735, *735*
Inpatient use of continuous glucose monitoring, 559
In-person counseling, support for physical activity and, 225
Institute of Medicine (IOM), 452, 748
Institutional settings, older adults with type 2 diabetes in, 441
Instructional strategies, 59–61, *60–61*
Insulin, 248–251, 510–520. *See also* Multiple daily injections (MDI)
  action mechanism, 511
  appropriate type for children and adolescents, 256–257
  basal-bolus regimen, 248
  breastfeeding and, 766
  for chronic kidney disease, 848, *851*
  determining hospital patient's total daily dose, 365, *366*
  for diabetes during pregnancy, 763–764
  dosing, 513
  dosing based on carbohydrate servings or total calories, 591–592
  education topics for persons taking, 249–250
  exercise-related hypoglycemia risk and, 203, 205
  fears of, 248–249
  fixed ratio combination of GLP-1 receptor agonists and basal, 251–252
  for gestational diabetes mellitus, 773–774
  hyperosmolar hyperglycemic state and restoration of normal glucose metabolism, 738
  inadequate, 723–724
  indications for use, 511
  instructions for persons with diabetes, 518–520
  key points on use of, 251
  metabolic effects of physical activity and, *201*
  monitoring use, 518
  normal production during pregnancy, 748, *748*
  overcoming administration problems, 250

physical activity and adjusting, 209, 210, *210*
physiology of insulin in diabetes, 510–511
precautions, 518
in pregnancy, 515–516
premixed, 411
regimens, 513–514, *514*
role in fuel metabolism, 383
side effects, 518
storage guidelines, 519
supplementation in diabetic ketoacidosis treatment, 730
tips for injections, *250*
transitioning from IV insulin to subcutaneous insulin injections, 366–367
for type 1 diabetes, 515
for type 2 diabetes, 514–515
types of, 511–513, *512, 517*
use in hospital, 364–365
use in older adults, 440
weight management and, 464

Insulin administration, 257
Insulin analogs, 512
for diabetes during pregnancy, 763–764
exercise-related hypoglycemia risk and, 203
introduction of, 4
Insulin aspart, 511
Insulin autoantibodies (IAAs), 391
Insulin delivery devices, 516–518. *See also* Insulin pumps
inhalation device, 516–518
jet injector, 516
pen device, 257, 440–441, 516
syringe, 516
Insulin glulisine, 511
Insulin injections, age able to give self, *353*
Insulin injection therapy
for adults, 409
for children and adolescents, 408–409, 409, 443–444
continuous subcutaneous insulin infusion, 411–412
during honeymoon period, 409–410
increased insulin needs with growth and puberty, 410
for infants and toddlers, 409
metabolic management, 410
premixed insulin, 410
regimen and dose determinations, 409–411
regimen flexibility, 410–411
for type 1 diabetes, 409–411
for type 2 diabetes, 436
Insulin lispro, 511–512, 764
Insulin mixing standards, 518
Insulin pens, 440–441, 516
needles, 257

Insulin pump initiation, 594–598
alcohol and, 596
dawn and Somogyi phenomenon, 596
fine-tuning basal and bolus ratios, 597–598
follow-up visits, 594, 596–597
during hospitalization, 595
initial outpatient visit, 595–596
Insulin pumps, 516, 586–587
children using, 257
correctional institutions and use of, 373
integrated with continuous glucose monitoring, 556–557
pediatric dosing calculations, *603*
pump insulin delivery, *587*
Insulin pump therapy, 4, 5
adjustments for physical activity, 210
benefits of, 587–588
candidate attributes for success with, 589–590
clinical indications for, *590,* 590–591
comprehensive education before pump initiation, 591–594
contraindications to, 588
for diabetes during pregnancy, 764
diabetic ketoacidosis and, 598–600
emergency pump supplies, *602*
gastric motility (gastroparesis) and, 601
how pumps work, 588–590
hyperglycemia and, 205, 598–600
hypoglycemia and, 593–594
insulins used in, 588
limitations of, 588
in older adults, 602
in pediatric population, 602–603, *603*
during pregnancy, 601
quality of life and, 600–602
sensor augmented, 589
sick days and, 733–734
starting basal, bolus, and correction bolus calculations, *593*
travel and, 601–602
type 2 diabetes and, 602
use of meditation while on, 705
Insulin requirements during pregnancy, 764, *764*
Insulin resistance, 489
in children and adolescents, 442
physical activity and, 183
psychological, 248–249
type 2 diabetes and, 391
Insulin secretion in persons without diabetes, *587*
Insulin sensitivity, physical activity and, 184
Insulin sensitivity factor (ISF), 456, 592
Insulin stacking, 562, 599
Insulin-to-carbohydrate ratios (ICRs), 454, 456, 588, 589, 592
Insurance coverage, coping and, 143

Integrated continuous glucose monitoring with glucose pumps, 556–557
Integrated delivery networks (IDNs), 13
Integrative health, defined, *648*
Integrative health care, 647
Integrative Health website, 255
Integrative medicine
complementary, alternative *vs.,* 703, 704
defined, *648*
Intellectual capacity, as factor influencing problem solving, 318–319
Intensity
of aerobic activity, 193–194, *194,* 195
of physical activity sessions, 190
Intermediate-acting insulin, 512, *512, 517*
Intermediate outcomes, 80, *81–86,* 171
Intermittent claudication, 806, 873
Intermittently scanned continuous glucose monitoring, 556
Intermittent peritoneal dialysis (IPD), 858
International Association for the Study of Pain, 877
International Association of Diabetes and Pregnancy Study Group (IADPSG), 389, 767
International Diabetes Center (IDC), 4
International Diabetes Federation, 2, 22, 580
International Federation of Clinical Chemistry (IFCC), 567
International Organization for Standardization (ISO), 536
International Protocol for the Validation of Automated BP Measuring Devices, 267
International SMBG Working Group, 580
International Society for Pediatric and Adolescent Disorders (ISPAD)
Clinical Practice Consensus Guidelines 2018: Nutritional Management in Children and Adolescents With Diabetes, 457
transition recommendations/guidelines, *359,* 361
Interpersonal barriers, 310
Interpersonal symptoms of stress, 146
Interventions, assessing need for, 41
Intima-media thickness (IMT), carotid, 784, 786
Intraepidermal nerve fiber density, 871–872, *872*
Intrauterine environment, type 2 diabetes in children and adolescents and, 442
Intravenous immunoglobulin therapy, 892
Intrinsic sympathomimetic activity (ISA), 636
Invokamet (canagliflozin/metformin), *524*
Irbesartan (Avapro®), 633
Ischemic optic neuropathy, 822
Ischemic stroke, 804

Islet cell antibodies (ICAs), 390, 391
Isometric exercise, 593
Isradipine controlled release (DynaCirc CR®), 638

J

Janumet® (sitagliptin/metformin), *524*
JDRF (Juvenile Diabetes Research Foundation), 22
Jeopardy!® Game, identifying knowledge deficit using, 316
Jet injector, 516
Joint Commission (JCAHO), 13, 70, 344
Joslin, Elliott P., 4, 6
Joslin Affiliated Programs, 341
Joslin Diabetes Mellitis, 381
Juvenile Diabetes Research Foundation, 361
Juvenile-onset diabetes, 257

K

Kaopectate, 254
Karvonen formula, 193
Kava, 690
Kemmis, Karen, 9
Ketones, 200
Ketone testing, 205, 567
  for gestational diabetes mellitus, 763, 773
  type 1 diabetes and, 408
Ketosis
  diabetic ketoacidosis and, *726,* 727
  hyperosmolar hyperglycemic state and absence of, 737
Kidney disease. *See* Chronic kidney disease (CKD); Diabetic kidney disease (DKD)
Kidney function, 838–839
Kidney transplantation, 856, 859–860
Knowledge content areas, 285–288
Knowles, Malcolm, 72
Kombiglyze XR (saxagliptin/metformin), *524*

L

Labeling requirements for dietary supplements, 649
Labetalol (Normodyne®), 636
Lab evaluation, 264
Labor and delivery, diabetes care during, 766
Lab panel, for initial monitoring, 265–266
Lactation, 752, 766
  nutrition recommendations for, 161–162
Lancets, 539–540
Lansoprazole (Prevacid®), 254
Lantus, 601
Large-nerve-fiber neuropathies, *874,* 877, *877*
Laser photocoagulation therapy, for diabetic retinopathy, 292, 829
Latent autoimmune diabetes in adults (LADA), 394–395, 425
  management of, 425
  misdiagnosis of, 266
  in older adults, 439
Laughter, 712
Laxatives, 254
Learner preferences, 57
Learning
  generational differences in, 64–65, *64–65*
  problem-based, 68–69
Learning objectives
  differentiating from behavioral objectives, *51*
  establishing collaboratively, 51
  guide for writing, *52*
  sample diabetes education plan, *58*
Learning theory, applying, 72
Lecture, *60*
"Legacy effect," 287
Lens, of the eye, 817, *817*
Leptin, role in fuel metabolism, 385
Levemir, 600, 601
LGBTQ community, 37
Lifespan, teaching across the, 63–65
Lifestyle changes, 797, 803
Lifestyle interventions, 434, 442, 443
Lifestyle issues, assessment and, 39
Lifestyle modifications
  for hypertension, 629
  reducing cardiovascular disease in diabetes and, 792–796
  reduction of lipids and, 291
Lifestyle physical activity, 187–188
Light therapy, 715
Likert scale, 90
Linagliptin (Tradjenta®), 247, 365, 435, *492,* 508, *508, 850*
γ-Linoleic acid, 893
Lipase inhibitors for obesity management, *481,* 485, *485*
Lipid management, 794–796
  for children and adolescents, 801
  dietary modification and, 795
  ezetimibe and PCSK9 inhibitors and, 796
  low-density lipoprotein monitoring and, 795–796
  monitoring, 267, *277*
  Standards of Care for, *286,* 290–291
  statins and, 794–795
  treating cardiovascular risk factors and, *790*
  triglyceride treatments and, 796
Lipids, 434
Lipid transport system, 613, *614*
Liraglutide (Saxenda®, Victoza®), 247, 257, 435, *482,* 485, *485, 493,* 505, *506,* 507, 786, *849*
Lisinopril (Prinivil®, Zestril®), 632, 797
Lispro, *517, 851*
Listeriosis, 751
Literacy, limitations in, 344
Lithium, diuretics and, 631
Lixisenatide (Adlyxin®), 247, *493,* 505, *506,* 507, *849*
Lomaira, *480*
Long-acting insulin, *512,* 512–513, *517*
Long-acting insulin analogs, 5
Long-term monitoring of metabolic management, 567–568
Long-term outcomes, 80, 171
Loop diuretics, 630, 631
Loop of Henle, 838
Loperamide (Imodium®), 254
Lorcaserin (Belviq®), *481,* 484
Losartan (Cozaar®), *620,* 633
Loss of protective sensation (LOPS), 294, 299
Lovastatin (Mevacor®, Altoprev®), 618, *620*
Low-carbohydrate/very low-carbohydrate eating pattern, 165–166, *167*
Low-density lipoproteins (LDL-C), 613, 614
  monitoring, 267
  monitoring for lipid management, 795–796
  as target of dyslipidemia treatment, 626
  targets, 290
Lower Extremity Amputation Prevention Program (LEAP), 294
Lower intestinal tract dysfunction, related to autonomic neuropathy, 887–888
Low-fat eating pattern, 165, *166*
Low-protein diet, for chronic kidney disease, 854
Low-vision evaluation, 830

M

Macronutrients, 455
Macrosomia, 757, 759
Macrovascular disease, monitoring, *266,* 266–268
Macular edema, 213, 821
Magnesium, hyperosmolar hyperglycemic state and, 738
Magnesium supplementation, 460
Magnet therapy, 715
Ma huang, 641
Maintenance stage
  for exercise behavior change, 226, 228
  of exercise progression, *191,* 192
Major depressive disorder (MDD), 133, 149
Maladaptive coping strategy example, 150–151
Male sexual dysfunction, related to autonomic neuropathy, 888–889
Marijuana, 136

Marketing diabetes self-management education and support program, 331, 339–340
Masked hypertension, 267
Massage therapy, 713, 716
Master certified health education specialist (MCHES), 12
Material self, 140, *141*
Maternal complications from pregnancy, 757–758
Maternal testing, *765*
Maturity-onset diabetes of the young (MODY), 388, 395
Mayo Clinic, 68, 712
Meal boluses, challenges in, 591–592
Meal plan
  for children with type 1 diabetes, 412–413
  in school setting, 418
Meal planning
  age and, *353*
  resources for, *173,* 173–174
  skills for, 174–176
Mealtime insulin, 515
Mean absolute relative deviation (MARD), 554
Meaning given transitional care, 356
Measurement of healthy coping, 144
Medicaid
  ACA and access to, 17
  diabetes care and, 4
  integrity provisions, 20
  prevention of chronic disease and, 19
Medical devices, diabetes, 13–14
Medical exam, pre-activity, 185–186, *186*
Medical nutrition therapy (MNT), 65
  blood pressure and, 289
  defined, 452
  for gestational diabetes mellitus, 770–771, *774*
  for hypertension, 629
  intensified insulin therapy and, 591
  nutrition recommendations and interventions for prevention of diabetes, 159–161
  nutrition recommendations for management of diabetes, 161–164
  for prediabetes and diabetes, 159
  pregnancy and, 298
  for pregnant women with preexisting diabetes, 754
  reducing risk for diabetic kidney disease, 292
  role in promoting healthy eating, 158–168
  standard of care for, *287*
  for type 1 diabetes, 412
  for type 2 diabetes, 434
Medicare
  coverage of glucose meters, 535
  for diabetes self-management education and support program, 340
  donut hole, 245
  exceptions to requirement for group education, 69–70
  financial impact of diabetes and, 4
  integrity provisions, 20
  Part D, 18, 245
  people with type 1 diabetes and, 426
  reimbursement for diabetes self-management education and support program, 328
Medication administration, 256–258
Medication assistance programs, 245
Medications, 241–262. *See also* Nonprescription medications
  See also specific types
  after myocardial infarction, 803
  for antihyperglycemic management, *490–493,* 490–504, *494, 496, 497, 498, 500, 501, 502, 503*
  barriers to taking, *312*
  barriers to use of, *243*
  basic clinical considerations, 245–252
  case study, 242, 252, 256, 320–322
  cautions in older adults, 440
  children and adolescents and, 256–258
  combination oral, *244*
  cost of, 244–245
  decision tree for, 317, *318, 319,* 323
  for diabetes during pregnancy, *760,* 763–764, *764*
  dietary supplements and, 689
  drug interactions, 242, 522, *524–527,* 527
  effects on blood glucose, *548*
  evaluating taking, *83*
  for gestational diabetes mellitus, 773
  home medication list, 370
  hypoglycemia risk and, 202–204, *203*
  nonprescription, 253–256
  for obesity management, *480–482*
  older adults and, 258–259
  oral glucose-lowering combinations, 244, *244*
  patient education, 245–252
  physical activity and adjustment to, 209–210
  preventing diabetic ketoacidosis and, *732*
  prevention of hyperosmolar hyperglycemic state and, *739*
  product aids, 244
  regimen flexibility in type 1 diabetes, 410–411
  for type 1 diabetes, 409–412
  for type 2 diabetes, 444
  use at discharge, 370–371
  use in hospital, 364–367
  weight loss, 464
Medication-taking behavior
  regimen changes and adjustments, 244
  relationships and communication to improve, 243–244
  warning signs, 242–243
Medication use aids, 258
Medihoney, 663
Meditation, 712
Mediterranean-style diet (MED), 165, *166,* 462, 465, 466, 792, 853
MedWatch, 14, 15, 649–650
Meglitinides, 248
  adjustments for physical activity, 209
  for chronic kidney disease, *850*
  for type 2 diabetes, 435, *490,* 495–497, *496*
  use in children and adolescents, 444
  use in older adults, 259
  weight management and, 464
Memory, education and, 72–73
Mental function, hypoglycemia and, 421
Mental health concerns, 131–138
  children with type 1 diabetes and, 417
  cognitive impairment, 132
Mercury-contaminated fish, avoidance by pregnant women, 750–751
Metabolic disorder
  diabetes diagnostic criteria, 385–387, *386*
  epidemiology, 380
  fuel homeostasis, 381–383
  gestational diabetes, 389
  normal fuel metabolism, 383–385
  other forms of diabetes, 388–389
  prediabetes, 387, *387*
  role of hormones, 383–385
  test selection, 388
  trends in, 380, *380, 381*
  type 1 diabetes, 387–388, *389*
  type 2 diabetes, 388
Metabolic disorder, pathophysiology of, 379–401, 389–395
  cancer risk and diabetes, 396, *397*
  pathogenesis of cardiovascular disease in diabetes, 395–396
  pathogenesis of diabetes-related complications, 395
  reducing risks for diabetes-related complications and role of diabetes care and education specialist, 396–397
  stress and diabetes, 396
  type 1 diabetes, 389–391
  type 2 diabetes, 391–395, *392, 393*
Metabolic equivalents (METs), 191, 195
Metabolic management
  for diabetic neuropathy, 893
  insulin injection therapy and, 410
  long-term monitoring of, 567–568

Metabolic surgery, 463, 464
Metabolic syndrome, 458, 842, *872*
Metaglip® (glipizide/metformin), *523*
Metformin (Glucophage®), 246
for adolescents with type 2 diabetes, 258
antihyperglycemic management and, 486
for children with type 2 diabetes, 257
for chronic kidney disease, 847, *849*
drug-drug interactions, *526*
effect on cardiovascular outcomes, 786
garlic combined with, 681
for gestational diabetes mellitus, 775
gut microbiota and, 665
starting, 243
for type 2 diabetes, 435, *491, 497,* 497–498, 579
use in children and adolescents, 257, 258, 443
use in hospital, 365
use in older adults, 259, 440
use in pregnancy, 764
weight management and, 464
Methyldopa (Aldomet®), 640, 641
Metoclopramide, 887
Metolazone, 631
Metoprolol succinate (Toprol XL®), 635
Metoprolol tartrate (Lopressor®), 635
Metronidazole, 887
mHealth, 13–15
mHealth evidence reporting and assessment checklist (mERA), 14
Michigan Neuropathy Screening Instrument, 870, 878
Microalbuminuria, 269, 799, 842
Microvascular disease, monitoring for, *268,* 268–272, *269, 270, 271, 272*
Midodrine, 886
Miglitol (Glyset®), 246, 435, *491–492, 500,* 500–501, *850*
Milk thistle *(Silybum marianum),* 664, *674*
Mind and body–based methods, 713–714
Mind and body practices, 647, *648,* 703
Mind-body interventions, 711–712
Mindfulness/meditation, 711–712
Mineral supplementation, glycemia and, 459–460
Minimal encouragers, 44
Minimed 670G, 589
Mini-Mental Status Exam (MMSE), 132, 144
Mini-Nutritional Assessment, 469
Minority populations, disparities in chronic complications in, 300
Modality variability of complementary health approaches, 705–706
Model, defined, 99
Modifications of resistance exercise, 196–197
Moexiptil (Univasc®), 632
Monitoring, *312. See also* Blood glucose meters; Blood glucose monitoring; Continuous glucose monitoring (CGM)
AADE7 Self-Care Behaviors®, *84*
baseline evaluation, 263
checklist for, *264, 277–278*
for complications and comorbidities, 265
comprehensive approach, 265–278
data management systems for, 263, 264
depression/cognitive assessment, 272–273
diabetes and pregnancy and, *760,* 761–763, *762*
of diabetes self-management education and support program, 340–341
diabetic ketoacidosis and, 265
dietary supplements and, 689
diuretics, 632
for gestational diabetes mellitus, 773
glucose levels in type 2 diabetes, 445
immunizations, 275–276
initial assessment for, 265–266
insulin use, 518
long-term, 263–264
for macrovascular disease, *266,* 266–268
for microvascular disease, *268,* 268–272, *269. 270, 271, 272*
noninvasive, 566
nutrition, 169
osteoporosis, 274–275, *276*
periodontal disease, 276–277
physical activity and, 207
preventing diabetic ketoacidosis and, *732*
prevention of hyperosmolar hyperglycemic state and, *739*
situations requiring more frequency, *277–278*
sleep apnea, 276, *276*
statin therapy and, 619
thyroid, 273–274
of type 1 diabetes, 407–409
vitamin D, 274
weight, 273
Monitor talk, 551
Monofilament testing, 871, *871,* 875
Mononeuropathies, 892
entrapment syndrome *vs., 892*
Month of Meals™ Diabetes Meal Planner, 173
Morning sickness, for women with diabetes, 764
Mortality, due to diabetes, 2–3, 5
Morton's neuroma, 873
Motivational interviewing (MI), 114–121
behavior change for exercise and, 228
DARN and, 48
evidence base, 119–120
example, *116*
person empowerment and, 120–121
primary communication principles of, 115–117
principles, skills, and strategies, 117–119
skills and micro skills, 115
Multidisciplinary team, successful use of pump therapy and, 591
Multifactorial treatment approach to modifying risk factors for cardiovascular disease, 789–791, *790–791*
Multiple daily injections (MDI), 4, 5
benefits of, 587
choices for, 586
insulins used in, 588
limitations of, 587
physical activity and, 592
pump failure and managing diabetes with, 590
switching back to, 600–601
Multiple-injection regimen, 513–514, *514*
Muscular fitness, 196
Music-assisted relaxation, 715–716
Music therapy, 715–716
Myocardial infarction (MI)
coronary artery disease and, 801
diabetes and risk of, 6783
educating patients after, 803
in persons with diabetes, 613
treatment of acute, 802–803
warning signs of, *801*

N

Nadolol (Corgard®), 635
Naltrexone/bupropion HCl (Contrave®), *481–482*
Naphazoline, 256
Naproxen, 253
Nateglinide (Starlix®), 209, 248, 435, *490,* 495–496, *496, 850*
National Academy of Medicine (Institute of Medicine), 21
National Alliance to Advance Adolescent Health, Got Transition, 357
National Cancer Institute, 8
National Center for Complementary and Integrative Health (NCCIH), 647, 650, 703, 704, 711
National Center for Complementary Medicine, 255
National Center for Telehealth & Technology, 316
National Committee for Quality Assurance, 344
National Diabetes Education Program, 119, 296, 301, 381, 418

National Diabetes Prevention Program (NDPP), 3, 16–17, 18, 19, 22, 102, 159, 453, 775–776
- certification by, 340
- Diabetes Prevention Recognition Program, 19
- Lifestyle Coaches, 98, 119

National Diabetes Statistics Report, 432
National Federation of the Blind, 541
National Glycohemoglobin Standardization Program (NGSP), 567
National Health and Nutrition Examination Survey (NHANES), 343
National Health Care Workforce Commission, 19
National Health Insurance Surveys (NHIS), 18
National Health Interview Survey (NHIS), 651, 704
National Health Service Corps, 20
National Health Service England, transition recommendations/guidelines, *359*
National Heart, Lung, and Blood Institute (NHLBI), 787, 801
National Institute for Health and Clinical Excellence (NICE), transition recommendations/guidelines, *359*
National Institutes of Health (NIH), 647, 650, 689, 703
National Kidney Foundation (NKF), 844
National Mail Order Program for Diabetes Testing Supplies, 535
National Practice Surveys, 9
National Quality Forum, 735, 790
National Standards for Diabetes Education, 10
National Standards for Diabetes Self-Management Education and Support (NSDSMES), 32, 76, 90, 98, 99, 328, *329*
- evaluation and, 77
- goal setting and, 46–47
- planning and, 54, 55

Native American medicine, 709–710
Native Americans
- complementary health approaches and, 651
- healthy coping and, 150

Natural Medicine Comprehensive Database, 653
Natural Medicines, 255, 653, 654, 689
Natural products, 647, *648,* 703
Natural Products Association, 649
Naturopathy, 710
Nebivolol (Bystolic®), 635
Needle anxiety, 420
Needle phobias, 409
Needles
- gauge of, 250, 516
- in infusion set, 589
- length of, 250
- size of, 516

NeedyMeds, 245
Neonatal hypocalcemia, 759
Neonatal hypoglycemia, 759
Neovascular glaucoma (NVG), 819, 820–821
Neovascularization elsewhere (NVE), 825
Neovascularization in the optic disc (NVD), 825
Nephrology referral, 854
Nephropathy
- exercise modifications for, *216*
- minority populations and, 300
- monitoring for, 268–269, *278*

Nephrotoxic agents, chronic kidney disease and avoidance, 853
Nerve conduction studies (NCS), 871
Nerve conduction velocity (NCV), 873, 877
Nerve Impairment Score, 870
Neuritis, 877
Neurological examination, 870–871
Neurologic changes, hyperosmolar hyperglycemic state and, 736–737
Neurologic Symptom Score, 870
Neuropathic pain
- case study, 881–882
- definition of, 877–878
- diagnosis of, 878–879
- laboratory tests to evaluate, 879
- nociceptive *vs.* non-nociceptive pain, 878–879
- pharmacologic therapeutic modalities for, 879–880

Neuropathic Pain Symptom Inventory (NPSI), 878
Neuropathy. *See also* Autonomic neuropathy (AN); Diabetic neuropathy (DN)
- acute sensory, 876
- assessment for, 293
- chronic inflammatory demyelinating, 893
- chronic sensorimotor, 874–875
- cranial, 892
- diabetic corneal, 822
- diabetic kidney disease and, 842
- distal symmetric diabetic polyneuropathies (DSPN), 874–877, 879
- entrapment syndromes, *892*
- exercise modifications for, 213–215, *214*
- focal limb, *869,* 892–893
- ischemic optic, 822
- large-fiber, 867, *874,* 877, *877*
- mixed, 877
- monitoring for, 269–271
- mononeuropathies, 892, *892*
- multifocal, *869,* 892–893
- ocular palsies, 822
- painful diabetic peripheral, 878
- peripheral, 269–271
- proximal-motor, 892
- rapidly reversible hyperglycemic, *869,* 875–877
- reducing risk for, 293
- small-fiber, 867, *874,* 875, *876,* 876–877
- standard of care for, *287*
- surgical treatment of, 894–895

Neuropathy Disability Score, 870, 878
Neuropathy Symptom Score, 870, 878
Neuropathy Total Symptom Score-6, 878
Neutral protamine Hagedorn (NPH), 512, *851*
"Never events," 735
Newest Vital Sign, 61
New Onset Diabetes After Transplant (NODAT), 859
Niacin, 624–625, 796
Niacin sustained release (Niaspan®), 624
Nicardipine sustained release (Cardene SR®), 638
Nicotine replacement therapy, 794, 853
Nicotinic acid immediate release (Niacin®), 624
Nicotinic acid sustained release (Slo-Niacin®), 624
Nifedipine long-acting (Adalat® CC, Procardia XL®), 638
Nifedipine (Procardia), *620*
Nisoldipine (Sular®), 638
Nociceptive pain, 878–879
Noctural penile tumescence (NPT), 888
Nocturnal hypertension, 267
Non-communicable diseases (NCD), 2
Noninsulin therapies for gestational diabetes mellitus, 774–775
Noninvasive blood glucose monitoring, 566
Non-nociceptive pain, 878–879
Nonnutritive and hypocaloric sweeteners, 458–459
- use during pregnancy, 750

Nonprescription medications, 253–256
- alcohol-free and sugar-free products, 253
- cough and cold products, 253
- dietary supplements, 255
- ophthalmologic products, 256
- oral hygiene and dental care products, 256
- pain and fever products, 253–254
- products for gastrointestinal ailments, 254–255
- products for genitourinary conditions, 255
- topical and dermatologic products, 255–256

Nonproliferative diabetic retinopathy (NPDR), 212, 825
Nonproliferative retinopathy, 823, *823*
Nonsteroidal anti-inflammatory drugs (NSAIDs), 253–254, *526,* 631, 633, 853
Nopal *(Opuntia streptacantha),* 664–665, *674–675*

Norepinephrine
metabolic effects of physical activity and, 200, *201*
Normalization, chronic disease and, 46
NovaMax®, 567
Novolin®, *517*
Novolog®, *517*
NSAIDs, 253–254, *526,* 631, 633, 853
Numeracy, 61, 344, 438
Nurse Education and Transition program, 70
Nutrient content claims, dietary supplements and, 649
Nutrition. *See also* Healthy eating; Medical nutrition therapy (MNT)
assessment, 168–169
breastfeeding and, 161–162
celiac disease and, 164
diagnosis, 169
for gastroparesis, 165
glycemia and personalized, 461
intervention, 169–170
for management of diabetes, 161–164
monitoring and evaluation, 170
during pregnancy, 161–162, 749–750, *750, 751*
for prevention, 159–161
recommendations and interventions for prevention of diabetes, 159–161
recommendations for management of diabetes, 161–164
Nutritional guidelines, 4
Nutrition assessment, 168–169
Nutrition Care Process, 452
Nutrition Care Process and Model (NCPM), 168–170
nutrition assessment, 168–169
nutrition diagnosis, 169
nutrition intervention, 169–170
nutrition monitoring and evaluation, 170
role of ethnicity and culture, 169
Nutrition diagnosis, 169
Nutrition intervention, 169–170
Nutrition labeling, 19
Nutrition monitoring and evaluation, 169
Nutrition Practice Guidelines (NPGs), 170
Nutrition therapy, 451–452
carbohydrate and glycemia, 455–459
cardiovascular disease and, 465–466
case study, 453–454, 461, 464, 468
in children and adolescents, 469
diabetic kidney disease and, 468
dyslipidemia and, 465–466
glycemic management and, 454–462
goals, 452–453
healthy eating pattern, 453–454
hypertension and, 467–468
macronutrients, 455
in older adults, 469–470
personalized nutrition and glycemia, 461
protein and fat and glycemia, 459
vitamin and mineral supplementation and glycemia, 459–460
weight management and, 451, 463–464
in youth, 469
Nutrition Therapy for Adults With Diabetes or Prediabetes, 158–159, 161, 452, 453–454, 462

O

OARS (Open-Ended Questions, Affirm, Reflect, and Summarize), 117
Obesity
exercise modifications for, 217
healthy eating and reduced risk for type 2 diabetes, 159–161
management approaches, 479–480
medications for management of, *480–482,* 480–485, *483, 484, 485*
pregnancy and complications associated with, 758
prevalence of diabetes and, 380, *381*
type 2 diabetes and, 5, 432, 438, 441
type 2 diabetes in children and adolescents and, 441
Observer contributor to problem solving, 313
Obstacles, common, 43. *See also* Barriers
Obstructive sleep apnea (OSA), 276, *276,* 291
Octreotide, 886
Ocular palsies, 822
Office of Disease Prevention and Health Promotion-National Clinical Care Commission, 21
Office of Minority Health and Health Disparities, 37
Off to College booklets, 361
Olanzapine (Zyprexa®), 253
Older adults
complementary health approaches and, 651
diabetes self-management education plan for, 64
dietary supplements and, 689–690
education strategies for, 440–441
exercise modifications for, 218–219
healthy coping and, 142
healthy eating in, 444
in institutional settings, 441
managing hypertension in, 641
medication administration for, 258–259
medication use in, 440
nutrition education for, 163
nutrition therapy in, 469–470
physical limitations and type 2 diabetes in, 439
polypharmacy in, 440
reducing sedentary time, 187–188
risk of hypoglycemia in, 440
self-care devices and, 440–441
type 2 diabetes in, 438–441
use of insulin pump therapy in, 602
Olmesartan (Benicar®), 633
Omega-3-acid ethyl esters (Lovaza®), 623
Omega carboxylic acids (Epanova®), 623
Omega-3 fatty acids, 623, 680–681, *686*
Omeprazole (Prilosec®), 254
Ominous octet of hyperglycemia, *392*
O'Neill, Tip, 22
Ongoing care for people with type 1 diabetes, 423–425
Online satisfaction surveys, 80
Online support for physical activity, 225
Open-ended questions, 43, 90
assessing diabetes distress using, 146–147
use in motivational interviewing, 114, 117–118
Operational policies, for diabetes self-management education and support program, 338
Ophthalmologic products, 256
Opioid agonist/aminoketone antidepressant, for obesity management, *481–482*
Optical coherence tomography, 830
Optimism, healthy coping and, 144
Oral agents, adjustments for physical activity, 209
Oral Glucose Challenge Test, 767
Oral glucose-lowering medications
breastfeeding and, 766
combination, 244, *244*
for diabetes during pregnancy, 764
for type 2 diabetes, 4
Oral glucose tolerance test (OGTT), 391, 439, 767, *767,* 860
Oral health, 297
Oral hygiene products, 256
Organizational structure, of diabetes self-management education and support program, 341–342
Orlistata, 464
Orlistat (Xenical®, Alli®), *481,* 485, *485*
Ornish eating pattern, 165, *167*
Orthorexia nervosa, 163
Orthostatic hypertension, 267, 641
Orthostatic hypotension, 886
Osmolality, diabetic ketoacidosis and increased, 727
Osteoarthritis, 218, 219, 873
Osteopathic medicine, 710
Osteoporosis, 274–275, *275*
Outpatient assessments, 40
Outpatient care, transition to, *367–368,* 367–371
Outpatient education, 70–71
"Over-basalization," 585
Overnight blood glucose levels, 407

Over-the-counter (OTC) drugs, 253
Overweight, exercise modifications for, 217
Oxidative stress, 390, 893–894
Oxymetazoline, 256

P

Paced learning and feedback, 440
Pacific Islanders
  complementary health approaches and, 651
  healthy coping and, 150
Pain and fever products, 253–254
Pain DETECT, 878
Painful diabetic peripheral neuropathy (PDPN), 878, 879
Pain intensity scales, 878
Pain mechanism, in small-fiber neuropathy, 877
Paleo eating pattern, 166, *167*
Pancreas, simultaneous transplant with kidney, 859
Pancreatic beta cell failure, 489
Pancreatic disorders, 388
Pancreatic (glucoregulatory) hormones, role in fuel metabolism, 383–384
Pandemic, 1–2
Paraphrasing, 44
Parathyroid hormone (PTH), 838–839
Parents
  fear of hypoglycemia in infants and toddlers, 416
  role in diabetes management, 417–418
  using complementary health approaches on their children, 706–707
PAR-Q+ (Physical Activity Readiness Questionnaire for Everyone), 186
Partial partner contributor to problem solving, 313
Participant satisfaction, measuring, 343
Parties, meals at, 176
Pathogenesis, 395–396
Pathophysiology
  of type 1 diabetes, *389*, 389–391
  of type 2 diabetes, 391–395
Pathways to Change, 107
Patient-centered medical home (PCMH), 5, 13
Patient education
  after myocardial infarction, 803
  for insulin, 248–251
  for medications, 245–252
Patient Health Questionnaire-2 (PHQ-2), 273
Patient Health Questionnaire (PHQ9), 133, *134*
Patient Protection and Affordable Care Act. *See* Affordable Care Act (ACA)
Patients
  agenda of, 48
  buy-in from, 48
  diabetes educator conflict with, *315*
  with disabilities, 73–74
  empowerment of, 110
  hearing impaired, 74
  insulin instructions for, 518–520
  keeping in the system, 339–340
  observing behavior of, 48
  problem-solving empowerment for, 315–316
  skill assessment, for goal planning, 49–50
  understanding and respecting as individual, 48
Pattern management, 575–576, 576–577
  attributes for effective, 577
  facilitating for intensifying therapy, 577, *578*
  records for, 581
PCSK9 inhibitors, 615, 616, 625, 626
Pediatric care, 352
Pediatric Endocrine Society, 361
Pedometers, 225, 226
Peer conflict, 149
Peer support, healthy coping and, 142, 414
Penbutolol (Levatol®), 635
Pennsylvania Project, 120
People, self-management decisions influenced by people in person's life, 310
Peptide YY (PYY), role in fuel metabolism, 385
% Daily Values, 175
Peridontal disease, monitoring for, 276–277
Perindopril (Aceon®), 632
Peripheral artery disease (PAD), 805–806
  A1C and, 784
  detection and diagnosis of, 805–806, *806*
  exercise modifications for, 212
  foot ulceration and, 294
  how presents in people with diabetes, 805
  monitoring for, 271–272
Peripheral nerve system, 869
Peripheral neuropathy
  exercise modifications for, *214*, 215
  foot ulceration and, 294
  monitoring for, 269–271, *278*
Peritoneal dialysis (PD), 856, 857–858
Permission to give advice or information, motivational interviewing and asking, 118
Persistent depressive disorder, 133
Personal barriers, 309–310
Personal care record, 299–300
Personal continuous glucose monitoring, 555–556, *556, 557, 558*
Personal identity, illness adjustment and, 140, *141*
Person-centered approach, 8, 38
Person empowerment
  behavior-change theories and, 109–110
  motivational interviewing and, 120–121
Pet therapy, 712
Phacoemulsification, 819
Pharmaceutical Research and Manufacturers of America, 245
Pharmacists, collaboration with and medication-taking behavior, 243
Pharmacodynamic interaction, 527
Pharmacokinetic interaction, 527
Pharmacologic interventions
  for chronic kidney disease, 847–848
  for diabetic dyslipidemia, 617–626, *618, 620*
  for diabetic neuropathic pain, 879–880
  for hypertension, 629–642, *630*
  for obesity treatment options, 479–485
  for type 2 diabetes, 435–436, 489–490
  for type 2 diabetes in children and adolescents, 443–444
  weight management and, 464
Pharmacotherapy for glucose management, 479–432
  amylin analog, 509–510, *510*
  approach to antihypertensive management, 486–489
  case study, 489, 509, 519
  combination oral medications for type 2 diabetes, 522, *523–524*
  diabetes treatment goals, 486
  drug interactions, 522, *524–527*, 527
  hypoglycemia, 520–522
  incretin-based therapies, 504–509, *505–506, 508*
  insulin, 510–520, *512, 514, 517*
  management of type 2 diabetes, 489–490
  medications for antihyperglycemic management, *490–493*, 490–504, *494, 496, 497, 498, 500, 501, 502, 503*
  medication side effects, 520
  obesity management, 479–485
Phendimetrazine (Bontril), *480, 483*
Pheniramine, 256
Phentermine (Adipex-P®), *480*, 482, *483*
Phentermine with topiramate (Qsymia™), *480–481*, 482–484, *483*
Phenylephrine, 256
Phosphate, 727, 730
Phosphorus, 738, 742, 838
PHQ-9, 144
Physical activity, *312*
  adoption and maintenance of, 221–229
  aerobic exercise prescription, 192–195, *194*
  after myocardial infarction, 803
  behavior-change rules, 229

benefits of, 183, 413
blood glucose monitoring and, 204–205, 207
carbohydrate requirements during, 207–208, *208*
cardiovascular disease management and, 212
case study, 184, 200, 209, 216, 222, 229
children and adolescent modifications, 220
for children with type 1 diabetes, 413–414
classification of, 187–188, *188*
comorbid health issues modifications, 211–221
cultural considerations, 220–221
defined, 185
developing structured program of, 188–189, *189*
for diabetes and pregnancy, *760,* 761, *762*
diabetes management and, 200–202
diabetic autonomic neuropathy and, 213–214, *214*
diabetic kidney disease, 215–216
diabetic neuropathy and, 213–215
dietary supplements and, 689
dyslipidemia/cardiovascular disease risk and, 211, 212, 466
energy systems during, 198–200, *199*
equivalent steps per activity, *227*
exercise training session format, 188–189
exercise (training) *vs.,* 185
flexibility and balance exercise, 197–198
general exercise prescription, 189–198, *191*
for gestational diabetes mellitus, 217–218, 773
glycemia and, 460
goal for diabetes prevention, 160
goal setting for, 224
hormonal responses, 198–200, *201*
hyperglycemia and, 202–206, *203*
hypertension and, 212
insulin adjustments and, 210, *210,* 211
insulin administration and, 210
insulin pump therapy and, 210
integrating daily activity before planned exercise, 221–222
intensified insulin therapy and, 592–594
kidney disease and, 852–853
lifestyle promoting, 187–188
medical evaluation for, 185–186, *186*
medication adjustments, 209–210
metabolic effects, *201*
monitoring and, 207
motivational interviewing, 228
nephropathy and, *216*
neuropathy and, 213–215, *214*
obesity modifications, 217
for older adults, *218,* 218–219, 470
overcoming barriers to, 184, 2220224
PAR-Q+ (self-assessment of physical activity readiness), 186
peripheral artery disease and, 212
physiological responses to, 202–204
pre-exercise stress testing, *186,* 186–187
during pregnancy, 217–218, 751–752, *752, 760,* 761, *762*
pregnancy modifications, 217–218
preventing diabetic ketoacidosis and, *732*
prevention of hyperosmolar hyperglycemic state and, *739*
prevention of type 2 diabetes and, 161
problem solving and, 210–211
program-design considerations, 187
promoting, 187–188
reducing cardiovascular disease in diabetes and, 794
regimen adjustment for, 211–221
resistance (strength) exercise prescription, 196–198
retinopathy and, 212–213, *213*
safety considerations, 211
self-efficacy and, 222
self-management strategies for, 206–207
snacking during, 207–209
social-environmental support for, 224–225
staged-matched interventions, 226–228
stages of change in behavior, 226–228
standards of care, *287*
type 1 diabetes and, 413–414
type 2 diabetes and, 161, 444
wearable activity technologies, 225–226
weight management and, 463–464, 467
Physical barriers to self-management, 300
Physical exam, for initial monitoring, 265
Physical inactivity, type 2 diabetes and, 432
Physical limitations
improving transitions for persons with diabetes with, *370*
in older adults, 439
Physical symptoms of stress, 146, 147
Physiologic reaction to stress, 147
Physiology of insulin, 510–511
Pindolol (Visken®), 635
Pioglitazone (Actos®), 248, 435, *491, 498,* 498–500, *850*
Pitavastatin (Livalo®), 618
Planning, 54–66
curriculum content, 55, *56*
a diabetes self-management education and support program, 333–336
DSME/S step, *35*
education plan components, *57,* 57–63, *58, 59, 60–61, 62*
engaging learner preference, 57
for problem-solving training and intervention, 315
program curriculum guiding individual education plan, 54–55
readiness to learn, 55–56
teaching across the lifespan, 63–65, *64–65*
technology and, 66
Planning transitional care, 356
Plantar fasciitis, 873
Plant stanols/plant sterols, 466
Play therapy, for preschoolers with diabetes, 416–417
Pneumococcal vaccination, 275–276, 296, 424
Pokes, blood, 541
Polycystic ovarian syndrome (PCOS), type 2 diabetes and, 441, 443
Polycythemia, 759
Polyhydramnios, pregnancy and, 758
Polypharmacy, 444
dietary supplements and, 690
in older adults, 440
Pooled Cohort Equation, 787, *788*
Population-based health, 35
Population health approach, 21
Portion sizes, 174
Post-immediate outcomes, of healthy eating, 171
Postpartum care and education, 766
after gestational diabetes mellitus, 775, *775*
for women with preexisting diabetes, 754–755
Postprandial blood glucose levels, 407, 581
Postprandial hyperglycemia
cardiovascular risk and, 784
preventing, 410
type 2 diabetes in older adults and, 438
Post-transplantation diabetes mellitus (PTDM), 859–860
Posttraumatic stress disorder (PTSD), healthy coping and, 149, 150
Postural hypotension, cardiac autonomic neuropathy and, 886
Potassium, 723
diabetic ketoacidosis and, 727, 730
hyperosmolar hyperglycemic state and, 738
Potassium-sparing diuretics, 630–631
PowerPoint® presentations, 71
Practice setting, assessment and, 40
Prader-Willi syndrome, 385
Pramlintide (Symlin®), 203, 246, 464, *493,* 509–510, *510, 850*
Prandial insulin, 586
Prandimet (repaglinide/metformin), *523*
Pravastatin (Pravachol®), 618
Prayer, 712
Prazosin (Minipress®), 639
Precision Xtra®, 567

Preconconception care and education, for women with diabetes, 752–757
Precontemplation stage for exercise behavior change, 226–227
Prediabetes, 2, 387
 categories of increased risk of, *387*
 defined, 385
 diabetes self-management education for, 32
 goals of medical nutrition therapy for, 159
 risk factors, 380–381, *387*
Predicting, 99
Preeclampsia, *758*
Pre-exercise stress testing, *186,* 186–187
Pregabalin, 879
Pregnancy. *See also* Gestational diabetes mellitus (GDM)
 AADE7 Self-Care Behaviors for diabetes and, *760,* 761–765
 alpha 1-receptor blockers and, 640
 angiotensin-converting enzyme inhibitors and, 632
 angiotensin receptor blockers and, 633
 beta-blockers and, 636
 bile acid resins and, 624
 blood pressure targets during, 289
 calcium channel blockers and, 638
 case study, 752–756
 central-acting alpha-adrenergic agonists and, 640
 complications with diabetes in, 757–761, *758*
 diabetes care during labor and delivery, 766
 diabetes in, 752–761
 diabetic retinopathy and, 292
 dietary supplements and, 689
 direct renin inhibitors and, 634
 diuretics and, 631
 exercise modifications for, 217–218
 fibrates and, 622
 healthy coping for women with preexisting diabetes, 765
 healthy eating, 761
 HMG-CoA reductase inhibitors (statins) and, 619
 influenza and, 759
 insulin pump therapy during, 601
 insulin therapy in, 515–516
 monitoring diabetes during, 761–763, *762*
 monitoring for retinopathy, 268
 niacin and, 625
 normal, 748–752
 nutrition during, 749–750, *750, 751*
 nutrition recommendations for, 161–162
 omega-3 fatty acids and, 623
 pathophysiology and diabetes in, 757
 PCSK9 inhibitors and, 621
 physical activity during, 751–752, *752,* 761, *762*
 physiology of, 748, *748*
 postpartum care, 766
 preconception care and education, 297–298, 752–757
 with preexisting diabetes, 747
 problem solving for women with preexisting diabetes, 764–765
 reducing risk of diabetes complications, 765, *765*
 requiring hospitalization, 755
 safe eating during, 750–751
 selective intestinal absorption inhibitors and, 621
 taking medications for diabetes, 763–764
 type 1 diabetes and, 747, 757
 type 2 diabetes and, 747, 757
 use of continuous glucose monitoring in, 558–559
 weight gain and, 748–749, *749*
Pregnancy planning, *287*
Preliminary prolonged starvation state, 382–383
Premixed insulins, 411, 513
Preparation stage for exercise behavior change, 226, 228
Preprandial blood glucose levels, 407
Prepregnancy counseling, 297–298
Preschoolers with type 1 diabetes
 education for, 406
 managing diabetes in, 352
 psychosocial issues, 416–417
Prevalence, defined, 3
Prevention
 of diabetic neuropathy, 893
 of hyperglycemia, 740–741
Prevention and Public Health Fund, 18
Preventive care services, 296–298
 dental care, 297
 immunizations, 296–297
 prepregnancy counseling, 297–298
PRIDE *(Partnership to Improve Diabetes Education)* toolkit, 62
Primary failure of therapy, 495
Primary open-angle glaucoma (POAG), 820
Prinizide®, 630
Print materials, *60*
Prioritizing, 313
Pritikin eating pattern, 165, *167*
Private insurance, coverage of glucose meters by, 535–536
Probiotics, 665–666, *675*
Problem analysis, 50
Problem Areas in Diabetes (PAID), 135, 146
Problem-based learning (PBL), 68–69
Problem-focused coping, 144–145
Problems, types of, 309
Problem solving, 134, 307–326
 anticipated situational opportunities for, 308
 barriers to physical activity, *223–224*
 blood glucose monitoring, *552*
 case study, 311, 320–322
 children and, 318
 components of, *308*
 defining, 307–308
 for diabetes and pregnancy, *760,* 764–765
 in diabetes education, 313–315, *315*
 in diabetes self-management, 308–313
 dietary supplements and, 689
 direct knowledge *vs.,* 308–309
 empowering person with diabetes as problem solver, 315–316
 environment encouraging, 311–313
 evaluating, *86*
 examples, 316–317
 facilitated, 313–314
 in group settings, 316–317
 identifying and assessing problems and barriers, 309–311, *312*
 individual options, 316
 to maintain euglycemia, 210–211
 pattern management and, 577
 physical activity and, 210–211
 preventing diabetic ketoacidosis and, *733*
 prevention of hyperosmolar hyperglycemic state and, *740*
 for sick days, 599, 733–734
 special considerations, 317–322, *318, 319*
 theoretical model for, 308
 type 2 diabetes and, 445
Process evaluation, 345
Product aids, 244
Productivity metrics, *344*
Profession, defined, 6
Professional continuous glucose monitoring, *556,* 557–558
Profile of Moods, 878, 879
Program goals, of diabetes self-management education and support program, 331
Program-level evaluation, 341
Program manager, 327–328
Program mission of diabetes self-management education and support program, 331
Program stages, physical activity, *191*
Progression, exercise, 191, *191*
Progressive resistance training (PRT), 713
Project Vision, 8
Proliferative diabetic retinopathy (PDR), 823, *823,* 825, 827
 exercise modifications for, 213, *213*
Proliferator-activated receptor gamma (PPAR-g), 499
Promotoras, 41

Promotoras de salud, 98
Propanolol extended release (Inderal LA®), 635
Propanolol (Inderal®), 635
Proprotein convertase subtilisin/kexin type 9 (PCSK9) inhibitors, 621–622, 796
Prose literacy, 61
Prostacyclin, 888
Prostaglandins, 843
Protamine, exercise-related hypoglycemia risk and, 203
Protein
  dietary, in older adults, 470
  glycemia and, 459
  recommended dietary allowance for pregnant women, 749, *751*
Proton pump inhibitors, 254–255
Proximal convoluted tubule, 838
Proximal-motor neuropathy (amyotrophy), 892
Pseudoephedrine, 641
Pseudohyponatremia, 730–731
Psychological self, 140, *141*
Psychosocial and emotional barriers to self-management, 300
Psychosocial assessment, *42*
  standard of care for, *286*
Psychosocial factors of social support, 142
Psychosocial issues
  for adolescents, 419–421
  after myocardial infarction, 803
  for infants and toddlers with type 1 diabetes, 416
  for preschoolers with type 1 diabetes, 416–417
  for school-aged children with type 1 diabetes, 417–418
Psychosocial Therapies Working Group, 151
Psyllium fiber, 666–667, *675,* 887
Public health interventions, type 2 diabetes in children and adolescents and, 442
Pupillomotor and visceral (metabolic) response related to autonomic neuropathy, 890–892
"Purity and potency" standards, 649

Q

Qigong/Qi Gong, 713, 716
Quality coordinator, 343
Quality of life (QOL)
  diabetic neuropathy and, 868
  insulin pump therapy and, 600–602
  measures, 873
  tools, 144
Quantitative sensory testing (QST), 871
Quinaptil (Accupril®), 632

R

Race
  cataracts and, 819
  prevalence of diabetes and, 380–383
  rate of diabetic kidney disease and, 842
  risk of CVD and, 789
Radiculopathy, 873, 893
Ramipril (Altace®), 632
Ranibizumab, 826, 827
Rapid-acting insulin, 511–512, *512, 517*
Rapidly reversible hyperglycemic neuropathy, 875–876
Rapidly reversible neuropathy, *869*
Rapport, developing, 49
Rating of perceived exertion (RPE), 193–194, *194*
Readiness for learning, planning diabetes self-management education curriculum and, 55–56
Readiness ruler, 119
Readiness to change, assessing, 41–42, *42*
Real-time continuous glucose monitoring (rtCGM), 556
  understanding trending, 561–562
Reassessment, 32
Recombinant human insulin (Exubera®), 516
Recommended Daily Allowance (RDA), 455
Red yeast rice (RYR), 682–683, *687*
Referral, therapist, 133, *134*
Referring providers, 339
Reflecting feelings, 44
Reflective listening, 114
Reflexology, 713
Regimen changes and adjustments, 244
Regiment review, 43
Registered dietitian nutritionist (RDN), medical nutrition therapy and, 452
Registered dietitian (RD)/registered dietitian nutritionist (RDN), healthy eating and, 158, 159
Rehabilitation facilities, transition to, 373–374
Rehydration, 728, *728,* 729–730, 737
Relapse prevention strategies, 148
Relatedness, Transtheoretical Model and, 108
Relaxation, 712
Religion, illness adjustment and, 140
Renal insufficiency, rehydration and, 737
Renal physiology, 838–839
Renal status, standard of care for, *286*
Renin, 839
Renin-angiotensin-aldosterone system (RAAS), 626–627, *627*
Repaglinide, 209, 248, 435, *490,* 495–496, *496, 850*
Reproductive health issues, in adolescence, 419–420
Research on complementary approaches, 708
Residential settings, transition of children to, 363
Resistance, motivational interviewing and rolling with, 115–116
Resistance exercise, 196–198, 197
  effect on diabetes management, 201–202
Resistance (strength) training
  combined with aerobic exercise, 198
  for older adults, 219
Resources
  for diabetes self-management education and support program, 329–330
  for ongoing support of diabetes self-management education and support program, 330–331
Resources, to manage diabetes, 310
Respiratory distress syndrome (RDS), 759
Retina, 817, *817*
Retinopathy. *See also* Diabetic retinopathy
  diabetic kidney disease and, 842
  exercise modifications for, 212–213, *213*
  minority populations and, 300
  monitoring for, 268, *278*
  risk factors for developing, *268*
Return on investment (ROI), 333
Revenue, 333
Reverse cholesterol transport, 614
Righting Reflex, 114–115, 117, 118
Riomet®, 246
Riomet ER™, 246
Risk factors
  for poor medication-taking behavior, 242–243
  for type 2 diabetes, 432–433
Risk reduction, 285–306
  barriers, 300–301
  children and adolescents and, 301
  for chronic complications, 288–294, *289, 290,* 300–301
  for diabetes and pregnancy, *760,* 765, *765*
  for diabetes-related complications and role of diabetes care and education specialist, 396–397
  dietary supplements and, 689
  disparities in behavior, 300–301
  evaluation of, *85*
  knowledge content areas, 285–288
  personal care record, 299–300
  preventing diabetic ketoacidosis and, *733*
  preventing hyperosmolar hyperglycemic state and, *740*
  preventive care services, 296–298
  skills, 298–300
  standards of care, *286–287,* 286–288
  standards of care for foot care, 294–296, *295*
  technology and, 301–302
  therapeutic goals, 287–288, *290*
  in type 2 diabetes, 394, 445

Risky behavior, dealing with, 148
Ritodrine, 764
Role-playing, *60*
Rosiglitazone (Avandia®), 248, 435, *491, 498,* 498–500, 786, *850*
Rosuvastatin (Crestor®), 616, 618, *620*
Roux-en-Y gastric bypass, 793
RULE (Resist the Righting Reflex, Understanding the Person's Perspective, Listen, and Empower), 117
Rydel-Seiffer tuning fork, 875

S

Safety
  of continuous glucose monitoring, 559–560, *561*
  general physical activity, 211
Safety categories for complementary health approaches, *654*
Saint Louis University Mental Status (SLUMS), 132, 144
St John's wort *(Hypericum perforatum),* 683, *688,* 690
Salmonella, 751
Satisfaction, outcome evaluation and, 80
Satisfaction surveys, 80, *87*
Saxagliptin (Onglyza®), 247, 259, 365, 435, *493,* 508, *508,* 509, 848, *850*
Scheduling, as barrier to diabetes management, 311
School-aged children with type 1 diabetes. *See also* Children
  education for, 406
  managing diabetes, 352–354
  psychosocial issues for, 417–418
School settings
  diabetes care in, 418
  insulin injection therapy at, 411
School Walk for Diabetes, 76
Screen for Early Eating Disorder Signs (SEEDS), 138, *139–140*
Screening questions
  for depression, anxiety, diabetes-related stress, *135*
  for eating disorders, *138*
SDPI (Special Diabetes Program for Indians), 709–710
Secoisolariciresinol diglucoside (SDG), 660
Secondary failure of therapy, 495
Secondary prolonged starvation state, 383
"Second sight," 819
Section 504, 418
Sedentary time, 184, 187, *188*
Selective intestinal absorption inhibitors, 620–621
Selective-serotonergic agents, *481, 484,* 484–485
Selective serotonin reuptake inhibitors (SSRIs), 690
Self-assessment, 35–39
Self-care
  dietary supplements and, 689
  taking medications and, 241
Self-care behaviors, type 2 diabetes and, 444–445
Self-care devices, older adults and, 440–441
Self-care skills, 58
Self-Determination Theory (SDT), 107–109, 120
Self-directed learning, 316
Self-efficacy, 133–134
  motivational interviewing and supporting, 117
  physical activity and enhanced, 222
  social cognitive theory and, 104
  Transtheoretical Model and, 105
Self-examination of feet and foot care, 299
Self-management, barriers that influence, 300–301
Self-management of healthy eating, 172–173
Self-management skills, 58–59
Self-management strategies for physical activity, 206–207
Self-monitoring
  of blood pressure, 298–299
  checklist for persons with diabetes, *264*
  goal setting and past experiences with, 50
Self-monitoring of blood glucose (SMBG), 4, 288, 298, 434, 533–534, *535. See also* Blood glucose monitoring
  barriers to, 536–542, *538*
  checklist for SMBG education, *535*
  continuous glucose monitoring *vs.,* 554–555
  diabetes care and education specialists and, 551–552, *553*
  for gestational diabetes mellitus, 773–774
  interpreting data, 542–552
  plan examples, *546–547*
  pregnancy and, 298, 761–762
  risk reduction and, 301–302
  sample record, *550*
  situations that may require more frequent monitoring, *542*
  standard of care for, *286*
  for type 1 and type 2 diabetes, 580
Semaglutide (Ozempic®), 247, *493,* 506, *506,* 507, 786, *849*
Semmes-Weinstein Monofilament exam, 270, *271,* 875
Sensory impairment, 295–296
Serenity Prayer, 712
Serotonin syndrome, 690
Sertraline, 690
Setting the tone for assessment, 38, *45*
Severe hypoglycemia, 520, 521
Sex, risk of cardiovascular disease and, 789
Sexual activity, after myocardial infarction, 803
Sexual dysfunction, related to autonomic neuropathy, 888–889
Shopping, 175
Short-acting insulin, 511–512, *512, 517*
Sick days
  insulin management on, 724, *725*
  pregnant diabetic women and, 764–765
  problem solving for, 599, 733–734
Sildenafil, 888
Simvastatin (Zocor®), 618, *620,* 800
Sitagliptin (Januvia®), 247, 259, 365, 435, *493,* 507–508, 786, *849*
Site changes, insulin pumps and, 600
Six Core Elements of Health Care Transition, 355
6 flavor tea, 710
Skilled nursing facility, transitioning to, 372
Skills
  assessment, 43
  motivational interviewing, 115
  outcome evaluation and, 80
  risk reduction, 298–300
Skills, Confidence and Preparedness Index, 144
Skill training, diabetes-specific problem-solving, 315–316
Skin biopsy, to investigate sensory nerves, 871–872
Sleep apnea, monitoring for, 276
Small-nerve-fiber neuropathy, *872, 874,* 875, *876,* 876–877
Small-nerve-fiber syndrome, 872
SMART goals, 51–53, 133, 224
SMES, reduction of diabetes distress and, 132–133
Smoking, diabetic retinopathy and, 825
Smoking cessation, 268, *278,* 291
  chronic kidney disease and, 853
  reducing cardiovascular disease in diabetes and, *791,* 794
  Transtheoretical Model and, 105
Snacking, 175
Snacks, 410
  bedtime, 208
  carbohydrate, 207
  composition of, 207–208
  self-management strategies for physical activity and, 206, 207–209
  timing of, 208–209
Social barriers to self-management, 300
Social cognitive theory (SCT), 102–104, 120
Social determinants of health (SDOH), 35
Social-environmental support for physical activity, 224–225

Social Learning Theory, 102
Social media, real-time updates on, 14
Social self, 140–141, *141*
Social support
for children and adolescents with type 2 diabetes, 444
psychosocial factors of, 142
social cognitive theory and, 102, 104
Society of Hospital Medicine, inpatient hyperglycemia management, 734–735, *735*
Socioeconomic factors
health disparities linked to, 37
in planning exercise, 220–221
Sodium
diabetic ketoacidosis and, 727
hyperosmolar hyperglycemic state and, 738
hypertension and, 467
hypertension and restriction of dietary, 852
restriction in older adults' diets, 470
Sodium bicarbonate, treating diabetic keto acidosis and, 730
Sodium-glucose co-transporter (SGLT) inhibitors, 5
Sodium-glucose co-transporter 2 (SGLT2) inhibitors, 247–248
antihyperglycemic management and, 486
for chronic kidney disease, 847–848, *849*
as diuretic, 631
effect on cardiovascular outcomes, 786
for female sexual dysfunction, 889
risk of euglycemic diabetic ketoacidosis, 265
for type 2 diabetes, 435, *492, 502,* 502–503, 579
use in hospital, 365
use in older adults, 259
weight management and, 464
Soliqua®, *517*
Somogyi phenomenon, 596
Space needs, for diabetes self-management education and support program, 335
Special needs people, self-monitoring of blood glucose and, 542
Special populations
assessment and, 40
diabetes self-management education for, 73–74
healthy coping and, 148–150
"Spirit of MI," 114, 115
Spironolactone (Aldactone®), 630, 631, 642
Sports, adjusting insulin injection therapy for, 412, 414
Sports drinks, 206, 209, 414
Staff
for diabetes self-management education and support program, 335–336
managing, 336–337
Stage-matched interventions for exercise behavior, 226–228
Standard of practice (SOP), 10, 66–67
Standards of Care, 285
complications, 288–294
foot care, 294–295
implementation resources, 296
preventive care services, 296–298
risk reduction, *286–287,* 286–294
Standards of care
blood glucose testing recommendations, 298
complications and, 288–294
Standards of Care and Clinical Practice Recommendations, 76
Standards of professional performance (SOPP), 10
Stanford Diabetes Self-Management Program, 104
Starches, 457
Static magnetic field therapy, 894
Statins, 794–795. *See also* HMG-CoA reductase inhibitors (statins)
for diabetic dyslipidemia, 465, 615–620, *616, 617*
intolerance to, 795
for prevention of cardiovascular disease, 852
safety of, 795
Steps per day
activity classification based on, *188*
tracking, 226, *227*
Steroids, 204, 803
Stigma, 121
STOP-Bang questionnaire, 276
Story catalog, 69
Storytelling, as teaching strategy, 69
Strengths-based language, 121
Stress, 135–136
diabetes and, 396
diabetic children and adolescents and, 148–149
gestational diabetes mellitus and, 775
screening questions, *135*
Stress management, 146–148
Stress testing, *186,* 186–187, 802
Stretching exercises, 189, 197–198
Stroke, 615
diabetes and risk of, 783
prevention of, 804
signs of, 804–805, *805*
Stroke Association, 805
Structure and function claims, dietary supplements and, 649
Structured monitoring, 545
Styles of coping, 144–146
Sudomotor dysfunction, related to autonomic neuropathy, 889–890
Sudomotor function, 872–873
SUDOSCAN, 872
Sugar alcohols, 458–459
Sugar-free nonprescription medications, 253
Sugars, 456–457
Sugar-sweetened beverages, 458
Sulfonylurea hypersensitivity reaction, 495
Sulfonylureas, 248
adjustments for physical activity, 209
aspirin and, 254
for chronic kidney disease, *850*
for type 2 diabetes, 435, *490, 494,* 494–495
use in children and adolescents, 444
use in hospital, 365
use in older adults, 259, 440
weight management and, 464
Summarizing, 46
Summative evaluation, 79, *79*
Supervision of physical activity, 225
Surgical cataract extraction, 819
Surgical treatment of neuropathy, 894–895
Surveys, 80, *87, 89*
Sweating disturbances, related to autonomic neuropathy, 889–890
Sweeteners, nonnutritive and hypocaloric, 458–459
Sympathomimetic agents, or obesity management, *480–481,* 482–484, *483*
Syndemic, 1, 2
Syringes, 516
Systematic approaches to facilitating self-directed behavior change, 109–114
System Usability Scale (SUS), 14

T

Tadalafil, 888
Tai Chi, 198, 202, 713–714, 716
"Talk Test," 193
Tamsulosin, 889
Tapentadol, 880
Target heart rate, 193
Tarsal tunnel entrapment syndrome (RRS), 894
Tarsal tunnel release, 894–895
Tarsal tunnel syndrome, 873
Teaching environment, 73
Teaching materials, 71–72
Teaching points for transitions, *357–358*
Teaching strategies, storytelling, 69
Technology
Diabetes Care and Education Specialist and, 14–15
diabetes self-management education and, 66
innovation in medical devices, 13–15
risk reduction and, 301–302
technical difficulties and, 71

transitional care and, 361–362
use in education, 73
wearable activity, 225–226
Teen T1D toolkit, 361
Telemedicine, 566
Telmisartan (Micardis®), 633
TENS units, 715
Terazosin (Hytrin®), 639
Terbutaline, 764
Tetanus boosters, 276
Tetracycline, 887
Tetrahydrozoline, 256
Theoretical approaches to behavior change, 100–109
Theoretical model, for problem solving, 308
Theory
applied to diabetes care and education, 99–100
choosing a theory that can be measured, 100
choosing theory that fits, 99–100
defined, 99
promoting healthy eating in practice and, 172–176
purposes of, 99
questions to answer to ensure theory appropriate to practice or program, 100
Theory-based approaches, 99
Theory-based practice, 100
Theory of Planned Behavior (TPB), 104–105
Theory of Reasoned Action (TRA), 104–105
Therapeutic alliance, 110
Therapeutic goals for adults, *290*
Therapeutic inertia, 576
Therapeutic relationship
medication-taking behavior and, 243–244
problem-solving approach and, 314–315, *315*
Therapist referral, 133, *134*
Therapy intensification, 575–576. *See also* Insulin pump therapy
case study, 582–585, 595
facilitating pattern management for, 577
initiating and advancing therapy in type 2 diabetes, 578–581
Thiazide-type diuretics, 629, 630, *630,* 631
Thiazolidinediones (TZDs), 248, 259, 848
for chronic kidney disease, *850*
for type 2 diabetes, 435, *491–492, 498,* 498–500
use in hospital, 365
use in older adults, 259, 440
weight management and, 464
Think Aloud Usability Test, 14
Third Injection Technique Workshop, 250
Thrombosis, diabetes and, 784
Thrombotic CVA, 805
Thyroid, monitoring function, 273–274
Thyroid disorders, type 1 diabetes and, 422–423, 425
Tidepool, 565
Time above range (TAR), 562
Time below range (TBR), 562
Time (duration)
of aerobic activity, 194, 195
of physical activity, 190
Time in range (TIR), 562, 575, 763
Time study, *89*
Timolol (Blocadren®), 635
Tinea pedis, 255–256
Tobacco use status, standard of care for, *287*
Tocolytic agents, 764
Toddlers with type 1 diabetes
coping and, 142
insulin injection therapy for, 409
managing diabetes in, 352
psychosocial issues, 416
Tolazamide, *850*
Tolbutamide, *850*
Topiramate, 482–483
Torsemide, 631
Total peripheral resistance (TPR), hypertension and, 626
Traditional Chinese Medicine (TCM), 704, 710–711
Trandolapril (Mavik®), 632
Transcendental meditation, 716
Transcutaneous electrical nerve stimulation (TENS), 894
Transformational Learning, 72
Transient hyperglycemia, 860
Transient ischemic attack (TIA), 804–805
Transitional care, 351
adolescence to young adulthood, 354–363, *357–358*
case study, 362, 371
to correctional institutions, 372–373
discharge to outpatient care, *367–368,* 367–371, *369, 370*
foster care/residential settings, 363
hospital admission, *363. 364,* 363–367, *367*
infancy through young adulthood, 351–354, *353*
physical limitations and, *370*
recommendations/guidelines, *359–360*
to rehabilitation facilities, 373–374
to skilled nursing facility or acute care hospital, 372
teaching points, *357–358*
technology and, 361–362
Transition Care Model (TCM), 70
Transition clinics, 356
Transtheoretical Model (TTM), 105–107, 171, 226
definitions and application, *108*
evidence base, 107, 108–109
stages of change, 106, *106*
Travel
insulin pump therapy and, 601–602
meals, 175–176
Treatment resistance hypertension, 641–642
Triamterene (Dytenium®), 630, 631
Tricare, 338–339
Trigger for development of type 1 diabetes, 390
Triglycerides (TGs), 613
lipid management and, 796
monitoring, 267
targets, 290
Trust, building, 37–38, *45,* 49
T-scores, 275, *275*
TSH screening, 274, 423
Turmeric, 667, *676,* 688
21st Century Cures Act (Cures Act), 13–15
Type 1 diabetes (T1DM), 2, 379, 387–388
in adults, 425
artificial pancreas technology and, 14
assessing risk for exercise-related hypoglycemia, 202
autoimmune disorders and, 422–423, 425
autoimmunity and, 390–391
blood glucose monitoring, 407–409
blood glucose targets for exercise, 204–205
blood glucose testing recommendations, 543, *544*
calorie consumption and normal growth in children, 412–413
care in school settings, 418
case studies, 405, 406, 410, 411, 420, 422, 423
celiac disease and, 266, 423
continuous subcutaneous insulin infusion, 411–412
diabetic ketoacidosis and, 422, 721–722
diagnosis, 404–407, *405,* 425
education first week after diagnosis, 406–407
exercise order for, 198
eye examination for persons with, 828
general exercise prescription for, 191
genetic propensity and, 389–390
geographic location and, 403
glucose levels above target and poor healthy outcomes, 420
glycemic targets for, 404, *404*
healthy coping and, 414–421, *415*
healthy eating and, 412
hypoglycemia and, 421–422, *422*
hypoglycemia prevention and, 413–414
hypoglycemia unawareness and, 890

insulin therapy for, 409–411, 515
meal plan and insulin regimen, 412–413
management of, 406
medical nutrition therapy, 412
medications for, 409–412
monitoring, 407–409
nutrition education for children with, 162–163, 469
nutrition recommendations for management of, 161
ongoing care, 423–425
oxidative stress and, 390
parent and child roles in diabetes management, 417–418
pathophysiology in, 389, *389,* 753
physical activity and, 413–414
physical activity and children with, 220
predictor of cardiovascular disease in people with, 786–787
pregnancy and, 162, 747, 757
prevalence and incidence, 403–404
primary treatment goals, 414, 425
progression of diabetic kidney disease and, 843
psychosocial issues during preschool years, 416–417
psychosocial issues for infants and toddlers, 416
psychosocial issues in adolescence, *419,* 419–421, *421*
psychosocial issues in school-aged children, 417–418
quarterly follow-up with healthcare provider, 423–424
regimen and dose determinations, 409–411
risk for cardiovascular events and, 784
risk of cardiovascular disease and, 288–289
self-management of physical activity and, 184
self-monitoring of blood glucose and, 580
thyroid disorders and, 422–423
transition to adult care, 424
treatment of hypoglycemia, 594
vaccinations and, 424
yearly assessments and screenings, 424

Type 2 diabetes (T2DM), 2, 379, 388, 431–449
AACE algorithm for medical management of, *487*
ADA algorithm for medical management of, *488*
aging and, 2
basal insulin for, 585–586
blood glucose management, 434
blood glucose testing recommendations, *544,* 544–547
case study, 435–436, 437–438
in children and adolescents, 3, 5, 257–258, 441–444
clinical presentation, 431–432
combination oral medications for, 522, *523–524*
continuous glucose monitoring and, 556
development of, 385
diagnosis, 433, *433,* 439, 441–443, *442*
education strategies, 440–441
eye examination for persons with, 828
general exercise prescription for, 191
genetics of, 392–393
gestational diabetes mellitus and risk of developing, 775
glycemic management and prevention of cardiovascular events in people with, 784–786
healthy coping and, 445
healthy eating and, 444
homeostasis of fasting and postload glucose during development of, *393*
hyperglycemia risk and, 440
incidence and prevalence, 3, 432, 438
individualized plan for, 435–36
initial therapy for, 579–580
initiating and advancing therapy in, 578–581
insulin pump therapy and, 602
insulin therapy for, 514–515
lifestyle interventions for, 434, 443
management of, 489–490
medications for, 4, 435, 440, 443–444
monitoring, 445
motivational interviewing dialog example, *116*
mulitfactorial treatment approach to modifying risk factors for cardiovascular disease and, 789–791, *790–791*
nutrition education for youth/adolescents with, 163, 469
nutrition recommendations for management of, 161
obstructive sleep apnea and, 291
in older adults, 438–441
oral medications for, 4
pathophysiology of, 391–395
pharmacologic interventions, 435, 440, 443–444
physical activity and, 183, 444
pregnancy and, 162, 747, 757
problem solving and, 445
progression of diabetic kidney disease and, 843
reducing complications, 434
risk factors, 159, 380–381, 432–433
risk for exercise-related hypoglycemia, 202, 204
risk reduction and, 394, 445
self-care behaviors, 444–445
self-management of physical activity and, 184
self-monitoring of blood glucose and, 580
social support, 444
treatment of, 433–438
treatment of hypoglycemia in, 522, 594
weight loss and, 792–793

Type of aerobic activity, 194–195
Type of physical activity, 190–191

U

Ubiquinone, 679–680
Ulceration, small-fiber neuropathy and risk of, 877
Ulcers, 215
Ultrasonography (echography), 829
UN Resolution on Diabetes, 22
United States
diagnosed and undiagnosed diabetes among adults in, *380, 381*
healthcare systems in, 13
incidence of diabetes in, 5
prevalence of diabetes in, 2

USDA Choose My Plate, 173, *173*
USDA Dietary Guidelines for Americans, 453
US Pharmacopeia (USP), 255, 649
US Preventive Services Task Force (USPSTF), 767
Universal design, 74
Upper gastrointestinal dysfunction, related to autonomic neuropathy, 886–887
Urinary albumin-to-creatinine ratio (UACR), 843
Urine testing for glucose, 566–567
Usability Problem Taxonomy (UPT), 14
Utilization review, 345

V

Vaginal candidiasis, 420
Valerian, 690
Valsartan (Diovan®), 633
Vardenafil, 888
Varenicline, 794, 853
Vascular dementia, 804
Vascular endothelial growth factor (VEGF), 820
Vegetarian and vegan eating patterns, 165, *166*
Verapamil (Calan®, Covera®, Verelan®), *620,* 636, 637, 638
Very low-density lipoproteins (VLDLs), 613, 614
Very low-fat eating pattern, 165, *167*
Veterans, healthy coping and, 149
Veterans Health Administration, 344
Vibration, 894

Vibratory sensation exam, 270–271
Visually impaired people, self-monitoring of blood glucose and, 541
Vinegar, 667–668, *676*
Viral triggers for type 1 diabetes, 390
Vision, blurred, 822
Vision loss, counseling for, 830
Visual Analogue Scale, 878
Visual changes, temporary, 822
Visual impairment, exercise modifications for, 212–213
Vitamin B1, 678
Vitamin B_{12} deficiency, 204, 498
Vitamin B_{12} malabsorption, in older adults, 470
Vitamin D, 839
  glycemia and, 459–460
  monitoring levels of, 274
  older adults and, 470
Vitamins
  dietary reference intake for pregnant women, 750, *751*
  glycemia and, 459–460
  to lower cardiovascular risk, 800
  supplementation in older adults, 470
Vitreous surgery for diabetic retinopathy, 829
Volume
  of aerobic activity, 195
  of exercise, 191
  of resistance exercise, 196
Vygotsky, Lev, 56

W

Warfarin (Coumadin®), *620,* 680
Warm-up exercises, 188–189
Warning signs of poor medication-taking behavior, 242–243
Weight
  gain during normal pregnancy, 748–749, *749*
  monitoring, 273
  standard of care for, *286*
Weight loss
  goal for diabetes prevention, 160
  healthy eating for, *172*
  hypertension and, 467
  for prevention of type 2 diabetes, 161
  reducing cardiovascular disease in diabetes and, 792–793
Weight management
  kidney disease and, 853
  skipped insulin injections and, 420, 723
Weight management, nutrition therapy and, 462–464
  anti-hyperglycemia therapy and, 464
  nutrition therapy for weight management, 463
  physical activity and weight management, 463–464
  weight loss effectiveness, 462–463
  weight loss medications and bariatric surgery and, 464
White-coat hypertension, 267, 797
Whole-body medical systems, 709–711
"Words matter" movement, 5
World Health Organization (WHO), 14, 21, 748, 798
  Expert Committee on Food Additives (JECFA), 667
Written agreement, on goals, 49

X

Xiaoke disease, 710
Xigduo XR (dapagliflozin/metformin), *524*
X-PERT, 113
Xuezhikang (red yeast rice), 682–683, *687*
Xultophy®, *517*

Y

Yi Ren Medical Qigong (YRMQ), 713
Yoga, 198, 202, 703, 704, 706, 716
Young adults
  developmental tasks, *353*
  healthy coping and, 142
  transitional care from adolescence to, 354–363
Youth, nutrition therapy in, 469

Z

Zone of Proximal Development (ZPD), 56

into the ACA, authorized the CDC to enhance surveillance of diabetes and to develop national quality standards for a national diabetes report card.[139] The *Diabetes Report Card* contains current information on the status of diabetes, gestational diabetes, prediabetes, preventive care practices, risk factors, quality of care, outcomes, and progress made toward meeting national goals.[4]

Diabetes-related provisions include wellness and prevention programs, Medicaid Health Homes for those with chronic conditions, the Medicaid Incentives to Prevent Chronic Disease Program, and the Medicare Independence at Home Demonstration Program.[139] The complete ACA contains 10 titles (or divisions), each addressing a particular aspect of reform. The next section contains a description of the 10 titles and offers a consolidated summary of the contents of the ACA, highlighting specific implications for the diabetes care and education specialist. The titles are summarized in Table 1.3. This brief summary is not intended to represent the entirety of this law.

Title I: Quality, Affordable Health Care for All Americans

Through shared responsibility, the ACA promises to transform healthcare coverage, access, and quality for all Americans as it is introduced incrementally, by 2020.[139] Persons with diabetes may particularly benefit from this important federal legislation, given the significant reforms for preventive services included in the act.[139] Borne out of the ACA is the National Diabetes Prevention Program, representing a partnership of public and private organizations working to reduce the growing problem of prediabetes and type 2 diabetes.[116,139]

This section discusses improvements in healthcare coverage for all Americans, including preventive health services. If the plan offers dependent coverage for an unmarried child, this coverage is available until the child turns 26. Wellness and prevention programs which include weight management, physical fitness, nutrition, heart disease, and diabetes prevention are specified. Subtitle B of this section elaborates actions to preserve and expand insurance coverage for those with preexisting conditions. Subtitle C describes quality health insurance coverage for all Americans, prohibiting preexisting condition exclusions or other discrimination based on health status. Covered essential health benefits include ambulatory services, emergency services, hospitalization, prescription drugs, lab services, preventive/wellness services with chronic disease management, as well as oral and vision care for children. Levels of coverage for Bronze (lowest level of coverage), Silver, Gold, and Platinum levels (highest level of coverage) are described. Flexibility in operation and enforcement of exchanges is permitted to vary by state, and states may establish alternative programs. Subpart B of this section describes procedures for determining eligibility. Title I addresses individual and small-business tax credits, individual and employer responsibilities, and a variety of miscellaneous provisions.

TABLE 1.3 The Affordable Care Act: Titles and Sections Addressing Aspects of Reform

Title	*Title Name*	*Sections of the ACA*
Title I	Quality, Affordable Health Care for All Americans	1001–2995
Title II	The Role of Public Programs	3001–3129
Title III	Improving the Quality and Efficiency of Health Care	3131–3602
Title IV	Prevention of Chronic Disease and Improving Public Health	4001–4402
Title V	Health Care Workforce	5001–5701
Title VI	Transparency and Program Integrity	6001–6801
Title VII	Improving Access to Innovative Medical Therapies	7001–7103
Title VIII	Community Living Assistance Services and Supports	8001–8002
Title IX	Revenue Provisions	9001–9023
Title X	Strengthening Quality, Affordable Health Care for All Americans	10101–10909

Source: Adapted from "An Act: The Patient Protection and Affordable Care Act." The Patient Protection and Affordable Care Act, Pub. L. No. 111-148, §2702, 124 Stat. 119, 318-319 (2010), US Government Printing Office. Because of myriad new bills and resolutions constantly occurring with the ACA, one may read the ACA by visiting this Web site: The Patient Protection and Affordable Care Act, 42 USC § 18001 (2010). US Government Printing Office. "HealthCare.gov" (cited 2020 March 12) on the Internet at: https://www.healthcare.gov/where-can-i-read-the-affordable-care-act/.

individual users) to build better tools to better manage life with diabetes. Many persons with diabetes are interested in directly improving diabetes technology by donating their data and sharing their experiences of living with do-it-yourself closed-loop systems.[134] Since these hybrid systems are not sold as medical devices, they are not subject to FDA regulation, creating some ethical concerns as to their safety.[134] The diabetes care and education specialist must be aware that the FDA has not evaluated the safety and effectiveness of unauthorized diabetes management devices or systems that combine devices in unintended ways, and that these devices or systems may give incorrect results and introduce unknown risks. Diabetes care and education specialists may be interested in subscribing to FDA Medical Device Safety Communication email alerts, which include clinical recommendations for self-management, by visiting the FDA Web site at https://www.fda.gov/medical-devices/safety-communications/2019-safety-communications.

Diabetes care and education specialists are in an ideal position to engage individuals in research and product development opportunities. Furthermore, they are ideally suited to encourage medical device adverse event reporting to MedWatch and advise patients to use only diabetes management devices the FDA has authorized for sale in the United States and to use these devices according to manufacturer instructions. To inquire about the FDA regulatory status of any product, the manufacturer can be contacted directly, or the FDA Division of Consumer Education can be reached at DICE@FDA.HHS.GOV, or by calling 800-638-2041 or 301-796-7100.[133] In an era of rapidly emerging technologies, the DCES may witness in clinical practice that which has not yet been published or reported by the FDA. Social media, even with its challenges and limitations, can offer noteworthy, real-time information of interest to all stakeholders in diabetes care and education.[136]

Diabetes Care and Education Specialists and the Affordable Care Act*

Although individuals with diabetes benefit from DSMES, many persons with diabetes have not had the advantage of receiving diabetes management guidance from a DCES. As healthcare delivery and payment structures in the United States evolve, diabetes care and education specialists are wondering what patterns will change and how comprehensive changes to the healthcare system will affect persons with diabetes. Health insurance coverage constitutes an important first step in obtaining access to care, managing disease, preventing complications, and reducing the likelihood of developing related conditions.[138] Moreover, lack of health insurance coverage results in increased out of pocket costs and delays in treatment, thereby substantially impacting the US economy. The Patient Protection and Affordable Care Act[139] plays an important role in the evolving healthcare system.

The Patient Protection and Affordable Care Act, also known as the Affordable Care Act (ACA), is sometimes called "Obamacare" because is became public law during the Obama administration (Pub. L. No. 111-148, 2010). The law contains 2 parts: the Patient Protection and Affordable Care Act and the Health Care and Education Reconciliation Act. The official and consolidated (unofficial) versions of these Acts are available in PDF or HTML formats on the HealthCare.gov Web site. This ACA has 3 primary goals:[139]

- Make affordable health insurance available to more people.
- Expand Medicaid programs to cover adults with an income below 138% of the federal poverty level.
- Support innovative medical care delivery methods designed to lower the costs of health care.

When the ACA passed, it represented an opportunity to decrease the toll of diabetes in the United States.[140] Many of the ACA provisions did not go into effect until 2014. During the 116th Congress (2019-2020), over 1700 bills which directly pertain to the ACA have been introduced or resolved. Numerous bills have been introduced to repeal the ACA (eg, H.R. 2536). Additional bills have been introduced to protect Americans with preexisting conditions (eg, H.R. 986), for lowering prescription drug costs (eg, H.R. 987), restoring access to medication (S.1089), and for protecting individuals from higher insurance premiums (eg, H.R. 2447).

The ACA expanded insurance coverage, consumer protections, and access to primary care services. The law contains several provisions of specific interest to persons with diabetes, policymakers, and healthcare providers, including the DCES. These provisions directly address gaps in diabetes prevention, screening, and care, creating a comprehensive approach toward improved treatment.[139] The Catalyst to Better Diabetes Care Act of 2009, built

*The following information on the Affordable Care Act is current as of January 19, 2020. Ongoing healthcare reform news updates are summarized and may be viewed at Health Markets Web site at: (https://www.healthmarkets.com/resources/health-insurance/trumpcare-news-updates/).[137]